PRINCIPLES AND PRACTICE OF
ENVIRONMENTAL MEDICINE

PRINCIPLES AND PRACTICE OF
ENVIRONMENTAL MEDICINE

Edited by
ALYCE BEZMAN TARCHER, M.D.

School of Medicine, University of California
San Francisco, California

Plenum Medical Book Company • New York and London

Library of Congress Cataloging-in-Publication Data

Principles and practice of environmental medicine / edited by Alyce
  Bezman Tarcher.
       p.   cm.
   Includes bibliographical references and index.
   ISBN 0-306-42893-8
   1. Environmental health.   I. Tarcher, Alyce Bezman.
   [DNLM: 1. Environmental Exposure--adverse effects.
   2. Environmental Pollutants--adverse effects.   WA 670 P957]
   RA565.P75 1992
   616.9'8--dc20
   DNLM/DLC
   for Library of Congress   92-49900
                                                                  CIP

ISBN 0-306-42893-8

©1992 Plenum Publishing Corporation
233 Spring Street, New York, N.Y. 10013

Plenum Medical Book Company is an imprint of Plenum Publishing Corporation

Printed in the United States of America

To Martin

CONTRIBUTORS

Kulbir S. Bakshi, Ph.D.

Senior Staff Scientist
Committee on Toxicology
National Academy of Sciences
Washington, DC 20418

John G. Banwell, M.D.

Professor of Medicine
Director of Gastroenterology
Case Western Reserve University
School of Medicine
Cleveland, Ohio 44106

Frank Bell, M.S.

Environmental Engineer Advisor (retired)
Criteria and Standards Division
Office of Drinking Water
U.S. Environmental Protection Agency
Washington, DC 20460

Ervin Bellack, Ph.D.

Chemist
Criteria and Standards Division
Office of Drinking Water
U.S. Environmental Protection Agency
Washington, DC 20460

Paul S. Berger, Ph.D.

Microbiologist
Criteria and Standards Division
Office of Drinking Water
U.S. Environmental Protection Agency
Washington, DC 20460

David R. Bickers, M.D.

Professor and Chairman
Department of Dermatology
Case Western Reserve University
School of Medicine
Cleveland, Ohio 44106

Edward J. Calabrese, Ph.D.

Professor of Toxicology
University of Massachusetts School of Public
  Health
Amherst, Massachusetts 01003

William A. Coniglio, M.S.

Biologist
Criteria and Standards Division
Office of Drinking Water
U.S. Environmental Protection Agency
Washington, DC 20460

Joseph A. Cotruvo, Ph.D.

Director, Health and Environmental Review
  Division
Office of Toxic Substances
U.S. Environmental Protection Agency
Washington, DC 20460

William F. Finn, M.D.

Professor of Medicine
University of North Carolina
School of Medicine
Chapel Hill, North Carolina 27514

Alf Fischbein, M.D.

Professor
Division of Occupational and Environmental Health
Department of Life Sciences
Bar Ilan University
Ramat Gan 52900
Israel

James E. Gadek, M.D.

Professor of Medicine
Director, Pulmonary Disease Division
Ohio State University
College of Medicine
Columbus, Ohio 43210

EDUARDO GAITAN, M.D.

Professor of Medicine
University of Mississippi
School of Medicine
Jackson, Mississippi 39216

G. GORDON GIBSON, Ph.D.

Senior Lecturer in Pharmacological Biochemistry
Department of Biochemistry
University of Surrey
Guildford, Surrey GU25XH
England

PHILIP S. GUZELIAN, M.D.

Professor of Medicine
Chief, Environmental Toxicology
University of Colorado
Health Sciences Center
Denver, Colorado 80262

DAVID E. HARTMAN, Ph.D.

Director of Neuropsychology
Cook County Hospital
Clinical Associate Professor
Department of Psychiatry
Chicago Medical School
Chicago, Illinois 60612

FRANZ HARTMANN, M.D.

Professor of Medicine
Head, Department of Internal Medicine
St. Marienkrankenhaus
Frankfurt, Germany

STEPHEN HESSL, M.D., M.P.H.

Associate Professor of Medicine
University of Illinois at Chicago
Chicago, Illinois 60612

HARRO JENSS, M.D.

Assistant Chief of Medicine
Department of Medicine
University of Tübingen
Tübingen, Germany

JAMES M. KAWECKI, Ph.D.

Visiting Professor of Medicine
Columbia University, School of Public Health
Center for Risk Assessment
Washington, DC 20007

HOWARD M. KIPEN, M.D., M.P.H.

Assistant Professor
Department of Environmental and Community
    Medicine
University of Medicine and Dentistry of New
    Jersey
Robert Wood Johnson Medical School
Piscataway, New Jersey 08854

RICHARD B. KURZEL, Ph.D., M.D.

Assistant Professor of Obstetrics and Gynecology
Division of Maternal and Fetal Medicine
School of Medicine
University of California, Los Angeles
Sylmar, California 91342

SI DUK LEE, Ph.D.

P.O. Box 13661
Research Triangle Park, North Carolina 27709

HOWARD I. MAIBACH, M.D.

Professor and Vice Chairman
Department of Dermatology
School of Medicine
University of California
San Francisco, California 94143

ANTHONY V. NERO, Jr., Ph.D.

Senior Scientist, Indoor Environment Program
Energy and Environment Division
Lawrence Berkeley Laboratory
University of California
Berkeley, California 94720

WILLIAM A. NEWTON, Jr., M.D.

Professor Emeritus of Pathology and Pediatrics
Ohio State University
College of Medicine
Columbus, Ohio 43210

JOHN D. OSTERLOH, M.D.

Associate Professor of Medicine and Clinical
    Laboratory Medicine
School of Medicine
University of California
San Francisco, California 94143

SUSHMA PALMER, D.Sc.

President of the Central European Center for
    Health and the Environment
Berlin, Germany

KENNETH D. ROSENMAN, M.D.

Associate Professor of Medicine
Department of Medicine
Michigan State University
East Lansing, Michigan 48824

DEAN SHEPPARD, M.D.

Associate Professor of Medicine
University of California
School of Medicine
San Francisco, California 94143

JOHN D. SPENGLER, Ph.D.

Professor of Environmental Health
Harvard School of Public Health
Boston, Massachusetts 02115

EMIL STEINBERGER, M.D.

President
Institute of Reproductive Medicine
Houston, Texas 77054

ROBERT D. STEPHENS, Ph.D.

Chief, Hazardous Materials Laboratory
California Department of Health Services
Berkeley, California 94704

ROBERT M. SUSKIND, M.D.

Professor and Chairman
Department of Pediatrics
Louisiana State University
School of Medicine
New Orleans, Louisiana 70112

ALYCE BEZMAN TARCHER, M.D.

Associate Clinical Professor
Department of Epidemiology and Biostatistics
Lecturer
Department of Medicine
School of Medicine
University of California
San Francisco, California 94143

JOHN R. TAYLOR, M.D.

Associate Professor
Department of Neurology
Medical College of Virginia
Richmond, Virginia 23298

JEFFREY E. WEILAND, M.D.

Associate Professor of Medicine
Ohio State University
College of Medicine
Columbus, Ohio 43025

I. BERNARD WEINSTEIN, M.D.

Director Comprehensive Cancer Center
Frode Jensen Professor of Medicine
Columbia University
College of Physicians and Surgeons
New York, New York 10032

RONALD C. WESTER, Ph.D.

Adjunct Associate Professor
School of Pharmacy
University of California
San Francisco, California 94143

PETER YANG, M.D.

Assistant Clinical Professor of Medicine
Case Western Reserve University
School of Medicine
Cleveland, Ohio 44106

PREFACE

Throughout the world, scientists and the general public are concerned about the adverse effects of toxic agents found in contaminated air, water, food, and soil. In the past, attention has focused on hazards originating in the workplace. As a consequence, occupational medicine has become a well-recognized and established clinical discipline. Much less attention has been paid to nonoccupational hazards. There is a growing awareness, however, of the dangers of exposure to toxic chemical and physical agents in the homes, community, and general environment, especially for the fetus, the infant, the very young, the elderly, and the chronically ill, those most susceptible. Environmental medicine, focusing on the study and care of individuals exposed in a nonoccupational setting, is an emerging discipline that will increasingly demand the attention of the medical and health professions.

I conceived and designed *Principles and Practice of Environmental Medicine* to address the need for a basic text in environmental medicine. It was organized to present the vast and complex body of data in a rapidly expanding field in a systematic manner. Its design is both theoretical and practical. Emphasis is placed on the basic theoretical and practical framework needed to assess and treat environmental illness and on the knowledge and skills required to incorporate environmental factors into clinical practice. The text is a collaborative effort of a number of noted authorities in their respective fields.

The work is aimed at a broad audience that includes medical students and physicians in all specialties who require the knowledge and skills necessary to recognize, diagnose, treat, and prevent environmental illness. It is also intended for other students and professionals concerned with environmental health and protecting the public from the adverse effects of hazardous exposure.

The book is organized into eight parts. Part I engenders a broad understanding of the relationship between environmental hazards and disease and provides a framework for assessing and dealing with environmental illness. Part II presents an overview of chemical and physical agents commonly found in contaminated air, water, food, and soil. The problem of hazardous wastes is also discussed. Part III characterizes the body's defense against such exposure. Defenses at the portals of entry are discussed, with emphasis placed on the role of nutrition. Detoxication and immunologic defense mechanisms are described. Part IV indicates the importance of and provides instruction on the method of including occupational and environmental factors in the routine medical history. The role of enhanced susceptibility as a factor in an individual's response to toxic exposure is discussed. Part V acquaints the reader with current medical information on the adverse health effects of common environmental contaminants. This section is organized by organ system. Part VI considers methods used to monitor exposure to environmental contaminants. Part VII discusses methods used by individuals and by society to control exposure to environmental chemicals and physical agents. Part VIII (Appendixes A–D) contains information on toxic chemicals and their adverse health effects and provides a comprehensive resource guide in the field of environmental and occupational medicine.

In the interest of keeping this book to a manageable size, a section organized according to type of hazard (e.g., metals, solvents, pesticides) was omitted. Instead, specific toxic agents are discussed in the chapters that deal with disorders of the various organ systems (Part V). In addition, Part VI contains, along with a discussion of environmental chemicals amenable to biological monitoring, information on their occurrence, metabolism, and health effects. Appendixes A, B, C, and D respond to questions related to the adverse effects of specific hazards. Although this arrangement results in some overlap, the reader has the advantage of consulting these sections without needing to refer to other sections of the book.

I am deeply indebted to all of the authors for

their outstanding contributions and for sharing the aims of this work. I am also grateful to many colleagues who assisted me by carefully reviewing manuscripts and offering valuable advice. I owe a great debt to the librarians of Mount Zion Medical Center of the University of California, San Francisco, for their extraordinary professionalism and dedication—in particular, Gail L. Sorrough, Gloria Y. Won, Sarah S. Stevens, and Angela Wesling. Many thanks are due to Mimi Horne, illustrator, for her expertise and commitment to this work. I wish to thank Richard M. Wright IV, Edwin N. Ali, and Ayyut Abdul Khalik at the Reprographics Department of Mount Zion Medical Center, University of California, San Francisco, for their technical assistance. It is a pleasure to acknowledge the support of the staff of Plenum Publishing Corporation, in particular the guidance of Mariclaire Cloutier and Eliot Werner and the production skills of Andrea Martin. During the many years this work was in preparation, my husband, Dr. Martin Tarcher, gave freely of his time. For his critical editorial·review of the entire work and his unwavering support, I am grateful beyond words.

CONTENTS

PART IV. CLINICAL CONSIDERATIONS

PART V. DISORDERS ASSOCIATED WITH EXPOSURE TO ENVIRONMENTAL CHEMICALS AND PHYSICAL AGENTS

PART VI.   ASSESSING EXPOSURE TO ENVIRONMENTAL CHEMICALS

PART VII.   CONTROLLING EXPOSURE TO ENVIRONMENTAL CHEMICALS AND PHYSICAL AGENTS

PART VIII.   APPENDIXES

Part I

FUNDAMENTALS OF ENVIRONMENTAL MEDICINE

1. PRINCIPLES AND SCOPE OF ENVIRONMENTAL MEDICINE

Alyce Bezman Tarcher

INTRODUCTION

Human health is determined by the interplay between heredity and the environment. The dimensions of the environment are vast, encompassing all external factors that impinge on humans. Air, water, food, and soil contain chemical, physical, and biological agents some of which are known to be harmful to health. In the past, the major cause of death was bacterial infection. With improved sanitation, biological factors (i.e., infections) pose a much smaller health threat in developed countries. With the microbial threat to health reduced, both medical scientists and clinicians have focused on changes within the body as a major source of disease. Investigators have made fundamental advances in the fields of biochemistry, physiology, pharmacology, and surgery, and clinicians have aimed at understanding the patient's symptoms and signs in terms of biochemical and physiological changes occurring within the body. Diagnostic tools became increasingly sophisticated, and therapeutic actions were directed to altering malfunctions within the body through medication and/or surgical intervention.

But the same technology that provided the clinician with sophisticated diagnostic and therapeutic tools also revolutionized industrial and agricultural development, creating a massive dependence on synthetic chemicals, pesticides, chemical fertilizers,

Principles and Practice of Environmental Medicine, edited by Alyce Bezman Tarcher. Plenum Medical Book Company, New York, 1992.

and other man-made agents. In 1984, it was estimated that some 5 million chemical compounds had been synthesized (40). In the United States alone, synthetic organic chemical production, coal tar, and primary products from petroleum and natural gas increased from about half a billion kilograms in 1940 to about 173 billion kilograms in 1989 (59) (Fig. 1-1). The more than 1000 new chemicals produced annually are added to the estimated 60,000 to 70,000 different chemicals currently being marketed (58). The synthetic organic chemicals provide a profusion of such products as plastics, solvents, fuels, synthetic fibers, pigments, and pesticides. Industrialization has increased the production of combustion products and organometallic compounds and altered the global distribution and conditions of exposure to such natural agents as asbestos, trace elements, and metals (17). These agents, now widely dispersed in the environment, have created new and often insufficiently understood health hazards.

Certain physical environmental agents also pose health risks. The adverse health effects of ionizing radiation have been understood for a number of years. Recently, radon gas and its decay products have caused concern because of their accumulation in residential dwellings. Nonionizing radiation in the ultraviolet range is also well known to be a health hazard. The potential health risks of electric and magnetic fields are currently being actively investigated. Increasing attention is also being directed to the health problems that may occur over the course of the next several decades as a result of global warming and depletion of the ozone layer.

3

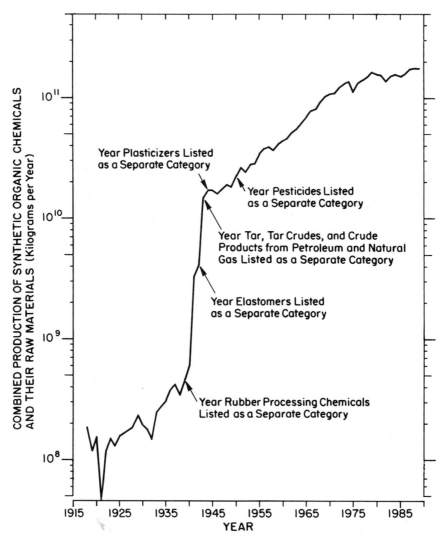

FIGURE 1-1. Combined production of all synthetic organic chemicals, coal tar, and primary products from petroleum and natural gas in the United States. Data obtained from U.S. International Trade Commission (59).

It should be appreciated that environmental degradation, including global warming, stratospheric ozone depletion, acid rain, air pollution, soil erosion, deforestation, and a decrease in ocean productivity, represent the ultimate threat to human health and the health of all species. The vast public health implications of such changes in the global environment are not fully apparent.

In many countries throughout the world, public concern with the chemical and physical agents in their midst was translated into the creation of new regulatory agencies and legislation charged with the task of protecting the populace from hazardous

toxic exposures. In the United States, right-to-know laws now inform workers and the populace at large about the nature and the potential health risks of chemical and physical agents in their midst (23).

Many individuals have also begun to turn to the medical community for guidance in these matters. The growing awareness of the potential risks of chemical and physical agents in the home, workplace, community, and general environment prompts physicians to gain skill in dealing with environmental health problems. Indeed, it is not surprising that the skill of the clinician who initially sees a patient is often crucial to the recognition, treatment, and prevention of disorders attributable to environmental or occupational exposures. Clinicians are required to (1) identify conditions induced by exposure to toxic substances in the home, the workplace, and the community; (2) provide appropriate treatment or referral for treatment; (3) identify occupational and environmental health risks; and (4) counsel or refer patients for counseling about preventive actions (1,26).

In addition to their clinical skills, physicians must also possess some knowledge of toxic exposures encountered in the workplace, home, and general environment and of their adverse effects. Of equal importance to a solid foundation in occupational and environmental medicine is an understanding of certain fundamental concepts and principles that are applicable to all environmentally and occupationally induced disorders. A major aim of this book is to provide such knowledge.

This book is designed to (1) engender a broad understanding of the relationship between environmental hazards and disease; (2) provide a framework for assessing and dealing with clinical problems in environmental and occupational medicine; (3) provide an overview of chemical and physical agents commonly found in contaminated air, water, food, and soil and characterize the body's defense against such exposure; (4) emphasize the importance of including occupational and environmental factors in the routine medical history; (5) indicate the significance of enhanced susceptibility as a factor in an individual's response to toxic exposure; (6) acquaint the reader with current medical information on the health effects of common environmental contaminants and consider the methods used to monitor such exposure; (7) discuss the methods used by individuals and by society to control exposure to environmental chemical and physical agents; and (8) provide the reader with a comprehensive resource guide in the field of environmental and occupational medicine.

Prior to discussing the basic principles underlying the relationship between toxic exposure and disease, it is essential to point out the fallacy in any attempt to create a distinction between environmental and occupational medicine. It is obvious that the workplace is an important part of the environment. The term "environment" must include the workplace as well as the home, neighborhood, community and general environment. The hazards found in all sectors are interrelated. Workers, for example, are often among the first, most heavily exposed, and severely affected by chemicals that subsequently put the community at risk. Many of the same chemicals cause concern in both the workplace and the community. Moreover, that facet of clinical medicine concerned with toxic hazards on the job and in the home and community share the same basic concepts and principles. This includes a concern for preven-

tion and the extent to which chemicals and physical agents present a health hazard.

Within this branch of clinical medicine, the focus or emphasis may favor one or more sectors. The sector that, to date, has received the greatest emphasis is "occupational medicine." Occupational medicine includes all aspects of the impact of work on health. It also considers the impact of health on a worker's ability to work. It is a well-recognized and established clinical specialty. Much attention has been paid to problems emanating in the workplace, and much is known about physical and chemical occupational hazards. Much less is known, however, about nonoccupational hazards found in the home, neighborhood, community, and general environment. "Environmental medicine," as discussed in this book, although including occupational hazards, focuses on the study and care of individuals in their homes and communities who are exposed to toxic agents through contaminated air, water, food, and soil. With this focus, environmental medicine is in the first stages of development as a clinical discipline. To date, its implications for and connections to clinical medicine are unclear (26). As more and more studies focus on the connection between environmental hazards and disease, the tie between environmental medicine and clinical medicine will undoubtedly continue to grow. In this context it is noteworthy that such susceptible groups as the fetus, the infant, the very young, the elderly, and the chronically ill all incur toxic exposure in a nonoccupational setting—through contaminated air, water, food, and soil.

In some cases, the health hazards of exposure to such agents as cigarette smoke, asbestos, benzene, vinyl chloride, lead, and carbon monoxide are quite well established. Moreover, in recent years it has become evident that low-level exposure to certain environmental chemicals causes subtle changes that are not clinically apparent. A prime example is the disturbance in neurobehavioral development seen in children as the result of low-level lead exposure (4,42,53).

For the majority of chemical agents in commercial use, the health effects are either poorly understood or still undetected and therefore generally unsuspected. We are dealing with so many unknowns that any tendency for complacency about the potential health effects of the chemical contamination of the environment is inappropriate. Our limited understanding of the problem is further dramatized by its dimensions. The pervasiveness and widespread human exposure to untold numbers of environmental agents, coupled with the possible inhibitory, additive, or synergistic effects of multiple exposures acting on individuals of different susceptibilities, offer some clues to the complexity of the relationship between exposure and disease.

As might be expected, identifying illnesses related to environmental exposures often tries the skills of the most adept physician. The problems encountered are many. Repeated exposure to a toxic agent in combination with other substances often makes it virtually impossible to identify a specific causal agent. The nonspecific and often delayed effects and symptoms of exposure to an environmental chemical present another dilemma in the identification of the causal agent(s). If the complexities of these problems are to be understood and countered in a meaningful and efficient manner, the clinician will require a basic grasp of the relationship between toxic exposure and disease.

BASIC PRINCIPLES OF TOXIC EXPOSURE AND DISEASE

Fundamental Relationships

The complexity and special conditions arising from the relationship between toxic exposure and disease contribute to the difficulties encountered in the recognition of environmentally and occupationally induced disease. The essential features of this relationship consist of an environmental agent acting on a host in a particular environmental setting. The agent is characterized by its intrinsic toxicity, potency, and such characteristics as its physical state, solubility, or wavelength (30). The host is characterized by such features as genetic make-up, age, gender, nutritional status, physiological status (including pregnancy and lactation), and general health status (60). The conditions of exposure, by influencing the extent to which an agent reaches the host, can modify the host's response. These basic interactions, well understood by pharmacologists and toxicologists, are also relevant to the clinician concerned with the health effects of toxic exposure. By being attentive to the agent and the host and by understanding the patterns, pathways, and conditions of human exposure, the clinician gains a broad overview. This overview is essential to understanding and diagnosing environmentally induced disease because it allows consideration and weight to be given to the various factors involved in its genesis.

Exposure and Effects

A fundamental part of environmental and occupational medicine is concerned with understanding and assessing exposure and its effects. Exposure refers to a contact with a substance that is described in terms of intensity, duration, frequency, time pattern (continuous or intermittent), and route(s). The dose gives information on the intensity of exposure in terms of the amount present. A quantitative description of the duration, frequency, and time pattern is also necessary (30).

An effect is the reaction or the response of an organism following exposure to a toxic agent. This reaction may vary with respect to quality strength, onset, and duration (30). Clearly, a "toxic effect" means one thing to a biochemist (e.g., enzyme inhibition) and another thing to a clinician (e.g., disease). For clinical purposes an "adverse effect" is a response that either impairs organ function at the subclinical level or results in disease or death (35).

An effect may be temporally related to exposure by onset and duration. An acute effect follows closely on an exposure and/or develops rapidly, whereas delayed or latent effects follow exposure within days, weeks, or sometimes decades. Chronic effects are long lasting.

Exposure–Response

Once environmental agents are absorbed, their exposure–response relationship generally follows one of three models: (1) for most agents the toxic manifestations are dose dependent. A safe threshold, or some minimal dose, appears to exist below which there is no demonstrable adverse effect. The concept of a threshold implies that there is some dose of a compound that is not capable of producing the adverse response (30). (2) For substances that are carcinogens, it is assumed that no safe threshold exists. The assumption of a linear, nonthreshold relationship implies that at any one molecule of dose, there is a risk of a response. No thresholds are known or presumed to exist for the mutagenic and carcinogenic effects of ionizing radiation and certain chemicals (57). (3) For substances producing hypersensitivity or allergic reactions, which are immunologic in nature, a previous sensitization is necessary. After this has occurred, allergic reactions develop from exposure to low doses of the inciting agent. For a specific allergic individual, allergic reactions are dose related (30).

The Host

It has long been recognized that many environmental substances are harmful only to certain members of a population. Thus, host factors are known to influence susceptibility. Many factors including genetics, age, gender, nutritional status, physiological status, health status, and prior exposures are important in determining susceptibility to toxic exposures (6–8,44,60,61) (see Chapter 12). Susceptibility is the result of many mechanisms that lead to differences in the movement of toxic agents from the environment into the body, to alterations in detoxification and immunologic reactions, and to variations in the responsiveness of target tissues. The diversity of host factors determining susceptibility coupled with the multiplicity of mechanisms underlying this condition means that the patterns of increased or decreased susceptibility to specific environmental agents undergo continuous change throughout an individual's lifetime (60).

The Genesis of Environmentally and Occupationally Induced Disease

A major determinant of the health or well-being of an individual is the balance between exposure to chemical or to physical agents and the body's biological responses. Put in another way, the body's defense against environmental assault is critical in maintaining health. There are three lines of defense against exposure to environmental agents: (1) the portals of entry, e.g., the skin, lung, and gastrointestinal tract, which provide the initial barrier against the entry of foreign agents; (2) the process of biotransformation, which chemically alters and thereby detoxifies many foreign compounds; and

(3) the immune response, which protects the body primarily from microbial invaders. Because of the critical roles these defense mechanisms play in protecting the body from the adverse effects of environmental exposures, the genesis of environmentally and occupationally induced disease can be viewed in the context of environmental exposures being opposed by the body defenses (Fig. 1-2). Moreover, it can be appreciated that susceptibility to the adverse effects of toxic exposure may be increased when defense mechanisms are compromised. There is evidence that certain defenses are compromised in such susceptible groups as the fetus, the infant, the very young, the aged, the malnourished, and those with impaired health or with particular genetic conditions (see Chapter 12).

Viewing the genesis of occupational and environmental illness in terms of the counterbalance between toxic exposure and host defenses directs attention to both sides of the equation in diagnostic and preventive efforts. It is noteworthy, for example, that infants and young children have structural and functional characteristics that compromise their de-

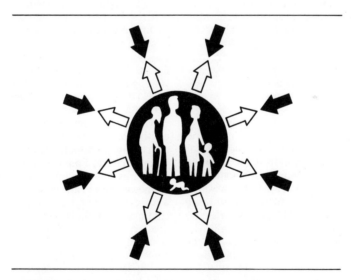

ENVIRONMENTAL EXPOSURES

Environmental Chemicals and
Physical Agents
• In Air, Food, Water
• In Home, Workplace, Community,
  General Environment

BODY DEFENSES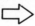

Defenses at Portals of Entry
• Skin, Lung,
  Gastrointestinal Tract
Detoxication Mechanisms
Immunologic Mechanisms

FIGURE 1-2. Factors operating in the genesis of environmentally and occupationally induced disease.

fenses against environmental exposures. It is therefore singularly important that they be given special consideration in terms of protection from toxic exposure (63).

Environmental exposures (i.e., chemicals and physical agents) in air, water, and food are discussed in Chapters 2–4. The body defenses against environmental exposures are discussed in Chapters 6–10. Chapter 12 focuses on susceptible groups, especially in relation to their defense against environmental exposures.

IMPORTANT CONCEPTS

Certain basic concepts can be applied to environmentally and occupationally induced disease. In large part, clinical skill in this area depends on understanding the clinical implications of such concepts as latency, multifactorial etiology, lack of specificity, and susceptibility to exposure.

Latency

Latency is concerned with the ability to relate exposure events causally with effects (e.g., disease) often distantly associated in time. In many instances the effects of toxic exposure occur long after the onset of exposure. Malignancies, for example, are well known to occur in some individuals exposed to a carcinogen only after a relatively long latent period. In the field of infectious disease, the concept of the incubation period is well established. However, in the main, this deals with days or weeks. Now, as we consider the effects of low-level exposures to chemical agents, many of which have only recently entered the environment, we are more and more often faced with the need to relate occurrences that are separated not by days, weeks, or months but by years. Understanding such a relationship is exceedingly complex, particularly if the interval between exposure to the causal agent and the evidence of disease is protracted and if the agent is no longer present when the disease becomes apparent. The longer the interval between the two events and the lower the frequency with which the secondary event follows the primary one, the more difficult it becomes to prove association, or indeed even to suspect it. This implies the necessity of viewing the entire human life span with an awareness that an individual's health status is influenced by all that went before and will in turn have an effect on all that follows.

Multifactorial Etiology

The genesis of environmental and occupational illness should be considered in the broadest pos-

sible context. In essence, this means that determining the effects of a particular toxic exposure is not an isolated problem. It exists in combination with other exposures and with the characteristics of the exposed host. Factors such as concomitant exposures, life style, underlying health, age, gender, and nutritional status may all act in concert to modify the body's response to a particular exposure. Preventive and therapeutic intervention should therefore consider both the modification of risk factors and a reduction of exposure. On this basis, potential risk factors should be considered in all cases of diseases suspected of being environmental in origin. This consideration is particularly important in cases of chronic disease. In some instances, the multiple factors involved are well defined and of major importance, as when asbestos and cigarette smoking act synergistically to cause an enormous increase in the risk of lung cancer (51,52). In other cases, the importance of host factors in combination with exposure is well documented and of major importance, as in the increased susceptibility of the fetus and very young to the toxic effects of lead exposure (4,42,53).

Lack of Specificity

For reasons that are unclear, some individuals hold the impression that diseases induced by chemical and physical agents can be distinguished from other diseases. Unfortunately, only in rare instances do toxic agents give rise to unusual patterns of illness (e.g., mesothelioma linked to asbestos and liver hemangiosarcoma linked to vinyl chloride) and to diagnostic laboratory findings (e.g., carboxyhemoglobin and methemoglobinemia). For the most part, there are few sets of clinical, laboratory, or pathological characteristics that would lead a clinician to suspect toxic exposure and exclude other causes. Even acute health effects may escape identification because chemical exposure may be only one of the potential causes of the patient's complaints. Toxic exposure, for example, can give rise to such common disorders as headache, nervousness, cardiac arrhythmias, asthma, infertility, and chronic renal disease (see Part V). It is only when the total context of disease pattern and the circumstances of its appearance are considered that a toxic etiology might be suspected.

Susceptibility to Exposure

Differences among individuals in exposure–effect curves are based on such factors as age, gender, intercurrent disease, genetic make-up, prior exposures, and nutritional and physiological status (7–10,35,44,60,61). Variability in susceptibility is readily appreciated when a group of people receive similar exposure to an agent but only some individuals show symptoms and signs of an effect. The large differences in response among individuals to a similar exposure indicate a variation in human susceptibility that insures a wide range in the threshold for any effect.

Variation in susceptibility has certain important clinical implications. Physicians, by the nature of their profession, are involved in caring for the more susceptible members of the population (e.g., the infant, the aged, the chronically ill). Indeed, at times, physicians see patients who require medical attention because they fall at the far end of the spectrum of susceptibility. Under such conditions, a patient's belief that his or her symptoms arise from a particular exposure or a type of exposure may be valid even though others with similar exposures do not offer similar complaints. Obviously similar complaints by other members of an exposed group strengthen a suspected association, but the absence of such findings does not rule it out. Moreover, by attending to the more susceptible members of the population, the alert clinician may be the first to identify new associations between exposure and disease.

DETERMINING THE HEALTH EFFECTS OF TOXIC EXPOSURE

Our current understanding of the risks to humans of toxic exposure comes from the efforts of many disciplines. Clinical observations, toxicological studies in animals, and epidemiologic investigations have all made their contributions (20,43,47, 54). Since each discipline has its strengths and limitations, they must be used in tandem to complement and reinforce each other (Table 1-1). Drawing from each discipline not only enhances a research program, it also strengthens the hand of clinicians in their attempt to decipher the link between exposure and disease.

Clinical Observations

Although it is frequently unrecognized, clinicians play a central role in providing the initial evidence of environmental causes of disease. Being in the "front line" gives clinicians the opportunity to monitor continuously the diseases within the community. As a consequence, they are in a unique position to get the first glimpse of new associations between exposure and disease and to note the appearance of unusual clusters of rare diseases linked to toxic exposure (38). It is relevant to recall that the dangers of such agents as polyvinyl chloride, Kepone, DES, and thalidomide were recognized not by a research laboratory or by a computerized medical record system but by astute clinicians in the course of their practice (12,14,27,36,37). Obviously, in light of their limited and biased purview, the findings noted in individual case reports are always suspect and require confirmation. Nonetheless, the early observations of environmental hazards by clinicians have generated useful etiological hypotheses that have given direction and impetus to epidemiologic and laboratory studies. Identifying unsuspected potential environmental causes of disease affords the clinician a rare challenge not easily found in other areas of medicine.

Controlled clinical studies have also contributed to our understanding of the acute effects of toxic exposure. Our grasp of the acute respiratory effects of certain air pollutants has benefitted from controlled human exposure in carefully monitored experimental settings. Indeed, such studies have contributed to such important observations as the acute effects of sulfur dioxide exposure on the respiratory function of asthmatics (see Chapter 16).

TABLE 1-1. The Role of Clinical, Toxicological, and Epidemiologic Approaches in Determining the Health Effects of Toxic Exposures

	Advantages	Disadvantages
Clinical observations	Cases well defined, generation of hypotheses	Limited perview, strong selection bias
Toxicology	Study of mechanisms of actions and toxicokinetics, exposure more exact, no delay for human experience to begin study	Quantitative extrapolation to humans uncertain, expensive
Classical epidemiology	Direct measurement of human experience, dose-response data can be calculated if exposures are measured	Time consuming, measurement of exposure difficult, does provide association, does not provide causation, insensitive, disease must exist for study to be done, expensive
Molecular epidemiology (incorporates biomarkers in analytic epidemiologic research)	Measures more precisely internal dose exposure and genetic predisposition, identifies susceptibility in an individual, identifies earliest phases of disease	Early stage of development, validation needed

Toxicology

Animal studies provide our major source of information related to the toxic effects of chemical exposure. The principal aims of such studies are twofold: (1) to identify toxic substances by finding out what happens to an animal at a given dose of a chemical and (2) to clarify the mechanism of action of the chemical after its identification. Many methods are used for the toxicological evaluation of a chemical. These include studies of structure–activity relations; determination of bioavailability; animal bioassays for carcinogenicity, neurotoxicity, and reproductive toxicity; and short-term tests for cytotoxicity and genotoxicity (40). A search for the mechanism of action involves a study of the metabolism and toxicokinetics of the chemical in question. Such studies identify metabolites and determine excretory rates and biological half-lives of the chemical agent and its metabolites. Animal studies also provide information on the development of pathological changes in the affected organs (16,30,47).

Assessing the toxicity of a chemical includes lifetime chronicity testing and, if indicated, multigenerational studies. The primary resource for conducting experimentally based toxicity testing in the United States is the National Toxicology Program, which was established in 1978 (47). Chemicals are evaluated by this program for their toxic and carcinogenic effects in laboratory animals. By this means, information on carcinogenicity has been gained for a number of important chemicals. For carcinogenicity studies, the National Toxicology Program recommends using lifetime exposures in rats and mice with up to maximally tolerated doses (i.e., doses that fail to produce an effect as assessed by the response of the whole animal). The presence of a carcinogenic effect in laboratory animals is inferred from dose–response relationships along with overall mortality rates and consistency with effects on other species (16,47).

The uncertainties in extrapolating the results of animal toxicity studies to humans are well known, e.g., differences in species, size, duration of life, susceptibility, duration of exposure, dose, and other concomitant exposures. Of major concern is the use of maximally tolerated toxic doses, which pose the potential problem of overwhelming the animal's defenses. This is coupled with the difficulty in interpreting data from experimental doses that greatly exceed those encountered by humans in occupational or environmental settings. High doses are used in animal experiments in order to perform studies of sufficient sensitivity without using the literally thousands of animals that would be required were lower doses used. The following references present a more detailed discussion of the design, use, and interpretation of animal studies (2,16,47).

In spite of the problems associated with animal studies, chronic animal bioassays are the most widely used tool for identifying and assessing carcinogens. Such studies have been of great value in identifying proven or probable causes of human cancer. When adequately tested, almost all of the specific chemicals known to be carcinogenic in humans are also positive in rodent bioassays. Moreover carcinogens subsequently discovered to cause cancer in humans were frequently initially identified in rodent studies (56). In light of the absence of human data for many known animal carcinogens, the International Agency for Research on Cancer (IARC) holds that "it is biologically plausible and prudent to regard agents for which there is sufficient evidence of carcinogenicity in experimental animals as if they presented a carcinogenic risk to humans" (25,56). The alternative to animal studies, awaiting the development of cancer in humans, is not consistent with sound preventive medicine.

Epidemiology

Epidemiology investigates the occurrence of disease in human populations. Environmental epidemiology focuses on the association between exposure and disease. The ultimate objective of an epidemiologic study concerned with disease etiology is to address the issue of causality. Thus, such studies attempt to discover if a causal relationship, not just an association, is likely between an agent and an adverse effect (28,33,34,49,62).

Advantages

The major advantage of epidemiologic studies is that they deal with humans in their natural surroundings. They thus offer the most direct means of assessing the health risks associated with chemical and physical exposures. Epidemiologic studies carry out several important functions (Table 1-2). As a part of addressing issues of causality, epidemiologic studies often evaluate the occurrence of disease at varying levels of exposure. They also play a role in assessing the course and characteristics of disease, investigating susceptibility factors, and providing a foundation for disease prevention and control (Table 1-2). In general, epidemiologic studies are most revealing when they deal with highly ex-

TABLE 1-2.   Role of Epidemiology in Investigating Environmentally Induced Disease

Evaluate causal relationships
Relate the occurrence of disease to exposure levels
Assess course and characteristics of illness
Investigate modifying or susceptibility factors

posed groups or a population having a high frequency of disease.

Limitations

A major limitation of the epidemiologic approach is that it is based on uncontrolled observations and can strongly support but not actually prove the existence of causal relationships. This is coupled with its lack of sensitivity and its inability to evaluate the impact of recent exposure. Thus, a negative study, even under favorable circumstances, will usually be compatible with a 20% increase in risk (13). The deficiencies of the epidemiologic method are most apparent in connection with evaluating the significance of low-level chemical hazards or in the analysis of complex life-style factors (22).

Descriptive and Analytic Epidemiology

Epidemiologic studies are often categorized as descriptive or analytic in nature. Descriptive studies focus on the patterns of disease occurrence and thereby may suggest the existence of relationships. Analytic studies focus on the detection of risk factors for disease. Epidemiologic terms commonly used are found in the Glossary at the end of this chapter.

In theory, the epidemiologic approach depends in large part on the information collected through descriptive studies to generate a particular hypothesis, which is then tested in an analytic study of appropriate design. In practice, however, hypotheses often come from clinical, experimental, or biological observations. In this context, ecological observations that show the consequences of exposure to environmental agents on such species as birds and fish may also provide important clues and direction for epidemiologic studies (15).

Descriptive Studies

Descriptive epidemiology notes the occurrence of disease in a population by incidence, prevalence rates, and mortality. The incidence rate of disease is defined as the ratio of the number of new cases to the population at risk during a specified time period. Mortality is defined similarly, with the number of deaths as the numerator. Prevalence rate, representing the proportion of population with disease at a particular time, is determined not only by the incidence rate but also by the duration of the disease.

In descriptive studies, incidence and mortality rates are derived from aggregates and from the use of such surrogates for exposure as location, drinking water source, and proximity to hazardous waste sites. Vital statistics may be linked to data derived

from environmental monitoring studies. Frequently, such studies do not consider the presence of important risk factors.

Cross-sectional studies in which disease is measured in an exposed and an unexposed group at a single time are commonly used because of their feasibility and low cost. Such studies are also limited. For example, the temporal relationship between exposure and disease may be obscured. However, such studies, apart from providing important information on the prevalence of specific diseases in the population, may also provide a guide to future research.

Analytic Studies

Analytic studies are of two types: cohort (prospective and retrospective) and case-control. In cohort studies, groups of exposed and unexposed are defined, and a comparison is made of their disease frequency. In a prospective cohort study, the disease is expected to occur in the future. In a retrospective cohort study, the disease already exists. The unexposed and the diseased populations should be similar except for the exposure factor under study.

The prospective cohort study has the advantage that both exposure status and disease status can be evaluated directly at the same time. Comprehensive exposure information can also be collected. Direct estimation of disease rates can be made for the exposed and nonexposed group. The costs, time, and difficulty associated with following a prospective cohort are substantial. Moreover, the loss of subjects introduces a source of potential bias. The retrospective cohort study has the advantage of rapidly evaluating the effects of an exposure because both the exposure and its effects have already occurred. Cohort studies, though of limited value when studying a disease that is rare, are the desired approach for evaluating the adverse effects of rare exposures.

A case-control (case-referent) study involves the identification of a group of individuals with a disease and a comparable group of individuals without the disease. These two groups are then compared with respect to their exposure histories. The retrospective case-control study is an important research strategy (21). In comparison to cohort studies, case-control studies are more easily performed, less costly, and less time consuming. Case-control studies, however, are not a feasible method for investigating the effects of an exposure that is rarely encountered.

Considerations Regarding the Validity and Interpretation of Epidemiologic Studies

An association between exposure and disease may truly reflect a causal relationship. It may also have occurred on the basis of uncontrolled bias or chance. A causal association can be accepted only after chance or bias has been excluded. Epidemiologists attempt to exclude bias by bringing extraneous variables under control. This can be done at the design stage of a study and at the stage of statistical analysis. An important part of an epidemiologic design and analysis is foreseeing which variables linked to exposure could also predispose to the disease (confounding factors).

Analytic studies of each design are accompanied by many methodological problems. These include bias in the selection of appropriate study groups, bias related to the ability or incentive of individuals to recall exposures, bias in terms of the susceptibility of the exposed and unexposed groups, and bias introduced by confounding factors.

An important factor to be considered in interpreting the findings of a study is whether the groups studied were large enough to permit a reasonable chance of detecting a statistically significant excess risk. It has been recommended that any negative epidemiologic report include a statement of the statistical power of the study to detect a particular increased frequency of a given disease (3). The power of a study to detect an effect depends on a number of factors. These include the size of the groups studied, the background prevalance of the disease or exposure, the length of time the subjects are followed, and the level of statistical significance required. A more detailed discussion of the principles of epidemiology is found in references 28, 33, and 49.

Criteria for Evaluating Disease Causation

With the observational methods of epidemiology in mind, Sir Austin Bradford-Hill proposed that certain criteria be considered in making inferences regarding a causal link between an agent or exposure and a disease (5) (Table 1-3). Temporal consistency is the only criterion absolutely essential for inferring causality. The strength of an association is a consideration. As the strength increases, a causal relationship is more likely; but this is not necessarily the case. A dose–response relationship strengthens the argument for causality. However, such a relationship may not always be biologically appropriate. Biological plausibility, though important, is not binding. Moreover, giving excessive weight to this criterion may reduce the observers' openness to unexpected relationships.

Consistency and coherence are of importance. Specificity is generally not relevant, especially in terms of chronic diseases, which are multifactorial in cause. There is no precise formula for assessing causality; the weight given to each criterion may vary with the particular association under consideration (35,48).

TABLE 1-3. Criteria for Evaluating Causation[a]

1. Temporal consistency: Exposure to a putative cause always precedes the outcome
2. Strength: An expression of the disparity between the frequency with which a factor is found in disease and the frequency with which it occurs in the absence of disease
3. Biological gradient: A dose–response relationship
4. Biological plausibility: The effect is predictable based on the effects known to be caused by the agent or by agents similar to it in actions
5. Consistency: Similar observations by multiple investigators in different populations under different circumstances
6. Coherence: Cause-and-effect intepretation for an association is not in conflict with other scientific data
7. Specificity: A unique exposure–response linkage
8. Analogy: Do other similar agents have similar effects?

[a]From references 5, 32, 48, and 49.

Although the criteria for evaluating causality are appropriately applied when evaluating the observational associations gleaned in an epidemiologic study, it is noteworthy that the methods used by clinicians to decipher the relationship between exposure and disease are also observational in nature. It is therefore important for clinicians to have some understanding of the criteria used for inferring causality. With this knowledge in hand, clinicians can more readily determine whether a causal relationship is likely to exist between a putative etiological agent and an adverse health effect. Clinicians will also have greater insight into the limitations that prevail when they attempt to make a "definitive" diagnosis of environmentally or occupationally induced disease.

Meta-Analysis

The method known as meta-analysis promises to play an increasingly important role in the assessment of health risks associated with environmental exposure. Epidemiologic and other studies dealing with the health effects of environmental and occupational exposures are now becoming the new target of such analyses. The term meta-analysis was introduced to deal with the issue of synthesizing large quantities of information on a particular subject. The method involves an analysis of previous analyses. It combines the findings of previous studies and then applies statistical techniques in an effort to draw conclusions that are thought to be more definite than what is known from the individual previous studies. With the combined studies, the larger numbers obtained provide a greater statistical power than any of the individual studies. They may also produce a unified concept and point to areas that need additional investigation. The value of meta-analysis is often contrasted to the weakness of a narrative review of a subject in which conclusions may be based on a simple tally of the findings of previous studies. However, meta-analysis, as with any research technique, has methodological problems. These include such issues as data quality of the studies used in the meta-analysis, sampling bias, variability between studies, and data retrieval. For a more extensive discussion of the strengths and weaknesses of meta-analysis and research issues in this area, the reader is referred to references 31, 50, and 55.

Biological Markers in the Pathway from Exposure to Disease

Biological markers (biomarkers) are cellular, biochemical, or molecular alterations that indicate that certain events have taken place in a biological system. The current emphasis on biomarkers stems from the remarkable advances that have taken place in molecular biology and in analytic techniques that permit us to glimpse inside the cell and identify and measure previously unrecognized molecular or biochemical alterations. These events have had a major impact on medicine, especially on the enormous advances made in the field of immunology, and they are now poised to have an impact on the disciplines concerned with the health effects of exposure to toxic agents. For the first time, the sequence of cellular, molecular, and biochemical alterations known or believed to occur between exposure and disease is being dissected. In theory, biomarkers relevant to these events should increase our understanding of the steps involved in the biological pathway from exposure to disease.

Although biomarkers can be classified in a number of ways, the scheme most useful in addressing issues related to exposure and disease classifies biological markers into three categories: exposure, effect, and susceptibility (46). This classification draws attention to the biological pathway from exposure to clinical disease (Fig. 1-3).

Once an exposure has occurred, a sequence of biological events may be detected. These events serve as markers of the continuum between exposure and disease. This pathway, at any point, may be modified by the susceptibility of the host and by environmental and life-style factors. As noted in Fig. 1-3, the pathway begins with the exposure or the external dose, which is the concentration of a chemical substance in an individual's immediate environment. After the dose is absorbed, the markers of the internal dose provide a direct measure of the exogenous chemical or its metabolites in cells, tissues, or body fluids. Pharmacological data such as half-life, circulating peak dose, or cumulative dose are often used in quantifying the internal dose. Next are the markers of the biologically effective dose. These indicate the amount of the absorbed chemical interacting with critical subcellular, cellular, and tissue targets, as measured in the target tissue or in an established surrogate tissue. Biological effective dose markers include the interaction of a chemical agent with such critical cellular targets as DNA, RNA, or protein.

Next are biological response markers, which include biological or biochemical changes in cells or tissues that are causally related to the action of the chemical. Such changes are presumed to be a critical stage in the genesis of disease. Markers of response, in contrast to markers of biological effective dose, represent more severe cellular and tissue changes. These changes include interactions of greater persistence and less reversibility. Biological response markers include chromosomal aberrations in response to exposure to mutagenic chemicals, and decreased acetylcholinesterase in response to organophosphate insecticide exposure.

Finally, the last stage in the pathway is exhib-

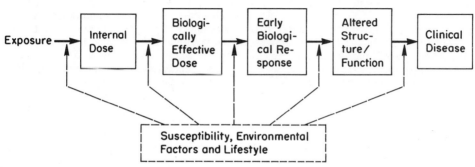

FIGURE 1-3. Biological markers (biomarkers) in the pathway from exposure to disease. Adapted from Committee on Biological Markers (9).

ited when the function of the target tissue is altered irreversibly by the chemical. A disease marker can represent a subclinical stage of disease or of the overt disease itself. Markers of subclinical disease include preclinical neoplastic lesions. Most biomarkers used to indicate disease have little if any relationship to the chemical or physical agents initiating the disease process (9,24). As advances are made, it is likely that any classification scheme currently in use will be modified.

Use of Biomarkers

Biomarkers are powerful tools that, apart from improving our understanding of disease pathogenesis, offer the potential advantage of improving the accuracy of exposure assessment; clarifying the dose–response relationship; estimating risks, especially for low-dose exposure; identifying the earliest phases of the disease process; and identifying individuals with increased susceptibility to certain exposures (19,24,46).

Biomarkers promise to play an important role in epidemiologic research and in clinical medicine. The incorporation of biomarkers into analytic epidemiologic research has been termed "molecular epidemiology" (24,46). Especially important is the potential for biomarkers to improve exposure assessment and thereby reduce exposure misclassification in epidemiologic research. Such errors result in random exposure misclassification and thereby produce erroneous and misleading results. The potential of biomarkers to detect very early evidence of a toxic endpoint offers clinicians increased opportunities for preventive action. For epidemiologists, it gains important time in identifying exposures that are implicated in diseases of long latency. The problems of latency may thereby be mitigated, especially in cancer epidemiology (44,45). Markers of early responses also hold promise as screening tools for the presence of subclinical occupational disease. The study of individual susceptibility may also be advanced through the use of biomarkers that identify variations indicative of individual susceptibility to chemicals (61).

It bears emphasis that the use of indicators of biochemical or molecular biological alterations has been an essential part of clinical medicine and epidemiology. Identical markers are often used by the two disciplines. For example, both physicians and epidemiologists studying cardiovascular disease may focus on serum concentrations of cholesterol, lipoprotein fractions, and lipids. Unfortunately, in their attempt to relate exposure causally to disease, both epidemiologists and clinicians have had to rely primarily on evidence from the far end of the exposure–disease pathway (Fig. 1-3). This promises to change as biomarkers of early changes in this pathway are developed and tested.

Limitations in the Use of Biomarkers

Certain biological markers of internal dose, biological effective dose, and biological response can now be measured by laboratory assays in human tissues, cells, or fluids. These include the agent itself or its metabolites, DNA and protein adducts, and chromosome aberrations. The use of biomarkers, however, is limited by the fact that they are largely in the developmental stage. Biomarkers are not fully evaluated. For the most part, biomarkers of exposure to environmental chemicals and their early adverse effects have not yet been correlated with future health outcomes. As with any new field of research, the initial high expectations must be tempered by the vast amount of time and effort needed before its potential can be realized.

RISK ASSESSMENT

Most of the health benefits that derive from the awareness of an environmental or occupational hazard come through action directed at population groups. Efforts to guide this action by the formulation of public health policy are directed to the assessment of human health risks. Risk assessment is basically an attempt to define the probability of an adverse health effect in an exposed population. In the past, risk assessment was largely concerned with carcinogenicity. Issues of reproductive and developmental toxicity, neurotoxicity, and immunotoxicity are now being addressed.

Risk assessment consists of (1) hazard identification—establishing whether the situation or exposure causes the adverse effect, (2) dose–response assessment—relating dose to the toxicological response, (3) exposure assessment—estimating the extent of human exposure, and (4) risk characterization—estimating the health risk expected in a defined population based on the information generated in the preceding steps (39). Risk assessment depends on data from clinical studies, epidemiologic studies, animal studies, and in vitro tests. Inevitably, such assessment requires the provisional acceptance of large numbers of assumptions and the use of estimates to circumvent the dilemmas posed by the lack of specific data. Each of the steps requires assumptions that are open to debate. An example is the extrapolation of data from animals to humans. A great deal of professional judgment is required at each step in the process. The expression of risk assessment may mask the degree of uncertainty underlying its formulation and thereby give a false sense of precision (29).

However, risk assessment is useful as a guide to regulatory agencies in setting exposure limits. It is tempting to extrapolate conclusions of a formal risk assessment and use them in the counseling of individuals concerned with specific environmental hazards. Such an exercise is inherently flawed, however, because risk assessments calculate risks in groups of peoples. Such variables as coexisting exposures that may increase or decrease an individual's risk are not assessed. Moreover, certain individuals fall outside the assumptions used in risk assessment. The subject of risk assessment is discussed in greater detail in Chapter 31. It has also been addressed by a National Academy of Sciences panel, and the interested reader is urged to consult a critical review of the subject (39).

RISK COMMUNICATION

A vital aspect of dealing with the topic of risk in relation to hazardous exposure is its communication to individuals and the public at large. This subject, in itself, is currently being explored with some intensity (11,18,41). Physicians, either by design or necessity, must often deal with this issue. A physician who becomes involved in this area must understand environmental issues and be aware that lay citizens may at times understand such issues and risks better than experts. Increasingly, citizens are becoming involved in environmental issues and the decisions that affect them. As they do so, it is important that they can draw on the medical community for information on the process of risk assessment and risk management.

SUMMARY

There is a growing awareness of the adverse health effects associated with exposure to toxic substances in the home, workplace, community, and general environment. A major challenge confronting the medical profession is the recognition and prevention of diseases linked to chemical and physical agents present in the environment. Clinical competence in the areas of environmental and occupational medicine requires clinical skills, an awareness of hazardous exposures and their effects, and an understanding of certain basic principles and concepts. Clinical observations, toxicology, and epidemiology have all contributed to our understanding of the adverse effects of toxic exposure. Drawing from each discipline strengthens the hand of the clinician in deciphering the link between exposure and disease. The process of risk assessment is a tool used, primarily by regulatory agencies, to define the probability of adverse health consequences of a specific hazardous situation. An understanding of this process will help the physician with the complex task of communicating risks to the public. The first step toward such understanding is the identification of the sources of the health risk—the toxic agents found in the air, water, and food. The next section of the book deals with these issues.

GLOSSARY*

Association: Statistical dependence between two or more events, characteristics, or other variables.

Bias: Deviation of results or inferences from the truth, or processes leading to such deviation. Any trend in the collection, analysis, interpretation, publication, or review of data that can lead to conclusions that are systematically different from the truth. The term "bias" does not necessarily carry an imputation of prejudice or other subjective factor.

Case: In epidemiology, a person in the population or study group identified as having the particular disease, health disorder, or condition under investigation.

Case-control study (Syn: case-referent study, retrospective study): A study that starts with the identification of persons with the disease and a suitable control group of persons without the disease. The relationship of an attribute to the disease is examined by comparing the diseased and nondiseased with regard to how frequently the attribute is present.

Causality: The relating of causes to the effects they produce. Most of epidemiology is concerned with causality; however, epidemiologic evidence by itself is insufficient to establish causality.

Cohort study (Syn: follow-up, longitudinal, prospective study): A method of epidemiologic study in which subsets of a defined population can be identified who are, have been, or in the future may be exposed or not exposed in different degrees to a factor thought to influence the occurrence of a disease or other outcome. The method entails the observation of a population for a sufficient number of person-years to generate reliable incidence or mortality rates in the population subsets.

Confounding: 1. A situation in which the effects of two processes are not separated; the distortion of the apparent effect of an exposure on risk brought about by the association with other factors that can influence the outcomes. 2. A relationship between the effects of two or more causal factors as observed in a set of data such that it is not logically possible to separate the contribution that any single factor has made to an effect. 3. A situation in which a measure of the effect of an exposure on risk is distorted because of the association of exposure with

*From Last (32).

other factors that influence the outcome under study.

Controls, matched: Controls who are selected so that they are similar to the study group, or cases, in specific characteristics. Some commonly used matching variables are age, sex, race, and socioeconomic status.

Cross-sectional study (Syn: disease frequency survey, prevalence study): A study that examines the relationship between diseases and other variables of interest as they exist in a defined population at one particular time.

Epidemiology: Study of the distribution and determinants of health-related states and events in populations and the application of this study to the control of health problems.

Incidence: The number of new cases of a disease in a defined population within a specified period of time.

Misclassification: The erroneous classification of an individual, a value, or an attribute into a category other than that to which it should be assigned.

Multivariate analysis: A set of techniques used when the variation in several variables has to be studied simultaneously.

Prevalence: The number of instances of a given disease or other condition in a given population at a designated time.

Random sample: A sample that is arrived at by selecting sample units such that each possible unit has a fixed and determinate probability of selection.

REFERENCES

1. American College of Physicians: Occupational and environmental medicine: The internist's role. A position paper. Annu Int Med 113:974, 1990.
2. Ames, BN: What are the major carcinogens in the etiology of human cancer? Six errors. In: Important Advances in Oncology, p 237, DeVita VT Jr, Hellman S, Rosenberg SA (eds.), JB Lippincott, Philadelphia, 1989.
3. Beaumont JJ, Breslow N: Power considerations in the evaluation of epidemiologic studies of vinyl chloride workers. Am J Epidemiol 114:725, 1981.
4. Bellinger D, Leviton A, Waternaux, C, et al: Longitudinal analyses of prenatal and postnatal lead exposure and early cognitive development. N Engl J Med 316:1038, 1987.
5. Bradford-Hill A: The environment and disease. Association or causation. Proc R Soc Med 58:295, 1965.
6. Calabrese EJ: Pollutants and High Risk Groups, John Wiley & Sons, New York, 1978.
7. Calabrese EJ: Nutrition and Environmental Health. The Influence of Nutritional Status on Pollutant and Carcinogenicity, Vol. I: The Vitamins, John Wiley & Sons, New York, 1980.
8. Calabrese EJ: Nutrition and Environmental Health. The Influence of Nutritional Status on Pollutant Toxicity and Carcinogenicity, Vol. II: Minerals and Micronutrients, John Wiley & Sons, New York, 1981.
9. Committee on Biological Markers in Environmental Health Research: Biological Markers in Environmental Health Research. Environ Health Perspect 74:3, 1987.
10. Conney AH, Burn JJ: Metabolic interactions among environmental chemical and drugs. Science 178:876, 1972.
11. Covello D, MacCallum M, Pavlova M (eds.): Effective Risk Communication, Plenum Press, New York, 1989.
12. Creech JL Jr, Johnson MN: Angiosarcoma of the liver in the manufacture of polyvinyl chloride. J Occup Med 16:150, 1974.
13. Day NE: Statistical considerations. In: Interpretation of Negative Epidemiological Evidence for Carcinogenicity. Scientific Publication No 65, p 13, Wald NJ, Doll R (eds.), International Agency for Cancer Research, Lyon, 1985.
14. Doll R: Pott and the prospects for prevention. Br J Cancer 32:263, 1975.
15. Goldsmith JR: The ecological imperative: Science as a protective system against unintended effects of technological change. In: Environmental Epidemiology: Epidemiological Investigation of Community Environmental Health Problems, p 247, Goldsmith JR (ed.), CRC Press, Boca Raton, FL, 1986.
16. Goodman DG: Animal testing of carcinogens. Occup Med 2:47, 1987.
17. Guthrie FE, Perry JJ (eds.): Introduction to Environmental Toxicology, Elsevier, Amsterdam, 1980.
18. Hadden S: Providing citizens with information about health effects of hazardous chemicals. J Occup Med 31:528, 1989.
19. Harris CC (ed.): Biochemical and Molecular Epidemiology of Cancer, Alan R. Liss, New York, 1986.
20. Hatch MC, Stein ZA: The role of epidemiology in assessing chemical-induced disease. In: Mechanisms of Cell Injury: Implications for Human Health, p 303, Fowler BA (ed.), John Wiley & Sons, New York, 1987.
21. Hayden GF, Kramer MS, Horwitz RI: The case-control study: A practical review for clinicians. JAMA 247:326, 1982.
22. Higginson J: Changing concepts in cancer prevention: Limitations and implications for future research in environmental carcinogenesis. Cancer Res 48:1381, 1988.
23. Himmelstein JS, Frumkin H: Right to know about toxic exposure—implications for physicians. N Engl J Med 312:687, 1985.
24. Hulka BS, Wilcosky TC, Griffith JD: Biological Markers in Epidemiology, Oxford University Press, London, 1990.
25. IARC: IARC Monographs on the Evaluation of Carcinogenic Risk to Humans, Supplement 7, International Agency for Research on Cancer, Lyon, 1987.
26. Institute of Medicine: Role of the Primary Care Physician in Occupational and Environmental Medicine, National Academy Press, Washington, 1988.
27. Jackson RS: Early testing and subsequent evaluation of the insecticide Kepone. Ann NY Acad Sci 392:318, 1979.
28. Kahn HA: An Introduction to Epidemiologic Methods, Oxford University Press, London, 1983.

29. Karatadt M: Quantitative risk assessment. Qualms and questions. Teratogen Carcinogen Mutagen 8:137, 1988.
30. Klaassen CD, Eaton DL: Principles of toxicology. In: Casarett and Doull's Toxicology. The Basic Science of Poisons, 4th ed., p 12, Amdur MO, Doull J, Claassen CD (eds.), Pergamon Press, New York, 1991.
31. L'Abbe KA, Detsky AS, O'Rourke K: Meta-analysis in clinical research. Ann Intern Med 107:224, 1987.
32. Last JM (ed.): A Dictionary of Epidemiology, 2nd ed., Oxford University Press, London, 1988.
33. Lilienfeld AM, Lilienfeld DE: Foundations of Epidemiology, 2nd ed., Oxford University Press, London, 1980.
34. Lilienfeld DE: Definitions of Epidemiology. Am J Epidemiol 107:87, 1978.
35. Mahaffey KR, Rapporteur: Human health effects. In: Mechanisms of Cell Injury: Implications for Human Health, p 431, Fowler BA (ed.), John Wiley & Sons, New York, 1987.
36. Miller RW: The discovery of human teratogen, carcinogens, and mutagens: Lessons for the future. In: Chemical Mutagens, p 101, Hollaender A, deSerres FJ (eds.), Plenum Press, New York, 1978.
37. Miller RW: Areawide chemical contamination: Lessons from case histories. JAMA 245:1548, 1981.
38. National Conference on Clustering of Health Events. Am J Epidemiol 132 (Suppl 1):S1–202, 1990.
39. National Research Council: Risk Assessment in the Federal Government: Managing the Process, National Academy Press, Washington, 1983.
40. National Research Council: Toxicity Testing Strategies to Determine Needs and Priorities, National Academy Press, Washington, 1984.
41. National Research Council: Improving Risk Communication, National Academy Press, Washington, 1989.
42. Needleman HL, Schell A, Bellinger D: The long-term effects of exposure to low doses of lead in childhood: An 11-year follow-up report. N Engl J Med 322:83, 1990.
43. Nelson N: Toxicology and epidemiology: Strengths and limitations. In: Epidemiology and Health Risk Assessment, p 39, Gordis L (ed.), Oxford University Press, London, 1988.
44. Omenn GS, Motulsky AG: Ecogenetics: Genetic variation in the susceptibility to environmental agents. In: Genetic Issues in Public Health and Medicine, p 83, Cohen BH, Lilienfeld AM, Huang PC (eds.), Charles C Thomas, Springfield IL, 1978.
45. Perera FP: Molecular cancer epidemiology: A new tool in cancer prevention. J Natl Cancer Inst 78:887, 1987.
46. Perera FP, Weinstein IB: Molecular epidemiology and carcinogen–DNA adduct detection. New approaches to studies of human cancer causation. J Chronic Dis 35:581, 1982.
47. Rall DP, Hogan MD, Huff JE, et al: Alternative to using human experience in assessing health risk. Annu Rev Public Health 8:355, 1987.
48. Rothman KJ: Causation and Causal Inference. In: Cancer Epidemiology and Prevention, Schottenfeld D, Fraumeni JF Jr. (eds.), p 15, WB Saunders, Philadelphia, 1982.
49. Rothman KJ: Modern Epidemiology, Little, Brown, Boston, 1986.
50. Sacks HS, Berrier J, Teitman D, et al: Meta-analyses of randomized controlled trials. N Engl. J Med 316:450, 1987.
51. Selikoff IJ, Hammond EC: Asbestos and smoking. JAMA 242:458, 1979.
52. Selikoff IJ, Hammond EC, Seidman H: Mortality experience of insulation workers in United States and Canada 1943–1976. Ann NY Acad Sci 330:91, 1979.
53. Smith M, Grant LD, Sors A (eds.): Lead Exposure and Child Development: An International Assessment, Kluwer Academic Publishers, Dordrecht, 1989.
54. Stallones RA: Epidemiology and environmental hazards. In: Epidemiology and Health Risk Assessment, p 7, Gordis L (ed.), Oxford University Press, London, 1988.
55. Thacker SB: Meta-analysis: A quantitative approach to research integration. JAMA 259:1685, 1988.
56. Tomatis L, Aitio A, Wilbourn J, et al: Human carcinogens so far identified. Review. Jpn J Cancer Res 80:795, 1989.
57. Upton AC: Are there thresholds for carcinogenesis? The thorny problem of low-level exposure. In: Living in a Chemical World, Proceedings of an International Conference on the Occupational and Environmental Significance of Industrial Carcinogens, p 863, New York Academy of Sciences, New York, 1988.
58. US Environmental Protection Agency, Office of Toxic Substances: Core Activities of the Office of Toxic Substances, Draft Program Plan. EPA Publication 560/4-760d05, US Environmental Protection Agency, Washington, 1976.
59. US International Trade Commission: Synthetic Chemicals. US Production and Sales, Annual Reports through 1989.
60. Vessell ES: Effects of human physiologic and genetic variability on the development and expression of pollutant-related diseases. In: Environmental Impacts on Human Health. The Agenda for Long-Term Research and Development, p 35, Draggan S, Cohrssen JJ, Morrison RE (eds.), Praeger, New York, 1987.
61. Vine MF, McFarland LT: Markers of susceptibility. In: Biological Markers in Epidemiology, p 198, Hulka BA, Wilconsky TC, Griffith JD (eds.), Oxford University Press, London, 1990.
62. World Health Organization: Guidelines on Studies in Environmental Epidemiology, Environmental Criteria 27. World Health Organization, Geneva, 1983.
63. World Health Organization: Principles for Evaluating Health Risks from Chemicals during Infancy and Early Childhood: The Need for a Special Approach, Environmental Health Criteria 59, World Health Organization, Geneva, 1986.

RECOMMENDED READINGS

Goodman DG: Animal testing of carcinogens. Occup Med 2:47, 1987.
Hernberg S: Introduction to Occupational Epidemiology, Lewis Publishers, Chelsea, Michigan, 1992.
Hulka BS, Wilcosky TC, Griffith JD: Biological Markers in Epidemiology, Oxford University Press, London, 1990.

Institute of Medicine: Role of the Primary Care Physician in Occupational and Environmental Medicine, National Academy Press, Washington, 1988.

National Research Council: Risk Assessment in the Federal Government: Managing the Process, National Academy Press, Washington, 1983.

National Research Council: Improving Risk Communication, National Academy Press, Washington, 1989.

Rall DP, Hogan MD, Huff JE, et al: Alternative to using human experience in assessing risk. Annu Rev Public Health 8:355, 1987.

Rothman KJ: Modern Epidemiology, Little, Brown, Boston, 1986.

Upton AC (guest ed.): Environmental medicine. Med Clin North Am 74:2, 1990.

World Health Organization: Our Planet, Our Health. Report of the WHO Commission on Health and Environment. World Health Organization, Geneva.

Part II

EXPOSURE TO ENVIRONMENTAL CHEMICALS AND PHYSICAL AGENTS

2. OUTDOOR AND INDOOR AIR POLLUTION

John D. Spengler

INTRODUCTION

Air pollution is a world problem afflicting densely populated urban centers and heavily industrialized areas. In recent years new data have changed our perception of air pollution. It is now recognized that air pollution crosses national boundaries to affect areas far distant from emission sources. In addition to its adverse health effects, air pollution also poses a danger to water, fish stocks, forests, natural vegetation, and agricultural crops. The evidence of pollutant transport across national boundaries now calls for increased international as well as national strategies for pollutant monitoring and control (46,86).

Air pollution is not new. It comes from such natural sources as smoke from forest fires, windblown dust from the soil and volcanoes, and such man-made sources as the burning of sulfur-containing fuel, the incomplete combustion of gasoline, and the evaporation of petroleum fuels. The concentrations of air pollutants depend on the combined effects of emission patterns, removal processes, climate, and weather conditions. Climate and weather conditions are particularly important in the generation, transformation, and dispersion of air pollution. In temperate regions, for example, domestic heating makes a considerable contribution to air pollution; in the tropics the photochemical conversion of auto exhaust gases is more prevalent. Turbulence and wind assist in the dispersion of pollutants. Their importance becomes readily apparent when the free flow of air is hindered by a temperature inversion that traps cool air with its pollutants near the ground. Episodes of air pollution have been de-

Principles and Practice of Environmental Medicine, edited by Alyce Bezman Tarcher. Plenum Medical Book Company, New York, 1992.

scribed throughout the centuries, the most famous being those that occurred in London, England, Donora, Pennsylvania, and the Meuse Valley of Belgium.

In past years outdoor air pollution was perceived as the major problem. Now, however, indoor air pollution in a nonmanufacturing setting has attracted the attention of scientists, policy makers and the public. Numerous studies have revealed that the concentrations of some air contaminants may be higher indoors than outdoors (30,83,87).

This chapter focuses on the sources, nature, and concentration of outdoor (ambient) and indoor air pollutants. It also includes a discussion of monitoring strategies and regulatory programs.

OUTDOOR AIR POLLUTION

Sources and Nature of Ambient Air Pollutants

Our ability to ascertain health and welfare effects and to prescribe effective standards and control strategies is directly dependent on our knowledge of pollutant sources and behavior. The major man-made sources of air pollution are (1) transportation, (2) fuel combustion in stationary sources (this includes fossel-fuel power plants and space heating), (3) industrial processes, and (4) waste disposal.

Air pollution stems from point sources and area sources. Point sources include such major industries as metallurgy, petroleum refineries, and chemical plants. Area sources include motor vehicle emissions and solvent use. Transportation sources, particularly the automobile, constitute a major source of air pollution (84). Gaseous pollutants from transportation sources include carbon monoxide, nitrogen oxides, and hydrocarbons. Particulate emissions from the automobile include unburned fuel or carbonaceous soot, fuel additives, lead, and other metal from engine use. Lead emissions for the most part have come from the use of tetraethyl lead in gasoline. This source has been sharply reduced in the United States.

Stationary combustion processes release sulfur and nitrogen oxides and particulate pollutants. Pollution emissions from industrial sources, which include petroleum refining and metal and chemical processes, are quite varied. Depending on the fuel, burning conditions and the facility, particles can be composed of soot, recondensed metal or organic vapors, and uncombusted mineral residues. Hazardous waste sites and the open burning of refuse can be a source of such pollutants as carbon monoxide, nitrogen oxides, hydrocarbons, solvents, volatile organic chemicals, aldehydes, toxic metals, and smoke.

Air pollutants may be classified as primary and secondary. A primary pollutant is defined as one that is emitted as such into the atmosphere. A secondary pollutant is one that is formed in the atmosphere by chemical or physical processes. The well-known problem of smog is an example of secondary pollutant formation. Photochemical oxidants are formed in the atmosphere in the presence of sunlight through a series of complex reactions that involve nitrogen oxides, organic compounds (hydrocarbons), and other reactive species. Ozone (O_3) is the major component of most photochemical smog. However, it is only one of the many oxidants present in photochemical pollution. Fine particles (typically less than 1 μm in size) are another example of secondary pollutants formed in the atmosphere from gaseous emissions that include recondensed metal vapors and oxidized sulfur and nitrogen compounds.

Air pollution is often a mixture of gases and particulate matter. The "traditional" gaseous pollutants—sulfur oxides, carbon monoxide, nitrogen oxides, and ozone—are well established as contributors to air pollution. More recently, attention has been directed to hazardous or toxic pollutants, which, in sheer numbers of compounds, make up the largest proportion of air pollutants (78). Toxic air pollutants include such agents as volatile organic chemicals (VOCs), metals, asbestos, radionuclides, and products of incomplete combustion (37). Many carcinogenic compounds are included in this list (61,78,80).

Gaseous Agents

Sulfur Dioxide Sulfur dioxide, a major air pollutant, is produced by the combustion of fossil fuels that contain sulfur. Ambient sulfur dioxide (SO_2) results largely from stationary-source coal and oil combustion, refineries, pulp and paper mills, and nonferrous smelters. Sulfur dioxide is emitted from industrial sources that use predominantly coal and fuel oil. Natural gas, gasoline, and diesel fuels have a relatively low sulfur content. Sulfur dioxide is a heavy, pungent, colorless gas that can easily oxidize in the atmosphere to form sulfuric acid and other sulfate aerosols.

Sulfur dioxide emissions are dominated by electric utilities. The combination of utilities and industrial sources that burn sulfur-containing coal and oil, and smelters that process sulfur-bearing ores, account for most of the SO_2 emitted in the United States.

Carbon Monoxide Carbon monoxide (CO) is an odorless, colorless gas emitted during incomplete combustion. Transportation (motor vehicles) sources account for approximately two-thirds of the CO emissions and thus are a major factor in the global increase. Increased concentrations of CO are found in urban areas with high concentrations of motor vehicles.

Nitrogen Dioxide Nitrogen oxides are emitted when combustion takes place at a high enough temperature to cause the thermal fixation of atmospheric nitrogen. Thus, almost any combustion process produces nitric oxide (NO), which subsequently undergoes oxidation to nitrogen dioxide (NO_2). The primary sources of nitrogen oxides are fuel combustion in gasoline engines, electric power plants, and other industrial processes. About half of the NO_2 is emitted from stationary fuel combustion, and the other half from transportation sources. As a result, NO_2 concentrations reflect the density of residential, commercial, and industrial fuel consumption as well as traffic patterns. Typically, higher NO_2 concentrations are found in the urbanized areas and in the vicinity of heavily traveled roads.

Oxides of nitrogen are an important precursor of other oxidants such as ozone, which is a major constituent of photochemical smog. Much of the nitrogen oxides coming from stationary sources is discharged through tall stacks and is thus subject to long-range transport. A portion of the nitrogen dioxide and sulfur dioxide released into the atmosphere is converted to nitric acids, which ultimately contribute to acid deposition in areas distant from the source (2,12,15). Acid precipitation has been observed in a number of locations including Canada, the United States, and Scandinavia (2,15).

Ozone Ozone, a principal component of photochemical smog, is one of the most pervasive pollutants. Ozone is not emitted directly into the air but is formed through complex chemical reactions between precursor emissions of volatile organic compounds and nitrogen oxides in the presence of sunlight. The photochemical formation of oxidant and ozone is the result of two coupled processes: (1) a physical process involving dispersion and transport of precursors to oxidants (e.g., hydrocarbons and nitrogen oxides) and (2) the photochemical reaction process. Both processes are strongly influenced by such meteorological factors as dispersion, solar radiation, temperature, and humidity. Since sunlight and temperature stimulate these reactions, peak ozone levels typically are reached during the summer. Both volatile organic compounds and nitrogen oxides are emitted by transportation and industrial sources.

Volatile Organic Chemicals

Volatile organic chemicals (VOC) make up a vast family of chemicals. Many polluting VOC are emitted into the atmosphere by incomplete combustion. Others are released by evaporation. The VOC are well recognized for their role in the formation of photochemical smog. These compounds are emitted by the chemical industry, by household and commercial solvent use, by incinerator plants, and by hazardous waste sites. In addition, VOC are likely to be emitted by new manufacturing processes involving the plastics and semiconductor industries. Many of the organic air pollutants were first discovered and identified as occupational hazards in the work environment.

Many of the organic compounds released into the atmosphere are recognized or suspected carcinogens (80). Specific organic compounds emitted include acrylonitrile, benzene, carbon tetrachloride, chloroform, ethylene oxide, formaldehyde, methylene chloride, naphthalene, perchloroethylene, trichloroethylene, toluene, and vinyl chloride (37).

Metals

The metals found in polluted air include arsenic, cadmium, chromium, copper, lead, mercury, and nickel. Arsenic is derived from coal and oil furnaces and from glass manufacturing. Cadmium is derived from such sources as electroplating, welding, smelters, and the plastic industry. Chromium is used for such processes as chrome plating, electroplating, and copper stripping. Copper is released from refuse incineration and electroplating operations. The major source of lead in the atmosphere has been motor vehicle emissions. Atmospheric mercury stems from the combustion of fossil fuels, including coal, and smelters. Sources of atmospheric nickel include smelters, fuel oil burning, electroplating, and stainless steel production.

Particulate Pollutants

Total suspended particulate matter (TSP) is the general term for particles found in the atmosphere. Particulate matter, as a pollutant class, apart from being exceedingly complex in its physical properties and chemical composition, varies greatly in size. It includes many organic and inorganic substances and ranges between <0.01 and >100 μm in diameter. Some particles are therefore large enough to be visible as soot or smoke. Others must be viewed with a microscope to be seen. Because of natural transformation and removal processes, the mass distribution of particles is usually bimodal. There is an accumulation mode peaking in the size range of 0.1 to 1.0 μm, and there is the coarse particle mode peaking around 10 μm in diameter (47).

The primary sources of particulate emissions include industrial processes, fuel combustion, transportation, and solid- waste incineration. Particulate emissions are often derived from such natural sources as forest fires, volcanoes, sea spray, and wind-blown soils.

Airborne particles arise from (1) large point sources such as smokestacks, (2) chemical reactions in the atmosphere that transform such gaseous emissions as sulfur and nitrogen oxides, ammonia, and volatile organic species into particulate matter, (3) combustion sources such as automobiles and trucks, residential furnaces, fireplaces, and wood stoves, (4) dust emissions stirred up by mechanical action or wind, as in dust storms, and (5) sporadic sources that can in some instances cause very high total suspended particulate values. These last two categories include agricultural tilling and burning and fires in forests, grasslands, and cities.

Fine Particles Fine particles, also referred to as aerosols, have diameters less than about 2 μm (82). Such particles, which can markedly reduce visibility, are more likely than large particles to be inhaled and to penetrate deep into the lungs. Fine particles, generally produced by burning fossil fuels, may contain such toxic substances as lead, vanadium, manganese, and polycyclic organic compounds (11,47). Sulfate, ammonium ions, organics, carbon, and combustion-associated metals are widely recognized to be the major components of fine particulate matter. A fraction of the sulfur oxide and nitrogen dioxide emissions oxidize further to particulate sulfate and nitrate particles, including strong acids (H_2SO_4 and NH_4HSO_4).

Most polycyclic organic compounds in ambient air are usually associated with particulate matter (11). Specific classes of organic compounds identified with airborne particulate matter include polycyclic aromatic hydrocarbons (PAH), aromatic and aliphatic hydrocarbons, aza-arenes, aliphatic and aromatic aldehydes and ketones, quinones, phenols, phthalic acid esters, aryl and alkyl halides, chlorophenols, nitro compounds, and alkylating agents (19,29).

Of all the airborne organic compounds, the polycyclic organic matter compounds—particularly the polycyclic aromatic hydrocarbons (PAHs)— have received the most attention. Many of these compounds are potent carcinogens in animals. Some of the polycyclic hydrocarbons identified in urban air include chrysene, benzo[a]anthracene, benzo[a]pyrene, benzo[b]fluoranthene, and alkyl derivates of these compounds (11,29,37,56).

Benzo[a]pyrene (BaP), a known animal carcinogen, was one of the earliest organic components of atmospheric particulate matter to be identified and routinely measured. Some measurements for BaP in the United States date to the early 1950s. Benzo[a]pyrene has been used as a surrogate for detecting the presence of airborne organic pollutants. It cannot be regarded as an adequate indicator of ambient polycyclic organic compounds or their carcinogenic properties. There is often a poor correlation between the release of polycyclic organic compounds and the release of benzo[a]pyrene. Auto emissions, for example, are low in benzo[a]pyrene, whereas such emissions from refuse burning are high (63).

Despite the intensive work that has been done on airborne organic particulates, especially the polycyclic aromatic hydrocarbons, it is estimated that over 99% of the atmospheric organic pollutants have never been determined (55). Today, more sophisticated techniques are being used in an attempt to determine the specific sources, concentrations, reactivity, and biological effects of airborne organic matter.

Large Particles Large particles are frequently generated by mechanical events of natural origin, i.e., wind-blown dust, agricultural tilling, and forest fires. Incinerator plants and the burning of refuse are responsible for the emissions of large particles into the atmosphere. Mining, milling, and mixing practices in many industries generate large particles. Examples of such industries include cement plants, iron and steel plants, smelters, coal-handling facilities, and asphalt-batching operations. A detailed discussion of particulate matter is found in Ambient Air Quality Criteria for Particulate Matter (73). Several comprehensive reviews of airborne organic particulate matter are also available (11,19,47).

Monitoring

The first federal legislation concerned exclusively with air pollution was enacted in 1955. It provided for research, data collection, and technical assistance to state and local governments. In 1957, a National Air-Sampling Network (NASN) began routine operation on a national basis. The U.S. Public Health Service, with cooperation from state health departments, has operated urban and nonurban stations for a number of years. In 1977, for example, over 4000 stations, mostly in state and local networks, reported to the National Aerometric Data Bank (NADB) of the U.S. EPA. The U.S. Environmental Protection Agency and its predecessor, the National Air Pollution Control Administration, have kept track of man-made pollutant emissions for over two decades.

Concern about air pollution has triggered national and international action. In 1973, the World Health Organization set up a global program to assist countries in air pollution monitoring. In 1976 this air-monitoring project became a part of United Nations Environmental Programme's Global Environmental Monitoring System (GEMS). By 1985, some 50 countries were participating in the GEMS air-monitoring project. Data are obtained from approximately 175 sites in 75 cities throughout the world, 25 of the sites in developing countries (26).

During the past 10 years great advances have been made in instruments and techniques for monitoring the airborne concentration of many air pollutants. Many types of sensitive instruments are now available for continuous and discrete-period measurements of such common gaseous pollutants as sulfur dioxide, ozone, nitrogen dioxide, and carbon monoxide. New instruments are able to provide and store data on cumulative exposure and on the frequency of periodic exposure peaks. Personal monitors are also available. They include small, inexpensive, lightweight devices that are sensitive enough to measure ambient concentrations of such pollutants as nitrogen dioxide, respiratory particles, sulfur dioxide, organic vapors, and carbon monoxide (58).

New techniques are currently being used to determine the specific chemical composition of particles. Many pollutant sources emit particles with an identifiable characteristic chemical signature. This information can be used to estimate the relative contributions of various pollutant sources. Particle analysis is increasingly used for this purpose. If an adequate description of the source signature is available, it is often possible to make approximate assignments of the relative amounts of suspended particulate matter derived from dust, power plants, automobiles, and other common sources.

Ultimately, the goal of measuring pollutant levels in ambient air lies in identifying and predicting undesirable effects. Until recently, epidemiologic studies investigating the relationship between air pollution and adverse health effects relied on such crude descriptions of outdoor air quality as annual averages or daily averages for total suspended particulates (TSP) or SO_2 to represent population exposures to air pollution. It is now recognized that these figures ignore such important considerations as the composition and size of particulate exposure, the contribution of pollutant exposure that is not measured by outdoor monitors, the influence of population mobility, the influence of peaks of pollutant exposure in addition to long-term low-level exposure, and the relationship between outdoor and indoor pollution levels. Considering the significance of indoor pollution to total exposure, the adequacy of using outdoor monitors to represent air pollutant exposure must be questioned (8,38).

It is clear that future epidemiologic studies concerned with the health effects of pollutant exposure must use more sophisticated exposure data than was used in the past. The noteworthy advances in instrumentation and techniques for monitoring air pollutants should be of help to future investigators.

Regulation

Air quality standards chosen to protect public health and welfare are a fundamental concept in air pollution management. The United States and several other countries have established National Ambient Air Quality Standards (NAAQS). The Clean Air Amendments of 1970 authorized the administrator of the United States Environmental Protection Agency to set primary standards and secondary standards. Primary air standards protect the public health; secondary standards protect welfare as measured by the effects of pollution on vegetation, on property, and on visibility.

The process of establishing air quality standards is lengthy. As a part of the process, the law requires EPA to prepare a "criteria document" that provides the scientific basis for the standard. Air quality standards are based on a wide range of toxicological, epidemiologic, and clinical research studies.

Since 1970, the Environmental Protection Agency has issued national ambient air quality standards for seven pollutants: sulfur dioxide, carbon monoxide, total suspended particulates, photochemical oxidants, hydrocarbons, nitrogen dioxide, and lead. The 1977 amendments to the Clean Air Act require EPA to review and revise, when appropriate, all existing ambient air quality standards (except for lead). Under this mandate, the standard for nonmethane hydrocarbons has been replaced by a guideline level, and the photochemical oxidant standard has been replaced by an ozone standard. These revisions were based on the rationale that adverse health effects could not be established from exposure to a class of nonspecific hydrocarbon compounds but were related to ambient photochemical reactions producing ozone and other oxidants.

The EPA has replaced TSP as the particle indicator for the primary standard with a new indicator that is based on a particle size of 10 μm (PM_{10}) (73). This was done in recognition of the fact that the averse health effects associated with exposure to suspended particulate matter are related not only to their concentration but also to their size. Smaller particles may pose a significant health risk because they penetrate deeply into the lungs. Table 2-1 presents the United States National Ambient Air Quality Standards criteria for various pollutants.

It is important to remember that the pollutants

TABLE 2-1. National Ambient Air Quality Standards (NAAQS)

Pollutant	Primary (health related)	
	Averaging time	Concentration
Ozone	1 h	0.12 ppm (235 μg/m³)
Carbon monoxide	8 h	9 ppm (10 mg/m³)
	1 h	35 ppm (40 mg/m³)
Nitrogen dioxide	Annual arithmetric mean	0.05 ppm (100 μg/m³)
Sulfur dioxide	Annual arithmetric mean	0.03 ppm (80 μg/m³)
	24 h	0.14 ppm (365 μg/m³)
Lead	Quarterly average	1.5 μg/m³
Suspended particulate matter (PM_{10})	Annual geometric mean	50 μg/m³
	24 h	150 μg/m³

embodied in the ambient air standards or emissions do not reflect the levels of toxic air pollutants found in our atmosphere. These pollutants are typically carcinogens, mutagens, and reproductive toxins. Acid aerosols, polynuclear aromatic hydrocarbons, chlorinated volatile organic vapors, and many toxic metals are examples of air contaminants not currently included in the national ambient air quality standards.

Unlike the criteria for pollutant standards that have developed over a number of years, a framework for regulating such toxic air pollutants as metals, radionuclides, and polycyclic organic compounds is emerging. Thus far, emission standards have been promulgated for mercury, asbestos, beryllium, vinyl chloride, benzene, arsenic, and radionuclides. The Clean Air Act of 1990 offers a comprehensive plan for achieving a significant reduction in the emissions of hazardous air pollutants from major sources. The law established a list of 189 hazardous air pollutants. The EPA must publish a list of source categories that emit certain levels of these pollutants within 1 year after the law is passed. The list of source categories must include (1) major sources emitting 10 tons/year of any one or 25 tons/year of any combination of those pollutants and (2) area sources (smaller sources, such as dry cleaners). EPA will describe Maximum Achievable Control Technology for industries emitting these 189 hazardous air pollutants (79).

Ambient Air Quality

Although air quality is affected by many factors, the determination of air quality and emissions trends in the United States focuses on the six "criteria" pollutants for which criteria documents are available and for which national ambient air quality standards are established. These are total suspended particulates (TSP), sulfur dioxide (SO_2), carbon monoxide (CO), nitrogen dioxide (NO_2), ozone (O_3), and lead (Pb). It should be noted that in 1987 the PM_{10} National Ambient Air Quality Standards (NAAQS) replaced EPA's earlier TSP standard. The ozone refers to ground-level ozone and not to stratospheric ozone.

Trends in the quality of the air in the United States for the 10-year period between 1979 and 1988 are encouraging for some pollutants but identify others that are still a problem. The overall concentrations of TSP, SO_2, and CO declined 20%, 30%, and 28%, respectively. During the same interval the composite average of NO_2 and lead decreased 7% and 89%, respectively, whereas O_3 increased 2% (77).

Between 1987 and 1988 improvement in air quality slowed, and air quality actually deteriorated for some major pollutants. In 1988, the ambient levels of PM_{10}, CO, and lead decreased 4%, 3%, and

15%, respectively. Ozone levels in 1988 were 8% greater than those measured in 1987; SO_2 and NO_2 levels increased 1% between 1987 and 1988 (77).

The improvements noted in air quality in the United States may in part be explained by pollution control programs started in the 1960s and early 1970s that were directed to the major sources of SO_2, CO, and particulate pollution. These include the restriction of sulfur in fuel, better controls on new and existing pollutant sources, the displacement of old sources and the building of new sources in less populated regions, energy conservation measures, and the construction of tall smoke stacks that increase the dispersion of pollutants. The improvement in CO levels reflects a reduction in emissions from new cars as a result of tighter federal standards for vehicle emissions and increased fuel economy. The downward trend in particulate emissions in the United States relates primarily to reducing stationary industrial emissions, converting to cleaner fuels, paving streets and roads, and restricting open burning. The reduction in lead emissions since 1970 in the United States is attributed to decreased lead in gasoline. Lead concentrations are expected to continue to decrease in the future because of the increased use of unleaded gasoline in new cars equipped with catalytic converters.

Although there have been significant improvements in U.S. air quality, the urban air pollution problems of ozone (smog), carbon monoxide (CO), and particulate matter (PM_{10}) persist. As seen in Fig. 2-1, about 121 million people in the United States reside in counties that did not meet at least one air quality standard during 1988. It is apparent that ozone is the most widespread and persistent urban air pollution problem. The diversity and number of urban air pollution sources that contribute to ozone formation help to explain the intractability of the problem. These sources include hydrocarbons from automobile emissions, petroleum refineries, chemical plants, dry cleaners, gasoline stations, house painting, and printing shops and nitrogen oxides from combustion of fuel for transportation, utilities, and industries.

In 1988 widespread violations of the O_3 standard occurred in 65 large metropolitan areas in the United States (77). Los Angeles still experiences some of the highest ozone concentrations in the country. Violations of the carbon monoxide standard occurred in many urban areas throughout the nation. The highest CO concentration recorded in 1988 was found in Los Angeles (77). Violations of the PM_{10} standard were recorded in 14 urban areas in the United States in 1988 (77).

Where records are available, they indicate that air quality for fine aerosols is deteriorating in suburban and rural regions of the eastern half of the United States, parts of the Southwest, and urban

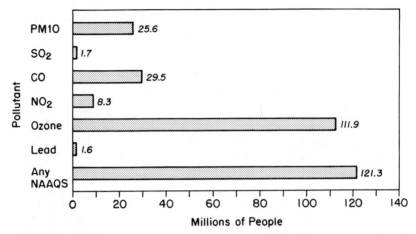

FIGURE 2-1. People in counties in the United States with 1988 air quality above primary National Ambient Air Quality Standards (NAAQS). From U.S. EPA (77).

areas of the west coast. Mountain-state cities, particularly those with increased domestic wood burning, are also affected (17). Thus, while the soot and dust in U.S. industrial and populated urban areas have decreased, the concentrations of fine atmospheric aerosols, which are likely to penetrate deeply into the lung, have increased over the last decade (1).

Toxics Release Inventory

The Toxics Release Inventory (TRI), compiled annually by the EPA, provides information on the release of toxic chemicals by manufacturing facilities. The report provides information on (1) amount of TRI chemicals released into air, land, and water or transported off-site, (2) where TRI chemicals are released, (3) which industries play major roles, and (4) which chemicals play major roles. The TRI is one of the cornerstones of the Emergency Planning and Community Right-to-Know Act of 1986. By providing information on toxic pollution, the TRI will undoubtly strengthen the regulation of toxic releases and assist in the development of pollution prevention programs.

The U.S. Environmental Protection Agency's TRI for 1988 showed that 19,762 industrial plants released 4.57 billion pounds of toxic chemicals into the nation's air, water, and land. Of this total, 2.43 billion pounds were emitted into the air (78). This information indicates that the control of toxic emissions into the air is inadequate. As with the initial TRI compiled in 1987, the 1988 TRI figures are entered into a national computerized data base that is available in over 4000 libraries and directly from EPA.

Ambient Air Quality Worldwide

The Global Environmental Monitoring System, assessing urban air quality (GEMS/Air report), selects cities that provide as broad a global coverage as possible. The cities were also chosen to represent different climatic condition, levels of development, and pollution situations. In most cities one monitoring station is located in an industrial zone, one in a commercial area, and one in a residential area. The data so obtained permit a reasonable evaluation of minimum and maximum levels and of long-term trends of urban air quality (26). The GEMS/Air report is based on data for sulfur dioxide (SO_2) and suspended particulate matter (SPM) that are fairly extensive. Data for nitrogen dioxide (NO_2), carbon monoxide (CO), and lead have come from national reports, the open literature, and through the use of a questionnaire.

The GEMS assessment of urban air quality has been carried out for all cities in the GEMS/Air network with 5 years or more of representative annual averages between 1973 and 1985 (26). As seen in Fig. 2-2, sulfur dioxide appears to be declining or remaining constant in 25 out of 33 cities assessed. With some notable exceptions, emissions of suspended particulate matter (SPM) have decreased in most industrialized nations from 1970 to 1985 (Fig. 2-3). Emissions of nitrogen oxides indicate an upward trend in several of the larger European cities, including London, Frankfurt, and Amsterdam (Fig. 2-4). A breakdown of the emission data by sector, where available, reveals that the upward trends are caused by increased emissions from motor vehicles. This is particularly noticeable for the Federal Republic of Germany and The Netherlands (26). Most

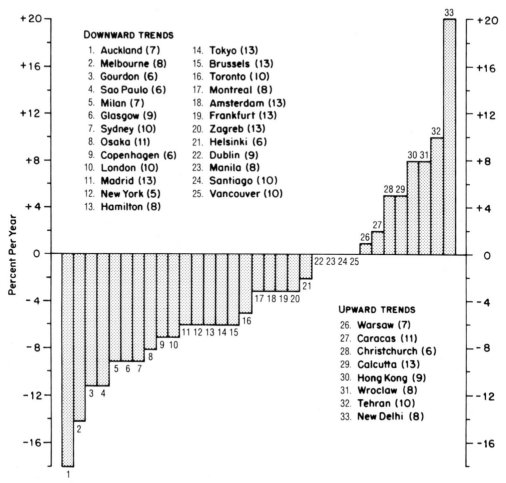

FIGURE 2-2. Trends in annual average SO_2 concentration in cities. The values in parentheses refer to the number of sampling years. All cities in the Global Environmental Monitoring Network (GEMS) with 5 years or more of representative annual averages between 1973 and 1985 were assessed for trends in SO_2 levels. From GEMS (26).

European countries do not have the stringent vehicular emission standards of the United States and Japan. Although the data are limited, it is probable that urban NO_x levels are increasing in the rapidly industrializing countries (26). Total carbon monoxide emissions have decreased in some countries including the United States, The Netherlands, and the Federal Republic of Germany. An increase in carbon monoxide emissions was noted in the United Kingdom between 1980 and 1985. Data from Hungary and Poland suggest that carbon monoxide emissions are also rising in at least some countries in eastern Europe (26). Environmental pollution, in general, is recognized to be a severe problem in eastern Europe (18). It is expected that an upward trend in the emissions of carbon monoxide will be found in some of the rapidly industrializing Asian and South American countries as a result of the increasing number of motor vehicles (26).

INDOOR AIR POLLUTION

Introduction

In recent years the problem of indoor air pollution in residential, office, and public buildings has come into sharp focus. Concerns about the potential health effects of indoor air pollution stem from three observations. (1) The levels of some pollutants are higher indoors than outdoors, in some cases exceeding the national standards set for exposure outdoors

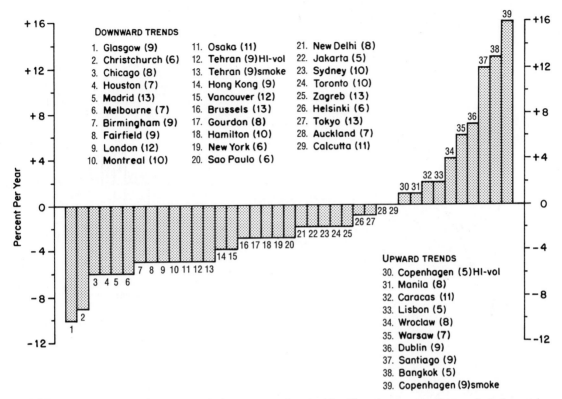

FIGURE 2-3. Trends in annual average particulate concentrations in cities. The values in parentheses refer to the number of sampling years. All cities in the Global Environmental Monitoring Network (GEMS) with 5 years or more of representative annual averages between 1973 and 1985 were assessed for trends in particulate levels. From GEMS (26).

(30,58,70). (2) Urban populations typically spend more than 90% of their time indoors; the single most important indoor location is the home, where individuals spend about 70% of their time. (3) It is the most susceptible groups—the young, the elderly, and the infirm—who spend the greatest amount of time indoors.

The indoor concentration of any given air pollutant depends on its source, strength, and rate of removal. A number of forces on both sides of this equation contribute to increased levels of indoor air pollution. In addition to infiltrating from the outdoor air, many indoor pollutants are released from the building and its contents and are generated by human activity (3,10,16,41,65).

A variety of construction materials, furnishings, and consumer products containing volatile chemicals provide sources of indoor contaminants. Synthetic organic materials are associated with emissions from walls, ceilings, carpets, draperies, plastics, paints, pesticides, cleaning materials, and

personal and household products. The wider use of cheaper fuels in home fireplaces, wood-burning stoves, and unvented kerosene space heaters has increased the indoor concentration of volatile organic compounds and such combustion products as carbon monoxide, sulfur dioxide, and nitrogen dioxide (27,41,65,83).

The worldwide energy crisis in 1973–1974 also contributed to the problem of indoor air pollution through efforts made to conserve fuel in commercial and residential buildings. Since approximately a third of the energy consumed in the United States and many other industrialized nations is used in heating and cooling indoor air, home owners and builders added insulation and reduced building ventilation to conserve fuel. These measures, which were actively promoted by electric utilities and federal programs, resulted in a buildup of indoor air pollutants.

As older buildings became better insulated and newer buildings were built with a thermal envelope,

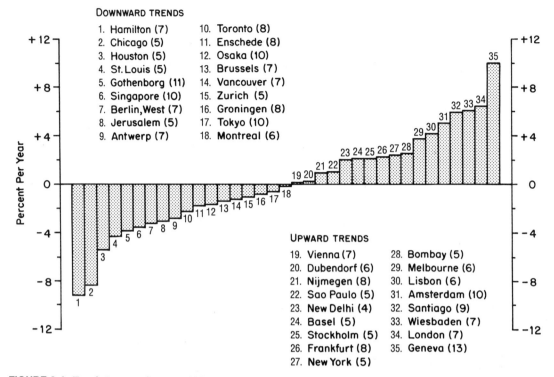

FIGURE 2-4. Trends in annual average NO_2 concentrations in cities. The values in parentheses refer to the number of sampling years. All cities in the Global Environmental Monitoring Network (GEMS) with 5 years or more of representative annual averages between 1973 and 1985 were assessed for trends in NO_2 levels. From GEMS (26).

less fresh air infiltrated into the structures. The natural ventilation provided by opening the windows was replaced by mechanical ventilation in most new office buildings. To further conserve energy, ventilation systems were often operated conservatively. To lower fuel costs, homes were caulked, weatherstripped, and sealed. The old-fashioned "leaky" home or office building with open windows, having a complete exchange of air every few hours, was replaced by energy-efficient buildings and homes having greatly reduced ventilation rates. During the heating season, modern homes in the United States have air changes of about 0.5 per hour. Modern office buildings generally recirculate about 80% or more of all indoor air (39).

The many sources of indoor pollution coupled with a reduction of air-exchange rates in existing and newly constructed buildings markedly increased the problem of indoor air pollution (Table 2-2). By 1980, the Department of Energy, the Environmental Protection Agency, and the National Institute of Occupational Safety and Health were involved in research programs related to the indoor air pollution in nonindustrial indoor environments. In 1981 the National Research Council's Committee on Indoor Pollutants published a comprehensive report on indoor air quality (10). A number of books and articles provide additional comprehensive reviews of indoor air pollution (25,65,68,81,83).

Sources and Nature of Indoor Air Pollutants

The sources of indoor air pollution may be divided into the following categories: (1) outdoor sources, (2) indoor sources, which include the building and its furnishings, and (3) indoor sources generated by human activities.

Outdoor Sources of Indoor Air Pollution

Although pollutants in outdoor air penetrate indoors, their average indoor concentration is less than that found outdoors. The levels of ozone, sulfate, aerosols, sulfur dioxide, and such metals as lead are typically lower indoors than outdoors. Indoor values 20% to 80% of the outdoor concentrations have been reported (6,21,87). Particles of respirable size will penetrate into indoor spaces with

TABLE 2-2. Influence of Changing Building Characteristics on Indoor Air Quality[a]

Since the mid-1960s, construction practices have changed:
Prefabricated exterior section mounted on steel frame
Inoperable windows
HVAC[b] systems with combined intake and exhaust systems located on roofs
Tight construction of homes
Greater use of organic-emitting building materials and furnishings
Energy conservation to save energy costs, resulting in reduced air infiltration and mechanical ventilation
Less maintenance as buildings become more complex
Changes in formulation of cleaning agents

[a]From American Thoracic Society (3).
[b]Heating, ventilation, air conditioning system.

the infiltrating air. Those particles that can be strictly termed "outdoor aerosols" typically have lower concentrations indoors. Particles primarily of outdoor origin are lead, vanadium, and sulfates.

Radon is an indoor contaminant that is derived primarily from the soil. In some homes, the source may be drinking water from a drilled well or, very rarely, building materials with high radium concentrations (44). Radon is a colorless, odorless, radioactive gas that occurs naturally from the breakdown of uranium deposits found in many types of rocks. Radon can seep into a home through the basement, through cracks in the foundation, or through the entrance utility service lines into the house below grade. Unless remedial action is taken, the soil under a building will continuously emit radon into the indoor air throughout the building's lifetime.

Radon production in soil is influenced by the distribution of uranium in the earth's crust and by soil and foundation conditions. The concentration of uranium varies widely. High concentrations of radon can be found in soils and rocks containing uranium, granite, shale, phosphate, pitchblende, and in some ground water supplies. Soils contaminated with industrial wastes from uranium or phosphate mining may also contain radon. Certain parts of the United States have high radon levels, which correlate with higher levels of radioactivity in the homes located in these areas. Information has been complied from a geological survey of the United States and Canada on deposits of four types of radon-bearing minerals: uranium, granite, phosphate, and shale. Areas known to have high levels of radon in the United States include the Reading Prong formation that cuts across New York, New Jersey, and Pennsylvania (44).

Since indoor levels of radon depend primarily on the concentration of radon in the underlying soil, the construction of the home or building, and the type of ventilation, home owners can often correct the problem by sealing cracks in the floor and by improving ventilation. Once radon enters a home, its fate is dependent on the ventilation and its radio

active decay. The major health risk of radon exposure stems primarily from the inhalation of radon decay products, which irradiate the surrounding tissue.

Concerns about the adverse health effects of indoor exposure to radon decay products are based on the higher incidence of lung cancer observed in uranium miners. The epidemiologic evidence also indicates a synergism between exposure to the products of radon decay and cigarette smoking. The extent of this synergism is unclear (7). Although indoor exposures are undoubtedly considerably less than those found in an occupational setting, risk is proportional to exposure (7).

In 1986, the United States Environmental Protection Agency issued guidance for naturally occurring indoor radon. The EPA recommended that homeowners consider taking action to reduce the level of radon if it exceeds 4 picocuries per liter (pCi/L) or 148 Bq/m^3 of air as an annual average concentration (72). Interpreting the measurements of indoor radon involves consideration of the risks associated with the measured concentration and the accuracy of the measurement. There is at present a great deal of scientific uncertainty in this area (51,52).

Building Sources of Indoor Air Pollution

A number of indoor air pollutants are emitted from such building materials as concrete, stone, plywood, particleboard, insulation, fire retardants, adhesives, and paints. Chemical contamination of indoor air is greater in new than in old buildings (59,60). The off-gassing of volatile chemicals from new building materials often continues for a number of months (59,60).

Such common earth-derived building materials as cinder block, aggregate, and building stone may contain radon. Particleboard and plywood that are made with formaldehyde-containing resin bonding agents can release formaldehyde. The emission rates from formaldehyde-containing pressed-wood products decline with age. During the first 6 to 12 months after manufacture, rapid declines in formaldehyde emissions were noted (40). However, recent manufacturing improvements in the pressed-wood product industry have reduced the indoor concentration of formaldehyde at least two- to threefold.

Asbestos and asbestos-containing products, such as ceiling and floor tiles, pipe insulation, spackling compounds, concrete, and acoustical and thermal insulating material, were formerly widely used in homes, office buildings, and schools. As these materials are displaced or deteriorate, asbestos fibers can be released into the air (Table 2-3). Paints can be the source of such solvents as toluene and xylene. A variety of contaminants may also be released from air-handling systems. These include microorganisms derived from condenser pans, air washer baffles, and composite material used in the manufacture of the duct material (3,9,25,27,41, 53,54,65).

Interior Furnishings as Sources of Indoor Air Pollution

A variety of furnishings, particularly those containing synthetic materials, can contribute to indoor air pollution. Wall-to-wall carpeting, often glued to the floor with adhesives, and draperies made of synthetic fibers can be the source of a variety of volatile chemicals. Organic dust and fibrous glass particles can arise from deteriorating foam cushions and curtains. Furniture constructed with particleboard can be a source of formaldehyde. Plastic and fabric-covered room dividers can emit volatile organic compounds. Office equipment can release a large number of pollutants. Photocopying machines, for example, may release ozone and volatile organic compounds. Small office refrigerators may become defective and leak Freon. Blueprint machines may release ammonia, and photographic equipment may release acetic acid (23,27,65,69,74–76) (Table 2-4).

Human Activities as Sources of Indoor Pollution

Human activities—ranging from cooking, heating, smoking, and hobbies to the use of office equipment—pesticides, and cleaning, personal, and household products can be important sources of indoor air pollutants (3,53,54,65) (Table 2-4).

The indoor combustion of fuels provides a source of CO, CO_2, SO_2, nitrogen oxides, a variety of volatile organic compounds (VOCs), and particulates. The major combustion sources in the home are gas- and oil-fired furnaces and gas cooking appliances. Numerous studies have reported elevated indoor levels of NO_2, NO, CO, and CO_2 in homes

TABLE 2-3. Asbestos Usage in Building Materials[a]

Building material	Likely asbestos presence	Ease of release by external damage
Thermal insulation		
Corrugated paper	High	Moderate
Molded pipe and boiler covering	High (fiber batting material is fibrous glass)	High
Cements	High	High
Corrugated paper air ducts or duct insulation	High	Low
Ceiling panels	Low (10% or less)	Moderate
Textured paints	High (unlikely in plasters)	Moderate
Wallboard	Relatively low	Moderate
Joint and spackle compounds used with wallboard	High	Low
Asbestos–vinyl floor tiles or linoleum	High, but fibers are not easily released	Very low
Asbestos–asphalt roofing	High, but release potential is low	Very low
Asbestos–cement shingles	High (some erosion potential from uncoated shingles)	Low
Flooring and roofing felts	Fairly high	Moderate, but generally inaccessible
Fire doors	Fairly high	Very low
Sheet insulation material in and about radiators	Fairly high	Low
Fireplace artificial ashes	High	High

[a]Refers to the probability of asbestos being present in building materials used prior to the mid-1970s. With the exception of flooring, roofing, or external siding materials, asbestos is no longer used in the listed materials. This list indicates the principal asbestos-containing materials used in residence buildings. Other materials or uses of asbestos may be present in such buildings, but their occurrence is less likely. From American Thoracic Society (3).

TABLE 2-4. Common Indoor Air Pollution Sources and Pollutants
in the Home and in Commercial Buildings[a]

Source	Pollutant
Tobacco smoking	Carbon monoxide
	Particles
	Organics
Standing water	Biological contaminants (e.g., *Legionella*, molds)
People	Carbon dioxide
	Odors (bioeffluents)
	Bacterial and viral contaminants
Furnishings, building materials	Formaldehyde
	Organics (e.g., solvents)
	Asbestos
Computers, copiers, white-out, typesetting equipment	Organics
	Particles
Garages, loading docks	Carbon monoxide
	Particles
	Organics
Outdoor air	Carbon monoxide, nitrogen dioxide, ozone, sulfur dioxide, particles, organics, pollen, allergens
Soil gas	Radon
	Biocides
	Organics
Gas boilers, furnaces, cookers, gas ranges, unvented kerosene and gas space heaters, coal and wood stoves	Carbon monoxide, nitrogen dioxide, particles
	Organics
Solvents, paints, glues, resins, personal care and household products	Organics

[a]Adapted from American Thoracic Society (3).

with unvented appliances (65). Elevated levels of NO$_2$ have also been measured routinely in kitchens during conventional gas cooking (49,64,68). When a gas stove is used for heating—a common practice among the urban poor—elevated levels of CO have been measured. Kerosene heaters, unvented gas heaters, and wood stoves provide important sources of NO$_2$ and CO (34). Faulty furnaces and attached garages in hotels, offices, homes, and apartments can cause increased levels of a variety of combustion products including NO$_2$ and CO (10,65) (Table 2-4).

Homecare and building maintenance materials, which include disinfectants, room deodorizers, carpet shampoos, cleaning solutions, furniture polish, and floor waxes, are additional sources of indoor air pollution. Consumer products such as aerosol sprays, shoe polish, air fresheners, moth crystals, fabric care products, and cosmetics contribute to the levels of indoor air contamination. Hobbies that call for the use of volatile hydrocarbons may at times increase exposures far beyond industrial guidelines. Residential contamination with pesticides may also be found in indoor environments (14,31,36,45,69). Measurements of indoor residential concentrations of chlordane made by the Armed Forces in more than 10,000 homes indicate that over 2% exceeded the guideline suggested by the National Academy of Sciences (36,45).

Recent studies of volatile organic compounds found indoors reveal a vast array of aliphatic hydrocarbons, halogenated hydrocarbons, aromatic hydrocarbons, alcohols, ketones, and aldehydes (3,42,83) (Table 2-5). These compounds emanate from such indoor sources as cooking and heating fuels, aerosol propellants, cleaning compounds, refrigerants, dry cleaning solvents, paints, varnishes, window cleaners, cosmetics, adhesives, fungicides, germicides, disinfectants, printed paper, and permanent-press textiles (83). Studies reveal that many volatile organic compounds have levels higher indoors than outdoors, and these levels are influenced by the use of consumer products (69,83).

Smoking indoors contributes to the levels of respirable particles, nicotine, polycyclic aromatic hydrocarbons, CO, acrolein, NO$_2$ and a variety of other substances (13). Tobacco smoke is the single most identifiable source of respirable particles indoors (58). As shown in Table 2-6, many substances formed in tobacco combustion are enriched in the sidestream smoke. As a result, hundreds of different compounds are present in the sidestream cigarette smoke (71).

Apart from smoking, the indoor sources of particles are varied and include combustion sources and the resuspension of dust by vacuuming, dusting, and other occupant activity. Pollen, molds, bac-

TABLE 2-5.   Common Organic Chemicals and Their Sources[a]

Chemicals	Measured peak nonoccupational exposures ($\mu g/m^3$)	Major sources of exposure
Volatile chemicals		
Benzene	100	Smoking, auto exhaust
Tetrachloroethylene	1,000	Passive smoking, driving, pumping gas, wearing or storing dry-cleaned clothes, visiting dry cleaners
p-Dichlorobenzene	1,000	Room deodorizers, moth cakes
Chloroform	250	Showering (10-min average)
	200 ng/L	Tap water, beverages
	50	Washing clothes, dishes
Methylene chloride	500,000	Paint stripping, solvent usage
1,1,1-Trichloroethane	1,000	Wearing or storing dry-cleaned clothes, aerosol sprays, fabric protectors
Trichlorethylene	100	Unknown (cosmetics, electronic parts)
Carbon tetrachloride	100	Industrial-strength cleansers
Aromatic hydrocarbons (toluene, xylenes, ethyl-benzene, trimethylbenzenes)	1,000	Paints, adhesives, gasoline, combustion sources
Aliphatic hydrocarbons (octane, decane, undecane)	1,000	Paints, adhesives, gasoline, combustion sources
Terpenes (limonene, Pinene)	1,000	Scented deodorizers, polishes, fabrics, fabric softeners, cigarettes, food, beverages
Semivolatile chemicals		
Chlorpyrifos (Dursban)	10	Household insecticides
Chlordane, heptachlor	10	Termiticide
Diazinon	10	Household insecticides
PCB[b]		Transformers, fluorescent ballasts, ceiling tiles
PAH[c]	<1	Combustion products (smoking, woodburning, kerosene heaters)

[a]From American Thoracic Society (3).
[b]Polychlorinated biphenyls.
[c]Polyaromatic hydrocarbons.

teria, mites, animal dander, fungi, algae, and insect parts are commonly found indoors. A ventilation system can be an important source of indoor air contamination with microorganisms. Humidification devices are another source of both allergic and pathogenic microorganisms (3).

Monitoring

It is now apparent that the evaluation of indoor as well as outdoor exposures is essential for assessing the health risk of air contaminants. Studies using direct personal monitoring have become possible with the development of passive sampling equipment and lightweight portable pump systems. Studies using these devices have established the importance of indoor sources of exposure to carbon monoxide, nitrogen dioxide, and respirable particulates (58,66). Although portable sampling devices have aided investigators, further advances in this field promise to increase our understanding of pollutant exposure.

Regulation

Although the United States and many other countries have established ambient (outdoor) air quality standards, the issue of indoor air pollution has only recently been considered (4,57). To date, in the United States, no overall government strategy exists to provide a coordinated approach to ensure adequate indoor air quality. In some cases, such as asbestos, many different federal agencies have jurisdiction; in other cases, such as combustion by-products and volatile organic emissions, responsibility is not defined (4).

The creation of a regulatory framework for indoor air quality poses special policy issues. As Sexton and Repetto (57) have pointed out, some fundamental differences exist between indoor and outdoor air. Outdoor air is a "public good" in the sense that members of a community breathe essentially the same ambient air. The situation is different for some indoor environments, especially private residences, where the costs and benefits of many pollution

TABLE 2-6.   Concentrations of Toxic and Carcinogenic Agents in Nonfilter Cigarette Mainstream Smoke and in Environmental Tobacco Smoke (ETS) in Indoor Environments[a]

Agent	Mainstream smoke		Inhaled as ETS constituents during 1 hour			
			Range		Episodic high values[b]	
	Weight	Concentration	Weight	Concentration	Weight	Concentration
Carbon monoxide	10–23 mg	24.9000–57,300 ppm	1.2–22 mg	1–18.5 ppm	37 mg	32 ppm
Nitrogen oxide	100–600 μg	230,000–1,400,000 ppb	7–90 μg	9–120 ppb	146 μg	195 ppb
Nitrogen dioxide	<5 μg	<7,600 ppb	24–87 μg	21–76 ppb	120 μg	105 ppb
Acrolein	60–100 μg	75,000–125,000 ppb	8–72 μg	6–50 ppb	110 μg	80 ppb
Acetone	100–250 μg	120,000–300,000 ppb	210–720 μg	150–500 ppb	3500 μg	2400 ppb
Benzene[c]	12–48 μg	11,000–43,000 ppb	12–190 μg	6–98 ppb	190 μg	98 ppb
N-Nitrosodimethylamine[d]	10–40 ng	9–38 ppb	6–140 ng	0.003–0.072 ppb	140 ng	0.072 ppb
N-Nitrosodiethylamine[d]	4–25 ng	3–17 ppb	<6–120 ng	<0.002–0.05 ppb	120 ng	0.05 ppb
Nicotine	1000–2500 μg	430,000–1,080,000 ppb	0.6–30 μg	0.15–7.5 ppb	300 μg	75 ppb
Benzo[a]pyrene[e]	20–40 ng	5–11 ppb	1.7–460 ng	0.0002–0.04 ppb	460 ng	0.04 ppb

[a]From U.S. DHHS (71).
[b]The designation "episodic high values" was chosen to classify those data in the literature that require confirmation.
[c]Human carcinogen according to the International Agency for Research on Cancer (IARC) (80).
[d]Animal carcinogen according to the IARC (80).
[e]Suspected human carcinogen according to the IARC (80).

control measures are internalized within households (57,65).

Concentration of Indoor Air Pollutants

In recent years a number of studies have assessed human exposure to a variety of indoor air pollutants. These studies indicate that outdoor measurements are generally poorly correlated with individual exposure to most air pollutants, especially those derived from indoor sources. Moreover, such agents as radon, asbestos, nitrogen dioxide, carbon monoxide, formaldehydes, volatile organic compounds, respirable particulates, aeropathogens, and aeroallergens can exceed outdoor concentration severalfold (Table 2-7) (3,65,87). This problem is particularly acute in developing countries, where large amounts of wood, crop residues, and dung are burned. These fuels are used by about half of the world's households for cooking and heating, often with little ventilation (62).

Volatile Organic Compounds

Investigators in a number of countries have measured volatile organic compounds (VOC) in hundreds of homes (20,32,35). The VOC are part of almost all materials and products in use. Over 500

TABLE 2-7. Main Indoor Pollutants[a]

Source and type	Indoor concentration	Indoor/outdoor ratio
Pollutants from outdoors		
Sulfur oxides	0–15 μg/m³	<1
Ozone	0–10 ppb	≪1
Pollutants from indoors and outdoors		
Nitrogen oxides	10–700 μg/m³	≫1
Carbon monoxide	5–50 ppm	≫1
Carbon dioxide	2000–3000 ppm	≫1
Particulate matter	10–1000 μg/m³	1
Pollutants from indoors		
Radon	0.01–4 pCi/L	≫1
Formaldehyde	0.01–0.5 ppm	>1
Synthetic fibers	0–1 fiber mL	1
Organic substances		>1
Polycyclic hydrocarbons		>1
Mercury		>1
Aerosols		>1
Microorganisms		>1
Allergens		>1

[a]From Spengler and Sexton (65).

different organic compounds have been identified in indoor air, but only 50 are commonly found. These are derived not only from building materials but also from cleaning agents and personal activities (Table 2-4) (3,69).

The Environmental Protection Agency has undertaken a long-term series of studies of human exposure, known generically as the total exposure assessment methodology (TEAM) studies. The goal of these studies is to determine the actual exposure of people to volatile organic compounds and pesticides during their normal daily activities. In 1989, the Environmental Protection Agency submitted a report to Congress that described the Agency's indoor air activities and recommended an appropriate federal response to the problem of indoor air pollution (74–76).

The major finding of the VOC study was that in every city evaluated (both rural and urban), personal exposures and indoor air concentrations exceeded outdoor air concentrations for essentially all of the 11 compounds measured. These include benzene, carbon tetrachloride, chloroform, ethylbenzene, tetrachloroethylene, trichloroethylene, and styrene (83).

The major finding of the nonoccupational pesticide study (NOPES), in which households were examined in two urban areas, shows that exposure to many pesticides occurred mainly through the indoor environment. The routine sampling of the public water supply of the urban areas involved did not identify any contamination by the pesticides under study. Food sources of pesticide exposure were not evaluated (31). Further investigation must be done to examine all potential routes of pesticide exposure within the home. Such information is particularly important with regard to infants, toddlers, and the elderly, who spend much of their time indoors.

The Environmental Protection Agency has also measured indoor pollutant concentrations in ten public access buildings, including schools, homes for the elderly, and office buildings. Since the buildings were not ones in which the occupants complained about the air quality, they are likely to be fairly representative of other buildings of their type. The results of this study revealed that new buildings may have levels of some VOC that start out as much as 100 times outdoor levels and gradually decrease to two to four times outdoor levels. Related studies show that building materials, including surface coating such as paints and adhesives, vinyl and hard rubber moldings, carpet, and particleboard emit in large quantities the same chemicals found at elevated levels in the new office buildings. It thus appears that building materials can cause high concentrations of a number of organic chemicals in new buildings for a number of months (59,60).

Respirable Particles

In an extensive indoor air quality survey, researchers at the Harvard School of Public Health monitored respirable particles with a diameter of less than 3.5 μm in over 80 homes in six U.S. cities. Twenty-four-hour samples were collected every sixth day for up to 2 years in each of the homes (67). On the average, the concentrations of respirable particles were generally higher indoors than outdoors. In addition, across the six cities under investigation, the variation in the concentration of respirable particles within the homes was far greater than the variation noted outdoors. This finding complicates attempts to investigate the health effects of respirable particles in ambient air without first defining exposure groups and delineating sources of indoor and outdoor particulate matter. The Harvard study indicates that smoking is a very important contributor to the indoor respirable-particulate fraction (Fig. 2-5). The study included a health survey of more than 10,000 children living in the six U.S. cities under investigation. The percentage of children living with one or more smoking adults was found to vary between 60% and 75% in these early studies. These figures reveal, however, the extensive nature of exposure to cigarette smoke in the general population (67). Fortunately, in the United States a substantial decrease in parental smoking has occurred in recent years.

Studies of personal exposure to particles have been performed by having subjects carry portable monitors and record their activities. In one such study in Topeka, Kansas, 45 nonsmoking adults carried portable monitors for 18 days. During the active 12-hour periods of the day, the subjects recorded the time and their activities in various locations. The results of this study point out the importance of home measurements in understanding the total personal exposure to particles. The outdoor concentrations of particles were poor predictors of personal exposure, since the indoor concentration of particles accounted for over 60% of such exposure (66).

Nitrogen Dioxide

Extensive field surveys in Portage, Wisconsin and Topeka, Kansas measured indoor and outdoor NO_2 in several hundred homes (22,48). Using passive diffusion tubes, week-long samples were collected in the kitchen, bedroom, and the outside of each home. In Portage, Wisconsin, a seasonal pattern was evident for the indoor concentration of NO_2 in homes using electricity, natural gas, and liquid propane for cooking. The effects of reduced air infiltration (and perhaps a greater amount of cooking) were reflected in elevated NO_2 concentrations during the winter months. In Portage, where the ambient level of NO_2 was 15 μg/m^3, gas cooking fuel

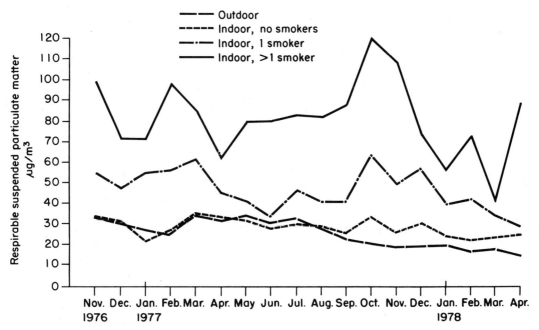

FIGURE 2-5. Monthly mean mass of respirable particulate concentrations across six cities. From Spengler et al. (67).

added, on average, 45 $\mu g/m^3$ to the indoor concentration of NO_2. Three percent of the homes monitored in Portage, Wisconsin exceeded the National Ambient Air Quality Standard set at 100 $\mu g/m^3$. Similar results were found in the Topeka study of 55 homes that used gas for cooking. During the summer months, when people typically spend more time outdoors and when the natural ventilation is greater, outdoor measurements more closely reflected individual exposure (49).

Problem Buildings

Complaints related to the indoor climate in nonindustrial buildings have increased markedly for nearly two decades. In some cases the illness can be defined and related to specific environmental factors. In other cases a diffuse set of symptoms are reported, but no specific cause has been identified (3,16,33). On the basis of this distinction, building-related health problems of known etiology are identified as building-related illness, whereas building-related health problems with no known etiology and without physical or laboratory findings are identified as sick (or tight)-building syndrome.

Building-Related Illness

Symptoms of building-related illness have toxic, allergic, or infectious manifestations that can be identified by the physician and the clinical laboratory. At times specific etiological agents can also be identified in the building in question. The types of building-related illness vary and include hypersensitivity pneumonitis, asthma, legionnaire's disease, influenza, and carbon monoxide poisoning (3,30,33). Resolution of the problem typically involved removal of the source of the problem rather than increasing the ventilation. The incidence of building-related illness may be relatively low, and therefore it may easily be missed by the examining physician.

Sick-Building Syndrome

The sick-building syndrome has generally been identified when a substantial number of individuals in a particular building or a portion of the building complain of a diffuse but often common set of symptoms. These symptoms, though nonspecific in isolation, form a recognizable pattern that has been repeatedly observed in connection with the sick-building syndrome (3,28,33,43,85). The common symptoms include eye, nose, and throat irritation, headache, recurrent fatigue, drowsiness, or dizziness, and reduced powers of concentration (3,16,42, 43,85). The symptoms generally begin slowly and progress. They are related to the time spent at work.

Most individuals report relief of symptoms on leaving the workplace and a recurrence on reentry.

Most documented cases of the sick building syndrome have been reported in newly constructed or newly remodeled energy-efficient buildings having a centrally controlled mechanical ventilation system. Such structures are almost always sealed air-conditioned buildings that do not permit the windows to be opened (85). Under these conditions a wide variety of pollutants may contaminate the indoor air (Tables 2-4 and 2-5) (3,35,42,85).

The sick building syndrome has been attributed to a variety of conditions, which include inadequate ventilation, pollutants such as volatile organic compounds, moisture conditions related to humidification and chilling systems, biological contamination or even outdoor contaminants brought in through the ventilation system (5,24,33,42). Early investigations of the sick-building syndrome often attributed the symptoms to mass hysteria. However, as the number of reports and outbreaks mounted, and as clinical and epidemiologic patterns emerged, attention was directed to searching for causal factors within the indoor air of problem buildings. British and Danish investigators have performed large epidemiologic studies of symptoms reported in relation to building characteristics. In some instances a specific cause was identified; in others none was discovered (5,25,68).

As might be imagined, diagnosing and evaluating building-related health problems can tax the abilities of even the most seasoned professional. From the foregoing it seems apparent that attention should be given to nonspecific symptoms, particularly those that arise somewhat suddenly and without an obvious cause. Under such conditions an occupational and environmental history is of utmost importance (see Chapter 11). Changes in the workplace and home environment in relation to the onset of symptoms may provide a necessary clue. A careful diary recording the onset of symptoms in connection with activities and environmental settings is essential. Once the physician suspects the presence of the sick-building syndrome, the building operator or management should be contacted about the suspected problem.

At times building-related health problems are resolved easily and quickly through a discussion between the physician and the building management. Under some circumstances, however, it becomes necessary to seek consultation with local or state public health agencies. Protocols that combine industrial hygiene and epidemiologic methods have been developed to study building-associated illnesses (3,9,50). This approach involves an interdisciplinary effort among health scientists, engineers, and architects. Protocols have been developed to examine heating, ventilation, and air-conditioning systems (3,9). Common problems in the operations of these systems are generally found in three areas: inadequate maintenance, load changes, and control modifications. Inadequate maintenance is reflected in such problems as missing or dirty filters, contaminated heating and cooling coils and drip pans, and disconnected exhaust fans. Load changes arise when the system is required to meet the needs of a higher occupant density, increased thermal demands (e.g., lighting and computers), or new sources of contaminants (e.g., copy machines and printers). Control-system problems may arise when, in a cost-cutting effort, the system is mistakenly adapted for a more simple operation (3).

SUMMARY

Air pollution from man-made sources has increased enormously during the past 50 years. Such emissions, now recognized as a world-wide problem, easily cut across national boundaries. The most common emissions are sulfur oxides, nitrogen oxides, particulate matter, volatile organic compounds, carbon monoxide, lead, and other trace compounds. Although regulatory efforts have resulted in significant improvements in the quality of air in the United States and certain other nations, the urban air pollution problems of ozone (smog), carbon monoxide, and particulate matter persist. The release of toxic air pollutants also represents a formidable problem that must be addressed.

Indoor air quality in residential settings has recently come under the scrutiny of investigators, policy makers, and the public. Many people, particularly those who are most vulnerable (the elderly and the young), spend more than 90% of their time indoors. Under these conditions it has been shown that indoor exposure to environmental pollutants can be substantial. Important pollutants found indoors include tobacco smoke, volatile organic compounds, formaldehyde, combustion products, radon decay products, asbestos fibers, microorganisms, and aeroallergens. Our increased understanding of the health effects of indoor exposures will eventually lead to a redefinition of ventilation codes and changes in building materials and design.

REFERENCES

1. Altshuller AP, Linthurst RA (eds.): The Acid Deposition Phenomenon and Its Effects: Critical Assessment Review Papers, Vols I and II, U.S. Environmental Protection Agency, Washington, 1984.
2. Altshuller AP, Johnson WB, Nader, JS, et al: Transport and fate of gaseous pollutants associated with National Energy Program. Environ Health Perspect 36:155, 1980.
3. American Thoracic Society: Environmental controls and lung disease. Am Rev Respir Dis 142:915, 1990.
4. Besch EL: Regulation and its role in the prevention of building-associated illness. Occup Med 4:741, 1989.
5. Burge S, Hedge A, Wilson S, et al: Sick building syndrome: A study of 4373 workers. Ann Occup Hyg 31:493, 1987.
6. Committee on Aldehydes, National Research Council: Formaldehyde and Other Aldehydes. National Academy Press, Washington, 1981.
7. Committee on the Biological Effects of Ionizing Radiation, National Research Council: Health Risks of Radon and Other Internally Deposited Alpha-Emitters. BEIR IV, National Academy Press, Washington, 1988.
8. Committee on the Epidemiology of Air Pollutants, National Research Council: Epidemiology and Air Pollution, National Academy Press, Washington, 1985.
9. Committee on Indoor Air Quality: Policies and Procedures for Control of Indoor Air Quality in Existing Buildings, National Academy Press, Washington, 1987.
10. Committee on Indoor Pollutants, National Research Council: Indoor Pollutants, National Academy Press, Washington, 1981.
11. Committee on Medical and Biological Effects of Atmospheric Pollutants, National Research Council: Particulate Polycyclic Organic Matter, National Academy Press, Washington, 1972.
12. Committee on Monitoring and Assessment of Trends in Acid Deposition, National Research Council: Acid Deposition: Long Term Trends, National Academy Press, Washington, 1986.
13. Committee on Passive Smoking, National Research Council: Environmental Tobacco Smoke: Measuring Exposures and Assessing Health Effects, National Academy Press, Washington, 1986.
14. Committee on Toxicology, National Research Council: Seven Pesticides Used for Termite Control, National Academy Press, Washington, 1982.
15. Committee on Atmospheric Transport and Chemical Transformation in Acid Precipitation, National Research Council: Acid Deposition: Atmospheric Processes in Eastern North America, National Academy Press, Washington, 1983.
16. Cone JE, Hodgson MJ (eds.): Problem buildings: Building-associated illness and the sick building syndrome. Occup Med. 4(4):575–797, 1989.
17. Cooper JA, Malek D (eds.): Residential Solid Fuels: Environmental Impacts and Solutions. Oregon Graduate Center, Beaverton, OR, 1982.
18. Crockett TR, Schultz CB: Environmental protection issues in eastern Europe, Int. Environ Rep 13:258, 1990.
19. Daisey JM: Organic compounds in urban aerosols. Ann NY Acad Sci 338:50, 1980.
20. DeBortoli A, Knoppel H, Pecchio E, et al: Measurements of Indoor Air Quality and Comparison with Ambient Air, Report EUR 9656 EN, Commission European Communities, Luxembourg, 1985.
21. Dockery DW, Spengler JD: Personal exposure to respirable particulates and sulfate. J Air Pollut Control Assoc 31:153, 1981.
22. Dockery DW, Spengler JD, Reed MP, et al: Relationships among personal, indoor and outdoor NO_2 measurements. Environ Int 5:101, 1981.

23. Esmen NA: Status of indoor air pollution. Environ Health Perspect 62:259, 1985.
24. Finnegan MJ, Pickering CAC, Burge PS: The sick building syndrome: Prevalence studies. Br Med J 289:1573, 1984.
25. Gammage RB, Kaye SV (eds.): Indoor Air and Human Health, Lewis Publishers, Chelsea, Michigan, 1985.
26. Global Environmental Monitoring System: Assessment of Urban Air Quality, United Nations Environmental Programme/World Health Organization, Geneva, 1988.
27. Godish T: Indoor air pollution in office and other non-residential buildings. J Environ Health 48:190, 1986.
28. Hodgson MJ: Clinical diagnosis and management of building related illness and the sick building syndrome. Occup Med 4:593, 1989.
29. Hoffman D, Wynder EL: Organic particulate pollutants. In: Air Pollution, Vol. II, 3rd ed., pp 1943, Stern AC (ed.), Academic Press, New York, 1977.
30. Hollowell CD, Miksch RR: Sources and concentrations of organic compounds in indoor air environments. Bull NY Acad Med 57:962, 1981.
31. Immerman FW, Schaum JL: Nonoccupational pesticide exposure study (NOPES), US EPA/600/S3-90/003, Washington, 1990.
32. Krause C, Mailahn W, Nagel R, et al: Occurrence of volatile organic compounds in the air of 500 homes in the Federal Republic of Germany. In: Indoor Air '87: Proceedings of the 4th International Conference on Indoor Air and Climate, p 102, Siefert B, Esdorn H, Fischer M, et al. (eds.), Institute for Water, Soil, and Air Hygiene, Berlin, 1987.
33. Kreiss K: The epidemiology of building-related complaints and illness. Occup Med 4:575, 1989.
34. Leaderer BP: Air pollutant emissions from kerosene heaters. Science 218: 1113, 1982.
35. Lebret E, Van der Viel HJ, Bos HP, et al: Volatile organics in Dutch homes. Environ Int 12:1371, 1986.
36. Lillie TH, Barnes ES: Airborne termiticide levels in houses on United States Air Force Installation. In: Indoor Air '87: Proceedings of the 4th International Conference on Indoor Air Quality and Climate, p 200, Siefert B, Esdorn H, Fischer M, et al. (eds.), Institute for Water, Soil, and Air Hygiene, Berlin, 1987.
37. Loiy PJ, Daisey JM (eds.): Toxic Air Pollution: A Comprehensive Study of Non-Criteria Air Pollutants. Lewis Publishers, Chelsea, Michigan, 1987.
38. Lippmann M, Lioy PJ: Critical issues in air pollution epidemiology. Environ Health Perspect 62:243, 1985.
39. Mage DT, Gammage RB: Evaluation of changes in indoor air quality occurring over the past several decades. In: Indoor Air and Human Health, Gammage RB, Kaye SV (eds.), Lewis Publishers, Chelsea, Michigan, 1985.
40. Matthews TB, Reed TJ, Tromberg BJ, et al: Formaldehyde emissions from combustion sources and solid formal dehyde-resin containing products: Potential impact on indoor air formaldehyde concentrations In: Formaldehyde: Analytical Chemistry and Toxicology, p 201, American Chemical Society, Washington, DC, 1985.
41. Meyer B: Indoor Air Quality, Addison-Wesley, Reading, MA, 1983.
42. Molhave L: Volatile organic compounds as indoor air pollutants. In: Indoor Air and Human Health, p 403, Gammage RB, Kaye SV (eds.), Lewis Publishers, Chelsea, Michigan, 1985.
43. Molhave L: The sick buildings—a subpopulation among the problem buildings. In: Indoor Air '87: Proceedings of the 4th International Conference on Indoor Air Quality and Climate, p 469, Seifert B, Esdorn H, Fischer M, et al. (eds.), Institute for Water, Soil, and Air Hygiene, Berlin, 1987.
44. Nazaroff WW, Nero AV Jr (eds.): Radon and Its Decay Products in Indoor Air, John Wiley & Sons, New York, 1988.
45. Olds KL: Indoor airborne concentration of termiticides in Department of the Army family housing. In: Indoor Air '87: Proceedings of the 4th International Conference on Indoor Air Quality and Climate, p 205, Siefert B, Esdorn H, Fischer M. et al. (eds.), Institute for Water, Soil, and Air Hygiene, Berlin, 1987.
46. Organisation for Economic Co-operation and Development: The State of the Environment 1985, OECD, Paris, 1985.
47. Perera FP, Ahmed AK: Respirable Particles, Ballinger, London, 1979.
48. Quackenboss JJ, Kanarek MS, Spengler JD, et al: Personal monitoring for nitrogen dioxide exposure: Methological considerations in a community. Environ Int 8:249, 1982.
49. Quackenboss JJ, Spengler JD, Kanarek MS, et al: Personal exposure to nitrogen dioxide: Relationship to indoor/outdoor air quality and activity patterns. Environ Sci Technol 20:775, 1986.
50. Quinlan P, Macher PM, Alevantis LE, et al: Protocol for the comprehensive evaluation of building-associated illness. Occup Med 4:771, 1989.
51. Samet JM: Radon and lung cancer. J Natl Cancer Inst 81:745, 1989.
52. Samet JM, Nero AV Jr: Indoor radon and lung cancer. N Engl J Med 32:591, 1989.
53. Samet JM, Marbury MC, Spengler JD: Health effects and sources of indoor air pollution, I. Am Rev Respir Dis 136:1486, 1987.
54. Samet JM, Marbury MC, Spengler JD: Health effects and sources of indoor air pollution, II. Am Rev Respir Dis 137:221, 1988.
55. Sawicki E: Airborne carcinogens and allied compounds. Arch Environ Health 14:46, 1967.
56. Sawicki E, Meeker JE, Morgan MJ: The quantitative composition of air pollution source effluents in terms of aza heterocyclic compounds and polynuclear aromatic hydrocarbons. Int J Air Water Pollut 9:291, 1965.
57. Sexton K, Repetto R: Indoor air pollution and public policy. Environ Int 8:5, 1982.
58. Sexton K, Ryan PB: Assessment of human exposure to air pollution: Methods, measurements, and models. In: Air Pollution, the Automobile, and Public Health, p 207, Watson AY, Bates RR, Kennedy D (eds.), Health Effects Institute, National Academy Press, Washington, 1988.
59. Sheldon LS, Handy RW, Hartwell TC, et al: Indoor Air Quality in Public Buildings, Vol. 1, EPA 600-6-88-009A, Washington, 1988.
60. Sheldon LS, Selon H, Sickles J, et al: Indoor Air Quality in Public Buildings, Vol. II, EPA 600-6-88-009B, Washington, 1988.

61. Shy CM, Struba RJ: Air and water pollution. In: Cancer Epidemiology and Prevention, p 336, Schottenfeld D, Fraumeni JF Jr, (eds.), WB Saunders, Philadelphia, 1982.

62. Skov P, Valbjorn O, Danish Indoor Study Group: The sick building syndrome in the office environment: The Danish Town Hall Study. Environ Int 13:339, 1987.

63. Smith KR: Biofuels, Air Pollution and Health: A Global Review, Plenum Press, New York, 1987.

64. Spengler JD, Cohen M: Emissions from indoor combustion sources. In: Indoor Air and Human Health, p 261, Gammage RB, Kaye SV (eds.), Lewis Publishers, Chelsea, Michigan, 1985.

65. Spengler JD, Sexton K: Indoor air pollution: A public health perspective. Science 221:9, 1983.

66. Spengler JD, Soczek ML: Evidence for improved ambient air quality and the need for personal exposure research. Environ Sci Technol 18:268A, 1984.

67. Spengler JD, Dockery WA, Turner JM, et al: Long-term measurement of respirable sulfates and particulates inside and outside homes. Atmos Environ 15:23, 1981.

68. Spengler JD, Hollowell C, Moschandreas D, et al. (eds.): Indoor air pollution (special issue). Environ Int 8:3–531, 1982.

69. Sterling DA: Volatile organic compounds in indoor air: An overview of sources, concentrations and health effects. In: Indoor Air and Human Health, p 387, Gammage RB, Kaye SV (eds.), Lewis Publishers, Chelsea, Michigan, 1985.

70. Turiel CD, Hollowell CD, Miksch RR, et al: The effect of reduced ventilation on the indoor air quality of an office building. Atmos Environ 17:51, 1983.

71. US Department of Health and Human Services: The Health Consequences of Involuntary Smoking: A Report of the Surgeon General, US Department of Health and Human Services, Public Health Service, Office on Smoking and Health, Washington, 1986.

72. US Environmental Protection Agency: A Citizen's Guide to Radon: What It Is and What to Do about It, DHHS publication no. EPA-86-004, Government Printing Office, Washington, 1986.

73. US Environmental Protection Agency: Ambient air quality standards for particulate matter, final rules. Fed Reg 52(126); 24634–24655, 1987.

74. US Environmental Protection Agency: Report to Congress on Indoor Air Quality, Vol. 1: Federal Programs Addressing Indoor Air Quality, EPA/400/1-89/001B, EPA, Washington, 1989.

75. US Environmental Protection Agency: Report to Congress on Indoor Air Quality, Vol. II: Assessment and Control of Indoor Air Pollution, EPA/400/1-89/001C, EPA, Washington, 1989.

76. US Environmental Protection Agency: Report to Congress on Indoor Air Quality, Vol III: Assessment and control of indoor air pollution, EPA/400/1-89/001D, EPA, Washington, 1989.

77. US Environmental Protection Agency: National Air Quality and Emissions Trends Report 1988, Office of Air Quality Planning and Standards, Research Triangle Park, NC, 1990.

78. US Environmental Protection Agency, Office of Pesticides and Toxic Substances: The Toxics in the Community, National and Local Perspectives, The 1988 Toxic Release Inventory National Report, EPA 560/4-90-017, EPA, Washington, 1990.

79. US Environmental Protection Agency: The Clean Air Act Amendments of 1990. Summary Materials, US EPA, Washington, 1990.

80. Vainio H, Hemminki K, Wilbourn J: Data on the carcinogenicity of chemicals in IARC monographs programme. Carcinogenesis 6:1653, 1985.

81. Wadden RA, Scheff PA: Indoor Air Pollution, Wiley–Interscience, New York, 1983.

82. Waggoner AP, Weiss RE, Ahlquist NC, et al: Optical characteristics of atmospheric aerosols. Atmos Environ 15:1891, 1981.

83. Wallace LA, Pellizzari ED, Gordon SM: Organic chemicals in indoor air: A review of human exposure studies and indoor air quality studies. In: Indoor Air and Human Health, p 361, Gammage RB, Kaye SV (eds.), Lewis Publishers, Chelsea, Michigan, 1985.

84. Watson AY, Bates RR, Kennedy D (eds.): Air Pollution, the Automobile, and Public Health, The Health Effects Institute, National Academy Press, Washington, 1988.

85. World Health Organization: Indoor Air Pollutants Exposure and Health Effects Assessment, EURO Reports and Studies 78, Working Group Report, WHO, Geneva, 1982.

86. World Health Organization, Regional Office for Europe: Air Quality Guidelines for Europe, WHO Regional Publications, European Series No 23, WHO, Geneva, 1987.

87. Yocum E: Indoor–outdoor air quality relationship. J Air Pollut Control Assoc 32:500, 1982.

RECOMMENDED READINGS

American Thoracic Society: Environmental controls and lung disease. Am Rev Respir Dis 142:915, 1990.

Cone JE, Hodgson MJ (eds.): Problem Buildings: Building-Associated Illness and the Sick Building Syndrome, Occup Med 4(4):575–797, 1989.

Nazaroff WW, Nero AV Jr (eds.): Radon and Its Decay Products in Indoor Air. John Wiley & Sons, New York, 1988.

Samet JM, Spengler JD (eds): Indoor Air Pollution: A Health Perspective, Johns Hopkins University Press, 1991.

Smith KR: Biofuels, Air Pollution and Health: A Global Review, Plenum Press, New York, 1987.

US Department of Health and Human Services: The Health Consequences of Involuntary Smoking: A report of the Surgeon General, US Department of Health and Human Services, Public Health Service, Office on Smoking and Health, Washington, 1986.

Watson AY, Bates RR, Kennedy D (eds.): Air Pollution, the Automobile, and Public Health, Health Effects Institute, National Academy Press, Washington, 1988.

World Health Organization, Regional Office for Europe: Air Quality Guidelines for Europe, World Health Organization, Regional Publications, European series no 23, WHO, Geneva, 1987.

3. CHEMICAL CONTAMINANTS IN FOOD

Sushma Palmer and Kulbir S. Bakshi

INTRODUCTION

Three categories of environmental contaminants generally occur in food: natural and synthetic organic compounds, traces of heavy metal, and certain natural and synthetic radioactive substances (51,69). This chapter summarizes the sources, occurrence, extent of exposure, and regulation of selected substances belonging to the first two categories, i.e., contaminants such as polycyclic aromatic hydrocarbons (PAH), residues of certain pesticides, traces of toxic metals, components of packaging materials such as polyvinyl chloride (PVC), and traces of industrial chemicals such as polychlorinated biphenyls (PCBs).

SOURCES OF CHEMICAL CONTAMINANTS IN FOOD

Environmental contamination in food can take several forms: long-term, low-level contamination resulting from gradual diffusion and reentry of agricultural and industrial chemicals through the environment and relatively shorter-term, higher-level contamination through industrial accidents and waste disposal. A well-documented example of high-level food contamination occurred in Michigan in 1973. At this time polybrominated biphenyls used as fire retardants were accidently mixed with animal feed. The milk produced by dairy cattle consuming

Principles and Practice of Environmental Medicine, edited by Alyce Bezman Tarcher. Plenum Medical Book Company, New York, 1992.

the contaminated feed was also contaminated, and the contamination spread to other animal products including meat (57).

Agricultural chemicals, especially pesticides, are a source of food contamination (8,12,16,69). Low-level contamination can occur through direct use of pesticides on food crops. Livestock, poultry, and fish may become contaminated when pesticides are applied or manufactured in their vicinity or when pesticides are transported through the environment. Improperly fumigated railroad cars, trucks, ships, or storage facilities for food and feed may also be a source of food contamination (58).

Another source of food contamination is the manufacture of organic chemicals that produce sludges, gases, and liquid effluents of varying chemical complexities. These chemicals can contaminate the environment through the atmosphere, soil, and surface or ground water and thus find their way into foods.

Finally, food may become contaminated with metals that are released into the environment. Mining and refining processes produce dust and gases that enter the atmosphere. Metallic salts formed during recovery and refining processes can escape as waste products into surface and ground water. The use of sewer sludge as fertilizer on agricultural land also poses the potential for contaminating food with metals (58).

In evaluating the significance of environmental contaminants in food, the fundamental question is the level of exposure and, accordingly, the magnitude of the risk. Measurable health effects depend on the toxicity of the substance, its concentration in food, the quantity of food consumed, and the vulnerability of the individual or population to the toxic effects (2).

MONITORING FOOD CONTAMINATION

Monitoring of Chemical Contaminants in Food in the United States

Responsibility for monitoring exposure to environmental contaminants in food primarily rests with the following federal agencies: the Food and Drug Administration (FDA) monitors the dietary intake of selected pesticides, toxic elements, industrial chemicals, and radionuclides (12,16,19); the Food Safety Inspection Service of the U.S. Department of Agriculture (USDA) (12) monitors residues in meat and poultry; and the Environmental Protection Agency (EPA), through its National Human Monitoring Program, estimates total body exposure to toxic substances, including pesticide residues (28).

The Total Diet Study or Market Basket Survey program initiated by the FDA in the early 1960s to monitor dietary intakes of selected pesticides, industrial chemicals, toxic elements, and radionuclides was modified in 1982. The program, which initially reflected quantities consumed by 16- to 19-year-old males, now estimates the dietary intake of eight age and sex groups ranging from infants to the elderly. It involves analyses of 234 items reflecting the diets of these population groups (19). The foods to be surveyed are collected simultaneously in three cities in four geographic areas of the United States. Seasonal items are collected when they become available. The Total Diet Study analyses are performed on foods prepared for consumption rather than on raw, unwashed commodities, as is the case in most FDA monitoring for enforcement of tolerances or other regulatory limits. Since food preparation may lower pesticide levels and the concentration of other chemical residues, analytic techniques used in the Total Diet Study are modified to assess quantities five to ten times lower than those used in the FDA programs for enforcement of regulatory limits (19).

Another pesticide-monitoring program established by the FDA is designed to monitor domestic and imported food and animal feed for pesticide residues and to gather information on the incidence and levels of pesticide residues in the food supply. This monitoring program assists the FDA in enforcing the pesticide residue tolerances established for a wide variety of raw agricultural food and feed (48).

Pesticide residue analyses are performed by analytic methods that determine a number of residues simultaneously. Although multiresidue methods allow the FDA to analyze a large number of samples for many pesticides, fewer than half of the pesticides that may leave residues in food are detected by this means. As shown in Table 3-1, a certain number of highly ranked pesticides cannot be monitored using multiresidue methods (12,58).

Under the pesticide-monitoring program, the FDA collects and analyzes samples of shipments of imported food to determine whether illegal residues are present. A huge number of food shipments that could potentially contain illegal pesticide residues enter the United States each year. Each year the FDA regulatory monitoring program samples and analyzes about 20,000 food shipments, about 60% of which are imports. This represents a very small fraction of imported food shipments. In 1988 the FDA analyzed 18,114 samples of food, 10,475 of which represented imports from 89 countries (67). The multiresidue methods used to test imported food samples for illegal residues are capable of testing for most pesticides banned for use in the United States. However, about 140 pesticides having some agricultural uses abroad have no EPA tolerances and no FDA reference standards and/or analytic methodology for determining the identity or concentration of their residues (67).

Global Monitoring of Chemical Contaminants in Food

Since the mid-1970s, food contamination in various parts of the world has been monitored by the World Health Organization in collaboration with the United Nations Environment Programme (UNEP) and the Food and Agricultural Organization (FAO). This monitoring is done through the Global Envi-

TABLE 3-1. Pesticides Detectable by the Methods Used
and Pesticides Detected in 1989 Regulatory Monitoring[a]

Acephate*	Amobam*	Benfluralin	Bromophos-ethyl*
Alachlor	Anilazine*	Benomyl*	Bromopropylate*
Aldicarb*	Aramite	Bensulide	Bufencarb
Aldoxycarb*	Aspon	BHC*	Bulan
Aldrin*	Atrazine*	Binapacryl	Butralin
Allethrin	Azinphos-ethyl	Biphenyl	Captafol*
Ametryn	Azinphos-methyl*	Bromacil	Captan*
Amitraz	Bendiocarb	Bromophos	Carbanolate

TABLE 3-1. *(Continued)*

Carbaryl*	Dicofol*	Maneb*	Profenofos*
Carbendazim*	Dicrotophos*	Mecarbam*	Profluralin
Carbofuran*	Dieldrin*	Mephosfolan	Prolan
Carbon disulfide	Dilan	Merphos	Promecarb
Carbon tetrachloride	Dimethoate*	Metalaxyl	Prometryn
Carbophenothion*	Dinitramine	Metasystox thiol	Pronamide*
Carboxin	Dinocap	Methamidophos*	Propanil
Chlorbenside	Dinoseb	Methidathion*	Propargite*
Chlorbromuron	Dioxacarb	Methiocarb*	Propazine
Chlordane*	Dioxathion	Methomyl*	Propham
Chlordecone	Diphenamid	Methoxychlor*	Propoxur
Chlordimeform	Diphenylamine*	Methyl bromide	Prothiofos*
Chlorfenvinphos*	Disulfoton*	Methyl trithion	Pyrazon
Chlornidine	Diuron	Methylene chloride	Pyrazophos
Chlornitrofen	Endosulfan*	Metiram*	Pyrethrins
Chlorobenzilate	Endrin*	Metobromuron	Quinalphos*
Chloroform	EPN*	Metolachlor*	Quintozene*
Chloroneb	EPTC	Metoxuron	Ronnel
Chloropicrin	Ethion*	Metribuzin	Salithion
Chloropropylate	Ethoprop*	Mevinphos*	Schradan
Chlorothalonil*	Ethoxyquin	Mirex	Simazine*
Chlorotoluron	Ethylene dibromide*	Mobam	Strobane
Chloroxuron	Ethylene dichloride	Monocrotophos*	Sulfallate
Chlorpropham*	Etrimfos	Monolinuron	Sulfotep
Chlorpyrifos*	Famphur	Monuron	Sulfur dioxide*
Chlorpyrifos-methyl*	Fenamiphos	Nabam*	Sulprofos
Chlorthion	Fenarimol	Naled	2,4,5-T
Chlorthiophos	Fenbutatin oxide	Napropamide	2,3,6-TBA
Clofentezine*	Fenitrothion*	Neburon	TDE*
Clomazone	Fensulfothion	Nitralin	Tecnazene*
Coumaphos	Fenthion*	Nitrofen	TEPP
Cyanazine	Fenuron	Norea	Terbacil
Cyanophos*	Fenvalerate*	Norflurazon	Terbufos
Cycloate	Fluchloralin	Omethoate*	Terbuthylazine
Cyhexatin*	Flucythrinate	Ovex*	Tetradifon*
Cypermethrin*	Fluometuron	Oxadiazon	Tetraiodoethylene
2,4-D	Fluvalinate	Oxamyl	Tetrasul
2,4-DB	Folpet*	Oxydemeton-methyl	Thiabendazole*
Daminozide*	Fonofos*	Oxyfluorfen	Thiodicarb
DCPA*	Formetanate	Oxythioquinox	Thionazin
DDT*	hydrochloride*	Parathion*	Thiophanate-methyl
DEF	Gardona	Parathion-methyl*	Tolylfluanid
Deltamethrin	Genite 923	Pendimethalin	Toxaphene*
Demeton*	Heptachlor*	Pentachlorophenol*	Triadimefon*
Dialifor	Hexachlorobenzene*	Permethrin*	Triadimenol*
Diallate	Imazalil*	Perthane	Triallate*
Diazinon*	Iprodione*	Phenkapton	Triazophos
Dibromochloropropane	Isobenzan*	Phenthoate	Tributyltin*
Dicamba	Isodrin*	Phenylphenol, ortho*	Trichlorfon
Dicapthon	Isofenphos	Phorate*	Trichloroethane*
Dichlobenil*	Isoprocarb	Phosalone*	Trichloronat
Dichlofenthion	Isopropalin	Phosmet*	Trifluralin*
Dichlofluanid*	Isoproturon	Phosphamidon*	Triforine
Dichlone	Jodfenphos	Phostex	Trimethacarb
Dichlorobenzene, ortho	Lead arsenate*	Phoxim	Triphenyltin hydroxide
Dichlorobenzene, para	Leptophos	Picloram	Vernolate
1,3-Dichloropropene	Lindane*	Pirimicarb	Vinclozolin*
Dichlorvos	Linuron*	Pirimiphos-ethyl	Zineb*
Diclofop-methyl	Malathion*	Pirimiphos-methyl*	Zytron
Dicloran*	Mancozeb*	Procymidone*	

[a]Some of these pesticides are no longer manufactured or registered for use in the United States. Those detected are indicated by asterisks.
From FDA (12).

ronment Monitoring System (GEMS). By 1988, 35 countries representing Australia, New Zealand, the whole of North America, large portions of Europe, South America, Asia, and a few countries in Africa, which include Egypt and Kenya, participated in the program (18). Air and water quality are also monitored through the GEMS program (see Chapters 2 and 4).

REGULATION OF FOOD ADDITIVES AND CONTAMINANTS

In 1984, a National Research Council committee determined that of the estimated universe of about 5 million known chemicals, humans are likely to be exposed to about 65,000 (53). Approximately 56,000 of these chemicals used in commerce are regulated under the Toxic Substances Control Act (TSCA) of 1976 and monitored by the Environmental Protection Agency (60). The TSCA excludes the majority of chemicals added to foods, food constituents, food contaminants, drugs, and pesticidal chemicals.

The federal laws governing food additives and contaminants in the United States are shown in Table 3-2. Categories of substances intentionally or unintentionally added to foods and those that may occur as contaminants are summarized in Table 3-3.

Considerable effort has been directed to controlling the use of pesticides. Federal jurisdiction over pesticide residues in food is divided among the Environmental Protection Agency (EPA), the U.S. Department of Agriculture (USDA), and the Food and Drug Administration (FDA). As noted, except for meat, poultry, and some egg products, which are under the USDA, monitoring and enforcement responsibilities for domestically produced and imported foods lie with the FDA. The EPA is responsible for regulating all pesticide products sold or distributed in the United States.

The regulation of pesticides began in 1947 with the enactment of the Federal Insecticide, Fungicide and Rodenticide Act (FIFRA). In order for a pesticide to be lawfully sold in the United States, it must be registered by the EPA. Under FIFRA, the EPA determines which pesticides can be registered. A pesticide must be used in accordance with the terms and conditions of its registration. The EPA is man-

dated to balance the benefits of using a pesticide against its potential risks to public health and the environment (8).

The registration of a pesticide by the EPA is linked to the establishment of tolerances, which place legal limits on the concentration of pesticide residues that can be present in foods sold in interstate commerce. Tolerances must be granted to cover pesticide residues expected to be found in or on raw and processed food before a pesticide can be registered. Tolerances are granted by the EPA under the aegis of the Federal Food, Drug and Cosmetics Act (FD&C). The Delaney Clause, contained in the FD&C Act, created a special rule for food additives that have been found to induce cancer when ingested by humans or animals. Under these conditions, no such additive can be approved, or in the case of a pesticide, granted a tolerance. The Delaney Clause applies specifically to the residues of those pesticides that are concentrated in a processed food or feed above the level allowed in the raw agricultural commodity (8). Though the Delaney Clause does not directly govern residues in raw food, it can have a significant effect on raw food tolerances. The Food and Drug Administration (FDA) has the responsibility for regulating pesticide residues that fall under the Delaney Clause.

The data required for the registration of a pesticide and the setting of its tolerance are defined by EPA regulations and guidelines. These data include a chemical description of the pesticide and identification and quantification of residues expected to be present in food. Information on food residues is generally derived through extrapolation from the data obtained on a limited number of field trials. Formidable problems are generally encountered in the process of gathering and interpreting the residue data. In most instances, complete residue data are not available for the pesticides that are currently registered (8).

The toxicity data currently required for pesticide registration and granting of a tolerance are quite extensive. For each active ingredient and for major impurities or metabolites, the following information is typically required: acute oral, dermal, and inhalation studies; two-generation reproduction studies; chronic feeding studies on rodents and nonrodents; oncogenicity studies on mice and rats; mutagenicity studies on gene mutation, structural chromosomal aberration, and other toxic effects on genetic material; teratogenicity studies on rats and rabbits; delayed neuropathy studies on chickens; and plant and animal metabolism studies (8).

In 1978, amendments to the FIFRA imposed new data requirements, many of which are listed above, for registering and granting tolerances for a new pesticide. Prior to this time, many pesticides were registered and had tolerances established

TABLE 3-2. Laws Governing Food Additives and Contaminants in the United States

Federal Food, Drug and Cosmetic Act (FDCA) (1938)
Federal Insecticide, Fungicide and Rodenticide Act (FIFRA) (1947)
Pesticide Monitoring Improvements Act (1988)

TABLE 3-3. The Federal Food, Drug, and Cosmetic Act: Categories of Food Constituents[a]

Category	Number of compounds in each category[b]	Example(s)	Applicability of Delaney Clause
Natural Food Constituents	?		NA[c]
Vitamins and minerals in foods	~70	Ascorbic acid in oranges; calcium in milk	
Other chemical components of foods	?	Caffeine in coffee; nitrate in spinach	
Intentionally added substances	~2,700		
Direct additives, e.g., stabilizers, leavening agents, emulsifiers, antioxidants, sweeteners	~400	Yeasts, sodium bicarbonate, sodium hydroxide, lecithin, butylated hydroxyanisole (BHA), saccharin	Yes
Previously sanctioned additives, e.g., preservatives	~100	Sodium nitrite	NA
GRAS (generally recognized as safe) substances, e.g., spices, seasonings, multipurpose substances	~600	Cumin, carrageenan, BHA, butylated hydroxytoluene (BHT), acetic acid, lecithin, sulfuric acid, hydrochloric acid, vanilla, caffeine, sodium chloride, sucrose	NA
Flavoring ingredients (many are GRAS)	~1,700	Monosodium glutamate, vanilla, licorice	NA
Color additives	~30	Food, Drug, and Cosmetic (FD&C) Blue #1, Orange B, Citrus Red #2, FD&C Yellow #5	Yes
Indirect additives	~12,000		
Indirect additives, e.g., processing aids, packaging components	~10,000	Acetone, methyl alcohol, methylene chloride, polystyrene	Yes, except for GRAS substances[d]
Drugs given to animals, e.g., synthetic hormones, antibiotics	~200	Dinestrol diacetate, tylosin	To residues only
Pesticide residues, e.g., organochlorine compounds, carbamates	~1,400	Hexachlorobenzene, lindane, carbaryl	NA
Unavoidable "added" constituents (contaminants)	?		NA
Fungi, microbial toxins, metal residues, industrial chemicals	?	Aflatoxin, patulin, polychlorinated biphenyls, mercury, beryllium	

[a]Code of Federal Regulations (1981). From Steering Committee (53).
[b]Information on the numbers of substances is derived partially from lists of additives published by the Food and Drug Administration in the Code of Federal Regulations and partly from estimates based on the opinion of experts in the field.
[c]NA, not applicable.
[d]Examples of indirect additives that are also GRAS substances are coconut oil, pulps, and sulfuric acid.

without data on oncogenicity and residue levels. Because of this policy, it is estimated that most of the carcinogenic risk associated with residues in food stems from pesticides, particularly herbicides and fungicides, granted tolerances before 1978 (8). FIFRA, however, mandates that all registered pesticides be reregistered using contemporary scientific standards and data. The EPA is now implementing this program.

The complex topic of regulating pesticide residues in food is examined in depth in a publication from the National Research Council. The Delaney Clause, its implications, and the methods used for estimating dietary oncogenic risk are considered in detail in this publication (8).

A critical aspect of the typical tolerance-setting process is the effort by the EPA to establish a safe level of exposure. A similar standard is established by the United Nations Food and Agriculture Organization (FAO) and the World Health Organization (WHO). The FAO/WHO establish Acceptable Daily Intakes (ADI), which represent daily intake of a chemical that, if ingested over a lifetime, appears to be without appreciable risk. The EPA standard, termed reference doses (RfDs), estimates total pesticide exposure to the human population (including sensitive subgroups) that are likely to be without appreciable risk of adverse effects over a lifetime. A safety factor of 100 is generally included in these calculations. Since the assumptions made by the EPA and the FAO/WHO are somewhat different, the RfDs can be higher or lower than ADIs. Both standards are revised as new data become available (12).

The Pesticide Monitoring Improvements Act of 1988 represents new legislation enacted by Congress to improve the FDA's coverage of pesticide residues in food, with an emphasis on imported foods (67). This legislation has three components dealing with pesticide monitoring and enforcement information, foreign pesticide usage information, and pesticide analytic methods. Briefly, the FDA is required to develop a computerized data management system that will record, summarize, and evaluate the results of pesticide-monitoring programs. Gaps in the program are to be identified, along with trends in pesticide residues in foods and public health problems arising from their presence. The FDA is also required to enter into cooperative agreements with the countries that are major sources of imported food or whose imports may be important in terms of volume, dietary significance, or potential pesticide problems. Finally, the Pesticide Monitoring Improvements Act of 1988 mandates that the FDA implement a long-range plan and timetable for research leading to new and improved multiresidue methods for analyzing pesticide residues. Such methods, it is hoped, will provide a cost-effective means of increasing the number of pesticides that can be measured (67).

CHEMICAL CONTAMINANTS IN FOOD

Polycyclic Aromatic Hydrocarbons

Approximately 100 types of polycyclic aromatic hydrocarbons (PAHs) have been identified in foods. Their presence in foodstuffs is of concern primarily because many of these compounds are known to be mutagenic and/or carcinogenic. There are two major sources of PAH contamination in foods: pyrolysis and contact with petroleum and coal tar products (24). Charbroiling of meats and fish over an open flame in which fat drippings can be pyrolyzed contributes substantially to diet-derived PAH exposure (7). Benzo[a]pyrene (BaP) constitutes 1% to 20% of the total carcinogenic PAH in the environment, and there are considerable data on the BaP content of foods. For example, levels as high as 50 μg/kg were found in thick T-bone steaks cooked close to the coals for long periods (30). In contrast, data on dietary exposure to other carcinogenic PAHs are fragmentary (55).

There are no comprehensive surveys of the BaP content of smoked foods in the United States. Commonly smoked foods include fish, meat, fowl, and cheeses. In one survey, Canadian smoked foods were reported to contain from 0.2 to 15 μg/kg of BaP (45). Domestically smoked products may often contain more PAHs than do commercially smoked foods. Conventional wood smoke may contribute more BaP than does liquid smoke, a condensate produced from wood smoke. The liquid smoke, having been cleansed, is thought to contain smaller amounts of PAHs (7).

Edible marine species may contain variable amounts of PAHs derived principally from polluted terrestrial runoff waters, from marine sediments, and from petroleum-contaminated aquatic environments. Bioaccumulation of PAHs in the marine food chain may be substantial. Furthermore, petroleum and coal tar products such as solvents used for refining edible oils or paraffin wax used for food packaging are another major source of PAH contamination (7). PAHs have also been detected in some alcoholic beverages (32). Vegetables and seafood, unless obtained from highly contaminated areas, are not considered to be major dietary sources of PAHs (4).

Table 3-4 shows the levels of PAHs in different categories of foods. The PAHs are not monitored by the FDA, and there is no acceptable daily intake (ADI) for PAHs. Their total daily intake in the United States, however, has been estimated to be 1.6–16 μg, of which 0.16–1.6 μg may come from benzo[a]pyrene (49). Human exposure to the PAHs

TABLE 3-4. Polycyclic Aromatic Hydrocarbons in Foods[a]

Compound	Foodstuff	Concentration (μg/kg)
Benz[a]an-thracene	Broiled sausage	0.2–1.1
	Smoked sausage	0.4–9.9
	Heavily smoked ham	12
	Spinach	16
	Crude coconut oil	98
	Refined vegetable oil	1
Benzo[a]pyrene	Broiled sausage	0.17–0.63
	Charcoal-broiled meat	2.6–11.2
	Smoked fish	2.1
	Spinach	7.4
	Tomatoes	0.2
	Crude coconut oil	43.7
	Roasted coffee	0.1–4
	Tea	3.9–21.3
	Cereals	0.2–4.1
Benzo[e]pyrene	Smoked ham	5.2
	Smoked fish	1.9
	Spinach	6.9
	Tomatoes	0.2
	Crude coconut oil	32.7
	Roasted coffee	0.3–7.2
	Roasted peanuts	0.4
Chrysene	Broiled sausage	0.5–2.6
	Heavily smoked ham	21.2
	Spinach	28
	Tomatoes	0.5
	Cereals	0.8–14.5
	Roasted coffee	0.6–19.1
	Black tea	4.6–6.3
Dibenz[a,h]anthracene	Spinach	0.3
	Tomatoes	0.04
	Cereals	0.01–0.6

[a]From Committee on Pyrene (7).

from dietary constituents is thought to greatly exceed that from any other source except specific occupational settings.

Epidemiologic observations in Europe and some studies in the United States have suggested an association between the consumption of high-PAH-containing food and gastrointestinal malignancies in selected populations (20,52,56). The lack of precise information about the PAH content of specific foods makes it difficult to extrapolate the findings to determine the level of risk to the general population in the United States or to define the health risks from exposure to PAHs in foods in more direct terms. Nevertheless, the quantitative dimensions of PAH exposure via the diet and the established carcinogenic potential of some of the compounds frequently identified in foods suggest that the health risk from this source of exposure, although still incompletely defined, may be important for certain populations (7).

Many of the orally ingested PAHs are rapidly absorbed and excreted in the feces and urine. Some of the absorbed material is retained in the adrenals, the ovaries, and in body fat and has been detected as long as 8 days later (11). Some PAHs, such as BaP and anthracene, have been detected in human liver (22–440 ng/kg) and in body fat (59–440 ng/kg) (41).

Pesticides

Vast amounts of pesticides, which include insecticides, herbicides, and fungicides, are used in the United States and throughout the world (44). Figure 3-1 shows pesticide use through 1985 and the projected increase to 1990. Residues of pesticides can remain on agricultural commodities after they have been harvested and prepared for consumer purchase. They are also found in processed foods derived from these commodities (Table 3-5). Traces of many fungicides and herbicides can also be detected in foods. Since many pesticides that have residues present in food are known or suspected of being carcinogenic in some animal species, there is basis for concern about their potential effects on human health. Three major categories of insecticides are discussed below.

Organochlorines

The use of several organochlorine compounds such as DDT and Kepone® has been suspended by the EPA in the past two decades. However, some concern is still warranted. These substances have a propensity to persist in the environment and to accumulate in the fat of such foods as meat, fish, poultry, and dairy products commonly consumed by humans (51). Because of their lipophilic nature, most of the chlorinated pesticides, including DDT, DDE, TDE, toxaphene, methoxychlor, and lindane,

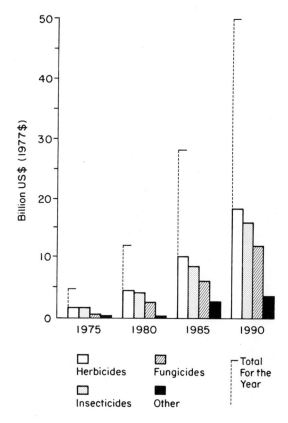

FIGURE 3-1. Sales and consumption of pesticides in the world. Adapted from Organisation for Economic Co-operation and Development (44).

also tend to accumulate in adipose tissues. Persistent pesticides such as DDT can be detected in exposed persons many years after the exposure has ceased. For example, although its use was banned in the United States in 1973, DDT or its metabolite DDE can still be detected in foods and in human and animal tissues and secretions (22,23,37). Many of the organochlorine pesticides have been replaced in recent years by organophosphates and carbamates.

Organophosphates

The most widely used organophosphorus insecticides are malathion, diazinon, parathion, and methylparathion. Generally, they are rapidly degraded to nontoxic chemicals after application and, unlike the chlorinated hydrocarbons, do not tend to accumulate in the environment. Their residues are primarily found in grains and cereals, whereas organochlorine insecticides are found primarily in meats and dairy products (16).

TABLE 3-5. Frequency of Occurrence of
Pesticides in Total Diet Study in 1989

Pesticide[a]	Total no. of findings[b]	Percentage occurrence
Malathion	185	20
DDT	124	13
Chlorpyrifos-methyl	93	10
Diazinon	80	9
Chlorpyrifos	71	8
Dieldrin	62	7
Methamidophos	58	6
Endosulfan	51	5
Chlorpropham	48	5
Hexachlorobenzene	47	5
Dicloran	39	4
Lindane	34	4
BHC, alpha & beta	31	3
Carbaryl[c]	31	3
Ethion	28	3
Quintozene	27	3
Acephate	26	3
Heptachlor	26	3
Dimethoate	24	3
Propargite[d]	23	2
DCPA	16	2
Dicofol	16	2
Toxaphene	14	1
Omethoate	13	1
Parathion	13	1
Permethrin	12	1
Pirimiphos-methyl	12	1
Thiabendazole[d]	11	1
Methomyl[c]	9	1

[a]Isomers, metabolites, and related compounds have not been listed
separately; they are covered under the generic or "parent" pesticide from which they arise.
[b]Based on 936 items.
[c]Reflects overall incidence; however, only 72 selected foods per
market basket (i.e., 288 total items) were analyzed for *N*-methyl-
carbamates.
[d]Analysis for propargite and thiabendazole began in FY89. Value
reflects overall incidence; however, only 39 selected foods per
market basket (i.e., 156 total items) were analyzed for these sulfur-
containing compounds.

Carbamates

Carbamates are among the most recent group
of pesticides to be introduced. The most widely
used carbamates include carbaryl, carbofuran, and
aldicarb. Their mode of action and environmental
persistence are similar to those of organophosphates (33).

Nitrogen Compounds

A large number of widely used herbicides and
fungicides are nitrogen compounds. Benomyl, for
example, is a widely used nitrogen heterocyclic
fungicide. Other nitrogen compounds used extensively as herbicides include the bipyridyls (i.e.,
paraquat and diquat), the anilides (i.e., alachlor and
propanil), the phenylureas (i.e., monuron and chlor-
oxuron), and the triazines (i.e., atrazine and simazine). The use of herbicides now rivals or exceeds
that of insecticides in amount and in expenditures
(Fig. 3-1).

Estimates of Exposure to Pesticide Residues

The general population is exposed to pesticidal
compounds principally through food and drinking
water (22,23). As noted, the U.S. FDA has the responsibility for enforcing tolerances for all pesticides used in food. Although thousands of domestic
and imported food shipments are monitored each
year, the number of samples analyzed from various
domestic and foreign pesticide–crop combinations
is limited, as are the pesticide detection capabilities
of the multiresidue methods used by the FDA. A
report of FDA monitoring of pesticide residues in
imported food reveals that violation rates for imports have not been significantly different from
those found for domestic foods (67).

The Market Basket Surveys conducted by the
FDA indicate that the levels of pesticides in food, in
general, are very low and tend to vary only slightly
from region to region (12,16). Table 3-6 presents
pesticide intakes found in total diet analyses in the
United States for three age and sex groups (12). The
intake of individual pesticides in the average U.S.
diet appears to be well within established acceptance levels. However, any estimate of the degree of
health risk associated with pesticide exposure
should consider the possible additive and/or potentiating effects of simultaneous exposure to several
pesticides and the fact that many pesticides currently in use in the United States were registered
with limited toxicity data, sometimes in the absence
of oncogenicity data.

In a large-scale 4-year study to estimate the
body burden of selected pesticides in the general
U.S. population, Murphy et al. (37) reported widespread exposure to several compounds. Residues or
metabolites of DDT were reported to occur in 99% of
serum samples and in 100% of adipose tissue samples, and other organochlorine pesticides occurred
in 4–14% of the serum and in 93–97% of the adipose
tissue samples.

Toxic Metals

Traces of toxic metals may be present in foods as
natural constituents, as contaminants, or as residues
of accidental contamination. Lead, cadmium, mercury, and arsenic in particular are frequently the
focus of concern because of their relatively high
toxicity to humans and animals. Table 3-7 shows the

Table 3-6. Pesticide Intakes (µg/kg body wt per day) Found in Total Diet Analyses and Their ADIs/RfDs for Three Age/Sex Groups in 1989

Pesticide	6–11 mo	14–16 yr M[a]	60–65 yr F[a]	FAO/WHO ADI[b]	EPA RfD[b]
Acephate	0.0046	0.0033	0.0054	30	4
Azinphosmethyl	0.0017	0.0050	0.0039	2.5	—[c]
BHC, alpha + beta	0.0009	0.0014	0.0006	—[c]	—
BHC, gamma (lindane)	0.0011	0.0020	0.0008	10	0.3
Captan	0.0129	0.0049	0.0160	100	130
Carbaryl	0.1004	0.0182	0.0343	10	—
Chlordane, total	0.0001	0.0001	0.0001	0.5	0.06
Chlorobenzilate	<0.0001	0.0001	0.0001	20	20
Chlorothalonil	<0.0001	<0.0001	<0.0001	3[d]	15
Chlorpropham, total	0.2700	0.4543	0.1496	—	200[e]
Chlorpyrifos	0.0131	0.0041	0.0043	10	3
Chlorpyrifosmethyl	0.0202	0.0236	0.0148	10	—
DCPA	0.0012	0.0007	0.0013	—	500
DDT, total	0.0287	0.0155	0.0079	20[f]	0.5[e]
DEF	<0.0001	0.0001	<0.0001	—	—
Diazinon	0.0031	0.0034	0.0017	2	—
Dicloran, total	0.1382	0.0337	0.0832	30[e]	—
Dicofol, total	0.0118	0.0088	0.0096	25	—
Dieldrin	0.0013	0.0015	0.0015	0.1[f]	0.05
Dimethoate	0.0114	0.0022	0.0045	10[f]	0.2
Endosulfan, total	0.0165	0.0088	0.0127	6[f]	0.05[e]
Endrin	<0.0001	<0.0001	0.0001	0.2	0.3
Ethion, total	0.0167	0.0060	0.0060	6[d,e]	0.5[e]
Fenitrothion	0.0008	0.0006	0.0009	5	—
Fenvalerate	0.0137	0.0080	0.0132	20	25
Folpet	0.0004	0.0002	0.0005	10[d]	100
Fonofos	<0.0001	0.0001	<0.0001	—	2
Heptachlor, total	0.0007	0.0008	0.0006	0.5[f]	0.5[e]
Hexachlorobenzene	0.0007	0.0009	0.0005	—	0.8
Iprodione, total	0.0045	0.0017	0.0026	300[e]	40[e]
Linuron	0.0004	0.0001	0.0002	—	2
Malathion	0.1151	0.0924	0.0529	20	20
Methamidophos	0.0112	0.0116	0.0264	0.6	0.05
Methomyl	0.0094	0.0055	0.0148	30	25
Methoxychlor, p, p'	<0.0001	0.0001	0.0001	100	—
Mevinphos, total	0.0032	0.0020	0.0049	1.5[f]	—
Omethoate	0.0072	0.0017	0.0039	0.3	—
Parathion	0.0091	0.0006	0.0011	5	—
Pentachlorophenol	0.0013	0.0012	0.0015	—	30
Permethrin, total	0.0387	0.0364	0.0497	50	50
Phosalone	0.0104	<0.0001	0.0001	6	—
Phosmet	0.0019	0.0008	0.0009	20[f]	20
Phosphamidon	0.0013	0.0039	0.0031	0.5[f]	—
Pirimiphosmethyl	0.0011	0.0013	0.0008	10	10
Profenofos	0.0001	<0.0001	0.0001	—	—
Propargite	0.5298	0.0613	0.0567	150	20
Quintozene, total	0.0005	0.0009	0.0002	7[f]	3[e]
Sulfur	0.0070	0.0018	0.0036	—	—
Tecnazene	<0.0001	0.0002	<0.0001	10	—
Tetradifon	0.0001	<0.0001	<0.0001	—	—
Thiabendazole	0.0854	0.0334	0.0581	300	—
Toxaphene	0.0059	0.0087	0.0046	—	—
Vinclozolin	0.0039	0.0016	0.0048	70	25

[a]M, male; F, female.
[b]ADIs and RfDs (EPA reference doses) are usually expressed as mg/kg body wt per day but are expressed here as µg/kg body wt per day for ease of comparison. The ADIs cited here reflect revisions made in 1988 and 1989. The RfDs cited here reflect April 3, 1990 EPA revisions and are reprinted with the permission of EPA.
[c]ADI or RfD not established.
[d]"Temporary" ADI.
[e]Parent chemical only.
[f]Includes other (related) chemicals.

TABLE 3-7. Daily Intake (µg/day) of Selected Elements (1982–1984)[a]

Element	Tolerable limit	Age/sex group							
		6–11 mo	2 yr	14–16 F	14–16 M	25–30 F	25–30 M	60–65 F	60–65 M
Arsenic (expressed as elemental As)	—[b]	4.9	12.2	23.0	27.7	31.0	45.3	35.2	43.8
Cadmium	57–72[c]	4.2	7.3	10.6	15.4	10.6	15.0	9.6	12.7
Lead	adults: 429[c] infants: 32 children: 46	16.7	23.0	28.7	41.3	29.6	40.9	30.4	37.6
Mercury	43[c]	0.49	1.3	2.4	2.6	2.9	3.9	3.1	3.6

[a]From Gunderson (19).
[b]There has been no agreement on the maximum acceptable intake to total (organic and inorganic) arsenic. However, FOA/WHO (Food and Agricultural Organization/World Health Organization) has estimated an adult provisional tolerable daily intake (PTDI) for ingested inorganic arsenic of 2 µg/kg body weight. (This PTDI may not be applicable to children.)
[c]PTDIs calculated from the provisional tolerable weekly intakes proposed by the FAO/WHO.

daily intake of selected metals for various age groups in the United States and their provisional tolerable daily intakes established by the Food and Agriculture Organization/World Health Organization (19).

Arsenic

Arsenic can be present in foods as a contaminant or as a residue of lead arsenate or calcium arsenate used in pesticides. The highest levels of arsenic in the U.S. food supply come from seafood. Meat may contain traces of arsanilic acid that is used as a growth additive in cattle and poultry feeds. Wine and cider may also contain arsenic, but it is usually removed during processing (27). The dietary intake of arsenic ranged between 4.9 and 45.3 µg/day (Table 3-7).

Trivalent arsenic compounds, including arsenic trioxide, are more toxic than other forms of arsenic. They are retained in tissues in greater amounts and are excreted more slowly. Arsenic in the pentavalent form in which it ordinarily occurs in foods, including the organically bound arsenic of shrimp, is easily absorbed and rapidly excreted in urine (5). Arsenic is distributed primarily to the liver, the kidneys, the intestinal wall, and the spleen, with the liver achieving the highest concentration. In humans, the average body content of arsenic, which apparently tends to increase with age, has been estimated at 3 to 4 mg (6).

The potential impact of acid rain on the environmental mobility of arsenic has not been thoroughly examined. Arsenic appears to be mobilized from household plumbing into tap water by the corrosive action of soft, mildly acidic water. Surface catchment systems, in areas with acidic deposition, may contain elevated levels of soluble arsenic. The acidification of aquatic ecosystems that provide drinking

water sources may enhance the release of arsenic into the water. The acidification of ground water may be of considerable concern since arsenic appears to be especially mobile near such water sources (40).

Changes in the acidity of soil and aquatic systems also pose a risk by changing biotransformation processes. With such changes the relative concentrations of the various chemical forms of arsenic may be altered and thereby affect its toxicity.

Cadmium

Food is the main source of cadmium intake in non-occupationally exposed persons (66). An extremely wide range of cadmium concentrations in food has been reported from various countries (15). Root crops and leafy vegetables, more than other food classes, tend to concentrate cadmium from the soil. Municipal sludges containing high levels of cadmium of industrial origin, applied to agricultural lands as fertilizer, are potentially important sources for the entry of cadmium into the human food chain (10). In Europe and possibly elsewhere, phosphate fertilizers provide a significant agricultural source of cadmium. Aquatic species—including fish, crabs, and shrimp—bioconcentrate cadmium, as do organ meats such as liver, kidney, and pancreas (39). The average intake of cadmium in the United States ranged between 4.2 and 15.4 µg/day (19).

Only a small proportion of ingested cadmium is absorbed, whereas the rest is excreted through the feces. Absorbed cadmium is stored principally in the liver and kidneys, and the total body burden is estimated at 1 mg at birth and 15–50 mg at age 50. In a recent cross-national study, cadmium levels ranged from 0.5 to 1.2 µg/kg in blood and 20 to 70 mg/kg wet weight of the kidney cortex (14). Human milk may be regarded as a minor excretory mechanism, but it is a source of intake for breast-fed infants (15).

The role of acid rain or acid precipitation in relation to cadmium exposure is difficult to assess. The pH of the soil appears to be an important factor in the uptake of cadmium in crops such as wheat or rice (40). Smelting operations, waste incineration, industrial activities, and the agricultural practice of using cadmium-containing phosphates and/or sewage sludge as fertilizers contribute to the soil load of cadmium that may be mobilized by acidification. Acid rain may thus increase the amount of cadmium in forage of game animals. Frank and Pettersson (13) observed elevated concentrations of cadmium in livers and kidneys of moose in Sweden in areas with high acid deposition. In areas where roof catchment cistern systems are used, a decrease in pH may cause an increase in cadmium concentrations of drinking water (46). Some increase in cadmium is also expected where galvanized water pipes are used.

Lead

Food accounts for 55% to 85% of a person's total daily exposure to lead (50). One-third of the dietary lead appears to be derived from migration of lead from the solder of cans into the food (25). Other handling or processing operations such as the grinding of meat can increase the lead content. Lead has also been detected in food wrappings (65). Vegetables and rice cooked in water may adsorb up to 80% of the lead in the water. The amount adsorbed varies with the concentration of lead in water, the hardness of water, the duration of cooking, and the surface area of the vegetables. Lead adsorbed on cooking utensils can also be subsequently desorbed into the food under acidic conditions (31). Contamination of crops with lead from soils treated with sewage sludge is generally not considered to be a problem because of the high pH of such soil (10).

The absorption of dietary lead is estimated at 5–10% in the adult and 40–50% in infants and children. Increased absorption is one of the factors that places infants and young children at especially high risk from lead toxicity. Total body lead is distributed among blood, soft tissues, and bone. Bone is the storage site for at least 90% of total body lead (47).

The impact of acid rain or acid precipitation on human exposure to lead depends on the source of exposure. The sources most affected by acid rain are drinking water and food. For example, high intakes of lead have been reported in Scotland because of the leaching of lead from pipes by acidified drinking water (36). In one town, maternal blood levels exceeded 35 µg/dL in 10% of the subjects after lead levels in drinking water had reached more than 1000 µg/L in some tap samples. Liming of the water

raised pH values and lowered blood lead levels so that none of the maternal samples examined exceeded 25 µg/dL.

In roof catchment systems containing lead, the influence of acid rain on lead intakes can also be considerable. Acid rain may also increase the exposure of children to lead by enhancing the corrosion of lead-containing materials in the child's environment. For example, acid rain may increase the weathering of lead-containing painted surfaces, which, in turn, may increase the ingestion of lead by children (40).

Mercury

Food is the main source of exposure to mercury in non-occupationally exposed populations. Fish, fish products, and other seafood account for most of this exposure. Mercury in foodstuffs is predominantly found in the form of methylmercury compounds, which are the most toxic forms of mercury, especially for the nervous system (43). The total intake of mercury in the United States (1982–1984) ranged between 0.49 and 3.9 µg/day (Table 3-7).

In humans, methylmercury concentrations in blood and hair provide an index of exposure. Blood concentrations of mercury more accurately reflect recent exposure. The content of mercury in the brain in unexposed persons is usually very low (about 0.3 µg/g), whereas up to 79 µg/g of methylmercury has been measured in persons poisoned with mercury (42).

Exposure to forms of mercury other than methylmercury usually does not reach toxic concentrations in air, water, and food (40). However, the methylmercury concentration in fish may be increased by acid precipitation. Data presented by Stokes et al. (54) suggest that acid precipitation increases the bioavailability of methylmercury in fish.

Food-Packaging Materials

Polyvinyl Chloride

Vinyl chloride is the parent compound or monomer for a series of thermoplastic resin polymers (e.g., PVC) and copolymers widely used for such food-packaging materials as containers, wrapping film, and coatings and for parts of food-processing equipment. In the United Kingdom several types of foods are packaged in PVC or may come in contact with PVC containers, for example: in bottles: cooking oil, concentrated fruit drink, gravy powder, and olives; in rigid containers: soft margarine, butter, potato salad, cakes, biscuits, and chocolates; in flexible films: fresh and cooked meats, sandwiches, fruit, vegetables, and cheese; in bottle closure liners: carbonated soft drinks and beer; in lacquered food cans: carbonated soft drinks and beer; in heat-sealed aluminum foil: chocolate and soft confectionaries (35).

Until recently, PVC was classified as an indirect additive in the United States, whereas vinyl chloride monomer was regulated as a contaminant. However, a subsequent proposal issued by the Food and Drug Administration would make residual vinyl chloride a constituent of PVC and therefore not subject to regulation under the Delaney Clause. As previously mentioned, the Delaney Clause was passed by the United States Congress in 1958 as part of an amendment to the FD&C Act. It forbids the addition to food of any substances shown to be carcinogenic in laboratory animals or in humans (64).

In 1973, Schenley Distillers in the United States noted significant organoleptic differences between various alcoholic beverages packaged in PVC containers and in glass. This was attributed to contamination with 0–20 mg/L vinyl chloride monomer, and as a result, PVC was banned from use in the packaging of alcoholic beverages (1). However, this ban did not extend to other foods.

Analysis of 28 samples of Canadian vinegars and ten samples of peanut oil packaged in PVC bottles contained 0 to 8.4 mg/L and 0.3 to 3.3 mg/L of vinyl chloride monomer, respectively (68).

The Working Party on Vinyl Chloride of the United Kingdom found that there was a gradual decline in the levels of vinyl chloride in foods packaged in PVC containers. An earlier investigation showed a level of 0.01 mg/kg vinyl chloride. By May 1976, this level had been reduced to 0.005 mg/kg (35).

There are no estimates of average daily dietary exposure to vinyl chloride in the United States.

Acrylonitrile

Acrylonitrile polymers are used for packaging a variety of foods. During the manufacturing process a small fraction of the unreacted monomer usually becomes physically entrapped in the polymer. It then can migrate slowly during storage and on contact with food. Just as with vinyl chloride, the FDA has proposed reclassifying acrylonitrile monomer in food-packaging materials as a "constituent" of the polymer (64). Thus, it may no longer be subject to banning under the Delaney Clause.

The Ministry of Agriculture, Fisheries and Food of Great Britain (35) conducted a number of surveys of acrylonitrile in soft margarine and ABS (acrylonitrile–butadiene–styrene resin) tubs. It detected 0 to 10 mg/kg of acrylonitrile in ABS tubs (mean of 6 mg/kg) and 0.01 to 0.02 mg/kg in soft margarine, with occasional samples containing up to 0.04 mg/kg. Similar levels were noted by Gilbert and Stratin (17) in food-packaging films used for

snack products. In the United States, D. Breder (unpublished data, 1980), in a survey of foods wrapped in packagings containing acrylonitrile polymer, found 13–45 μg/kg acrylonitrile in margarine and 38–50 μg/L in olive oil. None was detected in bologna or ham.

Until 1978, acrylonitrile was also used in the United States as a fumigant to protect grain, dried fruit, walnuts, and tobacco against insect pests. As a consequence, minute quantities had been detected in nuts as much as 38 days after fumigation (3).

There are no estimates for the average daily exposure to acrylonitrile in the United States.

Industrial Chemicals

Polychlorinated Biphenyls

Polychlorinated biphenyls (PCBs) have been used in a variety of industrial applications since 1929. However, because of concern over their environmental persistence and consequent health effects, the EPA in 1977 prohibited their manufacture, processing, and distribution in commerce. Currently, the use of PCBs is restricted to totally enclosed containers (59). Nevertheless, PCBs continue to be found as contaminants in foods and water, albeit at lower than previous levels. In the United States, the general population may be exposed to small amounts of PCBs through food, water, and air. Significant exposure may occur among sports fishermen who consume fresh-water fish from contaminated streams and lakes.

The FDA regulates PCBs as unavoidable contaminants in food and food-packaging materials under the Federal Food, Drug, and Cosmetic Act. As a first step to limit exposure from dietary sources, the FDA issued a notice that established 5 ppm as the temporary tolerance level for PCBs in foods and food-packaging materials (61). More recently, the tolerance levels were lowered in several food classes: in milk and dairy products (from 2.5 to 1.5 ppm fat basis), in poultry (from 5 to 3 ppm fat basis), and in seafood (from 5 to 2 ppm fat basis) (63).

The Interdepartmental Task Force on PCBs (21) outlined three major sources of food contamination: environmental contamination, i.e., background levels of PCBs in fish from lakes and streams; industrial accidents, i.e., isolated incidents involving direct leakage and spillage or contact of PCB fluids and other PCB-containing materials with animal feeds, feed ingredients, or food; and food-packaging materials, i.e., PCB migration to foods packaged in PCB-contaminated paper products. PCB contamination of packaging materials has for the most part been eliminated (51).

A national survey conducted by the FDA prior

to March 1972 found that 67% of the food-packaging material tested contained as much as 338 mg/kg PCBs and that 19% of the food exposed to such packaging was in turn contaminated, averaging 0.1 μg/g of PCB with a maximum of 5 μg/g (62).

Fresh-water fish is the major dietary source of PCBs, and PCBs tend to concentrate in fatty tissues. Because fish is also a source of feed for domestic animals, PCBs may be found in meat, milk, eggs, and poultry (34). On a national level, approximately 20% of all fish were found to contain some detectable amount of PCBs. Fewer than 2% were found to have reached or exceeded the FDA's temporary tolerance levels of 5 ppm in fish (34).

Jelinek and Corneliussen (26) reported a significant reduction of PCB contamination from 1969 to 1975 in the United States in all foods except fish, in which no trend was observed. Data from the FDA's program of sampling individual foods showed a substantial decline during 1973–1975 in milk, eggs, cheese, animal feeds, processed fruits, and baby foods. From October 1980 to March 1982, the dietary intake of PCBs was 0.196 μg/person per day (16).

Absorbed PCBs are excreted mainly through the feces, whereas only traces are found in urine. Kutz and Strassman (29) detected 1 μg/g or more of PCBs in 40.3% samples of human adipose tissues. More recently, in a large survey of the U.S. population, Murphy et al. detected PCBs in 23% of the samples of adipose tissue (37). Analysis of the lipid portions of samples of human milk from various areas of the United States showed the average range of PCBs from 1–7 μg/ml (38).

Polybrominated Biphenyls

The polybrominated biphenyls (PBBs) are flame retardants and, if used as intended, should not enter the food supply. However, in Michigan in 1973, instead of a feed additive, PBBs were accidentally added to animal feed. Consequently, cattle and poultry, and later humans, in surrounding areas were widely exposed; PBBs could be detected in human blood (up to 2.26 μg/dL), in breast milk (up to 22.7 μg/ml), and in adipose tissue (up to 174 μg/g) (9). Following the destruction of millions of chickens and thousands of cattle that were contaminated with PBBs, the levels of PBBs have been steadily declining.

Global Monitoring of Food Contamination

In 1988 information on the assessment of food contamination performed through the Global Environment Monitoring System (GEMS) was compiled, analyzed, and assessed (18). Unfortunately, at this time the available data on food contamination on a global or regional level do not permit comprehen-

sive and definitive assessment of its severity or trends. This is particularly true for developing countries, where little data are available.

Nonetheless, information obtained since the early 1970s, along with the findings of individual researchers, provides some clues to the overall conditions that exist with regard to the global problem of food contamination. Briefly summarized, it can be said that food contamination in industrialized countries in the total diet is generally well within established safety criteria, guidelines, or standards. The trend in food contamination is generally downward, particularly as the use of persistent pesticides and other toxic chemicals is banned or curtailed. In general, organophosphorus pesticides are uncommonly detected in food and usually occur in raw crops but not in food of animal origin. Sporadic episodes of organophosphorus contamination in cereal products, fruit, and vegetables have been recorded.

Under some conditions the levels of food contaminants exceed safety criteria or standards in certain countries. Included are levels of organochlorine pesticides and PCBs in human milk, mercury and PCBs in fish, lead in canned food, and aflatoxins in nuts and cereals. GEMS noted that the exposure of infants to organochlorine compounds in human milk occurs for only a limited period in a lifetime and that the alternative feeding methods for infants may well subject them to even greater health hazards. Limited data from developing countries suggests that in many areas the level of organochlorine pesticides and aflatoxins can be quite high and in excess of safety criteria.

The PCB content of food is generally low, with the highest concentration generally found in inland waters, estuaries, and enclosed seas. Where fish constitutes a major item in the diet, total intake of PCBs may be increased substantially.

In general, dietary lead intake by infants, children, and adults is well within established safety criteria. However, the intake of infants and children may sometimes approach or exceed the tolerance levels. Notable exposures above acceptable levels occur in heavily industrialized areas, in areas of high traffic density, and particularly in regions with high lead levels in the drinking water. A marked reduction in dietary lead intake has occurred in developed countries in connection with reduced auto emissions of lead and the increased use of non-lead-soldered cans.

The dietary intake of cadmium, although generally within the acceptable range, more closely approaches established standards or guidelines. One-fourth of the reporting countries indicate that exposure to certain subgroups in the population may exceed tolerable intake levels. The dietary intake of mercury is generally below established standards. However, populations consuming above-average quantities of contaminated fish may ingest quantities of mercury that exceed acceptable levels (18).

SUMMARY

Low levels of many PAHs are present in a variety of foods. Smoking and charcoal broiling of foods as well as consuming foods grown in contaminated areas make major contributions to the dietary PAH content. Minute quantities of some PAHs have also been detected in human tissues.

Residues of several classes of pesticides (e.g., organochlorine compounds, organophosphates, and carbamates) are commonly detected in the diet, but generally at levels that are one or two orders of magnitude below their acceptable daily intakes (ADI). Unlike the organophosphates and carbamates, the chlorinated hydrocarbons are metabolized slowly and tend to accumulate in body tissues.

Humans are exposed to traces of toxic metals such as arsenic, cadmium, lead, and mercury in a variety of foods. Among these, lead, because of its wider distribution and higher concentration, is probably the most significant and of greatest concern from the standpoint of human health.

Minute quantities of vinyl chloride and acrylonitrile are known to migrate from packaging materials into foods. However, in the United States, there are no adequate estimates of average daily dietary exposure to these substances.

Exposure to polychlorinated biphenyls in amounts that are well below the tolerance levels established by the FDA occurs primarily through fish, meat, and dairy foods. The PCBs are highly persistent in the environment and have been detected in human tissues. Barring accidental contamination, exposure of the general population to PBBs through diet is improbable.

In conclusion, very low levels of many environmental pollutants occur in the average diet. However, it should be emphasized that there is a sparsity of data on the complete range of contaminants, and thus the most significant exposures cannot necessarily be estimated with a high degree of confidence. The Committee on Diet, Nutrition, and Cancer of the National Research Council tentatively concluded that dietary exposure to individual environmental contaminants in the minute quantities in which they normally occur in the average diet probably does not contribute significantly to the overall cancer risk in the United States. However, the risk from simultaneous exposure to many such compounds **may** be significant. The committee recommended reduction of exposure to environmental contaminants to the extent feasible, establishment

of tolerance levels for unavoidable contaminants, and regular monitoring of the food supply to ensure that these tolerance levels are not exceeded (4).

REFERENCES

1. Anonymous: FDA to propose ban on use of PVC for liquor use. Food Chem News, 14 May, pp 3–4, 1973.
2. Archibald SO, Winter CK: Pesticides in our food. In: Chemicals in the Human Food Chain, p 1, Winter CK, Seiber JN, Nuckton CF (eds.), Van Nostrand Reinhold, New York, 1990.
3. Berck B: Retention of acrylonitrile and carbon tetrachloride by shelled walnuts fumigated with acrylon. J Agric Food Chem 8:128, 1960.
4. Committee on Diet, Nutrition and Cancer, National Research Council: Diet, Nutrition, and Cancer, National Academy Press, Washington, 1982.
5. Committee on Food Protection: Toxicants Occurring Naturally in Foods, National Academy of Sciences, Washington, 1973.
6. Committee on Medical and Biologic Effects of Environmental Pollutants: Arsenic. Medical and Biologic Effects of Environmental Pollutants, National Academy of Sciences, Washington, 1977.
7. Committee on Pyrene and Selected Analogues, National Research Council: Polycyclic Aromatic Hydrocarbons: Evaluation of Sources and Effects, National Academy Press, Washington, 1983.
8. Committee on Scientific and Regulatory Issues Underlying Pesticide Use Patterns and Agricultural Innovation, National Research Council: Regulating Pesticides in Food: The Delaney Paradox, National Academy Press, Washington, 1987.
9. Cordle F, Corneliussen P, Jelinek C, et al: Human exposure to polychlorinated biphenyls and polybrominated biphenyls. Environ Health Perspect 24:157, 1978.
10. Council for Agricultural Science and Technology: CAST Report No. 64: Application of Sewage Sludge to Cropland: Appraisal of Potential Hazards of the Heavy Metals to Plants and Animals, Office of Water Program Operations, US Environmental Protection Agency, EPA-430/9-76-013, Washington, 1976.
11. Daniel PM, Pratt OE, Prichard MM: Metabolism of labelled carcinogenic hydrocarbons in rats. Nature 215:1142, 1967.
12. Food and Drug Administration: Food and Drug Administration Pesticide Program, residues in foods, 1989. J Assoc Off Anal Chem 73:127A, 1990.
13. Frank A, Pettersson LR: Assessment of bioavailability of cadmium in the Swedish environment using the moose (Alces alces) as indicator. Z Anal Chem 317:652, 1984.
14. Friberg L, Vahter M: Assessment of exposure to lead and cadmium through biological monitoring: Results of a UNEP/WHO global study. Environ Res 30:95, 1983.
15. Friberg L, Piscator M, Nordberg GF, et al. (eds.): Cadmium in the Environment, CRC Press, Boca Raton, FL, 1974.
16. Gartrell MJ, Crann JC, Podrebarac DS, et al: Pesticides,

selected elements, and other chemicals in adult total diet samples. October 1980–March 1982. J Assoc Off Anal Chem 69:146, 1986.

17. Gilbert J, Stratin JR: Determination of acrylonitrile monomer in food packaging materials and in foods. Food Chem 9:243, 1982.

18. Global Environment Monitoring System: Assessment of Chemical Contaminants in Food, Report on the Results of the UNEP/FAO/WHO Programme on Health-Related Environmental Monitoring, United Nations Environment Programme, Food and Agriculture Organization, World Health Organization, Geneva, 1988.

19. Gunderson EL: FDA total diet study, April 1982–1984, Dietary Intakes of pesticides, selected elements, and other chemicals. J Assoc Off Anal Chem 71:1200, 1988.

20. Higginson J: Etiological factors in gastrointestinal cancer. J Natl Cancer Inst 37:527, 1966.

21. Interdepartmental Task Force on PCBs: Polychlorinated Biphenyls and the Environment, Interdepartmental Task Force on PCBs, Washington, 1972.

22. International Agency for Research on Cancer: IARC Monographs on the Evaluation of the Carcinogenic Risk of Chemicals to Man, Vol. 5, Some Organochlorine Pesticides, p 241, International Agency for Research on Cancer, Lyons, 1974.

23. International Agency for Research on Cancer: IARC Monographs on the Evaluation of the Carcinogenic Risk of Chemicals to Humans, Vol. 20, Some Halogenated Hydrocarbons, p 609, International Agency for Research on Cancer, Lyons, 1979.

24. International Chemical Congress of Pacific Basin Societies: Formation of mutagens—during cooking and heat processing of food. Environ Health Perspect 67:3, 1986.

25. Jelinek CF: Levels of lead in the United States food supply. J Assoc Off Anal Chem 65:942, 1982.

26. Jelinek CF, Corneliussen PE: Levels of PCBs in the US food supply. In: Proceedings of the National Conference on Polychlorinated Biphenyls, p 147, Office of Toxicological Substances, US Environmental Protection Agency, Washington, 1975.

27. Jelinek CF, Corneliussen PE: Levels of arsenic in the United States food supply. Environ Health Perspect 19:83, 1977.

28. Kutz FW: Chemical exposure monitoring. Residue Rev 85:227, 1983.

29. Kutz FW, Strassman SC: Residues of polychlorinated biphenyls in the general population of the US. In: US National Conference on Polychlorinated Biphenyls, Conference Proceedings, p. 139, Environmental Protection Agency, Washington, 1975.

30. Lijinsky W, Ross AE: Production of polynuclear hydrocarbons in the cooking of foods. Food Cosmet Toxicol 5:343, 1967.

31. Little P, Fleming RG, Heard MJ: Uptake of lead by vegetable foodstuffs during cooking. Sci Total Environ 17:111, 1981.

32. Masuda Y, Mori K, Hirohata T, et al: Carcinogenesis in the esophagus. III. PAH and phenols in whiskey. Gann 57:549, 1966.

33. McEwen FL, Stephenson GR: The Use and Significance of Pesticides in the Environment, John Wiley & Sons, New York, 1979.

34. McNally J: Polychlorinated biphenyls: Environmental contamination of food. In: Environmental Contaminants in Food, Vol. II Part A: Working Papers, pp CRS1–CRS131, Office of Technology Assessment, Washington, 1978.

35. Ministry of Agriculture, Fisheries, and Food: Survey of Vinyl Chloride Content of Polyvinyl Chloride for Food Content and of Foods. The Second Report of the Steering Group on Food Surveillance, Paper No. 2, Her Majesty's Stationery Office, London, 1978.

36. Moore MR: Influence of acid rain upon water plumbosolvency. Environ Health Perspect 63:121, 1985.

37. Murphy RS, Kutz FW, Strassmann SC: Selected pesticide residues or metabolites in blood and urine specimens from a general population survey. Environ Health Perspect 48:81, 1983.

38. New York State Health Planning Commission: Report to the Ad Hoc Committee on the Health Implications of PCBs in Mother's Milk, Health Advisory Council, Albany, NY, 1977.

39. Nordberg GF: Health hazards of environmental cadmium pollution. Ambio 3:55, 1974.

40. Nordberg GF, Goyer RA, Clarkson TW: Impact of effects of acid precipitation on toxicity of metals. Environ Health Perspect 63:169, 1985.

41. Obana H, Hori S, Kashimoto T, et al: Polycyclic aromatic hydrocarbons in human fat and liver. Bull Environ Contam Toxicol 27:23, 1981.

42. Okinaka S, Yoshikawa M, Mozai T, et al: Encephalomyopathy due to an organic mercury compound. Neurology 14:69, 1964.

43. Organisation for Economic Co-operation and Development: Mercury and the Environment. Studies of Mercury Use, Emission, Biological Impact and Control, OECD, Paris, 1974.

44. Organisation for Economic Co-operation and Development: State of the Environment 1985, OECD, Paris, 1985.

45. Panalaks T: Determination and identification of PAH in smoked and charcoal broiled foods by high pressure liquid chromatography and gas chromatography. J Environ Sci Health Bull (B) 11:299, 1976.

46. Piscator M: Dietary exposure to cadmium and health effects: Impact of environmental changes. Environ Health Perspect 63:127, 1985.

47. Rabinowitz MB, Wetherill GW, Koppel JM: Kinetic analysis of lead metabolism in healthy humans. J Clin Invest 58:260, 1976.

48. Reed DV, Lombardo P, Wessel JR, et al: The FDA pesticides monitoring program. J Assoc Off Anal Chem 70:591, 1987.

49. Santodonato J, Howard P, Basu D: Health and ecological assessment of polynuclear aromatic hydrocarbons. J Environ Pathol Toxicol (special issue) 5:1–366, 1981.

50. Schaffner RM: Lead in canned foods. Food Technol 35:60, 1982.

51. Seiber J: Organic chemicals. In: Chemicals in the Human Food Chain, p 183, Winger CK, Seiber JN, Nuckton CF (eds.), Van Nostrand Reinhold, New York, 1990.

52. Soos K: The occurrence of carcinogenic polycyclic hydrocarbons in foodstuffs in Hungary. Arch Toxicol Suppl 4:446, 1980.

53. Steering Committee on Identification of Toxic and Potentially Toxic Chemicals for Consideration by the

National Toxicology Program: Toxicity Testing Strategies to Determine Needs and Priorities, National Academy Press, Washington, 1984.

54. Stokes PM, Bailey RC, Groulx GR: Effects of acidification on metal availability to aquatic biota, with special reference to filamentous algae. Environ Health Perspect 63:79, 1985.

55. Suess MJ: The environmental load and cycle of polycyclic aromatic hydrocarbons. Sci Total Environ 6:329, 1976.

56. Tilgner DJ, Daun H: PAH (polynuclears) in smoked foods. Residue Rev 27:19, 1969.

57. US Congress, Office of Technology Assessment: Environmental Contaminants in Food. OTA-F-103, US Government Printing Office, Washington, 1979.

58. US Congress, Office of Technology Assessment: Pesticide Residues in Food: Technology for Detection, OTA-F-398, US Government Printing Office, Washington, 1988.

59. US Environmental Protection Agency: Polychlorinated biphenyls. Fed Register 44(106):31514–31568, 1979.

60. US Environmental Protection Agency: Toxic Substances Control Act, Chemical Substances Inventory, Cumulative Supplement II, US Government Printing Office, Washington, 1982.

61. US Food and Drug Administration: Polychlorinated biphenyls: Notice of proposed rulemaking. Fed Register 37:5705–5706, 1972.

62. US Food and Drug Administration: Polychlorinated biphenyls: Contamination of animal feeds, foods and food packaging materials and availability of supplement to environmental statement of rulemaking. Fed Register 38:18096, 1973.

63. US Food and Drug Administration: Polychlorinated biphenyls (PCBs): Reduction of tolerances. Fed Register 44(127):38330–38340, 1979.

64. US Food and Drug Administration: Policy for regulating carcinogenic chemicals in food and color additives: Advance notice of proposed rulemaking. Fed Register 47:14464–14470, 1982.

65. Watkins D, Corbyons T, Bradshow J, et al: Determination of lead in confection wrappers by atomic spectrometry. Anal Chim Acta 85:403, 1976.

66. Webb M: Cadmium. Br Med Bull 31:246, 1975.

67. Wessel JR, Yess NJ: Pesticide residues in food imported into the United States. Rev Environ Contamin Toxicol 120:83, 1991.

68. William DT, Miles WF: Gas–liquid chromatographic determination of vinyl chloride in alcoholic beverages, vegetable oils, and vinegars. J Assoc Off Anal Chem 58:272, 1975.

69. Winter CK, Seiber NJ, Nuckton CF (eds.): Chemicals in the Human Food Chain, Van Nostrand Reinhold, Washington, 1990.

RECOMMENDED READINGS

Winter CK, Seiber NJ, Nuckton CF (eds.): Chemicals in the Human Food Chain, Van Nostrand Reinhold, New York, 1990.

US Congress, Office of Technology Assessment: Pesticide Residues in Food: Technology for Detection, OTA-F-398, US Government Printing Office, Washington, 1988.

4. WATER POLLUTION AND CHEMICAL CONTAMINATION IN DRINKING WATER

William A. Coniglio, Paul S. Berger, and Joseph A. Cotruvo

INTRODUCTION

An ample supply of clean fresh water is essential for the well-being of all organisms. The quality of drinking water, often taken for granted in industrialized nations, is increasingly becoming a matter of concern. The original focus of most water quality improvement programs was on such conventional pollutants as dissolved oxygen, fecal coliform bacteria, suspended sediment, dissolved solids, and phosphorus. Although pathogens in inadequately treated drinking water are still the greatest public health concern related to drinking water, increased industrialization, the widespread use of chemicals in industry and agriculture, and the disposal of large volumes of industrial wastes have drawn attention to the importance of protecting drinking water from contamination with chemical agents. Over 60,000 chemicals are now being used by industry and agriculture. Accordingly, such substances as synthetic organic chemicals, solvents, pesticides, metals, cleaning preparations, and septic tank degreasers can pollute both surface and ground waters that are sources of drinking water.

The quality of drinking water can be compromised by a number of processes, which include leakage from underground storage tanks, agricultural runoff, improper industrial practices, mining operations, the subsurface injection of waste chemicals and brines, and corrosive water. The drinking water treatment process itself can create potentially hazardous byproducts. For example, drinking water is the principal route of human exposure for such disinfection byproducts as chloroform.

The quantity of a pollutant absorbed each day by an individual is the result of many personal choices and of several factors over which there is often little direct control. Where one works and lives and what one eats and drinks have a profound influence on exposure to pollutants. Personal preferences also determine the magnitude of exposure of family members to the pollutants entering the home through drinking water.

Chronic exposure to some substances can occur through the ingestion of drinking water and water used in cooking, through penetration of skin during bathing, and through inhalation if the contaminant becomes airborne as an aerosol or vapor (4). The degree of exposure of family members of different ages and activity patterns to drinking water pollutants can often be estimated based on standard values for respiration, fluid intake, pollutant concentration, volatility, and absorption.

It is estimated that approximately 255 gallons of water are used daily by the average household of two children and two adults in the United States, including washing, sanitation, and lawn (1). Two liters or less are actually consumed. Exposure to such volatile contaminants as chloroform and trichloroethylene in drinking water can be higher per unit of body weight among children than adults. Respiratory exposure during and immediately after showering can be similar to that occurring after

Principles and Practice of Environmental Medicine, edited by Alyce Bezman Tarcher. Plenum Medical Book Company, New York, 1992.

ingestion. Prolonged swimming, with its associated oral and dermal absorption, also has the potential for significantly increasing exposure to pollutants (5). Comprehensive discussions on the quality of drinking water, the processes for producing safe water, and the regulatory approaches for assuring the safety of drinking water are contained in several references (9,10,29).

The following discussion focuses on water pollution and chemical contaminants found in drinking water: their source and regulation. Selected regulated chemical contaminants are discussed.

WATER QUALITY IN THE UNITED STATES AND WORLDWIDE

Sources of Water Pollution

Sources of water pollution are shown in Table 4-1. They are commonly divided into point sources and nonpoint sources. A point source is an identified, contained source where flow and composition can be quite easily monitored. It includes such facilities as municipal sewage and industrial waste treatment plants. Nonpoint source pollutants are derived from such diffuse sources as runoff and seepage from agricultural and urban areas, silviculture, mining, livestock grazing, and construction sites. Pollutants from nonpoint sources do not discharge at a specific single location. They are generally carried above, over, and through the ground by rainfall, runoff, infiltration, and snow melt. It is difficult to quantify the volume and composition of nonpoint sources of pollution. As point-source discharges are reduced, attention is increasingly directed to nonpoint sources of water pollution. Failure to control nonpoint-source pollution is now a problem of

global importance (11,15,24,45). In particular, nonpoint-source pollution from modern intensive agricultural methods and urban runoff have increased dramatically and are far less easily controlled than is point-source pollution from industry (29,45,57).

Water Pollution in the United States

The National Water Quality Inventory

Information on the causes and sources of pollution found in U.S. rivers and streams is provided by The National Water Quality Inventory (57). Every 2 years, the states report to the U.S. Environmental Protection Agency (EPA) on the quality of their rivers, streams, lakes, estuaries, coastal water, wetlands, and ground water. The EPA then prepares a summary report to Congress (57). This information is used to assess the effect of current water quality protection policies and to help determine where improvements must be made.

The standard measure of water quality by the states is the degree to which waters support the uses for which they have been designated. For example, waters classified for the support of aquatic life and contact recreation should be usable for fishing and swimming. Waters designated for the drinking water supply should, after some treatment, be the source of water piped into homes for drinking and bathing.

After the States set the uses for their waters, regulatory scientists establish the criteria needed to protect those uses. These criteria establish conditions such as chemical or habitat requirements that must be met to be in compliance with the goals. If these criteria are not met, the uses they are protecting may be impaired. The status of U.S. waters is thus determined by assessing the degree to which

TABLE 4-1.   Sources of Water Pollution[a]

Category	Examples
Industrial	Pulp and paper mills, chemical manufacturers, steel plants, textile manufacturers, food-processing plants
Municipal	Publicly owned sewage treatment plants that may receive indirect discharges from small factories or businesses
Combined sewers	Storm and sanitary sewers combined, which may discharge untreated wastes during storms
Storm sewers/runoff	Runoff from streets, paved areas, lawns, etc., that enters a sewer, pipe, or ditch before discharge
Agricultural	Crop production, pastures, rangeland, feedlots
Silvicultural	Forest management, harvesting, road construction
Construction	Highway building, land development
Resource extraction	Mining, petroleum drilling, runoff from mine tailing sites
Land disposal	Leachate or discharge from septic tanks, landfills, hazardous waste disposal sites
Hydrologic modification	Channelization, dredging, dam construction, stream bank modification

[a]From U.S. EPA (57).

standards are met and designated uses are supported (57).

In the broadest sense water pollution encompasses changes in aquatic ecosystems that may endanger aquatic life, impair human health, and make recreational and esthetic pursuits impossible. The sources of water pollution are many and varied. Table 4-1 shows that water pollution stems from a variety of activities, which range from the discharge of wastes from industrial sources to hydrologic modification by channelization, dredging, dam construction, and stream bank modification (57).

The causes of water pollution are also varied. The leading causes of impaired water uses cited in the 1988 Water Quality Inventory were excessive nutrients and sediments. Nutrients are most commonly derived from fertilizers and phosphates found in detergents. These agents, by increasing the growth of aquatic plants and algae, which decrease the supply of available oxygen and light, adversely affect the aquatic ecosystem. Lakes and estuaries are especially vulnerable to the adverse effects of excessive nutrients. Sediments are suspended silt and solids that wash off plowed fields, construction and logging sites, urban areas, and strip-mined land. This process affects rivers, lakes, and coastal waters, thereby having an adverse effect on fish and aquatic habitats. Other causes of impaired water uses include toxic chemicals/heavy metals, pesticides/herbicides, organic enrichment, which includes sewage, leaves, the runoff from livestock feed lots and pastures, and habitat modification that occurs when streams and lakes are modified by grazing, farming, dredging, and the construction of dams. Figure 4-1 shows the sources of pollution in U.S. lakes, rivers, and estuaries. Figure 4-2 shows the top ten pollutants found in these waters (57).

As ground water is increasingly used, it has become apparent that this source, once thought to be quite safe from contamination, is also vulnerable. Depending on the activity (i.e., industry, agriculture, mining, etc.), the source of the groundwater contamination varies considerably (Fig. 4-3). The following major threats to the quality of ground water have been identified: (1) leaking underground storage tanks (i.e., gasoline storage tanks and heating oil supply tanks for schools and public buildings); (2) poorly operating septic systems; (3) agricultural activities such as pesticide and fertilizer usage; (4) poorly managed or poorly located municipal landfills used to dispose of nonhazardous waste products and household waste; (5) improperly located surface impoundments, pits, ponds, and other holding areas for hazardous wastes; and (6) abandoned and uncontrolled hazardous waste sites (Fig. 4-3) (6,7,56,57). When ground water is contaminated, the level of contamination may be far greater than that encountered in surface waters (49,50).

National Survey of Pesticides and Nitrate in Drinking Water Wells

The EPA completed a 5-year National Survey of Pesticides in Drinking Water Wells. This Survey was designed to provide statistically reliable estimates of the presence of pesticides and nitrate in the U.S. well-water supply. Between 1988 and 1990, the EPA sampled approximately 1300 wells in all 50 states, including both private rural domestic wells and wells that feed community water systems (community water systems serve a minimum of 15 service connections or an average of 25 people per day, year-round). These wells were surveyed for the presence of pesticides and nitrate (56). The EPA estimates that nitrate is present, at or above the analytical minimum reporting limit of 0.15 mg/L used in the Survey, in about 49,300 (52.1%) of the community water system wells and 5,990,000 (57.0%) of the rural domestic wells nationwide (56). About 1.2% of the community water system wells and 2.4% of the rural domestic wells are believed to have nitrate levels above 10 mg/L (as N), which could pose a health concern. Nitrate is derived from inorganic fertilizers that are used to enhance plant growth, animal wastes, septic systems, plant residues, and fixation from the atmosphere.

Pesticides were detected much less frequently than nitrate (56). The EPA estimates that 9850 (10.4%) of the community water system wells and 446,000 (4.2%) of the rural domestic wells contain at least one pesticide at or above the minimum reporting limits used in the Survey (subparts per billion). The two pesticides most frequently detected were dimethyltetrachloroterephthalate (DCPA) acid metabolites, a degradate of DCPA, and atrazine. The chemical DCPA is a broadleaf and grass weed killer used extensively on lawns, golf courses, and farms. Atrazine, also known as AAtrex or Atratol, is a weed killer widely used in agriculture, especially on corn and sorghum. Ten other pesticides were detected above Survey reporting limits. These include alachlor, bentazon, dibromochloropropane, dinoseb, hexachlorobenzene, prometon, simazine, ethylene dibromide, ethylene thiourea, and lindane. The EPA estimates that at most 750 (0.8%) community water system wells nationally and 60,900 (0.6%) rural domestic wells nationally contain at least one pesticide detectable above health-based standards (56).

The Toxics Release Inventory

In 1989 the first Toxics Release Inventory prepared by the EPA provided the public with information concerning the release of toxic chemicals into the nation's air, water, and land (58). Information on the release of toxic chemicals by manufacturing facilities is an important component of The Emer-

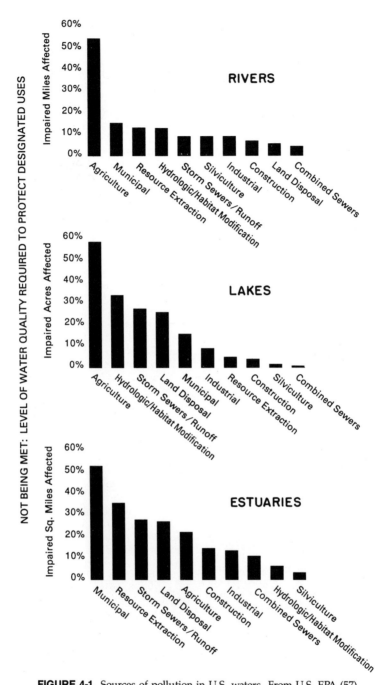

FIGURE 4-1. Sources of pollution in U.S. waters. From U.S. EPA (57).

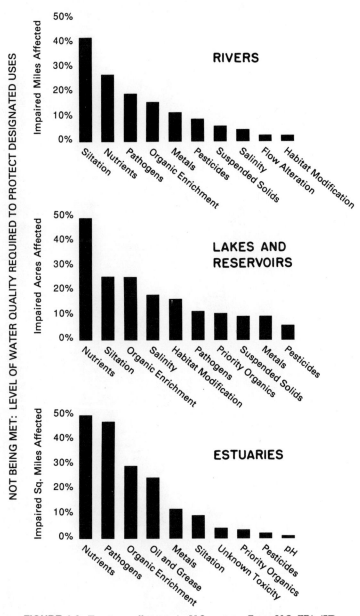

FIGURE 4-2. Top ten pollutants in U.S. waters. From U.S. EPA (57).

gency Planning and Community Right-to-Know Act of 1986. The law requires certain manufacturers to report to the EPA and to the states the amount of over 300 toxic chemicals that they release directly into the air, water, or land or that they transport to off-site facilities. This report, produced annually, analyzes where toxic chemicals are being released, along with the amounts and types of releases. Thus far the information provided by the Toxic Release Inventory has far exceeded all expectations as a tool for improving environmental management. A summary of the inventory collected in 1988 and published in 1990 showed that 0.36 billion pounds of toxic chemicals were released into U.S. rivers, lakes, streams, and other bodies of water (58). The Toxic Release Inventory is available from the U.S. Govern-

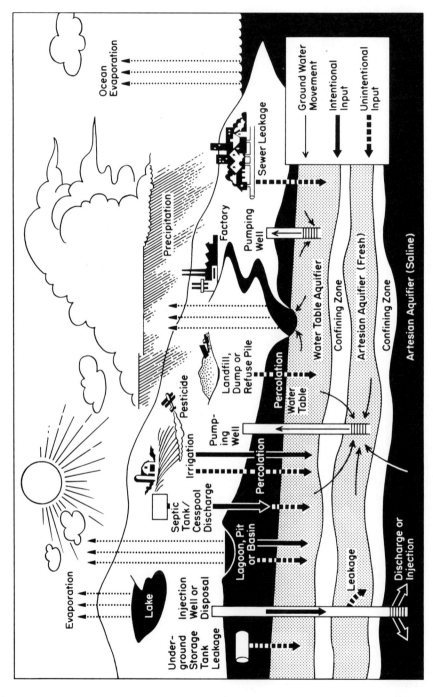

FIGURE 4-3. Sources of groundwater contamination. From U.S. EPA (57).

ment Printing Office. This information can also be accessed through the National Library of Medicine, where it is a component of the TOXNET system.

Water Pollution Worldwide

Organisation for Economic Co-operation and Development

A report from the Organisation for Economic Co-operation and Development (OECD), which includes European nations, Canada, and the United States, deals with the issue of water pollution by fertilizers and pesticides in OECD countries (28). This report cites the developments in agriculture occurring over the past few decades as the cause of ever-increasing nitrate pollution and eutrophication of water resources. As previously noted, most nitrogen from agricultural land is primarily derived from the application of inorganic and organic nitrogen fertilizer. The nitrate contamination in aquifers, observed to have grown rapidly both in extent and intensity, is viewed with concern, especially because aquifers provide a large proportion of drinking water resources in many countries.

Moreover, it is expected that surface waters also receiving agricultural runoff will, with increasing frequency, follow the same evolution as aquifers (see below). The general trend observed thus far is likely to continue because the use of fertilizers shows little sign of abating and because the long migration time (sometimes up to several decades) of the nitrogen-rich front in soil means that in many cases nitrates have not yet reached the aquifers (28).

The OECD report indicates that data from various OECD member countries, based on water-quality-monitoring systems and accident reports, provide evidence that episodes of pesticide pollution of the aquatic ecosystem are frequent (28). It is further noted that the commonly used technique of aerial application spraying of pesticides can cause some contamination of surface waters. In addition, pesticide residues from normal agricultural uses have been found to contaminate aquifers, particularly shallow ones, in various OECD member countries (28).

Global Monitoring of Water Quality

Within the framework of the United Nations Environmental Program's (UNEP) Global Environmental Monitoring System (GEMS), the World Health Organization (WHO) and UNEP have been working together since 1977 to monitor water quality worldwide. The project, known as GEMS/WATER, forms a part of the GEMS global monitoring efforts (15). Other activities include the measurement of urban air pollution (GEMS/AIR) and food contamination (GEMS/FOOD) (see Chapters 2 and 3). The GEMS water-monitoring project consists of 344 stations (240 river, 43 lake, and 61 groundwater stations) in 59 countries. Most stations are near industrial and urban centers. Unfortunately, this global assessment of water quality is limited by a lack of or limited data from such geographical regions as eastern Europe and Africa. In addition, surveillance programs are operational in only a few countries in Latin America and southeast Asia. About 50 different indicators of water quality are used in the GEMS water-monitoring program. These include dissolved oxygen, biological oxygen demand, fecal coliforms, nitrates, phosphorus, heavy metals, organochlorine pesticides, and polychlorinated biphenyls.

In the waters monitored by the GEMS/WATER network, the two most important nutrients, nitrogen and phosphorus, were found to be well above natural levels. The European rivers had the highest average nutrient levels. In some cases nitrate levels were 45 times higher than natural background concentrations. As noted, increased nitrate levels in ground waters are currently a severe problem in many western European countries as well as the United States. In many places the WHO guideline value for nitrate (10 mg/L as N) in drinking water has already been exceeded. Eutrophication, which is often directly related to organic waste, markedly affects many small lakes in Europe, the United States, and China (15).

Other global trends in water pollution reveal that in countries with a low level of development, water pollution in cities may be severe, but water resources in general do not suffer greatly from pollution. This is in contrast to regions where the large-scale exploitation of mineral resources results in mining waste deposits that severely pollute surface and ground water over a large area (15). Very severe pathogen pollution causing infant death occurs in many developing countries, especially when water availability is low.

Metal contamination of water resources has also been documented in such areas as the Jenzu and Elbe rivers. The Sudbury smelter in Canada represents one of the largest single-point sources of metal pollution of water resources in Ontario and Quebec provinces. This occurs through extensive atmospheric transport. Scandinavian rivers and North American rivers and lakes are affected by acid deposition with an associated increase in dissolved aluminum. Synthetic organic pollutants such as DDT, PCBs, chlorinated solvents, chlorophenols, and volatile aromatic compounds contaminate many rivers including the Jamuna river near Delhi and the Seine and Rhine rivers. Pesticides are also likely to be found in many southeast Asian and African rivers (15).

DRINKING WATER QUALITY

Drinking water may be derived from surface or ground water. Surface water includes lakes, ponds, creeks, streams, rivers, and oceans, which receive their water from snow and rain, overland runoff, and ground water. Ground water occurs in aquifers beneath the earth's surface. The source of ground water is precipitation. Aquifers provide water to wells and springs. The volume of ground water is vast, second only to that of the oceans and seas (11).

Over 50% of the United States population depends upon ground water for its drinking water. Nearly all of the rural population is dependent on untreated ground water for drinking purposes, and approximately 75% of American cities obtain all or some of their water from ground water (30,57). The heavy reliance on ground water as a source of drinking water in all regions of the United States is shown in Fig. 4-4. Certain other parts of the world also rely heavily on ground water for their drinking water (28).

Compared to surface water, which is continually flowing and mixing, ground water moves very slowly. Once ground water is contaminated, its slow movement provides little opportunity for dilution or mixing to resolve the problem. In many cases, ground water contamination may border on being essentially irreversible because of its inaccessibility and because of the long time required for aquifers to purge themselves of pollutants. Monitoring ground water contamination is difficult. Multiple test wells must be drilled. This process, apart from being time consuming and costly, often provides limited information on the extent of contamination because pollutant concentrations in ground water may vary greatly even within short distances (11,14).

DETERMINANTS OF DRINKING WATER QUALITY AND SAFETY

Experience has led to the recognition that drinking water quality and safety are affected by three factors: (1) the quality of the raw or untreated water; (2) the presence of water treatment additives and byproducts; (3) the introduction of contaminants during transit to the consumer's tap (Table 4-2); and (4) the effectiveness of the water treatment process.

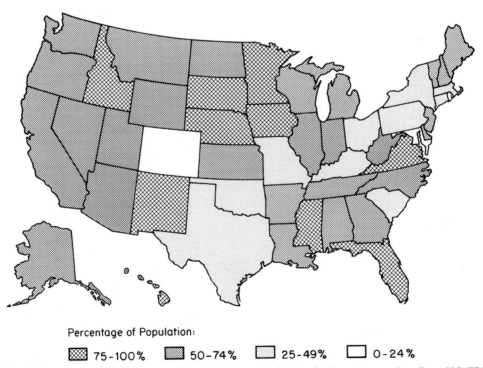

Percentage of Population:

▨ 75-100%   ▦ 50-74%   ▧ 25-49%   ☐ 0-24%

FIGURE 4-4. Percentage of the U.S. population served by ground water for domestic supplies. From U.S. EPA (57).

TABLE 4-2. Determinants of Drinking Water Quality and Safety, and Sources of Contamination

Source	Contaminants	Examples of specific contaminants
Raw or untreated water (surface and ground water)	Industrial wastes	Machine oils, tars, heavy metals, organic solvents, i.e., benzene, organochlorines, plastics, pesticides
	Municipal wastes	Food wastes, household cleaning solvents, soaps, detergents, suspended solids, inorganic chemicals, sewer sludge, pathogens
	Hazardous wastes	Heavy metals, solvents, toxic organic and inorganic chemicals
	Septic tank wastes	Bacteria, viruses, protozoa, nitrates, septic tank cleaners (trichloroethylene)
	Radioactive wastes	Radioactive materials
	Other pollution sources	
	Agricultural runoff	Pesticides, fertilizer, soil additives, sediments, animal wastes, pathogens
	Urban runoff	Oil, grease, heavy metals (cadmium, copper, lead, zinc), herbicides, pesticides, suspended solids, nutrients, animal wastes
	Underground storage tanks	Gasoline and other chemicals
	Silviculture	Herbicides
	Natural organic matter	Humic substances and their degradation products (resorcinol and phenolic compounds)
	Minerals	Sodium, chloride, arsenic, barium, asbestos, selenium, sulfate, etc.
	Radionuclides	Uranium, radium, radon
Water treatment additives	Disinfectants and byproducts	Chlorine, chlorine dioxide, chloramine, chloroform, bromoform
	Coagulation aids/corrosion control	Limes, clays, alum polyphosphates, polymers
	Impurities in the above	Acrylamide, epichlorohydrin, metals
Distribution of water after treatment	Sealants and coatings	Plasticizers from chlorinated rubber (PCBs), epoxy resins, coal tar, polyvinyl chloride
	Inorganics	Lead, cadmium, copper, zinc, asbestos
	Microbiological	Regrowth of bacteria, viruses, and protozoa; contamination from leakage and cross-contamination

Raw Water Quality

The quality of water derived from surface waters, i.e., rivers and streams, or drawn from underground aquifers varies. In some cases, natural deposits contribute asbestos and radioactivity to water. Such deposits also contribute suspended and dissolved inorganic and organic constituents to the water. These include discharges of sodium, chloride, calcium, heavy metals, crude oil, and natural materials. Living plant and animal communities contribute their wastes to surface streams. Chemical substances arise from the metabolic activity of living plants and animals and the decomposition of dead organisms. Man, in his management of the environment, has enhanced the movement of many natural chemicals into water. Currently study is directed to the potential role of acid rain in accelerating the leaching of certain metals from soil and rock (27,42). With industrialization, many synthetic chemicals have been released into surface waters. Pesticides and fertilizers run off fields during heavy rains. Combustion byproducts, oils, and other chemicals wash into rivers and streams. Effluents from factories and public waste treatment facilities enter rivers. The resultant mixture of biological and chemical contamination is unique to the segment of the stream.

Ground water is widely used for drinking water, irrigation, and rural and domestic livestock needs. As previously noted, ground water pollution in many cases may be essentially irreversible because the transport, dilution, and degradation processes capable of removing contaminants from surface waters are largely inoperative below the top layers of the soil (11,13). Dependence on ground water has increased markedly over the past 30 years. In some areas of the United States, it provides the only source of drinking water and is often used with little or no treatment. Although most ground waters are still not significantly contaminated, by 1988 normal agricultural usage of pesticides had contaminated ground water in most states (Fig. 4-5) (2,49,50,59).

Pollutant Contamination of Raw (Untreated) Water and Drinking Water

In general, the level of pollutants found in surface waters is low because of the large volume of water entering river systems. However, conditions may exist when natural organic or concentrated effluents from such sources as industry, agriculture, or mining enter a drinking water supply without the benefit of dilution or when environmental transport processes fail to purge the water supply. Higher levels of organic compounds may appear seasonally, and pesticides may be more prominent during periods of agricultural application and rainfall. Many of the chemical contaminants found in surface water supplies are also found at higher levels in contaminated ground waters (11,14,30,49,50,52).

Our present perspective on the chemicals in drinking water relies heavily on data from national monitoring surveys, which address groups of potential contaminants and regular monitoring of public water supplies for regulated substances (3,4,43, 45,48,62). In 1980 the Environmental Protection Agency prepared a national profile of organic chemicals detected in national drinking water surveys (8). The ranking of a chemical in this national profile was based on how frequently it was detected in community water supplies examined in National Monitoring Surveys (Table 4-3).

Volatile organic chemicals and radionuclides were found most often in communities using ground water. Pesticides and other organics were also detected on occasion. The 1980 chemical-ranking system may be used to provide a clue to the occurrence of selected organics in potable water. But it must be remembered that this perspective is based on limited data for a highly selective group of organic chemicals. In one case study, for example, more than 1000 unique chemicals were isolated from drinking water, usually at the parts-per-trillion level, from drinking water supplied to a large community along a highly industrialized river in the United States (23). The agents detected were not necessarily all industrial chemicals.

Water Treatment Byproducts

Drinking water treatment typically includes a number of processes. Water is moved from surface and ground water sources to storage areas. Copper sulfate may be added to control the growth of algae. A chemical such as alum is added to the water to coagulate particles. The water then moves through sedimentation basins, which allow particles to sink to the bottom. Final filtering is done as the water

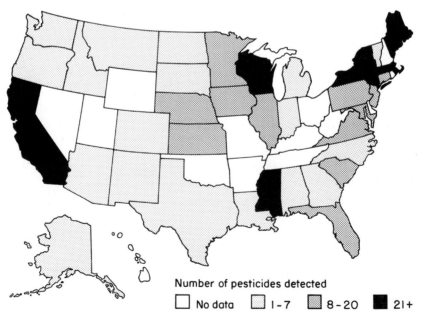

Number of pesticides detected

☐ No data   ▨ 1-7   ▨ 8-20   ■ 21+

FIGURE 4-5. Pollution of ground water in the United States from normal agricultural usage of pesticides. From U.S. EPA (59).

TABLE 4-3. A Relative Ranking of Selected Organic Chemicals in Drinking Water Based on the Frequency of Detection in National Monitoring Surveys[a]

Surface water supplies	Ground water supplies
Chloroform	Chloroform
Bromodichloromethane	Bromodichloromethane
Chlorodibromomethane	Chlorodibromomethane
Pentachlorophenol	Bromoform
Diethyl phthalate	Dichloroiodomethane
Dichloroiodomethane	Dibutyl phthalate
Dibutyl phthalate	Tetrachloroethylene
Atrazine	1,1,1-Trichloroethane
2,4-Dichlorophenol	1,1-Dichloroethane
Benzene	cis-1,2-Dichloroethylene
Phthalic acid	Phthalic acid
Toluene	2,4-Dichlorophenol
Tetrachloroethylene	Trichloroethylene
Carbon tetrachloride	Diethyl phthalate
Trichloroethylene	p-Dichlorobenzene
Simazine	bis(2-Chloroethyl)ether
p-Dichlorobenzene	Benzene
Bromoform	Ethyl chloride
1,3,4-Trichlorobenzene	Trichlorofluoromethane
Dichloromethane	1,1-Dichloroethylene
1,1,1-Trichloroethane	trans-1,2-Dichloroethylene
Disulfoton	Chlorobenzene
Benefin	Simazine
Malathion	Methyl parathion
Fluoranthene	Malathion
Phenylacetic acid	Pentachlorophenol
Cyanazine	Fluoranthene
Propazine	Dichloromethane
cis-1,2-Dichloroethylene	Carbon tetrachloride
Trichlorofluoromethane	bis(2-Chloroisopropyl)ether

[a]From Coniglio et al. (8).

moves through beds of gravel and sand. Chlorine or other disinfectants are then added. Treated water may be stored in reservoirs or, in some cases, go directly into the water system.

Disinfectants, such as chlorine, are highly reactive chemicals purposely added to water to render the water free of microbiological contaminants capable of causing disease. Chlorination has the potential of reacting with some organic compounds present in the water supply to create trihalomethanes (THMs) and other byproducts (31,41,46) (Table 4-2). Chloroform, bromodichloromethane, dibromochloromethane, and bromoform are major THMs formed as disinfectant byproducts. The level of total THMs in finished water is currently regulated at 100 μg/L. Surface water supplies, high in dissolved natural organic material (humics), are especially vulnerable to THM formation. When free chlorine is the disinfectant, THM levels are generally higher in com-

munities using rivers and streams as their source of drinking water than in communities using wells.

Clearly the major goal of disinfecting water supplies is to provide protection from waterborne diseases. Chlorination has performed admirably in this regard. However, concern for the potential carcinogenicity of the THMs and other chlorination byproducts has prompted the increased use of other disinfection methods to avoid or reduce this potential problem (12). Alternate methods of drinking water disinfection using chloramination, ozonation, and chlorine dioxide have been more widely used. Significant effort is currently directed to assessing the relative efficacy of alternatives to chlorination in eliminating resistant viruses and protozoan cysts. At the present time, however, chlorination continues to be the primary method of drinking water disinfection in the United States.

Distribution System Contaminants

In some instances the concentration of certain chemicals increases from the initial levels measured in untreated water entering the treatment plant to the levels found in the consumer's water glass. This can occur by several means. Some chemicals are introduced into potable water by extraction from pipes or coatings present in the distribution system. Other chemicals originate from physical or chemical erosion of such construction materials as metal, plastic, or asbestos cement (Table 4-2). In other cases, chemicals are derived from the impurities present in agents such as chlorine that are used in water treatment. The levels of asbestos, lead, and cadmium are strongly related to the chemical corrosivity of the potable water and its interaction with the distribution system (39). Microorganisms may increase in the distribution system due to water-main breaks, cross-connections, and growth on pipe surfaces.

DRINKING WATER REGULATIONS

In 1974, the Safe Drinking Water Act greatly expanded the government's role in providing safe drinking water. The act, which applied to all public water systems, mandated the development of primary (health-related) and secondary (esthetics) national drinking water regulations. In 1975, under this law, the National Interim Primary Drinking Water Regulations were first issued with maximum contaminant levels (MCLs) established.

In 1986 amendments added to the Safe Drinking Water Act called on the EPA to set maximum contaminant level goals (MCLGs) and National Primary Drinking Water Regulations (MCLs) for 83 specific contaminants, which include many organics, inorganics, radionuclides, and biological agents (Table 4-4). The MCLGs are nonenforceable health goals that are to be set at levels at which "no known or anticipated adverse health effects occur and which allow an adequate margin of safety." The MCLs must be set as close to MCLGs as is feasible.

TABLE 4-4. Contaminants Required to be Regulated under the Safe Drinking Water Act Amendments of 1986

Volatile organic chemicals	Organics
Trichloroethylene	Endrin
Tetrachloroethylene	Lindane
Carbon tetrachloride	Methoxychlor
1,1,1-Trichloroethane	Toxaphene
1,2-Dichloroethane	2,4-D
Vinylchloride	2,4,5-TP
Methylene chloride	Aldicarb
Benzene	Chlordane
Monochlorobenzene	Dalapon
Dichlorobenzene	Diquat
Trichlorobenzene	Endothall
1,1-Dichloroethylene	Glyphosphate
trans-1,2-Dichloro-ethylene	Carbofuran
cis-1,2-Dichloro-ethylene	Alachlor
	Epichlorohydrin
	Toluene
Microbiology and tur-bidity	Adipates
Total coliforms	2,3,7,8-TCDD (Dioxin)
Turbidity	1,1,2-Trichloroethane
Giardia lamblia	Vydate
Viruses	Simazine
Standard plate count	Polyaromatic hydrocar-bons (PAHs)
Legionella	Polychlorinated bi-phenyls (PCBs)
Inorganics	
Arsenic	Atrazine
Barium	Phthalates
Cadmium	Acrylamide
Chromium	Dibromochloropropane (DBCP)
Lead	
Mercury	1,2-Dichloropropane
Nitrate	Pentachlorophenol
Selenium	Pichloram
Silver	Dinoseb
Fluoride	Ethylene dibromide (EDB)
Aluminum	
Antimony	Dibromomethane
Molybdenum	Xylene
Asbestos	Hexachlorocyclopenta-diene
Sulfate	
Copper	Radionuclides
Vanadium	Radium-226 and -228
Sodium	Beta particle and photon radioactivity
Nickel	
Zinc	Radon
Thallium	Gross alpha particle ac-tivity
Beryllium	
Cyanide	Uranium

ᵃFrom Calabrese et al. (6).

The term feasible means with use of the best available technology, taking costs into consideration. Under the Safe Drinking Water Act amendments of 1986, granular activated carbon was considered a feasible means for controlling synthetic organic chemicals. Any technology found to be the best available for the control of synthetic organic chemicals must be at least as effective in controlling these substances as granular activated carbon (6).

Beginning in 1987, the Office of Drinking Water developed a six-phase regulatory phase schedule to implement the specified deadlines of the drinking water regulations under the Safe Drinking Water Amendments of 1986. A comprehensive review of the Safe Drinking Water Act and the importance and treatment of synthetic organic compounds in water supplies are found in several references (6,31,32). The philosophy and process for establishing national drinking water regulations, including risk-based considerations, are described elsewhere (9,10).

As mandated by the Safe Drinking Water Act, the National Academy of Sciences examined the health effects of drinking water contaminants. A series of nine volumes was published between 1977 and 1989 under the title "Drinking Water and Health." Volume 1 examines the health effects associated with microbiological, radioactive, particulate, and inorganic and organic chemical contaminants in drinking water. This volume deals with the complicated issue of risk assessment for cancer associated with ingesting chemical pollutants in drinking water (33). Volume 2 addresses the disinfection of drinking water and the chemistry of disinfectants in water. It also contains an evaluation of granular activated carbon for the reduction or removal of organic and other contaminants from drinking water (34). Volume 3 discusses epidemiologic studies on cancer frequency in relation to the presence of trihalomethanes, such as chloroform, in drinking water (35). Volume 4 identifies chemical and biological contaminants associated with drinking water distribution systems and the health implications of deficiencies in such systems (36). Volume 5 continues the assessment and evaluation procedures established in earlier volumes (37). Volume 6 contains the results of a two-part study on the toxicity of drinking water contaminants. The first part examines current practices in risk assessment, and the second part provides risk assessment for 14 specific compounds (38). Volume 7 addresses current and recent innovations in the methods of drinking water disinfection. The toxicity of selected disinfectants and their byproducts is discussed. In particular, the potential health effects of the long-term ingestion of low levels of such disinfection byproducts as the trihalomethanes are examined (46). Volume 8 reviews the risk assessment process and discusses the role of pharmacokinetic principles in evaluating risk

(47). Volume 9 focuses on possible uses of DNA adducts in risk assessment and also examines the issue of multiple toxic chemicals in drinking water and the assessment of their health risks (39).

The Academy did not make recommendations regarding MCLs for contaminants in drinking water because the Safe Drinking Water Act requires that MCLs be based not only on health effects but also on what is technologically and economically feasible. The health goal is embodied in the nonenforceable maximum contaminate level goal (MCLG). This number is derived primarily from health data and serves as a lower-limit goal for the MCLs.

As attested by the National Academy of Sciences reports noted above, our ability to relate the long-term use of drinking water with low levels of contaminants to the appearance of human disease is exceedingly limited. It is well recognized, however, that many recognized traditional toxicants such as lead and mercury along with known and suspected carcinogens can be drinking water contaminants (31,41,48). Statistics gathered from 1946 to 1980 indicate that 7% of the identified outbreaks of acute waterborne disease in the United States were caused by chemical agents (24). It is unlikely, however, that water meeting all national drinking water standards will be associated with adverse health affects.

Health Advisories

In response to the public need for guidance during emergency situations involving drinking water contamination, health advisories were prepared by the Criteria and Standards Division, Office of Drinking Water of the U.S. Environmental Protection Agency. They provide technical guidance to public health officials on health effects, analytic methodologies, and treatment technologies associated with drinking water contaminants. Each health advisory summarizes available data concerning the occurrence, pharmacokinetics, and health effects of a specific contaminant or mixture. A margin of safety is used to protect sensitive subgroups within the population (e.g., children, the elderly, pregnant women). As new information becomes available, the health advisories are subject to change. Thus far, health advisories have been published for 18 nonpesticide organic chemicals, numerous pesticides, inorganic chemicals, and the microbial genus *Legionella* (60,61).

Drinking Water Standards for Europe and Developing Countries

The World Health Organization (WHO) has adopted drinking water standards for Europe and the developing countries of Asia, Africa, and South America. These guidelines are periodically revised.

The WHO Guidelines for Drinking Water Quality comprise three volumes: Volume 1 includes recommended guidelines for all contaminants including synthetic organic chemicals and radionuclides; Volume 2 provides the toxicological, epidemiologic, and clinical evidence used in deriving the recommended guideline values; and Volume 3 provides guidelines for drinking water quality control for small community supplies (63–65). Volume 3 is concerned primarily with the bacteriological safety of water.

SELECTED REGULATED CHEMICAL CONTAMINANTS

A brief discussion of some chemical contaminants regulated under the Safe Drinking Water Act is presented. The health effects of exposure to these agents are discussed in detail in Part V of this book.

Inorganic Chemicals

Arsenic

Although arsenic compounds may occasionally contaminate water sources as the result of industrial discharges or pesticides, the occurrence of arsenic in drinking water is usually the result of ground water being drawn from mineral formations containing natural arsenic ores. The areas affected include the southwest, northwest, and northeast sections of the United States and Alaska. Arsenic occurs in both trivalent and pentavalent states as well as in organic forms. Trivalent compounds are generally more toxic than pentavalent compounds. The pentavalent state and organoarsenicals appear to predominate in foods, particularly seafood (33).

National U.S. projections made from the analysis of 835 groundwater samples and 263 surface water samples indicate that 14–28 million people are consuming drinking water that contains more than 5 µg/L of arsenic (18) (the drinking water MCL is 50 µg/L).

Exposure to inorganic arsenic compounds in drugs, drinking water, and occupational environments is causally associated with the development of skin cancer and neurological disorders in humans. The incidence of lung cancer was increased almost 10 times in smelter workers who inhaled high levels of arsenic trioxide (17).

Cadmium

The presence of cadmium in drinking water is normally the result of corrosion of galvanized pipes and fittings. Cadmium may occasionally be present as the result of contamination of the water sources.

Data available on the cadmium level at the consumer's tap are not adequate for national exposure estimates. Drinking water, however, is not considered to be a major exposure source. National U.S. projections made from the analysis of 835 groundwater and 90 surface water samples indicate that 0.2–1.1 million people are provided with drinking water that contains more than 2 µg/L of cadmium. The water supply of approximately 150 communities contains cadmium in excess of 5 µg/L. Studies reveal that within a particular system, 13–61% of the samples taken at household taps contain cadmium picked up from pipes and fixtures. Seldom has the concentration of cadmium in drinking water exceeded 10 µg/L (19). The current drinking water MCL is 5 µg/L.

Excessive intake of cadmium has been linked to proteinuria. Studies have suggested that human exposure to cadmium (primarily as the oxide) is associated with increased risks of prostatic and respiratory cancers (17).

Chromium

The occurrence of excess chromium in drinking water is relatively infrequent and may result from the contamination of raw water or the back siphonage of chromates used as corrosion inhibitors in pipes or boilers. Few people are exposed to drinking water that contains more than 120 µg/L of chromium (20).

Trivalent chromium is relatively nontoxic and is considered to be essential in man for efficient lipid, glucose, and protein metabolism. Hexavalent chromium has been shown to exert toxicity on the renal, hepatic, skin, and gastrointestinal systems. Hexavalent chromium is also carcinogenic and mutagenic. An increased incidence of lung cancer has been observed among workers in both the bichromate-producing industry and chromate-pigment manufacturing. There is evidence of a similar risk among chromium platers and chromium alloy workers (17). The current MCL (100 µg/L) for chromium is based on toxicity of the hexavalent form because Cr^{3+} may be converted to Cr^{6+} under oxidizing conditions created during chlorination (33).

Fluoride

Fluoride is a ubiquitous component of the earth's crust and therefore of potable water. It is incorporated into calcified tissue, where it may reduce dental caries and increase bone density. It exhibits dose-related toxicity at high levels of intake.

The mildest stages of cosmetic dental fluorosis have been noted at drinking water levels below 2 mg/L. Mild dental fluorosis is barely detectable. Moderate fluorosis is indicated by yellow to brown stain on the teeth. Severe dental fluorosis includes pitting of the dental enamel. Crippling fluorosis, growth retardation, and thyroid and kidney damage have been noted from chronic ingestion at levels above 10 mg/L. Radiologically detectable skeletal accumulation (osteosclerosis) can be observed in intermediate exposure conditions (33).

Very few drinking water supplies in the United States are known or expected to have fluoride concentration above 4 mg/L, and most of these use ground water. It has been projected that over 1300 water supplies in the United States contain over 2 mg/L fluoride. Virtually all of these are in small communities.

Lead

The occurrence of lead in drinking water is normally the result of corrosive action of water on pipes, fittings, and solder. The lead encountered in drinking water may be especially high when tap water is consumed without first flushing away the water that has been standing in the pipes overnight, especially the first 100 cc that has been in contact with brass faucets. In the United States this problem is most commonly encountered in the Northeast and Northwest. It may, however, be encountered in water supplies throughout the United States, especially where copper pipes are in use. This problem exists in other parts of the world as well.

Studies on humans have demonstrated that the fetus, infants, and young children are more susceptible than adults to the biochemical effects of lead (44). Excessive lead intake adversely effects the nervous, hematopoietic, gastrointestinal, renal, and immunologic systems. Of major concern are the teratogenic effects of lead exposure as well as its adverse effect on behavior in infants and young children (44). Lead-containing solders and pipe have been banned from future use in drinking water systems.

Mercury

Mercury may be found in water in organic and inorganic forms. The major source of mercury in drinking water is natural mineralization or effluent discharges (i.e., chloralkali manufacture), product disposal as a "solid" waste, and direct well contamination from such products as mercury-sealed well pumps. The reported occurrence of excess mercury in drinking water above the maximum contaminant level (MCL) is relatively rare.

National United States projections made from the analysis of 841 groundwater samples and 123 surface water samples indicate that 5–20 million people are consuming drinking water that at some times contains more than 1 µg/L of mercury (21).

The MCL for mercury of 0.002 mg/L is based on the neurological effects associated with the ingestion of alkyl mercury (33). Inorganic mercury can be converted into the alkyl form in the environment.

Nitrate

Most nitrate in drinking water stems from groundwater contamination by agricultural fertilizers, septic systems, and feed lots. Occasionally, groundwater contamination results from the decomposition of natural organic matter. Nitrate contamination is most frequent in the Midwest but may occur in other rural areas or in suburban areas where septic systems are used (33). Nitrate contamination is also well documented in surface and ground water in Europe and other parts of the globe (15,28).

As previously noted, a national survey conducted by the EPA based on the analysis of 1300 community water system wells and rural domestic wells reveals that an estimated 49,300 community water system wells and 5,990,000 rural domestic wells in the United States contain nitrate at or above the analytical reporting limit of 0.15 mg/L. The EPA estimates that 1130 (1.2%) community water system wells and 254,000 (2.4%) rural domestic wells nationwide contain nitrates that exceed federal health standards of 10 mg/L (as N) or about 45 mg/L as nitrate (56). Over a million people may well be using tap water that contains more than 10 mg/L of nitrate (as N).

Two health hazards are linked to drinking water containing high concentrations of nitrate or nitrite: the induction of methemoglobinemia, particularly in the newborn, and the potential formation of carcinogenic nitrosamines (33).

In 1945, nitrate in drinking water was first reported to be associated with methemoglobinemia in infants. The MCL for nitrate was intended solely to protect infants from methemoglobinemia or "blue baby" syndrome. The mechanism of toxicity involves the reduction of nitrate to nitrite by intestinal bacteria. The nitrite so formed affects the oxygen-carrying capacity of the blood. Infants in the first few months of life are particularly susceptible to this problem. Reported cases of methemoglobinemia have been related primarily to the ingestion of water from domestic wells. This problem often seems to correlate with concurrent biological contamination of the water (e.g., from septic tanks). The current standard appears to offer little margin of safety for some infants (33). Yet in recent years no known cases of infant methemoglobinemia have been associated with public drinking water supplies.

Selenium

Nearly all selenium in drinking water is extracted directly from natural mineral formations. In the United States high levels in potable water are generally limited to western states.

National U.S. projections made from the analysis of 835 groundwater samples and 310 surface water samples indicate that 1700–3200 systems are providing drinking water to consumers that contains more than 5 μg/L of selenium (22). Nearly 120,000 consumers are reportedly receiving drinking water than contains more than 45 μg/L of selenium.

The adverse health effects of chronic selenium ingestion, though not fully understood, range from gastric and intestinal problems to dental damage. Low levels of intake are essential for many animal species (33). The current MCL has been raised recently from 10 μg/L to 50 μg/L.

Radionuclides

Uranium

In 1991 National Primary Drinking Water Regulations were proposed for uranium in drinking water. Uranium occurs in both ground water and surface waters. Approximately 100 naturally occurring rocks contain 1% or more uranium, with a few ores containing 40–60% of this element. Uranium is found in phosphate deposits, tailings, and phosphate fertilizers. Few drinking water samples have been analyzed for uranium content, but its presence is inferred from analyses of nonpotable waters from nearby ground and surface sources. It is estimated that 5–13% of community water supplies contain a uranium concentration of 5 pCi/L (183 Bq/m^3) (16,55).

Radium-226/Radium-228

All but six states have reported known MCL violations for radium in drinking water. More than 200 groundwater supplies contain radium-226 activity in excess of 5 pCi/L (183 Bq/m^3). The radium content of surface water supplies is generally low. Ground water being drawn from carbonate aquifers and metamorphic rock aquifers is generally low in radium. Higher levels of radium-226/228 are found generally in igneous rock and sand aquifers.

National United States projections based on the analysis of 940 groundwater samples and 111 surface water samples indicate that 200–500 systems are providing drinking water to consumers that contains more than 5 μg/L of radium-226 (53). Occupational exposure to radium has been associated with increased risk of bone sarcoma and carcinoma of the sinus (53).

Radon

In 1991 National Primary Drinking Water standards were proposed for radon. Radon is a water-soluble inert gas found in many ground waters. It is thereby easily transferred from potable water to indoor air. Radon is produced from radium in soil and rock. Radon levels in water may be as high as 300,000 pCi/L (1.1×10^7 Bq/m³) in domestic wells from granitic zones in Maine to 46,000 pCi/L (1.7×10^6 Bq/m³) in North Carolina and 54,000 pCi/L (2×10^6 Bq/m³) in New Hampshire (11).

National U.S. projections based on the analysis of 2641 samples indicate that 33,000–36,000 systems that use ground water are providing drinking water containing more than 100 pCi/L (3.7×10^3 Bq/m³) of radon to 45 million consumers (54). It is estimated that about 10,000 pCi/L (370×10^3 Bq/m³) of radon in water would contribute about 1 pCi/L (0.0037×10^3 Bq/m³) to indoor air. Therefore, water is usually a very minor source of the radon in the home. There is concern that the enrichment of indoor air and subsequent inhalation of radon may be linked to an increased risk of lung cancer. The extent of this risk is unclear (26,40).

Organic Chemicals

Trihalomethanes

One or more of the trihalomethanes (THMs)—chloroform, bromodichloromethane, dibromochloromethane, and bromoform—have been detected in virtually every chlorinated water supply. Concentrations vary with the type and dose of chlorine being used as a disinfectant as well as the type and level of organic precursors found in the raw water (34,46). National regulations promulgated in 1979 limited the total THM level found in drinking water to 100 µg/L. This action was based on the toxicology of chloroform including the evidence of its carcinogenicity to animals as well as the formation of other undefined byproducts (17,46).

SUMMARY

Industrialization and the widespread use of chemicals coupled with modern intensive agricultural practices have raised a global concern about the quality of water resources. Increasingly, ground water, once thought to be protected from pollution, shows evidence of contamination with nitrates and pesticides. Improperly designed hazardous waste disposal sites are also important sources of groundwater contamination by organic chemicals. Corrosion-related byproducts such as lead can be significant contaminants in acidic waters (below pH 8). Synthetic organic chemicals at trace levels are being detected with greater frequency in drinking water. To a considerable degree this detection reflects the increased application of recently developed sensitive analytic techniques.

Although drinking water generally contributes relatively little to the daily pollutant exposure of the "average" adult in the United States, pollutant levels can be high for some specific communities where significant contamination exists. Groundwater levels of nitrate, volatile organics, radionuclides, or inorganics may be very high. Treated surface water may contain a high level of disinfection byproducts. Children may consume drinking water with high lead levels derived from pipes or solder. Infants and adults with a high water intake per unit of body weight may experience exposure levels above the average.

New U.S. national primary drinking water regulations have been published for 83 substances, including many organics, inorganics, radionuclides, and a number of biological agents. These regulations do not, in themselves, define the potability of a water supply, and they are not intended to be exhaustive. They assume the use of the best available source of water and the use of appropriate treatment systems that would remove virtually all significant contaminants to below the levels of concern. Thus public water supplies that meet all national standards are not likely to be associated with adverse health effects.

REFERENCES

1. Bailey JR, et al: A Study of Flow Reduction and Treatment of Waste Water from Households. Prepared by General Dynamics (Contract No. 14-12-428) for the Federal Water Quality Administration, Department of the Interior, Washington, 1962.
2. Board on Agriculture, National Research Council: Pesticides and Groundwater Quality: Issue and Problems in Four States, National Academy Press, Washington, 1986.
3. Boland PA: National Screening Program for Organics in Drinking Water. Prepared by SRI International (Contract No. 68-01-466) for Office of Drinking Water, US Environmental Protection Agency, Washington, 1981.
4. Brass HJ, Weisner MJ, Kingsley BA: The national organic monitoring survey: A sampling and analysis for purgeable organic compounds. In: Drinking Water Quality Enhancement through Source Protection, p 393, Pojasek RB (ed.), Ann Arbor Science, Ann Arbor, 1977.
5. Brown SH, Bishop DR, Rowan CA: The role of skin absorption as a route of exposure for volatile organic compounds (VOCs) in drinking water. Am J Public Health 74:479, 1984.
6. Calabrese EJ, Gilbert CE, Pastides H (eds.): Safe Drinking Water Act Ammendments, Regulations and Standards, Lewis Publishers, Chelsea, Michigan, 1989.
7. Committee on Groundwater Quality Protection, National Research Council: Ground Water Quality Protection State and Local Strategies, National Academy Press, Washington, 1986.

8. Coniglio W, Miller K, Mackeever D: The occurrence of volatile organics in drinking water—a briefing paper for the Environmental Protection Agency, Deputy Assistant Administrator for Drinking Water, Environmental Protection Agency, Washington, 1980.
9. Cotruvo JA: Risk assessment and control decisions for protecting drinking water quality. Adv Chem 214:693–733, 1987.
10. Cotruvo JA: Drinking water standards and risk assessment. Regul Toxicol Pharmacol 8:288, 1988.
11. Council on Environmental Quality: Environmental Quality, 15 Annual Report 1984, US Government Printing Office, Washington, 1986.
12. Drinking Water Health Effects Task Force: Health Effects of Drinking Water Treatment Technologies, Lewis Publishers, Chelsea, Michigan, 1989.
13. Freeze RA, Cherry JA: Groundwater. Prentice-Hall, Engelwood Cliffs, NJ, 1978.
14. Geophysics Study Committee, National Research Council: Groundwater Contamination. National Academy Press, Washington, 1984.
15. Global Environment Monitoring System: Assessment of Freshwater Quality, United National Environment Programme/World Health Organization, Geneva, 1988.
16. Hess CT, Michel J, Horton TR, et al: The occurrence of radioactivity in public water supplies in the United States. Paper presented before the Environmental Protection Agency-sponsored workshop on radioactivity in drinking water, 23–24 May 1983, Health Phys 48:553, 1985.
17. IARC: IARC Monographs on the Evaluation of Carcinogenic Risks to Humans, Suppl 7, International Agency for Research on Cancer, Lyon, 1987.
18. Letkiewicz F, Spooner C, Macaluso C, et al: Occurrence of arsenic in drinking water, food, and air. Prepared by JRB Associates (Contract No. 68-01-6388) for the Office of Drinking Water, US Environmental Protection Agency, Washington, 1987.
19. Letkiewicz F, Spooner C, Macaluso C, et al: Occurrence of cadmium in drinking water, food and air. Prepared by JRB Associates (Contract No. 68-01-6388) for the Office of Drinking Water, US Environmental Protection Agency, Washington, 1987.
20. Letkiewicz F, Spooner C, Macaluso C, et al: Occurrence of chromium in drinking water, food and air. Prepared by JRB Associates (Contract No. 68-01-6388) for the Office of Drinking Water, US Environmental Protection Agency, Washington, 1987.
21. Letkiewicz F, Spooner C, Macaluso C, et al: Occurrence of mercury in drinking water, food, and air. Prepared by JRB Associates (Contract No. 68-01-6388) for the Office of Drinking Water, US Environmental Protection Agency, Washington, 1987.
22. Letkiewicz, F, Spooner C, Macaluso C, et al: Occurrence of selenium in drinking water, food, and air. Prepared by JBR Associates (Contract No. 68-01-6388) for the Office of Drinking Water, US Environmental Protection Agency, Washington, 1987.
23. Lin DCK, Melton RG, Kopfler FC, et al: Glass capillary gas chromatographic/mass spectrometric analysis of organic concentrates from drinking and advanced waste treatment waters. In: Proceeding of Advances in the Identification and Analysis of Organic Pollutants in Water, p 861, Keith L (ed.), Ann Arbor Science, Ann Arbor, 1981.
24. Lippy EC, Waltrip SC: Waterborne disease outbreaks—1946–1980, a thirty-five year perspective. J Am Water Works Assoc 76:60, 1984.
25. Marrach D: Water and Health. In: Environment and Health, p 163, Trieff NM (ed.), Ann Arbor Science, Ann Arbor, 1980.
26. Mays CW, Rowland RE, Stehney AF: Cancer risk from the lifetime intake of Ra and U isotopes. Health Phys 48:1635, 1985.
27. Moore MR: Influence of acid rain upon water plumbosolvency. Environm Health Perspect 63:121, 1985.
28. Organisation for Economic Co-Operation and Development: Water Pollution by Fertilizers and Pesticides, OECD, Paris, 1986.
29. Pontius FW (ed.): Water Quality and Treatment, A Handbook of Community Water Supplies, McGraw-Hill, New York, 1990.
30. Pye VI, Patrick R: Ground water contamination in the United States. Science 221:713, 1983.
31. Ram NM, Calabrese EJ, Christman R (eds.): Organic Carcinogens in Drinking Water: Detection, Treatment and Risk Assessment, John Wiley & Sons, New York, 1986.
32. Ram MN, Christman RF, Cantor KP: Significance and Treatment of Volatile Organic Compounds in Water Supplies, Lewis Publishers, Chelsea, Michigan, 1990.
33. Safe Drinking Water Committee, National Research Council: Drinking Water and Health, Vol 1, National Academy Press, Washington, 1977.
34. Safe Drinking Water Committee, National Research Council: Drinking Water and Health, Vol 2, National Academy Press, Washington, 1980.
35. Safe Drinking Water Committee, National Research Council: Drinking Water and Health, Vol 3, National Academy Press, Washington, 1980.
36. Safe Drinking Water Committee, National Research Council: Drinking Water and Health, Vol 4, National Academy Press, Washington, 1982.
37. Safe Drinking Water Committee, National Research Council: Drinking Water and Health, Vol 5, National Academy Press, Washington, 1983.
38. Safe Drinking Water Committee, National Research Council: Drinking Water and Health, Vol 6, National Academy Press, Washington, 1986.
39. Safe Drinking Water Committee, National Research Council: Selected Issues in Risk Assessment, Vol 9, National Academy Press, Washington, 1989.
40. Samet JM: Radon and lung cancer. J Natl Cancer Inst 81:745, 1989.
41. Second International Symposium on Health Effects of Drinking Water Disinfectants and Disinfection By-Products. Environ Health Perspect 69:3–285, 1986.
42. Sharpe WE, DeWalle DR: Potential health implications for acid precipitation, corrosion, and metals contamination of drinking water. Environ Health Perspect 63:71, 1985.
43. Shy CM: Chemical contamination of water supplies. Environ Health Perspect 62:399, 1985.
44. Smith MD, Grant LD, Sors AI (eds.): Lead Exposure and Child Development, Kluwer Academic Publishers, Dordrecht, 1988.

45. Smith RA, Alexander RB, Wolman MG: Water-quality trends in the nation's rivers. Science 235:1607, 1987.
46. Subcommittee on Disinfectants and Disinfectant By-Products, National Research Council: Drinking Water and Health. Disinfectants and Disinfectant By-Products, Vol 7, National Academy Press, Washington, 1987.
47. Subcommittee on Pharmacokinetics in Risk Assessment, National Research Council: Pharmacokinetics in Risk Assessment, Vol 8, National Academy Press, Washington, 1987.
48. Symons JM, Bellar T, Carswell J, et al: National organics reconnaissance survey for halogenated organics. J Am Water Works Assoc 67:634, 1975.
49. US Congress, Office of Technology Assessment: Protecting the Nation's Groundwater from Contamination, Vol I, OTA-0-233, Washington, 1984.
50. US Congress, Office of Technology Assessment: Protecting the Nation's Groundwater from Contamination: Vol II, OTA-0-276, Washington, 1984.
51. US Environmental Protection Agency, Office of Water Supply and Solid Waste Management Programs: Waste Disposal Practices and Their Effects on Ground Water: Executive Summary, US Government Printing Office, Washington, 1977.
52. US Environmental Protection Agency, Office of Drinking Water: A Status Report on the National Public Water Supply Program, US Government Printing Office, Washington, 1981.
53. US Environmental Protection Agency: Radium 226 Occurrence in Drinking Water. Prepared by SAIC (Contract EPA No. 68-01-7166) for the Office of Drinking Water, US Government Printing Office, Washington, 1986.
54. US Environmental Protection Agency: Radon Occurrence in Drinking Water. Prepared by SAIC (Contract EPA No. 68-01-7166) for the Office of Drinking Water, US Government Printing Office, Washington, 1986.
55. US Environmental Protection Agency: Uranium Occurrence in Drinking Water. Prepared by SAIC (Contract EPA 68-01-7166) for the Office of Drinking Water, US Government Printing Office, Washington, 1986.
56. US Environmental Protection Agency: National Pesticide Survey, Phase 1 Report, EPA 570/9-90-015, US Government Printing Office, Washington, 1990.
57. US Environmental Protection Agency: National Water Quality Inventory: 1988 Report to Congress, EPA 440-4-90-003, US Government Printing Office, Washington, 1990.
58. US Environmental Protection Agency: Toxics in the Community—National and Local Perspectives, the 1988 Toxic Release Inventory National Report, EPA 560/4-90-017, US Government Printing Office, Washington, 1990.
59. US Environmental Protection Agency: EPA: The first twenty years. EPA J 16(5), 1990.
60. Ware GW (ed.): Review of Environmental Contamination and Toxicology. United States Environmental Protection Agency, Office of Drinking Water Health Advisories, Vol 104, Springer-Verlag, New York, 1988.
61. Ware GW (ed.): Review of Environmental Contamination and Toxicology. US Environmental Protection Agency, Office of Drinking Water Health Advisories, Vol 107, Springer-Verlag, New York, 1990.
62. Westrick JJ, Mello JW, Thomas RF: The Ground Water Supply, Summary of Volatile Organic Contaminant Occurrence Data, US EPA Technical Support Division, Office of Drinking Water, Cincinnati, OH, 1982.
63. World Health Organization: Guidelines for Drinking Water Quality. Vol 1. Recommendations. WHO, Geneva, 1984.
64. World Health Organization: Guidelines for Drinking Water Quality. Vol 2. Health Criteria and Other Supporting Information. WHO, Geneva, 1984.
65. World Health Organization: Guidelines for Drinking Water Quality. Vol 3. Guidelines for Drinking Water Quality Control for Small-Community Supplies. WHO, Geneva, 1985.

RECOMMENDED READINGS

Drinking Water Health Effects Task Force: Health Effects of Drinking Water Treatment Technologies, Lewis Publishers, Chelsea, Michigan, 1989.
Pontius FW (ed.): Water Quality and Treatment, A Handbook of Community Water Supplies, McGraw-Hill, New York, 1990.
Organization for Economic Co-Operation and Development: Water Pollution by Fertilizers and Pesticides, OECD, Paris, 1986.
Ram NM, Christman RF, Cantor KP: Significance and Treatment of Volatile Organic Compounds in Water Supplies, Lewis Publishers, Chelsea, Michigan, 1990.
US Environmental Protection Agency: National Water Quality Inventory, 1988 Report to Congress, EPA 440-4-90-003, US Government Printing Office, Washington, 1990.

5. HAZARDOUS WASTES

Robert D. Stephens

INTRODUCTION

The safe and economical disposal of hazardous waste is acknowledged to be one of our biggest environmental challenges. Problems relating to the management and disposal of hazardous waste afflict industrial nations throughout the world. It has been estimated that 20 to 24 million metric tons of hazardous waste are generated annually in Europe and another 7 to 8 million metric tons are generated annually from a group of Pacific countries that includes Japan, Australia, and New Zealand (18). The Environmental Protection Agency (EPA) estimates that about 255 to 275 million metric tons of hazardous waste are generated annually in the United States (8). By far the bulk of this waste is generated by the petrochemical industry. It is estimated that the production of synthetic organic chemicals has increased by over 400% since 1940. The EPA estimates that only 10% of all hazardous waste was properly disposed of in the past, most of it having been pumped into unlined lagoons on the generator's property (33).

Statistics reveal the size of the problem and something of its geographic scope. The EPA estimates that about 2000 hazardous sites will reach the National Priorities List. The sites on this list warrant the highest priority for remedial action (41). These sites are located throughout the United States, with the following states generating about 65% of all hazardous wastes: Texas, Ohio, Pennsylvania, Louisiana, Michigan, Indiana, Illinois, Tennessee, West Virginia, and California. The Office of Technology Assessment (OTA) estimates that 10,000 sites (or more) may require cleanup by the Federal Super-

fund program (35). By 1986 about 30% of the 703 sites on the National Priorities List had received remedial cleanup attention. Remedial cleanup in general has tended to be impermanent, often transferring environmental risks from one area to another (35). The passage of the reauthorized Comprehensive Environmental, Response, Compensation, and Liability Act of 1986 (CERCLA), better known as Superfund, has mandated a policy of permanent remedial solutions wherever possible.

Severe problems of soil and water contamination related to the uncontrolled disposal of toxic wastes occur in developing and developed countries. Little information is available from developing countries. However, heavily polluting resource-based industries are growing fastest in these countries (14). It is clear that a growing need for appropriate environmental and waste-management technologies exists in developing countries (14). In the 1980s, as controls tightened in some countries, the export of hazardous wastes from industrial nations to waste sites in developing nations also became a problem (5,13).

Industrial nations have reported problems stemming from the inappropriate disposal of toxic wastes. In Denmark, for example, over 3000 sites have been found. In The Netherlands about 350 of the 4000 sites discovered require immediate remedial action (25). In August 1978, Love Canal in the State of New York was declared a national disaster, the first from a man-made source. In some cases, e.g., Love Canal and Times Beach in Missouri, whole populations have been forced to relocate. Other serious incidents, mostly unpublicized, have also occurred.

Numbers do not convey the grim dilemma hazardous waste disposal poses for an industrial society. Hazardous substances have contaminated air, soil, and water. The contamination of ground water and surface waters has destroyed drinking water supplies. Fires and explosions have occurred. Natu-

Principles and Practice of Environmental Medicine, edited by Alyce Bezman Tarcher. Plenum Medical Book Company, New York, 1992.

78

II EXPOSURE

ral habitats such as rivers, streams, lakes, and fields have been compromised.

HAZARDOUS WASTES: THEIR SOURCE, NATURE, AND ADVERSE EFFECTS

Source of Hazardous Waste

Chemical Agents

Hazardous wastes are defined as discarded material that may, when improperly handled, pose a substantial threat or potential hazard to human health or the environment. Hazardous wastes are a product of the entire spectrum of the manufacturing, service, research, and academic industries. A significant percentage of the approximately 65,000 chemicals currently in commerce are represented within the generic classification of hazardous waste.

In 1989, the first Toxic Release Inventory (TRI) was published by the EPA. This report provided the public with information on the release of toxic chemicals by manufacturing facilities during 1987. For the first time, the TRI data analyzed where toxic chemicals were being released along with the types and amounts of releases. A second report, published in 1990, announced the results of the 1988 Toxic Release Inventory. This report showed that 0.36 billion pounds of toxic chemicals were released into rivers, lakes, streams, and other bodies of water; 2.43 billion pounds were emitted into the air; 0.56 billion pounds were disposed of in landfills; and 1.22 billion pounds were injected into underground wells. An additional 0.57 billion and 1.10 billion pounds were transferred to treatment and disposal facilities (43).

It is noteworthy that toxic chemical wastes are generated from many different sources, including manufacturing and nonmanufacturing industrial processes, use and disposal of consumer products, agricultural uses of chemicals, and mobile sources such as automobiles. The Toxic Release Inventory reporting requirements only cover manufacturing industries. Other businesses, such as warehouses, photographic processing plants, dry cleaners, and mining operations, are not included under Toxic Release Inventory reporting requirements. Moreover, households and small businesses that produce hazardous wastes containing many of the same chemicals as those used by large industries are not assessed.

The composition of hazardous wastes varies markedly from one industry to another. The composition of waste also varies among countries. As seen in Fig. 5-1, in the United States by far the greatest amount of hazardous waste is produced by the chemical industry (30). The wastes generated by the various sources include paint and organic residues used in paint production, organic and oily residues from petroleum products and machinery-manufacturing processes; metal sludges and pigments; cyanides and solvents generated during the manufacture of metal products; chlorinated organic compounds from the manufacture of plastics; oils and greases generated primarily from machinery, automobiles; solvents and organic compounds used during the manufacture of such products as rubber and organic chemicals; oils and greases coming primarily from machinery, automobiles, and other vehicles; and pesticides.

Although industry has generated hazardous wastes (e.g., heavy metals and acids) for decades, the modern hazardous waste problem can in large part be traced to the burgeoning petrochemical industry. Its production has grown from about a half billion kg of synthetic chemicals in 1940 to about 173

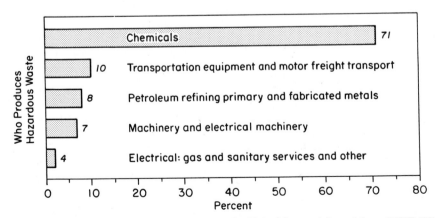

FIGURE 5-1. Production of hazardous wastes in the United States. Adapted from UNEP (30).

billion kg in 1989. This industry produces a host of products, which include synthetic fabrics, plastics, drugs, paints, solvents, and pesticides. Numerous petrochemical compounds have been found to be toxic, carcinogenic, or otherwise harmful (22). They are often stable for a long time, sometimes virtually forever. Petrochemical wastes include such unwanted byproducts as dioxin and such commercially useful compounds as polychlorinated biphenyls (PCBs), solvents, and pesticides.

Air and water pollution abatement programs are another increasingly important source of hazardous waste. These measures, which involve such control devices as filters, stack scrubbers, and waste water treatment, result in the accumulation of pollutants that must eventually be disposed of. The large amounts of hazardous sludges generated by these programs are frequently disposed of as cheaply as possible—often by simple burial.

Small businesses, in combination, generate significant amounts of hazardous waste. Such businesses typically include gas stations, auto paint and repair shops, photography studios, printing shops, dry cleaners, and metal manufacturers. Estimates of the quantity of hazardous wastes produced by small generators vary between 1% and 10% of all hazardous waste generated (10). Consumers also produce toxic wastes. Although no reliable estimates exist on the quantity of hazardous wastes produced by consumers, it is apparent that significant amounts of such toxic substances as paints, solvents, pesticides, and cleaning products are used in the home.

Radioactive Materials

The production of nuclear weapons has generated radioactive and hazardous waste since the 1940s. In the United States the various facilities in the weapons complex are owned by the federal government and operated by contractors subject to oversight by the Department of Energy (DOE). The DOE operates 17 major facilities to develop and produce nuclear weapons for the Department of Defense. These facilities are located throughout the United States. A report from the National Academy of Sciences indicates that virtually every facility has on-site contamination. In some cases the contamination is extensive and present off site as well (9). It has been estimated that it will take more than 20 years to process and dispose of the waste and clean up contaminated sites.

Low-level radioactive wastes originate from hospitals, laboratories, industries, and nuclear power plants. The issue of low-level radioactive waste, its sources, significance, strategies for disposal, and potential hazards, has been addressed in a recent symposium (29).

Nature of Hazardous Waste

Management strategies to deal with the vast array of hazardous materials and to cope with their public health and environmental threat require that hazardous wastes be classified. There are three basic approaches to the classification of hazardous waste: by origin and specific components; by physical, chemical, and toxic characteristics; and by composition and concentration. Each of these classifications best serves a particular objective (Table 5-1).

Defining hazardous waste by process or industrial origin expedites regulatory and compliance activities. Such definitions, however, because they are nonspecific, tend to make health and environmental impact assessments very difficult. Since the classification of waste, using this scheme, can be made with little or no testing, it reduces cost and complexity.

Defining hazardous wastes according to their characteristics, i.e., explosivity, corrosivity, reactivity, and toxicity, is particularly helpful in their proper handling and management. Using this classification for regulatory purposes poses problems because of the uncertainties that naturally occur in establishing acceptable toxicity levels—particularly for such chronic and irreversible effects as genetic damage, birth defects, and cancer. A report by the Office of Technology Assessment, U.S. Congress

TABLE 5-1. Classification Systems for Hazardous Wastes

Basis of classification	Primary purpose served
Process or industry source	Regulatory and litigation
Chemical and allied products	
Petroleum	
Metal-related	
Transportation equipment	
Motor freight transport	
Machinery	
Electrical machinery	
Electric, gas, and sanitary services	
Waste characteristics	Proper handling and management
Ignitability	
Corrosivity	
Reactivity	
Toxicity	
Chemical composition	Assessment of public health and environmental impacts
Heavy metals	
Synthetic organic chemicals	
Acids and bases	
Asbestos	
Flammables	
Radioactive materials	

discusses in detail the need for ranking hazardous wastes based on their degree of hazard (33).

Defining hazardous waste by chemical composition and concentration aids in the assessment of public health hazards and their environmental impact. Hazardous wastes fall into the following major chemical categories: heavy metals, synthetic organic chemicals, asbestos, acids and bases, flammables, and radioactive materials. Problems can arise when potentially toxic constituents are classified according to their composition and concentration. The comprehensive analytic characterization of complex mixtures can be expensive, time consuming, and uncertain. In spite of these drawbacks, hazardous wastes that have been thoroughly characterized are more readily assessed for their impact on the environmental and health.

Adverse Effects of Hazardous Waste

There is ample evidence that the improper disposal of hazardous wastes poses serious threats to the environment and public health. The wide range of well-documented ecological damage includes groundwater contamination, air pollution, soil contamination, damage to sewer systems, habitat destruction, fish kills, livestock losses, and damages to crops and wildlife. Recently, increasing concern has focused on groundwater contamination and volatilization of organic chemicals from hazardous

waste sites. Figure 5-2 shows the ways in which migrating contaminants from a hazardous waste landfill can contaminate air, water, and soil. There are many documented examples of environmental contamination stemming from specific hazardous waste sites (10,33,35).

Contamination of ground water, with the resultant loss of drinking water supplies, is a particularly disturbing corollary of certain waste disposal practices (7,15,27). Ground water provides approximately 50% of the drinking water and 20% of all water used in the United States. Of the contaminated sites targeted for remedial action by the EPA, approximately 75% pose a threat to ground water (35). Disposal methods linked to groundwater contamination include landfills and dumps, evaporation ponds or lagoons, septic systems, deep burial, and deep injection (35).

Although groundwater contamination from the improper disposal of hazardous waste represents an important problem, it should be recognized that such contamination also occurs unrelated to waste disposal. Accidental spills and leaks, atmospheric contaminants, highway deicing salts, mining operations, petroleum extraction, animal feedlot wastes, the field application of pesticides, herbicides, and fertilizers, and such natural events as the leaching of minerals and salt water intrusion are also important sources of groundwater contamination (21,34,35).

Public health risks from toxic waste require

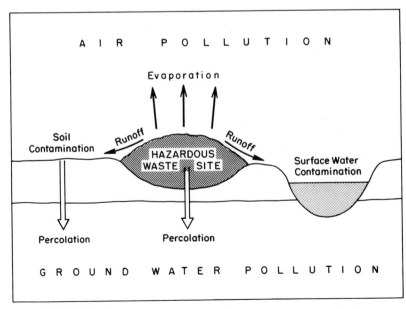

FIGURE 5-2. Environmental contamination from hazardous waste sites.

human exposure, which can occur through direct skin contact, the ingestion of contaminated water, breathing contaminated air, and ingesting contaminated food. Some wastes are flammable or prone to ignite or explode. Others are chemically very stable. The health hazards of toxic waste vary widely. Some wastes can be acutely toxic and produce immediate injury on inhalation, ingestion, or skin absorption. Others have chronic effects that are not immediately apparent. The long-term effects of particular concern include genetic damage, birth defects, and cancer. Populations living in proximity to poorly managed or improperly designed hazardous waste sites are at increased risk. To date, however, the health effects of exposure to the toxic agents found at hazardous waste sites have not been adequately investigated (18,23,32).

MONITORING

Monitoring hazardous waste sites provides information that serves as a technical basis for regulatory action and as a verification that public health and the environment are being protected (35). Both surveillance and assessment monitoring provide information about the operation of hazardous waste management facilities. Surveillance monitoring is used to verify compliance with regulatory requirements, whereas assessment monitoring is used to determine the extent of deterioration in environmental quality. Regulatory programs should require surveillance monitoring for all waste generating and management facilities, whereas assessment monitoring should be used only if there is evidence of health and/or environmental problems. Ambient monitoring, which provides information on the level of contaminants in air, soil, water, and biota, is of particular importance. Representative samples obtained from potentially contaminated areas and analyzed for a broad range of pollutants provide a means of assessing and minimizing the adverse effects of hazardous waste disposal.

All monitoring strategies are limited by problems inherent in sampling procedures, data comparability, and analytic methods. Decisions made regarding the frequency, location, and number of samples, for example, are critical in detecting contamination. A poor choice of sampling locations can mean that an area of high contamination is missed. Variances between laboratories and limitations in analytic techniques also pose problems.

REGULATION

Before 1976, there was no specific federal regulation of hazardous wastes in the United States. The Resource Conservation and Recovery Act of 1976 (RCRA) established the first comprehensive federal regulatory program for controlling present and future hazardous waste. The RCRA seeks to establish a "cradle-to-grave" system for regulating hazardous wastes from the point of generation through storage and transportation to treatment or disposal. Under RCRA, the U.S. Environmental Protection Agency is obliged to develop national standards and regulations for managing hazardous waste.

The Act is designed to protect public health and the environment by defining which wastes are hazardous, by tracking such wastes from the point of generation, and by seeing that hazardous waste management facilities meet minimum national standards of design and operation. In addition, RCRA is designed to assure that waste management facilities are properly maintained after closure and that the operators of such facilities are financially responsible for accidents that may occur at their facilities. The Act deals primarily with the operation of hazardous waste management facilities. It does not specify the process for selecting a hazardous waste site, apart from indicating what regulatory requirements must be met before the initiation of such activities.

Federal efforts thus far have focused on establishing the regulatory framework for hazardous waste management. Standards have been established for identifying and listing hazardous wastes, for the generators and the transporters of hazardous wastes, and for the managers of hazardous waste facilities. A detailed analysis of the federal program for the management of hazardous waste has been published by the Office of Technology Assessment (33). This report identifies many of the problems associated with the long-term containment of newly generated hazardous wastes.

Amendments to RCRA have significantly broadened its regulatory framework. In 1984 the Hazardous and Solid Waste Amendments focused on the protection of ground water by including requirements that landfills be protected with double liners beneath them and a system to monitor ground water and collect toxics that leak through the liners. Restrictions on the future land disposal of all dioxins and industrial solvents were mandated. In addition, severe restrictions were placed on the treatment, storage, and disposal of hazardous wastes in land management facilities. The 1984 amendments require a schedule for determining if the land disposal of untreated hazardous waste should be phased out. Congress states that "reliance on land disposal should be minimized or eliminated; and land disposal, particularly landfills and surface impoundments, should be the least favored method of handling hazardous waste." The statutory restrictions placed on the land disposal of hazardous waste reflect the concern that all land disposal facilities, even the most secure, may inevitably leak (10).

The 1984 amendments to RCRA established a new federal regulatory program to prevent health and safety problems arising from leaking underground storage tanks. This is the first time that RCRA has been extended to cover potentially hazardous products. Previously the law was restricted only to hazardous wastes. The millions of tanks containing liquid petroleum products and chemicals buried underground present a potential hazard to soils, to ground water and surface waters, to sewer systems, and to water treatment plants. Underground storage tanks are widely dispersed throughout the United States at service stations, manufacturing plants, military bases, hospitals, schools, and car rental agencies (10).

After federal legislation was enacted to deal with newly generated hazardous waste, it became apparent that a separate federal program was needed to deal with the cleanup of the large number of old hazardous wastes sites, many of which were abandoned and leaking large amount of toxic substances. In order to deal with the hazards posed by uncontrolled hazardous waste sites, Congress passed the Comprehensive Environmental Response, Compensation, and Liability Act of 1980 (CERCLA), better known as Superfund. The Superfund program also deals with the release of hazardous substances from leaking underground storage tanks, spills from transportation accidents, and ground water contaminated from pesticide use (21,35).

Because hazardous waste sites may vary markedly in their size and in the amount and the degree of hazardous substances they contain, Superfund mandated that the EPA establish a hazard-ranking system. This system is used by the EPA to set a National Priority List of sites that need remedial cleanup. To quality for remedial cleanup, a site must be placed on the National Priority List. Factors involved in estimating a waste site's hazard potential include the characteristics of the waste (e.g., quantity, toxicity, radioactivity, persistence, reactivity, solubility) and the distance to local populations, to drinking water sources, and to surface and ground water. The security of the hazardous waste site is also considered (e.g., the ratio of hazardous to nonhazardous waste, the use and conditions of containers, the use of leachate collection systems, and the use of liners (41). These factors are used to reflect the capacity of the waste site to cause harm, the probability that the contaminants would reach populated areas and critical environments, and the degree of potential damage. The EPA must regularly update the National Priority List. This list included 1207 sites in August 1990 (42).

At the inception of Superfund, the full magnitude of the uncontrolled sites requiring Superfund action was unclear. Most assessments have underestimated the cleanup needs. The Office of Technology Assessment has reviewed the Superfund program by projecting its likely size and examining the strategy used to cope with the problem (35).

MANAGEMENT

There are essentially three basic options in the management of hazardous waste: reducing the amount generated or reusing and recycling hazardous material; treating the hazardous waste to reduce its volume and to form nonhazardous or less hazardous material; and long-term storage (8,26,36) (Fig. 5-3). The proper use of these options substantially reduces the volume and toxicity of hazardous waste that must ultimately be permanently disposed of. The key to effective hazardous waste management is finding alternatives to land burial or disposal at sea (36).

Reduce Generation of Hazardous Waste

The first priority in hazardous waste management must be to reduce the generation of waste at the source. Many companies are actively pursuing ways to minimize the quantity and danger of hazardous wastes produced. It is generally agreed, however, that far greater resources should be committed to cutting the output of hazardous waste (36,40). Factors likely to affect waste reduction efforts include operating costs, concern over liability, technical feasibility, and stringent toxic-disposal laws.

Waste reduction can be done in many ways. Changing raw materials sometimes reduces waste generation. Changing industrial processes and retraining personnel to get rid of wasteful habits provide a means of reducing waste production (36,37). Wastes may also be recycled, reused, or otherwise processed to yield useful products (8).

Recycling and Reusing Hazardous Waste

Unfortunately, even with the adoption of stringent waste reduction techniques, many industries will continue to produce toxic wastes. Before these wastes are disposed of, the possibility of recycling and reusing such wastes must be considered. Recycling consists of recovering and treating waste byproducts, which are then used as raw material for the same or another process. Reuse involves the recovery of hazardous components of wastes without additional treatment. Such wastes can then be reused by the industry generating the waste or by another industry (16,19,28,36,44).

As the costs of raw materials, waste treatment,

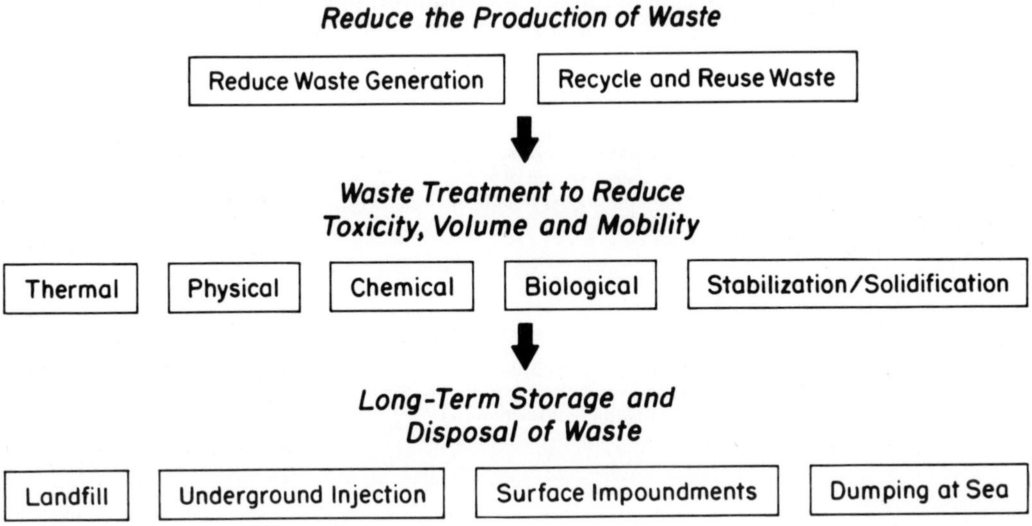

Reduce the Production of Waste

| Reduce Waste Generation | Recycle and Reuse Waste |

⬇

**Waste Treatment to Reduce
Toxicity, Volume and Mobility**

| Thermal | Physical | Chemical | Biological | Stabilization/Solidification |

⬇

**Long-Term Storage and
Disposal of Waste**

| Landfill | Underground Injection | Surface Impoundments | Dumping at Sea |

FIGURE 5-3. Management of hazardous waste. Adapted from Committee on Institutional Considerations (8).

and disposal rise, recycling and reusing chemicals from the waste stream becomes increasingly more profitable. Sometimes the potential for recycling is great. For example, before 1973, organic solvents were frequently used only once in many industrial processes and then discarded as waste. As the price of solvents rise, these agents are increasingly being recycled and reused until exhausted. Solvent recycling is one of the fastest growing markets. The reuse of waste, based on the concept that waste from one industry may be a useful raw material for another, is being implemented through the establishment of waste clearinghouses and waste-exchange organizations. In general, current efforts to recycle and reuse materials from hazardous waste are in an early stage of development.

Treatment Technologies for Hazardous Waste

A number of treatment technologies are available to immobilize toxic wastes and to reduce their bulk and toxicity (17). These include a variety of physical, chemical, biological, and thermal methods. The specific waste treatments used depend on a number of factors. These include the type of waste; its particular properties, in terms of both class (organic or inorganic) and physical properties; the available technology; the hazards involved; and cost considerations. Treatment technologies have become an integral part of hazardous waste management. Table 5-2 summarizes these technologies and points out their advantages and disadvantages (8,20,31,33,35).

Physical Treatment of Hazardous Waste

Physical treatment consists of nonchemical methods designed to separate and concentrate components in the waste stream. Physical treatment is often used to separate various hazardous components so that they can be reused or detoxified by chemical or biological means or destroyed by incineration. Physical treatment does not destroy the toxic components of the waste. The methods usually encountered include filtration, sedimentation, distillation, ion exchange, reverse osmosis, adsorption, coagulation, and centrifugation (16,28,44).

Chemical Treatment of Hazardous Waste

Chemical treatment is used to alter the chemical structure of the waste constituents. Such treatment renders the material nontoxic or less hazardous by modifying the chemical properties of the waste, e.g., reducing water solubility or neutralizing acidity or alkalinity. Chemical treatment can often be conducted on the site of the waste generator. In some cases, the chemical treatment of toxic waste can be carried out in mobile units.

Some of the common processes used in the chemical treatment of wastes are neutralization, precipitation, ion exchange, oxidation/reduction, and chemical dechlorination. Neutralization and precipitation are widely used to remove inorganic and some organic compounds from aqueous streams. Neutralization may be used alone to reduce the corrosivity of wastes. Precipitation, often used in

TABLE 5-2. Hazardous Waste Treatment Technologies[a]

Advantages	Disadvantages	Limitations
Destruction/detoxification processes		
Biological treatment		
• Conventional		
Applicable to many organic waste streams. High total organic removal. Inexpensive. Well understood and widely used in other applications.	May produce a hazardous sludge, which must be managed. May require pretreatment prior to discharge.	Microorganisms sensitive to oxygen levels, temperature, toxic loading, inlet flow. Some organic contaminants are difficult to treat. Flow and composition variations can reduce efficiency. Aeration difficult to depths >2 ft.
• In-situ biodegradation		
Destroys waste in place.	Limited experience. Extensive testing may be required. Containment also required.	Many common organic species not easily biodegraded. Needs proper combination of wastes and hydrogeological characteristics. Obtaining proper mix of contaminants, organisms, and nutrients. Organisms may plug pores.
Chemical treatment		
• Wet air oxidation		
Good for wastes too dilute for incineration or too concentrated or toxic for biological treatment.	Oxidation not as complete as thermal oxidation or incineration. May produce new hazardous species. Extensive testing is required. High capital investment. High level of operator skills required. May require posttreatment.	Poor destruction of chlorinated organics. Moderate efficiencies of destruction (40–90%).
• Chlorination for cyanide		
Essentially complete destruction. Well understood and widely used in other applications.	Specialized for cyanide.	Interfering waste constituents may limit applicability or effectiveness.
• Ozonation		
Can destroy refractory organics. Liquids, solids, mixes can be treated.	Oxidation not as complete as thermal oxidation or incineration. May produce new hazardous species. Extensive testing is required. High capital investment; high O&M.[b]	Not well understood.
• Reduction for chromium		
High destruction. Well understood and widely used in other applications.	Specialized for chromium.	Interfering waste constituents may limit applicability or effectiveness.
• Permeable treatment beds		
Limited excavation required. Inexpensive.	Developmental. Periodic replacement of treatment media required. Spent treatment medium must be disposed of.	Best for shallow plumes. Many reactants treat a limited family of wastes. Effectiveness influenced by groundwater flow variations.
• Chemical injection		
Excavation not required. No pumping required.	Developmental. Extensive testing required.	Best for shallow plumes. Need fairly homogeneous waste composition.

TABLE 5-2. (*Continued*)

Advantages	Disadvantages	Limitations
Incineration		
• Conventional incineration Destroys organic wastes (99.99+%).	Disposal of residue required. Test burn may be required. Skilled operators required. Expensive.	
• Onsite Destroys organic wastes (99.99+%). Transportation of wastes not required.	Disposal of residue required. Onsite feedstock preparation required. Test burn may be required. Skilled operators required. Expensive.	Mobile units have low feed rate.
• Thermal oxidation for gases Proven technology. High destruction efficiencies. Applicable to most organic streams.	May require auxiliary fuel. O&M cost can be high.	
Separation/transfer processes **Chemical treatment**		
• Neutralization/precipitation Wide range or applications. Well understood and widely used in other applications. Inexpensive.	Harzardous sludge produced.	Complexing agents reduce effectiveness.
• Ion exchange Can recover metals at high efficiency.	Generates sludge for disposal. Pretreatment to remove suspended solids may be required. Expensive.	Resin fouling. Removes some constituents but not others.
Physical treatment		
• Carbon absorption for aqueous streams Well understood and demonstrated. Applicable to many organics that do not respond to biological treatment. High degree of flexibility in operation and design. High degree of effectiveness.	Regeneration or disposal of spent carbon required. Pretreatment may be required for suspended solids, oil, grease. High O&M cost.	Many inorganics, some organics are poorly absorbed.
• Carbon absorption for gases Widely used, well understood. High removal efficiencies.	High capital and O&M costs.	More effective for low-molecular-weight, polar species. Disposal or regeneration of spent carbon required.
• Flocculation, sedimentation, and filtration Low cost. Well understood	Generates sludge for disposal.	—
• Stripping Well understood and demonstrated.	Air controls may be required.	Applicable only to relatively volatile organic contaminants.
• Flotation Well understood and demonstrated. Inexpensive.	Generates sludge for disposal.	—
• Reverse osmosis High removal potential.	Generates sludge for disposal. Pretreatment to remove suspended solids or adjust pH may be required. Expensive.	Variability in waste flow and composition effects performance.

^aFrom OTA (33).
^bO&M, operation and maintenance.

combination with neutralization, is used to reduce the concentration of metals from the waste stream. Ion exchange removes inorganic ions from a solution by using a resin bed. Oxidation/reduction processes are most often used to detoxify cyanide wastes from electroplating processes. Chemical dechlorination, a process currently being developed, is used to strip chlorine atoms from such compounds as polychlorinated biphenyls. The chemical treatment of waste is likely to result in residues that require further treatment or disposal (16,28,44).

Biological Treatment of Hazardous Waste

Biological treatment employs microorganisms to decompose wastes. Microorganisms, using waste constituents as food sources, decompose organic wastes, into water, carbon dioxide, and simple inorganic and organic molecules. Biological treatment may use indigenous microbial populations or microbial organisms adapted to act on a specific compound or group of compounds. Such treatment does not alter or destroy inorganic compounds. Biological waste treatment, used extensively in municipal wastewater treatment systems, is less widely used in the treatment of hazardous waste. Biological treatment methods include aerated lagoons, stabilization ponds, anaerobic digestion, and activated sludge (8,16,44).

Landfarming is a common technique that uses naturally occurring microorganisms in the soil to decompose organic compounds. In landfarming (or sludge farming), the waste is spread over the soil, and microorganisms biodegrade the organic waste as it moves through the soil. Only certain wastes can be used. Volatile and persistent organic compounds and metals that give rise to air pollution and groundwater and soil contamination should be treated by other methods. Thus far little attempt has been made to use genetically engineered organisms for the control and detoxification of hazardous waste. One of the difficulties associated with biological treatment is assuring the proper disposal of the sludge or residue from waste treatment (16,28,44).

Stabilization/Solidification and Fixation of Hazardous Waste

Stabilization/solidification and fixation processes employ physical and chemical methods to improve the handling and physical character of the waste and to make it more difficult for the waste constituents to migrate from the disposal site. Stabilizing waste prior to land disposal reduces the potential leaching of toxic materials by liquids that percolate through a landfill.

All industrial wastes are not amenable to chemical fixation. Those not readily solidified include organic solvents, oils, greases, and plastic components; those most suitable include inorganic compounds, heavy metals, and organic salts. In the solidification/stabilization process, wastes are mixed with a binding agent and then cured to a solid form. The processes used are cement-based, lime-based, thermoplastic, and encapsulation. Encapsulation is a process that encloses wastes in a stable water-resistant material (8,16,44). Many of the stabilization processes were originally developed for the containment of wastes having low-level radioactivity. Although solidification and stabilization methods offer promise in containing toxic wastes, their effectiveness over time is uncertain because of the lack of monitoring data.

Thermal Treatment of Hazardous Waste

Thermal treatment is designed to destroy waste by subjecting it to increased temperature. Incineration and pyrolysis are the two principal forms of thermal treatment. Incineration depends on the combustion of wastes in the presence of excess oxygen. Pyrolysis destroys waste through combustion in an oxygen-starved atmosphere. Incineration, the most common of the thermal treatment methods, is the controlled burning of wastes at a very high temperature. It reduces the volume and toxicity of organic wastes by converting them into nontoxic gaseous emissions and solid ash. One of the major criteria for using incineration in the treatment of hazardous waste is the virtually complete destruction of a given material. The EPA's current standard is 99.99%.

Many organic compounds, when subjected to elevated temperatures (usually between 425°C and 1650°C), are converted to less complex and less harmful compounds. The combustion byproducts generally include water, carbon dioxide, oxides of sulfur and nitrogen, hydrogen chloride, and ash. Noncombustible residues such as acids, metal oxides, and other inorganic compounds may accumulate in the ash. The following wastes have been treated in hazardous waste incinerators: solvent waste and sludges, waste mineral oils, varnish and paint wastes, plastics, rubber and latex waste sludges, phenolic wastes, mineral oil sludges, resin waste, grease and wax wastes, and pesticide waste (8,16, 19,20,44).

There are a number of high-temperature thermal processing systems. These include cement kilns, rotary kilns, liquid injection incinerators, and at-sea incinerators. The degree to which hazardous constituents are destroyed by incineration depends on the three important elements of good combustion: time, temperature, and turbulence. The type and amount of pollutants present in the flue gas depend primarily on the composition of the waste, the type of incineration system, control of the flue gas in the furnace, and the incineration temperature (44). Incinerators must be equipped to control the emission of hazardous air pollutants. Emission control equipment includes electrostatic precipitators for the removal of particulates and various types of scrubbers for the absorption of noxious gases. Residues from hazardous waste incinerators are at times hazardous and therefore require proper disposal.

Air pollution is a primary concern with the incineration of wastes. Flue gases may contain such substances as hydrogen chloride, nitrogen oxides, sulfur oxides, and lead and other metals (24). Of concern is the evidence that such toxic compounds as polychlorinated dibenzo-*p*-dioxins and polychlorinated dibenzofurans are emitted by municipal and industrial incinerators (24). Incinerating of wastes at sea causes atmospheric as well as marine pollution, since the atmospheric pollutants ultimately return to the marine environment. Between 1969 and 1978 approximately 600,000 metric tons of waste from western Europe were incinerated, primarily in the North Sea (44). In the fall of 1987, environmental ministers from eight European countries reached an agreement to stop this practice by the end of 1994 (12).

The design and operation of the incinerator greatly influences its emissions (11). High temperature and proper mixing appear to lower the concentration of some pollutants in the flue gas (2,6). Additional research must be directed to compounds that are released into the air from the incineration of waste.

Given the proper controls and the best available technology, the thermal destruction of toxic compounds offers an environmentally feasible treatment alternative for nonrecoverable hazardous wastes. If only short-term costs are considered, incineration is at present the most expensive waste treatment method. However, as greater restrictions are placed on the nature of the toxic waste that can be placed in a landfill, greater attention will be given to thermal processing methods. For a more detailed discussion of thermal treatment of hazardous waste the interested reader is referred to references (11,19,20,44).

Most of the technologies described above are not new but rather newly applied to the management of hazardous waste. Many innovative technologies are, however, currently in the developmental stage. The Office of Technology Assessment provides the interested reader with a summary of these emerging technologies and their advantages and disadvantages (35).

Disposal of Hazardous Waste

A means of waste disposal will undoubtedly always be needed. The treatment alternatives described above may reduce the volume and toxicity of a large percentage of hazardous waste, but they inevitably produce toxic residues that require disposal. In addition, many compounds are too cheap to recycle or reuse, too difficult to destroy, and too contaminated with heavy metals and other nonflammable material to incinerate. The last choice of optimal waste management is long-term storage (36). No method of hazardous waste disposal using long-term or indefinite storage offers absolute safety.

Long-term storage has been and continues to be the most common method of hazardous waste disposal in the United States. Landfills, surface impoundments (pits, ponds, and lagoons), and underground injection have been used for this purpose. In the United States as much as 80% of regulated hazardous waste is disposed of in or on land (13,33) (Fig. 5-4).

Landfills

Landfills, because they were cheap and simple, have long been the most common method for disposing of hazardous waste (33). In the past, a hole was dug in the ground, filled with untreated waste, and then covered with clay to keep out rainwater. The improper land disposal of toxic waste is responsible for scores of contaminated areas. Untreated waste landfills usually retain their toxicity and, even under optimum conditions, run the risk of eventually contaminating the soil, water, and air.

The growing concern regarding the safety of using land disposal in the management of hazardous waste resides in the inevitable potential for hazardous wastes to leak out of the disposal sites. This problem can be reduced if landfills are properly sited, designed, and constructed and have adequate operating standards. In an effort to physically isolate the waste from the environment, the design and operation of landfills have changed through the years. The current federally regulated secure landfills are required to have groundwater monitoring, double liners to contain hazardous materials, and a system for collecting toxics that leak through the liners (10). However, evidence that reasonably well designed landfills are leaking toxic substances suggests that current regulations and technologies are inadequate to protect the environment (19).

One of the major problems now facing industrial societies is the need to find additional sites for the disposal of newly generated hazardous wastes. Since most disposal methods used in the United States in the past are now either illegal or strictly controlled, the demand for legal disposal sites has increased. Federal involvement in siting disposal facilities is restricted to specifying design and operation criteria. Many states have therefore enacted

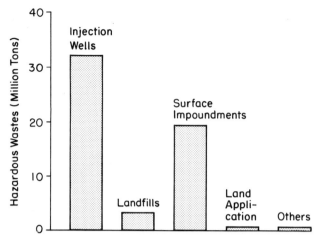

FIGURE 5-4. Disposal of hazardous wastes in the United States in 1981. Adapted from El-Hinnawi and Hashmi (13).

legislation to regulate the siting of hazardous waste facilities.

Given the strong public opposition to establishing new hazardous waste sites, it is doubtful that the legal disposal capacity at existing licensed landfills and treatment facilities (e.g., incinerators, treatment plants) is adequate to handle all of the newly generated toxic waste. Landfill capacity is highly variable throughout the United States. In many states, such as New Jersey and most of the New England states, there are no licensed chemical landfills. Wastes must be transported long distances to remote land disposal facilities or to treatment facilities.

Cleanup of Old, Abandoned, and Improperly Managed Waste Sites

Remedial action at abandoned and improperly managed waste sites can be divided into two categories: containment and treatment. Containment technologies arrest or prevent the movement of toxic waste and limit the extent of contamination that has already occurred. Treatment technologies detoxify waste by modifying or destroying its chemical structure or by separating hazardous materials from the medium (e.g., air, water, soil) that provides the route of exposure (35).

There are three basic options for the remedial cleanup of hazardous waste sites: (1) in situ treatment of soils or ground water; (2) removal of the hazardous waste solids, liquids, and/or sludges for disposal or storage for offsite (removals) or onsite treatment; and (3) control of contamination through the encapsulation and/or containment of waste or through the diversion of surface or ground water (35).

Most cleanup actions performed thus far under the Superfund legislation involved the removal and/or excavation of toxic waste followed by offsite disposal (39). Unless the removed wastes are destroyed, detoxified, treated, or stabilized, their relocation often results in the transfer of risk from one site to another. When containment is used as a method of handling old, uncontrolled dump sites, environmental monitoring is required for an indefinite period of time. Such monitoring should address all potential types of contamination, including surface water, ground water, soil, and air. Table 5-3 shows the substances found most often during the remedial treatment of abandoned or inactive waste sites (10).

Surface Impoundments

Surface impoundments are natural topographic depressions, man-made excavations, or diked areas to which liquid wastes are added. Surface impoundments known as lagoons, pits, treatment basins, or ponds have been a widely used and inexpensive method of disposing of toxic wastes. The risk of environmental contamination from leaching, overflow, and volatilization is great. Current regulatory requirements for surface impoundments include groundwater monitoring, the installation of two or more liners beneath the impoundment, and a leachate collection system.

Underground Injection Wells

Underground injection involves the use of specially designed wells to inject liquid wastes deep into the earth. Optimally, injection occurs below the lowest drinking water aquifer. The injection zone

TABLE 5-3. Substances Found Most Often at Waste Sites Undergoing Remedial Actions[a]

Substance	Percentage of remedial actions[b]
PCBs	23
Pesticides	14
Heavy metals	14
Unspecified organics	9
Toluene	9
Cyanide	7
Benzene	5
Paints	5
Caustic soda	5
Acids	5
Ethyl benzene	4
Trichloroethylene	4
Xylene	4
Information not available	6

[a]From Council on Environmental Quality (10).
[b]Figures add up to more than 100% because more than one type of substance may be found at a site.

may be 1000 to 10,000 feet down. Modern deep wells use such safety features as double or triple casings and leak detection systems. Detecting a leak in the system and remedying it, however, may be impossible because of the nature of the leak and its location. Underground injection wells pose a potential danger to groundwater supplies because of the possible migration of toxic wastes from the injection zone. The difficulty of monitoring the subsurface migration of toxic waste and the uncertainty of the effects of geological disturbances are also major problems associated with the underground injection of toxic wastes. Recent legislation discourages the disposal of hazardous waste in underground injection wells and mandates that the underground injection of hazardous wastes within a quarter mile of a drinking water source be prohibited (10).

Ocean Dumping

The four main types of waste currently being dumped at sea are dredge spoils, industrial waste, sludge from wastewater treatment plants, and radioactive waste (25). Marine disposal sites may be near shore or at deep-water locations. Concern about the disposal of toxic chemicals in the ocean focuses on the accumulation and transfer of metals and xenobiotic (foreign) compounds in marine food chains, on the toxic effects of contaminants on the survival and reproduction of marine organisms, and on the impact on the marine ecosystems (3).

Dredge spoils are dumped at sea near coastal areas. The need to dredge harbor channels regularly makes such dumping very large. Dredge soils cause pollution when the material contains toxic substances. This problem was evident when tests of dredge spoils in New York Harbor revealed high levels of PCBs (25).

The wastes dumped in the ocean include a wide range of inorganic and organic materials. These wastes, stemming from industrial and agricultural sources, include such hazardous agents as arsenic, cadmium, copper, lead, mercury, cyanides, fluorides, pesticides, halogenated organic compounds, resistant plastics, and acids and alkalis (25,38). The dumping of sludge from waste-water treatment plants is another source of marine pollution. Such sludge may contain such heavy metals as mercury, cadmium, and lead. There is also the outflow of waste from stormsewers and landfills. The long-standing practice by fishermen of dumping fishing nets at sea and the dumping of refuse by ships at sea present a significant environmental threat. This problem has intensified because of the worldwide trend of using plastic for fishing nets and for packaging materials. The dumping of low-level radioactive wastes is another source of marine pollution. There is currently a debate on the advisability of disposing radioactive waste in this manner (25,44). A report from the Office of Technology Assessment entitled *Wastes in Marine Environments* emphasizes the increasing problem of coastal marine pollution. This report indicates that unless vigorous efforts are made to bring it under control, marine pollution will continue to pose a significant threat to marine ecology and health (38).

SUMMARY

Virtually all industrial activity generates wastes, much of which pose a danger to health and the environment. The safe and economical disposal of hazardous waste is acknowledged to be a major global challenge. To date, most countries still rely on land disposal methods for hazardous wastes. Strategies to reduce waste generation include changing the manufacturing processes, reusing and recycling methods, and separating and concentrating the waste stream. Although a more vigorous approach is needed to develop waste minimization technologies, it is clear that waste prevention holds the greatest promise to diminish both the costs and the health and environmental hazards associated with hazardous waste production.

REFERENCES

1. Andelman JB, Underhill DW (eds.): Evaluation of Health Effects of Hazardous Waste Sites, Lewis Publishers, Chelsea, Michigan, 1986.

2. Befenati E, Gizzi F, Reginatro R, et al: Polychlorinated dibenzo-*p*-dioxins (TCDD) and polychlorinated dibenzofurans (PCDF) in emissions from an urban incinerator. Chemosphere 12:1151, 1983.

3. Board on Ocean Science and Policy, National Research Council: Disposal of Industrial and Domestic Wastes—Land and Sea Alternatives, National Academy Press, Washington, 1984.

4. Bumb RR, Crummett WB, Cutie SS, et al: Trace chemistries of fire: A source of chlorinated dioxins. Science 210:385, 1980.

5. Castleman BI: International mobility of hazardous products, industries, and wastes. Annu Rev Public Health 8:1, 1987.

6. Cavallaro A, Luciani L, Ceroni G, et al: Summary of results of PCDDs: Analysis from incinerator effluents. Chemosphere 11:859, 1982.

7. Committee on Ground Water Quality Protection, National Research Council: Ground Water Quality Protection, National Academy Press, Washington, 1986.

8. Committee on Institutional Considerations in Reducing the Generation of Hazardous Industrial Wastes: Reducing Hazardous Waste Generation—An Evaluation and a Call for Action, National Academy Press, Washington, 1985.

9. Committee to Provide Interim Oversight of the DOE Nuclear Weapons Complex: The Nuclear Weapons Complex, National Academy Press, Washington, 1989.

10. Council on Environmental Quality: Environmental Quality, 15th Annual Report 1984, US Government Printing Office, Washington, 1986.

11. Dellinger B: Theory and practice of the development of a practical index of hazardous waste incinerability. In: Hazard Assessment of Chemicals, Vol 6, p 293, Saxena J (ed.), Hemisphere Publishing, Washington, 1989.

12. Ditz D: The phase out of North Sea incineration. Int Environ Affairs 1:175, 1989.

13. El-Hinnawi E, Hashmi MH: The State of the Environment, United National Environment Programme, Butterworth, London, 1987.

14. Elkington J, Shopley J: Cleaning Up: US Waste Management Technology and Third World Development, World Resources Institute, Washington, D.C., 1989.

15. Geophysics Study Committee, National Research Council: Groundwater Contamination. National Academy Press, Washington, 1984.

16. Governors Office of Appropriate Technology: Alternatives to the Land Disposal of Hazardous Wastes: An Assessment for California, State of California, Sacramento, 1981.

17. Griffin RD: Principles of Hazardous Material Management. Lewis Publishers, Chelsea, Michigan, 1988.

18. Grisham JW (ed.): Health Aspects of the Disposal of Waste Chemicals. Pergamon, New York, 1986.

19. Harris RH, English CW, Highland JH: Hazardous waste disposal: Emerging technologies and public policies to reduce public health risks. Annu Rev Public Health 6:269, 1985.

20. Highland JH (ed.): Hazardous Waste Disposal, Ann Arbor Science, Ann Arbor, 1982.

21. Holden PW: Board on Agriculture, National Research Council: Pesticides and Groundwater Quality: Issues and Problems in Four States, National Academy Press, Washington, 1986.

22. Kimbrough RD, Jensen AA (eds.): Halogenated Biphenyls, Terphenyls, Naphthalenes, Dibenzodioxins and Related Products, 2nd ed. Elsevier, Amsterdam, 1989.

23. National Institute of Environmental Health Sciences (Sponsor): Research needs for evaluation of health effects of toxic waste dumps (special issue). Environ Health Perspect 48:1, 1983.

24. Oppelt ET: Incineration of hazardous waste. J Air Pollut Control Assoc 37:558, 1987.

25. Organisation for Economic Co-operation and Development: The State of the Environment 1985, OECD, Paris, 1985.

26. Peirce JJ, Vesilind PA: Hazardous Waste Management. Butterworth, London, 1981.

27. Pye VI, Patrick R: Ground water contamination in the United States. Science 221:713, 1983.

28. Senkan SM, Stauffer NW: What to do with hazardous waste. Technol Rev 84:34, 1981.

29. Symposium on Science and Society: Low-level radioactive waste, controversy and resolution: Committee on Public Health. Bull NY Acad Med 65:423–553, 1989.

30. United Nations Environment Programme: 1989 State of the World Environment, UNEP, Geneva, 1989.

31. United Nations Environment Programme: Environmental Guidelines for Handling, Treatment and Disposal of Hazardous Wastes. Environment Management Guidelines No. 18, United Nations Environment Programme, Geneva, 1990.

32. Upton AC, Kneip T, Toniolo P: Public health aspects of toxic chemical disposal sites. Annu Rev Public Health 10:1, 1989.

33. US Congress, Office of Technology Assessment: Technologies and Management Strategies for Hazardous Waste Control, OTA-M-197, US Government Printing Office, Washington, 1983.

34. US Congress, Office of Technology Assessment: Protecting the Nation's Groundwater from Contamination, OTA-8-233, US Government Printing Office, Washington, 1984.

35. US Congress, Office of Technology Assessment: Superfund Strategy, OTA-ITE-252, US Government Printing Office, Washington, 1985.

36. US Congress, Office of Technology Assessment: Serious Reduction of Hazardous Wastes, OTA-ITE-317, US Government Printing Office, Washington, 1986.

37. US Congress, Office of Technology Assessment: From Pollution to Prevention: A Progress Report on Waste Reduction—Special Report, OTA-ITE-347, US Government Printing Office, Washington, 1987.

38. US Congress, Office of Technology Assessment: Waste in Marine Environments, OTA-O-334, US Government Printing Office, Washington, 1987.

39. US Environmental Protection Agency: Remedial Actions at Hazardous Waste Sites: Survey and Case Studies, US Government Printing Office, Washington, 1981.

40. US Environmental Protection Agency: Minimization of Hazardous Wastes, EPA/520-SW-86 033A, US Government Printing Office, Washington, 1986.

41. US Environmental Protection Agency: National Priorities List Fact Book, US Government Printing Office, Washington, 1986.

42. US Environmental Protection Agency: National Priorities List: Supplementary Lists and Supporting Materials, HW10.14S, US Government Printing Office, Washington, 1990.
43. US Environmental Protection Agency: Toxics in the Community, National and Local Perspectives, The 1988 Toxic Release Inventory National Report, EPA 560/4-90-017, US Government Printing Office, Washington, 1990.
44. World Health Organization: Management of Hazardous Waste Policy Guidelines and Code of Practice, WHO Regional Publications, European Series No 14, WHO, Geneva, 1983.

RECOMMENDED READINGS

Committee on Environmental Epidemiology: Environmental Epidemiology, Vol. 1. Public Health and Hazardous Wastes, National Academy Press, Washington, 1991.
Griffin RD: Principles of Hazardous Materials Management, Lewis Publishers, Chelsea, Michigan, 1988.
US Congress Office of Technology Assessment: Superfund Strategy, OTA-ITE-252, US Government Printing Office, Washington, 1985.
US Congress Office of Technology Assessment: Serious Reduction of Hazardous Waste, OTA-ITE-317, US Government Printing Office, Washington, 1986.

Part III

BODY DEFENSE AGAINST EXPOSURE TO ENVIRONMENTAL CHEMICALS AND PHYSICAL AGENTS

6. THE SKIN

David R. Bickers

INTRODUCTION

The skin is a marvelous organ that functions as one of the body's major interfaces with the environment and, in that anatomic position, has at least two major functional requirements. First, it must provide a protective barrier that severely limits the ability of potentially toxic agents in the environment to penetrate into the body where injurious effects can occur. Conversely, the skin must also limit the egress of essential body constituents into the environment. The second major functional requirement for this organ is sufficient flexibility and elasticity to permit maximum freedom of movement while simultaneously possessing enough tensile strength to resist tearing by physical forces in the environment.

EPIDERMIS

Keratin

These functional requirements are well served by the structural components of human skin. This organ consists of two major compartments: the outermost epidermis and the underlying dermis (Fig. 6-1). The epidermis is a stratified squamous epithelium consisting of a basal layer of replicating cells and a spinous (prickle-cell) and granular layer of nonreplicating keratinocytes, which evolve into the stratum corneum on the surface. The stratum corneum (horny layer) is rich in keratins, a family of helical proteins of 40–70 kilodaltons (kd). A series of orderly changes in keratin polypeptide synthesis occurs during the differentiation of epidermal basal

Principles and Practice of Environmental Medicine, edited by Alyce Bezman Tarcher. Plenum Medical Book Company, New York, 1992.

cells into the acellular stratum corneum. Thus, it can be said that in normal human epidermis, keratin subunits of less than 60 kd are usually found in the basal epidermal cells; as the keratinocyte differentiates and migrates upward toward the stratum corneum, keratin polypeptides greater than 60 kd can be isolated. It is of interest that in both cultured keratinocytes and malignant epidermal tumors such as squamous cell carcinoma, the keratin patterns with regard to size distribution of subunits are quite similar to those observed in normal basal cells (25,31). The latter finding is consistent with the changes in terminal differentiation that characterize cultured keratinocytes and malignant epidermal tumors. Furthermore, it has now been shown that in epidermal neoplasms there are masked mRNA species coding for high-molecular-weight keratin polypeptides that are untranslatable. This could explain the failure of the tumors to express these higher-molecular-weight keratins that are present in normally differentiating epidermis.

In addition to keratin polypeptides, terminally differentiated keratinocytes also synthesize a protein envelope beneath the plasma membrane. In cultured cells, the envelope contains a soluble cytoplasmic precursor protein known as involucrin, which is stabilized by a cross-linking reaction catalyzed by the calcium-dependent enzyme transglutaminase (7). Intermolecular (L-glutamyl)-lysine bonds are produced in the granular layer, and this results in the synthesis of an insoluble envelope that is highly resistant to chemical degradation. A biochemically and immunochemically distinct protein has been identified in bovine and in human epidermis in vivo and has been called keratolinin (32). This soluble precursor of the envelope has a molecular weight of 36,000. Keratolinin and transglutaminase both participate in the elaboration of the insoluble envelope in vivo.

In addition to keratin filaments and the cell

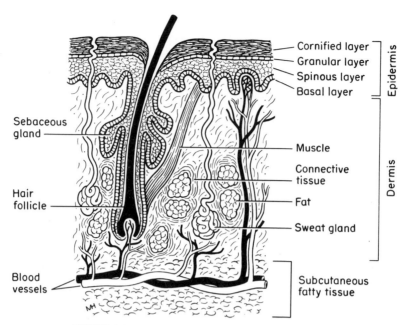

FIGURE 6-1. Diagram of a cross-section of human skin.

envelope, the stratum corneum contains a matrix protein known as filaggrin, within which the keratin filaments are embedded (18). This matrix material is an unusually polar cationic protein, rich in histidine, that aggregates with keratin filaments to form macrofibrils. Most believe that this structural pattern in the stratum corneum plays a major role in providing a barrier to percutaneous absorption of environmental chemicals into human skin.

Lipid

In addition to keratin, the epidermis is rich in a variety of polar and nonpolar lipids that are also thought to play an essential role in epidermal barrier function (8). The lipids found on the surface of human skin are predominantly elaborated by sebaceous glands with a small contribution by the epidermal cells themselves. The stratum corneum contains a complex mixture of polar and nonpolar lipids in its intercellular spaces that are important in protecting against water loss. These lipids evolve from lamellar granules in the granular layer (also known as Odland bodies or membrane-coating granules) that consist of polar non-phosphorus-containing lipids. The lamellar granules are extruded into the intercellular spaces, where they reassemble into sheets between the cells. In the terminally differentiated stratum corneum, the individual keratinocytes shrink and become dehydrated to contain

densely packed keratin embedded in filaggrin. Thus, the stratum corneum can be conceptualized as a multilayered stacking of dense keratinized cells embedded in lipid-rich matrix.

Although the predominant source of lipids in human skin is the sebaceous gland, it is now clear that epidermal cells themselves also elaborate a variety of lipids including ceramides, glucosylceramides, cholesterol, free fatty acids, and phospholipids. In the stratum corneum the vast majority of the lipids of epidermal origin consist of ceramides, cholesterol, and free fatty acids.

The critical importance of stratum corneum lipids in water homeostasis is illustrated by the effects of linoleic acid deficiency, in which the skin becomes scaly, the lamellar granules disappear, and the ability to preclude water transport across the epidermis is markedly diminished (30). Other studies have shown that an acyl-glucosylceramide-containing linoleic acid is a major constituent of normal epidermal lipid. In the linoleic-acid-deficient animal, linoleic acid is replaced by oleate, which undoubtedly plays an important role in the failure of the lamellar granules to assemble. This leads to impaired ability of the epidermis to inhibit water loss into the environment and gives the skin a "dry" and "scaling" appearance.

An additional role for these lipids is in stratum corneum cell adhesion. Free sterols are a major constituent of cell membranes (25–50% lipid by weight). Cholesterol as well as glucocorticosteroids, which are ultimately derived from cholesterol, exert important effects on membrane function. In the inherited disorder of keratinization known as recessive X-linked ichthyosis, there is increased adherence or "stickiness" of the cells in the stratum corneum. This results in the prolonged retention of these cells on the skin surface and increased scaliness of the skin. Patients with this disease are deficient in the enzyme known as steroid sulfatase, which normally desulfates various steroid moieties including cholesterol. This enzyme deficiency results in the accumulation of cholesterol sulfate in the skin and other tissues (10). The enhanced stickiness of the cells that accompanies increased cholesterol sulfate could result from an increase in electronegative charge imparted by the sterol. In normal individuals the enzyme catalyzes the gradual removal of sulfate groups from the cholesterol, rendering the membrane lipids in the intercellular space less electronegative and less sticky. This permits orderly shedding of corneocytes. These observations reemphasize that although cells in the stratum corneum have lost their nuclei and other organelles essential to life, they are not truly dead or inert as had previously been thought.

In addition to keratinocytes human epidermis contains two distinct types of cells that are of great importance in the interaction of body with its environment. These are Langerhans cells and melanocytes.

Langerhans Cells

It has become apparent in recent years that the skin is a major site of immunologic responsiveness in the body. Cutaneous tissue is provided with a unique collection of lymphoid cells, reticular cells, and organized lymphoid organs that have been given the name skin-associated lymphoid tissues (SALT) (28). A major function of this immunologic system is the processing and presentation of antigen to lymphocytes by dentritic cells known as epidermal Langerhans cells (12). Lymph nodes adjacent to the skin respond to immunogenic signals derived from these processed antigens. Subsets of circulating T lymphocytes exhibit a unique affinity for the skin that is determined, at least in part, by differentiation signals received in situ from resident cutaneous cells (28). Furthermore, epidermal cell-derived thymocyte-activating factor (ETAF), which is biochemically and functionally similar if not identical to interleukin 1 (IL-1), is known to be elaborated by keratinocytes (16). This coordinated system of keratinocytes, Langerhans cells, and imunocompetent lymphocytes provides the skin with an effective method of immune surveillance that likely plays a pivotal role in protecting the body against cutaneous

neoplasm and certain types of infections. This hypothesis is consistent with the concept that the immune system serves an important sensory function for the body. It possesses the capacity to recognize and to mount a response to a variety of noncognitive stimuli such as bacteria, viruses, and antigens (4).

For example, it is now appreciated that the interaction of the skin with solar radiation may evoke a variety of responses including the induction of suppressor T-cell activity in response to antigenic stimulation. This response may contribute to the strong association between ultraviolet radiation and skin cancer that occurs in human populations (14).

Melanocytes

The major epidermal cell, in addition to keratinocytes and Langerhans cells, that has important interactions with the environment is the melanocyte. The melanocyte is a dendritic cell that contains specialized organelles known as melanosomes within which the pigment melanin is produced. The melanosomes are transferred to adjacent keratinocytes by the dendritic processes that characterize the melanocyte. Melanin pigmentation is the major determinant of skin color in humans. It should be emphasized that the variability of human skin color derives not from differences in the number and distribution of melanocytes but rather from differences in the rate at which melanosomes are produced by these cells and the extent of their melanization (20). Melanin pigmentation or tanning is increased by exposure of the skin to environmental solar radiation. Tanning involves two distinct photobiological processes known as immediate pigment darkening and delayed tanning. Immediate pigment darkening occurs during or immediately after sun exposure and is induced primarily by ultraviolet A radiation (320–400 nm). It is not the result of new melanin synthesis but rather of the photooxidation of previously existing melanin pigment and changes in the distribution pattern of melanosomes. Delayed tanning, on the other hand, is an active process in which newly synthesized melanosomes are produced. This response is maximal 48–72 h after sun exposure, and the major action spectrum is in the ultraviolet B (UVB), 290–320 nm.

The major function of melanin pigmentation in the skin appears to be photoprotection against ultraviolet injury, both acute (e.g., sunburn) and chronic (e.g., skin cancer). This protective effect is related to one or more of the properties of the compound. Structurally, melanin is a complex polymer the synthesis of which begins with the amino acid tyrosine, which is converted by the enzyme tyrosinase into dihydroxyphenylalanine (DOPA), which in turn yields indole structures that polymerize into the complex pigment known as melanin. Melanin exerts its photoprotective effect by the attenuation of impinging radiation through a process of scatter and conversion to heat. Melanin has a very broad absorption in the ultraviolet and visible spectra and is an effective quencher of free radicals generated in the epidermis as a consequence of sun exposure. The critical importance of melanin for the photoprotection of human skin is dramatically illustrated by the exquisite sun sensitivity of individuals with various types of albinism in whom melanin synthesis is defective.

In addition to the stimulation of epidermal melanin synthesis, solar radiation is capable of enhancing the production of vitamin D_3 in the epidermis (19). This hormone, elaborated in the skin by solar radiation, then moves to the liver and kidney where subsequent metabolic modifications produce 1,25-dihydroxyvitamin D, which plays a critical role in calcium homeostasis.

From this brief description it can be appreciated that the epidermis possesses a complex array of structural components that play important roles in protecting the body against a variety of environmental toxins.

DERMIS

The dermis is the much thicker compartment of the skin that underlies the epidermis and essentially is the base on which the stratified squamous epidermal epithelium rests (Fig. 6-1). The epidermal–dermal junction is a complex structure that produces a tightly adherent bond between the two compartments and yet permits the transport of substances from the richly vascular dermis into the avascular epidermis. The major structural components of the dermis include the fibrous proteins collagen and elastin, which are embedded in a ground substance containing glycosaminoglycans. The dermal fibroblast is the major resident cell in the dermis and is capable of synthesizing the various components of this anatomic compartment of the skin.

Collagen

Collagen is the major structural protein of the skin and constitutes at least 90% of the protein in normal human dermis. The collagen molecule is a long and narrow (15Å) structure with an approximate molecular weight of 285,000. It consists of three polypeptides known as α chains, each of which contains approximately 1000 amino acids. These three polypeptide chains are wound ropelike around each other in a right-handed superhelix (29). There are multiple types of collagen depending on the constituent polypeptide chains, each of whose

structure is determined by a single gene. Type I collagen is the major form found in human dermis (9).

Elastin

The second major fibrous protein of the dermis is elastin. Elastin is a linear polypeptide with an approximate molecular weight of 72,000. A unique feature of elastin is the presence of desmosines, which are highly stable covalent cross-links (23).

Collagen and elastin simultaneously provide the skin with tensile strength and with elasticity. It is important to emphasize that these fibrous proteins are embedded in a supporting matrix that is rich in water and in glycosaminoglycans, including hyaluronic acid, chondroitin, chondroitin sulfate, dermatan sulfate, heparin, and heparin sulfate.

Sweat Glands

There are two major types of sweat glands in human skin—eccrine and apocrine. The eccrine sweat glands are widely distributed over the body and consist of two major portions, a secretory coil in the deep dermis or subcutaneous fat and a duct emptying onto the skin surface through which reabsorption can occur. Apocrine sweat glands have a much more limited distribution in the axillary and perineal areas. They are located in close relation to hair follicles and their associated sebaceous glands; their ducts open into the canal of the hair follicle superficial to the opening of the sebaceous gland.

The eccrine sweat rate increases with increasing core body temperature, probably as a result of changes in the preoptic hypothalamic area, which is crucial for the regulation of body temperature (13). The innervation of sweat glands consists primarily of sympathetic postganglionic fibers, but these are cholinergic rather than adrenergic fibers. The elaboration of eccrine sweat glands by changes in body temperature provides a major thermoregulatory system for the human body. Coupled with the exceedingly rich dermal vascular supply, which has an exquisitely sensitive mechanism for adjusting cutaneous blood flow, the skin provides a remarkably effective system for maintaining core body temperature in the face of widely fluctuating ambient temperatures in the environment.

The functional importance of eccrine sweat glands is fairly well understood (for excellent reviews see ref. 24), but that of aprocrine glands remains for the most part a mystery.

Sebaceous Glands

Sebaceous glands are holocrine glands located in the dermis immediately adjacent to hair follicles and are present over the entire skin surface except for the palms, soles, and dorsum of the feet. Sebaceous gland secretion is known as sebum and consists of a mixture of lipids that consists primarily of triglycerides (33%), wax esters (25%), and squalene (10%). Sebaceous secretion is enhanced by androgenic hormones and suppressed by estrogens. The functional significance of the surface lipid film (sebaceous lipids and epidermal lipids) in human skin remains unclear. Sebum has mild antibacterial and antifungal effects, but the relevance of these to human resistance to such microbes is unknown. The surface lipid film probably has little or no significance insofar as epidermal barrier function is concerned. However, it has been suggested that lipid-rich sebum could play a role in the excretion from the body of highly lipid-soluble metabolically inert environmental pollutants such as the halogenated hydrocarbons (6). This remains a controversial issue, and studies are needed to confirm or refute this interesting concept.

This brief introduction to the complexity of the skin's anatomy should serve to reemphasize the major importance of this body organ for homeostasis in the increasingly hostile and potentially toxic environment of today's world. In the remaining sections of this chapter the function of the skin as a barrier to percutaneous absorption and as a site of chemical metabolism is discussed. In particular, the role of the epidermal cytochrome P-450-dependent monooxygenase in the toxicology of selected environmental chemicals is considered.

PERCUTANEOUS ABSORPTION

A major functional role of human epidermis is to provide a structural barrier or interface between the environment and the body. As mentioned previously, the outermost layer of the epidermis is the stratum corneum, a thin but compact membrane-like structure some 10 μm in thickness. Several lines of experimental evidence support the concept that the epidermal barrier resides primarily in the stratum corneum. First, it has been shown that prior removal of the stratum corneum greatly enhances transepidermal water loss (5). Second, isolated epidermis in vitro is as effective a barrier to the penetration of a variety of chemicals as is epidermis in vivo (11).

Percutaneous absorption can be arbitrarily broken down into a series of steps or processes as follows. First, molecules of drug or chemical must be absorbed at the surface of the stratum corneum. Second, the molecules must diffuse through the stratum corneum. Third, they must reach the viable epidermis. Fourth, they must move through the viable epidermis into the upper dermis, where they reach the vasculature. Fifth, they must then be transferred into the circulation. Diffusion through the stratum corneum is the rate-limiting step in the sequence, since the remaining processes generally occur quite rapidly.

An appreciation for the factors that regulate percutaneous absorption requires that several terms be defined which can be expressed in an equation, based on the Fick principle, which follows:

$$J = K_p \cdot C$$

$$\text{where } K_p = D \times k_1$$
$$J = (D \times k_1/e) \cdot C$$

J = amount of drug absorbed per unit time and area
K_p = permeability constant
C = difference in concentration above and below the membrane (C_1 and C_2, respectively; C_2 is generally negligible)
D = diffusion constant of the drug in the stratum corneum
k_1 = partition coefficient of the drug between stratum corneum and the vehicle
e = thickness of the stratum corneum

From this equation, several generalizations can be made: (1) the extent of percutaneous absorption will be directly proportional to the diffusion constant of the drug in the stratum corneum, to the partition coefficient between drug and vehicle, and to the amount of drug applied to the skin; (2) the extent of percutaneous absorption will be inversely proportional to the thickness of the stratum corneum.

The diffusion constant is a measurement of the rate of transport of a drug through the stratum corneum. It is inversely proportional to both molecular size and viscosity of the cells. The extremely high viscosity of the stratum corneum renders the diffusion constant of most substances quite low (of the order of 10^{-9} cm^2 s^{-1} for alcohols and 10^{-12} to 10^{-13} cm^2 s^{-1} for steroids). In contrast, viable keratinocytes have diffusion constants closer to 10^{-6} cm^2 s^{-1}.

Because the stratum corneum behaves in many ways like a lipophilic membrane, drugs with relatively high lipid:water partition coefficients have relatively high permeability constants. Thus, when k_1 is high, the drug moves rapidly into the stratum corneum from the surface and is, therefore, adjacent to the viable keratinocytes of the epidermis, whence the drug can move rapidly across intercellular spaces and through the epidermis. Slight water solubility is also necessary for percutaneous absorption. Drugs that are purely lipid soluble or largely water soluble appear to be absorbed rather poorly.

Percutaneous absorption is also greatly influenced by a number of other factors including age, race, degree of hairiness, body region, and degree of hydration of the stratum corneum. The state of hydration of the stratum corneum plays a major role in determining the rate of percutaneous absorption. In general, hydration increases the rate of absorption of all substances, particularly water-soluble compounds, that can permeate the skin. Furthermore, it is known that elevated ambient temperatures and relative humidity both enhance the toxic effects of chemicals in occupational settings. Diseased skin in which barrier function is compromised is more susceptible to water loss and in general is thought to be more permeable to topically applied drugs.

At any given time the hydration of the stratum corneum is dependent on three factors: (1) the rate at which water moves into the stratum corneum from the underlying viable keratinocytes, (2) the rate at which water moves from the stratum corneum into the environment by evaporation, and (3) the capacity of the stratum corneum to retain moisture.

The movement of water through the skin (either from outside to inside or vice versa) is a purely passive process, and the diffusional resistance of the stratum corneum is 1000 times higher than that of the underlying epidermis.

Hydration of the stratum corneum also enhances the percutaneous absorption of many compounds, including salicylic acid and corticosteroids. Hydration is capable of enhancing absorption as much as tenfold, and increasing the temperature from 10°C to 30°C enhances absorption three- to fivefold. These in vitro observations have been confirmed by in vivo studies using occlusive films of thin plastic. The increase in humidity and temperature at the skin surface greatly enhances percutaneous absorption of topically applied compounds.

In addition to penetrating directly through the stratum corneum, drugs may also be capable of "short-circuiting" by way of sebaceous follicles or the sweat apparatus. Immediately following topical application of a drug, there is rapid movement through these shunts. The surface area of hair follicles represents only 0.1% to 0.5% of the surface area of the epidermis, and the diffusion constant through the epidermis is 100 to 10,000 times less than the diffusion constant through the hair follicles. In general, the flux by the two routes rapidly becomes constant so that each participates in absorption. The lag time for percutaneous absorption will, therefore, be determined by the diffusion constant of the agent (the greater the diffusion constant, the less the lag time).

One important consequence of the relative impermeability of the stratum corneum is known as the "reservoir effect." Certain drugs that are slowly released from the stratum corneum may exert pharmacological effects for prolonged periods, especially when the skin is occluded in such a way as to minimize loss of the topically applied compound into the environment.

Percutaneous absorption can also be altered by the solubility characteristics of the vehicle. Thus, drugs that have a relatively high stratum corneum/vehicle partition coefficient will in general have greater percutaneous absorption. Hydration of the stratum corneum with vehicles such as petrolatum will increase percutaneous absorption of drugs. Emulsions, both oil in water (O/W) and water in oil (W/O), alter percutaneous absorption. In general, it seems that the permeability constant is primarily dependent on the partition coefficient between the stratum corneum and the continuous phase of the emulsion.

It may seem ironic that a major area of current pharmacological research is aimed toward the development of drug delivery systems that enhance the percutaneous absorption of drugs. The advantages of this approach include remarkable precision of drug input and prolonged (1–7 days) therapy from a single application (26). In addition, new compounds such as Azone (1-dodecylagacycloheptan-Z-one) can enhance the skin penetration of a number of hydrophobic and hydrophilic drugs (27). The future potential of such agents appears to be substantial; yet, it should be obvious that caution must be exercised lest the indiscriminate use of such agents increase the risk of percutaneous absorption of known toxins.

Generally speaking, the percutaneous absorption of environmental pollutant chemicals causing substantial toxicity in humans has been relatively uncommon. However, there have been instances in which enhanced absorption of topically applied chemicals resulted in a serious health hazard. One example is an experience with the antibacterial compound hexachlorophene. This chemical was added to a variety of cosmetic and soap products for its antibacterial properties for decades with no known toxic effects. Then, suddenly and without warning, a number of infants in France who had been dusted with hexachlorophene-containing talcum powder died (17). As pointed out by Kligman, the lethal combination included (1) the fact that the treated infants were premature, supporting the concept that the epidermal barrier is incomplete until shortly before birth, and (2) the fact that the hexachlorophene was applied to the diaper area, which is generally wet and warm, both of which enhance percutaneous absorption as described above (15).

A second example of the unique susceptibility of the skin of premature infants to enhanced percutaneous absorption of a generally nontoxic substance is that of lindane. Lindane, or γ-benzene hexachloride, is a widely used scabicide that enjoys an excellent record of patient safety. However, application of a conventional formulation of the drug to a premature infant produced a blood level of lindane 17 times greater than that expected after a single topical application (22).

THE SKIN AS A SITE OF CHEMICAL METABOLISM

Skin, the largest organ in man, is commonly thought to function primarily as a passive barrier. Certainly its unique characteristics make it especially well suited for this role. However, in addition to impeding the entrance of noxious agents into the body, the skin also has the ability to metabolize endogenous substrates and exogenous chemicals.

Through its ability to metabolize such agents as drugs, steroid hormones, and chemicals the skin can modify their action. Experimental evidence indicates that xenobiotics entering the body by percutaneous absorption can be altered by the metabolic activity of the skin (3).

The implications of such metabolic activity are significant. Clearly, the skin may catalyze the biotransformation of topically applied drugs and other foreign compounds. In addition, there is strong evidence that the metabolism of certain polycyclic hydrocarbons is necessary for their cutaneous carcinogenic effects (3).

There is solid scientific evidence to show that mammalian epidermis possesses P-450-dependent microsomal enzyme activity required to convert polycyclic aromatic hydrocarbons such as benzo[a]-pyrene into reactive oncogenic metabolites (1,2,21). The enzyme system that carries out this activity is dependent on the heme-protein cytochrome P-450, which functions as its terminal oxidase. This membrane-bound system is capable of metabolizing a broad range of substrates, both endogenous such as hormones and exogenous such as drugs and environmental chemicals. Generally this type of enzyme activity yields metabolites with increased water solubility and enhanced excretability. This results in the pharmacological inactivation of its substrates. However, in some instances this same enzyme system potentiates the toxicity of certain chemicals by converting them into highly reactive metabolites that lead to the induction of cancer and other forms of tissue injury. Individual susceptibility to these forms of enzyme-mediated toxic injury will vary depending on both inherited characteristics and environmental exposure patterns.

The skin has an active P-450-dependent enzyme system, and since cutaneous tissue is a major portal of entry for environmental chemicals, this type of catalytic activity is likely to be a major determinant of the patterns of toxic injury in the skin.

SUMMARY

The skin is a remarkable organ that functions as a critical interface between the body and its environment. The skin is a complex tissue consisting of two major compartments, epidermis and dermis, each of which contains a variety of cell types and organelles. The outermost epidermis contains the stratum corneum, which is the major structural barrier to the percutaneous absorption of environmental chemicals. In addition, there is evidence that the skin has the metabolic capacity to alter chemicals that enter the body by percutaneous absorption. Such activity often results in increased water solubility and enhanced excretion of such agents. In some instances, however, such activity can enhance the toxic effect of certain chemicals.

REFERENCES

1. Akin FJ, Norred WP: Factors affecting measurement of aryl hydrocarbon hydroxylase activity in mouse skin. J Invest Dermatol 67:709, 1976.
2. Bickers DR, Kappas A: The skin as a site of chemical metabolism. In: Extrahepatic Metabolism of Drugs and Other Foreign Compounds, p 295, Gram TE (ed.), SP Medical & Scientific Books, New York, 1980.
3. Bickers DR, Kappas A, Alvares AP: Differences in inducibility of hepatic and cutaneous drug metabolizing enzymes and cytochrome P-450 by polychlorinated biphenyls and 1,1,1-trichloro-2,2-bis(p-chlorophenyl)ethane (DDT). J Pharmacol Exp Ther 188:300, 1974.
4. Blalock JE: The immune system as a sensory organ. J Immunol 132:1067, 1984.
5. Blank IH: Factors which influence the water content of the stratum corneum. J Invest Dermatol 18:433, 1952.
6. Charnetski WA, Stevens WE: Organochlorine insecticide residues in preen glands of ducks: Possibility of residue excretion. Bull Environ Contam Toxicol 12:672, 1974.
7. Cline PR, Rice RH: Modulation of involucrin and envelope competence in human keratinocytes by hydrocortisone, retinyl acetate and growth onset. Cancer Res 43:3203, 1983.
8. Downing DT, Stewart ME, Wertz PW, et al: Skin lipids. Comp Biochem Physiol 4:673, 1983.
9. Epstein EH Jr, Munderloh N: Human skin collagen. Presence of type I and type III at all levels of the dermis. J Biol Chem 253:1336, 1978.
10. Epstein EH Jr, Williams ML, Elias PM: Steroid sulfatase, X-linked ichthyosis, and stratum corneum cell cohesion. Arch Dermatol 117:761, 1981.
11. Franz RT: On the relevance of in vitro data. J Invest Dermatol 64:190, 1975.
12. Granstein RD, Lowy A, Greene MI: Epidermal antigen-presenting cells in activation of suppression: Identification of a new functional type of ultraviolet radiation-resistant epidermal cell. J Immunol 132:563, 1984.

13. Hammel HT: Regulation of internal body temperature. Annu Rev Physiol 30:641, 1968.

14. Hersey P, Haran G, Hasic E, et al: Alteration of T cell subsets and induction of suppressor T cell activity in normal subjects after exposure to sunlight. J Immunol 131:171, 1983.

15. Kligman AM: A biological brief on percutaneous absorption. Drug Dev Ind Pharm 9:521, 1983.

16. Luger TA, Stadler BM, Katz SI, et al: Epidermal cell (keratinocyte)-derived thymocyte activating factor (ETAF). J Immunol 127:1493, 1981.

17. Marzulli FN, Maibach HI: The hexachlorophene story. In: Animal Models in Dermatology, p 156, Maibach HI (ed.), Edinburgh, Churchill-Livingstone, 1975.

18. Meek RL, Lonsdale-Eccles JD, Dale BA: Epidermal filaggrin is synthesized on a large messenger ribonucleic acid as a high-molecular-weight precursor. Biochemistry 22:4867, 1983.

19. Nemanick MK, Whitney J, Arnaud S, et al: Vitamin D_3 production by cultured human keratinocytes and fibroblasts. Biochem Biophys Res Commun 115:444, 1983.

20. Pathak MA, Kowichi J, Szabo G, et al: Sunlight and melanin pigmentation. In: Photochemical and Photobiological Reviews, Vol 1, p 211, Smith KC (ed.), Plenum Press, New York, 1976.

21. Pohl RJ, Philpot RN, Fouts JR: Cytochrome P-450 content and mixed function oxidase activity in microsomes isolated from mouse skin. Drug Metab Dispos 4:442, 1976.

22. Pramanik AK, Hansen RC: Transcutaneous gamma benzene hexachloride absorption and toxicity in infants and children. Arch Dermatol 115:1224, 1979.

23. Rucker RB, Murray J: Cross-linking amino acids in collagen and elastin. Am J Clin Nutr 31:1221, 1978.

24. Sato K: The physiology and pharmacology of the eccrine sweat gland. In: Biochemistry and Physiology of the Skin, Vol 1, p 596, Goldsmith L (ed.), Oxford University Press, Oxford, 1983.

25. Scheweizer J, Winter H: Keratin biosynthesis in normal mouse epithelia and in squamous cell carcinomas. J Biol Chem 258:13268, 1983.

26. Shaw J: Development of transdermal therapeutic systems. Drug Dev Ind Pharm 9:579, 1983.

27. Stoughton RB, McClure WO: Azone: A new non-toxic enhancer of cutaneous penetration. Drug Dev Ind Pharm 9:725, 1983.

28. Streilein JW: Skin-associated lymphoid tissues (SALT): Origins and functions. J Invest Dermatol 80:12s, 1983.

29. Traub W, Piez KA: The chemistry and structure of collagen. Adv Protein Chem 25:243, 1971.

30. Wertz PW, Downing DT: Glycolipids in mammalian epidermis: Structure and function in the water barrier. Science 217:1261, 1982.

31. Winter H, Schweizer J: Keratin synthesis in normal mouse epithelia and in squamous cell carcinomas: Evidence in tumors for masked RNA species coding for high molecular weight keratin polypeptides. Proc Natl Acad Sci USA 80:6480, 1983.

32. Zettergren JG, Peterson LL, Wuepper KD: Keratolinin: The soluble substrate of epidermal transglutaminase from human and bovine tissue. Proc Natl Acad Sci USA 81:238, 1984.

RECOMMENDED READINGS

Blank IH: Protective role of the skin. In: Dermatology in General Medicine, 3rd ed, p 337, Fitzpatrick TB, Eisen AZ, Wolff K, et al. (eds.), McGraw-Hill, New York, 1987.

Bronaugh RL, Maibach HI (eds.): Percutaneous Absorption Mechanisms, Methodology and Drug Delivery, 2nd ed, Marcel Dekker, New York, 1989.

7. THE LUNG

Jeffrey E. Weiland and James E. Gadek

INTRODUCTION

The respiratory tract is unique in its dual role in the maintenance of health and prevention of disease. In addition to its function in gas exchange, the respiratory tract serves an important role in the body's first line of defense against environmental pollutants. Each day the lung is exposed to approximately 10,000 L of air containing large amounts of particulate matter and noxious gases. The manner in which the lung handles this burden influences the toxic injury it sustains and, to a great extent, the health of the entire body (54,75,131,152).

To counteract environmental assault the lung contains a complex integrated system of defenses (Table 7-1). This chapter focuses on those defenses and begins by defining the factors influencing the deposition of inhaled substances. This is followed by a description of the lung's defense mechanisms and an examination of the interactions between these defenses and exposure to various environmental pollutants.

Principles and Practice of Environmental Medicine, edited by Alyce Bezman Tarcher. Plenum Medical Book Company, New York, 1992.

FACTORS INFLUENCING THE DEPOSITION OF INHALED PARTICLES IN THE LUNG

Atmospheric particles that remain airborne for a length of time are defined as aerosols. Not all particles from an inhaled aerosol reach the lower respiratory tract. The most important factor influencing deposition of particles in the lung is particle size or diameter (Fig. 7-1). Although most suspended particles encountered in the environment are irregular in shape, studies on the deposition of particles in the respiratory tract are done using inhaled spheres of various diameters. This technique has revealed three mechanisms governing the deposition of inhaled particles: (1) inertial impaction, (2) sedimentation, and (3) diffusion.

Inertial Impaction

Inertia defines the tendency of particles to remain moving in a straight line despite a change in the direction of air flow. Inertial impaction is most relevant to the deposition of large particles (i.e., greater than 2 μm in diameter). The abrupt changes in direction of air flow in the nasopharynx and the branching tracheobronchial tree produce a baffle-like effect. As a result, most large particles impact in the upper respiratory tract and large airways.

TABLE 7-1.   The Lung's Defense against Environmental Pollutants

Nonspecific defenses
  Filtration and impaction
  Mucociliary system
  Sneezing and coughing
  Epithelial barriers
  Phagocytosis
    Performed by alveolar macrophages and polymorpho-nuclear leukocytes (ingesting particles, killing microbial organisms, presenting antigen to lymphocytes)

Specific immune defenses
  Humoral immunity
    Performed by B lymphocytes and mediated by specific antibodies (IgA, IgG, IgE)

  Cell-mediated immunity
    Performed by T lymphocytes; includes delayed hypersensitivity reaction and T-cell cytotoxicity

Biochemical defenses
  Protective proteins
    α_1-Antitrypsin, α_2-macroglobulin, etc.

  Antioxidant mechanisms
    Antioxidant enzyme systems, i.e., catalase, superoxide dismutases, enzymes of the glutathione redox cycle. Fat-soluble antioxidants, i.e., vitamin E, β-carotene, bilirubin
    Water-soluble antioxidants, i.e., vitamin C, uric acid, cysteine, etc.

  Pulmonary metabolism of xenobiotics
    Mixed-function oxidases present in type II, Clara, tracheal bronchial epithelial and ciliated cells and pulmonary macrophages

Sedimentation

Particles suspended in air fall or sediment under the influence of gravity. Each particle falls at a constant rate determined by the viscosity of the surrounding gas, the particle density, and the square of its diameter. This constant rate is defined as the terminal velocity. Although sedimentation is important in the deposition of all particles throughout the respiratory tract, it markedly influences particles of intermediate size (0.1 μm to 50 μm). Sedimentation is therefore a major factor in the deposition of particles in the small airways and alveoli.

Diffusion

The constant collisions between suspended air particles and molecules result in random movement termed Brownian motion. This motion causes particles to diffuse from one area or volume of gas to another. Since the distances involved are minute, diffusion is important in the deposition of small particles (less than 2 μm) in the terminal bronchioles and alveoli.

Other Factors

Other factors influencing the deposition of particles in the lung include air flow and patterns of breathing. Thus, the nature of air flow in the airways is complex. It has been shown that air flow in the nasopharynx and large airways is most likely turbulent, whereas flow in the small airways and alveoli is laminar (96,151). Turbulent air flow enhances deposition by inertial impaction and diffusion. Although

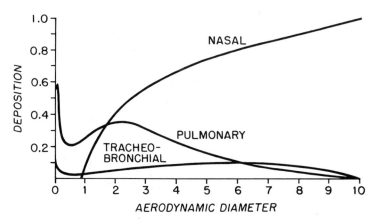

FIGURE 7-1. Deposition as a function of particle size for 15 respirations/min, 750-cm³ tidal volume. From Task Group on Lung Dynamics (133).

the airways become smaller with each successive division, the cross-sectional area actually increases enormously because of the increase in the number of airways. Therefore, for a given volume of inspired gas, velocity of air flow falls precipitously as respiratory bronchioles are approached. Thus, in the terminal elements of the respiratory tract, deposition of particles is a result of sedimentation and diffusion. The breathing pattern (tidal volume and frequency) affects the velocity of air flow and therefore the pattern of particulate deposition. For example, if minute ventilation is held constant, rapid, small tidal volumes decrease deposition in the distal airways and lung (decreased time for diffusion and sedimentation), whereas slow deep breathing increases deposition.

In summary, the physical properties of the particles, along with the anatomy of the respiratory tract and the type of breathing, are the principal determinants of the patterns and amounts of aerosols deposited within the lung.

FACTORS INFLUENCING THE UPTAKE OF POLLUTANT GASES

Nonparticulate pollutant gases behave to some extent as simple solutions. Therefore, several factors determine how much and at what location pollutant gases will be absorbed in the respiratory tract. These factors include solubility, flow rate, and duration of exposure.

Solubility

Solubility defines the tendency of a solute (pollutant gas) to dissolve in a solvent (fluid lining). In the context of gaseous effects on lung function, the "solvent" is the epithelial lining fluid. Thus, the more soluble a gas, the more likely it is to be absorbed in the more proximal portion of the respiratory tract. The solubility of many of the pollutant gases in water is known. However, until the characteristics and chemical composition of the fluid lining the respiratory tract are better defined, only rough estimates can be made regarding their solubility in this fluid.

Flow Rate

Aharonson's studies demonstrate that increasing rates of air flow increase the absorption of gases in the nose (1). Although the mechanism is unknown, it is possible that an increase in turbulent flow prolongs the contact of gases with the mucosal surface. Also, increased flow may cause a fall in temperature, thereby augmenting the solubility of pollutant gases.

Duration of Exposure

The duration of exposure may alter absorption by either of two mechanisms. First, the longer a gas is in contact with a liquid, the more time there is for equilibrium to occur and absorption to take place. Second, over time, pollutant gases may alter the chemical and ionic composition of the lining fluid and thereby increase absorption.

NONSPECIFIC DEFENSES

Mucociliary System

The mucociliary system is of prime importance in the lung's defense against inhaled particles (147). This system is largely responsible for cleansing the lung. Particles deposited on the mucus cover of the respiratory tract are propelled, by ciliary action, toward the pharynx. Here mucous, particulates, and cellular debris from the nasal cavity and lung meet and are mixed with saliva prior to being swallowed. The anatomy and physiology of the respiratory tract are well designed to support this cleansing action.

The respiratory epithelial cells most important for airway cleansing are the basal, ciliated columnar, epithelial mucous, and epithelial serous cells (Fig. 7-2). The luminal side of the epithelium is covered by a thin layer of mucous. The submucosal area containing abundant glands, both mucus and serous, is the main source of the mucus. The basal cell, being of endodermal origin, serves as the stem cell from which the overlying superficial cells develop. The ciliated columnar cells line the airways from the proximal trachea to the terminal bronchioles. Each cell contains approximately 200 cilia, which beat about 1000 times per minute in a craniad direction. The epithelial mucous (goblet) cell resembles the mucous cells of the submucosal glands. They are irregularly distributed through the airways, with the largest number located in the cartilage-containing airways. Goblet cells, containing large secretory granules, synthesize mainly acidic glycoproteins, an important constituent of mucus. Epithelial serous cells, having a distribution similar to the goblet cells, are thought to secrete neutral glycoproteins (a constituent of mucus), lysozyme, and the epithelial secretory component of IgA (11,69,127).

The submucosa, as previously noted, contains abundant secretory glands, which are located mainly in the cartilage-containing airways. They are not present in the bronchioles. These submucosal glands are the main source of mucus. They are also thought to be a source of lysozyme and the epithelial transfer factor for secretory IgA. Airway mucus is a complex mixture of water (95%), inorganic salts

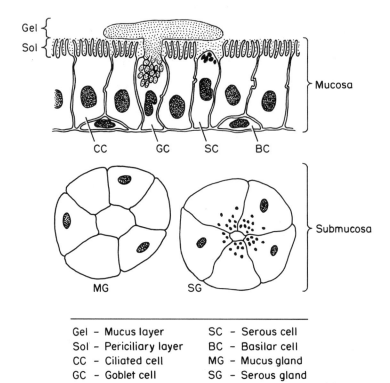

FIGURE 7-2. Diagram of airway mucosa. Adapted from Cong and Drage (25).

(1%), glycoproteins (2%), and other proteins and lipids (2%) (9,11,111).

In 1934 Lucas and Douglas proposed that airway mucus (93) is composed of two layers: a periciliary layer (sol) covered by a mucous layer (gel) (Fig. 7-2). The origin of the periciliary layer is not known. It may arise from liquefaction of the mucous layer from ciliary beating. More likely, it arises from the active transport of water and solute across the airway epithelium (107). The mucous layer arises primarily from the submucosal glands. Rather than being a continuous blanket, the mucous layer is thought to be discontinuous, with islands of mucus resting on the periciliary layer. Mucus is essential for particle transport. Functioning cilia are unable to transport particles in the absence of mucus. This requirement appears to be physical rather than chemical, since other substances with similar physical properties can substitute for the mucus (80).

Transport Mechanisms

The physical transport of inhaled particles from the lung can be divided into two distinct anatomic compartments. The first, mucociliary transport, involves particles deposited on the tracheobronchial tree. The second, alveolar transport, which is much more complex, involves particles deposited on the alveolar surface.

Studies on the removal of mucus from the lung have centered on two related mechanisms—transport and clearance. Transport is measured in anatomically defined lung units by depositing a marker substance on the respiratory epithelium and calculating the velocity of movement. Clearance is measured by determining the amount of an inhaled radioactive marker that is eliminated with time.

Animal studies show that mucociliary transport averages 10–20 mm min^{-1}. However, there are large variations. Transport is slowest in small bronchioles and fastest in the proximal trachea, where ciliated cells are more numerous and mucus is more abundant (12,66). These studies also show that mucus velocity is proportional to ciliary beat frequency and amplitude and therefore decreases with increasing viscosity of the periciliary layer (8). Studies of overall clearance show a biphasic pattern. An early rapid phase (24 h) represents mucociliary transport, and a late, prolonged phase (days to months) represents alveolar transport (111).

Alveolar transport appears to be much more

complex than airway transport. Removal of particles occurs by either of two routes, intracellular or extracellular. It is generally agreed that the intracellular pathway handles most of the inhaled particles deposited on the alveolar surface. The cell primarily involved in this pathway is the alveolar macrophage, which ingests the inhaled particle. After this process, most of the macrophages then migrate, or are carried by alveolar fluids, to the respiratory bronchiole, where they exit via the mucociliary ladder. This mode of removal is relatively rapid (less than 24 h) and efficient. A smaller number of macrophages ingest particles, migrate, and come to rest in the peribronchial and perivascular connective tissue. This route of migration is not well understood; however, it may involve crossing the walls of the alveoli and migrating toward the hilum. More likely, the macrophages may cross the epithelium of the bronchi or bronchioles (126). This mode of clearance is much slower, as particle-laden macrophages are found in the peribronchial connective tissue weeks to months after initial exposure.

Although the mechanism involved in the removal of extracellular particles from the alveolar surface has not been fully characterized, it probably occurs by either of two routes. The first is via the mucociliary ladder, and the second is via the lymphatics. Most particles are swept across the alveolar surface and deposited in the bronchioles. They exit via the mucociliary ladder. The fluid needed for the extracellular clearance of particles probably arises through transudation from alveolar capillaries and cellular secretions. The energy for fluid movement is thought to result from mechanical tension placed on alveolar septae by respiratory movements (50). It is postulated that as the pulmonary lobule expands during inspiration, mechanical tension is placed on the alveolar walls. Since the central lobular and subpleural areas are attached to fixed structures (airways and pleura), the mechanical tension is greatest in the midzonal areas of the lobule and least in the central lobular and subpleural areas. On this basis alveolar fluid and particles are forced centripetally towards the bronchioles and centrifugally towards the paraseptal and subpleural areas. This action could account for the patterns of particle clearance found in alveoli.

The second mode of exit, used by only a small percentage of extracellular particles, is via the pulmonary lymphatics. The pulmonary lymphatics play a more important role in the immunologic defense of the lung. This role is discussed in detail later. The lymphatic vessels begin as blind pouches in the area of the bronchoalveolar junction. These vessels gradually increase in size as they follow the bronchial tree and pulmonary artery (centrilobular) or the venous drainage (perilobular) and finally converge on the hilum.

Interspersed along the course of the lymphatics, particularly at branch points of bronchioles, are collections of lymphocytes and mononuclear cells resembling the Peyer's patches of the gastrointestinal tract. It has long been thought that these cellular collections served as sumps, processing material absorbed from the bronchial surface. However, Green has shown that the transfer of cell particles and lymph clearly occurs in both directions (49). Thus, the lymphoid nodules may serve as sumps to absorb fluid during times of bronchoalveolar flooding. Under normal conditions these nodules serve as exit pathways, allowing material to be deposited from the alveoli directly on the mucociliary ladder (13). Since there are no lymphatic vessels in the alveolar walls, the mechanism of lymph drainage from the alveoli and alveolar walls remain largely unknown (86).

Alveolar Fluids

The alveolar lining fluid is a complex mixture of phospholipids, neutralipids, protein, and carbohydrates. In addition, immunoglobulins G and A, transferrin, glutathione, α_1-antitrypsin, ceruloplasmin, and complement fragments are also found in the epithelial lining fluid (119). This fluid, in part, has surface active properties that prevent the alveoli from collapsing at low lung volumes (103). The alveolar lining fluid also undoubtedly plays an important role in the lungs' defense. It contributes to this defense by "nonspecific" and "specific" mechanisms, both of which aid the alveolar macrophage in its role of phagocytosis.

The marked difference in surface tension between an inhaled particle and the alveolar lining fluid increases the rapid and random movement of the particle. This action in turn increases the likelihood that the particle will come into contact with a phagocytic cell. In addition, specific immunoglobulin and complement factors present in the lining fluid facilitate the uptake of particles by the aveolar macrophage. Finally, ceruloplasmin, transferrin, and glutathione, proteins found in the alveolar lining fluid, may also provide protection against reactive oxidant species (16).

Cough

In general, cough is a symptom of disease in the respiratory tract. It is also a method of clearance for the lungs when other clearance mechanisms (mucociliary transport, lymphatic drainage) are overwhelmed. The mechanics of coughing achieve a high linear velocity by the expired air. This is accomplished by creating high initial expiratory flows coupled with a decreasing cross-sectional area of the airways. Cough originates primarily from irritation of one or more receptors located in the larynx, trachea, and bronchi. It may also originate in such diverse locations as the nose, ear, diaphragm, esophagus, stomach, and pericardium. The stimulus is carried, via the vagus nerve, to a "cough center" in the central nervous system. The efferent response returns via the vagus, phrenic, and other spinal motor nerves to the muscles of expiration.

Cough begins with a deep inspiration to a large lung volume. This tends to maximize expiratory flow rates by increasing the static recoil forces of the lung and decreasing airway resistance (by increasing the caliber of the airway). The glottis closes, and intercostal and abdominal muscles forcefully contract, dramatically increasing intrathoracic pressure. The glottis is forced open, producing a rapid flow of air. High linear velocity of flow is required to expectorate material from the airway wall. This condition, maintained by dynamic compression of the airways, is the result of the high intrathoracic pressures generated during cough (100).

Phagocytic Cells

The phagocytosis of inhaled particles is a major component of the lungs' defense mechanisms. Phagocytosis is important for keeping the airways and the alveolar surface free from debris. Phagocytosis may also exclude certain antigens from access to the immune system while helping others to be presented to this system. These functions are performed mainly by the alveolar macrophage and polymorphonuclear granulocytes (neutrophils).

The alveolar macrophage is the premiere phagocytic cell in the lung. The major functions of the macrophage in the lung's defense are to (1) isolate ingested particles by phagocytosis, (2) act as a vehicle for physical transport of particles through the lungs, and (3) detoxify inhaled and phagocytized material (52). However, as discussed below, the macrophage may, through elaboration of various substances into the extracellular environment, injure as well as protect the lung.

The origin of the alveolar macrophage has been debated for years. Langevoort proposed that this cell arose from the pleuripotential stem cell of the bone marrow (84). This concept is now generally accepted because of the evidence provided in 1976 by Thomas (136). Since alveolar macrophages are also capable of replication, a small percentage may arise in situ from other alveolar macrophages (46). The fate of the macrophage after phagocytosis depends to a large extent on the type of particle it ingests (123). Some particle-laden macrophages may be swept across the alveolar surface and rapidly exit via the mucociliary ladder. Other macrophages, after ingesting such toxic particles as silica dust, may die and leak cellular constituents onto the al-veolar surface. Finally, some macrophages may move through the alveolar well into the interstitium, thereby migrating to the bronchoalveolar junction and the associated lymphatic nodule. Here, the cells may exit onto the bronchiolar surface or pass into the lymphatic system. Though the lymphatic exit pathway is of minor importance for clearance, it has major implications for the immune defense of the lung.

The role of the macrophage in the immune defense is multifaceted (10). The macrophage not only minimizes the exposure of the lung cells to toxic or infectious agents but also plays a central role in the development of specific immunity. Its role in properly "presenting" antigen to lung lymphocytes makes the macrophage essential in both humoral and cell-mediated immune responses in the lung (85). This cooperation between the macrophage and lung lymphocyte appears to be reciprocal. The induction of specific immunity via aerosolized antigens results in enhanced metabolic activity ("activation") of the alveolar macrophage. This presumably occurs as a result of the interaction between the macrophages and antigen-specific lung T lymphocytes (74).

Phagocytosis can be divided into four separate steps: (1) chemotaxis, (2) attachment, (3) ingestion, and (4) digestion. Phagocytosis is facilitated by the physical properties of the alveolar lining fluid. It is also facilitated by the ability of the macrophage to move within the lung in response to various chemotactic stimuli (149). Once the macrophage is in close proximity to the foreign particle, attachment may occur either by electrostatic surface interaction or by cell binding via specific opsonins (129). Opsonins are broadly defined as molecules that enhance the attachment and subsequent phagocytosis of particles to which they are bound. Within the lung the most important opsonins are immunoglobulin G and the C3b fragment of complement. The surface of the alveolar macrophage contains specific receptors for both IgG and C3b, thus completing the "bridge" between the phagocytic cell and the inhaled particle (115).

Ingestion is an active energy-dependent process whereby the cell membrane gradually surrounds a particle and engulfs it. This segment of the membrane is then "pinched off" to form the phagosome. There is evidence that the macrophage cytoplasm contains microfilaments composed of actin and myosin. These play a role in the membrane changes associated with phagocytosis (130). The macrophage is well suited for the digestion of the ingested particles. It contains lysosomes with a full array of hydrolases and neutral proteases. After particles are ingested, the lysosomes gradually fuse with and empty their contents into the phagosomes. This leads to breakdown of the ingested material.

Since the macrophage is also rich in endoplasmic reticulum, it is capable of continuous enzyme and protein synthesis.

In the process of phagocytosis, the macrophage produces superoxide anion and hydrogen peroxide. These reactive species of molecular oxygen play a role in the killing of ingested microorganisms (56). Phagocytosis of either infectious or noninfectious particles leads to a generalized activation of the macrophage. This process is characterized by increased oxygen and glucose utilization and the release of various soluble mediators and enzymes useful in the lung's defense (10,56). In addition to its role in the "presentation" of antigens to lymphocytes, the macrophage may regulate lymphocyte function by secretion of a lymphocyte-activating factor (interleukin 1) (141). This soluble mediator appears to be one component of the interaction between the macrophage and lymphocyte in cell-mediated immune reactions. It is also thought that this macrophage product functions as an "endogenous pyrogen." The macrophage also secretes a colony-stimulating factor (a mediator that stimulates the clonal growth of bone marrow cells) and a chemotactic factor for neutrophils (46,62). This chemotactic factor activates and recruits neutrophils to the alveolar structures. By secreting a growth factor for lung fibroblasts, the macrophage may participate in maintaining the integrity of the lung's connective tissue matrix. Alternatively, this factor may contribute to the fibrosis resulting from the inhalation of certain toxic materials. Clearly, the macrophage, by secreting diverse soluble mediators, is able to amplify all phases of the lung's inflammatory and immune response to inhaled particles and gases.

Macrophages contain aryl hydrocarbon hydroxylase, a microsomal mixed-function oxidase that produces a mutagenic compound during the metabolism of certain aromatic polycyclic hydrocarbons present in cigarette smoke (22,33,48,97). It is now clear that this enzyme system found in the macrophage, initially thought to protect the lung against carcinogens, transforms the polycyclic aromatic hydrocarbon benzo[a]pyrene into a mutagenic compound (22,33,53). Macrophages also secrete collagenase and elastase (120; R. Senior, unpublished data). During inflammation, these connective tissue proteases may cause alterations of lung connective tissue. Since the macrophage contains relatively small amounts of these connective tissue proteases, it appears to exert an effect on connective tissue, primarily through the recruitment of neutrophils to the alveolar structures. Thus, the macrophage, by interacting with other inflammatory cells and by secreting a large number of mediators and enzymes, plays a critical role in the clearance and processing of inhaled particles. In addition, these functions allow the macrophage to direct and intensify the lung's immune and inflammatory responses and to contribute to connective tissue homeostasis.

In contrast to the alveolar macrophage, the neutrophil is not normally an inhabitant of the lower respiratory tract. The neutrophil, for example, constitutes fewer than 1% of cells recovered by bronchoalveolar lavage from healthy volunteers. The body does contain a large number of neutrophils, marginated within the vascular space, and these can be mobilized, activated, and recruited to the lung to aid in its defense.

The neutrophil arises from a pleuripotential stem cell of the bone marrow. The population of neutrophils in the body is divided among three compartments: bone marrow, vascular, and tissue. The bone marrow contains neutrophil precursors, some of which are actively replicating while others undergo maturation before their release to the vascular pool. The vascular compartment contains neutrophils that are divided between a circulating and a marginated pool. The tissue compartment contains mature neutrophils that have been recruited, by chemotactic stimuli, into areas of inflammation.

The life span of the mature neutrophil is brief, usually 2 to 3 days. Cell death, however, is markedly accelerated if the neutrophil enters an area of inflammation and is actively engaged in the phagocytosis of particles or other inflammatory agents.

The neutrophil's primary function in the lung's defense is to ingest and detoxify inhaled particles. To accomplish this the neutrophil contains fairly sophisticated mechanisms that respond to, recognize, and digest foreign particles. The neutrophil is activated and recruited to areas of inflammation by numerous chemotactic substances. These substances may arise from the complement cascade or be secreted directly by the alveolar macrophage during phagocytosis. The diffusion of any chemotactic compound from alveolar structures presumably creates a chemical gradient that directs the migration of the neutrophil. Once in the vicinity of an inhaled particle, the neutrophil attaches to and engulfs the particle. The neutrophil contains large quantities of highly efficient enzymes capable of processing digested particles. These neutrophil enzymes are formed and stored in cytoplasmic granules. In contrast, the alveolar macrophage, although able to generate and secrete many of the same enzymes (elastase, collagenase, β-gluconidase, etc.), does so only in small quantities (41).

The neutrophil's defense function defined most thoroughly is the oxygen-dependent system used to kill microorganisms. The neutrophil possesses an NADP-dependent enzyme system located on the external surface of the plasma membrane. This system is capable of reducing oxygen to superoxide anion (O_2^{-}), a potent form of molecular oxygen that is toxic to microorganisms and other cells present in the inflammatory milieu (3). If released within the cytoplasm in an acidic environment (such as within the phagosome), the O_2^- can spontaneously dismutate to hydrogen peroxide (H_2O_2), another bactericidal substance. At this point, the reaction may follow either of two routes. First, the O_2^- and H_2O_2 may form hydroxyl radical ($\cdot$OH) via the Haber–Weiss reaction. Second, the neutrophil, containing large quantities of myeloperoxidase, can convert H_2O_2 to hypochlorous acid (HOCl). Superoxide anion, H_2O_2, $\cdot$OH, and HOCl are not only potent bactericidal substances; they are also toxic to surrounding epithelial cells (73,81). The neutrophil, presumably to protect itself from oxidant injury as a result of the accidental leakage of these bactericidal substances, contains protective mechanisms. These include superoxide dismutase, an efficient scavenger of O_2^-, catalase, a scavenger of H_2O_2, and the glutathione enzyme system capable of preventing membrane lipid peroxidation (110).

Thus, through phagocytosis and mediator release, the alveolar macrophage and neutrophil make critical contributions to the lung's defense. The neutrophil, laden with preformed enzymes, can be mobilized to maximize the lung's ability to detoxify inhaled particles. The macrophage, with its sophisticated ability to recruit other inflammatory cells, stands as the guardian to the lung. As the first line of cellular defense, the alveolar macrophage orchestrates the lung's defense. It can ingest particles, amplify the immune and inflammatory response, and permit the lung to adapt to its constantly changing environment.

SPECIFIC IMMUNE DEFENSES

Humoral Mechanisms

The body's antigen-specific response to inhaled particulates is provided by immunoglobulins (Table 7-1). These antibodies are derived from two distinct sources: (1) local production by lung lymphocytes and (2) ultrafiltration from the plasma immunoglobulin pool. The principal immunoglobulins found in the lower respiratory tract are IgA, IgG, and IgE. IgE mediates the degranulation of mast cells in response to inhaled allergens (immediate hypersensitivity). Although IgE may function in the lung's defense against environmental pollutants, any such role remains speculative. To date, IgD has not been found in alveolar fluid (117). As anticipated, IgM is not present in the alveolar fluid of normal individuals. Its large molecular size (900,000) impedes its transudation from the systemic circulation (116). However, lymphocytes capable of secreting IgM are present in the lower respiratory tract (87). Immunoglobulin M may play a role in the lung's defense,

especially when inflammation and increased permeability are present. Under these conditions this large immunoglobulin can diffuse across the alveolar capillary membrane. However, any unique role for this class of antibody in the lung host defense system is uncertain.

Immunoglobulin A exists in two molecular forms, dimeric and monomeric. It is the most abundant immunoglobulin found in the upper respiratory tract (i.e., above the larynx) and is also found in substantial quantities in the lower respiratory tract (101). Serum IgA circulates in the monomeric form, but most of the IgA found in the respiratory tract is in the dimeric form. Since a significant proportion of IgA in the respiratory tract is found in the monomeric form, it presumably is derived by transudation from the systemic circulation. Dimeric IgA is probably produced locally from cells arising in the bronchial-associated lymphatic tissue in response to specific antigenic stimulation. Once produced, this secretory IgA enters the lung epithelial cells, where the addition of a secretory piece enables it to be secreted onto the surface of the airway lumen (140). Secretory IgA does not appear to share the conventional properties of other immunoglobulin classes: IgA does little to enhance bacterial phagocytosis, nor does it initiate complement fixation. Its ability to "neutralize" a wide variety of viruses, however, is well established (118,140,146). Immunoglobulin A is thought to exert its protective role in viral infections by binding to surface receptors required for pathogenicity. It is possible that this function is relevant to the lung's defense against bacterial pathogens, for IgA may block the attachment of a pathogen to the respiratory epithelium. Although the precise role of IgA in defending the lung against inhaled particles is unknown, there is evidence that specific antibody in the respiratory tract markedly decreases the transmural absorption of inhaled antigen. This protection is probably achieved by the formation of an impenetrable antigen–antibody complex (32).

Immunoglobulin G is found in relatively high concentrations in the lower respiratory tract (116). Because of its relatively small molecular size (180,000), the major source of IgG appears to be the intravascular pool (via transudation across the alveolar epithelium). However, IgG-secreting cells do exist in the lower respiratory tract of man (87). By forming antigen–antibody lattices, IgG is an exceedingly efficient agglutinator of particles. By thus impeding transepithelial transport of these complexes, this mechanism may restrict access of antigen to systemic distribution. Immunoglobulin G also acts as an opsonin by binding to antigenic sites on an inhaled particle. The IgG facilitates phagocytosis by interacting with the Fc receptor on the alveolar macrophage membrane. Finally, following its binding to antigenic sites, IgG presents an efficient template for initiation of the classical complement cascade. This process amplifies the processing of infectious particles via direct lysis. Complement activation also generates peptide fragments that mediate changes in permeability and stimulate the chemotaxis of phagocytes, as discussed earlier.

Cell-Mediated Mechanisms

Specifically sensitized T lymphocytes are responsible for cell-mediated immunity in the lungs (Table 7-1). Two mechanisms are involved in cell-mediated immunity. First, direct cell-mediated lysis of targets (microbial pathogens, tumor cells, etc.), and second, lymphokine-mediated reactions. Using the first mechanism, T lymphocytes destroy cells that possess membrane antigens to which the lymphocyte has been previously sensitized. This action is believed to be the basis of allograft rejection and tumor cell destruction (18).

It is the second mechanism, however, involving lymphokine-mediated reactions, that appears to be the major manifestation of cell-mediated immunity in the lung. Lymphokines are biologically active soluble factors released by sensitized T lymphocytes in the presence of specific antigens. Although a myriad of lymphokines have been described, those important for this discussion include monocyte chemotactic factor (MCF), migration inhibition factor (MIF), macrophage-activating factor (MAF), and interleukin 2 (IL-2) (23). The MCF is a factor capable of recruiting macrophages to the alveolar structures (62); MIF and MAF function to maintain and activate those macrophages already present within the lung (105). Interleukin 2 is a mediator that specifically stimulates other T lymphocytes (and probably nonspecifically B lymphocytes) to proliferate (59, 124). Since macrophages are important for phagocytosis as well as for antigen presentation in the normal immune response, it is clear that the secretion of these lymphokines can significantly amplify the inflammatory and immune responses.

Bronchus-Associated Lymphoid Tissue

Although aggregations of lymphoid tissue in the bronchial wall were first described by Arnold in 1880, they were poorly characterized until Bienenstock published his observations in 1973 (2,7). He observed airway lymphoid tissue in follicles of small and medium-sized lymphocytes. Although these follicles lack the germinal centers and plasma cells typical of lymph nodes, they bear a strong morphological resemblance to the gut-associated lymphoid tissue (GALT) of the intestine. These follicles are distributed along the mucosal surface of the large and medium-size bronchi, particularly at points of bifurcation. The follicles are covered by an epithelium conspicuously lacking ciliated and mucus-secreting cells but interspersed with lymphocytes. These epithelial cells contain numerous microvilli, a feature common to cells specially adapted for absorption.

The physiological function of bronchus-associated lymphoid tissue (BALT) is not well understood. T lymphocytes constitute a small proportion (fewer than 20%) of cells present, and there are no mature plasma cells capable of producing immunoglobulins (121). Subsequent studies, however, indicate that the BALT may be the source of immunoglobulin A immunoblasts. These cells, which circulate in the lung and other organs, establish B-cell regions capable of maintaining generalized mucosal immunity after antigenic stimulation (99). In this context, the specialized lymphoepithelium overlying BALT may intercept and absorb inhaled antigens (113). The immune mechanisms present in the lung have been reviewed (61,75,76).

BIOCHEMICAL DEFENSES

Protective Proteins

There are numerous proteins in the lower respiratory tract that provide specific protection against the adverse effects of inhaled pollutants. Of the proteins protecting alveolar structures, α_1-antitrypsin is probably the most plentiful. There are, however, others such as α_2-macroglobulin, bronchial mucous inhibitor, and various lung antioxidants. Inflammatory cell products released at the alveolar surface during particle phagocytosis could potentially lead to lung cell death or derangement of the connective tissue matrix in the lung. For this reason, a sophisticated molecular basis exists in the lung for protecting normal alveolar structures from inflammation-cell proteases and oxidants.

Clinical and experimental observations concerning the pathogenesis of emphysema in α_1-antitrypsin deficiency demonstrate the importance of protease–antiprotease homeostasis in the lung (40, 77,82,89). Basically, this theory holds that because of the lung's unique interface with the environment, it is constantly subject to protease activity from inflammatory cells. Under normal circumstances, the lung's structural proteins are adequately protected by an antiprotease screen within the lower respiratory tract. However, when the balance is shifted in favor of protease activity, as occurs with the inhalation of cigarette smoke, there is destruction of the alveolar structures (4,24,39,68).

α_1-Antitrypsin (α_1-AT) is a glycoprotein that constitutes 90% of the α_1-globulins present in normal human serum. The primary source of α_1-AT is the hepatocyte. Because of its relatively low molecular weight (52,000), the α_1-AT freely diffuses through to the alveolar surface. Here it is found in concentrations similar to those in serum (referable to a protein standard, i.e., albumin) (42,108). α_1-Antitrypsin functions primarily as an antiprotease (a molecule that combines with proteolytic enzymes to render them inactive). In addition to trypsin, α_1-AT is able to inhibit thrombin, chymotrypsin, and plasmin. Its primary function in the lung, however, is to inhibit neutrophil elastase, a broad-spectrum protease capable of degrading most structural proteins of the extracellular matrix (40,68). α_1-Antitrypsin interacts with elastase by forming a tight "pseudoirreversible" complex in a 1:1 molar ratio (5,72,104). The elastase binding site α_1-AT is centered around a methionine residue. Once this binding occurs, there is limited proteolytic cleavage of α_1-AT, and it is unable to function again as an antiprotease (71). To bind with elastase it is critical that the methionine residue at the active site on α_1-AT be in reduced form. If it is oxidized, the association constant is reduced by a factor of 2000 (5). This factor is particularly relevant to situations in which the alveolar structures are exposed to oxidants such as those produced by cigarette smoke and other air pollutants.

α_2-Macroglobulin (α_2-M), a large-molecular-weight (725,000) glycoprotein synthesized by the liver, has a wide range of antiprotease activity. It inhibits neutrophil elastase, collagenase, and other proteases involved in clotting and fibrinolysis (128). Because of its large size, α_2-M probably remains in the intravascular space unless inflammation and increased permeability allow it to leak into tissue sites. Studies using sensitive assays show that α_2-M is undetectable or present in very small amounts in the lower respiratory tract of normal human volunteers (42). Thus, α_2-M is a minor component of the antiprotease screen in the normal lung. However, during times of inflammation it may supplement the role of α_1-AT.

Hochstrasser in 1972 described a low-molecular-weight (11,000) inhibitor in bronchial secretions (bronchial mucus inhibitor; BMI) with an antiprotease profile similar to α_1-AT (inhibits elastatse and cathepsin G but not collagenase) (55). This inhibitor, present in most mucosal secretions, is secreted by the epithelial and/or mucous acinar cells for the upper respiratory tract (135). Studies by Tenger show that BMI accounts for approximately 90% of the antielastase activity in the epithelial fluid of the large airways. The remainder is supplied by α_1-AT (134). Although there are large amounts of BMI in central airway secretions and purulent sputum, this antiprotease does not appear in fluid recovered from the distal airways and parenchyma (42). These studies suggest that BMI provides an important antiprotease screen for the large airways and the

upper respiratory tract, while α_1-AT provides a similar function in the lung parenchyma.

Antioxidant Mechanisms

The lung is subjected to large amounts of oxidant stress imposed by two distinct mechanisms: (1) direct environmental sources (ozone, NO_2, radiation, cigarette smoke) and (2) endogenous oxygen radicals released from phagocytic cells in response to inhaled particulates. Even increased levels of oxygen, which until recently were only encountered in the therapy of hypoxemic patients, have—with space travel and the undersea exploration for oil—become a potential occupational hazard.

Any compound with an unpaired electron has the potential to serve as an oxidant. This process may occur directly, as with the oxidation of protein sulfhydryl groups by ozone, or indirectly, by the transfer of the free electron to O_2 to form superoxide anion (O_2^-). This anion may exert a toxic effect itself, or it may combine with H_2O_2 to produce hydroxyl radical ($\cdot OH$) via the Haber–Weiss reaction. This anion is extremely toxic to host as well as to microbial cells. Oxygen, so essential for cellular function, is also involved in toxic oxygen radical production. Thus, toxic oxygen radical production can be viewed as an unavoidable byproduct of oxidative metabolism. In an effort to cope with this biological paradox, the lung has evolved sophisticated mechanisms for containing oxidant stress (37,38,54,125). These include such enzyme systems as superoxide dismutase, glutathione enzymes, and catalase as well as such nonspecific antioxidant systems as the vitamin E component of lipid cell membranes and several of the protein constituents of alveolar lining fluid (94) (Table 7-2).

Superoxide dismutase is an enzyme ubiquitous in cells that metabolize oxygen. It markedly accelerates (by a factor of 10) the slow but naturally occurring dismutation of the superoxide radical: $2O_2^- + 2H^+ \rightarrow H_2O_2 + O_2$ (54). Superoxide dismutase, an extremely efficient scavenger of O_2^-, also indirectly prevents the production of $\cdot OH$. This is done by scavenging O_2^- before it can react with H_2O. The activity of this enzyme is increased in the lungs of rats exposed to sublethal levels of O_2. Such animals survive longer when transferred to a 100% O_2 environment (27). This adaptive mechanism, however, has not been clearly demonstrated in the human lung.

There is indirect evidence that the glutathione system plays a role in protecting the lung from oxidants by one of two mechanisms. The first depends on the ability of reduced glutathione to convert toxic lipid peroxides (produced through free radical attack on unsaturated lipid membrane components) to nontoxic products (54). This reaction,

TABLE 7-2.   Major Pulmonary Oxidant Scavengers[a]

Category	Structure	Tissue site	Actions
Enzyme systems			
Catalase	Tetrameric hemoprotein	Peroxisomes	Catalyzes dismutation of H_2O_2, reduces methyl and ethyl hydroperoxides.
Superoxide dismutases	CuZn-SOD[b]	Primarily cytosol, also nucleus	Catalyze dismutation of O_2^- to H_2O_2
	Mn-SOD	Primarily mitochondria	
	Cu-SOD	Primarily plasma	
GSH[b] redox cycle			
GSH peroxidase	Selenoprotein	Primarily cytosol, also mitochondria	Catalyzes reduction of H_2O_2 and other hydroperoxides (lipid peroxides, lipoxygenase products).
GSH reductase	Dimeric protein	Primarily cytosol, also mitochondria	Catalyzes reduction of low-molecular-weight disulfides.
G-6-PD and 6-phosphogluconate dehydrogenase	NADP-dependent enzymes	Extramitochondrial cytosol	Supply NADPH to the GSH redox cycle.
Fat-soluble compounds			
Vitamin E	Fat-soluble vitamin	Lipid membranes, extracellular fluids (including alveolar)	Converts O_2^-, ·OH, and lipid peroxyl radicals to less reactive forms. Breaks lipid peroxidation chain reactions.
β-Carotene	Metabolic precursor to vitamin A	Membranes of tissues	Scavenges O_2^-, reacts directly with peroxyl radicals.
Bilirubin	Product of hemoprotein catabolism	Bloodstream, tissue	Chain-breaking antioxidant. Reacts with ROO·.
Water-soluble compounds			
Vitamin C	Water-soluble vitamin	Wide distribution in intracellular and extracellular fluids	Directly scavenges O_2^- and ·OH. Neutralizes oxidants from stimulated neutrophils. Contributes to regeneration of vitamin E.
Uric acid	Oxidized purine base	Wide distribution	Scavenges ·OH, O_2^-, oxoheme oxidants, and peroxyl radicals. Prevents oxidation of vitamin C. Binds transition metals.
Glucose	Carbohydrate	Wide distribution	Scavenges ·OH.
Cysteine	Amino acid	Wide distribution	Reduces various organic compounds by donating electron from sulfhydryl groups.
Cysteamine	Amino acid	Wide distribution	Same as cysteine.
GSH	Tripeptide	Largely intracellular, also in alveolus	In addition to role as substrate in GSH redox cycle, reacts directly with O_2^-, ·OH, and organic free radicals.
Taurine	β-Amino acid	Intracellular in cells with high rates of oxygen radical generation	Conjugates xenobiotics, reacts with HOCl.
High-molecular-weight antioxidants			
Tracheobronchial mucus	Protein and glycoprotein	Upper airways	Scavenges inhaled oxidants.
Albumin	Protein	Wide distribution	Binds transition metals. Reacts with oxidants as a "sacrificial" antioxidant.

[a]From Heffner and Repine (54).
[b]Definition of abbreviations: GSH, glutathione; H_2O_2, hydrogen peroxide; ·OH, hydroxyl radical; O_2^-, superoxide anion; Cu, copper; Zn, zinc; Mn, manganese; SOD, superoxide dismutase; G-6-PD, glucose-6-phosphate dehydrogenase; NADPH, nicotinamide adenine dinucleotide phosphate; O_2, singlet oxygen; HOCl, hypochlorous acid.

catalyzed by glutathione peroxidase, has been studied almost exclusively in erythrocytes. A continuous supply of reduced glutathione is derived from the transfer of reducing equivalents (supplied by the hexose monphosphate shunt) to oxidized glutathione (90). This process is catalyzed by the enzyme glutathione reductase. A second mechanism, proposed by McCay and Fong, suggests that membrane lipid peroxidation may actually be prevented by the direct scavenging of $\cdot OH$ by glutathione peroxidase (35,98). This theory is based on indirect evidence that shows a correlation between oxygen tolerance and the activity of these enzyme systems within the lung (19,20,79).

Catalase, by catalyzing the reaction $2H_2O_2 \rightarrow 2H_2O + O_2$, is an efficient scavenger of H_2O_2. Catalase is important not only for the removal of H_2O_2 but also for decreasing the generation of $\cdot OH$ by the abovementioned Haber–Weiss reaction. What role catalase plays in the lung's antioxidant defense is unclear. Recent evidence, however, suggests that increased catalase activity is present in the lungs of animals that survived exposure to both hyperoxia and NO_2 (28,36,153).

Vitamin E, a lipid constituent of the cell membrane, is an important antioxidant. It is thought that vitamin E donates reducing equivalents to lipid peroxides formed through oxidation in the cell membrane. Through its function as an antioxidant, vitamin E limits the chain reaction between the lipid peroxides and their neighboring polyunsaturated fatty acids. Breaking this chain reaction is thought to limit lipid peroxidation and confine the resultant membrane damage (58,132). In this regard, alveolar lining fluid from patients under oxidant stress (cigarette smoking) has been reported to be deficient in vitamin E (109). To date, the evidence that supports the aggravation of oxidant injury in vitamin-E-deficient animals is much stronger than the evidence that demonstrates its protective effect when given prior to or with oxidant stress.

As discussed in the section on nonspecific defense mechanisms, recent evidence shows that constituents of alveolar lining fluid may protect the lung from oxidant stress (16). Although the exact mechanism is uncertain, oxidant protection of the lung seems to be provided by transferrin, ceruloplasmin, and glutathione, all of which are present in alveolar lining fluid (16,54). Theoretically, any protein with a sulfhydryl group could reduce oxidant injury by donating reducing equivalents to a free oxygen radical, thereby preventing sulthydryl oxidation of cellular proteins.

Pulmonary Metabolism of Xenobiotics

There is evidence that the lung possesses measurable levels of the microsomal P-450-dependent monooxygenase (mixed-function oxidase) activity required to metabolize a broad range of substrates. These substrates include such exogenous compounds as drugs and environmental pollutants. Generally this type of enzyme activity yields metabolites that are water soluble and therefore easily excreted by the kidney. By this means the body detoxifies and excretes many xenobiotics. Although the major site of xenobiotic metabolism occurs in the liver, considerable interest has developed in the metabolism of xenobiotics by extrahepatic organs, particularly at the portal of entry (i.e., the skin, lung, or intestine; see Chapters 6 and 8). It is now abundantly evident that the enzyme system that transforms many xenobiotics into excretable metabolites also potentiates the toxicity of certain chemicals by converting them into reactive metabolites that may lead to the induction of cancer and other types of tissue injury (22,33,48). (See Chapter 9 for a detailed discussion of detoxication mechanisms.)

THE LUNG'S INTERACTIONS WITH SPECIFIC ENVIRONMENTAL CHEMICALS

Many compounds have been identified as constituents of polluted air. These include such agents as carbon monoxide, oxides of sulfur and nitrogen, ammonia gas, polycyclic aromatic hydrocarbons, formaldehyde, lead, and zinc (88). The presence and concentration of these agents in a given area depend to a large extent on the industries present, control measures, and local meteorological conditions. In this section, the discussion focuses on the commonly occurring air pollutants (sulfur dioxide, nitrogen dioxide, photochemical oxidants, and cigarette smoke) that may have specific interactions with components of the lung's defense mechanisms.

Sulfur Dioxide

Sulfur dioxide (SO_2), a major constituent of polluted air, arises from the combustion of impurities in various fossil fuels (coal, oil, gas). A large fraction of SO_2 in the atmosphere may be transformed into particulate sulfate compounds (H_2SO_4, metal sulfate salts). Because SO_2 is a fairly soluble gas, it primarily affects the nasopharynx and proximal airways. This is in contrast to particulate sulfate compounds, which may penetrate farther into the lung, reaching the distal airways and parenchyma. Acute exposure to SO_2 decreases tracheal ciliary beating and mucus transport in animals. Chronic exposure leads to goblet cell hyperplasia (29,30,83). Subsequent in vitro and in vivo studies on rats demonstrate that exposure to varying concentrations of SO_2 increases the mucosal permeability of the trachea and bronchi (143). Although the increased permeability diminished with time, it was still present 3 months after termination of exposure. Studies by Skornik show that inhaling various metal sulfate aerosols is toxic to hamster alveolar macrophages. The toxicity is reflected in a significant depression of phagocytosis (123). There is also evidence that mice, after prolonged exposure to SO_2, suffer a significant decrease in local and systemic antibody formation after antigenic challenge (154). These studies suggest that inhalation of sulfur byproducts of fossil fuel combustion may significantly alter the lung's defense mechanisms.

Nitrogen Dioxide

Nitrogen dioxide (NO_2) arises from the high-temperature combustion of fossil fuels such as occurs in the internal combustion engine. Since NO_2 is poorly soluble, it may penetrate to the distal airways and alveoli before producing its effect. Because NO_2 contains an unpaired electron, it probably produces toxic effects by serving as an oxidant. Exposure to NO_2 results in the formation of atypical cilia in the airway mucosa of mice and guinea pigs. It also increases the permeability of the respiratory epithelium (114). Studies by Gordon et al. reveal that NO_2 exposure increases both the permeability of the respiratory epithelium and endocytosis by alveolar type I pneumocytes (47). On this basis NO_2 exposure may make the lung more susceptible to the effects of other pollutants. Nitrogen dioxide reduces the number and phagocytic capabilities of the alveolar macrophage, and it may also inhibit interferon production by the macrophage in response to viral infection (44,144). Immunologic studies in mice exposed to NO_2 demonstrate enhancement of T and B lymphocyte functions with short exposure and suppression with chronic exposures (57).

Photochemical Oxidants

Ozone is the most abundant photochemical oxidant in polluted air. Although it arises mainly from photochemical reactions in smog, ozone is also generated by the solar irradiation of oxygen. This agent may reach high concentrations in the atmosphere (106). Many studies document the adverse effects of ozone on pulmonary structure and function. Little is known, however, about ozone's interaction with the lung's defense mechanism. Numerous studies indicate that inhalation of ozone increases the severity of bacterial pneumonia in laboratory animals. A recent study in sheep demonstrates that exposure to a combination of ozone and SO_2 significantly decreases tracheal mucus velocity but not ciliary beat frequency (102,112). There are many animal studies dealing with the direct effect of inhaling various ozone concentrations on the

lung cell population and function. For example, Coffin et al. demonstrate a marked influx of neutrophils into rabbit lungs after ozone exposure (21). Ozone, in concentrations as low as 0.3 ppm, reduces the phagocytic function of alveolar macrophages. Ozone also depresses the activity of alveolar macrophage acid hydrolases and inhibits the "cell-stabilizing activity" of lipoproteins in the alveolar fluid (45,64,65). Finally, ozone inactivates α_1-antitrypsin both in vitro and in vivo. This is very likely the result of oxidation of the methionine residue on the elastase binding site (70). Taken together, these studies suggest that ozone may subvert the lung's defenses. The precise mechanisms, however, remain speculative.

Cigarette Smoke

The effects of the inhalation of cigarette smoke on the lung's defense mechanisms have been studied extensively. It appears that cigarette smoke significantly alters the lung response to other environmental pollutants. Although there is disagreement on the effects of short-term cigarette smoke inhalation on mucociliary clearance, there is general agreement that chronic exposure to cigarette smoke decreases mucociliary transport (15,91). In addition, human studies show that inhaling cigarette smoke increases epithelial permeability and the deposition of aerosols in the respiratory tract (78). Cigarette smoke also has deleterious effects on cells involved in the lung's defense. For example, the alveolar macrophages of animals exposed to cigarette smoke are less able to ingest and kill bacteria in vitro. This is accompanied by a decrease in protein synthesis by the alveolar macrophages (51). This decreased synthesis may be caused by the oxidant gas acrolein, which is present in large amounts in cigarette smoke (92). Although in vitro studies of human macrophages have not supported this observation, there is a consensus suggesting that alveolar macrophage migration and adherence are reduced by exposure to cigarette smoke (51,148,147).

Studies have demonstrated that smokers have an increased number of macrophages and neutrophils in their lungs (53,60,95). In addition, the macrophages of cigarette smokers secrete greater amounts of superoxide anion and a neutrophil chemotactic factor (56,60). These studies suggest that the net effect of cigarette smoking on the lung's host defense may be to initiate an inflammatory response that is deleterious to the lung structure and function.

Epithelial cells in the respiratory tract are also subject to the adverse effects of cigarette smoke. The frequency and severity of epithelial lesions observed in smokers contrast sharply with the respiratory epithelium of nonsmokers.

Examination of lymphocyte function after exposure to cigarette smoke reveals several relevant observations. Studies in animals indicate a biphasic response. Moderate exposure to cigarette smoke enhances both the humoral and cell-mediated immune response, whereas prolonged exposure depresses these reactions (137–139). Although studies in man are less conclusive, they do indicate that exposure to cigarette smoke increases the number of lung T lymphocytes while significantly diminishing normal T-cell function (31,150).

Clinical studies demonstrate that smokers, compared to nonsmokers, have a reduced serum antibody response to influenza infection or vaccination (34). In addition, this specific immunity is less sustained. The detrimental influence of cigarette smoke on the biochemical defense mechanisms have only recently been elucidated. In vitro studies show that cigarette smoke inactivates both α_1-antitrypsin and the bronchial mucus inhibitor (1,7,67). Although the structure of the bronchial mucus inhibitor has yet to be determined, it appears that like α_1-antitrypsin, it is inactivated by the oxidative effects of cigarette smoke. In vivo studies in rats and man demonstrate that cigarette smoke, by inactivating α_1-AT, produces functional antiprotease deficiency in the lower respiratory tract (42,68). Finally, the antioxidant activity of ceruloplasmin is decreased in the serum of smokers. This finding suggests that ceruloplasmin is also inactivated by the oxidants present in cigarette smoke. It has been postulated that ceruloplasmin, a major serum antioxidant also found in the alveolar fluid, may serve to protect α_1-AT from oxidation (6,26,43). In this context, it seems that cigarette smoke subverts the lung's antiprotease defense by direct (α_1-antitrypsin oxidation) and indirect (antioxidant inactivation) mechanisms.

The inhalation of cigarette smoke may adversely affect both the nonspecific (mucociliary clearance, phagocytosis) and specific (immune, biochemical) defense mechanisms of the lung. These alterations may in turn lead to a greater deposition of particulates as well as an increased incidence of infection, destructive lung disease, and cancer in those exposed to cigarette smoke.

SUMMARY

Virtually every component of the lung's defense is subverted, to some degree, by pollutants found in ambient air. In most instances, however, the defense appears to hold, as each of the defense mechanisms undoubtedly has considerable functional reserve. The apparent adequacy of the lung's defense is no cause for complacency, for this important barrier can be weakened and/or overpowered by pollutant exposure.

Cigarette smoking, in particular, is capable of compromising the lung's defense at many levels. Recent studies suggest that "passive smoking" plays a role in the development of respiratory illness in children (142). Clearly, the potential effects of "passive smoking" should receive great scrutiny. The lung's defense in individuals with preexisting disease or particular susceptibility is undoubtedly more easily overpowered. It follows that the young, the aged, individuals with asthma or chronic lung or cardiovascular disease, or those with congenital defects are all likely to have a lower pulmonary barrier to the adverse effects of pollutant exposure.

The increased susceptibility of certain individuals with congenital defects has provided unique evidence for the distinct and important role played by many components of the lung's defenses. For example, the recurrent lower respiratory tract infections in individuals with dysmotile cilia syndrome, hypogammaglobulinemia, deficiencies of complement components, and abnormalities of T-lymphocyte function in the acquired immunodeficiency syndrome (AIDS) and neutropenia clearly demonstrate that the lung's defenses require the intimate cooperation of many functional components. In every instance, when the threshold of the host's defense is exceeded, opportunistic pathogens gain access to the respiratory tract.

REFERENCES

1. Aharonson EF, Menkes H, Gurtner G, et al: Effect of respiratory airflow rate on removal of soluble vapors by the nose. J Appl Physiol 37:654, 1974.
2. Arnold J: Uber das Vorkommen lymphatischen Gewebes in den Lungen. Virchows Arch Pathol Anat 80:315, 1880.
3. Babior BM: Oxygen-dependent microbial killing by phagocytes. N Engl J Med 298:659, 1978.
4. Bearn AG: Alpha$_1$-antitrypsin deficiency: A biological enigma. Gut 19:470, 1978.
5. Beatty K, Bieth J, Travis J: Kinetics of association of serine proteinases with native and oxidized α_1-proteinase inhibitor and α_1-antichymotrypsin. J Biol Chem 255:3931, 1980.
6. Bell DY, Haseman JA, Spock A, et al: Plasma proteins of the bronchoalveolar surface of the lungs of smokers and nonsmokers. Am Rev Respir Dis 124:72, 1981.
7. Bienenstock J, Johnston N, Perey DYE: Bronchial lymphoid tissue: Morphologic characteristics. Lab Invest 28:686, 1973.
8. Blake J: On the movement of mucus in the lung. J Biomech 8:179, 1975.
9. Bowes D, Corrin B: Ultrastructural immunocytochemical localization of lysozyme in human bronchial glands. Thorax 32:163, 1977.
10. Brain JD, Golde DW, Green GW, et al: Biologic potential of pulmonary macrophages. Am Rev Respir Dis 118:435, 1978.

11. Brandtzaeg P: Mucosal and glandular distribution of immunological components: Differential localization of free and bound SC in secretory epithelial cells. J Immunol 112:1553, 1974.

12. Breeze RG, Wheeldon EB: The cells of the pulmonary airways. Am Rev Respir Dis 116:705, 1977.

13. Brundelet PJ: Experimental study of the dust clearance mechanism of the lung. Acta Pathol Microbiol Scand 175:1, 1965.

14. Camner P: Clearance of particles from the human trachiobronchial tree. Clin Sci 59:79, 1980.

15. Camner P, Philipson K, Arvidsson T: Withdrawal of cigarette smoking: A study on tracheobronchial clearance. Arch Environ Health 26:90, 1973.

16. Cantin AM, North SL, Hubbard RC, et al: Normal alveolar epithelial lining fluid contains high levels of glutathione. J Appl Physiol 63:152, 1987.

17. Carp H, Janoff A, Harel S: Inactivation of human bronchial mucous inhibitor (BMPi) by cigarette smoke. Am Rev Respir Dis 121:227, 1980.

18. Cerottini JC, Brunner KT: Cell mediated cytotoxicity, allograft rejection and tumor immunity. Adv Immunol 18:67, 1974.

19. Chow CK: Biochemical responses in lung of ozone-tolerant rats. Nature 260:721, 1976.

20. Chow CK, Tappel AL: Activities of pentose shunt and glycolytic enzymes in lungs of ozone exposed rats. Arch Environ Health 26:205, 1973.

21. Coffin DL: Influence of ozone on pulmonary cells. Arch Environ Health 16:633, 1968.

22. Cohen GM: Pulmonary metabolism of foreign compounds: Its role in metabolic activation. Environ Health Perspect 85:31, 1990.

23. Cohen S, Pick E, Oppenheim JJ (Eds.): Biology of the Lymphokines, Academic Press, New York, 1979.

24. Committee on Diagnostic Standards for Nontuberculous Respiratory Disease: Chronic bronchitis, asthma, and pulmonary emphysema: Statement of the American Thoracic Society. Am Rev Respir Dis 85:762, 1962.

25. Cong H, Drage CW (eds.): The Respiratory System: A Core Curriculum, Appleton-Century-Crofts, New York, 1982.

26. Cranfield LM, Gollan JL, White AG, et al: Serum antioxidant activity in normal and abnormal subjects. Ann Clin Biochem 16:299, 1979.

27. Crapo JD: Tierney DF: Superoxide dismutase and pulmonary oxygen toxicity. Am J Physiol 226:1401, 1974.

28. Crapo JD, Sjostrom K, Drew RT: Tolerance and cross-tolerance using NO_2 and O_2. I. Toxicology and biochemistry. J Appl Physiol 44:364, 1978.

29. Dalhamm T: Mucous flow and ciliary activity in the trachea of healthy rats exposed to respiratory irritant gases (SO_2, NH_3, HCHO). Acta Physiol Scand 36:1, 1956.

30. Dalhamm T: Studies on the effect of sulfur dioxide on ciliary activity in rabbit trachea in vivo and in vitro and on the resorptional capacity of the nasal cavity. Am Rev Respir Dis 83:566, 1961.

31. Daniele RP, Dauber JH, Altose MD, et al: Lymphocyte studies in asymptomatic cigarette smokers. Am Rev Respir Dis 116:997, 1977.

32. Dawson CA, Braley JF, Moore VL: Influence of immunity on the absorption of inhaled antigen. Chest 75 (Suppl):276, 1979.

33. Duncan CA: Lung metabolism of xenobiotic compounds. Clin Chest Med 10:49, 1989.

34. Finklea J, Hasselblad V, Riggan WB, et al: Cigarette smoking and hemagglutination inhibition response to influenza after natural disease and immunization. Am Rev Respir Dis 104:368, 1971.

35. Fong KL, McCay PB, Poyer JL: Evidence that peroxidation of lysozomal membranes is initiated by hydroxyl free radicals produced during flavin enzyme activity. J Biol Chem 248:7792, 1973.

36. Frank L, Bucher JR, Roberts RJ: Oxygen toxicity in neonatal and adult animals of various species. J Appl Physiol 45:699, 1979.

37. Fridovich I: The biology of oxygen radicals. Science 201:875, 1978.

38. Fridovich I, Freeman B: Antioxidant defenses in the lung. Annu Rev Physiol 48:693, 1986.

39. Gadek JE, Fells GA, Crystal RG: Cigarette smoking induces functional antiprotease deficiency in the lower respiratory tract in humans. Science 206:1315, 1979.

40. Gadek JE, Fells GA, Wright DG, et al: Neutrophil elastase functions as a type III collagenase. Biochem Biophys Res Commun 95:1818, 1980.

41. Gadek JE, Hunninghake GW, Fells GA, et al: Evaluation of the protease–antiprotease theory of human destructive lung disease. Bull Eur Physiopathol Respir 16:27, 1980.

42. Gadek JE, Fells GA, Zimmerman RL, et al: Antielastases of the human alveolar structures. J Clin Invest 68:889, 1981.

43. Galdston M, Levytska V, Schwartz MS, et al: Ceruloplasmin. Am Rev Respir Dis 129:258, 1984.

44. Gardner DE, Holzman RS, Coffin DL: Effect of nitrogen dioxide on pulmonary cell population. J Bacteriol 98:1048, 1969.

45. Gardner DE, Pfitzer EA, Christian RT, et al: Loss of protective factor for alveolar macrophages when exposed to ozone. Arch Intern Med 127:1078, 1971.

46. Golde DW, Finley TN, Cline MJ: The pulmonary macrophage in acute leukemia. N Engl J Med 290:875, 1974.

47. Gordon RE, Case BW, Kleinerman J; Acute NO_2 effects on penetration and transport of horseradish peroxidase in hamster respiratory epithelium. Am Rev Respir Dis 128:543, 1983.

48. Gram TE, Okine LK, Gram RA: The metabolism of xenobiotics by certain extrahepatic organs and its relationship to toxicity. Annu Rev Pharmacol Toxicol 26:259, 1986.

49. Green GM: Alveolo-bronchiolar transport: Observations and hypothesis of a pathway. Chest 59(Suppl): 1S, 1971.

50. Green GM: Alveolobronchiolar transport mechanisms. Arch Intern Med 131:109, 1973.

51. Green GM, Carolin D: The depressant effect of cigarette smoke on the in vitro antibacterial activity of alveolar macrophages. N Engl J Med 276:422, 1967.

52. Green GM, Jakab GJ, Low RB, et al: Defense mechanisms of the respiratory membrane. Am Rev Respir Dis 115:479, 1977.

53. Harris CC, Hsu IC, Stoner GD: Human pulmonary

alveoli macrophages metabolize benzo[a]pyrene to proximate and ultimate mutagens. Nature 272:633, 1978.

54. Heffner JE, Repine JE: Pulmonary strategies of antioxidant defense. Am Rev Respir Dis 140:531, 1989.

55. Hochstrasser K, Teichert R, Schwarz S, et al: Isolierung und Charakterisierung eines Proteaseninhibitors aus dem menschlichen bronchial Sekret. Hoppe-Seylers Z Physiol Chem 353:221, 1972.

56. Hoidal JR, Fox RB, LeMarbe PA, et al: Altered oxidative metabolic response in vitro of alveolar macrophages from asymptomatic smokers. Am Rev Respir Dis 123:85, 1981.

57. Holt PG, Finlay-Jones LM, Keast D, et al: Immunological function in mice chronically exposed to nitrogen oxides (NO_x). Environ Res 19:154, 1979.

58. Horwitt MK: Vitamin E. A reexamination. Am J Clin Nutr 29:569, 1976.

59. Hunninghake GW, Crystal RG: Mechanisms of hypergammaglobulinemia in pulmonary sarcoidosis. J Clin Invest 67:86, 1981.

60. Hunninghake GW, Crystal RG: Cigarette smoking and lung destruction. Am Rev Respir Dis 128:833, 1983.

61. Hunninghake GW, Gadek JE, Kawanami O, et al: Inflammatory and immune processes in the human lung in health and disease: Evaluation by bronchoalveolar lavage. Am J Pathol 7:149, 1979.

62. Hunninghake GW, Gadek JE, Fales HM, et al: Human alveolar macrophage-derived chemotactic factor for neutrophils. Stimuli and partial characterization. J Clin Invest 66:473, 1980.

63. Hunninghake GW, Gadek JE, Young RC, et al: Maintenance of granuloma formation in pulmonary sarcoidosis by T-lymphocytes within the lung. N Engl J Med 302:594, 1980.

64. Hurst DJ, Coffin DL: Ozone effect on lysosomal hydrolases of alveolar macrophages. Arch Intern Med 127:1059, 1971.

65. Hurst DJ, Gardner DE, Coffin DL: Effect of ozone on acid hydrolases of the pulmonary alveolar macrophage. Res J Reticuloendothel Soc 8:288, 1970.

66. Iravani J, Melville GN: Mucociliary function in the respiratory tract as influenced by physiochemical factors. Pharmacol Ther 2:471, 1976(B).

67. Janoff A, Carp H: Possible mechanisms of emphysema in smokers. Cigarette smoke condensate suppresses protease inhibitor in vitro. Am Rev Respir Dis 116:65, 1977.

68. Janoff A, White R, Caro H, et al: Lung injury induced by leukocytic proteases. Am J Pathol 97:111, 1979.

69. Jeffrey PK: The respiratory mucous membrane. In: Respiratory Defense Mechanisms, Part I, p 193, Brain JD (ed.), Marcel Dekker, New York, 1977.

70. Johnson DA: Ozone inactivation of human α_1-proteinase inhibitor. Am Rev Respir Dis 121:1031, 1980.

71. Johnson DA, Travis J:Human alpha I-antiproteinase inhibitor mechanism of action: Evidence for activation by limited proteolysis. Biochem Biophys Res Commun 72:33, 1976.

72. Johnson D, Travis J: Structural evidence for methionine at the reactive site of human α_1-proteinase inhibitor. J Biol Chem 253:7142, 1978.

73. Johnston JR, Keele BB Jr, Misra HP, et al: The role of superoxide anion generation in phagocytic bactericidal activity. J Clin Invest 55:1357, 1975.

74. Jurgensen PF, Olsen GN, Johnson JE 3rd, et al: Immune response of the human respiratory tract II. Cell mediated immunity in the lower respiratory tract to tuberculin and mumps and influenza viruses. J Infect Dis 128:730, 1973.

75. Kaltreider HB: Expression of immune mechanisms in the lung. Am Rev Respir Dis 113:347, 1976.

76. Kaltreider HB: Phagocytic, antibody and cell-mediated immune mechanisms. In: Textbook of Respiratory Medicine, p 322, Murray JF, Nadel JA (eds.), WB Saunders, Philadelphia, 1988.

77. Karlinsky JB, Snider GL: Animal models of emphysema. Am Rev Respir Dis 117:1109, 1978.

78. Kennedy SM, Elwood RK, Wiggs BJR, et al: Increased airway mucosal permeability of smokers. Am Rev Respir Dis 129:143, 1984.

79. Kimball RE, Reddy K, Peirce TH, et al: Oxygen toxicity: Augmentation of antioxidant defense mechanisms in rat lung. Am J Physiol 230:1425, 1976.

80. King M, Gilboa A, Meyer A, et al: On the transport of mucus and its rheologic simulants in ciliated systems. Am Rev Respir Dis 110:740, 1974.

81. Klebanoff SJ, Clark RA: The Neutrophil: Function and Clinical Disorders, Elsevior/North-Holland, Amsterdam, 1978.

82. Kuhn C, Senior RM: The role of elastases in the development of emphysema. Lung 155:461, 1977.

83. Lamb D, Reid L: Mitotic rates, goblet cell increase and histochemical changes in mucus in rat bronchial epithelium during exposure to SO_2. J Pathol Bacteriol 96:97, 1968.

84. Langevoort HC: The nomenclature of mononuclear phagocytic cells. In: Mononuclear Phagocytes, p 1, van Furth R (ed.), FA Davis, Philadelphia, 1970.

85. Laughter AH, Martin RR, Twomey JJ: Lymphoproliferative responses to antigens mediated by human pulmonary alveolar macrophages. J Lab Clin Med 89:1326, 1977.

86. Lauweryns JM, Boussauw L: The ultrastructure of pulmonary lymphatic capillaries in newborn rabbits and human infants. Lymphology 1:108, 1968.

87. Lawrence EC, Blaese RM, Martin RR, et al: Immunoglobulin secreting cells in normal human bronchial lavage fluids. J Clin Invest 62:832, 1978.

88. Lawther JPL: Air pollution and tobacco smoke. In: Clinical Aspects of Inhaled Particles, Muir DCF (ed.), p 21, Heineman, London, 1972.

89. Lieberman J: Elastase, collagenase, emphysema and alpha I-antitrypsin deficiency. Chest 70:62, 1976.

90. Little C, Olinescu R, Reid KG, et al: Properties and regulation of glutathione peroxidase. J Biol Chem 254:3632, 1970.

91. Lourenco RV, Klimer MF, Borowski CJ: Deposition and clearance of 2 particles in the tracheobronchial tree of normal subjects: Smokers and nonsmokers. J Clin Invest 50:1411, 1971.

92. Low RB: Effects of acrolein on in vitro protein biosynthesis and substrate transport by rabbit pulmonary alveolar macrophages. Am Rev Respir Dis 111:924, 1975.

93. Lucas AM, Douglas LC: Principles underlying ciliary activity in the respiratory tract. Arch Otolaryngol 20: 518, 1934.

94. Lucy JA: Functional and structural aspects of biological membranes: A suggested structural role for vitamin E in the control of membrane permeability and stability. Ann NY Acad Sci 204:4, 1972.

95. MacNee W, Wiggs B, Belzberg AS, et al: The effect of cigarette smoking on neutrophil kinetics in human lungs. N Engl J Med 321:924, 1989.

96. Martin D, Jacobi W: Diffusion of small-sized particles in the bronchial tree. Health Phys 23:23, 1972.

97. Mason RJ: Metabolism of alveolar macrophages. In: Respiratory Defense Mechanisms, p 893, Brain JD, Proctor DF, Reid LM (eds.), Marcel Dekker, New York, 1977.

98. McCay PB, Gibson DD, Fong KL, et al: Effect of glutathione peroxidase activity on lipid peroxidation in biological membranes. Biochim Biophys Acta 431: 459, 1976.

99. McDermott MR, Bienenstock J: Evidence of a common mucosal immunologic system. I. Migration of B immunoblasts into intestinal, respiratory, and genital tissues. J Immunol 122:1982, 1979.

100. Mead J, Turner JM, Macklem PT, et al: Significance of the relationship between lung recoil and maximum expiratory flow. J Appl Physiol 22:95, 1967.

101. Merrill WW, Goodenberger D, Strober W, et al: Free secretory component and other proteins in human lung lavage. Am Rev Respir Dis 122:156, 1980.

102. Miller S, Ehrlich R: Susceptibility to respiratory infections of animals exposed to ozone. J Infect Dis 103: 145, 1958.

103. Morgan TE: Pulmonary surfactant. N Engl J Med 284:1185, 1971.

104. Nakajima K, Powers JC, Ashe BM, et al: Mapping the extended substrate binding site of cathepsin G and human leukocyte elastase. J Biol Chem 254:4027, 1979.

105. Nathan CF, Karnovsky ML, David JR: Alterations of macrophage functions by mediators from lymphocytes. J Exp Med 133:1356, 1971.

106. National Research Council: Atmospheric Ozone Studies, National Academy of Sciences, Washington, 1966.

107. Negus VE: Function of mucus. Acta Otolaryngol (Stockh) 56:204, 1963.

108. Olsen GN, Harris JO, Castle JR, et al: Alpha I-antitrypsin content in the serum alveolar macrophages and alveolar lavage fluid of smoking and non-smoking normal subjects. J Clin Invest 55:427, 1975.

109. Pacht ER, Kaseki H, Mohammed JR, et al: Deficiency of vitamin E in the alveolar fluid of cigarette smokers: Influence on alveolar macrophage cytotoxicity. J Clin Invest 77:786, 1986.

110. Patriarca P, Dri P, Rossi F: Superoxide dismutase in leukocytes. FEBS Lett 43:247, 1974.

111. Phipps RJ: The airway mucociliary system. In: Respiratory Physiology III, p 215, Widdicombe JG (ed.), University Park Press, Baltimore, 1981.

112. Purvis MR, Miller S, Ehrlich R: Effect of atmospheric pollutants on susceptibility to respiratory infections. J Infect Dis 109:238, 1961.

113. Racz P, Tenner-Tacz K, Myrvik QN, et al: Functional architecture: Bronchial associated lymphoid tissue and lymphoepithelium in pulmonary cell mediated reactions in the rabbit. J Reticuloendothel Soc 22:59, 1977.

114. Ranga V, Kleinerman J, Collins AM: The effect of nitrogen dioxide on tracheal uptake and transport of horseradish peroxidase in the guinea pig. Am Rev Respir Dis 122:438, 1980.

115. Reynolds HY, Atkinson JP, Newball HH, et al: Receptors for immunoglobulin and complement on human alveolar macrophages. J Immunol 114:1813, 1975.

116. Reynolds HY, Newball HH: Analysis of proteins and respiratory cells obtained from human lungs by bronchoalveolar lavage. J Lab Clin Med 84:559, 1974.

117. Reynolds HY, Newball HH: Fluid and cellular milieu of the human respiratory tract. In: Immunologic and Infectious Reactions in the Lung, Vol 1, p 3, Kirkpatrick CH, Reynolds HY (eds.), Marcel Dekker, New York, 1976.

118. Reynolds HY, Thompson RE: Pulmonary host defenses. II. Interaction of respiratory antibodies with *Pseudomonas aeruginosa* and alveolar macrophages. J Immunol 111:369, 1973.

119. Robertson J, Caldwell JR, Castle JR, et al: Evidence for the presence of components of the alternative (properidim) pathway of complement activation in respiratory secretions. J Immunol 117:900, 1976.

120. Rodriquez RJ, White RR, Senior RM, et al: Elastase release from human alveolar macrophages: Comparison between smokers and nonsmokers. Science 198: 313, 1977.

121. Rudzik O, Clancy RL, Perey DYE, et al: The distribution of a rabbit thymic antigen and membrane immunoglobulins in lymphoid tissue, with special reference to mucosal lymphocytes. J Immunol 114:1, 1975.

122. Serafini SM, Wanner A, Michaelson ED: Mucociliary transport in central and intermediate size airways: Effect of aminophylline. Bull Eur Physiopathol Respir 12:415, 1976.

123. Skornik WA, Brain JD: Relative toxicity of inhaled metal sulfate salts for pulmonary macrophages. Am Rev Respir Dis 128:297, 1983.

124. Smith KA, Gillis S, Baker PE, et al: T-cell growth factor mediated T-cell proliferation. Ann NY Acad Sci 332:423, 1979.

125. Smith LL: The response of the lungs to foreign compounds that produce free radicals. Annu Rev Physiol 48:681, 1986.

126. Sorokin SP, Brain JD: Pathways of clearance in mouse lungs exposed to iron oxide aerosols. Anat Rec 181: 581, 1975.

127. Spicer SS, Frayser R, Virella G, et al: Immunocytochemical localization of lysozyme in respiratory and other tissues. Lab Invest 36:282, 1977.

128. Starkey PM, Barrett AJ: α_2-Macroglobulin, a physiologic regulator of proteinase activity. In: Proteinases in Mammalian Cells and Tissues, p 663, Barret AJ (ed.), Elsevier/North-Holland, Amsterdam, 1977.

129. Stossel TP: Phagocytosis: Recognition and ingestion. Semin Hematol 12:83, 1975.

130. Stossel TP, Hartwig JH: Interactions of actin, myosin and new actin-binding protein of rabbit pulmonary

macrophages II. Role in cytoplasmic movement and phagocytosis. J Cell Biol 68:602, 1976.

131. Symposium on chemicals and lung toxicity—to study the agent or the disease. Environ Health Perspect 85:3–331, 1990.

132. Tappel AL: Vitamin E. Nutrition Today 8:4, 1973.

133. Task Group on Lung Dynamics: Deposition and retention models for internal dosimetry of the human respiratory tract. Health Phys 12:179, 1966.

134. Tegener H: Quantitation of human granulocyte protease inhibitors in non-purulent bronchial lavage fluids. Acta Otolaryngol 85:282, 1978.

135. Tegner H, Ohlsson K: Localization of a low molecular weight protease inhibitor to tracheal and maxillary sinus mucosa. In: Neutral Proteases of Human Polymorphonuclear Leukocytes, p 208, Havemann K, Janoff A (eds.), Urban & Schwarzenberg, Baltimore, 1978.

136. Thomas ED, Ramberg RE, Sale GE: Direct evidence for a bone marrow origin of the alveolar macrophage. Science 192:1016, 1976.

137. Thomas WR, Holt PG, Keast D: Cellular immunity in mice chronically exposed to fresh cigarette smoke. Arch Environ Health 27:372, 1973.

138. Thomas WR, Holt PG, Keast D: Effect of cigarette smoking on primary and secondary responses in mice. Nature 243:240, 1973.

139. Thomas WR, Holt PG, Keast D: Humoral immune response of mice chronically exposed to fresh cigarette smoke. Arch Environ Health 30:78, 1975.

140. Thomasi TB, Grey HM: Structure and function of immunoglobulin A. Prog Allergy 16:81, 1972.

141. Ulrich F: Studies of lymphocyte activating factor from alveolar macrophages. Res J Reticuloendothel Soc 21:33, 1977.

142. US Public Health Service: The Health Consequences of Involuntary Smoking. A Report of the Surgeon General, Department of Health and Human Services, Washington, 1986.

143. Vai F, Fournier MF, LaFuma JC, et al: SO$_2$-induced bronchopathy in the rat: Abnormal permeability of the bronchial epithelium in vivo and in vitro after anatomic recovery. Am Rev Respir Dis 121:851, 1980.

144. Valand SB, Acton JP, Myrvik QN: Nitrogen dioxide inhibition of viral-induced resistance in alveolar monocytes. Arch Environ Health 20:303, 1970.

145. Vassallo CL, Domm BM, Poe RH, et al: NO$_2$ gas and NO$_2$ effects on alveolar macrophage phagocytosis and metabolism. Arch Environ Health 26:270, 1973.

146. Waldman RH, Ganguly R: The role of the secretory immune system in protection against agents which infect the respiratory tract. Adv Exp Med Biol 45:283, 1974.

147. Wanner A: Clinical aspects of mucociliary transport. Am Rev Respir Dis 116:73, 1977.

148. Warr GA, Martin RR: In vitro migration of human alveolar macrophages: Effects of cigarette smoking. Infect Immun 8:222, 1973.

149. Warr GA, Martin RR: Chemotactic responsiveness of human alveolar macrophages: Effects of cigarette smoking. Infect Immun 9:769, 1974.

150. Warr GA, Martin RR, Holleman C, et al: Classification of bronchial lymphocytes from non-smokers and smokers. Am Rev Respir Dis 113:96, 1976.

151. West JB: Observation on gas flow in the human bronchial tree. In: Inhaled Particles and Vapours, p. 3, Davies CN (ed.), Pergamon Press, New York, 1961.

152. Witschi DH: Responses of the lung to toxic injury. Environ Health Perspect 85:5, 1990.

153. Yam J, Frank L, Roberts RJ: Oxygen toxicity: Comparison of lung biochemical responses in neonatal and adult rats. Pediatr Res 12:115, 1978.

154. Zarkower A: Alterations in antibody response induced by chronic inhalation of SO$_2$ and carbon. Arch Environ Health 25:45, 1972.

RECOMMENDED READINGS

Heffner JE, Repine JE: Pulmonary strategies of antioxidant defense. Am Rev Respir Dis 140:531, 1989.

Kaltreider HB: Phagocytic, antibody and cell-mediated immune mechanisms. In: Textbook of Respiratory Medicine, p 332, Murray JF, Nadel JA (eds.), WB Saunders, Philadelphia, 1988.

Symposium on Chemicals and Lung Toxicity—To study the agent or the disease. Environ Health Perspect 85:3–331, 1990.

8. THE GASTROINTESTINAL TRACT

Franz Hartmann and Harro Jenss

INTRODUCTION

With its mucosal surface thought to be 200 times the body surface area, the gastrointestinal tract is a major route of exposure to pathogenic organisms and environmental chemicals. Food- and water-borne chemicals enter the body via the gastrointestinal tract. Most agents are ingested; however, some inhaled substances are swallowed after being trapped in the mucus of the respiratory tract. Thus, apart from its classic role of nutrient absorption, the gastrointestinal tract must also protect the body from environmental assault (83,89,109,137,166).

Three categories of environmental agents affect the intestine: bacterial, viral, and parasitic agents; food and plant substances; and toxic agents in food, water, and the environment (8). The gastrointestinal tract is exposed to a wide variety of foreign chemicals (xenobiotics). These include such environmental contaminants as polycyclic aromatic hydrocarbons, pesticide residues, toxic metals, plasticizers, and such industrial chemicals as polychlorinated biphenyls (138). The scope of the problem is illustrated by the fact that about 63,000 chemicals are estimated to be in common use.

Principles and Practice of Environmental Medicine, edited by Alyce Bezman Tarcher. Plenum Medical Book Company, New York, 1992.

HOST DEFENSE MECHANISMS IN THE GASTROINTESTINAL TRACT

A variety of mechanisms have evolved in the gastrointestinal tract to defend the body from invasion by pathogens and toxins. These defenses include nonimmune and immune mechanisms (Table 8-1). Nonimmune defenses protecting the host are found in the intestinal secretions, enzymes, mucus, microflora, and epithelium. Such normal intestinal functions such as digestion, metabolism, detoxication, secretion, elimination (motility), and the shedding of mucosa cells also modify the absorption of noxious agents. Immune defenses are present in antibodies that are secreted into the intestine and in cell-mediated responses in gut-associated lymphoid tissue (GALT). Since the effectiveness of each component is limited, the strength of the intestinal defense depends on the integration of all components.

This chapter discusses the nature of the intestinal mucosal defense against noxious assault. It begins with an examination of the nonimmune luminal and mucosal components of the defense system, and it concludes with a discussion of the immune defense.

A number of conditions may alter intestinal defenses. These include (1) the quantity and concentration of the environmental agent ingested; (2) the amount of food, digestive enzymes, acid, and bile salts present in the intestinal lumen; (3) the nutrient status of the host; (4) the vascular state of the mucosal surface; (5) the sensitivity of the individual; and (6) the current state of the epithelial cell (126).

TABLE 8-1.   Host Defense Mechanisms
in the Gastrointestinal Tract

Luminal factors
  Secretions
  Enzymes
  Mucus
  Microflora
  Motility
Mucosal factors
  Cell walls and cytoplasm
  Metabolism
  Excretion
  Cell exfoliation
Immune factors
  Humoral antibody responses
    Secretory IgA
    Other immunoglobin classes (IgG, IgM, IgE)
  Cell-mediated responses

LUMINAL FACTORS

Ingested xenobiotics are subjected to a number of forces prior to reaching the intestinal mucosa. After first being engulfed by the aqueous secretions of the intestine and then being stirred by intestinal motility, the xenobiotics must transit three different fluid layers within the lumen of the intestine before reaching the mucosa. These layers are the unstirred water layer, the mucus layer, and the proton-rich sheet called the acid microclimate (Fig. 8-1). In addition, ingested chemicals are subjected to the metabolic action of the intestinal microflora. The following section deals with the nature of the luminal factors that modify the exposure of the intestinal mucosa to environmental agents.

Intestinal Secretions

In the path from the pharynx to the colon, the luminal concentration of noxious agents is markedly changed by the large volume of liquid that enters the alimentary tract (136). This liquid, containing water, ions, enzymes, and bile, includes about 2 L/day of ingested fluid, 6 L/day of salivary, gastric, biliary, and pancreatic secretions, and 6 L/day of small intestinal secretions. When the contents of the intestine enter the colon, this large volume is reduced about tenfold. The volume of water found in the feces is further reduced to 0.1–0.2 L/day. On this basis the concentration of unabsorbed chemicals reaches its highest level in the colon.

Within the gut lumen there are many molecular and ionic changes that affect environmental agents. A xenobiotic may be solubilized, oxidized, reduced, complexed, precipitated, or metabolized. Gastrointestinal secretions contain a number of agents that act on ingested chemicals. For example, the stomach contains the proteolytic enzyme pepsin, which is active only at a low pH. Acid hydrolysis also occurs in the stomach. The main site of enzymatic activity, however, is found in the duodenum, jejunum, and ileum, where the pH of the intestinal contents gradually increases to 7 or 8. The luminal contents of the small intestine contain proteases, carbohydrases, lipases, glucuronidases, and bile acids that act on ingested chemicals as well as on ingested nutrients (136). Hydrolysis also occurs in the distal small intestine. Because of the chemical and/or enzymatic

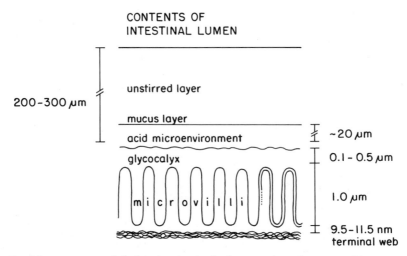

FIGURE 8-1. Conditions encountered during the transit of substances from the intestinal lumen to the microvilli.

action taking place in the intestine, many drugs may have greater activity when given parenterally, i.e., erythromycin, β-lactam antibiotics, and acetylcephalosporins (116,160,184).

The Unstirred Layer

The unstirred layer is the first layer luminal xenobiotics must cross prior to reaching the mucosal surface. This layer is formed in the intestinal lumen because of the following conditions. It is well known that solid surfaces, when immersed in a moving fluid, create a stationary layer of adherent fluid. This condition also applies to the luminal contents of the intestine. Thus, although intestinal secretions within the lumen can be mixed, the flow closer to the mucosal surface becomes increasingly slower and more laminar until there is a layer of immobile fluid abutting the mucosa (155).

The relatively immobile fluid layers adjacent to the intestinal mucosa, together with the mucus and glycocalyx, constitute the "unstirred layer" (99). The thickness of this unstirred layer has been investigated in animals (29) and humans (128). In healthy subjects, the functional unstirred layer exhibited a thickness of 500–600 μm, which is similar to the height of an intestinal villus.

This stagnant aqueous layer is now a well-recognized component of the barrier to the mucosal permeation of xenobiotics. The unstirred water layer is not in equilibrium with the remainder of the luminal contents (178). Thus, the diffusion of molecules through this layer, which abuts the mucosa, may be slower than through the bulk water phase of the luminal contents. The unstirred layer can be rate limiting to absorption (150). This occurs when the rate of diffusion through this layer is slower than the rate of penetration into the cell membrane. Studies demonstrate that the unstirred layer can retard the intestinal absorption of nonpolar compounds, particularly xenobiotics in micellar solution (174,179). Thus, for many nonpolar environmental agents such as pesticides, dyes, and food additives, the unstirred layer may be an important intestinal defense mechanism.

Intestinal Mucus

Gastrointestinal mucus is the second layer that xenobiotics must cross prior to reaching the mucosal surface. Mucus has several important functions. It protects the intestinal mucosa from the physical and chemical injury that might occur with the movement and digestion of food and the elimination of fecal material. It provides a lubricant, which eases the movement of intestinal contents. It aids in the removal of parasites by binding and entrapment (45, 78,117). It has also been suggested that the mucus

layer provides a barrier to the penetration of the mucosal surface. Reviews by Forstner et al. (46,117) describe in detail the clinical importance of gastrointestinal mucus.

Mucus, produced throughout the entire gastrointestinal tract, forms a continuous gelatinous mantle over its mucosal surface. An extensive array of cell types produces mucus along the length of the gastrointestinal tract. These include esophageal mucous glands, the stomach's cardiac, fundic, and pyloric glands, Brunner's glands of the duodenum, and goblet cells present in the small and large intestine.

Glycoproteins or mucins, which impart the viscous gel-forming properties to intestinal mucus, make up between 1% and 10% by weight of the gel. Up to 95% by weight of mucus is water, with the remainder consisting of salts, proteins, and nucleic acids (80). Mucus glycoproteins from secretions of the gastrointestinal tract have been characterized by a number of investigators. Generally all nonproteolytically derived mucins from the stomach, small intestine, and colon behave as extremely large molecules with estimated molecular weights ranging from 1.5×10^6 to 15×10^6 (107). Eighty percent of the dry weight is carbohydrate; the rest are lipids and probably membrane proteins. The qualities of mucus are well suited to its unique function. Its gel structure with its elastic qualities is resistant to solubilization, and it flows. In addition, since mucus glycoproteins are sticky molecules, they stick to each other, to other molecules, and to the mucosal surface (117). Variations in mucus may occur with changes in its thickness, the secretory state, the ionic environment, and the presence of cross-linking or viscotropic agents.

Gastric mucus constitutes a major diffusion barrier for hydrogen ions (177). Several studies suggest that mucus is an important barrier to water, electrolytes, and small molecules. Toxic heavy metals, for example, may be trapped and held tightly by mucin for later excretion in the feces. In the case of tetracycline, cations may also favor secondary binding reactions by forming a drug–calcium–mucin complex (2).

Mucus may retard adherence of bacteria to the mucosal surface—a precondition for colonization of the upper small intestine. A number of mechanisms may be involved in this process. Mucus may form a viscous barrier entrapping the bacteria, which are then moved through the intestinal tract. Mucus may provide false binding sites that compete with those present on the mucosal surface. It may also furnish a semistable matrix in which immunoglobulins and intestinal enzymes are embedded (46). Mucins also bind viruses more or less specifically. For example, the sialic acid and sulfate residues present on mucus glycoproteins form a well-known ligand for influenza virus and some human enteroviruses (30). Mucus secretion may also provide a nonspecific mucosal defense by aiding in the elimination of intestinal parasites. This has been shown for *Nippostrongylus brasiliensis*, a helminth that invades the small intestine of rats (111), and *Giardia muris*, a protozoan studied in mice (162).

Acid Microclimate

The third luminal layer that foreign chemicals must cross before reaching the mucosal surface is the acid microclimate. This proton-rich sheet is in close proximity to the coating of the intestinal surface. Lucas et al. (104,105), using pH-sensitive microelectrodes, detected this layer. These investigators, using rat small intestine and fresh human biopsy samples, discovered a layer approximately 20 μm thick with a microclimate of pH 5.9. This pH is in sharp contrast to the pH of 7.3 that is found in the lumen of the small intestine. The permeability of weak acid and bases may be influenced by this acid microclimate layer.

Intestinal Flora

The role of the gastrointestinal microflora in the metabolism of organic compounds received little attention until the past decade. It is now appreciated that microorganisms located within the intestinal lumen play an important role in the metabolism of drugs and environmental agents (139,140,176). The interested reader is referred to comprehensive reviews on this subject (35,146,147).

Soon after birth, the lumen of the gastrointestinal tract, which is sterile in the fetus, develops an enormously complex bacterial system, particularly in the colon (34,135). Detailed bacteriological studies show that more than 400 aerobic and anerobic bacterial species are present in the colonic flora (112). Data related to the species and numbers of bacteria that inhabit the various portions of the bowel are presented in Table 8-2.

Normally the stomach and proximal small intestine are relatively free of bacteria. Most of the ingested bacteria are destroyed by the acidic environment of the stomach (39). Some streptococci, lactobacilli, and fungi, however, may survive. In many normal subjects, the jejunum is free of bacteria or contains fewer than 10^4 organisms per gram of contents. If gastric acidity is compromised and the pH is maintained at 5 or higher, as many as 10^4 to 10^8 microorganisms per gram of contents can be recovered from the stomach and jejunum (35). Thus, the stomach and small intestine of patients who are achlorhydric or have undergone partial gastrectomy may contain significant numbers of aerobic and anaerobic bacteria (38,55). Impaired gastrointestinal motility also increases bacterial concentration (164).

The ileum represents a zone of transition between the few aerobic bacteria found in the stomach and proximal small intestine and the very dense population of anaerobic microorganisms found in the colon. The most dramatic change in the enteric flora occurs distal to the ileocecal valve, where there is an increase in bacterial concentration to 10^9–10^{12} microorganisms per gram of feces. Fastidious anaerobes such as *Bacteroides*, anaerobic lactobacilli, and *Clostridia* outnumber aerobes and facultative anaerobes 10,000 to one. A variety of substances such as short-

TABLE 8-2. Normal Microbial Populations of the Alimentary Tract[a]

	Stomach	Jejunum	Ileum	Cecum
Total bacterial counts[b]	0–10^3	0–10^4	10^5–10^8	10^{10}–10^{12}
Aerobes and facultative anaerobes				
Streptococci	0–10^3	0–10^4	10^2–10^5	10^4–10^9
Lactobacilli	0–10^3	0–10^4	10^2–10^5	10^6–10^{10}
Staphylococci	0–10^2	0–10^2	10^2–10^5	10^2–10^5
Enterobacteria	0–10^2	0–10^3	10^3–10^8	10^5–10^8
Fungi	0–10^2	0–10^2	10^2–10^4	10^4–10^6
Anaerobes				
Bacteroides	0	0	10^3–10^7	10^9–10^{12}
Bifidobacteria	0	0	10^3–10^6	10^8–10^{10}
Clostridia	0	0	10^2–10^4	10^8–10^9
Eubacteria	0	0	0	10^9–10^{12}
Redox potential	$+150$	-50	-150	-200
pH	3.0	6.0–7.0	7.5	6.8–7.3

[a]From Donaldson and Toskes (35). Data compiled from Donaldson (34), Savage (135), and Simon and Gorbach (146).
[b]Viable microorganisms per gram of contents.

chain fatty acids and colicines, produced by the organisms themselves, limit their growth in the colon (16,81).

Studies in man indicate that although dietary changes affect the metabolic activity of the intestinal bacterial enzymes, they have little effect on the composition of the fecal flora (70). It bears emphasis, however, that such studies were performed using standard methods of identifying and counting fecal microorganisms. In view of the vast numbers of aerobic and anaerobic species found in the gut, dietary changes could have caused marked but undetected alterations in colonic flora. Nonetheless, the complex bacterial system present within the intestine appears to be capable of resuming its original composition shortly after a variety of environmental insults (146). Clearly much work remains to be done in this important area.

The metabolism of foreign compounds by gastrointestinal microorganisms has received considerable scrutiny (39,40,139,140,149). Drugs such as lactulose, sulfasalazine, L-dopa, isonictinuric acid, salicyluric acid, and digoxin are extensively metabolized (17,101,139,140). Endogenous compounds such as sex steroid hormones (37,86) and bile acids (69,134) are also metabolized by the intestinal microflora.

Although the reactions in bacteria are diverse, most transformations are hydrolytic, reductive, or involve the removal of various chemical groups. The following metabolic reactions may occur in bacteria: hydrolysis, dehydroxylation, decarboxylation, O-demethylation, heterocyclic ring fission, reduction of double bonds, nitroreduction, azoreduction, aromatization, dehalogenation, reduction of ketones, deacylation, deamination, acetylation, and esterification (139).

The metabolism of foreign compounds by the gastrointestinal flora, however, is very often the reverse of that occurring in mammalian tissues. Whereas the metabolic reactions in mammalian tissue convert lipophilic, nonpolar compounds to polar, water-soluble (and therefore excretable) compounds, microbial metabolism frequently reduces the polarity of drugs and other foreign compounds. The hydrolysis of glycosides, in which a highly water-soluble compound is converted to a nonpolar aglycon, is an example of this process.

Epidemiologic (91,114,183) and experimental (68,96,118,163) studies show that the incidence of colon cancer is strongly correlated with meat and animal fat consumption. The following observations suggest that this link may be, in part, related to the enzyme activity of the intestinal microflora. It is well established that dietary factors affect intestinal bacterial enzyme activity and that such activity can produce mutagenic substances (28,140,146,147).

The studies of Goldin and Gorbach (52) illustrate the importance of diet on the intestinal microflora. These investigators discovered that glucuronidase, azoreductase, and nitroreductase enzymes in the fecal flora of rats were altered by diet. Changing the diet from grain to one high in beef increased the activity of all three enzymes. Supplementing the diet with 30% beef fat caused similar enzymatic changes. Additional experiments revealed that rats fed such diets were more susceptible to carcinogens. Variation in diet has been shown to have similar effects on enzyme activity of fecal flora of humans. Thus, omnivores who ate a mixed Western diet had higher fecal levels of glucuronidase, nitroreductase, and 7-dehydroxylase than did lactovegetarians or strict vegetarians (147).

Reddy and Wynder (129) demonstrate that a Western-style diet is correlated with a high fecal excretion of secondary bile acids, i.e., hepatically formed or primary bile acids that are subjected to further changes by the action of the intestinal bacteria. Bile acids have been the focus of many studies because of their structural similarity to polycyclic aromatic hydrocarbons, which are known carcinogens (68,69,114,118). Additional studies reveal that the fecal flora of North Americans and Western Europeans have higher dehydroxylase activity than those of Ugandans or Indians (71). Bacterial β-glucosidase activity was also higher in subjects eating a Western-type diet (130).

It has been postulated that a Western-type diet plays a role in carcinoma of the colon, in part by influencing the metabolic activity of the intestinal flora, which produces carcinogens or cocarcinogens from bile acids (5). In addition, it is possible that such bacterial enzymes as β-glucuronidase, β-glucosidase, β-galactosidase, nitroreductase, azoreductase, 7-α-dehydroxylase, and cholesterol dehydrogenase may mediate the transformation of the procarcinogenic substances in natural products, food preservatives, dyes, additives, or pollutants into carcinogens within the gut lumen. The role of the bacterial flora in promoting mutagenicity has been reviewed (28,140,148).

Achlorhydria is associated with an increased incidence of gastric cancer (185). A proliferation of nitrate-reducing bacteria that can occur with gastric hypoacidity has been implicated in the development of gastric dysplasia and gastric cancer (28,33,148, 152). Such bacterial activity can contribute to increased levels of nitrite, which have induced gastric tumors in rats (173).

As early as 1900 the intestinal flora was thought to have a role in the prevention of human disease. At that time Metchnikoff attributed the longevity and good health of Bulgarian peasants to their predilection for yogurt, a cultured dairy product produced by fermentation with lactobacilli (110). This subject was recently investigated in a study of the incidence of colon cancer in Danes and Finns (131), which revealed that Finns had a low risk of colon cancer while Danes are at high risk. The Finns, with a higher intake of dairy products, have significantly higher counts of lactobacilli in their feces than do the Danish group. Because the Finns also consume more dietary fiber, the cause of the protective effect is uncertain. Nevertheless, experimental data in humans (54) as well as in rats (53) demonstrate a decrease of fecal bacterial β-glucuronidase, nitroreductase, azoreductase, and 7-α-dehydroxylase activity with the ingestion of dairy products. Under these conditions, the incidence of dimethylhydrazine-induced colon tumors in rats was significantly reduced after 20 weeks but not after 36 weeks. These results suggest that feeding lactobacilli might provide some protection from ingested carcinogens.

MUCOSAL FACTORS

Before foreign chemicals penetrate the mucosal surface and enter the circulation, they must deal with the physical barrier of the epithelium, the process of absorption, and the metabolic action of the mucosa.

Physical Barriers to Absorption

The small intestine, with its major function the absorption of nutrients, has the largest intestinal surface area exposed to foreign agents. The surface area of the small intestine is magnified many times by the millions of small villi that project from the surface of the mucosa. Each villus, covered by an epithelium one cell thick, contains goblet cells that secrete mucus and absorptive cells that carry out the main functions of digestion and absorption. The most distinctive feature of the absorptive cell is its brush border composed of microvilli. Covering the microvillus is a cell membrane or apical membrane. This membrane is, in turn, covered by a continuous filamentous-appearing coat called the glycocalyx (Fig. 8-1).

Prior to entering the body from the small intestine, xenobiotics must cross the glycocalyx, the apical membrane, the absorptive cell, and the basolateral membrane.

Glycocalyx

A filamentous surface coat composed of acidic mucopolysaccharides is applied directly to the surface of the microvillus (82). This layer, called the glycocalyx or "fuzzy layer," is firmly attached to the microvillus membrane and is resistant to mucolytic and proteolytic agents.

Disaccharidases, some dipeptidases, and binding sites for glucose, iron, and intrinsic factor are localized in the glycocalyx (24). Very little is known about what role the glycocalyx plays in the absorption of xenobiotics. The glycocalyx may bind foreign chemicals, which may be a prerequisite for their absorption. It has also been postulated that this layer acts as a filter to protect the epithelial cell against bacteria and such macromolecules as endotoxins.

Apical Membrane

Underlying the glycocalyx is the cell membrane of the microvillus. This apical membrane, 9.5–11.5 nm thick, is similar in structure to other biological membranes (15). It consists of two molecular layers of lipid in opposition. Each lipid molecule is composed of a hydrophilic portion coated with protein facing outward and a hydrophobic portion directed inwards. The fusion of the outer layer of two adjacent cell membranes forms a tight junction, which provides an effective barrier between the intestinal lumen and the intercellular space. A number of studies have shown that a range of enzymes and transport systems are present in the membrane of the microvillus (63). These enzymes are capable of digesting a wide variety of foodstuffs.

Epithelial Cell Contents

In addition to the apical membrane, the epithelial cell contents may also present a barrier to the transfer of xenobiotics. To reach the blood, molecules penetrating the apical membrane of the epithelial cell must diffuse approximately 30 μm across its cytoplasm. The cytoplasm contains a number of structures that may impair the movement of xenobiotics. These include the rough and smooth endoplasmic reticulum, Golgi material, mitochondria, lysosomes, and fine filaments for ribosomes as well as the cell water, which may itself be highly structured (64,65). The barrier afforded by the cell contents may in part consist of bilayer membranes within the cytoplasm. It is possible that some permeability properties of the cell content are similar to those of the apical and basal membrane. This, however, remains controversial (108).

Basal Barriers

The next barrier separating a foreign molecule from the blood is the basal membrane of the epithelial cell. This bilayer membrane probably has permeability properties similar to other cell membranes. Another bilayer membrane, the basement membrane, lies close to the basal cell membrane. The basal and basement membranes are separated by a narrow water-filled extracellular space.

The last layer separating the absorbed xenobiotic from the circulation is the membrane of the villus capillaries. It is about 1 nm thick (41). The capillary membrane, containing fenestrae 40–50 nm wide, is covered with a 2- to 4-nm thick mucopolysaccharide membrane that contains practically no lipid. The surface area of these fenestrae represents approximately 10% of the total surface area of the capillary wall. Much of the exchange across the capillary wall is apparently handled by these circular openings (41).

Mucosal Absorption

Ingested xenobiotics are subjected to the same processes used for the absorption of nutrients. Accordingly, the following mechanisms are available for absorbing foreign chemicals: diffusion, facilitated diffusion, active transport, and pinocytosis. The absorption of xenobiotics is also dependent on such factors as lipid versus water solubility, the degree of ionization, and molecular size. A mechanism termed "solvent drag," wherein absorbed water carries along dissolved molecules, also affects the absorption of xenobiotics (119,120). In general, xenobiotics do not undergo digestion in the intestinal lumen. They must, however, be solubilized before coming in contact with the gut mucosa. It appears that the processes of absorption offer the body little specific protection from the mucosal penetration of foreign chemicals.

Many factors influence the intestinal absorption of xenobiotics. These include such conditions as gastric emptying time, intestinal motility, the surface area of the small intestine, intestinal blood flow, diet, genetic factors, and age (20,36,75,113,180,186).

Diffusion

Most foreign substances are absorbed by simple diffusion, whereas nutrients are actively absorbed (20,75). Simple diffusion is not energy dependent; it is dependent on physiochemical factors. Absorption by simple diffusion is proportional to the concentration gradient and to the lipid–water partition coefficient of the xenobiotic. Facilitated diffusion, a more complex form of diffusion, depends on carrier proteins. There are data to suggest that such heavy metals as lead and cadmium are absorbed by this mechanism (20,75).

Active Transport

Active transport, a complex energy-requiring mechanism, moves chemicals against an electrochemical gradient and is substrate specific. This system, which is Na^+, K^+-ATPase dependent, is responsible for the transport of such compounds as

amino acids, sugars, low-molecular-weight peptides, and bile acids (20,75).

Iturri and Wolff (84) showed that ATPase activities as well as transport capacities may be influenced by environmental agents. For example, DDT [2,2-bis-(p-chlorophenyl)-1,1,1-trichloethane] and DDE [2,2-bis-(p-chlorophenyl)-1,1-dichloroethylene] inhibit the active transport of D-glucose and L-tyrosine as well as the membrane-bound Na^+, K^+-ATPase in the rat small intestine.

Pinocytosis

Pinocytosis, the process of engulfing particles by invagination of the absorptive cell membrane, is used for the absorption of some large foreign molecules. There is evidence that such particulate materials as colloidal silver, starch particles, and endotoxins are absorbed in significant quantities by this process (98). After absorption, these particles may accumulate in large numbers in the reticuloendothelial system. The toxicological implications of such absorption are unknown at this time.

Mucosal Metabolism of Xenobiotics

Until recently, it was assumed that the intestinal mucosa functioned exclusively to digest and absorb nutrients and to absorb foreign chemicals. It is now well established that the intestinal mucosa also has the capacity to metabolize foreign chemicals (1,21, 60,65,142,181). Because the intestine is directly exposed to a wide variety of foreign chemicals, this capacity may protect the mucosa from injury and influence the bioavailability of absorbed xenobiotics. With the intestinal metabolism of xenobiotics, it is possible that some absorbed compounds are detoxified in the mucosa and never reach the circulation. The biotransformation system within the intestine is similar to that in the liver (20). Detailed reviews of the biotransformation of xenobiotics by the gastrointestinal mucosa are available (48,60,73,74,182).

Xenobiotic metabolism within the enterocyte is catalyzed by enzymes bound to the smooth endoplasmic reticulum. This metabolism, although similar to that found in the liver, generally proceeds at a slower rate (20). The biochemical defense provided by the enterocyte, basically similar to that found in the liver, depends on a series of reactions that transform nonpolar lipophilic compounds to polar and more readily excretable metabolites. The principle behind this transformation is that most toxic compounds, being nonpolar, are not excreted through the usual water-based pathways until they are transformed into polar compounds.

Two processes are used to convert nonpolar lipophilic chemicals to polar water-soluble products. Phase I converts the chemical into a relatively polar compound by adding a polar or reactive group. Phase II consists of conjugation reactions. Phase I requires a mixed-function oxidase system with cytochrome P-450 as oxygen activator and NADPH–cytochrome c reductase to supply electrons (51). In phase II, compounds undergo conjugation with such endogenous substances as glucuronic acid, sulfate, or glutathione.

The specific enzymes involved in these metabolic conversions (i.e., cytochrome-P-450/448-dependent mixed-function oxidases, uridine diphosphoglucuronyltransferases, sulfotransferases, or glutathione S-transferase) have all been identified in the intestinal mucosa of various animal species and man (26,61,74,94,95,127,153). Hartiala (60) and Caldwell (17) have reviewed the metabolic reactions occurring within the gut wall.

A number of drugs and environmental toxins are known to undergo extensive metabolic conversion in the intestinal mucosa (Table 8-3). This phenomenon has been termed the "intestinal first-pass effect" (49), to distinguish it from the first-pass metabolism by the liver or metabolism by the intestinal microflora (139). Because of its clinical importance, particularly in the metabolism of ingested drugs, the intestinal first-pass metabolism is receiving attention (74,85,92,133).

Biotransformation of a lipophilic xenobiotic by the intestinal mucosa generally produces a water-soluble compound with lower pharmacological activity or toxicity than the parent compound. The gut microsomal enzyme system reaction is, however, capable of generating active metabolites with increased toxicity or carcinogenicity (7). Such activation has been shown for N-nitrosamines, aflatoxin, and 1,2-dimethylhydrazine (7) and for such polycyclic hydrocarbons as benzo[a]pyrene, 1-methylcholanthrene and 7,12-dimethylbenz[a]anthracene (6,100). It appears that in the intestine, as in other organs that metabolize xenobiotics, a balance exists between metabolic detoxication and activation of carcinogens and toxins. (See Chapter 9 for a detailed discussion of metabolic detoxication and activation.)

The activity of the mucosal mixed-function oxidase system is highest in the duodenum. Its activity decreases from the duodenum to the colon in parallel with intestinal absorptive capacity (77). The mature enterocytes at the mucosal villus tips have the highest cytochrome P-450 content and mixed-function oxidase activity. There is very little activity in the undifferentiated crypt cells.

Effects of Diet and Xenobiotic Exposure on Mucosal Metabolism

Wattenberg and his co-workers first noted that dietary factors affected the ability of the intestine to metabolize xenobiotics (170). These workers used the aryl hydrocarbon hydroxylase (AHH) system to study the effect of dietary modification on intestinal xenobiotic-metabolizing enzymes in the rat. Benzo[a]pyrene was used as a representative substrate. Starvation and a semisynthetic diet resulted in the

TABLE 8-3. Metabolism of Drugs and Environmental Agents by Intestinal Mucosa

Compound	Reaction	Reference
Flurazepam	N-Dealkylation	Mahon et al. (1977) (106)
Phenacetin	O-Deethylation	Pantuck et al. (1974) (123)
		Klippert et al. (1982) (92)
Isoproterenol	Sulfation	Conolly et al. (1972) (23)
	O-Methylation	
Chlorpromazine	Demethylation	Hartmann et al. (1983) (62)
	Sulfoxidation	
Pentobarbital	Oxidation	Knodell et al. (1980) (93)
Morphine	Oxidation	Iwamoto and Klassen (1977) (85)
	Glucuronidation	
Stilbestrol	Glucuronidation	Fischer and Millburn (1970) (44)
Testosterone	Oxidation	Farthing (1982) (43)
Ethanol	Oxidation	Seitz et al. (1979) (141)
Tetrahydrocannabinol	Hydroxylation	Green and Saunders (1974) (56)
1-Naphthol	Glucuronidation	Wollenberg (1983) (182)
Benzo[a]pyrene	Oxidation	Hietanen (1980) (66)
Propranolol	—	Shand and Rangno (1972) (142)
Clonazepam	—	Colburn et al. (1980) (22)
Methyldigoxin	—	Hinderling et al. (1977) (72)

loss of all intestinal AHH activity. Oral iron deprivation provides another example of the effect of nutrient exposure on intestinal enzyme activity. A
marked reduction in intestinal cytochrome P-450
activity occurs within 24 h of oral iron deprivation.
At this time plasma iron levels are unchanged (77).

Hietanen et al. (67) demonstrated that such
chemicals as phenoxyacid herbicides and glyphosphate, widely used in agriculture and forestry to
control the growth of weeds and brush, can change
intestinal biotransformation activities. Rats given
glyphosphate or 4-chloro-2-methylphenoxyacetic
acid (MCPA) orally showed a marked decrease in
intestinal aryl hydrocarbon hydroxylase activity.
The activities of ethyoxycoumarin O-deethylase and
epoxide hydrolase were increased after such exposure. Intestinal exposure to polycyclic aromatic hydrocarbons (cigarette smoke and charcoal-broiled
meat) increases intestinal xenobiotic metabolism (124).

A report by Pascoe et al. (125) demonstrates that
cytochrome P-450 synthesis and assembly require
the presence of selenium in the intestinal lumen. A
reduction in glutathione peroxidase activity also
occurs with selenium deprivation. A reduction in
peroxidase activity may impair the intestinal detoxification of toxic organic peroxides and hydroxy-
peroxides and thereby promote chemical carcinogenesis.

Subsequent work by Wattenberg and co-workers (151,169,171,172) illustrates another important aspect of dietary control of xenobiotic metabolism.
Cruciferous plants (i.e., Brussels sprouts, cabbage,
cauliflower, and broccoli) and such compounds as
benzylisothiocyanate, β-naphtoflavone, coumarin,
and disulfiram inhibit carcinogen-induced neoplasia in experimental animals. They also increase
the activity of xenobiotic-metabolizing enzymes in
the liver and the small intestine. These findings
suggest that dietary nutrients may alter the intestinal response to chemical carcinogens in favor of the
host. Intestinal xenobiotic metabolism and its potential role in protecting against colon cancer have
recently been reviewed (73). The findings noted
above, as well as those of other workers, indicate
that dietary factors play a unique role in controlling
the intestinal metabolism of foreign chemicals (4,67,
125,151,159).

The work of Hoensch et al. suggests that nutritional conditions may also influence the intestinal
metabolism of foreign compounds in man (76). These
investigators, using jejunal biopsy specimens, studied the effect of semisynthetic diets on intestinal
function and morphology. They report that eating a
semisynthetic diet caused a marked reduction in
intestinal xenobiotic metabolism and villus height.
This reduction was eliminated when the subjects
resumed their normal eating pattern. It is of interest
that jejunal enzyme activity was markedly lower in
female than in male subjects. This difference was
not explained by the use of hormonal contraception.

It appears that diet affects intestinal enzyme
activity more than it affects liver enzyme activity.
For example, Wattenberg et al. (170) and Hoensch et
al. (77) report that rats that are switched from Purina
Rat Chow to a balanced purified diet show a rapid
decrease in intestinal cytochrome P-450 activity. Hepatic cyctochrome P-450 activity, however, remains
unchanged.

Age may also be a factor in the intestinal metabolism of foreign compounds. The intestines of the
young and the old may be less able to metabolize
environmental agents. This subject needs further
investigation.

Our understanding of the biological impact and
mode of regulation of the intestinal metabolism of
foreign compounds is nascent. The capacity of the
intestine to metabolize foreign compounds undoubtedly offers the body an important defense
against invasion by foreign chemicals.

Mucosal Secretion of Chemicals and Shedding of Mucosal Cells

Two important, and often overlooked, processes modulating the effect of noxious exposure are
the intestinal secretion of xenobiotics and the shedding of mucosal cells (97,102,103).

Thus far the discussion has focused on the
entry of xenobiotics from the gastrointestinal tract.
The gut, however, can also act as an excretory organ
for such agents. For example, such compounds as
quaternary ammonium compounds, strong acids,
and cardiac glycosides are actively secreted into the
intestinal lumen (8). In addition, the fecal elimination of such lipophilic toxins as hexachlorobenzene
and chlordecone (Kepone®) is increased by giving
paraffin or cholestryamine (60,132). The secretory
capacity of the intestine, amplified by giving cholestyramine, has been used to detoxify individuals
with chlordecone poisoning (58). The physiological
importance and the clinical application of these secretory processes, possibly as excretory mechanisms for endogenous as well as exogenous compounds, have yet to be evaluated.

The shedding of mucosal cells is another important intestinal defense mechanism. It is well established that the turnover rate of intestinal cells is very
fast (102). The epithelial cells of the intestinal tract
are among the most rapidly proliferating cells in the
body. Studies by Lipkin et al. reveal that the epithelial cells of the gut are produced at a mean rate close
to 1 cell per 100 cells per hour (102). It is estimated
that billions of cells per day are discarded along the
length of the human intestine. It is likely that cell

exfoliation is associated with the elimination of xenobiotics. Heavy metals and highly lipophilic agents, in particular, may be eliminated from the intestine by this method.

IMMUNE FACTORS

The intestinal immune system plays a role in protecting the host from bacteria, viruses, protozoa, and foreign chemicals. During the last decade, remarkable advances have been made in our understanding of this system (10,31,32,47,59,83,89,145).

The gastrointestinal tract and liver contain one of the major components of the immune system, the gut-associated lymphoid tissue (GALT) (11,42,47, 83,89,109). Approximately one-quarter of the intestinal mucosa is composed of lymphoid tissue (9,109). The GALT has a number of components. It includes nodular lymphoid tissues scattered throughout the intestinal submucosa (Peyer's patches), solitary mucosal lymphoid follicles, and solitary lymphoid cells found throughout the entire gastrointestinal mucosa.

Peyer's patches, aggregates of lymphoid follicles located directly under the epithelium of the intestinal lumen, are of major importance in the initiation and expression of intestinal immunity. Studies in humans demonstrate that Peyer's patches increase from a few follicles in the duodenum to more than 900 in the terminal ileum. There are several distinct regions within Peyer's patches: the follicle, the dome, and the region between the follicles. The follicles are populated by B lymphocytes. T-cell-dependent regions are located between the follicles and in the dome area overlying the follicles. Columnar epithelium densely infiltrated with lymphocytes and interspersed with specialized M cells overlies the Peyer's patches. This specialized epithelium, containing few mucus-producing goblet cells and lacking fully developed micovilli, seems necessary for antigen presentation to the intestinal immune system. Antigen absorption from the bowel lumen to Peyer's patches is attributed to the M cells (122).

Lymphoid cells are found between the intestinal epithelial cells lining the villous surface. They are also diffusely scattered throughout the lamina propria. T lymphocytes are found in the intraepithelial population along with mast cells and their precursors. The lamina propria contains T and B lymphocytes as well as macrophages, mast cells, and polymorphonuclear leukocytes. The dense concentration of lymphoid cells within the epithelium and lamina propria of the intestine along with its large surface area make these sites a major source of lymphoid cells in the intestine. Indeed, it has been estimated that the B-cell population of the intestinal

lamina propria makes up about 25% of the lymphoid pool in normal adults (9).

Antigen Uptake and Stimulation of Gut-Associated Lymphoid Tissue

Peyer's patches are capable of absorbing such particulate antigens as macromolecules and bacteria from the bowel lumen (87,122). Interaction occurs between luminal antigens and T and B cells in Peyer's patches. After antigen challenge, activated lymphocytes in Peyer's patches follow a migration pathway (12). They migrate from Peyer's patches into the mesenteric lymph nodes, the thoracic duct, and then into the circulation. After entering the circulation, a portion of these cells return to the lamina propria of the intestine, where they may perform a role in immune defense (57,165). Lymphoid cells from Peyer's patches can also disseminate to other mucosa sites and mediate immune responses. The determinants of the migratory pathways of intestinal lymphoid cells are not well understood at this time.

The migration of IgA precursor cells from the mucosa of the intestine to other mucosal sites in the intestine, breast, lung, or reproductive tract helps to clarify the finding that immunization at one mucosa surface often results in the production of identical antibodies at other mucosal sites. The evidence of the migratory pathway of intestinal lymphoid cells supports the concept of a common mucosa-associated lymphoid system (12,13). Immunity in mucosal tissues depends on mucosa-associated lymphoid tissues (MALT), which are widely distributed in the intestine, the lung, part of the urogenital tract, the mammary gland, the conjunctiva, the middle ear, and the lacrimal and salivary glands.

The exchange of information between one mucosal site and another can be of considerable practical importance. It has been shown that after oral immunization, IgA with antibodies against intestinal antigens is found in breast milk. Oral immunization with a nonpathogenic strain of Escherichia coli during the last month of pregnancy results in colostrum containing antibodies to Escherichia coli (167). Antibodies in mammary secretions are thus provided when the newborn infant is deficient in intestinal antibodies. These events do not occur when immunization is given parenterally.

Mucosal Antibodies

It is well established that a prominent feature of the immunologic defense at the intestinal mucosal surface is the presence of antibodies in intestinal secretions (109,156,157,161). Evidence of this defense was reflected in the observation by Davies, in 1922, that subjects with a bacterial infection possessed fecal antibodies when antibodies were not present in the blood (25). This observation, along with the findings of other workers, revealed that resistance to local infection can occur in the absence of a systemic response. The discovery by Tomasi and co-workers that IgA was the major antibody in external secretions and that its structure differed markedly from that of serum antibodies suggested that the gut's immunologic defenses were uniquely suited to guard the host from environmental assault (158). Although IgA remains the hallmark of local immunologic response, other cellular and humoral elements are also involved in mucosal defenses.

The IgA found in intestinal secretions (secretory IgA) differs structurally from the IgA present in the serum. About 85% of human serum IgA is monomeric, whereas secretory IgA (sIgA) consists of two IgA monomers linked together by a polypeptide J chain (J) and a secretory component (SC) (156,157). The entire immunoglobulin dimer with the J chain is derived from plasma cells in the lamina propria (90). Following its synthesis, sIgA is transported across the intestinal epithelial cell into the intestinal lumen by a unique transport system involving a glycoprotein called secretory component (SC). The secretory component, synthesized by the epithelial cells, mediates the transport of IgA across the epithelial cell into the intestinal lumen. Similar events occur in the bronchi and the mammary, salivary, and tear ducts. The IgA bound to the secretory component is ingested by receptor-mediated endocytosis, transported across the epithelial cell, and secreted into the lumen (Fig. 8-2). The addition of secretory component to secretory IgA appears to protect this immunoglobulin from the action of proteolytic enzymes.

Immunoglobulin A is found in bile. In man, IgA is transported across bile duct epithelial cells by means of secretory component, whereas transport across hepatocytes depends on a mechanism other than secretory component (79,115).

The importance of the secretory IgA system for the protection of the mucous membranes and for efficient defense against potential antigens is well documented. Intestinal antibodies function to bind antigens in the intestine and limit their absorption (89,168). They also prevent bacteria from adhering to the intestinal surface, control their proliferation and mucosal penetration, and protect the bowel mucosa from injury that can arise from continuous antigen exposure (89,175). Secretory IgA can directly neutralize viruses in the absence of complement. After oral poliovaccine immunization, for example, IgA antipolio virus neutralizing antibody can be detected in intestinal secretions (121).

The most common primary immunodeficiency is a selective IgA deficiency. Many individuals with this immune deficiency apparently suffer no ill effects; however, a certain number have an increased incidence of mucosa infections, allergy, and autoimmune disease (166).

Although IgA predominates, all classes of immunoglobulins are found in the intestinal secretions. Precursors to IgG and IgM have been shown to be derived from the mesenteric lymph nodes. Relatively little is known, however, about the part played by IgM or IgG in mucosal defenses. The intestinal tract is also rich in IgE-producing cells. Sensitization by the intestinal route may therefore be one element in the pathophysiology of certain allergic diseases.

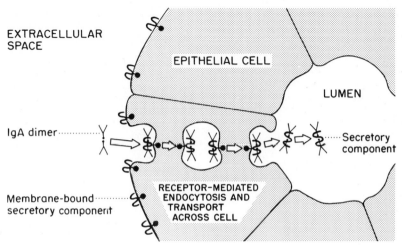

FIGURE 8-2. The transport of secretory IgA across an intestinal epithelial cell. From Alberts et al. (3).

Mucosal Cell-Mediated Immune Mechanisms

The intestinal mucosa contains all ingredients needed for a cellular immune response. As mentioned, the intestinal lymphoid population includes an abundance of regulatory T cells. T-cell regulatory functions include enhancement of the mucosal production of IgA. After oral immunization, helper T cells facilitate the production of IgM and IgG. Suppressor T cells have been described in the development of oral tolerance. Oral tolerance involves the suppression of systemic immune responses to parenteral immunization (42).

In addition to its regulatory function, the mucosal cellular immune system participates in cytotoxic reactions. Cytotoxic cells have been identified in Peyer's patches, lamina propria, and the mucosal epithelium after oral or intraperitoneal immunization (88). Natural killer (NK) cell activity has been reported in cells from the intestinal lamina propria (154). These cells are thought to be important in the recognition and killing of tumor cells (14). The intestine is also rich in mast cells. These cells, by releasing such potent mediators as histamine, serotonin, and the leukotrienes, may cause edema of the oral mucosa and pharynx as well as contraction of smooth muscle of the gastrointestinal tract and diarrhea (36,113). Although a great deal is known about the secretory IgA system, far less is known about the role cell-mediated responses and IgE, IgM, and IgG play in the interaction between the host and intestinal antigens.

Effects of Diet and Xenobiotic Exposure on the Intestinal Immune System

It is well established that nutrition plays a critical role in intestinal structure and function (19). Malnutrition is associated with changes in the intestinal immune system (18). Children dying of severe protein–energy malnutrition have atrophy of the tonsils and of the gut-associated lymphoid tissue (19). The concentration and specific antibody response of secretory IgA are reduced in the mucosal secretions of malnourished individuals (19). The proportion of intraepithelial lymphocytes is also reduced. Although these findings indicate that nutritional deficiency alters mucosal immunity, our understanding of this relationship and its clinical implications is limited. Impaired intestinal mucosal immunity, however, is often associated with increased susceptibility to enteral infections and septicemia (19).

The literature is replete with studies investigating the effects of xenobiotic exposure on the immune system (27,50,143,144). Many such studies reveal that environmental chemicals have a deleterious effect on the immune system. Thus far, however, little attention has been given to the effects of xenobiotic exposure on the immune system in the gastrointestinal tract.

SUMMARY

The gastrointestinal tract contains an elaborate system to defend the body from environmental assault. This system includes the intestinal secretions, enzymes, mucus, microflora, epithelium, and the immune system. Mucosal metabolism, excretion, and cell exfoliation are also important parts of this defense system. Many conditions, including age, sex, nutrition and, xenobiotic exposure, influence the responsiveness of intestinal mucosal defenses.

REFERENCES

1. Aitio A, Marniemi J: Extrahepatic glucuronide conjugation. In: Extrahepatic Metabolism of Drugs and Other Foreign Compounds, p 365, Gram TE (ed.), MTP Press, Lancaster, 1980.
2. Albert A, Rees CW: Avidity of the tetracyclins for the cations of metals. Nature 177:433, 1956.
3. Alberts B, Dennis B, Lewis J, et al: Molecular Biology of the Cell, Garland Publishing, New York, 1983.
4. Anderson KE, Schneider J, Pantuck EJ, et al: Acetaminophen metabolism in subjects fed charcoal-broiled beef. Clin Pharmacol Ther 34:369, 1983.
5. Aries VC, Crowther JS, Drasar BS, et al: Bacteria and the etiology of cancer of the large bowel. Gut 10:334, 1969.
6. Autrup H: Use of explant cultures to study the metabolism of polycyclic aromatic hydrocarbons in the human gastrointestinal tract. In: Advances in Physiological Sciences, Vol 29, Gastrointestinal Defense Mechanisms, p 385, Mozik G, Hanninen O, Javor T (eds.), Pergamon Press, New York; Akademiai Kiado, Budapest, 1981.
7. Autrup H: Carcinogen metabolism in human tissues and cells. Drug Metab Rev 13:603, 1982.
8. Banwell JG: Environmental contaminants and intestinal function. Environ Health Perspect 33:107, 1979.
9. Barnik V, ReMine SG, Chiba M, et al: Isolation and characterization of colonic intraepithelial and lamina proprial lymphocytes. Gastroenterology 78:976, 1980.
10. Bienenstock J, Befus AD: Mucosal immunology. Immunology 41:249, 1980.
11. Bienenstock J, Befus AD: The gastrointestinal tract as an immune organ. In: Gastrointestinal Immunity for the Clinician, p 1, Sorter RG, Ku JB (eds.), Grune & Stratton, Orlando, 1985.
12. Bienenstock J, McDermott M, Belfus AD: A common mucosal immune system. In: Immunology of Breast Milk, p 91, Ogra PL, Dayton DH (eds.), Raven Press, New York, 1979.
13. Bienenstock J, McDermott M, Befus AD, et al: Mucosal immunology. Monogr Allergy 16:1, 1980.
14. Bloom BR: Natural killers to rescue immune surveillance? Nature 300:214, 1982.

15. Bretscher MS: Membrane structure: Some general principles. Science 181:622, 1973.
16. Byrne BM, Dankert J: Volatile fatty acids and aerobic flora in the gastrointestinal tract of mice under various conditions. Infect Immun 23:559, 1979.
17. Caldwell J: The metabolism of drugs by the gastrointestinal tract. In: Presystemic Drug Elimination, George CF, Shand DG, Renwick AG, et al. (eds.), Butterworths, London, 1982.
18. Chandra RK: Mucosal immune responses in malnutrition. Ann NY Acad Sci 409:345, 1983.
19. Chandra RK: Nutritional modulation of intestinal mucosal immunity. Immunol Invest 18:119, 1989.
20. Chhabra RS, Eastin WC Jr: Intestinal absorption and metabolism of xenobiotics in laboratory animals. In: Intestinal Toxicology, p 145, Schiller CM (ed.), Raven Press, New York, 1984.
21. Clifton G, Kaplowitz N: The glutathion S-transferase of the intestine in the rat. Cancer Res 37:788, 1977.
22. Colburn WA, Bekersky I, Min BH, et al: Contribution of gut contents, intestinal wall and liver to the first pass metabolism of clonazepam in the rat. Res Commun Chem Pathol Pharmacol 27:73, 1980.
23. Conolly ME, Davies DS, Dollery CT, et al: Metabolism of isoprenaline in dog and man. Br J Pharmacol 46:458, 1972.
24. Creamer B: Biomembranes. In: Intestinal Absorption, Vol 4A, p 1, Smyth DH (ed.), Plenum Press, London, 1974.
25. Davies A: Investigation into the serological properties of dysentery stools. Lancet 2:1009, 1922.
26. Dawson JR, Bridges JW: Guinea-pig intestinal sulphotransferases: An investigation using the cytosolic fraction. Biochem Pharmacol 30:2409, 1981.
27. Dean JH, Cornacoff JB, Luster MI: Toxicity of the immune system: A review. In: Immunopharmacology Reviews, Vol 1, p 377, Hadden JW, Szentivanyi A (eds.), Plenum Press, New York, 1990.
28. Deschner EE, De Cosse JJ, Sherlock P: Chemical and environmental agents in gastrointestinal carcinogenesis. Clin Gastroenterol 10:755, 1981.
29. Desnam ES, Levin RJ: An experimental method of identifying and quantifying the active transfer electrogenic component from the diffuse component during sugar absorption measured in vivo. J Physiol (Lond) 246:181, 1975.
30. Di Girolamo R, Liston J, Matches J: Ionic binding: The mechanism of viral uptake by shellfish mucus. Appl Environ Microbiol 33:19, 1977
31. Dobbins WO: Gut immunology and immunodeficiency. Curr Concepts Gastroenterol 1/2:6, 1983.
32. Doe WF: An overview of intestinal immunity and malabsorption. Am J Med 67:1077, 1979.
33. Domellof L, Erikson S, Janunger DG: Carcinoma and possible precancerous changes of the gastric stump after Billroth II resection. Gastroenterology 73:462, 1977.
34. Donaldson RM: Role of indigenous enteric bacteria in intestinal function and disease. In: Handbook of Physiology, Sec. 9, p 301, Code CF (ed.), American Physiological Society, Washington, 1968.
35. Donaldson RM Jr, Toskes PP: The relation of enteric bacterial populations to gastrointestinal function and disease. In: Gastrointestinal Disease. Pathophysiol-

ogy, Diagnosis, Management, 4th ed., p 107, WB Saunders, Philadelphia, 1989.
36. Donowitz M, Charney AN, Hefferman T: Effect of serotonin treatment on intestinal transport in the rabbit. Am J Physiol 232:85, 1977.
37. Dossetar J: Drug interaction with oral contraceptives. Br Med J 4:467, 1975.
38. Drasar BS, Hill MJ: Human Intestinal Flora, Academic Press, New York, 1974.
39. Drasar BS, Shiner M, McLeod GM: Studies on the intestinal flora. I. The bacterial flora of the gastrointestinal tract in healthy and achlorhydric persons. Gastroenterology 56:71, 1969.
40. Drasar BS, Hill MJ, Williams RED: The significance of the gut flora in safety testing of food additives. In: Metabolic Aspects of Food Safety, p 245, Roe FJC (ed.), Blackwell Scientific Publications, London, 1970.
41. Eade MN: Gut circulation and absorption, a review, part I. NZ Med J 84:10, 1976.
42. Ernst PB, Scicchitano R, Underdown BJ, et al: Oral immunization and tolerance. In: Immunology of the Gastrointestinal Tract and Liver, Heyworth MF, Jones AL (eds.), p 125, Raven Press, New York, 1988.
43. Farthing MJG, Vinson GP, Edwards CR, et al: Testosterone metabolism by the rat gastrointestinal tract, in vitro and in vivo. Gut 23:226, 1982.
44. Fischer LJ, Millburn P: Stilbesterol transport and glucuronide formation in everted sacs of rat intestine. J Pharmacol Exp Ther 175:267, 1970.
45. Florey H: Mucins and the protection of the body. Proc R Soc Lond [Biol] 143:147, 1955.
46. Forstner G, Wesley A, Forstner J: Clinical aspects of gastrointestinal mucus. In: Mucus in Health and Disease II, p 189, Chantler EN, Elder JB, Elstein M (eds.), Plenum Press, New York, 1982.
47. Gallin JI, Fauci AS (eds.): Advances in Host Defense Mechanisms, Mucosal Immunity, Raven Press, New York, 1985.
48. George CF: Drug metabolism by the gastrointestinal mucosa. Clin Pharmacokinet 6:259, 1981.
49. Gibaldi M, Perrier D: Route of administration and drug disposition. Drug Metab Rev 3:185, 1974.
50. Gibson GG, Hubbard R, Parke DV (eds.): Immunotoxicology, Academic Press, New York, 1983.
51. Gilette R, David DC, Sesame HA: Cytochrome P-450 and its role in drug metabolism. Ann Rev Pharmacol 12:57, 1972.
52. Goldin BR, Gorbach SL: The relationship between diet and rat fecal bacterial enzymes implicated in colon cancer. J Natl Cancer Inst 57:371, 1976.
53. Goldin BR, Gorbach SL: Effect of lactobacillus acidophilus dietary supplements on 1,2-dimethylhydrazine dihydrochloride induced intestinal cancer in rats. J Natl Cancer Inst 64:263, 1980.
54. Goldin BR, Swenson L, Dwyer J, et al: Effect of diet and lactobacillus supplements on human fecal bacterial enzymes. J Natl Cancer Inst 64:225, 1980.
55. Gray JDA, Shiner M: Influence of gastric pH on gastric and jejunal flora. Gut 8:574, 1967.
56. Green ML, Saunders DR: Metabolism of tetrahydrocannabinol by the small intestine. Gastroenterology 66:365, 1974.
57. Guy-Grand D, Griscelli C, Vassali P: Peyer's patches, gut IgA plasma cells and thymic function: Study in

nude mice bearing thymic grafts. J Immunol 115:361, 1975.

58. Guzelian PS: Chlordecone poisoning: A case study in approaches for detoxification of humans exposed to environmental chemicals. Drug Metab Rev 13:663, 1982.

59. Hanson LA, Ahlstedt S, Andersson B, et al: Mucosal immunity. Ann NY Acad Sci 409:1, 1983.

60. Hartiala KJW: Metabolism of hormones, drugs and other substances by the gut. Physiol Rev 53:496, 1973.

61. Hartmann F, Bisell DM: Metabolism of heme and bilirubin in rat and human small intestinal mucosa. J Clin Invest 70:23, 1982.

62. Hartmann F, Gruenke LD, Craig JC, et al: Chlorpromazine metabolism in extracts of liver and small intestine from guinea pig and from man. Drug Met Dispos 11:244, 1983.

63. Hayton WL: Rate-limiting barriers to intestinal drug absorption: A review. J Pharmacokin Biopharm 8:321, 1980.

64. Hazlewood CF: Bound water in biology. Acta Biochim Biophys 12:263, 1977.

65. Hechter O: Intracellular water structure and mechanisms of cellular transport. Ann NY Acad Sci 195:625, 1972.

66. Hietanen E: Oxidation and subsequent glucuronidation of 3,4-benzopyrene in everted intestinal sacs in control and 3-methyl-cholanthrene-pretreated rats. Pharmacol 21:233, 1980.

67. Hietanen E, Linnainmaa K, Vainio H: Effects of phenoxyherbicides and glyphosphate on the hepatic and intestinal biotransformation activities in the rat. Acta Pharmacol et Toxicol 53:103, 1983.

68. Hill MJ: Bacteria and etiology of colonic cancer. Cancer 34:815, 1974.

69. Hill MJ: The role of colon anaerobes in the metabolism of bile acids and steroids and its relation to color cancer. Cancer 36:2387, 1975.

70. Hill MJ: Diet and the human intestinal flora. Cancer Res 41:3778, 1981.

71. Hill MF, Drasar BS, Aries V, et al: Bacteria and aetiology of cancer of large bowel. Lancet 1:95, 1971.

72. Hinderling PH, Garrett ER, Webster RC: Pharmacokinetics of b-methyldigoxin in healthy humans. II. Oral studies and bioavailability. J Pharm Sci 66:314, 1977.

73. Hoensch H, Hartmann F: The intestinal enzymatic biotransformation system: Potential role in protection from colon cancer. Hepato-gastroenterol 28:221, 1981.

74. Hoensch H, Hutt R, Hartmann F: Biotransformation of xenobiotics in human intestinal mucosa. Env Health Perspect 33:71, 1979.

75. Hoensch HP, Schwenk M: Intestinal absorption and metabolism of xenobiotics in humans. In: Intestinal Toxicology, p 169, Schiller CM (ed.), Raven Press, New York, 1984.

76. Hoensch HP, Steinhardt JH, Weiss G, et al: Effects of semisynthetic diets on xenobiotic metabolizing enzyme activity and morphology of small intestinal mucosal in humans. Gastroenterology 86:1519, 1984.

77. Hoensch H, Woo CH, Raffin SB, et al: Oxidative metabolism of foreign compounds in rat small intes-

tine. Cellular localization and dependence on dietary iron. Gastroenterology 70:1063, 1976.

78. Hollander F: The two-component mucus barrier. Arch Int Med 93:107, 1954.

79. Hopf U, Brandtzaeg P, Hutteroth TH, et al: In vivo and in vitro binding of IgA to the plasma membrane of hepatocytes. Scand J Immunol 8:543, 1978.

80. Horowitz MI: Gastrointestinal glycoproteins. In: The Glycoconjugates, Vol I, p 189, Horowitz MI, Pigman W (eds.), Academic Press, New York, 1977.

81. Iglewski WJ, Gerhardt NB: Identification of an antibiotic producing bacterium from the human intestinal tract and characterization of its antimicrobial product. Antimicrob Agents Chemother 13:81, 1978.

82. Ito S: The enteric surface coast on cat intestinal microvilli. J Cell Biol 27:475, 1965.

83. Heyworth MF, Jones AL (eds.): Immunology of the Gastrointestinal Tract and Liver, Raven Press, New York, 1988.

84. Iturri SJ, Wolff D: Inhibition of the active transport of D-glucose and L-tyrosine by DDT and DDE in the rat small intestine. Comp Biochem Physiol 71:131, 1982.

85. Iwamoto K, Klassen CD: First pass effect of morphine in rats. J Pharmacol Exp Ther 200:236, 1977.

86. Jarvenpaa P, Kosunen T, Fotsis T, et al: In vitro metabolism of estrogens by isolated intestinal microorganisms and by human foecal microflora. J Steroid Biochem 13:345, 1980.

87. Joel DD, Sordat B, Hess MW, et al: Uptake and retention of particles from the intestine by Peyer's patches in mice. Experientia 26:694A, 1970.

88. Kagnoff MF: Effects of antigen-feeding on intestinal and systemic immune responses. I. Priming of precursor cytotoxic T cells by antigen feeding. J Immunol 120:395, 1978.

89. Kagnoff MF: Immunology of the digestive system. In: Physiology of the Gastrointestinal Tract, 2nd ed., p 1699, Johnson LR (ed.), Raven Press, New York, 1987.

90. Kagnoff MF, Donaldson RM Jr, Trier JS: Organ culture of rabbit small intestine: Prolonged in vitro steady-state protein synthesis and secretion and secretory IgA secretion. Gastroenterology 63:541, 1972.

91. Kinlen LJ: Meat and fat consumption and cancer mortality: A study of strict religious orders in Britain. Lancet I:946, 1982.

92. Klippert P, Borm P, Noordhoek J: Prediction of intestinal first-pass effect of phenacetin in the rat from enzyme kinetic data correlation with in vivo data using mucosal blood flow. Biochem Pharmacol 31:2545, 1982.

93. Knodell RG, Spector MH, Brooks DA, et al: Alterations in pentobarbital pharmacokinetics in response to parenteral and enteral alimentation in the rat. Gastroenterology 79:1211, 1980.

94. Koster AS, Noordhoek J: Similarity of rat intestinal and hepatic microsomal 7-HO-coumarin-UPP-glucuronyltransferase. Biochem Pharmacol 31:2701, 1982.

95. Koster AS, Noordhoek J: Glucuronidation in the rat intestinal wall. Biochem Pharmacol 32:895, 1983.

96. Laquerur GL, Spatz M: Toxicology of cycasin. Cancer Res 28:2262, 1968.

97. Lauterbach F: Intestinal secretion of organic ions and

drugs. In: Intestinal Permeation, p 173, Kramer M, Lauterbach F (eds.), Excerpta Medica, Amsterdam, 1974.

98. Le Fevre ME, Joel DD: Minireview: Intestinal absorption of particulate matter. Life Sci 21:1403, 1977.

99. Levin RJ: Assessing small intestinal function in health and disease in vivo and in vitro. Scand J Gastroenterol 17 (Suppl 74):31, 1982.

100. Levin W, Jagi H, Conney A, et al: Oxidative metabolism of polycyclic aromatic hydrocarbons to ultimate carcinogens. Drug Metab Rev 13:555, 1982.

101. Lindenbaum J, Rund DG, Butho VP, et al: Inactivation of digoxin by the gut flora: Reversal by antibiotic therapy. N Engl J Med 305:789, 1981.

102. Lipkin M: Proliferation and differentiation of gastrointestinal cells. Physiol Rev 53:891, 1973.

103. Lipkin M: Proliferation and differentiation of normal and diseased gastrointestinal cells. In: Physiology of the Gastrointestinal tract, 2nd ed., p 255, Johnson LR (ed.), Raven Press, New York, 1987.

104. Lucas ML: The association between acidification and electronic events in the rat proximal jejunum. J Physiol (Lond) 257:645, 1976.

105. Lucas ML, Schneider W, Haberich FJ, et al: Direct measurement by pH microelectrode of the pH microclimate in rat proximal jejunum. Proc R Soc Lond [Biol] 192:39, 1975.

106. Mahon WA, Inoba T, Stone RM: Metabolism of flurazepam by the small intestine. Clin Pharmacol Ther 22:228, 1977.

107. Marshall T, Allen A: The isolation and characterization of the high-molecular-weight glycoprotein from pig colonic mucus. Biochem J 173:569, 1978.

108. McElhaney RN: Membrane lipid, not polarized water, is responsible for the semipermeable properties of living cells. Biophys J 15:777, 1975.

109. McNabb PC, Tomasi TB: Host defense mechanisms at mucosal surfaces. Annu Rev Microbiol 35:477, 1981.

110. Metchnikoff E: The prolongation of life, GP Putnam, New York, 1908.

111. Miller HRP, Nawa J: *Nippostrongylus brasiliensis*: Intestinal goblet cell response in adoptively immunized rats. Exp Parasitol 47:81, 1979.

112. Moore WEC, Holdeman CV: Discussion of current bacteriologic investigations of the relationships between intestinal flora, diet and colon cancer. Cancer Res 35:3418, 1975.

113. Mortillardo NA, Granger DN, Kuietys PR, et al: Effects of histamine and histamine antagonists on intestinal capillary permeability. Am J Physiol 240: G381, 1981.

114. Mower HF, Ray RM, Shoff R: Fecal bile acids in two Japanese populations with different colon cancer risks. Cancer Res 39:328, 1979.

115. Nagura H, Smith PD, Nakane PK, et al: IgA in human bile and liver. J Immunol 126:587, 1981.

116. Nelson E: Physicochemical factors influencing the absorption of erythromycin and its esters. Chem Pharm Bull 10:1099, 1962.

117. Neutra MR, Forstner JF: Gastrointestinal mucus: Synthesis, secretion, and function. In: Physiology of the Gastrointestinal Tract, 2nd ed., p 975, Johnson LR (ed.), Raven Press, New York, 1987.

118. Nigro ND: Animal studies implicating fat and fecal steroids in intestinal cancer. Cancer Res 41:3769, 1981.

119. Ochsenfahrt H, Winne D: The contribution of solvent drag to the intestinal absorption of the basic drugs amidopyrine and antipyrine from the jejunum of the rat. Arch Pharmacol 281:175, 1974.

120. Ochsenfahrt H, Winne D: The contribution of solvent drag to the intestinal absorption of the acidic drugs benzoic acid and salicylic acid from the jejunum of the rat. Arch Pharmacol 281:197, 1974.

121. Ogra PL, Karzon DT, Righthand F, et al: Immunoglobulin response in serum and secretions after immunization with live and inactivated poliovaccine and natural infection. N Engl J Med 279:893, 1968.

122. Owen RL: Sequential uptake of horseradish peroxidase by lymphoid follicle epithelium of Peyer's patches in the normal unobstructed mouse intestine: An ultrastructural study. Gastroenterology 72:440, 1977.

123. Pantuck EJ, Hsiao KC, Kaplan SA: Effects of enzyme induction on intestinal phenacetin metabolism in the rat. J Pharmacol Exp Ther 191:45, 1974.

124. Pantuck EJ, Hsiao KC, Kuntzmann R: Intestinal metabolism of phenacetin in the rat: Effect of charcoalbroiled beef and rat chow. Science 187:744, 1975.

125. Pascoe GA, Wong IS, Soliven E, et al: Regulation of intestinal cytochrome P-450 and heme by dietary nutrients. Biochem Pharmacol 32:3027, 1983.

126. Pfeiffer CA: Gastroenterologic response to environmental agents—absorption and interactions. In: Handbook of Physiology, Sec 9, p 349, Lee DHK (ed.), American Physiological Society, Bethesda, 1977.

127. Pinkus LM, Kutly JN, Jakoby WB: The glutathione S-transferase as a possible detoxification system of rat intestinal epithelium. Biochem Pharmacol 26: 2359, 1977.

128. Read NW, Barber DC, Levin RJ, et al: Unstirred layer and kinetics of electronic glucose absorption in the human jejunum in situ. Gut 18:865, 1977.

129. Reddy BS, Wynder EL: Large-bowel carcinogenesis: Fecal constituents of populations with diverse incidence rates of colon cancer. J Natl Cancer Inst 50:1437, 1973.

130. Reddy WS, Weisburger JH, Wynder EL: Fecal bacterial glucuronidase: Control by diet. Science 183:416, 1974.

131. Report from the International Agency for Research on Cancer, Intestinal Microecology Group: Dietary fibre transit-time, fecal bacteria, steroids and colon cancer in two Scandinavian populations. Lancet 2: 207, 1977.

132. Richter E, Fichtl B, Schafer SG: Effects of dietary paraffin, squalene and sucrose polyester on residue disposition and elimination of hexachlorobenzene in rats. Chem Biol Interact 40:335, 1982.

133. Rontledge PA, Shand DG: Presystemic drug elimination. Annu Rev Pharmacol Toxicol 19:447, 1979.

134. Salviolo G, Salata R, Bondi M, et al: Bile acid transformation by the intestinal flora and cholesterol saturation in bile. Digestion 23:80, 1981.

135. Savage DC: Microbial ecology of the gastrointestinal tract. Annu Rev Microbiol 31:107, 1977.

136. Schedl HP: Water and electrolyte transport: Clinical aspects. Med Clin North Am 58:1429, 1974.
137. Schedl HP: Environmental factors and the development of disease and injury in the alimentary tract. Environ Health Perspect 20:39, 1977.
138. Schedl HP: Intestinal disease and the urban environment. Environ Health Perspect 33:115, 1979.
139. Scheline RR: Metabolism of foreign compounds by gastrointestinal microorganisms. Pharmacol Rev 25:451, 1973.
140. Scheline RR: Drug metabolism by the gastrointestinal microflora. In: Extrahepatic Metabolism of Drugs and Other Foreign Compounds, p 551, Gram TE (ed.), MTP Press, Lancaster, 1980.
141. Seitz HK, Korsten MA, Lieber CS: Ethanol oxidation by intestinal microsomes: Increased activity after chronic ethanol administration. Life Sci 25:1443, 1979.
142. Shand DG, Rangno RE: The disposition of propranolol. I. Elimination during oral absorption in man. Pharmacology 7:159, 1972.
143. Sharma RP (ed.): Immunologic Considerations in Toxicology, Vol I, CRC Press, Boca Raton, 1981.
144. Sharma RP (ed.): Immunologic Considerations in Toxicology, Vol 2, CRC Press, Boca Raton, 1981.
145. Shorter RG, Tomasi TB: Gut immune mechanisms. Ann Intern Med 27:247, 1982.
146. Simon GL, Gorbach SL: Intestinal flora in health and disease. Gastroenterology 86:174, 1984.
147. Simon GL, Gorbach SL: Intestinal flora in health and disease. In: Johnson LR (ed.), Physiology of the Gastrointestinal Tract, 2nd ed., p 1729, Raven Press, New York, 1987.
148. Sinrala M, Lehtola J, Ihamaki T: Atropic gastritis and its sequelae. Results of 19–23 years follow-up examinations. Scand J Gastroenterol 9:441, 1974.
149. Smith RL: The role of the gut flora in the conversion of inactive compounds to active metabolites. In: Symposium on Mechanisms of Toxicity, p 229, Aldridge WN (ed.), Macmillan, New York, 1971.
150. Smithson KW, Millar DB, Jacobs LR, et al: Intestinal diffusion barrier: Unstirred water layer or membrane surface mucous coat. Science 214: 1241, 1981.
151. Sparnins VL, Venegas PL, Wattenberg LW: Glutathione S-transferase activity: Enhancement by compounds inhibiting chemical carcinogenesis and by dietary constituents. J Natl Cancer Inst 68:493, 1982.
152. Stockbrugger RW, Cotton PB, Eugenides N, et al: Intragastric nitrites, nitrosamines and bacterial overgrowth during cimetidine treatment. Gut 23:1048, 1982.
153. Stohs SJ, Grafstrom RC, Burke MD, et al: The isolation of rat intestinal microsomes with stable cytochrome P-450 and their metabolism of benzo(a)pyrene. Arch Biochem Biophys 177:105, 1976.
154. Tagliabue A, Befus AD, Clark DA, et al: Characteristics of natural killer cells in the murine intestinal epithelium and lamina propria. J Exp Med 155:1785, 1982.
155. Thomas ABR: Unstirred water layers: A basic mechanism of gastrointestinal mucosal cell cytoprotection. In: Basic Mechanisms of Gastrointestinal Mucosal Cell Injury and Protection, p 327, Harmon JW (ed.), Williams & Wilkins, Baltimore, 1981.
156. Tomasi TB, Bienenstock J: Secretory immunoglobulins. Adv Immunol 9:1, 1968.
157. Tomasi TB, Grey HM: Structure and function of immunoglobulin A. Prog Allergy 16:81, 1972.
158. Tomasi TB, Tan EM, Solomon A, et al: Characteristics of an immune system common to certain external secretions. J Exp Med 121:101, 1965.
159. Tredger JM, Chhabra RS: Factors affecting the properties of mixed-function oxidases in the liver and small intestine of neonatal rabbits. Drug Metab Dispos 8:16, 1980.
160. Tsuj A, Miyamoto E, Kagami I, et al: GI absorption of β-lactam antibiotics I: Kinetic assessment of competing absorption and degradation in GI tract. J Pharm Sci 67:1701, 1978.
161. Underdown BJ, Schiff JM: Immunoglobin A: Strategic defense initiative at the mucosal surface. Annu Rev Immunol 4:389, 1986.
162. Underdown BJ, Roberts-Thomson IC, Anders RF, et al: Giardiasis in mice: Studies on the characteristics of chronic infection in C3H/He mice. J Immunol 126:669, 1981.
163. Vango D, Moskowitz M, Floch MH: Faecal bacterial flora in cancer of the colon. Gut 21:701, 1980.
164. Vimmo WS: Drugs, diseases and altered gastric emptying. Clin Pharmacokinet 1:189, 1976.
165. Waksman BH: The homing pattern of thymus-derived lymphocytes in calf and neonatal mouse Peyer's patches. J Immunol 111:878, 1973.
166. Walker WA: Host defense mechanisms in the gastrointestinal tract. Pediatrics 57:901, 1976.
167. Walker WA, Isselbacher KJ: Intestinal antibodies. N Engl J Med 297:767, 1977.
168. Walker WA, Isselbacher KJ, Block KJ: Intestinal uptake of macromolecules: Effect of oral immunization. Science 177:608, 1972.
169. Wattenberg LW: Inhibition of neoplasia by minor dietary constituents. Cancer Res 43 (Suppl):2448s, 1983.
170. Wattenberg LW, Leong JC, Strand PJ: Benzo(a)pyrene hydroxylase activity in the gastrointestinal tract. Cancer Res 22:1120, 1962.
171. Wattenberg LW, Coccia JB, Cam LKT: Inhibitory effects of phenolic compounds of benzo(a)pyrene-induced neoplasia. Cancer Res 40:2820, 1980.
172. Wattenberg LW, Borchert P, Destafney CM, et al: Effects of p-methoxyphenol and diet on carcinogen-induced neoplasia of the mouse forestomach. Cancer Res 43:4747, 1983.
173. Weisburger JH, Marwuardt H, Hirota N, et al: Induction of cancer in the glandular stomach in rats by an extract of nitrite-treated fish. J Natl Cancer Inst 64:163, 1980.
174. Westergaard H, Dietschy JM: Delineation of the dimensions and permeability characteristics of the two major diffusion barriers to passive mucosal uptake in the rabbit intestine. J Clin Invest 54:718, 1974.
175. Williams RC, Gibbons RJ: Inhibition of bacterial adherence by secretory immunoglobin A: A mechanism of antigen disposal. Science 177:697, 1972.
176. Williams RT: Toxicological implications of biotransformation by intestinal microflora. Toxicol Appl Pharmacol 23:769, 1972.
177. Williams SE, Turnberg LA: Retardation of acid diffu-

sion by pig gastric mucus: A potential role in mucosal protection. Gastroenterology 79:299, 1980.

178. Wilson FA, Dietschy JM: The intestinal unstirred layer: Its surface area and effect on active transport kinetics. Biochim Biophys Acta 363:112, 1974.

179. Winne D: Rat jejunum perfused in situ: Effect of perfusion rate and intraluminal radius on absorption rate and effective unstirred layer thickness. Naunyn-Schmiedebergs Arch Pharmacol Exp Pathol 307:265, 1979.

180. Winne D: Influence of blood flow on intestinal absorption of xenobiotics. Pharmacology 21:1, 1980.

181. Wollenberg P, Ullrich V: The drug monooxygenase system in the small intestine. In: Extrahepatic Metabolism of Drugs and Other Foreign Compounds, p 267, 1980, Gram TE (ed.), SP Medical & Scientific Books, London, 1980.

182. Wollenberg P, Ullrich V, Rummel W: Conjugation of 1-naphthol and transport of 1-naphthol-conjugates in the vascularly perfused small intestine of the mouse. Biochem Pharmacol 32:2103, 1983.

183. Wynder EL: The epidemiology of large bowel cancer. Cancer Res 35:3388, 1975.

184. Yamana T, Tsuji A: Comparative stability of cephalosporins in aqueous solution: Kinetics and mechanisms of degradation. J Pharm Sci 65:1563, 1976.

185. Zamcheck N, Grable E, Ley A, et al: Occurrence of gastric cancer among patients with pernicious anemia at the Boston City Hospital. N Engl J Med 252:1103, 1955.

186. Zeigler EE, Edwards BB, Jensen RL, et al: Absorption and retention of lead by infants. Pediatr Res 12:29, 1978.

RECOMMENDED READINGS

Brostoff J, Challacombe SJ (eds.): Food Allergy and Intolerance: Part I. Basic Mechanisms, Bailliere Tindall, London, 1987.

Koster AS, Richter E, Hartmann F, et al: Intestinal Metabolism of Xenobiotics, Gustav Fisher Verlag, Stuttgart, 1989.

9. DETOXICATION MECHANISMS AND THE ROLE OF NUTRITION

G. Gordon Gibson

INTRODUCTION

Humans living in a highly industrialized society are increasingly exposed to many environmental chemical pollutants deliberately or accidentally introduced into the biosphere. Approximately 65,000 chemicals are in use today. This includes about 1500 active ingredients of pesticides, drugs, and food additives. Although many of these chemicals represent little danger to public health, the scientific community has become increasingly concerned about the adverse health effects of widespread chemical pollution. This awareness has stimulated much research into the exposure, metabolism, and toxicity of chemical pollutants. This chapter discusses one aspect of the bodily defense against pollutant exposure—detoxication mechanisms, with particular emphasis on their relationship to nutrition. The discussion focuses on several key environmental chemicals (Table 9-1) that represent a problem because of their ubiquitous environmental disposition, their potential toxicity, or their long persistence within the body.

Principles and Practice of Environmental Medicine, edited by Alyce Bezman Tarcher. Plenum Medical Book Company, New York, 1992.

DETOXICATION DEFENSE MECHANISMS: BASIC CONSIDERATIONS

Once they have been absorbed, the body deals with offending chemicals by using an elegant interacting system consisting of distribution, metabolism, and excretion (Fig. 9-1). The distribution and metabolism of the chemical play a central role in determining its residence time in the body. In many cases this factor may determine the chemical's toxic effects. One of the major concerns associated with pollutant exposure is the abnormal persistence of many of these agents within the body. Environmental chemicals tend to persist in the body for two reasons. First, most of the pollutants, being highly lipophilic, tend to distribute in organs and tissues such as adipose tissue and cellular membranes that are themselves hydrophobic. Second, many of the pollutants are complex chemical structures resistant to metabolism and excretion (9).

Tissue Distribution and Retention of Environmental Chemicals

The high lipid solubility of most environmental chemicals clearly favors their partition away from aqueous body tissues and into cellular lipids. A well-documented example is the tissue distribution and persistence of the polychlorinated biphenyl 2,2'4,4',5,5'-hexachlorobiphenyl (6CB). After the intravenous administration of a single dose of this

TABLE 9-1. Environmental Chemicals

Classification	Example	Use or occurrence
Halogenated hydrocarbons	2,3,7,8-Tetrachlorodibenzo-p-dioxin (TCDD), polychlorinated biphenyls (PCBs), polybrominated biphenyls (PBBs)	Contamination of herbicides and defoliants (2,4,5-T), insulator in capacitors and transformers, flame retardant
Pesticides	DDT (dichlorodiphenyltrichloroethane), chlordecone (Kepone®), piperonyl butoxide	Agricultural pesticide, organochlorine pesticide, insecticide synergist
Polycyclic aromatic hydrocarbons	3-Methylcholanthrene, phenanthrene, chrysene, 1,2-benzanthracene, benzo[a]pyrene	Environmental pollutants found in industrial and domestic combustion products, cigarette smoke, and oil contaminants
Solvents	Benzene, toluene, xylenes	Solvents, cleaning agents, and degreasers

agent, the pollutant is cleared from the blood, muscle, liver, and skin but remains in the adipose tissue. The persistence of a polychlorinated hydrocarbon is a function of the lipid solubility of the compound itself. For example, as the chlorination of this chlorinated biphenyl increases from 1 to 6, the lipid solubility also increases, resulting in a body half-life of months or years. This avid retention of the polychlorinated biphenyls is in stark contrast to therapeutic drugs, which often have a half-life of hours.

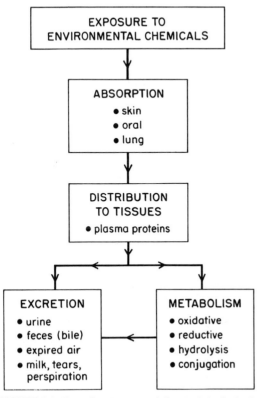

FIGURE 9-1. Fate of environmental chemicals in the body.

Detoxication Reactions

The fate of drugs and environmental chemicals in the body depends, in part, on their physicochemical nature (112). The metabolism of pollutants and most foreign compounds (xenobiotics), including drugs, is strongly governed by the lipid solubility of the compound. Polar, nonlipophilic compounds may be excreted unchanged or after undergoing some very simple alteration. In contrast, lipid-soluble compounds, in order to be excreted by the kidney, must undergo a two-step transformation to convert the nonpolar lipophilic chemicals to polar hydrophilic products (Fig. 9-2). The biochemical defense thus depends largely on a series of reactions that convert a nonpolar lipophilic agent to a polar hydrophilic one. These biochemical processes, termed biotransformations, are usually enzymatic in nature.

Although the enzymes that catalyze the metabolism of drugs and pollutants are widely distributed in the body, they are localized primarily in the liver and in such portals of entry as the skin, lung, and intestine. The detoxication reactions are carried out largely in the endoplasmic reticulum or in the microsomes of the cell. The term microsomal enzyme system, another commonly used name, is derived from the location of the enzymes within the cell. This system catalyzes a wide variety of reactions that have been classified as phase I and phase II reactions (Table 9-2 and 9-3).

Phase I metabolism converts a nonpolar chemical into a relatively polar compound by exposing or adding a polar or reactive group. It includes such reactions as oxidation, reduction, dehalogenation, and desulfuration. The microsomal mixed-function oxidases are involved in many aspects of phase I metabolism. In phase II metabolism, conjugation with such endogenous compounds as glucuronic acid, sulfate, glutathione, glycine, and other amino acids occurs. The overall result of phase I and phase II metabolism is the conversion of a lipophilic, nonpolar compound into a more polar, readily excret-

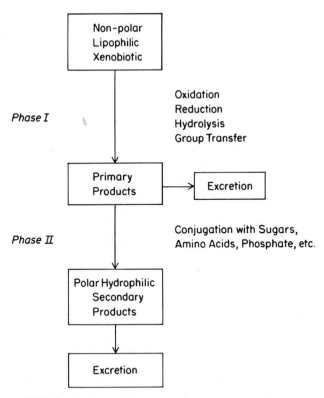

FIGURE 9-2. Steps in the biotransformation of xenobiotics.

able metabolite. On the basis of this series of biochemical reactions, a pathway exists for the removal of drugs and environmental pollutants; hence the term "detoxication reactions." Since the enzymes that transform xenobiotics were first encountered in connection with the metabolism of drugs, they may also be referred to as the drug-metabolizing enzymes.

As shown in Table 9-4, many enzymes, including cytochrome P-450, contribute to the overall process of xenobiotic metabolism. The highest concentration of cytochrome P-450 is found in the liver, the most active site of xenobiotic metabolism. Cytochrome P-450, a hemoprotein localized primarily in the endoplasmic reticulum membrane, catalyzes many reactions, including those listed as microsomal mixed-function oxidase reactions in Table 9-2. Multiple forms of cytochrome P-450 catalyze the oxidation (phase I) of literally hundreds of drugs and environmental pollutants (52,71,87). During recent years much attention has been directed to a detailed study of the cytochrome P-450 superfamily of mixed-function oxidase enzymes (42,47,68,103). Environmental chemicals metabolized by this microsomal enzyme system include the polycyclic aro-

matic hydrocarbons (benzo[a]pyrene), organometals (the organotins), pesticides (DDT and parathion), and the halogenated biphenyls (polychlorinated and polybrominated biphenyls).

It bears emphasis that the detoxication enzymes are relatively nonspecific. Thus, in addition to drugs, such endogenous compounds as steroids, fatty acids, cholesterol, prostaglandins, and vitamin D_3 are efficiently metabolized by this system (25).

In many instances the series of reactions that facilitate the excretion of drugs and pollutants from the body decrease the toxicity of the chemical (115). At times, however, the detoxifying enzymes activate innocuous chemicals and environmental pollutants to yield metabolites that are clearly more toxic than the parent compounds from which they came. Indeed, many chemicals are nontoxic until they are metabolized by the liver. Potent mutagens, teratogens, and carcinogens can result from such metabolism (74,75,119). For example, the polycyclic aromatic hydrocarbon benzo[a]pyrene, a potent mutagen and carcinogen found in air, water, food, and soil, is biologically inert until it undergoes metabolic activation (119). This metabolic activation, carried out by the mixed-function oxidases and related enzymes,

TABLE 9-2. Phase I Reactions[a]

Microsomal mixed-function oxidations	
Aliphatic oxidation	$R-CH_3 \longrightarrow R-CH_2OH$
Aromatic oxidation	
Epoxidation	$R-CH=CH_2 \longrightarrow R-CH-CH_2$ (epoxide, O bridging)
Oxidative deamination	$R-CH\begin{smallmatrix}NH_2\\CH_3\end{smallmatrix} \longrightarrow \left[R-C\begin{smallmatrix}NH_2\\OH\ \ CH_3\end{smallmatrix}\right] \longrightarrow R-C(=O)-CH_3 + NH_3$
N-Dealkylation	$R-N\begin{smallmatrix}CH_3\\CH_3\end{smallmatrix} \longrightarrow \left[R-N\begin{smallmatrix}CH_2OH\\CH_3\end{smallmatrix}\right] \longrightarrow R-N\begin{smallmatrix}H\\CH_3\end{smallmatrix} + HCHO$
O-Dealkylation	$R-O-CH_3 \longrightarrow R-OH + HCHO$
S-Dealkylation	$R-S-CH_3 \longrightarrow R-SH + HCHO$
N-Oxidation	$R_3 \equiv N \longrightarrow R_3 \equiv N \rightarrow O$
N-Hydroxylation	
Sulfoxidation	$\begin{smallmatrix}R\\R\end{smallmatrix}S \longrightarrow \begin{smallmatrix}R\\R\end{smallmatrix}S\rightarrow O \longrightarrow \begin{smallmatrix}R\\R\end{smallmatrix}S=O$
Desulfuration	$\begin{smallmatrix}R\\R\end{smallmatrix}C=S \longrightarrow \begin{smallmatrix}R\\R\end{smallmatrix}C=O$
Dehalogenation	$R-CH_2Cl \longrightarrow R-CH_2OH$
Nonmicrosomal oxidations	
Monoamine and diamine oxidation	$R-CH_2NH_2 \xrightarrow{O_2} R-CH-NH \xrightarrow{H_2O} R-CHO + NH_3$
Alcohol dehydrogenation	$R-CH_2OH \longrightarrow R-CHO$
Aldehyde dehydrogenation	$R-CHO \longrightarrow R-COOH$
Microsomal reductions	
Nitro reduction	$R-NO_2 \longrightarrow R-NO \longrightarrow R-NHOH \longrightarrow R-NH_2$
Azo reduction	$RN-NR^1 \longrightarrow RNH-NHR^1 \longrightarrow R-NH_2 + R^1-NH_2$
Reductive dehalogenation	$R-CCl_3 \longrightarrow R-CHCl_2$
Nonmicrosomal reductions	
Aldehyde reduction	$\begin{smallmatrix}R\\R\end{smallmatrix}C=O \longrightarrow \begin{smallmatrix}R\\R\end{smallmatrix}CHOH$
Hydrolyses	
Ester hydrolysis	$RCO-OR^1 \xrightarrow{H_2O} RCOOH + R^1OH$
Amide hydrolysis	$RCO-NH_2 \xrightarrow{H_2O} RCOOH + NH_3$
Epoxide hydration	$RCH-CH_2 \text{ (epoxide)} \xrightarrow{H_2O} RCH(OH)CH_2OH$

[a] Derived from Parke (113).

TABLE 9-3. Phase II Reactions[a]

UDPGA[b]-mediated glucuronylations		
Ether glucuronide	ROH	$\longrightarrow$ RO-C$_6$H$_9$O$_6$
Ester glucuronide	RCOOH	$\longrightarrow$ RCOO-C$_6$H$_9$O$_6$
N-Glucuronide	RNH$_2$	$\longrightarrow$ RNH-C$_6$H$_9$O$_6$
S-Glucuronide	RSH	$\longrightarrow$ RS-C$_6$H$_9$O$_6$
PAPS[c]-mediated Sulfate ester formation		
Alkyl or aryl sulfate	ROH	$\longrightarrow$ RO-SO$_3$H
Sulfamate	RNH$_2$	$\longrightarrow$ RNH-SO$_3$H
S-Adenosylmethionine-mediated methylations		
O-methylation	ROH	$\longrightarrow$ RO-CH$_3$
N-Methylation	RNH$_2$	$\longrightarrow$ RNH-CH$_3$
S-Methylation	RSH	$\longrightarrow$ RS-CH$_3$
Acetylations	RNH$_2$	$\xrightarrow{\text{acetyl CoA}}$ RNH-COCH$_3$
Peptide conjugations	RCOOH	$\xrightarrow{\text{CoA + glycine}}$ RCO-NHCH$_2$COOH
	RCH-CH$_2$ \ O /	$\xrightarrow{\text{GSH}}$ RCHOH-CH$_2$-SG

[a]Derived from Parke (113).
[b]Uridine diphosphate glucuronic acid.
[c]Phosphoadenosine phosphosulfate.

results in the formation of an epoxide metabolite, benzo[a]pyrene-7,8-diol-9,10-epoxide. This compound can initiate the complex processes of mutagenesis and carcinogenesis by binding covalently to DNA. The biochemical process of detoxication must therefore be considered a "double-edged sword" with the potential to either increase or decrease the toxicity of environmental pollutants (114,117). Which it will be depends on the inherent biological potency of the metabolic products formed during the biotransformation process.

Biotransformation is the sum of the processes by which the body subjects a foreign chemical to chemical change. It is of interest that recent studies on the cytochrome P-450 superfamily of mixed-function oxidase enzymes have indicated that one major family, namely, the cytochromes P-448 (P-450-I), are primarily responsible for the activation of carcinogens and toxic chemicals (67,117).

Before we proceed to a discussion of specific environmental chemicals, there is an important feature of the detoxication system that requires consideration. This complex enzyme system located in the endoplasmic reticulum is highly inducible. Thus

TABLE 9-4. Enzymes of Xenobiotic Metabolism

Enzyme	Catalytic function or reaction type
Phase I	
Monooxygenases (including cytochrome P-450)	Mixed-function oxidations
Dehydrogenases	Dehydrogenations
Nitroreductases	Aromatic nitro group reduction
Azoreductases	Azo linkage reduction
Hydrolases	Hydrolysis
Monoamine oxidase	Amine oxidation
Epoxide hydrolase	Forms dihydro-diols from epoxide substrates
Phase II	
UDP-Glucuronyltransferases	Conjugation of a phase I metabolite with glucuronic acid
Sulfotransferases	Formation with sulfate esters of phase I metabolites
Methyltransferases	Amine methylation
Gluthathione-S-transferases	Condensation of glutathione with electrophiles
Acetyltransferases	Amine acetylation
Acyltransferases	Conjugation of organic acids with amino acids

[a]Derived in part from Juchau (74).

with prolonged or repeated exposure to a specific environmental chemical, the concentration of enzymes in this system can increase. The metabolism of the offending chemical is thereby also increased. Since these detoxication enzymes are relatively nonspecific, their induction by one chemical almost invariably enhances the metabolism of other compounds acted on by these enzymes. This fact first alerted investigators to the inducibility of the cytochrome P-450 enzymes. It was noted that rats whose cages had been recently sprayed with the insecticide chlordane were much less susceptible to the soporific effects of hexobarbital. Further study revealed that the chlordane had induced the liver enzymes that metabolize hexobarbital as well as chlordane.

The enzymatic induction caused by pollutant exposure is exceedingly complex. Intense investigation is currently directed to elucidating this important process. It is clear, however, that one environmental pollutant can have a significant effect on the metabolism of other agents. For this reason it is difficult to predict the toxic effects of xenobiotic exposure in a natural setting, where multiple exposures are present.

METABOLIC DETOXICATION AND ACTIVATION OF ENVIRONMENTAL CHEMICALS

The process of pollutant metabolism, as previously mentioned, often represents a balance between metabolic detoxication and activation. The following discussion focuses on these processes as well as on the pollutant's inherent susceptibility to

metabolism. The particular environmental pollutants selected for discussion represent a range of chemical agents whose metabolic pathways are relatively well understood.

Monocyclic Aromatic Hydrocarbons

The simplest and most extensively studied member of this series of compounds is benzene. Benzene has a long history of industrial use as a solvent, as an anti-knock reagent in gasoline, and as an indispensable chemical in the synthesis of many compounds including polystryrene. Because benzene has a significant vapor pressure at ambient temperatures, the compound is relatively volatile. It therefore constitutes a significant environmental hazard via inhalation exposure. Benzene toxicity can be reflected in such blood disorders as aplastic anemia and leukemia, which have been found in exposed workers (66,133).

Man's exposure to benzene raises two critical questions. First, what is his ability to metabolize this hydrocarbon? Second, does this metabolism lead to detoxication or activation? Detailed animal experiments (134) have shown that benzene is readily metabolized to a variety of products (Fig. 9-3), all of which may bind covalently to tissue macromolecules, producing toxicity. A limited number of studies in man indicate that low concentrations of benzene are metabolized by similar pathways (59), with phenol being the major metabolite excreted. Although the tissue retention and half-life of benzene in man are clearly difficult to ascertain, animal experiments reveal the half-life of benzene (and its

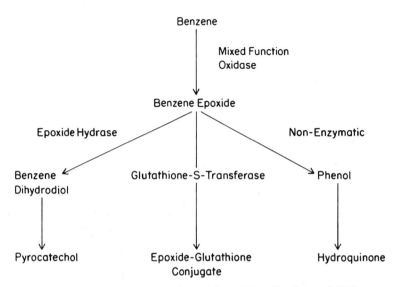

FIGURE 9-3. Benzene metabolism. Adapted from Snyder et al. (134).

metabolites) to be in the range of 1 to 13 h. Elimination occurs primarily via the lung (unchanged benzene) and urine (metabolites). Studies of tissue distribution show that certain tissues (including fat, bone marrow, and kidney) exhibit higher benzene levels than occurs in blood. Such findings suggest preferential uptake and storage by these organs.

Although benzene is readily metabolized in experimental animals and man, this metabolism has divergent effects. Some of its polar, innocuous metabolites are readily excreted, whereas other oxidation products appear to be responsible for the development of blood dyscrasias. Both the liver and bone marrow can metabolize benzene to electrophilic species that are thought to initiate the complex series of events leading to the blood disorders. The nature of these metabolites, however, is uncertain (134,135).

Many other environmentally derived monocyclic hydrocarbons undergo multiple routes of biotransformation similar to those described for benzene. These include bromobenzene (72,139), substituted benzaldehydes and benzyl alcohol (131,157), styrene (85,140) toluene (6,8), and phthalate diesters (1,84).

Any appraisal of the metabolism of the moncyclic hydrocarbons should be done on an individual basis with consideration being given to the toxicity of the parent compound and its various metabolites. The complexity of the detoxification process highlights the problem of arriving at an "overall conclusion" concerning the protective or deleterious role of metabolism.

Polycyclic Aromatic Hydrocarbons

The polycyclic aromatic hydrocarbons (PAH), a ubiquitous group of environmental pollutants, are produced by the incomplete combustion of fossil fuels. They are found in automobile exhaust, cigarette smoke, industrial effluents, and in some charcoal-broiled foods. The structure of the polycyclic hydrocarbons reveals an absence of sites of high chemical reactivity. Because they are lipophilic, these compounds tend to sequester in adipose tissue.

The PAH benzo[a]pyrene is, however, metabolized to a mixture of epoxides, diol-epoxides, and their conjugation products (Fig. 9-4). In addition, phenols, quinones, and their corresponding conjugates are also formed. It might appear from the extensive metabolism and excretion of many of its metabolites that PAHs are an innocuous group of environmental pollutants. Unfortunately, the inherent biological activity of their metabolities prevents this from being so. In the metabolism of benzo[a]-pyrene, benzo[a]pyrene-7,8-diol-9,10-epoxide is formed. This represents a biological activation of the parent compound to produce the diol-epoxide metabolite, a potent mutagen and carcinogen (46,70). The recognition of benzo[a]pyrene-7,8-diol-9,10-epoxide as a toxic metabolite is the basis for the evolution of the "bay region" hypothesis. This affords a molecular description of chemical carcinogenesis based on the bay region of the sterically hindered position of benzo[a]pyrene (i.e., the 9,10 position). The initial oxidation product (7,8-epox-

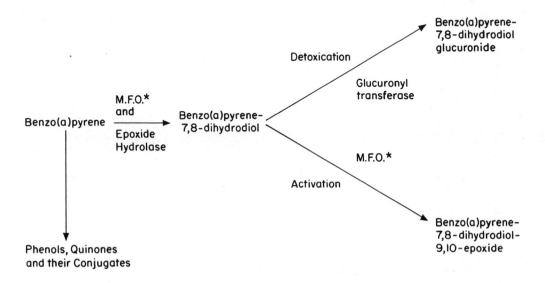

*Mixed function oxidase activity

FIGURE 9-4. Metabolism of benzo[a]pyrene. Adapted from Guenther and Oesch (55).

ide), which is a substrate for the enzyme epoxide hydrolase, is transformed into 7,8-dihydrodiol, which in turn is oxidized to the 7,8-diol-9,10-epoxide. This metabolite represents the end product of this particular pathway, as steric hindrance in the bay region of the molecule precludes further metabolism. This metabolic pathway therefore represents an activation reaction. The metabolic activation of PAHs that results in carcinogenic products has been widely studied. The interested reader is referred to the review by Pelkonen and Nebert (119).

In addition to the classical phase-I- and phase-II-dependent metabolism of polycyclic aromatic hydrocarbons, as described above, benzo[a]pyrene and congeners can be metabolized by the prostaglandin synthetase system (77,111,124). In this reaction benzo[a]pyrene is activated by being oxidized to the potent 7,8-diol-9,10-epoxide carcinogen.

The metabolism of benzo[a]pyrene clearly demonstrates that the "detoxication" enzymes have diametrically opposed biological functions: activation and detoxication. The function that emerges depends on the relative toxicity of the parent compound and its metabolites.

The relative concentrations of the phase I and phase II enzymes are also an important factor in the production of reactive intermediates during PAH metabolism. The phase I isoenzymes of cytochrome P-450, which themselves are induced by environmental pollutants, have varying abilities to oxidize benzo[a]pyrene (46). In addition, modulation of the phase II enzyme epoxide hydrolase by environmental pollutants has been shown to have a significant influence on the binding of benzo[a]pyrene metabolites to DNA (106). These findings indicate that the relative concentrations of the enzymes involved in the detoxication reactions are important. The enzymatic balance may influence the body's susceptibility or resistance to the carcinogenic effects of such widely dispersed pollutants as PAHs.

Halogenated Biphenyls

The two major groups of compounds classified as halogenated biphenyls are the polychlorinated biphenyls (PCBs) and the polybrominated biphenyls (PBBs). These compounds are mixtures of isomers containing 12–68% halogen. Because of their chemical and physical stability, these agents have been extensively used in industry in transformers and capacitors as coolants, as additives to hydraulic oils (PCBs), and as flame retardants (PBBs).

Polychlorinated Biphenyls

Among the polyhalogenated biphenyls, both metabolism and kidney excretion decrease as the extent of halogenation increases. This is in agreement with the findings of Hutzinger et al. (64), who

identified metabolites of 4-mono-, 4,4'-di-, and 2,5,2',5'-tetrachlorinated isomers of biphenyl but not of 2,4,5,2',4',5'-hexacholorbiphenyl (6CB). The metabolic resistance of the highly chlorinated biphenyls is further reflected in the PCBs retained in human adipose tissue. Studies have clearly demonstrated that the single most abundant PCB in adipose tissue is the 6CB isomer. This is in marked contrast to the lower-chlorine-containing-PCBs, which are quite readily excreted. The interested reader is referred to a review describing the elimination of PCBs from the body (90).

Polybrominated Biphenyls

Millions of pounds of PBBs have been manufactured. Sold under the trade name of FireMaster™, these compounds were used mainly as a flame retardant in thermoplastics. Great concern was raised about the environmental and public health impact of PBB exposure after some 500–1000 pounds of these compounds were inadvertently mixed with cattle feed. This event, occurring in the State of Michigan during the summer of 1973, resulted in serious contamination of the food chain.

As with PCBs, the extent of PBB metabolism depends on the degree and position of halogen substitution. Thus, an unsubstituted *para* position on the biphenyl nucleus increases susceptibility of the PBBs to metabolism and excretion. When both *para* positions are blocked, there is little metabolism and substantial tissue accumulation.

Although the metabolism of PBBs is difficult to assess in man, animal studies have demonstrated that 2,4,5,2',4',5'-hexabromobiphenyl is very slowly metabolized. During a 42-day period after exposure to this PBB, only 6–7% of the dose was recovered in urine and feces. It has been estimated that during its lifetime the rat is able to excrete only 10% of the total dose (91).

Little is known about the nature of the lower-brominated PBB metabolites. The monobrominated biphenyls appear to be metabolized primarily by aromatic hydroxylation. Small amounts of debrominated metabolites have been tentatively identified in the urine of experimental animals (99).

It is of interest that many bacteria are able to dehalogenate the polyhalogenated biphenyls. Since mammals (including man) appear to be devoid of this pathway, the limited metabolism and excretion of PBBs occurs primarily via phase I and phase II reactions at unsubstituted positions in the molecule.

Chlorinated Dibenzodioxins

Unlike the PCBs and PBBs, the chlorinated dibenzodioxins have never been used in an industrial context. They are present as contaminants or impurities of industrial or agricultural chemicals. The

most extensively studied chemical of this series is
2,3,7,8-tetrachlorodibenzo-*p*-dioxin (TCDD or Dioxin) (80). This chlorinated hydrocarbon has been
found as a contaminant of the herbicide 2,4,5-T
(2,4,5-trichlorophenoxyacetic acid), trichlorophenol,
pentachlorophenol (a wood preservative and fungicide), PCBs, and hexachlorophene (a disinfectant).
Dioxin came as an ecological and toxicological surprise in that prior to its identification as a contaminant of the above products, its toxicity was not
generally recognized. A classic example of dioxin
contamination is reflected in the herbicide 2,4,5-T,
which was extensively used by the United States as
a defoliant in Vietnam. Although 2,4,5-T is a toxic
compound, much of its previously described toxicity was clearly related to its contamination with
dioxin. The acute toxicity of dioxin in species like
the rat or guinea pig is approximately 100 times
greater than that of the nerve gas sarin and around
10,000 times greater than that of sodium cyanide (9).
On this basis dioxin is the most acutely toxic low-
molecular-weight compound known. There are,
however, marked species differences in the degree
of dioxin's toxicity (80). It causes such problems as
liver and skin damage (chloracne) and compromised immune function (92,125,142).

Because of the high degree of chlorination at
positions 2, 3, 7, and 8 and the sterically hindered
1, 4, 6, and 9 positions, TCDD is very resistant to
metabolic deactivation by the detoxication enzymes.
Only very small amounts of dioxin metabolites
(phenolic products and/or their glucuronide conjugates) have been detected in animals (120). Animal
studies indicate that, as with the PCBs and PBBs, the
adipose tissue concentration of TCDD is much
higher than that in other organs. The liver also has
a high affinity for dioxin, which slowly declines
with time (9).

Although many environmental accidents involving TCDD are on public record, limited information is available regarding the tissue retention,
metabolism, or toxicity of TCDD in man. The interested reader is referred to an excellent review of this
problem edited by Coulston and Pocchiari (31). This
review includes a detailed analysis of the episode of
dioxin contamination that occurred at Seveso, Italy
in 1976. A subsequent publication by Mocarelli et al.
reported on the clinical laboratory findings in children exposed to dioxin (96). They noted that the observed abnormalities were slight and disappeared
with time.

Pesticides

In contrast to the dioxins, pesticides were deliberately introduced into the environment. Since the
introduction of DDT (dichlorodiphenyltrichloreth-
ane) in 1939, many other polychlorinated hydrocarbon pesticides have been put to agricultural use.

These include such compounds as chlordane, aldrin, dieldrin, endrin, heptachlor, toxaphene, chlordecone, and Mirex®.

In general, the organochlorine insecticides are
lipophilic compounds that have the tendency to be
stored in adipose tissue. Although the metabolic susceptibility of these pesticides can vary (34,38,83),
they all undergo so little metabolism that they are
classed as persistent pollutants that accumulate in
body tissues.

The metabolic fate of insecticides often varies
with the species exposed. The polycyclic perchlori-
nated hydrocarbon Mirex®, which is both an insecticide and fire retardant, reflects this finding. In the
rat, Mirex® has a biological half-life of about 2 years,
whereas in the rhesus monkey most of a given dose
accumulates in the adipose tissue and remains there
for up to 1 year (48,156).

Aromatic Amines

Aromatic amines are compounds of considerable industrial and commercial importance. Used as
intermediates in the synthesis of many azo dyes and
as antioxidants in the rubber industry, the aromatic
amines pose a potential threat to occupationally exposed workers. This discussion focuses on one of
this heterogeneous group of compounds, 2-naph-
thylamine, a potent human bladder carcinogen (155).

Animal experiments have shown that 2-naph-
thylamine requires metabolic activation to exhibit its
carcinogenic potential. Such activation results in the
formation of the two potent carcinogens 2-amino-1-
naphthol and 2-naphthylhydroxylamine. The metabolism of 2-naphthylamine proceeds via the
phase I oxidative and phase II conjugative pathways. Glucuronidation of the carcinogenic metabolites in the liver represents a detoxication reaction.
By this means the toxic oxidative products of the
phase I reaction are detoxified. Unfortunately, the
excretion of the glucoronides is not the final fate of
2-naphthylamine. In certain species (including
man) the renal tubules contain a β-glucuronidase
enzyme, which, by hydrolyzing the 2-naphthyl-
amine glucuronide, releases carcinogenic metabolites into the bladder. The metabolism of 2-naph-
thylamine is clearly a complex process that follows
the sequence of activation, detoxication, and finally
reactivation by renal hydrolases. The detoxication or
activation of 2-naphthylamine therefore depends on
both the present and relative amounts of the enzymes involved in the overall metabolic fate of this
aromatic amine (122).

Haloethylenes

The haloethylenes are halogen derivatives of
ethylene. They include important industrial chemicals such as vinyl chloride, dichlorethylene, vinyli-

dene chloride, and trichloroethylene. Trichloroethylene has been widely used as a solvent, degreaser, and dry cleaning agent. The half-life of trichloroethylene in man is approximately 36 h. It is extensively metabolized to various products including trichloroacetic acid and trichloroethanol. The beneficial effect of this metabolism must be counterbalanced by the toxicity of an as yet unidentified metabolite (probably the epoxide) of trichloroethylene (126). The metabolic fates of other haloethylenes such as *cis*- and *trans*-1,2-dichloroethylenes and vinylidene chloride are probably similar to that of trichloroethylene. This includes epoxidation, hydrolysis, and conjugation reactions (29,30,93).

Alkyl Halides

Alkyl halides have been extensively used in industry as solvents, organic intermediates, and pesticides. This group includes such compounds as carbon tetrachloride, dichloromethane, and chloroform. The alkyl halides are toxic to many different tissues, including liver, kidney, and lung. There is also concern about their mutagenic and carcinogenic properties, which presumably are the result of their potency as alkylating agents (43,151). The alkyl halides are metabolized by oxidation, reduction, and conjugation. This pattern is exemplified by the metabolism of 1,2-dichloroethane. The extensively halogenated alkyl halides (such as carbon tetrachloride) undergo cytochrome-P450-catalyzed reductive metabolism. Under anaerobic conditions or when there is low oxygen tension, this pathway is particularly favored with the easily reduced alkyl halides (58). As with the PAHs, it appears that the metabolism of alkyl halides encompasses both activation and detoxication reactions. The ultimate biological response depends on the predominance of each pathway and on the alkyl halide in question.

Nonnutritive Heavy Metals

Human exposure to environmentally derived, nonnutritive heavy metals, such as cadmium, mercury, and lead, is a major problem. These metals, widely used in industry, have no effective metabolic pathway for excretion from the body. Unlike organic compounds, heavy metal ions are refractory to biological oxidation processes. Their accumulation in such tissues as the kidney and nervous system can be associated with toxicity (7).

Cadmium disposition has been extensively studied in mammals. The metal, bound to a low-molecular-weight protein called metallothionein, is found predominantly in the kidney and liver. It was originally thought that the binding of cadmium by metallothionein represented a detoxication reaction. However, this concept is the subject of debate, especially since cadmium-complexed metallothionein is almost completely reabsorbed from the renal tubules (150).

Mercury, with its many and varied industrial and domestic uses, has numerous opportunities to contaminate our food and water. Elemental mercury is absorbed primarily by the respiratory tract. Less than 0.01% of this element is absorbed from the gastrointestinal tract. Organic mercury, however, because of its lipid solubility, is readily absorbed from the gastrointestinal tract. The overall capacity of the body to eliminate mercury is poor. Mercury has great affinity for the kidney regardless of its form, and the avid retention of mercury is a result of the high tissue affinity for the metal. Mercury is highly reactive with tissue proteins and nucleic acids. It must be emphasized that the rate and route of mercury elimination are highly dependent on the form of the metal (elemental, organic, or inorganic) that is absorbed.

Despite the medical awareness of lead toxicity, and despite legislation designed to reduce environmental contamination, lead is one of the most widely used heavy metals. Significant human exposure occurs from automobile exhaust fumes, cigarette smoke, lead-based paints, and plumbing systems. Lead is present in two major forms. The first is inorganic lead as various salts and oxides. The second is alkyl or organic lead, which includes tetraethyl lead and tetramethyl lead. Lead is a cumulative poison affecting multiple systems within the body. Most notably lead affects the central and peripheral nervous system, the kidney, and hematopoiesis and heme synthesis. It can also affect the gastrointestinal tract and the reproductive system. The ability of lead to be absorbed varies dramatically with age. Adults absorb about 10% of an oral dose. Young children can absorb up to 50%. The marked difference in absorption predisposes young children to lead toxicity. Lead is stored primarily in the bone. Minimal excretion occurs in the bile and urine.

ROLE OF NUTRITION IN THE METABOLISM OF ENVIRONMENTAL CHEMICALS

Much energy is required in the metabolic detoxication of chemical pollutants. Many enzymes and cofactors must be synthesized to achieve the goal of pollutant metabolism and excretion. The process of detoxication is therefore linked to protein, carbohydrate, and lipid metabolism and the availability of vitamins and minerals. It is not surprising that the composition of the diet markedly influences the metabolism of such xenobiotics as drugs and environmental pollutants (19,53,141). Evidence of the role of nutrition in human drug metabolism is readily available, but much less is known about nutritional influences on pollutant metabolism in man. Clearly, the toxic nature of most environmental chemicals imposes ethical constraints on human experimentation. It is, however, becoming increasingly apparent from animal and epidemiologic studies that a poor nutritional status can seriously compromise the detoxication defense against pollutant exposure (16). Such impairment may substantially increase the toxicity of pollutant exposure (116).

The influence of nutritional status on the toxicity of environmental chemicals has received the attention of many investigators (21,23,41,94). It has been shown that many compounds naturally present in foods can alter the metabolism, and hence the toxicity, of foreign compounds. Investigators have demonstrated that many organic compounds contained in foods inhibit carcinogenesis (60,145). Among these compounds are phenols, indoles, and aromatic isothiocyanates (143–146,148,149). The phenols studied thus far include cinnamic acid derivatives, which are common constituents of plants. Phenolic compounds have an inhibiting effect on benzo[a]pyrene-induced neoplasia (143,147,149).

Cruciferous vegetables such as Brussels sprouts, cabbage, cauliflower, and broccoli inhibit benzo[a]-pyrene-induced neoplasia when added to the diet of mice before and during administration of benzo[a]-pyrene. When certain indoles contained in these vegetables were added to the diet of experimental animals, they were found to inhibit benzo[a]pyrene-induced neoplasia (146). Aromatic isothiocyanates are other constituents of cruciferous plants that have been shown to inhibit neoplasia induced by polycyclic aromatic hydrocarbons when they were given to experimental animals (143). Because of the complexity and variation of the human diet, it is clear that the influence of dietary components in chemical toxicity and carcinogenicity in man is extremely difficult to evaluate at present. There is, however, evidence that such dietary components as fruits and vegetables exhibit a natural protective effect against cancer.

The following discussion focuses on the role of lipids, protein, vitamins, and trace elements in pollutant metabolism. The interested reader is referred to the many surveys already published (2,3,5,12,19, 23,24,36,78,94,116). Particular attention is drawn to the excellent material reviewed by Calabrese (13,14), who gives extensive consideration to the influence of nutritional status on pollutant toxicity and carcinogenicity.

Lipids

The majority of the enzymes responsible for pollutant metabolism, particularly cytochrome P-450, are embedded in membranes of the lipid-rich endo-plasmic reticulum. These cellular lipids, especially phospholipids with a high percentage of unsaturated fatty acids, play an obligatory role in the metabolism of xenobiotics (88). The most important member of this group is phosphatidylcholine.

Animal studies have demonstrated that altering dietary lipids affects the ability of the membrane-bound enzymes to metabolize environmental pollutants. Rats fed herring oil supplements metabolized the environmental carcinogen benzo[a]pyrene almost twice as fast as those given lard (10% in the diet). The rate of metabolism was dependent on the unsaturated fatty acid content of the endoplasmic reticulum membrane, particularly linoleic ($C_{18:2}$) eicosapentaenoic ($C_{20:5}$), and decosahaenoic ($C_{22:6}$) acids (148). These findings underline the importance of polyunsaturated fatty acids in environmental carcinogen metabolism.

The studies in vitro noted above have been complemented by in vivo chemical carcinogenicity studies. Animals fed high- (15%) and low-fat diets (2%) were subsequently challenged by a chemical carcinogen, 2-acetylaminofluorene. A high-fat diet (containing saturated and unsaturated fatty acids) significantly increases the tumor incidence induced by 2-acetylaminofluorene. An indirect-acting carcinogen, 2-acetylaminofluorene requires metabolic activation to express its carcinogenicity. It is possible, in this instance, that modulation of the fat content of the diet has an appreciable influence on carcinogen metabolism. The precise mechanism, however, remains obscure. Of note is the evidence that diets high in fat have been implicated in cancer of the breast, colon, and prostate (61).

The fate of dietary lipids is influenced by nutritional factors, in particular, the cofactors needed for phospholipid methylation. Diets deficient in L-methionine interfere with the transport and synthesis of lipids. As a result the triglyceride concentration in the liver increases. There is evidence that a fatty liver, so induced, has a reduced capacity to metabolize aflatoxin B_1 (a hepatocarcinogen). In this context, choline deficiency also decreases drug metabolism. This decrease is paralleled by a decrease in phosphatidylcholine in the liver.

Overall it appears that the capacity of the liver to metabolize pollutants and drugs is related to any factor that influences the amount and fatty composition (saturated or unsaturated) of microsomal phosphatidylcholine. Dietary fat may therefore play an important role in the hepatic metabolism of xenobiotics.

Protein

Many studies show that a protein-deficient diet leads to inhibition of hepatic xenobiotic metabolism (18,94). This inhibition may in part be secondary to the catabolism of tissue protein necessary to meet the body energy requirements. This catabolism is associated with decreased concentrations of drug-metabolizing enzymes, amino acids, and peptides (glutathione) required for the phase II conjugation reactions (123). Protein–calorie malnutrition thus affects pollutant metabolism by reducing biotransformation reactions. This response, depending on the toxicity of the pollutant metabolite(s), may be beneficial or detrimental. Animals on low-protein diets may be more susceptible to the toxic effects of pollutants, as reported with chlordane (11). They may be protected, however, if the toxicity of the agent is expressed through its metabolic intermediate, as in the case of aflatoxin B_1 (89,127).

In vitro experiments have helped delineate the relationship between dietary protein and the enzymes involved in pollutant metabolism. A low-protein diet, for example, reduces mixed-function oxidase and epoxide hydrolase activities. The activities of these two enzymes are intimately and sequentially involved in the biotransformation of many environmental pollutants (53). There is additional evidence that the inhibition of mixed-function oxidase is more pronounced at low substrate concentrations than at higher levels. Epoxide hydrolase activities, however, are inhibited to the same extent at low and high substrate concentrations. These findings assume importance when it is realized that most pollutants are present in the environment in low concentrations. Under such conditions the body's mixed-function oxidase system would tend to be subsaturated. These results also highlight the crucial interplay between sequential enzymes participating in pollutant metabolism. Clearly, in regard to the effects of protein–calorie malnutrition on pollutant metabolism, the relationships among multiple enzymes must be considered.

Many investigators have studied the influence of low- or high-protein diets on the initiation or promotion of carcinogenic environmental pollutants. Studies with the breast carcinogen 7,12-dimethylbenzanthracene show that increasing dietary protein fed prior to (but not following) administration of this environmental polycyclic aromatic hydrocarbon results in fewer tumors (116). These findings may result from an increase in hepatic carcinogen metabolism, which in turn reduces mammary gland exposure to the toxic metabolic products. Dietary protein deficiency may thus influence polycyclic aromatic hydrocarbon-induced carcinogenesis by its effect on cancer initiation rather than cancer promotion.

Vitamins and Trace Elements

Vitamins and trace elements constitute an important part of the diet. They are necessary for the synthesis of proteins and lipids, which are vital

components of the pollutant-metabolizing enzyme systems. It is not surprising, therefore, that changes in vitamin levels, particularly deficiencies, cause changes in the body's ability to metabolize pollutants. The role of vitamins and minerals on drug and pollutant metabolism has recently been extensively reviewed (13,14,94), and the interested reader is encouraged to consult these references. In general, vitamin deficiency results in a reduction in the activity of the xenobiotic-metabolizing enzymes, although the information is sometimes contradictory. The precise effect depends on many factors including the age, sex, species, and hormonal status of the experimental animal involved.

Some of the vitamins involved in drug and pollutant metabolism are vitamins A, C, E, and those of the B group including niacin, riboflavin, and thiamine. A riboflavin derivative is an essential component of a flavoprotein linked to cytochrome P-450. When rats are fed a diet deficient in riboflavin, a 90% drop in hepatic azo-reductase (a flavoprotein) is observed. In vitamin-B_2-deficient rats, the azo-reductase activity was paralleled by a fall in the azo-reduction of the carcinogen 4-dimethylaminoazobenzene.

The most widely studied vitamin, in terms of drug metabolism, is vitamin C. This is in part because of its nutritional requirement in man, monkey, and guinea pig. Vitamin C deficiency has been particularly well studied in the guinea pig, because this species is unusually sensitive to such drugs as pentobarbital and procaine. As might be expected from this increased sensitivity, vitamin C deficiency in the guinea pig markedly reduces xenobiotic metabolism, including the metabolism of the carcinogen benzo[a]pyrene. This finding probably relates to lower levels of cytochrome P-450 in vitamin-C-deficient animals. Although the specific role of vitamin C in drug and pollutant metabolism is debatable, it is clear that this vitamin forms an essential dietary component in the maintenance of xenobiotic biotransformation pathways.

Vitamin E is reported to inhibit xenobiotic metabolism. Vitamin E, an antioxidant, can inhibit lipid peroxidation initiated by many toxic pollutants such as carbon tetrachloride. In addition, vitamin E may act to inhibit pollutant metabolism by virtue of its postulated requirement in heme biosynthesis.

Trace elements, including iron, zinc, magnesium, copper, and selenium, can influence pollutant metabolism. In magnesium-depleted animals, thyroid hormone levels are depressed. This change is known to be associated with decreased xenobiotic metabolism. Magnesium-depleted diets are also linked to a marked reduction in hepatic microsomal lipid concentrations, further decreasing xenobiotic metabolism. Iron-deficient diets cause a marked decrease in intestinal xenobiotic metabolism. This effect may be important, particularly with respect to the carcinogenicity of polycyclic aromatic hydrocarbons. (See Chapter 8 for a further discussion of this subject.) Parathion toxicity is greater in copper-deficient than normal mice. The increased toxicity is linked to a lowered production of 4-nitrophenol, a nontoxic metabolite. This impairment of metabolism allows more parathion to be converted to paraoxon, the active anticholinesterase formed from parathion.

Delineating the precise role of vitamins and trace elements in xenobiotic metabolism is a formidable task. Experiments designed to manipulate their levels, although easily accomplished, are difficult to interpret. For example, because of their nutritional nature, a deficiency or excess of vitamins and trace elements can influence intermediary metabolism. The variation in such metabolism between different species, sexes, etc. makes comparative studies extremely difficult to analyze.

METABOLIC INTERACTIONS OF ENVIRONMENTAL CHEMICALS

Up to this point consideration has been given to pollutant metabolism and its relationship to dietary factors. Specific emphasis has been placed on the ability of the body to detoxify or activate these xenobiotics. Another aspect of pollutant metabolism that bears emphasis is the propensity of some pollutants to induce or inhibit the metabolism of other pollutants and drugs. These important interactions will now be considered.

Induction of Metabolism

Induction of the detoxifying enzymes is best characterized by the action of dioxin and the polycyclic aromatic hydrocarbons (PAHs) (102,107). Such PAHs as benzo[a]pyrene also have the ability to induce the enzymes responsible for their own metabolism. The interested reader is referred to published material (10,20,46,59,119).

Dioxin and PAHs are thought to increase the concentration of microsomal enzymes by interacting with the Ah receptor. This interaction switches on the Ah structural genes and these in turn induce the mixed-function oxidases, cyctochrome P-450, and many other proteins, including the phase II enzyme UDP-glucuronyltransferase (100). The presence of the Ah receptor is thought to be necessary, as genetically responsive strains of mice have at least 50 times more detectable Ah receptor than nonresponsive strains (108). The induction of the microsomal enzymes appears to be an adaptive response, since their concentration falls once the exposure to the inducing chemicals is reduced.

The extensive investigation of PAH induction of the drug-metabolizing enzymes seems well justified in view of the wide human exposure to these carcinogens. It has been shown, for example, that ambient benzo[a]pyrene concentrations in industrial/urban areas may be as high as 6×10^6 µg/1000 m^3 of air (coal-tar roofing area). This figure is in stark contrast to the equivalent figure of 0.04 in the Grand Canyon Park, Arizona (57).

Polybrominated biphenyls (PBBs) and polychlorinated biphenyls (PCBs) are excellent inducers of cytochrome P-450 isoenzymes and epoxide hydrolase (33,118,128) and also influence the metabolism of other environmental pollutants (128). For example, pretreating rats with Arochlor 1254 (a commercial mixture of PCBs) increases the metabolism of benzo[a]pyrene by liver and lung microsomal fractions about nine and four times, respectively. The induction of benzo[a]pyrene metabolism by PCBs, however, may be species dependent. The same treatment performed on rabbits increases benzo[a]pyrene metabolism only 1.3 times in the liver and reduces it 50% in the lung.

Additional studies show that the individual PCB isomers differ markedly in their ability to induce the enzymes of pollutant metabolism. For example, various PCB isomers (such as the 6,2',3', 4',6'-penta-, 2,4,2',4',6'-penta-, and 4,2',3',4',5',6'-hexachlorobiphenyls) increase the formation of dieldrin, the epoxide of the insecticide aldrin, about sixfold. This reaction relies on the activity of the cytochrome-P-450-dependent mixed-function oxidase system (129).

Although animal data on pollutant induction of the enzymes of pollutant metabolism are extensive, data available in man are exceedingly limited. In light of the species differences noted above, obvious dangers exist in extrapolating animal data to man.

Induction of Drug and Endogenous Compound Metabolism

Since phase I and II enzymes usually exhibit very broad substrate specificities, it is not surprising that some environmental pollutants effect the metabolism of many drugs that are used in clinical practice (26). Extensive animal and human experiments clearly show that some pollutants increase the metabolism of therapeutic agents and drugs (Table 9-5). Although the data in man are scant, several environmental pollutants have been shown to induce hepatic enzymes and to modify drug levels in environmentally or occupationally exposed populations. These pollutants include PCBs (10), PBBs (4), DDT (121), chlordecone (39), and TCDD (dioxin) (65).

The pollutant-dependent increase in drug-metabolizing activity is well exemplified by the decrease in the hexobarbital narcosis that occurs when

TABLE 9-5. Environmental Chemicals That Induce Microsomal Enzyme Activity

Chemical	Drug whose metabolism is increased	References
Halogenated insecticides[a]	Aminopyrine demethylation	20,82
Nicotine and cigarette smoking	Meprobamate oxidation, phenacetin dealkylation, antipyrine hydroxylation, theophylline demethylation and oxidation, imipramine demethylation, pentazocine hydroxylation	76,153
Polycyclic aromatic hydrocarbons	Hexobarbital oxidation	95
Polybrominated biphenyls	Aminopyrine demethylation	50,99,128
Polychlorinated biphenyls	Aminopyrine demethylation, zoxazolamine hydroxylation, warfarin hydroxylation, barbiturate hydroxylation, ethylmorphine demethylation, benzphetamine demethylation	49,110,128,159
2,3,7,8-Tetrachlorodibenzo-*p*-dioxin	Zoxazolamine hydroxylation, acetaminophen hydroxylation, phenacetin deethylation	100
Urea herbicides[b]	Aminopyrine demethylation	81
Volatile oils[c]	Amphetamine oxidation, zoxazolamine hydroxylation, pentobarbital oxidation, aminopyrine demethylation	73

[a]Including Mirex, DDT, toxaphene, and chlordecone.
[b]Including herban and diuron.
[c]Eucalyptol.

rats are pretreated with PCB. The reduced response to hexobarbital is related to the PCB-dependent induction of the hexobarbital oxidase enzymes, which increase the metabolism and clearance of the barbiturate. Similar experiments in rabbits resulted in no change in hexobarbital sleeping times (159).

Induction of cytochrome-P-450-dependent mixed-function oxidase activities by such environmental pollutants as polychlorinated biphenyls and polychlorinated dibenzofurans can result in marked changes in steroid metabolism (152). For example, 3,4,5,3′,5′-pentachlorobiphenyl selectivity induces the 7α-hydroxylation of both testosterone and progesterone by about threefold but dramatically suppresses the 2α-, 6β- and 16α-hydroxylation and 5α-reduction of both steroids (160). Similarly, PBBs and TCDD have been shown to modulate progesterone metabolism (35,56). Finally, both DDT and PCB exposure results in a change in the biotransformation of testosterone, 4-androstene-3,17-dione, and estradiol-17β in experimental animals (104).

Insecticides such as parathion, malathion, chlorthione, DDT, and chlordane have also been shown to inhibit testosterone hydroxylation in the liver (158). In addition, carbon tetrachloride inhibits the hepatic metabolism of estradiol-17β and estrone in rat liver (86).

Inhibition of Drug Metabolism

Since cytochrome P-450 functions as the terminal hemoprotein responsible for drug oxidations, much attention has focused on the ability of xenobiotics to inhibit drug metabolism pathways (137). Many of the structurally diverse environmental pollutants have the ability to decrease drug metabo-lism. They do this by altering the synthesis or degradation of cytochrome P-450 or by forming functionally inactive complexes with this hemoprotein (Table 9-6).

SUMMARY

The body is exposed to an unending variety of potentially toxic chemicals. This exposure poses a considerable challenge to the body's defense mechanisms. A most important defense is based on a series of biochemical reactions that protect the body against naturally occurring as well as man-made chemicals. Since most toxic chemicals are nonpolar, they cannot be excreted through the normal water-based excretory mechanisms. The biochemical defense thus depends on a series of reactions that convert the nonpolar, lipophilic chemicals to polar products. This biotransformation facilitates their excretion by the kidney. In many cases the poorly metabolized lipophilic pollutants are sequestered in adipose tissue. This sequestration often leads to an indefinite retention of some pollutants within the body.

For those environmental chemical pollutants that are metabolized, the process of metabolism can be beneficial or detrimental depending on the relative toxicities of the parent chemical and its metabolic products. There are many examples of innocuous environmental pollutants being metabolically activated to potent chemical carcinogens, thus dispelling the myth that the "detoxication" enzymes always play a beneficial role on pollutant disposition and metabolism. An important determinant of pollutant metabolism and toxicity is the contribution

TABLE 9-6. Environmental Chemicals That Inhibit Microsomal Enzyme Activity

Chemical class	Examples	References
Chemicals altering the synthesis or degradation of cytochrome P-450		
Acetylenic derivatives	Acetylene, dactylyne	79,154
Alkyl halides	Carbon tetrachloride, bromotrichloromethane	37,51,97,98
Metals	Co^{2+}, Cd^{2+}, Pb^{2+}, Zn^{2+}, Cr^{2+}, Mn^{2+}	40,51,130,132
Olefin derivatives	Vinyl chloride, trichloroethylene, ethylene	54,109,138
Thionosulfur derivatives	Carbon disulfide, disulfiram, diethylphenylphosphorothionate	62, 105
Chemicals that form inactive complexes with cytochrome P-450		
Alcohols	Methanol, ethanol, benzyl alcohol	22,136
Gases	Carbon monoxide, cyanide	27,28,101
Insecticide synergists	Piperonyl butoxide and sesamex	32,44,45,69

made by the various enzymes involved in the detoxication process. This process may be affected by the ability of pollutants themselves to induce or decrease the concentration of specific detoxication enzymes.

The role of nutrition in the metabolism of environmental pollutants must not be underestimated. Factors that adversely influence nutrition usually decrease the ability of the organism to metabolize chemicals. An impaired nutritional state, by reducing the metabolism of pollutants that express their toxicity through their metabolites, may be of benefit. Conversely, an impaired nutritional state may be detrimental if it reduces the excretion of toxic agents. Under these conditions, retention of the chemical may dispose the body to toxic insult.

Finally, it should be remembered that the basis of our knowledge of pollutant disposition, metabolism, and toxicity comes primarily from controlled animal experiments using single or repeated doses of a chemical agent. Man, however, is exposed simultaneously to a heterogeneous mixture of environmental pollutants whose interactions are not clearly defined. These conditions clearly add an important dimension to pollutant exposure that needs careful exploration.

REFERENCES

1. Albro PW, Moore B: Identification of the metabolites of simple phthalate diesters in rat urine. J Chromatogr 94:209, 1974.
2. Alvares AP, Kappas A, Anderson KE, et al: Nutritional factors regulating drug biotransformations in man. In: Advances in Pharmacology and Therapeutics, Vol 8, pp 43–51, Olive G (ed.), Pergamon Press, New York, 1979.
3. Alvares AP, Pantuck EJ, Anderson KE, et al: Regulation of drug metabolism in man by environmental factors. Drug Metab Rev 9:185, 1979.
4. Anderson HA, Wolff MS, Lilis R, et al: Symptoms and clinical abnormalities following ingestion of polybrominated-biphenyl contaminated food products. Ann NY Acad Sci 320:684, 1979.
5. Anderson KE, Conney AH, Kappas A: Nutritional influences on chemical biotransformations in humans. Nutr Rev 40:161, 1982.
6. Angerer J: Occupational chronic exposure to organic solvents. Metabolism of toluene in man. Int Arch Occup Environ Health 43:63, 1979.
7. Bach PH, Bonner FW, Bridge JW, et al (eds.): Nephrotoxicity: Assessment and Pathogenesis. John Wiley & Sons, New York, 1982.
8. Baselt RC, Cravey RH: Disposition of Toxic Drugs and Chemicals in Man. Year Book Medical Publishers, Chicago, 1989.
9. Bickel MH, Muehlebach S: Pharmacokinetics and ecodisposition of polyhalogenated hydrocarbons: Aspects and concepts. Drug Metab Rev 11:149, 1980.
10. Blumberg WE: Enzymic modification of environmental intoxicants: The role of cytochrome P450. Q Rev Biophys 11:481, 1978.
11. Boyd EM, Taylor FI: The acute oral toxicity of chlordane in albino rats fed for 28 days from weaning on a protein-deficient diet. Ind Med Surg 38:434, 1969.
12. Bridges JW, Back PH, Bonner FW, et al: The effects of nutritional factors on renal response to toxins. In: Nephrotoxicity: Assessment and Pathogenesis, p 182, Bach PH, Bonner FW, Bridges JW, et al. (eds.), John Wiley & Sons, New York, 1982.
13. Calabrese EJ: Nutrition and Environmental Health. The Influence of Nutritional Status in Pollutant Toxicity and Carcinogencity, Vol 1, The Vitamins, John Wiley & Sons, New York, 1980.
14. Calabrese EJ: Nutrition and Environmental Health. The Influence of Nutritional Status in Pollutant Toxicity and Carcinogencity, Vol 2, Minerals and Macronutrients, John Wiley & Sons, New York, 1981.
15. Campbell TC: Nutrition and drug metabolising enzymes. Clin Pharmacol Ther 22:699, 1977.
16. Campbell TC: Influence of nutrition on metabolism

of carcinogens. In: Advances in Nutrition Research, Vol 2, p 29, Draper HH (ed.), Plenum Press, New York, 1979.

17. Campbell TC, Hayes JR: Role of nutrition in the drug-metabolising enzyme system. Pharmacol Rev 26:171, 1974.

18. Campbell TC, Hayes JR: The effect of quantity and quality of dietary protein on drug metabolism. Fed Proc 35:2470, 1976.

19. Campbell TC, Hayes JR, Merrill AH Jr, et al: The influence of dietary factors on drug metabolism in animals. Drug Metab Rev 9:173, 1979.

20. Chambers JE, Trevathan CA: Effect of Mirex, dechlorinated Mirex derivatives and chlordecone on microsomal mixed function oxidase activity and other hepatic parameters. Toxicol Lett 16:109, 1983.

21. Clayson DB: Nutrition and experimental carcinogenesis: A review. Cancer Res 35:3292, 1975.

22. Cohen GM, Mannering GJ: Involvement of a hydrophobic site in the inhibition of the microsomal *para*-hydroxylation of aniline by alcohols. Mol Pharmacol 8:383, 1973.

23. Committee on Diet, Nutrition, and Cancer, National Research Council: Diet Nutrition and Cancer, National Academy Press, Washington, 1982.

24. Conference on Nutrition on the Causation of Cancer: Cancer Res 35:3301–3303, 1975.

25. Connelly JC, Bridges JW: The distribution and role of cytochrome P450 in extrahepatic organs. In: Progress in Drug Metabolism, Vol 5, p 1, Bridges JW, Chasseaud LF (eds.), John Wiley & Sons, New York, 1980.

26. Conney AH, Burns JJ: Metabolic interactions among environmental chemicals and drugs. Science 178:576, 1972.

27. Cooper DY, Levin S, Narasimhulu S, et al: Photochemical action spectrum of the terminal oxidase of mixed function oxidase systems. Science 147:400, 1965.

28. Cooper DY, Schleyer H, Levin SS, et al: A re-evaluation of the role of cytochrome P450 as the terminal oxidase in hepatic microsomal mixed function oxidase-catalysed reactions. Drug Metab Rev 10:153, 1979.

29. Costa AK, Ivanetich KM: Vinylidene chloride: Its metabolism by hepatic microsomal cytochrome P450 in vitro. Biochem Pharmacol 21:2083, 1982.

30. Costa AK, Ivanetich KM: The 1,2-dichloroethylenes: Their metabolism by hepatic cytochrome P450 in vitro. Biochem Pharmacol 31:2093, 1982.

31. Coulston F, Pocchiari F (eds.): Accidental Exposure to Dioxins. Human Health Aspects. Ecotoxicity and Environmental Quality Series, Academic Press, Orlando, 1983.

32. Dahl AR, Hodgson E: The interaction of aliphatic analogues of methylenedioxyphenyl compounds with cytochromes P450 and P420. Chem Biol Interact 27:163, 1979.

33. Dannam GA, Guengerich FP, Kaminsky LS, et al: Regulation of cytochrome P450. Immunochemical quantitation of eight isozymes in liver microsomes of rats treated with polybrominated biphenyl congeners. J Biol Chem 258:1282, 1983.

34. Dauterman WC: The role of hydrolases in insecticide metabolism and the toxicological significance of the metabolites. J Toxicol Clin Toxicol 19:623, 1983.

35. Derr SK: In vivo metabolism of exogenous progesterone by polychlorinated biphenyl-treated female rats. Bull Environ Contam Toxicol 19:729, 1978.

36. Dickerson JWT: The inter-relationship of nutrition and drugs. In: Nutrition in the Clinical Management of Disease, p 308, Dickerson JWT, Lee HA (eds.), Edward Arnold, London, 1978.

37. Dingell JV, Heimberg M: The effects of halogenated hydrocarbons on hepatic drug metabolism. Biochem Pharmacol 17:1269, 1964.

38. Dorough HW: Toxicological significance of pesticide conjugates. J Toxicol Clin Toxicol 19:637, 1983.

39. Dossing M: Changes in hepatic microsomal enzyme function in workers exposed to mixtures of chemicals. Clin Pharmacol Ther 32:340, 1982.

40. Drummond GS, Kappas A: The cytochrome P450-depleted animal; an experimental model for in vivo studies in chemical biology. Proc Natl Acad Sci USA 79:2384, 1982.

41. Environmental Chemicals and Nutrition. Relationship to Metabolism, Action and Toxicology of Drugs: Clin Pharmacol Ther 22(5, part 2):623–824, 1977.

42. Estabrook RW, Lindenlaub E, Oesch R, et al: Toxicological and Immunological Aspects of Drug Metabolism and Environmental Chemicals, Symposia Medica Hoechst 22, FK Schattauer Verlag, Stuttgart, 1988.

43. Fishbein L: Industrial mutagens and carcinogens. I. Halogenated aliphatic derivatives. Mutat Res 32:267, 1976.

44. Franklin MR: Inhibition of mixed function oxidations by substrates forming reduced cytochrome P450 metabolic–intermediate complexes. Pharmacol Ther A 2:227, 1979.

45. Fujji K, Jaffe H, Bishop Y, et al: Structure–activity relationships for methylenedioxyphenyl and related compounds on hepatic microsomal enzyme function, as measured by prolongation of hexobarbital narcosis and zoxazolamine paralysis in mice. Toxicol App Pharmacol 16:482, 1970.

46. Gelboin HV: Benzo(a)pyrene metabolism, activation and carcinogenesis. Role and regulation of mixed function oxidases and related enzymes. Physiol Rev 60:1107, 1980.

47. Gibson GG: Comparative aspects of the mammalian cytochrome P450 IV gene family. Xenobiotica 19:1123, 1989.

48. Gibson JR, Ivie GW, Dorough HW: Fate of Mirex and its major photodecomposition product in rat. J Agric Food Chem 20:1246, 1972.

49. Goldstein JA, Hickman P, Bergman H, et al: Separation of pure polychlorinated biphenyl isomers into two types of inducers on the basis of induction of cytochrome P450 or cytochrome P448. Chem Biol Interact 17:69, 1977.

50. Goldstein JA, Linko PC, Levy LA, et al: A comparison of a commercial polybrominated biphenyl mixture 2,4,5,2',4',5'-hexabromobiphenyl and 2,3,6,7-tetrabromonaphthalene as inducers of liver microsomal drug metabolising enzymes. Biochem Pharmacol 28:2947, 1979.

51. Gregus Z, Watkins JB, Thompson TN, et al: Resistance of some phase II biotransformation pathways to hepatotoxins. J Pharmacol Exp Ther 222:471, 1982.

52. Guengerich FP: Isolation and purification of cytochrome P450 and the existence of multiple forms. Pharmacol Ther 6:99, 1979.

53. Guengerich FP: Effects of nutritive factors on metabolic processes involving bioactivation and detoxication of chemicals. Annu Rev Nutr 4:207, 1984.

54. Guengerich FP, Mason RS, Scott WT, et al: Roles of 2-haloethylene oxides and 2-haloacetaldehydes derived from vinyl bromide and vinyl chloride in irreversible binding to protein and DNA. Cancer Res 41:4391, 1981.

55. Guenther TM, Oesch F: Metabolic activation and inactivation of chemical mutagens and carcinogens. In: Drug Metabolism and Distribution, p 30, Lamble JN (ed.), Elsevier-North Holland, Amsterdam, 1983.

56. Gustafsson JA, Ingleman-Sundberg M: Changes in steroid hormone metabolism in rat liver microsomes following administration of 2,3,7,8-tetrachlorodibenzo-p-dioxin (TCDD). Biochem Pharmacol 28:497, 1979.

57. Hammond EC, Selikoff IJ, Lawther PL, et al: Inhalation of benzo(a)pyrene and cancer in man. Ann NY Acad Sci 271:116, 1977.

58. Hanzlik RP: Reactivity and toxicity among halogenated methanes and related compounds. A physicochemical correlate with predictive value. Biochem Pharmacol 30:3027, 1981.

59. Harvey RG: Polycyclic hydrocarbons and cancer. Am Sci 70:386, 1982.

60. Hayatsu H, Arimoto S, Negishi T: Dietary inhibitors of mutagenesis and carcinogenesis. Mutat Res 202:429, 1988.

61. Hopkins GJ, West CE: Possible roles of dietary fats in carcinogenesis. Life Sci 19:1103, 1976.

62. Hunter AL, Neal RA: Inhibition of hepatic mixed function oxidase activity in vitro and in vivo by various thiono-sulphur-containing compounds. Biochem Pharmacol 24:2199, 1975.

63. Hunter CG: Aromatic solvents. Ann Occup Hyg 9:193, 1966.

64. Hutzinger O, Nash DM, Safe S, et al: Polychlorinated biphenyls: Metabolic behaviour of pure isomers in pigeons, rats and brook trout. Science 178:312, 1972.

65. Ideo G, Bellati G, Bellobuono A, et al: Increased urinary D-glucaric acid excretion by children living in an area polluted with tetrachlorodibenzoparadioxin (TCDD). Clin Chim Acta 120:273, 1982.

66. Infante PF, Wagoner JF, Rinsky RA, et al: Leukemia in benzene workers. Lancet 2:76, 1977.

67. Ionannides C, Parke DV: The cytochromes P-448—a unique family of enzymes involved in chemical toxicity and carcinogenesis, 36:4197, 1987.

68. Ionannides C, Parke DV: The cytochrome P450 I gene family of microsomal hemoproteins and their role in the metabolic activation of chemicals. Drug Metab Rev 22:1, 1990.

69. Jaffe H, Fujii K, Sengupta M, et al: In vivo inhibition of mouse liver microsomal hydroxylating systems by methylene dioxyphenyl insecticide synergists and related compounds. Life Sci 7:1051, 1968.

70. Jerina DM, Yagi H, Lehr RE, et al: The Bay-Region theory of carcinogenesis by polycyclic aromatic hydrocarbons. In: Polycyclic Hydrocarbons and Cancer. Vol 1 Environment, Chemistry and Metabolism, p

173, Gelboin HV, Ts'O POP (eds.), Academic Press, New York, 1978.

71. Johnson EF: Multiple forms of cytochrome P450: Criteria and significance. In: Reviews in Biochemical Toxicology, p 1, Hodgson E, Bend JR, Philpot RM (eds.), Elsevier-North Holland, Amsterdam, 1979.

72. Jollow DJ, Mitchell DR, Zampaglione H, et al: Bromobenzene-induced liver necrosis. Protective role of glutathione and evidence of 3,4-bromobenzene oxide as the hepatoxic metabolite. Pharmacology 11:151, 1974.

73. Jori A, Bianchett A, Prestini PE, et al: Effect of eucalyptol (1,8-cineole) on the metabolism of other drugs in rats and in man. Eur J Pharmacol 9:362, 1970.

74. Juchau MR: Enzymatic bioactivation and inactivation of chemical teratogens and transplacental carcinogens/mutagens. In: The Biochemical Basis of Chemical Teratogenesis, p 63, Juchau MR (ed.), Elsevier-North Holland, Amsterdam, 1981.

75. Juchau MR: Bioactivation in chemical teratogenesis. Annu Rev Pharmacol Toxicol 29:165, 1989.

76. Jusko WJ: Influence of cigarette smoking on drug metabolism in man. Drug Metab Rev 9:221, 1979.

77. Kadlubar FF, Frederick CB, Weis CC, et al: Prostaglandin endoperoxide synthetase-mediated metabolism of carcinogenic aromatic amines and their binding to DNA and proteins. Biochem Biophys Res Commun 108:253, 1982.

78. Kato R: Drug metabolism under pathological and abnormal physiological states in animals and man. Xenobiotica 7:25, 1977.

79. Kaul PM, Kulkami SK: New drug metabolism inhibitor of marine origin. J Pharm Sci 67:1293, 1978.

80. Kimbrough RD, Jensen AA (eds.): Halogenated Biphenyls, Terphenyls, Naphthalenes, Dibenzodioxins and Related Products, 2nd ed., Elsevier, Amsterdam, 1989.

81. Kinoshita FK, Du Bois KP: Induction of hepatic microsomal enzymes by Herban, Diuron and other substituted urea herbicides. Toxicol App Pharmacol 17:406, 1970.

82. Kinoshita FK, Frawley JP, Du Bois KP: Quantitative measurement of induction of hepatic microsomal enzymes by various dietary levels of DDT and toxaphene in the rat. Toxicol Appl Pharmacol 9:505, 1966.

83. Kulkarni AP, Hodgson E: The metabolism of insecticides—the role of monooxygenase enzymes. Annu Rev Pharmacol Toxicol 24:19, 1984.

84. Lake BG, Phillips JC, Linnell JC, et al: The in vitro hydrolysis of some phthalate diesters by hepatic and intestinal preparations, from various species. Toxicol Appl Pharmacol 39:239, 1977.

85. Leibman KC: Metabolism and toxicity of styrene. Environ Health Perspect 11:115, 1975.

86. Levin W, Welch RM, Conney AH: Effect of carbon tetrachloride and other inhibitors of drug metabolism on the metabolism and action of estradiol-17β and estrone in the rat. J Pharmacol Exp Ther 173:247, 1970.

87. Lu AYH, West SB: Multiplicity of mammalian microsomal cytochromes P-450. Pharmacol Rev 31:277, 1980.

88. Lu AYH, Levin W, Kuntzman R: Reconstituted liver microsomal enzyme system that hydoxylates drugs, other foreign compounds and endogenous substrates. VII. Stimulation of benzphetamine N-de-

methylation by lipid and detergent. Biochem Biophys Res Commun 60:266, 1974.

89. Madhaven TV, Gopalan C: The effect of dietary protein on carcinogenesis of aflatoxin. Arch Pathol 85: 133, 1968.

90. Mathews HB, Dedrick RL: Pharmacokinetics of polychlorinated biphenyls. Annu Rev Pharmacol Toxicol 24:85, 1984.

91. Mathews HB, Kato S, Morales NM, et al: Distribution and excretion of 2,4,5,2',4',5'-hexabromobiphenyl, the major component of Firemaster BP-6. J Toxicol Environ Health 3:599, 1977.

92. McConnell EE: Acute and chronic toxicity and carcinogenesis in animals. In: Halogenated Biphenyls, Terphenyls, Naphthalenes, Dibenzodioxins and Related Products, 2nd ed., p 161, Kimbrough RD, Jensen AA (eds.), Elsevier, Amsterdam, 1989.

93. McDonald TL: Chemical mechanisms of halocarbon metabolism. CRC Crit Rev Toxicol 11:85, 1983.

94. Meydani M: Dietary effects on detoxification process. In: Nutritional Toxicology, Vol II, p 1, Hathcock JN (ed.), Academic Press, Orlando, 1987.

95. Mizokami K, Inouie K, Sunouchi M, et al: 3-Methylcholanthrene induces phenobarbital-induced cytochrome P-450 haemoprotein in fetal liver and not cytochrome P-448 haemoprotein induced in maternal liver of rats. Biochem Biophys Res Commun 107:6, 1982.

96. Mocarelli P, Marocchi A, Brambilla P, et al: Clinical laboratory manifestations of exposure to dioxin in children. JAMA 256:2687, 1986.

97. Moody DE, James JL, Smuckler EA: Cytochrome P-450-lowering effect of alkyl halides, correlation with decrease in arachidonic acid. Biochem Biophys Res Commun 97:673, 1980.

98. Moody DE, Clawson GA, Woo CH, et al: Cellular distribution of cytochrome P-450 loss in rats of different ages treated with alkyl halides. Toxicol App Pharmacol 66:278, 1982.

99. Moore RW, Dannan GA, Aust SD: Structure–function relationships for the pharmacological and toxicological effects and metabolism of polybrominated biphenyl congeners. In: Molecular Basis of Environmental Toxicity, p 173, Bhatnagar RS (ed.), Ann Arbor Science, Ann Arbor, 1980.

100. Nebert DW, Jensen NM: The Ah locus: Genetic regulation of the metabolism of carcinogens, drugs and other environmental chemicals by cytochrome P-450-mediated monooxygenases. CRC Crit Rev Biochem 6:401, 1979.

101. Nebert DW, Kumaki K, Sato M, et al: Association of type I, type II and reverse type I difference spectra with absolute spin state of cytochrome P-450 iron. In: Microsomes and Drug Oxidations, p 224, Ullrich V, Roots A, Hildebrandt A, et al. (eds.), Pergamon Press, New York, 1977.

102. Nebert DW, Eisen HK, Negishi M, et al: Genetic mechanisms controlling the induction of polysubstrate monooxygenase (p-450) activities. Annu Rev Pharmacol Toxicol 21:431, 1981.

103. Nebert DW, Nelson DR, Adesnik M, et al: The P450 superfamily: Updated listing of all genes and recommended nomenclature for the chromosomal loci. DNA 8:1, 1989.

104. Nowicki HG, Norman AW: Enhanced hepatic metabolism of testosterone, 4-androstene-3,17-dione and oestradiol-17β in chickens pretreated with DDT or polychlorinated biphenyls. Steroids 19:85, 1972.

105. Obreska MJ, Kentish P, Parke DV: The effects of carbon disulphide on rat liver microsomal mixed function oxidases, in vivo and in vitro. Biochem J 188: 107, 1980.

106. Oesch F, Guenthner TM: Effects of the modulation of epoxide hydrolase activity on the binding of benzo[a]pyrene metabolites to DNA in the intact nuclei. Carcinogenesis 4:57, 1983.

107. Okey AB, Vella LM: Binding of 3-methylcholanthrene and 2,3,7,8-tetrachlorodibenzo-p-dioxin to a common Ah receptor site in mouse and rat hepatic cytosols. Eur J Biochem 127:39, 1982.

108. Okey AB, Bondy GT, Mason ME, et al: Regulatory product of the Ah locus. Characterisation of the inducer–recepter complex and evidence for its nuclear translocation. J Biol Chem 254:11636, 1979.

109. Ortiz de Montellano PR, Mico BA: Destruction of cytochrome P-450 by ethylene and other olefins. Mol Pharmacol 18:128, 1980.

110. Ozawa N, Yoshihara S, Yoshimura H: Selective induction of rat liver microsomal cytochrome P-448 by 3,4,5,3',4'-pentachlorobiphenyl and its effect on liver microsomal drug metabolism. J Pharm Dyn 2:309, 1979.

111. Panthananickal A, Weller P, Marnett LJ: Stereoselectivity of the epoxidation of 7,8-dihydrobenzo[a]pyrene by prostaglandin H synthase and cytochrome P-450 determined by the identification of polyguanylic acid adducts. J Biol Chem 258:4411, 1983.

112. Parke DV: The Biochemistry of Foreign Compounds, Pergamon Press, New York, 1968.

113. Parke DV: The disposition and metabolism of environmental chemicals by mammalia. In: Handbook of Environmental Chemistry, p 141, Hutzinger O (ed.), Springer-Verlag, New York, 1982.

114. Parke DV: Activation mechanisms to chemical toxicity. Arch Toxicol 60:5, 1987.

115. Parke DV: The role of enzymes in protection mechanisms for human health. Regul Toxicol Pharmacol 7: 222, 1987.

116. Parke DV, Ioannides C: The role of nutrition in toxicology. Annu Rev Nut 1:207, 1981.

117. Parke DV, Ioannides C, Lewis DFV: Metabolic activation of carcinogens and toxic chemicals. Human Toxicol 7:397, 1988.

118. Parkinson A, Safe SH, Robertson LW, et al: Immunochemical quantition of cytochrome P-450 isoenzymes and epoxide hydrolase in liver microsomes from polychlorinated or polybrominated biphenyl-treated rats. A study of structure–activity relationships. J Biol Chem 258:5967, 1983.

119. Pelkonen O, Nebert DW: Metabolism of polycyclic aromatic hydrocarbons: Etiologic role in carcinogenesis. Pharmacol Rev 34:189, 1982.

120. Poiger H, Schlatter C: Biological degradation of TCDD in rats. Nature 281:706, 1979.

121. Poland A, Smith D, Kuntzman R, et al: Effect of intensive occupational exposure to DDT on phenylbutazone and cortisol metabolism in human subjects. Clin Pharmacol Ther 11:724, 1970.

122. Radomski JL: The primary aromatic amines: Their biological properties and structure–activity relationships. Annu Rev Pharmacol Toxicol 19:129, 1979.

123. Reed DJ, Beatty PW: Biosynthesis and regulation of glutathione: Toxicological implications. Rev Biochem Toxicol 2:213, 1980.

124. Reed GA, Marnett LJ: Metabolism and activation of 7,8-dihydrobenzo(a)pyrene during prostaglandin biosynthesis. Intermediacy of a bay region epoxide. J Biol Chem 257:11368, 1982.

125. Reggiani G: An overview of the health effects of halogenated dioxins and related compounds—the Yusho and Taiwan episodes. In: Accidental Exposure to Dioxins. Human Health Aspects, p 39, Coulston F, Pocchiari F (eds.), Academic Press, Orlando, 1983.

126. Reynolds ED, Moslen MT: Metabolic activation and hepatotoxicity of trichloroethylene. In: Biological Reactive Intermediates, 2, Chemical Mechanisms and Biological Effects (Part A), p 693, Snyder R, Parke DV, Kocsis JJ, et al. (eds.), Plenum Press, New York, 1982.

127. Rogers AE, Newberne PM: Diet and aflatoxin B_1 toxicity in rats. Toxicol Appl Pharmacol 20:113, 1971.

128. Safe S: Polychlorinated biphenyls (PCBs) and polybrominated biphenyls (PBBs): Biochemistry, toxicology and mechanism of action. CRC Crit Rev Toxicol 13:319, 1984.

129. Safe S, Campbell MA, Lambert I, et al: Polychlorinated biphenyls as phenobarbital-type inducers: Structure activity correlations. In: Cytochrome P-450, Biochemistry, Biophysics and Environmental Implications, p 341, Hietanen E, Laitinen M, Hanninen O (eds.), Elsevier-North Holland, Amsterdam, 1982.

130. Sasame HA, Boyd MR: Paradoxical effects of cobaltous chloride and salts of other divalent metals on tissue levels of reduced glutathione and microsomal mixed function oxidase components. J Pharmacol Exp Ther 205:718, 1978.

131. Seutter-Berlage F, Rietveld EC, Plate R, et al: Mercapturic acids as metabolites of aromatic aldehydes and alcohols. In: Biological Reactive Intermediates 2. Chemical Mechanisms and Biological Effects, Part A, p 359, Snyder R, Parke DV, Kocsis JJ, et al. (eds.), Plenum Press, New York, 1982.

132. Sinclair JF, Sinclair PR, Healey JF, et al: Decrease in hepatic cytochrome P-450 by cobalt. Biochem J 204:103, 1982.

133. Snyder R, Lee EW, Kocsis JJ, et al: Bone marrow depressant and leukemongenic actions of benzene. Life Sci 21:1709, 1977.

134. Snyder R, Longacre SL, Witmer CM, et al: Biochemical toxicology of benzene. In: Reviews in Biochemical Toxicology 3, p 123, Hodgson E, Bend JR, Philpot RM (eds.), Elsevier-North Holland, Amsterdam, 1981.

135. Snyder R, Longacre SL, Witmer CM, et al: Metabolic correlate of benzene toxicity. In Biological Reactive Intermediates 2. Chemical Mechanisms and Biological Effects, Part A, p 245, Snyder R, Parke DV, Kocsis JJ, et al. (eds), Plenum Press, New York, 1982.

136. Testa B: Structural and electronic factors influencing the inhibition of aniline hydroxylation by alcohols and their binding to cytochrome P-450. Chem Biol Interact 12:1, 1976.

137. Testa B, Jenner P: Inhibitors of cytochrome P-450 and their mechanism of action. Drug Metab Rev 12:1, 1981.

138. Testai E, Citti L, Gervasi PG, et al: Suicidal inactivation of hepatic cytochrome P-450 in vitro by some aliphatic olefins. Biochem Biophys Res Commun 107:633, 1982.

139. Thor H, Svensson SA, Hartzell P, et al: Biotransformation of bromobenzene to reactive metabolites by isolated hepatocytes. In: Biological Reactive Intermediates 2. Chemical Mechanisms and Biological Effects, Part A, p 287, Snyder R, Parke DV, Kocsis JJ, et al. (eds.), Plenum Press, New York, 1982.

140. Vainio H, Norppa H, Hemminki K, et al: Metabolism and genotoxicity of styrene. In: Biological Reactive Intermediates 2. Chemical Mechanisms and Biological Effects. Part A, p 257, Snyder R, Parke DV, Kocsis JJ, et al. (eds.), Plenum Press, New York, 1982.

141. Vessell ES: Complex effects of diet on drug disposition. Clin Pharmacol 36:285, 1984.

142. Vos JG, Luster MI: Immune alterations. In: Halogenated Biphenyls, Terphenyls, Naphthalenes, Dibenzodioxins and Related Products, 2nd ed, p 295, Kimbrough RE, Jensen AA (eds.), Elsevier, Amsterdam, 1989.

143. Wattenberg LW: Inhibitors of chemical carcinogens. In: Environmental Carcinogenesis, p 241, Emmelot P, Kriek E (eds.), Elsevier/North-Holland Biomedical Press, Amsterdam, 1979.

144. Wattenberg LW: Inhibition of chemical carcinogens by antioxidants. In: Carcinogens, Vol 5, Modifiers of Chemical Carcinogenesis, p 85, Slaga TJ (ed.), Raven Press, New York, 1980.

145. Wattenberg LW: Inhibition of carcinogenesis by naturally occurring and synthetic compounds. Basic Life Sci 52:155, 1990.

146. Wattenberg LW, Loub WD: Inhibition of polycyclic hydrocarbon-induced neoplasia by naturally occurring indoles. Cancer Res 38:1410, 1978.

147. Wattenberg LW, Leong JC, Strand PJ: Benzo(a)pyrene hydroxylase activity in the gastrointestinal tract. Cancer Res 22:1120, 1962.

148. Wattenberg LW, Coccia JB, Cam LKT: Inhibitory effects of phenolic compounds on benzo(a)pyrene-induced neoplasia. Cancer Res 40:2820, 1980.

149. Wattenberg LW, Borchert P, Destafry CLM, et al: Effects of p-methoxyphenol and diet on carcinogen-induced neoplasia of the mouse forestomach. Cancer Res 43:4747, 1983.

150. Webb M: Role of metallothioneins and other binding proteins in the renal handling and toxicity of heavy metals. In: Nephrotoxicity: Assessment and Pathogenesis, p 296, Bach PH, Bonner FW, Bridges JW, et al. (eds.), John Wiley & Sons, New York, 1982.

151. Weisburger E: Carcinogenicity studies on halogenated hydrocarbons. Environ Health Perspect 21:7, 1977.

152. Welch RM, Levin W, Conney AH: Insecticide inhibition and stimulation of steroid hydroxylases in rat liver. J Pharmacol Exp Ther 155:167, 1967.

153. Wenzel DG, Broadie LL: Stimulatory effect of nicotine on the metabolism of meprobamate. Toxicol Appl Pharmacol 8:455, 1966.

154. White INH: Metabolic activation of acetylenic substituents to derivatives in the rat causing the loss of hepatic cytochrome P-450 and haem. Biochem J 174:853, 1980.

155. World Health Organization: Evaluation of carcino-genic risk of chemicals to man. Some aromatic am-ines, hydrazine and related substances, N-nitroso compounds and miscellaneous alkylating agents. IARC Monogr 4:27, 1974.

156. Wiener M, Pittman KA, Stein V: Mirex kinetics in the rhesus monkey. I. Disposition and Excretion. Drug Metab Dispos 4:281, 1978.

157. Williams RT: Detoxication Mechanisms, 2nd ed., Chapman and Hall, London, 1959.

158. Wills ED: The role of polyunsaturated fatty acid com-position of the endoplasmic reticulum in the regula-tion of the rate of oxidative carcinogen metabolism. In: Microsomes, Drug Oxidations and Chemical Car-cinogenesis. Vol I, p 545, Coon MJ, Conney AH, Esta-brook RW, et al. (eds.), Academic Press, Orlando, 1980.

159. Wolff T, Hesse S: Species differences of mixed func-tion oxidase induction between rabbits and rats after pretreatment with polychlorinated biphenyls. Bio-chem Pharmacol 26:783, 1977.

160. Yoshihara S, Nagata K, Wada I, et al: A unique change of steroid metabolism in rat liver microsomes induced with a highly toxic polychlorinated biphenyl and polychlorinated dibenzofuran. J Pharm Dyn 5: 994, 1982.

RECOMMENDED READINGS

Gibson GG, Skett P: Introduction to Drug Metabolism, Chapman and Hall, London, 1986.

Meydani M: Dietary Effects on Detoxification Processes. In: Nutritional Toxicology, Vol II, p 1, Hathcock JN (ed.), Academic Press, Orlando, 1987.

Parke DV: Activation mechanisms to chemical toxicity. Arch Toxicol 60:5, 1987.

Parke DV: The role of enzymes in protection mechanisms for human health. Regul Toxicol Pharmacol 7:222, 1987.

Parke DV, Ioannides C: The role of nutrition in toxicology. Annu Rev Nutr 1:207, 1981.

Timbrell JA: Principles of Biochemical Toxicology, 2nd Ed. Taylor & Francis, London, 1991.

10. IMMUNOLOGIC MECHANISMS AND THE ROLE OF NUTRITION

Robert M. Suskind

INTRODUCTION

The objectives of this chapter are twofold: to emphasize the role of the immune system in protecting the body against environmental assault and to increase the reader's awareness of the critical relationship between immunity and nutrition.

THE IMMUNE SYSTEM

Major advances have been made in understanding the immune system's structure and function (17,117,118,126,158). This complex system is composed of a network of organs and cells that act to defend the host against invasion by foreign agents and to protect the host against the development and spread of cancer. Immune function is maintained and regulated by the lymphoid system in conjunction with the macrophages and related cells. The lymphoid system is composed of primary lymphoid tissue, the thymus and bone marrow, and secondary lymphoid tissue, the lymph nodes, spleen, and gut-associated lymphoid tissue. Macrophages along with monocytes, fixed tissue histiocytes, and Kupffer and Langerhans cells have a common origin and function. These cells, which make up the mononuclear phagocyte system, are found in all tissues but are highest in concentration in the lymph nodes and spleen. The primary lymphoid organs, the bone marrow and thymus, are responsible for lympho-

cyte development and maturation. Here lymphoid stem cells differentiate via two pathways into lymphocytes capable of reacting with antigen. One population of stem cells differentiates into B lymphocytes and plasma cells that are responsible for the production of antigen-specific antibodies. Another population of stem cells, under the influence of the thymus gland, become thymus-derived or T lymphocytes involved in antigen recognition in cell-mediated immune reactions including delayed hypersensitivity. The cellular components of the immune system and their development are shown in Fig. 10-1 (153).

The immune response has two functional but interrelated divisions, the innate or nonspecific immune response and the adaptive or specific immune response (Table 10-1). Innate immune mechanisms, being nonspecific, represent the first line of defense against invading microorganisms. The skin and mucous membranes, mucus, and cilia on epithelial surfaces also provide a variety of physical and biochemical barriers that have been discussed in Chapters 6, 7, and 8. The innate immune response is initiated when the surface barriers are penetrated by microorganisms. This nonspecific response includes phagocytosis and the inflammatory response with the involvement of the complement, coagulation, and kinin systems. Invading microorganisms thus encounter phagocytic cells and natural killer cells. With the development of the inflammatory response, a number of acute-phase proteins rapidly increase in the serum. These include C-reactive protein and other complement components.

The adaptive immune response, which provides a specific assault on each infectious agent, comes into play when the nonspecific immune defenses are

Principles and Practice of Environmental Medicine, edited by Alyce Bezman Tarcher. Plenum Medical Book Company, New York, 1992.

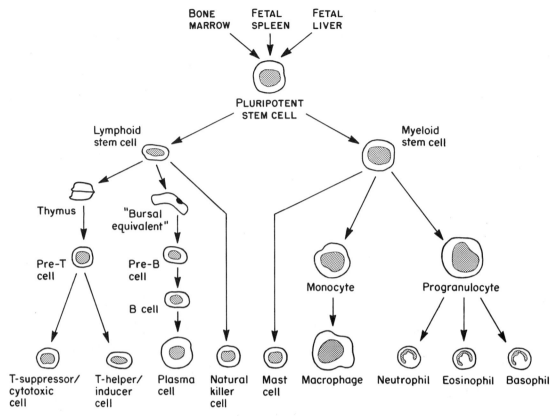

FIGURE 10-1. Origin and development of immune cells. Adapted from Vos and Luster (153).

breached. The specificity is based on two forms of adaptive immunity, humoral and cell-mediated, which employ different populations of lymphocytes. Humoral immunity depends on the production of antigen-specific antibodies by plasma cells, which are mature cells of the B-lymphocyte series. Antibodies are immunoglobulins that have a wide range of specificity for different antigens. In humans, there are five major classes of immunoglobulins, designated IgG, IgA, IgM, IgD, and IgE. Although the basic structures of the immunoglobulins are similar, they differ in the type of amino acid heavy chain, in molecular weight, and in function. A deficiency or defect of B lymphocytes is associated with bacterial and viral infections. Cell-mediated immunity depends on thymus-derived or T lymphocytes. T cells are divided into two major subpopulations: CD8 or T8$^+$ suppressor/cytotoxic lymphocytes and CD4 or T4$^+$ helper/inducer lymphocytes. These regulatory T cells, influenced by the genetic structure of the host, modify the immune response. In general CD4$^+$ T cells provide a helper or regulatory function on immune responses, whereas CD8$^+$ T cells have suppressive effects on immune responses. T-cell

TABLE 10-1.   Differences between Nonspecific and Specific Immune Responses

Type of response	Characteristics	Cells involved
Nonspecific	Effective against a wide range of infectious agents	Polymorphonuclear leukocytes, natural killer cells, macrophages/monocytes
Specific	Depends on specific reaction to each infectious agent	T and B lymphocytes, macrophages/monocytes

functions facilitate antibody production by plasma cells, amplify cell-mediated cytotoxicity, and modulate many aspects of the immune response through the release of lymphokines. T cells also suppress immune responses, thereby down-regulating the immune system. Because of their vital control of immunity, T cells are fundamental governors of immune function. Impaired cell-mediated immunity is associated with infectious diseases caused by certain pathogenic bacteria, mycobacteria, viruses, fungi, and parasites.

An immune response entails the production of antibody, the stimulation of cytotoxicity, and the release of a variety of immunoregulatory factors. These events involve a cascade of closely regulated complex collaborative intercellular interactions and immunoregulatory processes (17,114,117,126,160). For a further discussion of immune function and its relationship to exposure to environmental chemicals, the reader is referred to Chapter 23.

TESTS OF IMMUNOCOMPETENCE

Assessment of immunocompetence includes evaluation of both nonspecific and specific immune responses (Table 10-2) (17). Tests of nonspecific immune function evaluate aspects of the inflammatory response and phagocytic cell function, whereas tests of specific immune function measure those responses associated with cell-mediated immunity and humoral immunity (see Chapter 23 for further discussion).

Nonspecific Immune Response

Phagocytosis

Polymorphonuclear leukocytes (PMN) are an essential and integral part of the nonspecific immune response. A principal function of the PMN is the phagocytosis of invading bacteria. When the number of PMN is decreased or their function is impaired, severe recurrent infections may occur. Tests of phagocyte function can be divided into the following sequential steps: (1) chemotaxis (directed cell movement), (2) phagocytosis (attachment and ingestion), (3) metabolic changes associated with phagocytosis, and (4) microbial killing. In vitro assays to determine the chemotactic, phagocytic, and bactericidal capabilities of the leukocytes can be performed in specialized laboratories. The metabolic

TABLE 10-2. Tests of Immune Function[a]

Nonspecific (primary) immune response	Specific (secondary) immune response
Tests of inflammatory response and phagocytic cell function WBC count and differential Sedimentation rate C-reactive protein Complement activity Rebuck skin window technique Quantitative or histochemical NBT test Chemiluminescence Chemotactic assay Phagocytic index Bactericidal activity Phagocytic cell adherence Measurement of specific WBC enzymes	Enumeration of B lymphocytes (EA and EAC rosettes, monoclonal antibodies) Enumeration of T lymphocytes and subsets (E rosettes, monoclonal antibodies) Tests of humoral (antibody) function Quantitation of immunoglobulins and IgG subclasses Specific antibody responses: prior sensitization, isohemagglutinins (IgM), DPT, poliovirus, or measles (IgG Schick and Dick tests (IgG) Specific antibody responses: de novo sensitization, *Salmonella* O (IgM); H (IgG) Tests of cell-mediated (delayed hypersensitivity) function In vivo Skin tests (prior sensitization), *Candida*, *Trichophyton* Skin tests (de novo sensitization); DNCB Skin grafts In vitro Lymphocyte stimulation: nonspecific (PHA); specific (antigen) Measurement of effector molecules (MIF) Mixed lymphocyte culture (MLC) Natural killer (NK) cell activity Antibody-dependent cellular cytotoxicity (ADCC) or killer (K) cell activity Lymph node biopsy

[a]From Bellanti (17).

changes associated with phagocytosis can also be measured.

Complement System

The complement system consists of an extremely complex group of plasma proteins and glycoproteins whose sequential interaction is vital to the initiation and regulation of inflammation, the opsonization of foreign agents in preparation for phagocytosis, and the mediation of cytotoxicity against various cells and microorganisms (82). The use and interpretation of the laboratory assessment of the complement system have been reviewed (72).

Specific Immune Response

Cell-Mediated Immunity

Cell-mediated immunity is assessed in vivo by delayed-hypersensitivity-type (DTH) intradermal skin tests. Such testing can measure prior sensitization or de novo sensitization. In vitro tests of cell-mediated immunity include the enumeration of lymphocytes and lymphocyte subpopulations and antigen- and mitogen-induced lymphoproliferative responses.

The traditional delayed-type hypersensitivity skin test is still the first line of investigation for detecting cell-mediated immune deficiency. Within 48 h, over 80% of normal individuals respond with both erythema and induration to the intradermal injection of small amounts of antigen. The common antigens applied to the skin include purified protein derivative (PPD), mumps, *Candida*, streptococci, and fungus antigens (17).

The use of monoclonal antibodies has permitted the identification and enumeration of subsets of T cells (161). As previously noted, CD4[+] T cells express helper or inducer functions in immune responses, whereas CD8[+] T cells have the capacity to suppress immune responses (114). Assays of lymphocyte subsets are useful in evaluating disorders of immunoregulation (72).

The most commonly used in vitro correlate of delayed hypersensitivity testing is measurement of mitogen- or antigen-induced lymphocyte proliferation. This test is based on the transformation, proliferation, and replication responses of normal lymphocytes to stimulation. Lymphocytes from peripheral blood are gathered, cultured in vitro, and tested to determine whether they are stimulated by exposure to appropriate mitogens or antigens. The assay uses nonspecific mitogens such as phytohemagglutinin (PHA), or specific antigens. Although the degree of lymphocyte proliferation has been determined by lymphoblasts present in the culture, a more accu-

rate measure uses radiolabeled thymidine, a nucleoside precursor incorporated into newly synthesized DNA (86).

Humoral Immunity

The competency of the humoral immune system is determined by enumerating the number of B cells, by measuring circulating immunoglobulins, by measuring the antibody response to antigenic stimulation, and by studying secretory immunoglobulins (17).

It is noteworthy that attention has focused on the value of including tests of immunocompetence as a functional index of nutritional status. This concept developed because nutritional deficiency so consistently impairs immune responsiveness and results in a marked susceptibility to infection (38, 57,121). Several authors have recently introduced the concept of the functional assessment of nutritional status as a means of enhancing the more traditional measurements of nutritional status (28,88,143,144). Although evaluation of the usefulness of immunologic testing as an index of the nutritional state is far from complete, there is evidence that immune function may be a sensitive marker of nutritional status and disease vulnerability. The presence of anergy, in particular, is associated with a high risk of sepsis and death. Thus patients who are both nutritionally compromised and anergic prior to surgery are at increased risk for postoperative sepsis or death (29,40,57). Although immunologic testing may provide a broad index of nutritional adequacy, immune responses are also influenced by such factors as age, infections, drugs, and the presence of various disease states.

IMMUNITY AND NUTRITION

Worldwide, malnutrition is the most common cause of secondary immunodeficiency. It is well recognized that nutritional status is a critical determinant of immunocompetence and the risk of illness (13,30,48,49,54,68,86,146,148,156). Early studies investigating the relationship between nutrition and immunity focused on the impaired immune responses found in children in developing countries who suffered from generalized protein–energy malnutrition. It is estimated that at least 10 million children are severely malnourished and an additional 200 million are inadequately nourished (65, 77). More recently it has been recognized that mild to moderate undernutrition and deficiencies of vitamins, minerals, and trace elements may lead to subtle deficits in the immune response (37,54,107, 162). Immune function was found to be compromised in many malnourished hospitalized patients, those with chronic disease, small-for-gestational age infants, and the elderly. Conditions associated with overnutrition such as obesity and diabetes may also adversely affect immune function (26,37,68,110, 112,121).

FACTORS AFFECTING THE RELATIONSHIP BETWEEN IMMUNE FUNCTION AND NUTRITION

The complex relationship between nutritional status and immune function is influenced by such factors as age; the type, severity, and duration of malnutrition; specific nutrient deficiencies; and the presence of infection and underlying disease.

Age

When one considers the effect of nutrition on immunity, the age of the host often becomes a critical factor. The rapid growth and development sustained by the young make them more susceptible to nutritional deprivation. Nutritional deficiencies that have relatively little effect on the adult may lead to stunted growth, learning deficits, and compromised immune function in the fetus, neonate, and young child. Immunologic studies of young children with protein–energy malnutrition have amply demonstrated the susceptibility of their immune system to nutritional deficiencies (33,40,137, 146,150,156). The developing immune system of the fetus and neonate is also profoundly affected by nutritional deprivation. If malnutrition occurs during the critical early stages of immunologic development, the adverse effects may be prolonged or even permanent (53,86). It has been observed, for example, that infants who display intrauterine growth retardation as the result of such insults as maternal malnutrition or infection have impaired cell-mediated immunity, which may persist for several months or years (33,46,80). In contrast, most preterm low-birth-weight infants usually recover normal immunoresponsiveness by the age of 3–4 months (39,81). Malnutrition occurring early in postnatal life has also been linked to persistent immune dysfunction. A number of studies have shown that infants malnourished early in postnatal life continue to have long-term evidence of impaired humoral and cell-mediated immunity (4,86,87).

The two ends of the age spectrum present certain similarities in their vulnerability to infection and other environmental insult. The fetus and neonate have a developmentally immature immune system, whereas the elderly suffer a progressive loss of immunocompetence, particularly cell-mediated immunity (18,159). Although the impact of nutritional deprivation on immune function has, to some extent, been characterized in the very young, the role of poor nutrition in the decline of immune function in the elderly has not yet been adequately evaluated.

A number of factors indicate that it is pertinent to ask if the decline in immune function seen in the elderly may, in part, be related to nutritional deficiencies. It is well established that nutritional status plays a critical role in immunity. It is also well established that the aged are among the most poorly nourished in industrialized countries. Nutritional surveys in the United States suggest that dietary deficiencies exist in about one-third of the elderly who live independently (132,151). Moreover, there is a marked similarity between the age-related declines in cell-mediated immunity, T-cell number, and thymic factor activity and those seen in protein–calorie malnutrition (48,51). To date only a few studies have simultaneously looked at both nutrition and immunocompetence in the elderly.

Type, Severity, and Duration of Malnutrition

Malnutrition may include a broad spectrum from life-threatening conditions seen in children in developing countries to subclinical deficiencies of selected nutrients and overnutrition found in developing countries and in industrial societies.

Protein–Energy Malnutrition

Generalized malnutrition is often called protein–energy (or protein–calorie) malnutrition. When severe protein–energy malnutrition occurs in children, it leads to kwashiorkor or marasmus. Kwashiorkor is the result of protein loss or deprivation. It is characterized by edema, skin lesions, hair changes, apathy, anorexia, enlarged fatty liver, and decreased total serum protein and albumin. Marasmus is the result of severe deprivation of both protein and calories. This condition leads to growth retardation, weight loss, muscular atrophy, and loss of subcutaneous tissue. Serum proteins, including transferrin, albumin, lipase, amylase, esterase, and others, are significantly depressed in children with kwashiorkor (147).

Generalized malnutrition, though more common in developing countries, is also an important consequence of severe medical or surgical illnesses. Patients who have major trauma, burns, surgery, or who are septic are especially likely to become malnourished. For example, the caloric needs of patients with severe trauma, infections, or burns can be increased by 10–50%. Patients with cancer may also markedly increase their metabolic demands (13,25,63,115,125).

In contrast to the dramatic appearance of severe malnutrition, moderate undernutrition may go virtually undetected. In terms of the public health hazard, moderate nutritional deprivation is of great importance in developing countries (65). Growth failure and small stature in young children are often accepted as the norm in some developing countries. Mild to moderate malnutrition is frequently encountered in industrialized nations, particularly in the elderly, the poor, and those with chronic disease. Although the impact of moderate and marginal malnutrition on immunity is less well defined, there is growing evidence that even mild or moderate deficits may alter the immunologic response (30,32,37,162).

Specific Nutrient Deficiencies

Recent work has established that deficiencies of single nutrients impair immunocompetence. Specific deficiencies most intensely studied are those of iron, zinc, vitamin A, vitamin B_6, copper, and selenium (10,16,23,43,56,85,86,90). Although many studies have documented the role of single nutrients on immune function, most of the data on the effects of protein and amino acids, vitamins, minerals, and trace elements generally come from controlled experiments in laboratory animals. Far less has been deciphered in humans. Human malnutrition is a complex mosaic of many nutrient deficiencies occurring in different combinations. Thus, in clinically evident malnutrition it is virtually impossible to define the part played by individual nutrient deficiencies in the development of impaired immune function. Though uncommon in humans, imbalances of single nutrients are most likely to occur in the elderly, the pregnant woman, the obese, the food faddist, and the growth-retarded or premature child. Patients with chronic anemias, alcoholism, recurrent or chronic diarrhea, chronic renal, liver, or biliary disease, regional enteritis, or other malabsorptive states may have single or multiple deficiencies. Patients who have had intestinal bypass surgery or those receiving long-term hemodialysis or intravenous alimentation may also develop deficiencies of single or multiple nutrients (16,125).

Overnutrition

There is increasing evidence that obesity may impair the immune response. This form of "malnutrition" is most frequently found in industrialized societies. Data in both humans and laboratory animals indicate that obesity is associated with decreased cell-mediated immunity, antibody response to T-dependent antigens, and phagocyte bactericidal activity. The relationship between overnutrition and immunity has been reviewed (37,40,50).

Infection and Disease

The historic association between malnutrition and infection has been supported by epidemiologic studies, which invariably link malnutrition to an increased susceptibility to infection. The risk of death correlates with nutritional status (37,64,106,109,134, 146). It is well recognized that infection itself is often a major factor in precipitating nutritional deficiencies (3,6–9,14,86,134,141,146). Diarrheal diseases in particular pose a major health threat (128). This mutually aggravating interaction means that malnutrition makes the host more prone to infection, and infection exacerbates malnutrition. This destructive synergism and its immunologic consequences often prove fatal to the growing infant and young child in developing nations (6,15,102,133,141). The relationship between these forces and diminished immune responsiveness has been widely observed (30,130, 134,148).

Most diseases, whether infectious, degenerative, malignant, acute, or chronic, lead to significant nutritional and metabolic changes. It has been observed that the marked weight loss associated with severe disease, cancer, or trauma often leads to fatal infections with organisms that might otherwise not be pathogenic. There is evidence that the infectious complications seen in cachectic patients are, in part, a manifestation of impaired immunocompetence (11,12,54,86,125,145,146).

THE RELATIONSHIP BETWEEN IMMUNE FUNCTION AND NUTRITIONAL DEFICIENCIES

The long-recognized association between malnutrition and infectious disease, repeatedly confirmed by clinical and epidemiologic observations, led to intense investigation of the interaction between nutrition and immunity (54,109,134,156). During the past decade and a half, a number of investigators have systematically investigated the link between nutrition and immunocompetence (10,36, 54,90,146).

Protein–Energy Malnutrition

Protein–energy malnutrition represents a broad spectrum of nutrient deficits, not only of protein and calories but also of vitamins, minerals, and trace elements. Deficiencies of many specific nutrients including iron, zinc, folate, pyridoxine, and vitamin A have been associated with alterations in the immune response. The immune alterations noted in protein–energy malnutrition cannot be related to any specific nutrient deficiency. One can only document the changes in the immune response and determine whether these changes are reversible with improved nutrient intake.

Protein–energy malnutrition broadly modifies immune function by affecting the cell-mediated immune response, the humoral immune response, the complement system, and leukocyte function. The most commonly observed effects of nutritional deprivation on immunity include an absent or reduced delayed cutaneous hypersensitivity response to microbial antigens, a decline in the number of T lymphocytes in the peripheral blood, a reduction in the phagocytic and bactericidal capacity of leukocytes, a decreased concentration of secretory IgA, and a reduced level and activity of various complement proteins (2,35,36,62,73,76,78,140). There have been many extensive reviews of this subject (10,49,62, 90,146,156).

Specific Immune Response

Cell-Mediated Immune Response

The cell-mediated immune response, mediated through the thymus-dependent lymphocyte or T cell, plays a major role in host defenses against most viruses, mycobacteria and fungi. As noted, cell-mediated immunity is evaluated in vivo by intradermal skin testing and in vitro by enumeration of T lymphocytes, antigen and mitogen stimulation of isolated lymphocytes, and by changes in the production of lymphokines.

Anatomic and Histologic Changes Significant protein–energy malnutrition is evidenced by involution of the lymphoid system (96). In addition to atrophy of the thymus, the lymph nodes, tonsils, and spleen are smaller in malnourished children (111). In the lymph nodes, the thymus-dependent areas are depleted of lymphoid cells. Of interest, a reduction in tonsil size has proved a useful clinical indicator of malnutrition (142). In light of the lymphoid atrophy observed in cases of protein–energy malnutrition, it is not surprising that investigators have noted an increased susceptibility to those infections commonly controlled by the cell-mediated response.

Delayed Cutaneous Hypersensitivity Response Jayalakshmi and Gopalan were the first to note that the percentage of positive tuberculin skin tests was significantly lower in children with protein–energy malnutrition than in a control population (97). They were also the first to suggest that nutritional rehabilitation could lead to repair of a defective skin test response. Harland found that the malnourished child was able neither to be sensitized when exposed to a new antigen nor to develop a normal inflammatory response to a skin test irritant (92). Both of these functions normalized with an improvement in the patient's nutritional status. Other investigators have confirmed the defect in skin test responsiveness to various antigens, including *Monilia*, streptococcal antigen, *Tricophyton*, PHA, and mumps virus. Anergy to a battery of different antigens is commonly found (30,79,103,160). Additional studies have noted an absent or impaired delayed cutaneous hypersensitivity response in moderately malnourished subjects (107,162).

Law et al. were the first to describe a depression of delayed cutaneous hypersensitivity in malnourished adults (103). Following intravenous hyperalimentation, their patients demonstrated a significant improvement in delayed hypersensitivity. Though only a few studies have investigated the relationship between immunocompetence and nutrition in the elderly, the data suggest that correcting nutritional deficiencies in the aged is linked to an improved immune response (46,55,74). Whether the decline in immune function noted in healthy elderly individuals is related, in part, to nutritional deficiencies is not resolved. Nor is it clear if the maintenance of good nutrition and immunocompetence will affect morbidity and mortality (46,51,104,152).

Thymus-Dependent T Lymphocytes In protein–energy malnutrition, there is a lymphopenia and a reduction in the number of circulating T lymphocytes. The number of T4+ helper cells is decreased, sometimes quite markedly. Because the change in number of T8+ suppressor cells is less marked, the helper/suppressor ratio is significantly decreased (44,59).

Peripheral blood lymphocytes from children with protein–energy malnutrition respond poorly to stimulation with such mitogens as PHA and pokeweed (33,101,103,135,142,160).

In a study of the etiology of the depressed cell-mediated immunity found in protein–energy malnutrition, the presence of infection must be evaluated along with the degree and type of malnutrition. Sellmeyer et al. observed that well-nourished children with measles and gastroenteritis had a profound depression of lymphocyte transformation (135). Further studies reveal that the serum from malnourished children contains certain factors that may interfere with in vitro lymphocyte transformation (32,108,142). Many factors thus play a role in the depression of cell-mediated immunity, which often improves long before the malnourished child has completely recovered nutritionally (101).

Lymphokines and Monokines Cytokine is the general term used to describe the soluble molecular mediators released by cells during the immune response. Cytokines produced by monocyte/macrophages are termed monokines, whereas lymphokines are produced by lymphocytes. Lymphokines are the molecular mediators of many T-cell functions. A number of T-cell-derived lymphokines (e.g., interleukin 2, interleukin 3, interleukin 4, interferon, granulocyte–macrophage colony-stimulating factor) and monocyte/macrophage-derived monokines have been identified [e.g., interleukin 1, tumor necrosis factor (TNF), interleukin 6, interferon] (75,93). The effects of malnutrition on the production of these important immune-regulating substances have not been well studied. The limited data available have been reviewed (95). Thus far, it appears that protein–energy malnutrition may have different effects on lymphokine and monokine production. Interleukin 1 production and functional activity on target cells is depressed, whereas interleukin 2 production may be normal (95).

Humoral Response

Serum Immunoglobulins Circulating IgA, IgM, and IgG levels are normal or elevated in children with protein–energy malnutrition (4,100). Increased serum IgD and IgE have also been observed in malnourished children (98,113). Elevated IgE levels may be secondary to an increased parasitic load or decreased T-cell function (35).

Antibody Response to Antigen Stimulation Although antibody responses to such antigens as yellow fever vaccine, influenza vaccine, and typhoid vaccine are impaired in malnourished children, their response to many antigens, including measles, polio virus, tetanus, and diphtheria toxoid, appears to be adequate (27,99,123,134). It has not been determined which of the specific nutrient deficiencies in the malnourished child is responsible for the depressed response. The presence of associated infection may profoundly suppress antibody synthesis (99). Of importance is the finding that, as the nutritional state improves, the antibody response to antigenic stimulus also improves. Antibody affinity was shown to be decreased (60).

B Cells In contrast to circulating T cells, which are depressed in malnourished children, B-cell numbers are normal or elevated (101). Several investigators have speculated that the elevated immunoglobulin levels found in children with protein–energy malnutrition may result from their increased exposure to infectious agents and their inability to respond to many of these agents as the malnutrition becomes more severe. Other investigators have speculated that, as a part of the depressed T-cell population, there may be suppression of the T-suppressor cell population, resulting in uncontrolled nonspecific antibody production (149).

Mucosal Immunity A number of studies indicate that protein–energy malnutrition leads to a reduction in mucosal immunity (35,41,42,52,149). A decreased concentration of secretory IgA was noted in the nasopharyngeal and salivary secretions of malnourished children (34,124,139). In addition, the secretory IgA antibody response to live attenuated measles and polio vaccines is reduced (34). These observations suggest that in the malnourished child there is either a failure to synthesize IgA normally or a block in the passage of IgA from the mucosal surface. The possibility of IgA returning to the circulation has been excluded by the fact that no reactive anti-SC was detected in the serum. It is unclear if the secretory component is the limiting factor. Some workers find lower levels of secretory component, but others do not (71,157). The mucosal immune response in protein–energy malnutrition has been summarized (52,61). Other changes that accompany the decreased secretory immunoglobulins are an atrophied gut wall, reduced digestive enzymes, and an impaired hepatic reticuloendothelial system. All of these may play a role in increasing the host's susceptibility to gram-negative organisms, especially from the gastrointestinal tract (35). Intestinal immune defenses are discussed in detail in Chapter 8.

Nonspecific Immune Response

Polymorphonuclear Leukocyte and Macrophage Function

The chemotactic response of leukocytes in vitro in infected and noninfected children with protein–energy malnutrition appears to be no different from that found in infected or noninfected well-nourished children. However, the infected children in both groups showed a smaller response than the noninfected children (127). Phagocytosis of various particles by circulating neutrophils or monocytes isolated from malnourished children was normal, but the intracellular bactericidal capacity of polymorphonuclear leukocytes was often reduced (73). The glycolytic activity in leukocytes during the postphagocyte period was also diminished (136).

The Complement System

Defects in the complement system have been associated with increased susceptibility to bacterial infection. Therefore, it is not unreasonable to expect that the complement system in malnourished individuals may be affected by their nutritional status. Activation of the complement system leads to production of complement fragments that are involved in host defenses. These include the induction and control of inflammation, the opsonization of foreign materials for phagocytosis, and the mediation of direct cytotoxicity of microorganisms and various cells (82). Investigation of the complement system in protein–energy malnutrition generally reveals a reduced serum concentration of almost all components (67,113,138). In addition to a depression of the complement proteins, there is a depression of the hemolytic complement activity in children with protein–energy malnutrition (140). The lowered hemolytic activity in some patients is associated with anticomplement activity, which may be the result of the action of endotoxin. It appears that complement activity in protein–energy malnutrition is affected not only by decreased nutrient availability but also by an increased activation of the system.

Vitamin and Trace Element Deficiencies

As the field of nutritional immunology evolved, the focus has shifted from assessing the immunologic effects of generalized protein–energy malnutrition to determining the effects of single nutrient deficiencies on the immunologic response. It is now established that many vitamins and trace elements are key factors in the generation, maintenance, and amplification of the immune response (10). Since imbalances of single nutrients are relatively rare in humans, much of our knowledge in this area comes from animal studies. The following discussion presents a selected overview of the subject. The interested reader is encouraged to consult a number of excellent reviews (16,23,36,43,47,54,56,81,84,90, 120,146).

Trace Elements

Iron Iron deficiency is a major health problem worldwide. It is the single nutrient deficiency that is most likely to occur in the absence of other forms of malnutrition. Women in the reproductive years, particularly those who are pregnant or lactating, infants, adolescents, and the elderly are most likely to develop iron deficiency. Because of its varied and important role in metabolic processes, iron deficiency adversely affects many tissues including the immune system. Immune functions have been studied in patients and experimental animals with varying degrees of iron deficiency. Iron deficiency, in most cases, was found to impair the lymphocyte proliferative response to antigens and mitogens (10,24,40). In addition, a number of investigators have also reported decreased intracellular bacterial killing activity of phagocytic cells in cases of iron deficiency (3,31,105). Little change in serum immunoglobulin and serum complement levels was noted in iron-deficient subjects (16). The effect of iron deficiency on immunity has been reviewed by Vyas and Chandra (155).

Zinc Zinc has long been recognized as an essential cofactor for a large number of enzymes. However, the first evidence of its importance in human nutrition came from epidemiologic surveys that in-

dicated that patients with low serum zinc levels had immune abnormalities and increased susceptibility to infectious disease (129). Zinc deficiency has been shown to be a factor in the impaired immunity observed in protein–energy malnutrition. Zinc deficiency occurs in an inherited disease, acrodermatitis enteropathica, which results from a diminished ability of intestinal cells to absorb zinc. With this deficiency there are multiple immunodeficiencies and increased susceptibility to infection. Increased ingestion of zinc reverses these processes (91). Clinical and laboratory evidence of zinc deficiency has also been observed in patients receiving total parenteral nutrition (89,119).

A number of studies performed in both humans and experimental animals reveal that zinc has a critical role in immune function. Zinc deficiency results in lymphoid atrophy, impaired delayed cutaneous hypersensitivity, decreased lymphocyte proliferative response to mitogen stimulation, low lymphocyte counts, and a reduction in the proportion of T4$^+$ helper cells. Phagocytic function is also impaired (1,66,70,83,119). The effects of zinc on the immune response have recently been reviewed (69). Of importance is the observation that excessive ingestion of zinc in human subjects impairs immune responses (45).

Selenium Severe selenium deficiency in humans is unlikely except in cases of prolonged unsupplemented intravenous hyperalimentation and in populations who live in areas where the selenium content of the soil is low, e.g., the Keshan region of China and some areas of New Zealand. Selenium is essential for the activity of glutathione peroxidase, which functions as a powerful antioxidant. It also functions as an activator of vitamin E in cell membranes. Selenium deficiency, particularly in association with vitamin E deficiency, reduces antibody production and decreases phagocytic bactericidal activity. Thymic hormone activity is also reduced (81).

Vitamins

Isolated vitamin deficiencies are rarely found in human populations. Therefore, much of the data supporting the importance of vitamins in maintaining immune function have come from laboratory animals.

Fat-Soluble Vitamins

Vitamin A Although isolated vitamin deficiencies are rare in industrial countries, vitamin A deficiency associated with malnutrition is frequently found in developing countries (154). Because of this, vitamin A is an important micronutrient. Vitamin A deficiency is associated with an increased susceptibility to infection. Animals fed a diet devoid of vitamin A developed multiple septic foci and had a high mortality rate (5). Vitamin A deficiency also results in atrophy of lymphoid tissue, a decreased number of lymphocytes in peripheral blood, decreased function of B and T cells, and lowered complement levels. These findings were summarized by Vyas and Chandra (154).

Vitamin E In addition to its intracellular antioxidant functions, vitamin E is a major antioxidant component of lipid membranes, protecting them from lipid peroxidation. The dietary requirement of vitamin E, in part, depends on the level of oxidizable fatty acids ingested (122). Animal studies indicate that vitamin E is required for optimal function of lymphocytes and mononuclear cells (19). Vitamin E supplements appear to have an immunostimulatory effect, whereas megadose supplements inhibit the immune response (10).

Water-Soluble Vitamins

B-Group Vitamins Although the incidence of isolated deficiency of the various B vitamins is rare, generalized malnutrition undoubtedly includes deprivation of some of the B vitamins. The B vitamins are critical factors in a wide range of metabolic events, including the metabolism of sugars, proteins, and lipids and the synthesis of nucleic acids. Because of their fundamental importance, deficiencies of various B vitamins have been shown to affect a large number of immune functions. Deficiencies of thiamin, riboflavin, pantothenic acid, and biotin can lead to depressed antibody responses after the injection of vaccines (10,94). Pyridoxine deficiency undoubtedly has a more profound effect on immune function than other B vitamins because of its role in nucleic acid and protein synthesis. Pyridoxine deficiency results in atrophy of lymphoid tissue and decreased cell-mediated and humoral responsiveness to a variety of test antigens (10). Deficiencies of folic acid and B_{12} also depress humoral and cell-mediated immunity (10). A review of the B vitamins and their effects on immunity can be found in several references (10,22,90).

Antioxidant Nutrients

A number of investigators have given special consideration to the antioxidant nutrients. These nutrients, which include vitamins A, C, and E, the provitamin β-carotene, and trace elements zinc, copper, and selenium, function in large part to prevent oxidative damage to cells. It is widely recognized that intracellular oxygen has a high potential for toxicity because of the ease with which it is reduced to reactive compounds. As an unavoidable result of aerobic respiration, a number of highly

reactive free radicals are generated from oxygen. Without oxygen-detoxification mechanisms, the generation of free-radical forms of oxygen would rapidly destroy biological macromolecules and biological membranes (116). Antioxidant nutrients help to overcome free radicals and damaging oxidative effects on cell membranes (23). A recent review of the role of antioxidant nutrients in immune responses indicates that these agents may enhance various aspects of cell-mediated and humoral immunity. A detailed discussion of the mechanisms by which antioxidants may enhance immunity is found in two references (20,21).

SUMMARY

The immune system provides the body with a major defense against environmental assault, particularly invasion by microorganisms. Nutrition, through its modulation of specific and nonspecific immune responses, is a critical determinant of optimum immune function. It is well recognized that both severe and moderate nutritional deprivation are associated with impaired immune responses. Indeed, malnutrition is the most frequent cause of immunodeficiency throughout the world. Correction of nutritional deficiencies has been shown to improve immune function and thereby enhance the body's defense against environmental assault.

REFERENCES

1. Allen JL, Kay NE, McClain CJ: Severe zinc deficiency in humans: Association with a reversible T-lymphocyte dysfunction. Ann Intern Med 95:154, 1981.
2. Alvarado J, Luthringer DG: Serum immunoglobulins in edematous protein–calorie malnutrition. Clin Pediatr 10:174, 1971.
3. Arbeter A, Echeverri L, Franco D, et al: Nutrition and infection. Fed Proc 30:1421, 1971.
4. Aref GH, El-Din K, Hassan AJ: Immunoglobulins in kwashiorkor. J Trop Med Hyg 73:186, 1970.
5. Bang FB, Bang BG, Foard M: Acute Newcastle virus infection of the upper respiratory tract of the chicken. II. The effect of diets deficient in vitamin A on the pathogenesis of the infection. Am J Pathol 78:417, 1975.
6. Beisel WR: Metabolic response to infection. Annu Rev Med 26:9, 1975.
7. Beisel WR: Malnutrition as a consequence of stress. In: Malnutrition and the Immune Response, p 21, Suskind R (ed.), Raven Press, New York, 1977.
8. Beisel WR: Nonspecific host factors—a review. In: Malnutrition and the Immune Response, p 341, Suskind R (ed.), Raven Press, New York, 1977.
9. Beisel WR: Magnitude of the host nutritional response to infection. Am J Clin Nutr 30:1206, 1977.
10. Beisel WR: Single nutrients and immunity. Am J Clin Nutr 35 [Suppl]:417, 1982.

11. Beisel WR: Nutrition, infection, specific immune responses, and nonspecific host defenses: A complex interaction. In: Nutrition, Disease Resistance, and Immune Function, p 3, Watson RR (ed.), Marcel Dekker, New York, 1984.

12. Beisel WR: Nutrition and infection. In: Nutritional Biochemistry and Metabolism, with Clinical Applications, p 369, Linder MC (ed.), Elsevier, New York, 1985.

13. Beisel WR: Role of nutrition in immune system diseases. Compr Ther 13:13, 1987.

14. Beisel WR, Blackburn GL, Feigin RD, et al: Impact of infection on nutritional status of the host. Am J Clin Nutr 30:1203, 1977.

15. Beisel WR, Cockerell GL, Janssen WA: Nutritional effects on the responsiveness of acute-phase reactant glycoproteins. In: Malnutrition and the Immune Response, p 395, Suskind R (ed.), Raven Press, New York, 1977.

16. Beisel WR, Edelman R, Nauss K, et al: Single-nutrient effects on immunologic functions. JAMA 245:53, 1981.

17. Bellanti JA: Immunology III, WB Saunders, Philadelphia, 1985.

18. Bellanti JA, Boner AL, Valletta E: Immunology of the fetus and newborn. In: Neonatology, 3rd ed., p 850, Avery GB (ed.), JB Lippincott, Philadelphia, 1987.

19. Bendich A: Antioxidant vitamins and immune responses. In: Nutrition and Immunology, p 125, Chandra RK (ed.), Alan R Liss, New York, 1988.

20. Bendich A: Antioxidant nutrients and immune functions: Introduction. In: Antioxidant Nutrients and Immune Functions, p 1, Bendich A, Phillips M, Tengerdy RP (eds.), Plenum Press, New York, 1990.

21. Bendich A: Effects of antioxidant vitamins on cellular immune function. In: Antioxidant Nutrients and Immune Functions, p 105, Bendich A, Phillips M, Tengerdy RP (eds.), Plenum Press, New York, 1990.

22. Bendich A, Cohen M: B vitamins: Effects on specific and nonspecific immune responses. In Nutrition and Immunology, p 101, Chandra RK (ed.), Alan R Liss, New York, 1988.

23. Bendich A, Phillips M, Tengerdy RP (eds.): Antioxidant Nutrients and Immune Functions, Plenum Press, New York, 1990.

24. Bhaskaram P: Immunology of iron-deficient subjects. In: Nutrition and Immunology, p 149, Chandra RK (ed.), Alan R Liss, New York, 1988.

25. Bistrian BR, Blackburn GL, Scrimshaw NS: Cellular immunization in semistarved states in hospitalized adults. Am J Clin Nutr 28:1148, 1975.

26. Bistrian BR, Blackburn GL, Vitale J, et al: Prevalence of malnutrition in general medical patients. JAMA 235:1567, 1976.

27. Brown RE, Katz M: Failure of antibody production to yellow fever vaccine in children with kwashiorkor. Trop Geogr Med 18:125, 1966.

28. Calloway DH: Functional consequences of malnutrition. Rev Infect Dis 4:736, 1982.

29. Casey J, Flinn WR, Yao JST: Correlation of immune and nutritional status with wound complications in patients undergoing vascular operations. Surgery 93:822, 1983.

30. Chandra RK: Immunocompetence in undernutrition. J Pediatr 81:1194, 1972.

31. Chandra RK: Reduced bactericidal capacity of polymorphs in iron deficiency. Arch Dis Child 48:864, 1973.

32. Chandra RK: Rosette-forming T lymphocytes and cell-mediated immunity in malnutrition. Br Med J 3:608, 1974.

33. Chandra RK: Fetal malnutrition and postnatal immunocompetence. Am J Dis Child 129:450, 1975.

34. Chandra RK: Reduced secretory antibody response to live attenuated measles and poliovirus vaccine in malnourished children. Br Med J 2:583, 1975.

35. Chandra RK: Immunoglobulins and antibody response in protein–calorie malnutrition. In: Malnutrition and the Immune Response, p 155, Suskind R (ed.), Raven Press, New York, 1977.

36. Chandra RK: Immunology of Nutritional Disorders, Edward Arnold, London, 1980.

37. Chandra RK: Immunodeficiency in undernutrition and overnutrition. Nutr Rev 39:225, 1981.

38. Chandra RK: Immunocompetence as a functional index of nutritional status. Br Med Bull 37:89, 1981.

39. Chandra RK: Serum thymic hormone activity and cell-mediated immunity in health neonates, preterm infants and small-for-gestational-age infants. Pediatrics 67:407, 1981.

40. Chandra RK: Nutrition, immunity, and infection: Present knowledge and future directions. Lancet 1: 688, 1983.

41. Chandra RK: Mucosal immune responses in malnutrition. Ann NY Acad Sci 409:345, 1983.

42. Chandra RK: Nutritional regulation of immunity and infection in the gastrointestinal tract. J Pediatr Gastroenterol Nutr 2(Suppl 1):S181, 1983.

43. Chandra RK: Trace elements and immune responses. Immunol Today 4:322, 1983.

44. Chandra RK: Numerical and functional deficiency in T helper cells in protein–calorie malnutrition. Clin Exp Immunol 51:126, 1983.

45. Chandra RK: Excessive intake of zinc impairs immune responses. JAMA 252:1443, 1984.

46. Chandra RK: Nutritional regulation of immune function at the extremes of life: In infants and in the elderly. In: Malnutrition: Determinants and Consequences, p 245, White PL, Selvey N (eds.), Alan R Liss, New York, 1984.

47. Chandra RK: Trace element regulation of immunity and infection. J Am Coll Nutr 4:5, 1985.

48. Chandra RK (ed.): Nutrition, Immunity and Illness in the Elderly, Pergamon Press, New York, 1985.

49. Chandra RK (ed.): Nutrition and Immunology, Alan R Liss, New York, 1988.

50. Chandra RK: Effects of overnutrition on immune responses and risk of disease. In: Nutrition and Immunology, p 315, Chandra RK (ed.), Alan R Liss, New York, 1988.

51. Chandra RK: Nutritional regulation of immunocompetence and risk of disease. In: Nutrition in the Elderly, p 203, Horwitz A, Macfadyen DM, Munro H, et al. (eds.), Oxford University Press, Oxford, 1989.

52. Chandra RK: Nutritional modulation of intestinal mucosal immunity. Immunol Invest 18:119, 1989.

53. Chandra RK, Matsumura T: Ontogenic development

of the immune system and effects of fetal growth retardation. J Perinat Med 7:279, 1979.

54. Chandra RK, Newberne PM: Nutrition, Immunity and Infection: Mechanisms of Interactions, Plenum Press, New York, 1977.

55. Chandra RK, Purl S: Nutritional support improves antibody response to influenza virus vaccine in the elderly. Br Med J 291:705, 1985.

56. Chandra RK, Purl S: Trace element modulation of immune responses and susceptibility to infection. In: Trace Elements in Nutrition of Children, p 87, Chandra RK (ed.), Raven Press, New York, 1985.

57. Chandra RK, Scrimshaw NS: Immunocompetence in nutritional assessment. Am J Clin Nutr 33:2694, 1980.

58. Chandra RK, Tejpar S: Review/commentary: Diet and immunocompetence. Int J Immunopharmacol 5:175, 1983.

59. Chandra RK, Gupta S, Singh H: Inducer and suppressor T cell subsets in protein–energy malnutrition: Analysis by monoclonal antibodies. Nutr Res 2: 21, 1982.

60. Chandra RK, Chandra S, Gupta S: Antibody affinity and immune complexes after immunization with tetanus toxoid in protein–energy malnutrition. Am J Clin Nutr 40:131, 1984.

61. Chandra RK, Puri S, Vyas D: Malnutrition and intestinal immunity. In: Immunopathology of the Small Intestine, p 105, Marsh MN (ed.), John Wiley & Sons, New York, 1987.

62. Chandra S, Chandra RK: Nutrition, immune response and outcome. Prog Food Nutr Sci 10:1, 1986.

63. Charpentier B, Branco D, Paci L, et al: Deficient natural killer activity in alcoholic cirrhosis. Clin Exp Immunol 58:906, 1983.

64. Chen LC, Chowdhury AKMA, Huffman SL: Anthropometric assessment of energy–protein malnutrition and subsequent risk of mortality among preschool aged children. Am J Clin Nutr 33:1836, 1980.

65. Children and the Environment: The State of the Environment—1990. United Nations Environmental Programme and United Nations Children's Fund, New York, 1990.

66. Chvapil M, Stankova L, Weldy P, et al: The role of zinc in the function of some inflammatory cells. In: Zinc Metabolism: Current Aspects in Health and Disease, p 103, Brewer GJ, Prasad AS (eds.), Alan R Liss, New York, 1977.

67. Coovadia HM, Parent MA, Loening WEK, et al: An evaluation of factors associated with the depression of immunity in malnutrition and in measles. Am J Clin Nutr 27:665, 1974.

68. Cunningham-Rundles S: Nutritional factors in immune response. In: Malnutrition: Determinants and Consequences, p 233, White PL, Selvey N (eds.), Alan R Liss, New York, 1983.

69. Cunningham-Rundles S, Cunningham-Rundles WF: Zinc modulation of immune response. In: Nutrition and Immunology, p 197, Chandra RK (ed.), Alan R Liss, New York, 1988.

70. Cunningham-Rundles C, Cunningham-Rundles S, Garafolo J, et al: Increased T lymphocyte function and thymopoietin following zinc repletion in man. Fed Proc 38:1222, 1979.

71. Darip MD, Sirisinha S, Lamb AL: Effect of vitamin A deficiency on susceptibility of rats to Angiostrongylus cantonensis. Proc Soc Exp Biol Med 161:600, 1979.

72. deShazo RD, Lopez M, Salvaggio JE: Use and interpretation of diagnostic immunologic laboratory tests. JAMA 258:3011, 1987.

73. Douglas SR, Schopfer K: The phagocyte in protein–calorie malnutrition. In: Malnutrition and the Immune Response, p 231, Suskind R (ed.), Raven Press, New York, 1977.

74. Duchateau J, Delepesse G, Vrijens R, et al: Beneficial effects of oral zinc supplementation on the immune response of old people. Am J Med 70:1001, 1981.

75. Durum SK, Oppenheim JJ: Macrophage-derived mediators: Interleukin 1, tumor necrosis factor, interleukin 6, interferon and related cytokines. In: Fundamental Immunology, 2nd ed., p 639, Paul WE (ed.), Raven Press, New York, 1989.

76. Dutz W, Rossipal E, Ghavami H, et al: Persistent cell-mediated immune-deficiency following infantile stress during the first 6 months of life. Eur J Pediatr 122:117, 1976.

77. Ebrahim GJ: Social and Community Paediatrics in Developing Countries, Macmillian, London, 1985.

78. Edelman R: Cell-mediated immune response in protein–calorie malnutrition—a review. In: Malnutrition and the Immune Response, p 47, Suskind RM (ed.), Raven Press, New York, 1977.

79. Feldman G, Gianantonio CA: Aspectos inmunologicos de la desnutricion en el nino. Medicina 32:1, 1972.

80. Ferguson A, Lawlor G, Neumann L, et al: Decreased rosette-forming lymphocytes in malnutrition and intrauterine growth retardation. Trop Pediatr 85:717, 1974.

81. Fletcher MP, Gershwin ME, Keen CL, et al: Trace element deficiencies and immune responsiveness in human and animal models. In: Nutrition and Immunology, p 215, Chandra RK (ed.), Alan R Liss, New York, 1988.

82. Frank MM, Fries LF: Complement. In: Fundamental Immunology, 2nd ed., p 679, Paul WE (ed.), Raven Press, New York, 1989.

83. Frost P, Chen JC, Rabbani I, et al: The effect of zinc deficiency on the immune response. In: Zinc Metabolism: Current Aspects in Health and Disease, p 143, Brewer GJ, Prasad AS (eds.), Alan R Liss, New York, 1977.

84. Gershwin ME, Hurley L: Trace metals and immune function in the elderly. Compr Ther 13:18, 1987.

85. Gershwin ME, Beach R, Hurley L: Trace metals, aging and immunity. J Am Geriatr Soc 31:374, 1983.

86. Gershwin ME, Beach RS, Hurley LS: Nutrition and Immunity, Academic Press, Orlando, 1985.

87. Ghavami H, Dutz W, Mohallatee M, et al: Immune disturbances after severe enteritis during the first six months of life. Isr J Med Sci 15:364, 1979.

88. Gibson RS: Principles of Nutritional Assessment, Oxford University Press, Oxford, 1990.

89. Golden MHN, Golder BE, Harland PSEB, et al: Zinc and immunocompetence in protein–energy malnutrition. Lancet 1:1226, 1978.

90. Gross RL, Newberne PM: Role of nutrition in immunologic function. Physiol Rev 60:188, 1980.

91. Hambridge KM: The role of zinc in the pathogenesis

and treatment of acrodermatitis enteropathica. In: Zinc Metabolism: Current Aspects in Health and Disease, p 329, Brewer GJ, Prasad AS (eds.), Alan R Liss, New York, 1977.

92. Harland PSEB: Tuberculin reactions in malnourished children. Lancet 2:719, 1965.

93. Hodes RJ: T-cell-mediated regulation: Help and suppression. In: Fundamental Immunology, 2nd ed., p 587, Paul WE (ed.), Raven Press, New York, 1989.

94. Hodges RE, Bean WB, Ohlson MA, et al: Factor affecting human antibody response V. Combined deficiences of pantothenic acid and pyridoxin. Am J Clin Nutr 11:187, 1962.

95. Hoffman-Goetz L: Lymphokines and monokines in protein–energy malnutrition. In: Nutrition and Immunology, p 9, Chandra RK (ed.), Alan R Liss, New York, 1988.

96. Jackson CM: The Effects of Inanition and Malnutrition upon Growth and Structure, P Blakiston's Son, London, 1925.

97. Jayalakshmi VT, Gopalan C: Nutrition and tuberculosis I. An epidemiological study. Indian J Med Res 46:87, 1958.

98. Johansson SG, Melbin T, Vahlquist B: Immunoglobin levels in Ethiopian preschool children with specific reference to high concentration of immunoglobulin E(IgND). Lancet 1:1118, 1968.

99. Jose DG, Welch JS, Doherty RL: Humoral and cellular immune responses to streptococci, influenza and other antigens in Australian Aboriginal school children. Aust Paediatr J 6:192, 1970.

100. Keet MP, Thom H: Serum immunoglobulins in kwashiorkor. Arch Dis Child 44:600, 1969.

101. Kulapongs P, Suskind R, Vithayasai V, et al: In vitro cell mediated immune response in Thai children with protein–calorie malnutrition. In: Malnutrition and the Immune Response, p 99, Suskind R (ed.), Raven Press, New York, 1977.

102. Latham MC: Nutrition and infection in national development. Science 188:561, 1975.

103. Law DK, Dudrick SJ, Abdou NI: Immunocompetence of patients with protein–calorie malnutrition. The effects of nutritional repletion. Ann Intern Med 79: 545, 1973.

104. Lipschitz DA: Nutrition, aging, and the immunohematopoietic system. Clin Geriatr Med 3:319, 1987.

105. Macdougall LG, Anderson R, McNab GM, et al: The immune response in iron-deficient children: Impaired cellular defense mechanisms with altered humoral components. J Pediatr 86:833, 1975.

106. Mata LF: Malnutrition–infection interactions in the tropics. Am J Trop Med Hyg 24:564, 1975.

107. McMurray DN, Loomis SA, Casazza LJ, et al: Development of impaired cell-mediated immunity in mild and moderate malnutrition. Am J Clin Nutr 34:68, 1981.

108. Moore DL, Heyworth B, Brown J: PHA-induced lymphocyte transformation in leukocyte-cultures from malarious malnourished and control Gambian children. Clin Exp Immunol 17:647, 1974.

109. Morehead CD, Morehead M, Allen DM, et al: Bacterial infections in malnourished children. Environ Child Health 20:141, 1974.

110. Morley JE (moderator): Nutrition in the elderly. Ann Intern Med 109:890, 1988.

111. Mugerwa JW: The lymphoreticular system in kwashiorkor. J Pathol 105:105, 1971.

112. Mullen JL: Consequences of malnutrition in the surgical patient. Surg Clin North Am 61:465, 1981.

113. Neumann CG, Lawlow GJ, Stiehm ME, et al: Immunologic responses in malnourished children. Am J Clin Nutr 89:104, 1975.

114. Nossal GJV: Current concepts in Immunology. The basic components of the immune system. N Engl J Med 316:1320, 1987.

115. Orr JW Jr, Shingleton HM: Importance of nutritional assessment and support in surgical and cancer patients. J Reprod Med 29:635, 1984.

116. Parke DV: Mechanisms of chemical toxicity—a unifying hypothesis. Regul Toxicol Pharmacol 2:267, 1982.

117. Paul WE (ed.): Fundamental Immunology, 2nd ed., Raven Press, New York, 1989.

118. Paul WE: The immune system: An introduction. In: Fundamental Immunology, 2nd ed., p 3, Paul WE (ed.), Raven Press, New York, 1989.

119. Pekarek RS, Sandstead HH, Jacob RA, et al: Abnormal cellular immune responses during acquired zinc deficiency. Am J Clin Nutr 32:1466, 1979.

120. Prasad AS: Trace element status of the elderly. In: Nutrition, Immunity and Illness in the Elderly, p 62, Chandra RK (ed.), Pergamon Press, New York, 1985.

121. Puri S, Chandra RK: Nutritional regulation of host resistance and predictive value of immunologic test in assessment of outcome. Pediatr Clin North Am 32: 499, 1985.

122. RDA, Committee on Dietary Allowances, Food Nutrition Board, National Research Council: Recommended Dietary Allowances, 9th ed., National Academy Press, Washington, 1980.

123. Reddy V, Srikantia SG: Antibody response in kwashiorkor. Indian J Med Res 53:1154, 1964.

124. Reddy V, Raghuramulu N, Bhaskaram C: Secretory IgA in protein–calorie malnutrition. Arch Dis Child 51:871, 1976.

125. Rogers AE, Newberne PM: Nutrition and immunological responses. Cancer Detect Prev 1 [Suppl]:1, 1987.

126. Roitt V, Brostoff J, Male D: Immunology, 2nd ed., Gower Medical Publishing, London, 1989.

127. Rosen EU, Geefhuysen J, Anderson R, et al: Leukocyte function in children with kwashiorkor. Arch Dis Child 50:220, 1975.

128. Rosenberg IH, Solomons NW, Schneider RE: Malabsorption associated with diarrhea and intestinal infections. Am J Clin Nutr 30:1248, 1977.

129. Sandstead HH, Vo Khactu KP, Solomons NW: Conditioned zinc deficiencies. In: Trace Elements in Human Health and Disease, Vol 1, p 33, Prasad AS (ed.), Academic Press, New York, 1976.

130. Schlesinger L, Stekel A: Impaired cellular immunity in marasmic infants. Am J Clin Nutr 27:615, 1974.

131. Scrimshaw NS: Significance of the interactions of nutrition and infection in children. In: Textbook of Pediatric Nutrition, p 229, Suskind RM (ed.), Raven Press, New York, 1981.

132. Scrimshaw NS: Epidemiology of nutrition of the aged. In: Nutrition in the Elderly, p 3, Horwitz A, Macfadyen DM, Munro H, et al. (eds.), Oxford University Press, Oxford, 1989.

133. Scrimshaw NS, Taylor CE, Gordon JE: Interactions of nutrition and infection. Am J Med Sci 237:367, 1959.

134. Scrimshaw NS, Taylor CE, Gordon JE: Interactions of Nutrition and Infection. WHO Monograph Series 57, WHO, Geneva, 1968.

135. Sellmeyer E, Bhettay E, Truswell AS, et al: Lymphocyte transformation in malnourished children. Arch Dis Child 47:429, 1972.

136. Selvaraj RJ, Bhat KS: Metabolic and bactericidal activities of leukocytes in protein–calorie malnutrition. Am J Clin Nutr 25:166, 1972.

137. Seth V, Chandra RK: Opsonic activity, phagocytosis, and bactericidal capacity of polymorphs in undernutrition. Arch Dis Child 47:282, 1972.

138. Sirisinha S, Edelman R, Suskind R, et al: Complement and C3-proactivator levels in children with protein–calorie malnutrition and effect of dietary treatment. Lancet 1:1016, 1973.

139. Sirisinha S, Suskind R, Edelman R, et al: Secretory and serum IgA in children with protein–calorie malnutrition. Pediatrics 55:166, 1975.

140. Sirisinha S, Suskind R, Edelmen R, et al: The complement systems in protein–calorie malnutrition. In: Malnutrition and the Immune Response, p 309, Suskind R (ed.), Raven Press, New York, 1977.

141. Smith H. Biochemical challenge of microbial pathogenicity. Bacteriol Rev 32:164, 1968.

142. Smythe PM, Brereton-Stiles GG, Grace HJ, et al: Thymolymphatic deficiency and depression of cell-mediated immunity in protein–calorie malnutrition. Lancet 2:939, 1971.

143. Solomons NW: Assessment of nutritional status: Functional indicators of pediatric nutriture. Pediatr Clin North Am 32:319, 1985.

144. Solomons NW, Allen LH: The functional assessment of nutritional status: Principles, practice and potential. Nutr Rev 41:33, 1983.

145. Stinnett DJ: Nutrition and the Immune Response, CRC Press, Boca Raton, 1983.

146. Suskind R (ed.): Malnutrition and the Immune Response, Raven Press, New York, 1977.

147. Suskind R: The immune response in the malnourished child. In: Nutrition, Disease Resistance, and Immune Function, p 149, Watson RR (ed.), Marcel Dekker, New York, 1984.

148. Suskind R, Sirisinha S, Vithayasai V, et al: Immunoglobulin and antibody response in children with protein–calorie malnutrition. Am J Clin Nutr 29:835, 1976.

149. Suskind R, Sirisinha S, Edelman R, et al: Immunoglobulins and antibody response in Thai children with protein–calorie malnutrition. In: Malnutrition and the Immune Response, p 185, Suskind R (ed.), Raven Press, New York, 1977.

150. Tanphiachitr P, Meknanandha V, Valyasevi A: Impaired plasma opsonic activity in malnourished children. J Med Assoc Thai 56:118, 1973.

151. Ten State Nutrition Survey 1968–1970: US Department of Health Education and Welfare, Publications 72:8131, 8132, 8133, Center for Disease Control, Atlanta, 1972.

152. Thompson JS, Robbins J, Cooper JK: Nutrition and immune function in the geriatric population. Clin Geriatr Med 3:309, 1987.

153. Vos JC, Luster MI: Immune alterations. In: Halogenated Biphenyls, Terphenyls, Naphthalenes, Dibenzodioxins and Related Products, 2nd Ed., p 275, Kimbrough RD, Jensen AA (eds.), Elsevier, Amsterdam, 1989.

154. Vyas D, Chandra RK: Vitamin A and immunocompetence. In: Nutrition, Disease Resistance, and Immune Function, p 325, Watson RR (ed.), Marcel Dekker, New York, 1984.

155. Vyas D, Chandra RK: Functional implications of iron deficiency. In: Iron Nutrition in Infancy and Childhood, p 45, Stekel A (ed.), Raven Press, New York, 1984.

156. Watson RR (ed.): Nutrition, Disease Resistance, and Immune Function, Marcel Dekker, New York, 1984.

157. Watson RR, McMurray DN, Martin P, et al: Effect of age, malnutrition and renutrition on free secretory component and IgA in secretions. Am J Clin Nutr 42:281, 1985.

158. Weir DM: Immunology, 6th Ed. Churchill Livingstone, Edinburgh, 1989.

159. Weksler ME: Biological basis and clinical significance of immune senescence. In: Clinical Geriatrics, 3rd ed., p 57, Rossman I (ed.), JB Lippincott, Philadelphia, 1986.

160. Work TH, Ifewunigwe A, Jelliffe DB, et al: Tropical problems in nutrition. Ann Intern Med 79:701, 1973.

161. Young M, Geha RS: Human regulatory T-cell subsets. Annu Rev Med 37:165, 1986.

162. Ziegler HD, Ziegler PB: Depression of tuberculin reaction in mild and moderate protein calorie malnourished children following BCG vaccination. Johns Hopkins Med J 137:59, 1975.

RECOMMENDED READINGS

Abbas AK, Lichtman AR, Pober JS: Cellular and Molecular Immunology, WB Saunders, Philadelphia, 1991.

Chandra RK (ed.): Nutrition, Immunity and Illness in the Elderly, Pergamon Press, New York, 1985.

Chandra RK (ed.): Nutrition and Immunology, Alan R Liss, New York, 1988.

Gershwin ME, Beach RS, Hurley LS: Nutrition and Immunity, Academic Press, Orlando, 1985.

Paul WE (ed.): Fundamental Immunology, 2nd ed., Raven Press, New York, 1989.

Part IV

CLINICAL CONSIDERATIONS

11. THE OCCUPATIONAL AND ENVIRONMENTAL HEALTH HISTORY

Alyce Bezman Tarcher

INTRODUCTION

In recent years, public understanding of occupational hazards and the extent to which environmental chemical and physical agents can adversely affect health has increased enormously. Figure 11-1 illustrates the complex nature of human exposure to these agents. This awareness has encouraged patients to consult their physicians about the safety of their workplace, home, and community environment and to consider a possible relationship between hazardous exposure and their health status. The importance of discovering environmentally related illness cannot be overemphasized (2,9,15). Benefits may accrue not only to the patient but also to coworkers and to family members with similar exposures.

The occupational and environmental health history is fundamental in assessing the health effects of chemical and physical agents in the environment and workplace (7,16). In the broadest sense, it must be interwoven into all components of the medical history. Its purpose is to (1) diagnose and treat occupational and environmental illness, (2) prevent the development of such problems by identifying occupational and environmental hazards, (3) counsel patients in preventive behavior, and (4) discover new relationships between exposure and disease.

Expanding the scope of the medical history to include a search for diseases of environmental origin requires a system of inquiry. Emphasis must be placed on a potential connection between environ-

mental exposure(s) and patient health; symptoms and disease must be evaluated in terms of present and past exposure(s); and sources of exposure must be analyzed in terms of their health impact (2,7,16,19).

Obviously, a fund of knowledge is required to search effectively for environmentally related illness. Physicians with some understanding of agents that have toxic potential and of where they are found in occupational and environmental settings will more easily and quickly investigate such clinical problems (Tables 11-1 through 11-3; Appendixes A, B, and C).

Clinicians are also called on to be familiar with the specific environmental and work hazards existing in their communities. Certain communities and localities have particular health risks. For example, in agricultural areas relying on private wells for drinking water, an increased incidence of methemoglobinemia may be seen in infants. This problem arises from the ingestion of ground water contaminated with nitrate from chemical fertilizers and manure (see Chapter 21). Individuals living in agricultural areas may experience farmer's lung following exposure to moldy compost or have increased exposure to pesticides, particularly from the aerial spraying of these agents. In the central city, young children living in old dilapidated housing with flaking lead paint have an increased risk of lead toxicity. Office workers may be faced with health problems associated with exposures found in sealed office towers. Some communities may be affected by important sources of industrial and air pollution. Still others may be faced with such issues as hazardous waste sites, contaminated ground water, or radon emanating from the soil.

Physicians in certain specialities are faced with special clinical problems related to toxic exposure. For example, obstetricians and urologists require

Principles and Practice of Environmental Medicine, edited by Alyce Bezman Tarcher. Plenum Medical Book Company, New York, 1992.

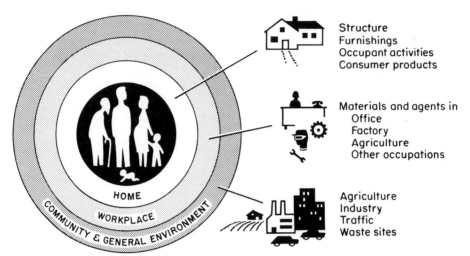

Structure
Furnishings
Occupant activities
Consumer products

Materials and agents in
   Office
   Factory
   Agriculture
   Other occupations

Agriculture
Industry
Traffic
Waste sites

FIGURE 11-1. Humans in the environment: a complex multimedia exposure to chemicals and physical agents in air, food, and water.

some understanding of the effects of hazardous exposure on reproduction and fetal development. Pediatricians should be familiar with the effects of hazardous exposure on the the fetus, infant, and young child. Both psychiatrists and neurologists require an understanding of the neurobehavioral effects of certain toxic agents.

SEARCHING FOR OCCUPATIONAL AND ENVIRONMENTAL ILLNESS

A medical history that embodies a systematic search for occupational and environmental illness has three components: (1) the general medical history (e.g., present illness and review of systems), which includes queries looking for a link between symptoms and exposure; (2) the occupational and environmental health history, which provides an assessment of likely sources of toxic exposure; and (3) the evaluation of factors that modify an individual's response to occupational and environmental hazards.

General Medical History

In taking a medical history that explores the link between symptoms and their underlying etiology, it is wise to ask patients if they suspect that their symptoms are related to toxic exposure. In the case of infants and children, the parents may be so queried. Under some circumstances, such questioning may lead the physician directly to the offending agent or the offending conditions. At the very least,

such questioning will serve to alert both physician and patient to the presence of potentially hazardous exposures.

A major problem in identifying illness related to toxic exposure is that the symptoms are nonspecific and can involve any organ system. The body's response generally gives few clues to the inciting agent. The questions listed in Table 11-4 may help the clinician uncover health problems related to occupational and environmental exposure. It is important to determine the chronology of events. For example, did the symptoms appear soon after moving into a new home, refurbishing an old one, or taking a new job. A positive response to such queries indicates the need for a more complete evaluation.

The questions noted in Table 11-4 are helpful only when changes in the patient's symptoms can be connected to environmental factors. Many illnesses of environmental origin become chronic and thereby show no variation with exposure patterns. Other environmentally and occupationally induced conditions, such as the effects of exposure to chemical carcinogens, develop after a long latent period, and thereby are uncovered by epidemiology studies.

Occupational and Environmental Health History

The occupational and environmental health history contains specific information about present and past exposures in the workplace, the home, and the general environment. This history should be obtained even in the absence of specific complaints that suggest a work- or environmentally related ill

TABLE 11-1. Categories of Potentially Hazardous Agents[a]

Aerosols, vapors, gases (A)	Metals, metal fumes (H)
Carbon monoxide	Aluminum
Formaldehyde	Arsenic
Hydrogen sulfide	Cadmium
Ethylene oxide	Chromium
Nitrogen dioxide	Cobalt
Ozone	Iron
Phosgene	Lead
Smoke	Mercury
Sewer gas	Nickel
Sulfur dioxide	Organic dust (I)
Inert gases	Cotton dust
Welding fumes	Wood dust
Biological inhalants (B)	Poison oak
Bacteria	Petrochemicals (J)
Fungi	Asphalt and tar
Molds	Creosote
Spores	Coal tar
Corrosive substances (C)	PBB (polybrominated biphenyls), PCB
Acids	(polychlorinated biphenyls)
Alkalis	Petroleum distillates
Ammonia	Physical agents (K)
Chlorine	Heavy lifting
Phenol	Noise
Dyes, stains (D)	Thermal stress
Aniline dyes	Vibration
Azo dyes	Plastics (L)
Benzidine	Vinyl chloride
Inorganic dusts, powders (E)	Epoxy resins
Asbestos	Acrylonitrile
Beryllium	Styrene
Coal dust	Methyl ethyl ketone peroxide
Fiberglass	Sensitizing agents (M)
Nickel	Aliphatic amines
Silica	Methane diisocyanate
Talc	Toluene diisocyanate
Insecticides, herbicides (F)	Nickel
Carbamates	Platinum
Halogenated hydrocarbons	Proteolytic
Organophosphates	(detergent) enzymes
Phenoxyherbicides	Solvents (N)
Ionizing and nonionizing radiation (G)	Benzene
X ray	Carbon disulfide
Ultraviolet radiation	Carbon tetrachloride
Electromagnetic radiation	Chloroform
	Methanol
	Perchloroethylene
	Trichloroethylene
	Xylene
	Glycol ethers (cellusolves)

[a]From Occupational and Environmental Health Committee (16).

ness. Obtaining such information, even in asymptomatic individuals, may uncover risk factors that open the way to preventive action and greater clinical scrutiny. An example of an occupational and environmental health history form along with general questions that can be asked by the physician are shown in Fig. 11-2.

Occupational History

It is noteworthy that a work history that includes only job titles may miss important clues to specific exposures. Therefore, patients should be asked to describe the nature of their work, and efforts should be made to get some idea of the

TABLE 11-2. Major Hazardous Exposures by Occupation[a]

Occupation or activity	Exposure[b]
Agriculture and pest control	A, B, F, K
Automobile, aircraft manufacturing and repair	A, C, E, H, K, M
Bakers, food handlers	B, L, M
Boiler operations and cleaning	A, C, E, K
Ceramics and masonry	E, H
Carpentry, woodworking, and lumber industry	B, I, J, K, N
Chemical industry and users	A, N
Construction work, demolition, road work, maintenance, and plastering	C, D, E, K, J, N
Dry cleaning and laundry	J, M, N
Electric, electronics	C, E, H, J, M
Foundry work	A, C, E, H, K
Health care, laboratory work, dental work	A, B, C, D, E, G, K, L, M, N
Machinery, grinding, and metal work	A, C, H, K, M, N
Mining	A, E, G, K
Oil industry, petrochemical	A, C, J, K, N
Paper industry	E, N
Plastic manufacturing	E, J, L
Plumbing, pipefitting, shipfitting	A, C, E, H, K
Printing, lithography	D, I, K, N
Sandblasting, spray painting	A, E, H, K, N
Shipyard, dock work, transportation	A, C, E, H, J, K, N
Textile industry	A, D, E, I, N
Welding	A, E, H, M
X-ray occupations	G

[a]From Occupational and Environmental Health Committee (16).
[b]See Table 11-1 for exposure categories.

TABLE 11-3. Sources of Common Indoor Air Pollutants in Homes and Commercial Buildings[a]

Source	Pollutant
Tobacco smoking	Carbon monoxide
	Particles
	Organics
Standing water	Biological contaminants (e.g., *Legionella*, molds)
People	Carbon dioxide
	Odors (bioeffluents)
	Bacterial and viral contaminants
Furnishings, building materials	Formaldehyde
	Organics (e.g., solvents, paints, glues, etc.)
	Asbestos
Computers, copiers, white-out, typesetting equipment	Organics
	Particles
Garages, loading docks	Carbon monoxide
	Particles
	Organics
Outdoor air	Carbon monoxide, nitrogen dioxide, ozone, sulfur dioxide, particles, organics, pollen, allergens
Soil gas	Radon
	Biocides
	Organics
Gas boilers, furnaces, cookers, gas ranges, unvented kerosene and gas space heaters, coal and wood stoves	Carbon monoxide, nitrogen dioxide, particles
	Organics
Solvents, paints, glues, resins, personal care and houshold products	Organics

[a]Adapted from American Thoracic Society (3).

TABLE 11-4. Questions to Evaluate the Relationship between the Patient's Illness and Occupational and Environmental Exposures

General questions
- Are your symptoms linked in any way to your exposure pattern?
- Do your symptoms appear with any specific activity or in a particular location?

Questions related to occupational exposure
- Are your symptoms related to certain activities on the job?
- Did you begin a new job?
- Did you move into a new building?
- Did a manufacturing process change? Are new chemicals being used?
- Was there a change in the location of your work station?
- Was there any change in ventilation? Does the ventilation seem adequate?
- Did you move into an area with heavy smoking?
- Do your symptoms change when you are off from work for a few days or on vacation?
- Do your symptoms return when you return to work?
- Is there a temporal relationship between your symptoms and your work during the course of a day or a week?
- Are your co-workers ill?
- Did an incident or accident occur at work that resulted in exposure to chemicals?

Questions related to environmental exposure
- Did you move into a newly built home or a mobile home?
- Was your home or apartment recently remodeled or repainted?
- Did you refurnish your home or apartment?
- If your home heating system is gas, is it vented?
- Do you have a hobby involving the use of chemicals?
- If you garden or have plants indoors, do you use pesticides?
- Was your home or apartment fumigated?
- If you have a pet, what is used for flea control?
- Did you have an accident at home that resulted in exposure to chemicals?
- Do you live near industry, a smelter or refinery, or a construction or hazardous waste site?

intensity, frequency, duration, and route of toxic exposure on the job. For example, higher exposure occurs with spray painting than when one uses a brush. The use or nonuse of protective equipment may offer important clues to the intensity of exposure.

Commonly, patients are unaware of or deny potential workplace or environmental hazards. Specific questions regarding exposures to dust, fumes, gases, chemicals, and radiation are indicated. There is often a mixture of toxic exposures, especially in an industrial setting. Understanding the total picture is therefore important. Inquiries should be made regarding illness in co-workers. Though such information is helpful, a negative response does not rule out occupational illness.

Environmental History

An environmental history includes questions related to the home or apartment, including its construction and furnishings, the method of heating, the use of household and garden chemicals, hobbies, and pets. Such questioning is particularly important in the case of infants, young children, the elderly, and the infirm, who spend the greatest

amount of time indoors. Potential hazards in the neighborhood and community and possible contamination of water, air, and soil must also be considered. As seen in Tables 11-5 and 11-6, household chemicals and hobbies are sources of a long list of potentially hazardous exposures. Hazardous materials can also be brought into the home through contaminated clothing or shoes (10). Exposures in school to such items as chalk, solvents, and asbestos may need investigation. Potential toxic exposures in parks and playground sites should not be overlooked. At least two parks are on the EPA's list of top-priority hazardous waste sites (6).

Factors That Modify an Individual's Response to Occupational and Environmental Hazards

The medical history supplies important information and clues regarding a patient's risk of developing environmental and occupational illness. This includes genetic, physiological, health, and behavioral factors than can predispose or modify an individual's response to toxic exposure. These factors must be considered in any clinical evaluation of the problem (Table 11-7) (see Chapter 12 for a discussion of this issue).

Occupational and Environmental Health History Form

I. IDENTIFICATION

Name _____

Address _____

_____ Zip _____

Telephone: home _____ work _____

Soc. Sec. _____ - _____ - _____

Sex: M _____ F _____

Birthday _____

II. OCCUPATIONAL HISTORY

Fill in the table below listing all jobs at which you have worked, including short-term, seasonal, and part-time employment. Start with your present job and go back to the first. Use additional paper if necessary.

Workplace (Employer's name and address or city)	Dates worked From	To	Type of Industry (Describe)	Your job duties (Describe)	Health hazards in workplace (Gases, dust, metals, solvents, radiation, infectious agents, etc.)	Protective equipment used (Describe)	Health problems related to work (Describe)

FIGURE 11-2. Occupational and environmental health history form. The questionnaire is adapted from Occupational and Environmental Health Committee (16).

Occupational Exposure

1. Describe any health problems or injuries related to present or past jobs.

2. Have you or your coworkers had health problems or injuries?

3. Do you believe you have health problems related to your present or past work?

4. Have you been off of work because of a work-related illness or injury? If so, describe:

5. Have you worked with a substance that caused a skin rash? What was the substance? Describe your reaction.

6. Have you had trouble breathing, coughing, or wheezing while at work? If so, describe:

7. Do you have any allergies? If so, describe:

8. Have you had difficulty conceiving a child?

9. Do you have any children who were born with abnormalities?

10. Do you smoke or have you ever smoked cigarettes, cigars, or pipes? For how long and how many per day?

11. Do you smoke on the job?

12. Have you ever worked at a job or hobby in which you came into direct contact with any of the following substances through breathing, touching, or direct exposure? If so, please place a checkmark beside the substance.

Acids	Halothane
Alcohols (industrial)	Heat (severe)
Alkalis	Isocyanates
Ammonia	Ketones
Arsenic	Lead
Asbestos	Manganese
Benzene	Mercury
Beryllium	Methylene chloride
Cadmium	Nickel
Carbon tetrachloride	Noise (loud)
Chlorinated naphathalenes	PBBs
Chloroform	PCBs
Chloroprene	Perchloroethylene
Chromates	Pesticides
Coal dust	Phenol
Cold (severe)	Phosgene
Dichlorobenzene	Radiation
Ethylene dibromide	Rock dust
Ethylene dichloride	Silica powder
Fiberglass	Solvents

FIGURE 11-2. (*Cont.*)

Styrene	Trinitrotoluene
Talc	Vibration
Toluene	Vinyl chloride
TDI or MDI	Welding fumes
Trichloroethylene	X rays

If you have answered "yes" to any of the above, please describe your exposure on a separate sheet of paper.

Environmental Exposure

1. Do you live in the central city or in a rural, urban, or suburban area?

2. Have you ever changed your residence or home because of a health problem? If so, describe:

3. Do you live in the immediate vicinity of a refinery, smelter, factory, battery recycling plant, hazardous waste site, or other potential pollution source?

4. Do you (and your child) live in or regularly visit a building with peeling or chipped lead paint (e.g., built before 1960)? Has there been recent, ongoing, or planned renovation or remodeling of this structure(s)?

5. Do any members of your household have contact with dusts or chemicals in the workplace that are then brought into the home?

6. Do you have a hobby that you do at home? If so, describe:

7. Do you fumigate your home or use pesticides in and around your home and on a pet? Do you use mothballs?

8. What cleaning agents and solvents are used in your home?

9. Is there evidence of mold in your home?

10. Which of the following do you use in your home?

Air conditioner	Humidifier
Electric stove	Wood stove
Air purifier	Gas stove
Fireplace	Unvented kerosene heater or gas heater

11. What is your source of drinking water?

    Community water system
    Private well
    Bottled water

FIGURE 11-2. (*Cont.*)

TABLE 11-5. Examples of Common Dangerous Household Products[a]

Product	Potentially hazardous agents
Disinfectants	Cresol; phenol; hexachlorophene
Cleaning agents and solvents	
Bleaches	Sodium hypochlorite (bleach)
Window cleaner	Ammonia
Carpet cleaner	Ammonia, turpentine, naphthalene; 1,1,1-trichloroethane
Oven and drain cleaners	Potassium hydroxide, sodium hydroxide
Dry-cleaning fluids, spot removers	1,1,1-Trichloroethane, perchloroethylene, petroleum distillates
Paint and varnish solvents	Turpentine, xylene, toluene, methanol, methylene chloride, acetone
Pesticides	Malathion, dichlorvos, carbaryl, methoxychlor
Emissions from heating or cooling devices	
Gas stove pilot light	Nitrogen oxides
Indoor use of charcoal grill	Carbon monoxide
Leaks from refrigerator or air conditioner cooling systems	Freon

[a]From Goldman and Peters (7).

TUTORING THE PATIENT

A clear and precise exposure history usually comes from a well-tutored patient. Clinicians must tell their patients what information is needed and then provide guidance in obtaining such informa-tion. Often, patients must be instructed to keep a diary of their activities and to include the dates, times, places, intensity, duration, and route of exposure. The diary should also include responses to exposure by the patient and others: e.g., was an odor detected, was there coughing, difficulty in breath-

TABLE 11-6. Examples of Hazards in Hobbies[a]

Activity	Potential hazard
Painting	Toxic pigments, e.g., arsenic (emerald green), cadmium, chromium, lead, mercury; acrylic emulsions; solvents
Ceramics	
Raw materials	Colors and glazes containing barium carbonate; lead, chromium, uranium, cadmium
Firing	Fumes of fluoride, chlorine, sulfur dioxide
Gas-fired kilns	Carbon monoxide
Sculpture and casting	
Grinding silica-containing stone	Silica (silicon dioxide)
Serpentine rock with asbestos	Asbestos
Woodworking	Wood dust
Metal casting	Metal fume, sand (silica) from molding, binders of phenol formaldehyde or urea formaldehyde
Welding	Metal fume, ultraviolet light exposure, welding fumes, carbon dioxide, carbon monoxide, nitrogen dioxide, ozone or phosgene (if solvents nearby)
Plastics	Monomers released during heating (polyvinyl chloride), methyl methacrylate, acrylic glues, polyurethanes (toluene 2,4-diisocyanate), polystyrene (methyl chloride release), fiberglass, polyester of epoxy resins
Woodworking	Solvents, especially methylene chloride
Photography	
Developer	Hydroquinone, metal
Stop bath	Weak acetic acid
Stop hardener	Potassium chrome alum (chromium)
Fixer	Sodium sulfite, acetic acid-sulfur dioxide
Hardeners and stabilizers	Formaldehyde

[a]From Goldman and Peters (7).

TABLE 11-7. Factors That Modify an Individual's Response
to Occupational and Environmental Hazards[a]

Modifying factor	Known or probable effects
General factors	
Age	Fetus, infant, young child, and elderly generally more susceptible to toxic exposure
Gender	Gender differences in toxicity exist for some conditions, reproductive effects
Nutrition	Malnutrition affects susceptibility to certain toxic agents
Smoking status	
Current smoker	Confers additive risk in some situations
Smoker at time of exposure	Confers synergistic risk in some situations
Smoking during exposure	Modifies toxic exposure in some situations, such as polymer fume fever
Alcohol use	May increase the effects of hepatotoxins
Exercise at time of exposure	Increases exposure to air pollution
Family history	Certain hereditary conditions associated with increased susceptibility to toxic exposure
Medical conditions	
Atopy	Tendency toward sensitization
Asthma	Increased bronchial reactivity
Neurological conditions	
Diminished mental capacity	May affect judgment and response to exposure situation
Neurological disease	Neurotoxic effects may be additive
Seizure disorder	Certain toxic exposures may alter threshold
Impaired perceptions	Impaired ability to avoid hazard
Dermatological conditions	Skin rashes may increase dermal absorption
Respiratory disease	
Respiratory insufficiency	Diminished pulmonary reserve
Bronchitis	Increased bronchial reactivity, increased bronchial irritation
Cardiovascular disease	
Cardiac insufficiency	Increased susceptibility to toxic agents affecting the heart
Coronary artery disease	Angina under certain conditions such as carbon monoxide and methylene chloride exposure
Renal disease	
Renal insufficiency	Increased susceptibility to toxic agents excreted by the kidneys; increased susceptibility to renal toxins
Liver disease	Increased susceptibility to agents detoxified by the liver; increased susceptibility to hepatotoxins
Immune deficiency states	Increased susceptibility to infections and to toxic agents affecting the immune system
Hereditary	
Immunosuppressive therapy	
Infections	
Acute viral illness	Increases susceptibility to bronchial irritation; may depress host resistance
Chronic infection	May depress host resistance

[a]Adapted from Occupational and Environmental Health Committee (16).

ing, nausea, headache, or altered mentation? What responses occurred immediately, and which were delayed?

CHARACTERIZING THE TOXIC EXPOSURE

If the medical history gives a strong suspicion that toxic exposure has taken place, and its source and route of exposure have been determined, the next step is to identify the chemical(s) by its generic name. The patient's assistance is often needed, e.g.,

to look at labels on containers. It should be noted that federal legislation in the United States now mandates that workers have the right to Material Data Safety Sheets, which list the names and potential health effects of hazardous exposures in the workplace. With the permission of the patient, physicians may also request such data.

If a specific chemical(s) is identified, its toxicology can be researched to determine if such exposure can be linked to the clinical findings. A number of references give information on the toxicity of individual substances (5,11–14,17–24).

SEEKING CONSULTATION

Consultation is usually in order if further assessment of exposure is needed, if there is concern about the health status of the patient's co-workers, or if it seems likely that the patient must change his or her job or living conditions for reasons of health.

Consultants in such subspecialities as occupational medicine, neurology, and dermatology may prove helpful. Many university medical centers offer consultative services through a department of occupational and environmental medicine. The patient may also be referred to one of the many occupational and environmental clinics located throughout the United States (see Appendix D for locations of these clinics). Other sources of consultation are also listed in Appendix D.

UNCOVERING OCCUPATIONAL AND ENVIRONMENTAL ILLNESS

Diagnostic Criteria

The following criteria, though not always met, should be considered when making a diagnosis of environmental illness: (1) the temporal pattern is consistent, e.g., the putative exposure always preceeds the onset of disease; (2) the symptoms, signs, and laboratory findings are predictable based on the effects known to be caused by the exposure; (3) the nature and extent of the exposure are sufficient to cause the disease; and (4) epidemiologic data, if available, support the effects of exposure observed in the individual. Toxicologic information may also provide corroborative evidence. It would be useful for the reader to consider how these criteria apply to specific cases.

Case Reports

The importance of the clinician's awareness of toxic exposure as a source of illness is reflected in the following case reports from the literature. The cases were chosen to illustrate the importance of asking the right questions, having a store of knowledge or a means of obtaining that knowledge, and remaining alert to a possible link between disease and exposure. In somes instances the practioner was alert to this relationship; in others the causal relationship was missed.

Case 1: Recurrent Respiratory Symptoms in an Infant

A 7-month-old infant was repeatedly hospitalized for cough, wheezing, and respiratory distress (8). The past history revealed that the child had been in good health until 3 months of age, when episodes of cough and wheezing began. There were no smokers in the household and no family history of asthma, tuberculosis, or other chronic respiratory disease. Evaluation by an allergist gave no positive findings for allergies.

Subsequent treatment with antihistamines, decongestants, and antibiotics did not help. The child's respiratory symptoms continued in spite of bronchodilatory therapy. Numerous hospitalizations were necessary. During his fourth hospitalization, after vigorous treatment with bronchodilators, postural drainage, and antibiotics, the patient was free of respiratory distress. He was sent home on a regimen of theophylline, but within 12 h of returning home, he began coughing and wheezing. The symptoms abated when he was taken to a neighbor's home. It was then noted that the neighbor used a fuel oil furnace, whereas the child's home contained a wood-burning stove. A chronological history then revealed that the patient's symptoms began several weeks after his family had purchased and installed the wood-burning stove as the primary source of heat. Prior to this, a fuel oil furnace, vented to the outside, had been used. The history also revealed that the child had frequently stayed with his grandparents, who also used a wood-burning stove as a primary source of heat.

With this discovery, the child's family reverted to the use of the fuel oil furnace. The patient was then free of symptoms until he again visited his grandparents. Two separate visits were associated with a recurrence of his respiratory symptoms. Without exposure to a wood-burning stove, the patient was well. An examination 1 year later indicated that the patient had remained well without any need of medication.

This case illustrates the value of relating the chronology of the patient's illness to noxious exposure. The repeated onset and worsening of symptoms associated with exposure to a wood-burning stove and the absence of symptoms when the stove was removed clearly indicate a link between the patient's illness and the wood-burning stove. The case also emphasizes the importance of asking if the patient's initial illness was associated with a new exposure. If the clinicians had been alerted to this possibility early in the course of the patient's illness, a recurrence of symptoms would have directed their attention to the wood-burning stove. The case also emphasizes the vulnerability of the infant to the adverse effects of indoor air pollution.

Case 2: A Retired Executive with Acute Myocardial Infarctions

A 66-year-old retired executive with no prior history of cardiac disease was admitted to the hospital for severe crushing substernal chest pain (25). Six hours prior to admission he had worked for 3 h applying a commercial liquid gel paint and varnish remover to a chest of drawers. His chest pain began 1 h after leaving his basement workshop. After being admitted to the hospital with a diagnosis of a myocardial infarction, the patient showed his physician the can of paint remover he had been using prior to the onset of his chest pain. The label cautioned that the product contained 80% methylene chloride and was to be used only with adequate ventilation. The physician drew no causal relationship between the patient's recent exposure to the paint remover vapor and his acute myocardial infarction. Two weeks after discharge, the patient again worked for 3 h in his basement workshop, applying paint remover. The substernal pain recurred, and he was readmitted with a severe myocardial infarction, this time complicated by cardiogenic shock, dysrhythmia, and heart failure. Six months after his second myocardial infarction, the patient returned to his basement workshop to complete the paint-stripping job. Two hours after he commenced work, he developed chest pain and died.

The case illustrates the tragic consequences when an attending physician is not attuned to looking for a link between toxic exposure and disease. A simple investigation of the toxic properties of methylene chloride would have revealed that it is metabolized to carbon monoxide, an agent that places substantial stress on the cardiovascular system. The amount of carbon monoxide produced has been shown to be directly related to the amount of methylene chloride absorbed.

Case 3: A Young Worker with a Cardiac Arrhythmia

A 24-year-old man was admitted to the hospital with a 6-month history of "skipping heart beats," dizziness, and headaches (1). On his admission to the hospital, the electrocardiogram showed sinus rhythm and multiple premature ventricular contractions. There was no other clinical, electrocardiographic, radiologic, or echocardiographic evidence of heart disease. The premature ventricular contractions noted on admission did not respond to lidocaine therapy. On the second day of hospitalization, without further therapy, the premature ventricular contractions became less frequent. By the fourth hospital day, the patient's heart rate was normal, and he was free of headache and dizziness. Since the patient gave a 7-month history of working in a dry cleaning plant and using perchloroethylene (a dry cleaning agent), a plasma level of this agent was obtained on the fifth day of hospitalization and showed 0.15 ppm.

A few days after leaving the hospital the patient returned to the dry cleaning plant and soon began again to notice headaches, dizziness, and "skipping heart beats." Two weeks later he was seen as an outpatient; again the cardiogram revealed frequent premature ventricular beats. The plasma level of perchloroethylene at this time was 3.8 ppm. The patient was then advised to leave his present occupation and was assisted in finding a suitable job. A month later the patient was found to be free of all symptoms.

This case illustrates how an alert clinician, investigating the patient's occupation, can establish a causal link between symptoms and exposure. It demonstrates how the measurement of toxic substances in the body can provide some assessment of exposure. It also alerts the treating physician to the presence of an occupational hazard that may be affecting the patient as well as his or her co-workers.

Case 4: Lead Poisoning in a Child

A 2-year-old child was discovered to have an elevated blood level of lead (4). The child lived in an area where there was concern that the water supplies contained excessive amounts of lead. When this proved to be unfounded, it was thought that the patient's increased lead absorption might have resulted from exposure to lead-containing paint. This was not supported by the medical history. The child's home was newly built, made primarily of cinderblock and synthetic building materials, and painted only with latex paints. Analysis of the water, soil, and paint did not reveal any sources of lead.

On further investigation, the child's father stated that he was a brass cutter. (Brass may contain 5–10% lead.) The wife then volunteered the following information: she stated that her husband came home covered from head to toe with metal filings, and before washing or changing his clothes, he would play with the child. In addition, she stated that the family car was full of metal filings. Once the nature of the lead exposure became apparent, the parents thoroughly washed down the home and automobile. The father also stopped contaminating his home with workplace hazards. Although the child initially required chelation therapy, he spontaneously improved once the lead exposure stopped. A 2-year follow-up revealed a normal lead absorption state.

This case points out the importance of obtaining a detailed occupational history of the adults living in the home. It demonstrates that the hazards of the workplace frequently extend into the home. It also illustrates that, in contrast to an adult, the child has a far greater susceptibility to the toxic effects of lead.

Case 5: Anemia in a Young Child

A 2-year-old boy taken to a pediatrician because of a fall was discovered to have a hemoglobin value of 7 g/dL (26). He was given oral iron for 3 weeks. On return visit to his physician, the hemoglobin and hematocrit values were 4g/dL and 12%, respectively. The white blood count was 5000 cu/mL, and the platelet count was 470,000 cu/mL. The differential white blood count showed 35% lymphocytes, 64% segmented neutrophils, and 1% eosinophils. The patient otherwise appeared to be well. When the patient had first been seen, there was no history of blood loss or exposure to toxins. The patient's parents and a 9-year-old brother were in good health.

The patient was admitted to the hospital for further evaluation. The physical examination was normal except for pallor. Bone marrow examination revealed an almost complete absence of red blood cell precursors and a normal number of myeloid cells and megakaryocytes. Blood chemistries, which included blood urea nitrogen, total protein, and lactic dehydrogenase, were normal. A Coombs test was negative. Serum iron was 207 µg/dL. A bone survey, chest x ray, and intravenous pyelogram were normal.

The patient was given 175 mL of packed red blood cells, which raised his hemoglobin value to 10 g/dL. Ten days later his hemoglobin had fallen to 7.1 g/dL. A second bone marrow examination showed that total cellularity was reduced but erythroid precursors were now present. The patient was given 100 mL of packed red blood cells, and his hemoglobin rose to 11.6 g/dL.

It was discovered during his second hospitalization that the patient had been exposed to benzene hexachloride (lindane). About 3 months before the anemia was diagnosed, the patient's father had been dipping their pet dog in a solution of a product called Sarcoptic Mange Treatment®. The label contained no information about the formulation of the product. The dog had been treated with this agent at weekly intervals for 8 weeks, received no treatment for 1 month, and had been dipped again at 2-week intervals. After the dog was dipped, the chemical dried on the animal's fur. Since the dog was kept in the house, the 2-year-old child had been in close contact with the animal.

Once the composition of the Sarcoptic Mange Treatment® was determined by checking with the manufacturer, no further dipping occurred. During the ensuing year, the patient's hemoglobin remained at normal levels without need for further treatment.

This case illustrates a number of points. First, even with proper inquiry, the source of toxic exposure can be missed, particularly if it is inconspicuous; second, the importance of the exposure may not be appreciated until the specific agent is known; and finally, the range of individual susceptibility to toxic exposure is reflected in the absence of any hematological problems in the patient's 9-year-old brother, who also played with the dog, and in the patient's father, who had dipped the dog.

REFERENCES

1. Abedin Z, Cook RC, Milberg RM: Cardiac toxicity of perchloroethylene (a dry cleaning agent). South Med J 73:1081, 1980.
2. American College of Physicians: Position paper. Occupational and environmental medicine: The internist's role. Ann Intern Med 113:974, 1990.
3. American Thoracic Society: Environmental controls and lung disease. Am Rev Respir Dis 142:915, 1990.
4. Chisolm JJ Jr: Management of increased lead absorption—illustrative cases. In: Lead Absorption in Children, p. 171, Chisolm JJ Jr, O'Hara DH (eds.), Urban & Schwarzenberg, Baltimore, 1982.
5. Daugaard J: Symptoms and Signs in Occupational Disease: A Practical Guide, Year Book Medical Publishers, Chicago, 1978.
6. Environmental Protection Agency: Hazardous Waste Sites, National Priorities List, August 1983, EPA, Washington, 1983.
7. Goldman RH, Peters JM: The occupational and environmental health history. JAMA 246:2831, 1981.
8. Honicky RE, Akpom CM, Osborne JS: Infant respiratory illness and indoor air pollution from a woodburning stove. Pediatrics 7:126, 1983.
9. Institute of Medicine: Role of the Primary Care Physician in Occupational and Environmental Medicine, National Academy Press, Washington, 1988.
10. Knishkowy B, Baker EL: Transmission of occupational disease to family contracts. Am J Ind Med 9:543, 1986.
11. LaDou J (ed.): Occupational Medicine, Appleton & Lange, Norwalk, Connecticut, 1990.
12. Levy BS, Wegman DH (eds.): Occupational Health, 2nd ed., Little, Brown, Boston, 1988.
13. Mackison FW, Stricoff RS, Partridge LJ Jr (eds.): NIOSH/OSHA Pocket Guide to Chemical Hazards, US Department of Health and Human Services, US Government Printing Office, Washington, 1978, reprinted 1980.
14. McCann M: Health Hazards Manual for Artists, Nick Lyons Books, New York, 1985.
15. Miller RW: Area-wide chemical contamination: Lessons from case histories. JAMA 245:1548, 1981.
16. Occupational and Environmental Health Committee of the American Lung Association of San Diego and Imperial Counties: Taking the Occupational History. Ann Intern Med 99:641, 1983.
17. Procter NH, Hughes DJP, Fischman ML: Hazards of the Workplace, 2nd ed. JB Lippincott, Philadelphia, 1988.
18. Raffle PAB, Lee WR, McCallum RI, et al (eds.):

Hunter's Diseases of Occupations, Hodder & Stoughton, London, 1987.

19. Rosenstock L: Occupational medicine: Too long neglected. Ann Intern Med 95:774, 1981.
20. Rosenstock L, Cullen MR (eds.): Clinical Occupational Medicine, Blue Books Series, WB Saunders, Philadelphia, 1986.
21. Rutstein DD, Mullan RJ, Frazier TM, et al: Sentinel health events (occupational): A basis for physician recognition and public health surveillance. Am J Public Health 73:1054, 1983.
22. Sax I, Lewis RJ: Hazardous Chemicals Desk Reference, Van Nostrand Reinhold, New York, 1987.
23. Schardein J: Chemically Induced Birth Defects, Marcel Dekker, New York, 1985.
24. Sittig M: Handbook of Toxic and Hazardous Chemicals and Carcinogens, 3rd ed, Noyes Data Corporation, Park Ridge, New Jersey, 1990.
25. Stewart RD, Hake CL: Paint-remover hazard. JAMA 235:398, 1976.
26. Vodopick H: Cherchez la chienne. JAMA 234:850, 1975.

RECOMMENDED READINGS

Goldman RH, Peters JM: The occupational and environmental health history. JAMA 246:2831, 1981.
Occupational and Environmental Health Committee of the American Lung Association of San Diego and Imperial Counties: Taking the occupational history. Ann Intern Med 99:641, 1983.
Rutstein DD, Mullan RJ, Frazier TM, et al: Sentinel health events (occupational): A basis for physician recognition and public health surveillance. Am J Public Health 73:1054, 1983.

12. ENHANCED SUSCEPTIBILITY TO ENVIRONMENTAL CHEMICALS

Alyce Bezman Tarcher and Edward J. Calabrese

INTRODUCTION

Individuals differ widely in their susceptibility to the adverse effects of occupational and environmental chemicals (28,183,185,186). During the past several decades considerable effort has been directed to studying the occurrence and biochemical bases of individual differences in susceptibility to toxic substances (28,32,36,37,50,61,94,110,169,170,176,184–187,227,230,248,251). Efforts have also been made to develop simple, accurate, and cost-effective methods of identifying individuals with enhanced risks to toxic exposure (28,32,54,171,180,231).

This chapter focuses primarily on host factors that may influence an individual's susceptibility to chemical exposure in the workplace and general environment. These factors include genetic background, age, gender, nutritional status, physiological status (including pregnancy), presence of disease, behavioral/lifestyle considerations, and exposure patterns (Table 12-1). Some factors, such as those related to age (i.e., stages of development and senescence), nutrition, physiological status, behavior, and life style affect all individuals. Other factors, such as genetically inherited conditions and pregnancy, effect a portion of the population. The overall population dose-response curve, by masking the more vulnerable subgroups of the population, may be misleading (Fig. 12-1) (182).

With changes in the relative roles of the various host and environmental factors, there are times when each individual becomes either more or less vulnerable to toxic exposure. The changes in susceptibility that accompany circadian rhythmicity, for example, affect all individuals (165,166). Factors affecting susceptibility may interact to increase or decrease the adverse effects of toxic exposure(s). They may be independent or interdependent. The factors that increase the susceptibility of the aged, for example, are often interdependent and include changes in nutritional status, exercise, medication, and the functional reserve of all organs. A more detailed representation of host and environmental factors that can influence an individual's response to foreign chemicals is shown in Fig. 12-2 (247,248).

In many instances, enhanced susceptibility to the toxicity of foreign chemicals can be traced to impaired or altered bodily defenses. Complex host defenses reside at the portals of entry, i.e., the skin, lung, and gastrointestinal tract, in the processes of biotransformation and excretion, and in the immune response. The bodily defenses, discussed in detail in Chapters 6–10, are vital to the survival of the organism. Compromised host defenses may thus play a role in the development of pollutant-related or environmentally induced disease. Although the causes of unusual susceptibility are generally multiple and complex, viewing the problem within the framework of impaired host defenses can be of value. Having an awareness of host defenses against environmental exposure can be of special help to physicians as they attempt to unravel the complex effects of exposure to toxic chemicals.

Because individuals with enhanced susceptibility are often in need of medical attention, physicians must be especially aware of individual differences in susceptibility and in the factors that predispose

Principles and Practice of Environmental Medicine, edited by Alyce Bezman Tarcher. Plenum Medical Book Company, New York, 1992.

TABLE 12-1. Factors Influencing Susceptibility to Occupational and Environmental Chemicals

Genetic traits	Physiological status
Age	Behavior/life-style factors
Gender	Coexisting exposures
Nutritional status	Presence of disease

individuals to the adverse effects of environmental exposures. Identifying unusually susceptible individuals and the factors that contribute to their condition can lead to more accurate diagnoses, a greater mindfulness of toxic exposures, a modification of host factors that increase susceptibility, and enhanced preventive services (182).

The terms susceptible and hypersusceptible are increasingly being applied to individuals who are more responsive to the adverse effects of chemical exposure. It has been suggested that such individuals should be considered to have a predisposition or an unusual susceptibility to chemical exposure (183). This predisposition relates to specific agents. Individuals who are unusually susceptible to a certain chemical may evidence little susceptibility to other chemicals. The young, the aged, the sick, and those with certain genetic conditions may display varying degrees of susceptibility to varying numbers of agents.

Hypersensitivity or allergy is one form of increased susceptibility; it describes a state of altered reactivity to an antigen that can result in pathological reactions on exposure of a sensitized host to that particular antigen (17). The term sensitivity or hypersensitivity, however, is often used without implying an immunologic etiology.

FACTORS ENHANCING SUSCEPTIBILITY TO CHEMICAL EXPOSURE

Genetic Factors

It has long been suspected that genetic factors affect susceptibility to occupational illness. In 1938, the famous geneticist J. B. S. Haldane suggested a possible role for genetic constitution in the occurrence of bronchitis among certain potters (90). Beginning in the early 1960s, numerous articles cited the potential importance of genetically related differences in susceptibility to industrial chemicals (204,231,232).

The term ecogenetics was coined to describe genetically determined differences among individuals in their susceptibility to the actions of environmental agents (29,170,187). Historically, ecogenetics evolved from the study of pharmacogenetics, which deals with genetically determined differences in the response to drugs (170,184,187,250). Individual and ethnic differences in the response to drugs, now widely recognized, have been studied for a number of years (110,127,245,246,252). In contrast, the role of genetic factors in affecting susceptibility to environmental agents, though based on excellent theoretical foundations, is supported by remarkably few animal or epidemiologic studies (35). Our ability to identify and quantitate genetic factors that might

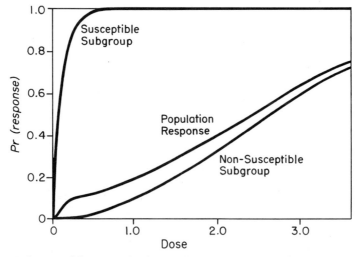

FIGURE 12-1. Schematic diagram of the potential inclusion of a susceptible or high-risk subgroup in a large population. From Omenn and Gelboin (186).

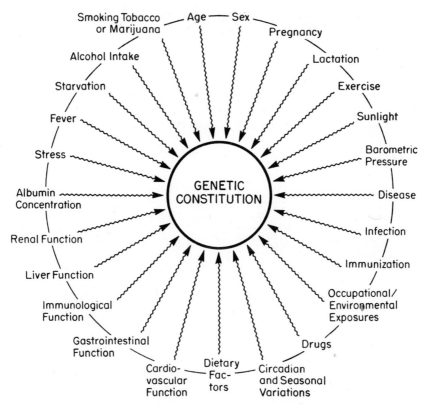

FIGURE 12-2. Host and environmental factors that can influence an individual's response to foreign chemicals. From Vesell (247).

predispose an individual to develop job-related and/or environmentally induced disease is in its infancy (38,180,249).

Genetic variation among individuals represents a basic attribute of living matter. All levels of inquiry have revealed evidence of individual variation (e.g., blood groups, enzyme variants, protein variants, chromosomal variants). The biochemical mechanisms underlying individual differences are varied. They include differing rates of biotransformation and excretion of foreign chemicals and differing responses of tissue enzymes and receptors to such exposure (115,245,246,248). Genetic variation exists within populations and between populations. Measurement of intrapopulation differences is termed "average heterozygosity," whereas the equivalent measure between populations is called the "genetic distance." It appears that the genetic difference among the three major human races (Caucasian, Mongoloid, and Negro) are much smaller than the "average heterozygosity" (77). Ethnic differences in reactions to drugs and xenobiotics have been reviewed (110).

Given the marked differences in gene frequencies among individuals and populations for many genetic traits, some observers have suggested that the genetic variation in susceptibility to drugs and environmental chemicals detected thus far represents the tip of the iceberg (184). It has been postulated that as humans are increasingly exposed to new chemical agents, greater numbers of individuals may exhibit unusual susceptibility to the adverse effects of such exposure (77). To date, our insight into what effects genetic variation may have on susceptibility to occupational and environmental chemicals is drawn primarily from the differences observed in the response to drugs (98,109,127,245, 246,248,249).

Although one's genetic constitution may influence the body's response to environmental chemicals, it must be appreciated that this response is modified by many other host and environmental factors. These factors (Fig. 12-2), always superimposed on the genetic backdrop, may reduce or increase an individual's susceptibility to chemical exposure (248).

Most of the approximately 50 known inherited traits that could potentially enhance an individual's susceptibility to environmental chemicals are exceedingly rare and often difficult to detect. Table 12-2 lists some inherited traits and notes their influence on susceptibility to certain occupational and environmental chemicals. Few studies have investigated the relationship between inherited traits and enhanced susceptibility to pollutant exposure. There is evidence that individuals with immotile cilia syndrome and α_1-antitrypsin deficiency are unusually vulnerable to cigarette smoke (56,168,233). In the case of G-6-PD deficiency, a few observations suggest that such individuals may be unusually susceptible to oxidizing chemicals in the workplace (64, 128,234). Without question many genetic conditions associated with enhanced susceptibility to environmental chemicals remain to be discovered. Some of the genetic conditions listed in Table 12-2 are discussed.

Glucose-6-Phosphate Dehydrogenase Deficiency

Glucose-6-phosphate dehydrogenase deficiency was first noted in individuals who developed severe hemolytic episodes after receiving the anti-malarial drug primaquine. Although there are many genetic variants of this X-linked genetic abnormality, it occurs most frequently in two forms. The mild and more common form is the African variant (A−), which affects approximately 12% of African-American males. The more severe form is the Mediterranean variety (B−) (139).

G-6-PD-deficient erythrocytes have limited capacity to reduce NADP to NADPH and to maintain glutathione (GSH) in the reduced state. This condition makes the G-6-PD-deficient red cell particularly susceptible to oxidant stress. There is evidence that, on exposure to an offending drug or chemical, the G-6-PD-deficient red cell accumulates peroxides, which damage the cell membrane and shorten its life span (139).

Glucose-6-phosphate dehydrogenase deficiency predisposes affected males to develop hemolytic anemia on exposure to a number of oxidizing drugs (22). Such individuals may also be at risk when exposed to oxidizing chemicals in the workplace. Exposure to trinitrotoluene (TNT) has been associated with hemolytic episodes in at least six workers. In some instances the hemolysis recurred with reexposure to TNT (64,128). Beutler comments that the temporal relationship between TNT exposure and

TABLE 12-2. Genetic Factors and Susceptibility to Occupational and Environmental Chemicals[a]

Predisposing factor	Incidence	Chemical(s)	Status of genetic environmental interaction
Glucose-6-phosphate dehydrogenase deficiency	About 12% among African-American males; very high in tropical and subtropical countries	Oxidizing chemicals	Likely
Sickle-cell trait	7–13% among African-Americans; 30% of population in parts of Africa	CO, aromatic amino compounds	No clear evidence
Methemoglobin reductase deficiency	About 1% of population are heterozygotes	Nitrites, aniline	Definite
Aryl hydrocarbon hydroxylase induction	High-induction-type Caucasians about 30%	Polycyclic aromatic hydrocarbons	Possible
Slow acetylator phenotype	Caucasians and Negroes about 60%; Orientals about 10–20%	Aromatic amine-induced cancer	Possible
Paraoxonase variant	Caucasians about 50%, Orientals about 30%, Negroes about 10%	Parathion	Possible
Acatalasia	Mainly Japan and Switzerland, reaching 1% in some areas of Japan	Hydrogen peroxide	Definite
Nontaster status	30% Caucasians, 10% Chinese, 3% Negroes	Goitrogens (thiourea, etc.)	Definite
α_1-Antitrypsin deficiency	Homozygotes about one in 6700 North American Caucasians	Respiratory irritants Smoking	Most likely Definite
Immotile cilia syndrome	About 1:40,000 in all major races	Respiratory irritants, smoking	Most likely
Immunologic hypersensitivity	Unknown, 2% in some occupational populations	Isocyanate	Definite

[a]From references 2, 33, 35, 38, 56, and 77.

the development of severe hemolysis is strongly suggestive of a cause-and-effect relationship (22). Szeinberg et al. reported a mild reticulocytosis in a G-6-PD-deficient individual exposed to TNT (234). It has also been noted that a few Iraqi Jews with G-6-PD deficiency developed severe acute hemolytic anemia while working in a trinitrotoluene (TNT) plant (182). A report by Linch suggests that workers with G-6-PD deficiency who are exposed to aromatic nitro and amino compounds may be more susceptible than normals to cyanosis (135). Although there has been no systematic study of this problem, the limited data presented thus far suggest that G-6-PD-deficient individuals may be at risk, particularly when exposed to nitro-aromatic and nitro-amino compounds in the workplace.

Sickle-Cell Anemia and Sickle-Cell Traits

These genetic conditions result from the presence of an abnormal hemoglobin molecule, hemoglobin S (HbS), located in the erythrocytes of affected persons. Hemoglobin S differs from the normal adult hemoglobin A (HbA) only by the substitution of valine for glutamine at a single location in the hemoglobin chain. Hemoglobin S polymerizes at low oxygen tension. When this occurs, the red cells assume their typical sickle shapes. An individual with sickle-cell anemia is homozygous for HbS, whereas one with sickle-cell trait is heterozygous for HbS. In general, the homozygous person has nearly 100% HbS, whereas the heterozygous person has from 20–40% HbS.

Although individuals with sickle-cell anemia have increased morbidity and mortality, those with sickle-cell trait have few if any clinical problems. The overall life expectancy of hemoglobin S heterozygotes is no different from that of individuals with hemoglobin A. Thus, although it has been suggested that such individuals may be at increased risk when exposed to benzene, lead, cadmium, aromatic amino or nitro compounds, carbon monoxide, and cyanide, there is no evidence to support this view (38,180,232). Individuals with sickle cell trait should not be considered unusually susceptible to the adverse effects of chemical exposure.

Acetylator Phenotype

The observation that some patients excrete the antituberculosis drug isoniazid rapidly, whereas others excrete it relatively slowly led to the discovery of a pharmacogenetic polymorphism. The differences noted were linked to the activity of an enzyme that acetylates isoniazid in the liver. The activity of N-acetyltransferase differs markedly among individuals. A single gene determines the rate of acetylation; rapid acetylation is an autosomal dominant trait. Population studies reveal that about 60% of Caucasians and Negroes and about 10%–20% of Orientals are slow acetylators (77,95). A number of drugs are metabolized by the acetylation of an amino or hydrazino group. These include isoniazid, hydralazine, procainamide, and a number of sulfa drugs. With the long-term administration of isoniazid, adverse effects tend to occur more frequently in slow acetylators, who develop higher blood levels of the drug. As isoniazid interacts with pyridoxine, the principal form of toxicity is a peripheral neuritis caused by a pyridoxine deficiency.

The rate of acetylation may be important in relation to exposure of industrial chemicals. The detoxication of arylamines, which include such potent bladder carcinogens as 2-naphthylamine and benzidine, involves acetylation. The hypothesis that slow acetylators are at increased risk to arylamine-induced bladder cancer has excellent support from animal studies. Epidemiologic evidence, though meager, also suggests that slow acetylators may have a predisposition to arylamine-induced bladder cancer (43). Additional observations are needed.

Aryl Hydrocarbon Hydroxylase

A wide variety of xenobiotics such as drugs, chemical carcinogens, and environmental contaminants, as well as such endogenous compounds as steroids, fatty acids, and prostaglandins, are metabolized by the cytochrome-P-450-containing mixed-function oxidase system. Cytochrome-P-450-dependent monooxygenases are a large family of enzymes with markedly different substrate specificities and biological activities. In many cases cytochrome-P-450-catalyzed metabolism is beneficial, leading to detoxified metabolites that are safely excreted. Sometimes, however, the metabolites so formed are mutagenic, carcinogenic, or more toxic than the original compound. Both environmental and genetic factors have been shown to affect variations in mixed-function oxidase activity (74,175,250).

Particular attention has been directed to the mixed-function oxidase, aryl hydrocarbon hydroxylase (AHH). This enzyme, present in most mammalian tissues, displays increased activity following exposure to such agents as polycyclic aromatic hydrocarbons, insecticides, steroids, and drugs. Aryl hydrocarbon hydroxylase is known to catalyze the first step in the metabolism of benzo[a]pyrene and other polycyclic aromatic hydrocarbons (PAHs). When AHH acts on the polycyclic aromatic hydrocarbons found in cigarette smoke, many of the resulting products are carcinogenic; AHH has therefore been extensively studied to determine if the inducibility of this enzyme correlates with susceptibility to chemically induced cancer, particularly lung cancer, in humans.

The role of genetically regulated AHH inducibility in affecting susceptibility to PAH-induced cancer is well documented in animal studies (174, 176). In animal models, AHH activities vary among inbred strains of mice. With this genetically controlled variation, an excellent correlation has been demonstrated between high AHH levels and PAH-induced tumors (124,125,174,176). In humans, the association between high inducibility of AHH and susceptibility to cigarette-smoke-induced lung cancer is not clearly established. Some reports demonstrate a good correlation between high levels of AHH inducibility in mitogen-stimulated lymphocytes isolated from patients with lung cancer, laryngeal carcinoma, and cancer of the oral cavity, but others do not (66,114,125,134,254). It is also possible that the high inducibility of AHH may be a consequence of the cancer rather than one of the causative factors (11). Most such studies in humans measure AHH activity in peripheral blood lymphocytes, which is easily obtained. It has been suggested that differences in assay techniques may play a role in producing inconsistent results (125). Numerous studies indicate that differences in AHH levels in humans are under genetic control (10,26,124,133). The high-inducibility AHH phenotype is thought to represent about one out of ten of the U.S. population.

It is of interest that epidemiologic studies support a tendency for lung cancer to cluster in families (240,241). Increased attention is being directed to the role of genetic factors in susceptibility to cancer (11,13,94,211,216,227).

Immotile Cilia Syndrome

The immotile cilia syndrome (ICS) is a hereditary disease characterized by the congenital malfunction of cilia in the airways and elsewhere. The estimated prevalence of this syndrome is about 1 : 40,000. Inherited as a recessive autosomal trait, the syndrome has been described in all major races and in most countries (2).

The upper and lower respiratory tract is well supplied with ciliated epithelium and mucus-secreting cells. Under normal conditions inhaled noxious particles and bacteria are removed by being carried on mucus that is propelled along the air passages on the tips of beating cilia. When the mucus reaches the pharynx, it is swallowed along with the transported particles. Mucociliary clearance represents the lung's primary defense against inhaled irritants. When effective mucociliary clearance is compromised, as in the case of the immotile cilia syndrome, increased vulnerability to environmental exposure, especially to inhaled particles, can be expected (118,233). Among individuals with immotile cilia syndrome, smokers appears to have a greater deterioration of lung function than nonsmokers (168).

In the immotile cilia syndrome, respiratory symptoms appear shortly after birth. Although the severity of pulmonary symptoms may vary from patient to patient, all subjects develop chronic bronchitis characterized by chronic cough and the production of thick, purulent sputum. Chronic sinusitis and otitis media are commonly present. Bronchiectatic changes may develop slowly as the disease progresses (2).

Serum α_1-Antitrypsin Deficiency

α_1-Antitrypsin, a circulating glycoprotein produced in the liver, accounts for 90% of the α_1-globulins in human serum. α_1-Antitrypsin is a broad-spectrum protease inhibitor that acts in the tissues against the proteolytic enzymes released from white blood cells. The major protective role of α_1-antitrypsin depends on its ability to prevent the proteolytic enzymes from attacking the alveolar structures in the lung. It is well established that in cases of profound α_1-antitrypsin deficiency, the destruction of alveolar tissue produces emphysema, which is usually diagnosed during the fourth and fifth decades of life (56).

The level of α_1-antitrypsin is under genetic control. A marked genetic heterogeneity has been demonstrated. The variants form the basis for the protease inhibitor (PI) system of classifying α_1-antitrypsin phenotypes. Most normal individuals in the U.S. population, designated as PIMM, have two M genes. It is estimated that one in 6700 Caucasians has a homozygous deficiency (PIZZ) (56).

Individuals with the homozygous deficiency are clearly at increased risk of developing emphysema. It is a matter of some controversy whether the heterozygote is also at increased risk. It appears that there may be a critical level of α_1-antitrypsin below which the development of emphysema is likely and above which it is unlikely. Heterozygotes who are nonsmokers are usually asymptomatic. However, heterozygotes who smoke and who have a serum α_1-antitrypsin level that is roughly one-third of normal are likely to develop destructive lung disease (56,129). Because smoking depletes α_1-antitrypsin, individuals who already suffer from an α_1-antitrypsin deficiency are particularly vulnerable to cigarette smoke (56). Such individuals may also be unusually vulnerable to high levels of air pollution (15).

Allergy/Hypersensitivity

There are very strong genetic factors predisposing individuals to develop allergic and autoimmune reactions to chemicals. To date, our knowledge of allergy/hypersensitivity and immunologically induced environmental disease is relatively limited.

However, the application of sophisticated immunologic methods has increased our understanding of drug-induced allergy, chemically induced autoimmunity, environmentally induced asthma, and other immunologically induced lung disease (24,76,80, 81). For example, the immunopathological basis of respiratory disorders induced by occupational exposure to such agents as trimellitic anhydride and toluene diisocyanate has been revealed by the evidence that simple low-molecular-weight chemicals acquire sensitization potential after combining with carrier proteins (21,84).

More recently, environmental pollution has been implicated in allergic reactions. Researchers working in widely different parts of the world report that the blood of people living in highly polluted areas contains IgE concentrations significantly higher than those found in people living in less-polluted areas. The studies, performed in school children and adults, excluded smokers and individuals with known allergies (20,91,111).

Reports from Japan indicate that allergic rhinitis from Japanese cedar pollen is now the most common allergic disease. Prior to 1950, allergic pollinosis was quite rare in Japan. Epidemiologic surveys show that the incidence of allergic rhinitis among school children living in areas with high levels of air pollution from auto exhaust is markedly higher than that found in less polluted areas. In some areas with high levels of air pollution, one-third of the children were found to have allergic rhinitis (111). The increase in allergic pollinosis observed in Japan appeared to be related to an increase in the number of diesel cars being used. To investigate this relationship, Miyamoto et al. measured the IgE response in mice immunized intraperitoneally or intranasally with antigens and diesel exhaust particles (162). The results of this study suggest that diesel exhaust particles in the atmosphere have adjuvant activity with respect to IgE antibody production. These findings may, in part, explain the relationship between air pollution and inhalant allergies. The Japanese study will undoubtedly be the forerunner of much additional research. (See Chapter 23 for a discussion of the adverse effects of pollutant exposure on the immune system.)

Age

Unusual susceptibility to environmental assault is exhibited at the two extremes of the life cycle. Much of our awareness of the importance of age-related responses to chemical agents is derived from the study of drugs. However, as foreign chemicals increasingly permeate our environment, concern must be directed to the unique vulnerability of the fetus, the child, and the aged to these agents (9, 12,50,193).

The Fetus, Neonate, Infant, and Young Child

Since developmental immaturity is an important determinant of susceptibility to chemical exposure, the fetus is particularly vulnerable. It is well established, for example, that chemicals may interfere directly with embryonic or fetal development at levels that cause no apparent toxicity to the mother (267). Chemical exposure during fetal development can cause malformations, delays in growth, or death of the embryo/fetus. In addition, altered development and cancer occurring after birth may stem from prenatal exposure. The stage of fetal development at the time of chemical exposure greatly influences its effect. Of note is the unique vulnerability of the fetus to such environmental chemicals as lead, mercury, and polychlorinated biphenyls (68, 210,267). The effects of chemical exposure on fetal development are discussed in detail in Chapter 24.

Chemical exposure during infancy and childhood also poses unusual hazards (107,167,193). The infant and young child are structurally and functionally different from the older child and adult. Many of these differences, which represent normal stages of growth and development, increase the vulnerability of the fetus, infant, and young child to chemical exposure. These differences include rapid cell division, larger body surface area in relation to weight, higher metabolic rate and oxygen consumption, and immature host defenses.

Conditions Underlying Enhanced Susceptibility

Factors Related to Growth and Development

Rapid Cell Division. Rapid cell division during the fetal period was thought to be linked to enhanced susceptibility to radiation-induced cancer (229). Although there is evidence that malignant disease is increased following prenatal x rays, subsequent studies have cast uncertainty on the conclusion that radiation was the primary cause (140,163). It should be noted, however, that diagnostic abdominal x rays during pregnancy irradiate the entire fetus and are thus more carcinogenic (163).

Large Body Surface Area in Relation to Weight. The large surface area available for absorption in the premature infant and newborn (about three times that of the adult) increases their susceptibility. Topically applied agents of similar strengths have more than 2.5 times the systemic availability in the newborn than in the adult. Infants and young children undergoing rapid growth and having large surface areas have a higher resting metabolic rate and oxygen consumption than do adults. On this basis, the volume of inspired air in the resting infant is twice that of the resting adult per unit body weight. Exposure to pollutants in air, per unit body weight, is therefore significantly greater in the infant than in the adult (223).

Immature Host Defenses

In many instances, the increased vulnerability of the young to drugs and environmental chemicals can be traced to immature bodily defenses. Host defenses against environmental assault, discussed in detail in Chapters 6–10, depend on the body surfaces at the portals of entry, the biotransformation and excretion of xenobiotics, and the immune system.

The Body Surfaces at the Portals of Entry. The permeability barrier of the skin provides a defense against the percutaneous absorption of noxious agents. The thickness of the stratum corneum in large part determines the adequacy of the barrier. At birth the stratum corneum appears to be fully developed. Although the skin's barrier function appears to be fully developed in the full-term infant, there are a number of factors that may affect percutaneous absorption in the very young. Apart from the large surface area already mentioned, absorption is greatly enhanced when the skin barrier is damaged or when the site of application is under an occlusive dressing. Occlusion affects absorption by producing changes in the hydration and temperature of the skin. These conditions occur in infants when diapers and rubber pants are used. Thus, a chemical applied to the buttocks of infants, particularly when the skin is irritated, is more likely to have systemic effects (263).

Unlike that of the full-term infant, the skin of the premature infant is more permeable than the skin of the adult. Studies on the development of the stratum corneum reveal that preterm infants lack an intact barrier (224). Studies by Nachman and Esterly reveal that premature infants have increased skin permeability (148,173).

The gastrointestinal tract represents an important site of entry of foreign chemicals for the infant and young child. Breast milk is often a source of foreign chemicals for the young infant. Nearly all chemicals to which the mother is exposed may, to some extent, be excreted in human milk (103,268). The chemicals most frequently found are organochlorine industrial chemicals and pesticides (e.g., DDT and PCBs). It has been suggested that the absorption of some chemicals is greater in the young than in the adult. Much of the evidence comes from studies of drug and metal absorption (97). It has been shown, for example, that suckling rats absorb a greater percentage of ingested lead than do older rats (72). Alexander et al. and Ziegler et al. demonstrated that infants and young children absorb substantially more lead than do adults. Of note is the finding that absorption and retention of lead, expressed as a percentage of intake, increases significantly with increasing lead intake. Absorption and retention of lead were inversely correlated with calcium intake (3,4,272).

Little information is available concerning the relationship between the absorption of inhaled chemical atmospheric pollutants and the continuing postnatal development of the respiratory tract.

Immature Detoxication Processes. Considerable evidence indicates that the activities of many of the enzymes involved in the bioactivation and detoxifying of foreign chemicals are markedly lower in the fetus and neonate than in the adult (191). However, studies indicate that the bioactivation of foreign organic chemicals in the fetus during organogenesis may be of some importance (106).

During the perinatal period, the newborn takes on its own defense against exposure to environmental chemicals. This complex task begins suddenly after birth, when the mother's detoxifying system is no longer available. Immaturity of the detoxifying enzymes increases the neonate's vulnerability to the toxic actions of drugs and environmental chemicals (9,191).

The elimination of xenobiotics from the body involves a number of biochemical reactions, the sum of which is termed biotransformation. These reactions are divided into two phases: in phase I, oxidation, reduction, and hydrolysis of the foreign compounds take place; in phase II, the intermediates produced in phase I are hydrated or conjugated with endogenous compounds to produce soluble end products that can be excreted through the kidney. The endogenous moieties may be glutathione, sulfate, or glucuronic acid. Conjugation with glucuronic acid, or glucuronidation, is used in the detoxication of a wide range of compounds, especially secondary and tertiary compounds of a phenolic nature. A large number of xenobiotics such as polychlorinated biphenyls (PCBs) and hexachlorophene are conjugated with glucuronic acid. Glucuronidation is an excellent example of a biochemical process involved in detoxication that is not fully developed in the neonate. From a developmental perspective, the process of glucuronidation does not become fully mature in the adult sense until about 3 months after birth (188). The biotransformation of drugs and other xenobiotics during postnatal development has been reviewed in detail by Klinger (117).

Impaired Renal Excretion. Immaturity of kidney resulting in impaired renal clearance can be a factor in the newborn's vulnerability to chemical exposure. The function of the renal tubules of the neonate is less mature than that of the glomeruli. This lack of development is particularly important for those chemicals that depend on tubular secretion for their elimination from the body (65).

Immature Immune System. At birth the immune system is not fully developed. Immunocompetence develops relatively quickly, in part as a response to environmental assault. Of the components of the immune system not fully developed at birth, most notable are elements of the nonspecific immune response and circulating immunoglobulins. The course of development of serum immunoglobulins during maturation has been well defined (18). The IgG immunoglobulins are passively transferred during gestation and fall rapidly immediately after birth. They reach very low levels between the second and fourth months. Adult levels of IgG are attained by 5 to 6 years of age. The IgM globulins reach adult levels by 1 year. The serum levels of IgA reach adult levels after 10 to 14 years in contrast to the secretory IgA concentration, which develops rapidly. It seems likely that the relative immaturity of the immune system in the newborn and young child plays a role in their increased susceptibility to infection. It has been demonstrated, for example, that some adults with genetically determined IgA deficiency are at increased risk for respiratory infections. Caution has been advised regarding the potential adverse effects of pollutant exposure on the developing immunologic system (18).

Examples of the Enhanced Susceptibility of the Fetus, Infant, and Young Child to the Toxic Effects of Environmental Chemicals

Data collected over the past 30 years leave little doubt that the fetus, infant, and young child have a special susceptibility to the harmful effects of chemical pollutants (79,99,177,193). Numerous studies provide evidence of their unique vulnerability (19,49,71,99,104,107,152,161,177,181,193,243). In some instances the adverse effects were noted after episodes of environmental contamination. In others the adverse effects were noted after exposure to low levels of environmental chemicals.

Methyl Mercury

The unusual vulnerability of the fetus to methyl mercury exposure was demonstrated by an episode of environmental contamination that occurred in Japan in the mid-1950s. At that time an epidemic of congenital cerebral palsy related to environmental contamination with methyl mercury occurred in villages along Minamata Bay, Japan. The disease was attributed to intrauterine exposures, which resulted when pregnant women ate fish contaminated with methyl mercury. The contamination was traced to the dumping of waste in Minamata Bay by a

vinyl plastics factory. In many cases, severe neurological disorders were seen in the offspring of mothers who suffered no adverse neurological effects (93). In other parts of the world where grain, treated with methyl mercury-containing fungicide, was mistakenly used for animal feed or baking, there were similar consequences.

Polychlorinated Biphenyls

A study by Fein et al. reveals that the fetus may be vulnerable to ordinary maternal dietary levels of PCBs (69). Evidence of fetal PCB exposure was based on a maternal history of eating contaminated fish and on the detection of PCBs in umbilical cord blood. This study suggests that increased fetal exposure to PCBs may be associated with lower birth weight and smaller head circumference.

Lead

A study by Bellinger et al. provides evidence that prenatal exposure to very low levels of lead can cause slower mental growth than expected by the age of 2 (19). The authors performed a prospective cohort study of 249 children from birth to 2 years of age that assessed the relationship between prenatal and postnatal lead exposure and early cognitive development. The results reveal that infants with umbilical cord blood lead levels between 10 and 25 $\mu g/dL$ (0.5–1.2 $\mu mol/L$), when compared with infants with levels under 10 $\mu g/dL$ (0.5 $\mu mol/L$), had stable performance deficits during the first 2 years of life. (For further discussion see Chapter 14.)

Nitrate Exposure

During the first few months of life, infants are uniquely prone to develop acquired methemoglobinemia. This problem was vividly portrayed by Comly in a case report published in 1945. In this early report the young pediatric resident described methemoglobinemia-caused cyanosis in two infants, which resulted from the ingestion of well water containing large amounts of nitrate compounds (49). Subsequent work revealed that the unusual susceptibility of infants to methemoglobinemia depends on two special conditions, one residing in the gastrointestinal tract and the other in the metabolism of neonatal red blood cells.

Young infants characteristically exhibit a low acidity in their gastric juice. This condition allows the growth of sufficient numbers of nitrate-reducing bacteria high in the gastrointestinal tract to convert the generally innocuous ingested nitrate to the much more toxic nitrite (55). The nitrite, once absorbed, converts hemoglobin to methemoglobin. In contrast to hemoglobin, methemoglobin cannot reversibly transport O_2. In addition to their enhanced ability to convert nitrate to nitrite because of the favorable environment for nitrate-reducing bacteria in the stomach, infants also have a decreased capacity to convert methemoglobin back to hemoglobin. The most important pathway for reducing methemoglobin to hemoglobin is dependent on the generation of NADH. The NADH-dependent enzyme previously identified as methemoglobin reductase is now identified as NADH-cytochrome b_5 reductase. The activity of this enzyme, in its soluble form in the red blood cells of neonates, is reduced by 50%. Adult capacity of this enzyme is reached at about 6 months of age (138).

It is suggested that cases of methemoglobinemia in infants are much more common than suspected, particularly in rural areas where individual wells are a major source of drinking water. Farm wells, especially shallow ones, are often contaminated with nitrates and microorganisms. Such contamination occurs during periods of flooding, when runoff may contain chemical fertilizers from nearby fields. Wells are also contaminated by feed lots, barnyards, and septic tank systems (104). Over the last decade, ground water has become increasingly contaminated with nitrate. This pollution stems from the application of chemical fertilizer, which builds up in the soil and then leaches into the groundwater.

Hexachlorophene Exposure

The chlorophenol hexachlorophene was widely used as an antiseptic in soaps and baby powders to prevent *Staphylococcus* infections until it was discovered to cause neurotoxicity and death in premature and neonatal infants. Evidence of brain damage was most evident in small premature infants who received repeated whole-body bathing with 3% hexachlorophene soap and in infants and young children who, because of a manufacturing error, were exposed to baby powder containing over 6% hexachlorophene (220). An outbreak of hexachlorophene poisoning in France affected 204 children, of whom 36 died (151).

Underdeveloped barrier defenses of the skin, the large surface area available for absorption, immature detoxifying mechanisms, and an underdeveloped blood-brain barrier undoubtedly contributed to the unusual susceptibility of the premature infant and neonate to the neurotoxic effects of topically applied hexachlorophene. In addition, the practice of applying talc-containing hexachlorophene to babies' buttocks, which were often inflamed, undoubtedly increased its absorption (115, 116,148,152,178,191).

There were a body of toxicological data and a number of clinical observations that might have alerted the scientific community to the hazards of hexachlorophene exposure (115,116,148,152,178,191, 220). The outbreaks of hexachlorophene poisoning reflect the danger of exposing a susceptible population to a relatively high concentration of a chemical agent without first taking into account the results of toxicological studies and the findings of experienced clinical observers.

Indoor Air Pollutants

A number of epidemiologic studies suggest that the infant and young child may be at increased risk of developing acute respiratory illnesses from air pollution. Indoor air pollution, in particular, poses a risk. There is much evidence that the children of parents who smoke have an increased incidence of a variety of acute respiratory illnesses (243). In addition, a few investigators have noted an association between respiratory illnesses in the young and gas stove emissions (71,155,181).

The Aged

Aging processes can be identified at all levels of biological organization. With increasing age, physiological changes impair the maintenance of homeostasis. Although there are wide individual variations, the cardiac, renal, pulmonary, and immune functions decrease progressively with advancing age. These and other normal physiological changes, coupled with the increased incidence of disease in the aged, work in concert to increase vulnerability to environmental assault. Thus, the aged, though often able to function adequately under resting conditions, are less capable of withstanding environmental stress. They exhibit increased vulnerability to infection, a greater susceptibility to heat and cold, and a predisposition to exhibit toxicity after the administration of drugs (78,85,101,120,149,205,228, 242). Although it is reasonable to assume that the elderly would be more susceptible to the adverse effects of environmental chemicals, the subject of environmental toxicity and the aging process has only recently come under view (12,37,50). Our current understanding of the response of the aged to foreign chemicals is based primarily on their response to drugs (47,85,86).

Background

The relationship between the aging process and exposure to environmental chemicals is complex. It involves the response of the aged to toxic exposure as well as the effects of toxic exposure on the aging process. Little attention has been given to this subject. However, as the population continues to age in all industrial societies, inquiry will be directed to what effects such environmental factors as diet, exercise, pharmaceutical use, and life style have on people as they age. Increasingly, investigators will study the effects of exposure to environmental pollutants on the life span and on the quality of life of an aging population.

As clinicians see larger numbers of elderly patients, they must be aware of the relationship between aging and exposure to environmental chemicals. The gradual age-dependent deterioration of all organ systems means that performance in the elderly is based on fragile reserves. The implications of the waning functional reserves in the aged may be displayed to physicians in two ways: previously masked toxic disorders may become clinically evident, and toxic exposures that cause no apparent problems in the healthy adult may cause clinically evident toxicity in the aged.

Of interest is the proposal by Calne et al. that Alzheimer's disease, Parkinson's disease, and motoneuron disease are linked to environmental damage to specific regions of the central nervous system that are particularly susceptible to age-related neuronal attrition. These workers postulate that environmentally induced damage to the central nervous system remains subclinical for many years and becomes clinically apparent only after the aging process has substantially reduced the structural and functional reserves of the nervous system. This hypothesis stems from the association between environmental factors and certain neurodegenerative diseases (e.g., methylphenyltetrahydropyridine and parkinsonism, poliovirus infection and postpoliomyelitis syndrome, chickling pea ingestion and lathyrism, and trauma and pugilist's encephalopathy) that have long latent periods between the initial exposure and the appearance of clinical symptoms (40). A similar phenomenon may take place in other organs of the body as their functional reserve wanes with increasing age.

Conditions Underlying the Enhanced Susceptibility of the Aged

Many of the structural and functional changes in the elderly that impair their performance also serve to increase their vulnerability to chemical exposure. These changes include reduced host defenses, deteriorating physiological processes, and changes in body composition.

Impaired Host Defenses. It appears that the aged, like the neonate, suffer from impaired host defenses, which are found at the portals of entry, e.g., the skin, lung, and gastrointestinal tract; in the processes of biotransformation and excretion; and within the immune system (see Chapters 6–10).

The Body Surfaces at the Portals of Entry. Age-associated skin changes can increase the vulner-

ability of the elderly to environmental insult. The studies of Roskos et al. indicate that changes in the stratum corneum in the aged skin can increase the percutaneous absorption of drugs and other foreign chemicals (207). Structural and functional changes found in the aged lung, including the loss of elastic recoil, decreased mucus secretion, impaired ciliary action, and decreased cough reflex, all act to reduce pulmonary defenses against environmental assault (194,253,261).

Possible Changes in Detoxication. A decrease in the metabolic clearance of a number of drugs that are biotransformed by oxidative mechanisms has been noted in the elderly. In contrast, the metabolic clearance of drugs biotransformed primarily by conjugative pathways does not appear much changed in the aged. Whether these findings indicate a reduction in the oxidative drug-metabolizing enzymes in the elderly is unclear (47,85,86). It has been suggested that age-associated changes in the metabolism of foreign chemicals might be linked to the increased incidence of cancer in the elderly. No human data are available, however. Animal studies thus far provide limited and conflicting data (25).

Impaired Immune Function. Senescence of the immune system, a well-recognized phenomenon, is associated with a reduction in cell-mediated immunity, T lymphocytes, and thymic factor activity (1,262). Most notable is the involution of the thymus gland, which is complete by the age of 45–50 years.

Impaired Physiological Functions. The particular susceptibility of the aged to the toxic effects of therapeutic drugs can be linked, in part, to their reduced capacity to eliminate these agents. A number of factors including the age-related deterioration of the liver, kidney, and cardiovascular function account for this. Hepatic blood flow declines with age, in part because of reduced cardiac output. The aged have as much as 50% less hepatic blood flow than do young adults. It has been shown that the glomerular filtration rate declines approximately 0.5% per year after the age of 20. It is also well established that there is a 1% annual decline in cardiac output after the age of 30 (12,50,120).

Changes in Body Composition. Alterations in body composition and protein binding affect drug disposition in the aged. With age, there is a marked increase in adipose tissue mass with a decline in lean body mass. As a result, water-soluble drugs have smaller volumes of distribution and greater serum levels in the aged, whereas lipid-soluble agents have an increased volume of distribution. An age-related decline in serum albumin is observed. The degree of drug binding to protein is thereby reduced in the elderly, particularly for extensively bound drugs (86,242).

As noted, virtually all of the data available on the effects of old age on the absorption, distribution, metabolism, and elimination of chemicals have come from the study of drugs. These agents, though distinct in many ways from environmental pollutants, also represent a class of foreign chemicals that must be metabolized and excreted by the body. Information on the response of the elderly to therapeutic drugs may thus provide important clues to their response to environmental pollutants.

Gender-Related Factors

It has long been recognized that the sexes differ in their response to toxic substances. This gender-related difference, best documented in the rat, has been observed in a wide range of species, including the mouse, gerbil, squirrel, hamster, guinea pig, chicken, dog, and human. In humans, male-female differences in the response to toxic exposure have been detected for a few environmental chemicals, which include benzene, lead, and cigarette smoke (36).

A number of authors have noted male-female differences in susceptibility to benzene. Human and animals studies reveal that females are likely to be more susceptible to the effects of benzene (27,60, 100,150,209).

There is evidence that females show a greater hematopoietic response to lead than do males. Studies by Roel et al. and Yamada et al. reveal that lead-exposed nonpregnant women are likely to show an increase in free erythrocyte protoporphyrin at blood lead levels of 20–30 μg/100 mL (1–1.5 μmol/L). In males this increase occurs at blood lead levels of 30–40 μg/100 mL (1.5–1.9 μmol/L). Increases in aminolevulinic acid (ALAU) in females began at blood lead levels less than 35 μg/100 mL (1.8 μmol/L), whereas this response was noted at less than 45 μg/100 mL (2.16 μmol/L) in males. These differences were not explained by lower serum iron levels in the females. Roels et al. indicate that there is no evidence that the slight gender differences in response to lead exposure are associated with a greater susceptibility to lead toxicity in the female (206,270).

Gender differences in response to inhaled pollutants, particularly as related to cigarette smoke, are observed. Numerous studies reveal that men have a higher incidence of cigarette-related pulmonary disease than do women (14,67,235). For equal cigarette usage, men often exhibit as much as twice the difference in cough and phlegm production as do women (87,235). Whether the greater susceptibility to the adverse effects of cigarette smoke observed in men is influenced by their occupational exposures is unclear. Pulmonary function studies reveal that males also differ from females in their response to cigarette smoke. Evidence of small airway disease was found in young male smokers but not in young female smokers (67,159).

Nutritional Factors

Over the past 50 years, there has been a continuing interest in the notion that susceptibility to toxic chemicals can be modified by nutrition. A number of animal studies and a few human studies have investigated the influence of nutrition on the toxicity of environmental pollutants (33,34,46,130, 142,143,192,217). Particularly noteworthy are studies that reveal that dietary deficiencies increase susceptibility to the toxic effects of certain environmental pollutants. These pollutants include such heavy metals as lead and cadmium, such pesticides as carbamate, carbaryl, and parathion, and such atmospheric pollutants as ozone and nitrogen dioxide (46,144,172,262).

Conditions Underlying the Effect of Nutrition on the Toxicity of Environmental Chemicals

Many investigators have looked for biological mechanisms underlying the effects of nutrition on the toxicity of foreign chemicals (52,158,160,192, 259). The interested reader is urged to consult these references. Chapter 9 contains a detailed discussion of the role of nutrition in the metabolism of environmental chemicals.

The relationship between nutrition and toxicity includes the effect of nutrition on the toxicity of environmental chemicals. It also includes the effect of added nutritional demands imposed on the host by the metabolism of environmental chemicals (192). The action of toxic chemicals is dependent on their rate of absorption, on their tissue distribution and reaction with tissue receptors, and on their rate of detoxication and excretion from the body. Although much of our information in this area comes from experiments in laboratory animals, human studies have also provided data.

Alterations in Host Defenses

It appears that changes in nutrition may affect the toxicity of environmental chemicals in part by altering host defenses. As discussed in Chapters 6–10, the body's defenses against environmental insult are found at the portals of entry, e.g., the skin, lung, and gastrointestinal tract; within the immune system; and in the processes of biotransformation and excretion. It has been pointed out earlier that impairment of the host defenses plays a role in the unique susceptibility of the young and the aged to foreign chemicals.

The Body Surfaces at the Portals of Entry. The work of Flanagan et al. demonstrated that dietary factors can be important in the absorption of toxic metals. These workers, using labeled cadmium in the study of human subjects, showed that the absorption of dietary cadmium is increased in subjects with iron deficiency (70). Females were found to have higher cadmium absorption than males, a finding that was in keeping with their lower body stores of iron. Zeigler et al., using metabolic balance techniques, demonstrated that the absorption and retention of lead by infants and young children were inversely related to their intake of calcium (272).

Tissue Distribution. The toxicity of certain xenobiotics may be influenced by their sequestration in bone and adipose tissue. Because of this sequestration, relatively less of the toxic agent is available to reach such important sites as the liver, kidney, and brain. Compounds affected by this process include lead and certain chlorinated hydrocarbons. The size of body adipose tissue stores has been shown, in animals, to affect the toxicity of the chlorinated hydrocarbon dieldrin (113). When this agent was given to dogs, its concentration in fat was inversely related to the total weight of adipose tissue.

Detoxication. Changes in diet can profoundly affect the toxicity of xenobiotics by altering the body's chemical defenses. These defenses hinge on a number of biochemical reactions dependent on mixed-function oxidases, including cytochrome P-450, which are localized in the intracellular endoplasmic reticulum (microsomes). These reactions convert lipophilic compounds into polar metabolites, which are more readily excreted by the kidney. Without this biotransformation, most of the xenobiotics, including chemical carcinogens, would accumulate in the body (see Chapter 9).

Dietary changes may increase or decrease the toxicity of environmental chemicals by altering the levels of key compounds involved in biotransformation (see Chapter 9). For example, protein-deficient diets and specific changes in the type of dietary protein reduce the concentration of cytochrome P-450 (112). Studies indicate that the effect of protein-calorie malnutrition on chemical toxicity is linked to this reduction (45). The reduced activity of the hepatic mixed-function oxidase system inhibits the metabolism of foreign chemicals. This need not always result in greater toxicity, however, for it is now recognized that the same enzyme system that functions to detoxify compounds can also cause the reverse effect, activation. The metabolites of certain xenobiotics may thereby be more toxic than the parent compound. Protein-calorie deficiency thus has a variable effect on the ultimate toxicity of foreign compounds. Animals fed low-protein diets

were more susceptible to the toxic effects of most pesticides (e.g., chlordane, lindane, malathion, DDT, carbaryl, parathion, captan) (126). In contrast, these animals were protected against the toxic effects of such agents as heptachlor and carbon tetrachloride, which are converted to highly reactive metabolites.

The absolute amount of dietary fat affects the activity and induction of the mixed-function oxidase system and the rate of oxidative demethylation. These reactions are lowest in animals on a fat-free diet; they increase with the addition of 10% lard to the diet and are highest when 10% corn oil (50% linoleic acid) is added to the diet. The effect of dietary fat was more pronounced after treatment with phenobarbital, a substance known to induce the activity of mixed-function oxidases (208). It has been shown that a high-fat diet (saturated and unsaturated fatty acids) promotes the incidence of 7,12-dimethylbenz[a]anthracene (DMBA)-induced tumors (42). The tumor-promoting action of a high-fat diet in animals has been recognized for many years (158). Epidemiologic studies also suggest a link between diets high in fat and the incidence of cancer of the breast, prostate, and large intestine (52).

Only recently have investigators focused their attention on the effects of dietary changes on the metabolism of foreign chemicals in humans. A number of investigators have assessed the effects of nutrition on drug metabolism (5,41). The metabolic clearance rates of antipyrine and theophylline were found to be similar in subjects on a high-fat and on a high-carbohydrate diet. In contrast, a high-protein diet increased the clearance of these drugs. Substituting saturated and unsaturated fat in the diet of normal subjects had little effect on the clearance of antipyrine and theophylline (8). Of interest is the finding that drug metabolism may be impaired in cases of protein-energy malnutrition (7,154).

The Antioxidant Effect of Certain Nutrients

The relationship between nutrition and pollutant injury to the lung has been extensively studied in animals. Particular attention has been given to ozone (O_3) and nitrogen dioxide (NO_2), two of the most common oxidant components of photochemical smog. The toxicity of ozone and nitrogen dioxide is based on the ability of these gases to form free radicals. Other compounds such as carbon tetrachloride, paraquat, and silica-containing dust also cause oxidant damage to the lung (225). The lung contains a number of mechanisms to deal with oxidant stress (73); these are discussed in detail in Chapter 7.

Animal studies have shown that the antioxidant action of vitamins E, A, and C protects the lung against oxidant damage (172). Vitamin E, in particular, appears to be an important antioxidant. A number of animal studies demonstrate that a vitamin-E-deficient diet increases the lung's vulnerability to ozone and nitrogen dioxide toxicity. A deficiency of dietary selenium also results in increased oxidant injury to the lung in animals (45,156,172,261).

Thus far, there is no evidence to suggest that, in the case of adequately nourished human subjects, supplemental vitamin E offers protection against exposure to toxic substances (23). It should be recognized, however, that in developed countries frank vitamin E deficiency is most likely to exist in small premature infants and in children with malabsorption of fat. Vitamin E supplementation in premature infants has therefore been proposed for two conditions associated with the delivery of high levels of oxygen: bronchopulmonary dysplasia and retrolental fibroplasia. In the first case, there is no clear evidence that vitamin E administration protects against bronchopulmonary dysplasia. In the second case, it is of interest that Hittner et al. reported a significant decrease in the severity of retrolental fibroplasia in neonates receiving oral supplements of vitamin E (96).

Examples of the Relationship between Nutritional Status and Enhanced Susceptibility to Environmental Pollutants

Perhaps one of the best-documented relationships between nutritional status and altered susceptibility to pollutant toxicity is in the case of lead exposure. Many investigators have demonstrated, in animals and in humans, that lead toxicity in the young is altered by diet, particularly one low in calcium and iron (82,141).

Epidemiologic studies and balance studies in children provide information on the link between their nutrition and their susceptibility to lead toxicity. Balance studies performed after the ingestion of dietary lead reveal that children absorb a greater percentage of ingested lead than do adults (3). Additional studies by Ziegler et al. show not only that children absorb a greater percentage of ingested lead than do adults but that the degree of lead absorption can be influenced by the calcium content of the diet (272). Lead absorption and retention were inversely correlated with the amount of calcium in the diet. Similar effects are noted in rats (157). These findings are particularly important because there is evidence that the developing nervous system suffers most severely from the effects of lead exposure (19,177) (see Chapter 14).

Epidemiologic studies performed by Mahaffey et al. and Sorrell et al. show that dietary calcium intake is lower in children with elevated blood lead levels than in matched controls (105,146,226). A neg-ative correlation between blood lead levels and dietary calcium intake was noted by Sorrell et al. (226). Children with elevated blood lead levels had low serum 1,25-hydroxycholecalciferol concentrations, which returned to normal after chelation therapy (226).

Animal studies reveal that iron deficiency also plays a role in susceptibility to lead intoxication. Studies in rats demonstrate that iron deficiency increases their susceptibility to lead toxicity, whereas increased dietary iron reduces lead concentration in blood, bone, and kidney (146). Iron appears to prevent the accumulation of lead within the body rather than increasing its excretion.

The role of iron deficiency in relation to the severity of lead toxicity has not been well defined in humans. However, many believe that iron deficiency is potentially more important than calcium deficiency in increasing the susceptibility of children to lead exposure. A number of surveys in the United States reveal that iron is the most common nutrient deficiency in the diet of infants and young children. The deficiency occurs most frequently in children under the age of 2 years (189). Mahaffey and Annest show that hematopoiesis is severely interrupted by lead exposure in individuals with a low iron status. Using data obtained from the second National Health and Nutrition Examination Survey, these workers noted a strong association between elevated blood lead levels and low iron status and erythrocyte protoporphyrin levels. Persons with both a low iron status and high blood lead levels were more than six times as likely than other individuals to have an elevated erythrocyte protoporphyrin (143).

The evidence that the quality of nutrition plays a role in the prevention of lead toxicity in children has important clinical and public health implications. Good nutrition must clearly be added to environmental management as a means of preventing lead toxicity. Clinicians should be aware that young children among the urban poor not uncommonly have prolonged lead exposure and diets deficient in both calcium and iron (144).

Nutrition and Carcinogenesis

Although the mechanism of cancer is not fully understood, numerous instances of chemically induced cancer have been documented in animals and man (102,244). This topic is discussed in detail in Chapter 26.

Animal studies provide considerable evidence that foods and components of foods can afford protection against chemically induced neoplasia (255,256,257,259). These components include phenols, indoles, aromatic isothiocyanates, and flavones, which are found in plants, in fruits, and in such cruciferous vegetables as Brussels sprouts, cabbage, cauliflower, and broccoli. When the foods or the specific compounds are added to the diet of experimental animals, they inhibit neoplasia that is induced by such chemical carcinogens as benzo[a]pyrene (BaP), 7,12-dimethylbenz[a]anthracene (DMBA), and polycyclic aromatic hydrocarbons (PAHs) (256,258,260). Vitamin A and many of the retinolds also inhibit the development of cancer in animals exposed to chemical carcinogens (164,179). Epidemiologic studies provide evidence of the role of dietary factors in the development of cancer (50,265,266). Several investigators have found an inverse relationship between the incidence of stomach and colon cancer and the consumption of green and yellow vegetables and members of the cruciferous family (e.g., cabbage, Brussels sprouts, and broccoli) (83,89).

In 1982, the Committee on Diet, Nutrition, and Cancer of the National Research Council published a comprehensive review of the epidemiologic and animal evidence pertaining to the role of diet and nutrition in relation to cancer (52). The Committee emphasized the constraints imposed by a limited data base and by our poor understanding of the mechanistic link between diet and cancer. Nonetheless, on the basis of their in-depth assessment, the National Research Council Committee concluded that "the differences in the rates at which various cancers occur in different human populations are often correlated with differences in diet. The likelihood that some of these correlations reflect causality is strengthened by laboratory incidence that similar dietary patterns and components of food also affect the incidence of certain cancer in animals" (52). Specifically, the Committee concluded that of all the dietary components, the relationship between dietary fat and neoplasia is most convincing. They also concluded that the frequent consumption of certain fruits and vegetables, especially those rich in carotene (i.e., dark green and deep yellow) and cruciferous vegetables (e.g., cauliflower, broccoli, cabbage, and Brussels sprouts) is associated with a decreased risk of cancer of the lung, esophagus, stomach, large intestine, bladder, and larynx (50,190).

In 1989, a publication from the National Research Council explored the relationship between diet and health with particular reference to the role of nutrition in the development of chronic disease (51). In this comprehensive review, evidence for dietary influences on arteriosclerosis, hypertension, obesity, cancer, osteoporosis, diabetes, mellitus, hepatobiliary disease, and dental caries was evaluated. Conclusions are drawn on the effects of nutrient, food, and dietary patterns on health. Dietary recommendations having the potential for reducing the risk of chronic disease are presented. The interested reader is urged to consult this publication.

Behavior/Life Style and Coexisting Exposure to Toxic Chemicals

Enhanced susceptibility depends not only on an altered responsiveness; it also can be affected by exposure to toxic chemicals. There is good evidence that susceptibility to one environmental exposure may be altered by exposure to other environmental agents. Life style and occupation, therefore, as determinants of a particular environmental insult, may modify an individuals's susceptibility to other agents. A most important and obvious example of exposure to toxic chemicals based on life style is smoking. By smoking, many individuals increase their risk of developing such diseases as chronic bronchitis, emphysema, and lung cancer. They may also increase their susceptibility to the toxic effects of industrial and environmental chemicals.

By far the best-documented example of enhanced susceptibility linked to smoking is in the case of asbestos toxicity. Lung cancer is the major disease of asbestos workers, resulting in about 20% of all deaths (92,215). Epidemiologic studies show that the relative risk of death from lung cancer is about 5 with asbestos exposure alone; 10 with smoking, independent of asbestos exposure; and 50 with combined exposure (92). When mortality ratios were calculated for the amount smoked, a gradient in risk was observed. Heavily smoking asbestos workers experience nearly 90 times the risk of succumbing to lung cancer as individuals who were not exposed to tobacco or asbestos. The possible mechanisms underlying this increased susceptibility have been reviewed (48).

The Presence of Disease

It is reasonable to assume that the presence of disease impairs one's ability to withstand the adverse effects of exposure to pollutants. Thus, individuals with impaired renal function may have a reduced capacity to excrete toxic metabolites; those with impaired liver function may have a reduced capacity to detoxify certain pollutants and/or to excrete them in the bile; and those suffering from cardiovascular diseases would be at greater risk from the effects of carbon monoxide than are healthy individuals. Thus far, however, few studies have investigated this problem. The best evidence obtained to date indicates that pulmonary disease, especially asthma, increases one's vulnerability to air pollution (44,75,119,137,218,219,222,264,271).

Two acute episodes of severe air pollution illustrate the unique susceptibility of individuals with preexisting disease, particularly among the elderly. The episodes, occurring in Donora Pennsylvania in 1948 and in London in 1952, resulted in excess morbidity and mortality. Large numbers of people suffered from symptoms of pulmonary disease, and an excessive number of deaths were recorded. Most deaths occurred in the elderly who suffered from heart and lung disease (137,214).

Since asthma is a disease characterized by an increased responsiveness of the airways to a wide variety of stimuli, it is not surprising that asthmatics tend to become symptomatic when confronted with increased levels of air pollution. Several studies have reported increased symptoms and emergency room visits for persons with asthma during times of increased air pollution (44,75,222,264,271).

There is considerable evidence that, under conditions of short-term controlled exposure, asthmatics are more susceptible to inhaled SO_2 than are normal subjects. Sulfur dioxide has repeatedly been shown to be a potent stimulus to bronchoconstriction in asthmatics. This response occurs in concentrations that may at times be found in polluted outdoor air (119,136,218,219).

Enhanced Susceptibility to Chemical Exposure Occurring without Known Cause: Multiple Chemical Sensitivities

The foregoing discussion demonstrates that wide differences exist among individuals in their response to toxic exposure based on such host factors as nutritional and physiological status, age, concurrent disease, and genetic background. In recent years, a number of physicians, particularly those specializing in occupational medicine and allergy, have encountered patients who develop multiple symptoms on exposure to any or a combination of many diverse chemicals at levels far below those observed to cause an adverse response in the general population. The symptoms involve multiple organ systems and commonly include such complaints as fatigue, insomnia, inability to concentrate, dizziness, depression, irritability, and mood swings (53,57,59,153,212). The clinical response cannot be explained by traditional allergic or toxicological principles. Moreover, the increased responsiveness to chemical exposure does not appear to arise from factors currently understood to be associated with enhanced susceptibility. In the absence of identifiable physical, laboratory, and pathological findings, a great deal of confusion and controversy surround those individuals who react so diffusely to very low levels of environmental and occupational exposures.

Controversy has centered specifically on the concepts and practices of a group of physicians known as clinical ecologists. A major concept of clinical ecology states that the wide range of symptoms noted in susceptible individuals is dependent on the "total environmental load." The total environmental load goes beyond exposure to environmental chemicals to include food intolerances, inhalant allergens, and psychosocial stresses. It is further postulated that symptoms involving multiple organ systems occur when the body fails to adapt adequately to ongoing low-level chemical exposure. Chemical agents commonly cited as inducing symptoms in susceptible individuals include tobacco smoke, diesel and vehicle exhaust, paint, organic solvents, pesticides, natural gas fuel, plastics, perfumes, synthetic fabrics, household cleaners, new building material, and poorly ventilated new buildings (16,62,63,195–197,199–203).

Since a major hypothesis of clinical ecology is based on the concept of total environmental load, the term "environmental illness" has been used to identify patients whose symptoms are provoked by a wide range of low-level environmental exposures. However, in the absence of a uniform definition of the clinical disturbance, many other terms such as environmentally induced disease, chemical hypersensitivity syndrome, multiple chemical sensitivities, 20th century disease, total allergy syndrome, ecologic illness, and food and chemical sensitivities have also been used (6). The theories and the methods of diagnosis and treatment used by clinical ecologists have been the subject of several critical reviews (6,39,108,236,238,239).

To gain further insight and spur serious research into the health problems of patients who respond so diffusely to low levels of environmental chemicals, Cullen and the staff of the Yale-New Haven Occupational Medicine Program initiated a dialogue among the various observers of this complex clinical condition (57). At the outset, Cullen defines a syndrome of "multiple chemical sensitivities" (MCS). (The term sensitivities is used without any immunologic or allergic implications.) The designation, applied to a fairly narrow diagnostic group, is proposed as an initial step in studying the problem. MCS is defined "as an acquired disorder characterized by recurrent symptoms, referable to multiple organ systems, occurring in response to demonstrable exposure to many chemically unrelated compounds at doses below those established in the general population to cause harmful effects. No single widely accepted test of physiologic function can be shown to be correlated with symptoms" (58). The discussion that follows presents the various theories and modes of treatment used in patients with multiple chemical sensitivities. The interested reader is urged to consult the review of this complex problem (57).

Widely divergent theories involving psychiatric, immunologic, or toxicologic mechanisms are held regarding the cause of the symptoms encountered in patients with multiple chemical sensitivities (30,31,131,133,198). Some observers believe that many, if not all, of these individuals are suffering from a psychiatric disorder and/or psychosocial disruptions (30,31,212). The constellation of subjective complaints offered by such patients, for the most part, meets the diagnostic criteria for a somatoform disorder or a posttraumatic stress disorder. The extent to which a psychiatric diagnosis is appropriate is uncertain. The role of the immune system in the development of symptoms has also been questioned. Given the specificity of the immune response, the symptomatology noted is considered too wide-ranging, nonspecific, and variable to be based on immunologic mechanisms. In addition, the specific patterns of tissue inflammation and corresponding organ dysfunction known to be associated with immunologically mediated forms of hypersensitivity have not been demonstrated in such patients (237).

Although controversy exists as to the etiology of the clinical condition, there is little disagreement that physicians are seeing patients with multiple chemical sensitivities with some frequency (53,57, 58,153). It is likely that the syndrome will prove to have many manifestations and multiple etiologies. Moreover, it appears that there are many subgroups of patients who are currently identified as having multiple chemical sensitivities (53,88,153,213,221) (see Chapter 14).

IMPLICATIONS OF ENHANCED SUSCEPTIBILITY TO ENVIRONMENTAL AND INDUSTRIAL CHEMICALS

Clinical Implications

The issue of individual differences in susceptibility comes as no great surprise to physicians who have, in practice, observed the unique vulnerability of the fetus, the neonate, the elderly, and those who are ill. Enhanced susceptibility has long been considered in relation to administered drugs. Now, as toxic chemicals increasingly pervade our environment, these agents must also be included as sources of increased risk to susceptible populations. Indeed, it seems likely that the problem will be on the rise as large populations with vast differences in susceptibility are exposed to vast numbers of new environmental and industrial chemicals.

Few specific clinical guidelines or screening tests are available to assist physicians in identifying individuals who are uniquely susceptible to chemical exposure. Yet there is a body of knowledge that should help physicians to deal with this problem. A good working knowledge of the genetic and environmental factors that modify susceptibility will increase the physician's powers of observation and the likelihood that differences in responsiveness will be recognized. A good working knowledge of the vastly complex interrelationship between host factors and susceptibility to toxic chemicals will alert physicians to unexpected and/or unusual responses to toxic exposure. An awareness of individual differences in response to toxic exposure encourages physicians to recommend that uniquely susceptible individuals avoid excessive exposures.

Assessing susceptibility to toxic assault requires a highly individualized approach, an approach used by physicians in the care of patients. Historically, the case report was often used by physicians to provide the first sophisticated observation of a clinical event. It bears emphasis, therefore, that clinical observations are widely recognized to play a critical role in providing the initial evidence of the toxicity of a chemical exposure (161,193). Such observations may also provide important information on individual differences in susceptibility to toxic exposure.

Regulatory Implications

The extent to which society should protect susceptible populations represents a major public policy issue. This complicated issue is far from resolved. Far too little attention has been given to the matter of individual variation in susceptibility to environmental pollutants. This should change, however, as techniques to measure subtle differences in individual response to toxic chemicals become available and as regulatory efforts place greater emphasis on susceptible groups (269).

The EPA has considered the issue of special susceptibility in the standard-setting process for air and water pollutants. Attention has been given to the enhanced susceptibility of the young in the case of nitrate exposure and the formation of methemoglobinemia and in the case of lead exposure and the development of lead toxicity. The enhanced risk of individuals with preexisting disease has also been considered for those with various pulmonary diseases who are exposed to respiratory irritants. In general, however, a more specific and consistent approach is needed in utilizing our knowledge about susceptible groups, particularly in the formulation of environmental health policy and the setting of standards for pollution control. The government's role in the regulation of exposure to environmental chemicals is discussed in Chapter 31.

SUMMARY

Although statistics focus on commonality and its variation, it is well recognized that variability is a major theme in all biological processes. Convincing evidence has emerged that individuals differ markedly in their susceptibility to toxic chemicals. Enhanced susceptibility may stem from a particular inherited trait. It also resides in conditions associated with growth and development and in the process of aging. Host factors such as nutritional, physiological, and health status, gender, life style, and coexisting exposures also influence susceptibility to environmental chemicals. Thus, individuals throughout their lives exhibit greater or lesser degrees of susceptibility to specific toxic exposures.

Of interest is the evidence that nutrition may influence susceptibility to chemical exposure. This information is of considerable significance for the field of environmental and occupational medicine. The basis is now established for an active and consistent research program to evaluate the effect of nutrition, including the use of vitamin and mineral supplements, on the absorption, distribution, detoxication, and excretion of various industrial and environmental chemicals.

REFERENCES

1. Adler WH, Nagel JE: Clinical immunology. In: Principles of Geriatric Medicine, p 413, Andres R, Bierman EL, Hazzard WR (eds.), McGraw-Hill, New York, 1985.
2. Afzelius BA, Mossberg B: The immotile-cilia syndrome (primary ciliary dyskinesia), including Kartagener's syndrome. In: Metabolic Basis of Inherited Disease, 6th ed. p 2739, Scriver CR, Beaudet AL, Sly WS, et al. (eds.), McGraw-Hill, New York, 1989.
3. Alexander FW, Delves HT, Clayton BE: The uptake and excretion by children of lead and other contaminants. In: Proceedings of the International Symposium. Environmental Health Aspects of Lead, Amsterdam, 2–6 October, p 319, Commission of the European Communities, Luxembourg, 1972.
4. Alexander FW, Clayton BE, Delves HT: Mineral and trace-metal balances in children receiving normal and synthetic diets. Q J Med 43:89, 1974.
5. Alvares AP, Anderson KE, Conney AH, et al: Interactions between nutritional factors and drug biotransformations in man. Proc Natl Acad Sci USA 73:2501, 1976.
6. American College of Physicians: Position paper: Clinical ecology. Ann Intern Med 111:168, 1989.
7. Anderson KE, Conney AH, Kappas A: Nutritional influences on chemical biotransformations in humans. Nutr Rev 40:161, 1982.
8. Anderson KE, Conney AH, Kappas A: Nutrition as an environmental influence on chemical metabolism in man. In: Ethnic Differences in Reactions to Drugs and Xenobiotics, p. 439, Kalow W, Goedde HW, Agarwal DP (eds.), Alan R. Liss, New York, 1986.
9. Aranda JV, Stern L: Clinical aspects of developmental pharmacology and toxicology. Pharmacol Ther 20:1, 1983.
10. Atlas SA, Vesell ES, Nebert DW: Genetic control of interindividual variations in the inducibility of aryl hydrocarbon hydroxylase in cultured human lymphocytes. Cancer Res 36:4619, 1976.
11. Autrup H: Host factors in carcinogenesis: Carcinogen metabolism and DNA damage. In: Biochemical and Molecular Epidemiology of Cancer, p 359, Harris CC (ed.), Alan R. Liss, New York, 1986.
12. Baker SR, Rogul M (eds.): Environmental Toxicity and the Aging Processes, Progress in Clinical and Biological Research, Vol. 228, Alan R. Liss, New York, 1987.
13. Bartsch H, Armstrong B (eds.): Host Factors in Human Carcinogenesis, International Agency for Research on Cancer, Lyon, 1982.
14. Beck BD, Weinstock S: Gender. In: Variations in Susceptibility to Inhaled Pollutants, p 127, Brain JD, Beck BD, Warren AJ, et al. (eds.), The Johns Hopkins University Press, Baltimore, 1988.
15. Beckman G, Beckman L, Mikaelsson B, et al: Alpha$_1$ types and chronic obstructive lung disease in an industrial community in northern Sweden. Hum Hered 30:299, 1980.
16. Bell IR: Clinical Ecology, Common Knowledge Press, Bolinas, California, 1982.
17. Bellanti JA (ed.): Immunology III, WB Saunders, Philadelphia, 1985.
18. Bellanti JA, Boner AL, Valletta E: Immunology of the fetus and newborn. In: Neonatology, 3rd ed. p 850, Avery GB (ed.), JB Lippincott, Philadelphia, 1987.
19. Bellinger D, Leviton A, Waternaux C, et al: Longitudinal analyses of prenatal and postnatal lead exposure and early cognitive development. N Engl J Med 316:1037, 1987.
20. Berciano FA, Crespo M, Bao CG, et al: Serum levels of total IgE in nonallergic children. Allergy 24:276, 1987.
21. Bernstein IL: Occupational asthma. Clin Chest Med 2:255, 1981.
22. Beutler E: Hemolytic Anemia in Disorders of Red Cell Metabolism, Plenum Press, New York, 1978.
23. Bieri JG, Corash L, Hubbard VS: Medical uses of vitamin E. N Engl J Med 308:1063, 1983.
24. Bigazzi PE: Autoimmunity induced by chemicals. Clin Toxicol 26:125, 1988.
25. Birnbaum LS: Age-related changes in carcinogen metabolism. J Am Geriatr Soc 35:51, 1987.
26. Borresen AI, Berg K, Magus P: A twin study of aryl hydrocarbon hydroxylase (AHH) inducibility in cultured lymphocytes. Clin Genet 19:281, 1981.
27. Bowditch M, Elkins HB: Chronic exposure to benzene (benzol) 1. The industrial aspects. J Ind Hyg Toxicol 21:321, 1939.
28. Brain JD, Beck BD, Warren AJ, et al. (eds.): Variations in Susceptibility to Inhaled Pollutants, The Johns Hopkins University Press, Baltimore, 1988.
29. Brewer GJ: Annotation: Human ecology, an expanding role for the human geneticist. Am J Hum Genet 23:92, 1971.
30. Brodsky CM: "Allergic to everything": A medical subculture. Psychosomatics 24:731, 1983.
31. Brodsky CM: Multiple chemical sensitivities and other "environmental illness": A psychiatrist's view. Occup Med 2:695, 1987.

32. Calabrese EJ: Pollutants and High Risk Groups, John Wiley & Sons, New York, 1978.
33. Calabrese EJ: Nutrition and Environmental Health. The Influence of Nutritional Status on Pollutant Toxicity and Carcinogenicity, Vol 1: The Vitamins, John Wiley & Sons, New York, 1980.
34. Calabrese EJ: Nutrition and Environmental Health. The Influence of Nutritional Status on Pollutant Toxicity and Carcinogenicity, Vol II: Minerals and Macronutrients, John Wiley & Sons, New York, 1981.
35. Calabrese EJ: Ecogenetics: Genetic Variation in Susceptibility to Environmental Agents, John Wiley & Sons, New York, 1984.
36. Calabrese EJ: Toxic Susceptibility: Male/Female Differences, John Wiley & Sons, New York, 1985.
37. Calabrese EJ: Age and Susceptibility to Toxic Substances. John Wiley & Sons, New York, 1986.
38. Calabrese EJ: Ecogenetics: Historical foundation and current status. J Occup Med 28:1096, 1986.
39. California Medical Association Scientific Board Task Force on Clinical Ecology: A critical appraisal. West J Med 144:239, 1986.
40. Calne DB, Eisen A, McGeer E, et al: Alzheimer's disease, Parkinson's disease, and motoneurone disease: Abiotrophic interaction between ageing and environment? Lancet 2:1067, 1986.
41. Campbell TC, Hayes JR: The effect of quantity and quality of dietary protein on drug metabolism. Fed Proc 35:2470, 1974.
42. Carroll KK, Khor HT: Dietary fat in relation to tumorigenesis. Prog Biochem Pharmacol 10:308, 1975.
43. Cartwright RA, Glashan RW, Rogers JH, et al: Role of N-acetyltransferase phenotypes in bladder carcinogenesis: A pharmacogenetic epidemiological approach to bladder cancer. Lancet 2:824, 1982.
44. Chiaramonte LT, Bongiorno JR, Brown R, et al: Air pollution and obstructive respiratory disease in children. NY State J Med 70:394, 1970.
45. Chow CK: Nutritional influence on cellular antioxidant defense systems. Am J Clin Nutr 32:1066, 1979.
46. Chowdhury BA, Chandra RK: Biological and health implications of toxic heavy metal and essential trace element interactions. Prog Food Nutr Sci 11:55, 1987.
47. Cohen JL: Pharmacokinetic changes in aging. Am J Med 80(Suppl 5A):31, 1986.
48. Collins M, Schenker M: Susceptibility to neoplasia altered by tobacco smoke exposure. In: Variations in Susceptibility to Inhaled Pollutants, p 269, Brain JD, Beck BD, Warren AJ, et al. (eds.), The Johns Hopkins University Press, Baltimore, 1988.
49. Comly HH: Cyanosis in infants caused by nitrates in well water. JAMA 129:112, 1945.
50. Committee on Chemical Toxicity and Aging, National Research Council: Aging in Today's Environment, National Academy Press, Washington, 1987.
51. Committee on Diet and Health, National Research Council: Diet and Health, National Academy Press, Washington, 1989.
52. Committee on Diet, Nutrition, and Cancer, National Research Council: Diet Nutrition and Cancer, National Academy Press, Washington, 1982.
53. Cone JE, Harrison R, Reiter R: Patients with multiple chemical sensitivities: Clinical diagnostic subsets among an occupational health clinic population. Occup Med 2:721, 1987.
54. Cooper WC: Indicators of susceptibility to industrial chemicals. J Occup Med 15:355, 1973.
55. Cornblath M, Hartmann AF: Methemoglobinemia in young infants. J Pediatr 33:421, 1948.
56. Cox DW: α_1-Antitrypsin deficiency. In: The Metabolic Basis of Inherited Disease, p 2409, Scriver CR, Beaudet AL, Sly WS, et al (eds.), McGraw-Hill, New York, 1989.
57. Cullen MR (ed.): Workers with Multiple Chemical Sensitivities, Occup Med 2:655–806, 1987.
58. Cullen MR: Workers with multiple chemical sensitivities: An overview. Occup Med 2:655, 1987.
59. Cullen MR: Multiple chemical sensitivities: Summary and directions for future investigators. Occup Med 2:801, 1987.
60. Deichmann WB, MacDonald WE, Bernal E: The hemopoietic tissue toxicity of benzene vapors. Toxicol Appl Pharmacol 5:201, 1963.
61. de Serres FJ, Pero RW (eds.): Individual Susceptibility to Genotoxic Agents in the Human Population, Plenum Press, New York, 1984.
62. Dickey LD: Clinical genitourinary allergy. Cutis 15:854, 1975.
63. Dickey LD (ed.): Clinical Ecology, Charles C Thomas, Springfield, IL, 1976.
64. Djerassi LS, Vitany L: Haemolytic episode in G6PD deficient workers exposed to TNT. Br J Ind Med 32:54, 1975.
65. Edelmann CM Jr, Spitzer A: The kidney. In: The Physiology of the New Born Infant, p 416, Smith CA, Nelson NM (eds.), Charles C. Thomas, Springfield, IL, 1976.
66. Emery AEH, Anand R, Canford N, et al: Aryl-hydrocarbon-hydroxylase inducibility in patients with cancer. Lancet 1:470, 1978.
67. Enjeti S, Hazelwood B, Permutt S, et al: Pulmonary function in young smokers: Male-female differences. Am Rev Respir Dis 118:667, 1978.
68. Fabro S, Scialli AR (eds.): Drug and Chemical Action in Pregnancy, Marcel Dekker, New York, 1986.
69. Fein GG, Jacobson JL, Jacobson SW, et al: Prenatal exposure to polychlorinated biphenyls: Effects on birth size and gestational age. J Pediatr 105:315, 1984.
70. Flanagan PR, McLeelan JS, Haist J, et al: Increased dietary cadmium absorption in mice and human subjects with iron deficiency. Gastroenterology 74:841, 1978.
71. Florey C du V, Melia RJW, Chinn S, et al: The relationship between respiratory illness in primary school children and the use of gas for cooking III. Nitrogen dioxide, respiratory illness and lung function. Int J Epidemiol 8:347, 1979.
72. Forbes GB, Reina JC: Effect of age on gastrointestinal absorption (iron, strontium, lead) in the rat. J Nutr 102:647, 1972.
73. Fridovich I, Freeman B: Antioxidant defenses in the lung. Annu Rev Physiol 48:693, 1986.
74. Gelboin HV: Editorial retrospectives: Carcinogens, drugs, and cytochromes P-450. N Engl J Med 309:105, 1983.
75. Glasser M, Greenberg L, Field F: Mortality and mor-

bidity during a period of high levels of air pollution. Arch Environ Health 15:684, 1967.

76. Gleichmann E, Kimber I, Purchase IFH: Immunotoxicology: Suppressive and stimulatory effects of drugs and environmental chemicals on the immune system: Review article. Arch Toxicol 63:257, 1989.

77. Goedde HW: Ethnic differences in reactions to drugs and other xenobiotics: Outlook of a geneticist. In: Ethnic Differences in Reactions to Drugs and Xenobiotics, p 9, Kalow W, Goedde HW, Agarwal DP (eds.), Alan R. Liss, New York, 1986.

78. Goidl EA (ed.): Aging and the Immune Response, Marcel Dekker, New York, 1987.

79. Golding J: Child health and the environment. Br Med Bull 42:204, 1986.

80. Goldstein RA, Patterson R: Occupational immunologic lung disease. J Allergy Clin Immunol 70:1, 1982.

81. Goldstein RA, Patterson R: Drug allergy: Prevention, diagnosis and treatment. J Allergy Clin Immunol 74:549, 1984.

82. Goyer RA, Mahaffey KR: Susceptibility to lead toxicity. Environ Health Perspect 1:73, 1972.

83. Graham S, Schotz W, Martino P: Alimentary factors in the epidemiology of gastric cancer. Cancer 30:927, 1972.

84. Grammer LC, Patterson R: Occupational immunologic lung disease. Ann Allergy 58:151, 1987.

85. Greenblatt DJ, Shader RI: Pharmacokinetics in old age: Principles and problems of assessment. In: Clinical Pharmacology and the Aged Patient, p 27, Jarvik LF, Greenblatt DJ, Harman D (eds.), Raven Press, New York, 1981.

86. Greenblatt DJ, Sellers BM, Shader RI: Drug disposition in old age. N Engl J Med 306:1081, 1982.

87. Gulsvik A: Prevalence of respiratory symptoms in the city of Oslo. Scand J Respir Dis 60:275, 1979.

88. Gyntelberg F, Vesterhauge S, Fog P, et al: Acquired intolerance to organic solvents and results of vestibular testing. Am J Ind Med 9:363, 1986.

89. Haenszel W, Kurihara M, Segi M, et al: Stomach cancer among Japanese in Hawaii. J Natl Cancer Inst 49:969, 1972.

90. Haldane JBS: Heredity and Politics, George Allen and Unwin, London, 1938.

91. Hallauer JF, Krämer U, Stiller-Winkler R, et al: Concentration of IgE in sera of children from residential areas with different air pollution. Zentralbl Bakt Hyg 184:432, 1987.

92. Hammond EC, Selikoff IF, Seidman H: Asbestos exposure, cigarette smoking and death rates. Ann NY Acad Sci 330:473, 1979.

93. Hargada M: Chronology and medical report. In: Minamata, p 51, Smith WE, Smith AM (eds.), Holt Rinehart & Winston, New York, 1975.

94. Harris CC: Interindividual variation among humans in carcinogen metabolism, DNA adduct formation and DNA repair. Carcinogenesis 10:1563, 1989.

95. Harris HW, Knight RA, Selin MJ: Comparison of isoniazid concentration in the blood of Japanese and European descent—therapeutic and genetic implications. Am Rev Tuberculosis 78:944, 1958.

96. Hittner HM, Godio LB, Rudolph AJ, et al: Retrolental fibroplasia: Efficacy of vitamin E in a double-blind clinical study of preterm infants. N Engl J Med 305:1356, 1981.

97. Hoffman H: Absorption of drugs and other xenobiotics during development in experimental animals. Pharmacol Ther 16:247, 1982.

98. Human pharmacogenetics and new directions in pharmacogenetics: Fed Proc 43:2295, 1984.

99. Hunt VR, Smith MK, Worth D: Environmental Factors in Human Growth and Development, Banbury Report 11, Cold Spring Harbor Laboratory, New York, 1982.

100. Hunter FT: Chronic exposure to benzene (benzol) II. The clinical effects. J Ind Hyg Toxicol 21:331, 1939.

101. Hurwitz N: Predisposing factors in adverse reactions to drugs. Br Med J 1:536, 1969.

102. International Agency for Research on Cancer: IARC Monographs on the Evaluation of Carcinogenic Risk of Chemicals to Humans, IARC Monographs, Vols 1–42, IARC Monographs Supplement 7, IARC, Lyon, 1987.

103. Jensen AA: Chemical contaminants in human milk. Res Rev 89:1, 1983.

104. Johnson CJ, Bonrud PA, Dosch TL, et al: Fatal outcome of methemoglobinemia in an infant. JAMA 257:2796, 1987.

105. Johnson NE, Tenuta K: Diets and lead blood levels of children who practice pica. Environ Res 18:369, 1979.

106. Juchau MR: Bioactivation in chemical teratogenesis. Annu Rev Pharmacol Toxicol 29:165, 1989.

107. Kacew S, Reasor MJ (eds.): Toxicology and The Newborn, Elsevier, Amsterdam, 1984.

108. Kahn E, Letz G: Clinical ecology: Environmental medicine or unsubstantiated theory. Ann Intern Med 111:104, 1989.

109. Kalow W: Pharmacogenetics: Heredity and the Response to Drugs, WB Saunders, Philadelphia, 1962.

110. Kalow W, Goedde HW, Agarwal DP (eds.): Ethnic Differences in Reactions to Drugs and Xenobiotics, Alan R. Liss, New York, 1986.

111. Kaneko S, Shimada K, Horiuchi H, et al: Nasal allergy and air pollution. Oto-Rhino-Laryngology (Tokyo) 23(Suppl 4):270, 1980.

112. Kato R, Chiesara E, Vassanelli P: Factors influencing induction of hepatic microsomal drug-metabolizing enzymes. Biochem Pharmacol 11:211, 1962.

113. Keane WT, Zabon MR: Dieldrin poisoning in dogs: Relation to obesity and treatment. Br J Ind Med 26:338, 1969.

114. Kellermann G, Luyten-Kellermann M, Shaw CR: Aryl hydrocarbon hydroxylase inducibility and bronchogenic carcinoma. N Engl J Med 289:934, 1973.

115. Kimbrough RD: The toxicity of polychlorinated polycyclic compounds and related chemicals. CRC Crit Rev Toxicol 2:445, 1973.

116. Kligman AM: A biological brief on percutaneous absorption. Drug Dev Ind Pharm 9:521, 1983.

117. Klinger W: Biotransformation of drugs and other xenobiotics during postnatal development. Pharmacol Ther 16:377, 1982.

118. Koenig JQ, Omenn GS: Factors affecting susceptibility to nonneoplastic pulmonary disease: Genetics. In: Variations in Susceptibility to Inhaled Pollutants, p 59, Brain JD, Beck BD, Warren AJ, et al.

(eds.), The Johns Hopkins University Press, Baltimore, 1988.

119. Koenig JQ, Pierson WE, Horike M, et al: Effects of SO₂ plus NaCl aerosol combined with moderate exercise on pulmonary function in asthmatic adolescents. Environ Res 25:340, 1981.

120. Kohn RR: Aging and age-related diseases: Normal processes. In: Relations between Normal Aging and Disease, p 1, Johnson HA (ed.), Raven Press, New York, 1985.

121. Kouri RE, Nebert DW: Genetic regulation of susceptibility to polycyclic hydrocarbon-induced tumors in the mouse. In: Origins of Human Cancer, p 811, Hiatt HH, Watson JD, Winsten JA (eds.), Cold Spring Harbor Laboratory, New York, 1977.

122. Kouri RE, Schectman LM, Nebert DW: Metabolism of chemical carcinogens. In: Genetic Differences in Chemical Carcinogenesis, p 21, Kouri RE (ed.), CRC Press, Boca Raton, 1980.

123. Kouri RE, McKinney GE, Slomiany DJ, et al: Positive correlation between high aryl hydrocarbon hydroxylase activity and primary lung cancer as analyzed in cryopreserved lymphocytes. Cancer Res 42:5030, 1982.

124. Kouri RE, Lubet RA, McKinney GE, et al: Aryl hydrocarbon hydroxylase activity of mice and humans. In: Application of Biological Markers to Carcinogen Testing, p 79, Milman H, Sell S (eds.), Plenum Press, New York, 1983.

125. Kouri RE, Levine AS, Edwards BK, et al: Source of individual variation in aryl hydrocarbon hydroxylase in mitogen-activated human lymphocytes. In: Genetic Variability in Responses to Chemical Exposure, Banbury Report 16, p 132, Omenn GS, Gelboin HV (eds.), Cold Spring Harbor Laboratory, New York, 1984.

126. Krijnen CJ, Boyd EM: The influence of diets containing from 0 to 81 percent of protein on tolerated doses of pesticides. Comp Gen Pharmacol 22:373, 1971.

127. LaDu BN: Pharmacogenetics: Defective enzymes in relation to reactions to drugs. Annu Rev Med 23:453, 1972.

128. Larizza P, Brunetti P, Grignani F: Anie Emolitiche Enzimopenishe. Haematologica (Pavia) 45:1, 1960.

129. Larsson C: Natural history and life expectancy in severe alpha₁-antitrypsin deficiency, PiZ. Acta Med Scand 204:345, 1978.

130. Levander OA, Cheng L (eds.): Micronutrient interactions: Vitamins, minerals, and hazardous elements. Ann NY Acad Sci 355:1, 1980.

131. Levin AS, Byers VS: Environmental illness: A disorder of immune regulation. Occup Med 2:669, 1987.

132. Levine SA, Reinhardt JH: Biochemical pathology initiated by free radicals, oxidant chemicals, and therapeutic drugs in the etiology of chemical hypersensitivity disease. Orthomol Psychiatry 12:166, 1983.

133. Levine AS, McKinney CE, Echelberger CK, et al: Aryl hydrocarbon hydroxylase inducibility among primary relatives of children with leukemia or solid tumors. Cancer Res 44:358, 1984.

134. Lieberman J: Aryl hydrocarbon hydroxylase in bronchogenic carcinoma. N Engl J Med 298:686, 1978.

135. Linch AL: Biological monitoring for industrial exposure to cyanogenic aromatic nitro and amine compounds. Am Ind Hyg Assoc J 35:426, 1974.

136. Linn WS, Venet TG, Shamoo DA, et al: Respiratory effects of sulfur dioxide in heavily exercising asthmatics. Am Rev Respir Dis 127:278, 1983.

137. Logan WPD: Mortality in London fog incident. Lancet 1:336, 1953.

138. Lukens JN: The legacy of well-water methemoglobinemia. JAMA 257:2793, 1987.

139. Luzzatto L, Mehta A: Glucose-6-phosphate dehydrogenase deficiency. In: The Metabolic Basis of Inherited Disease, p 2237, Scriver CR, Beaudet AL, Sly WS, et al. (eds.), McGraw-Hill, New York, 1989.

140. MacMahon B: Some recent issues in low-exposure radiation epidemiology. Environ Health Perspect 81: 131, 1989.

141. Mahaffey KR: Nutrient lead interactions. In: Monograph on Lead Toxicity, p 425, Singhal RL, Thomas JA (eds.), Urban & Schwarzenberg, Baltimore, 1980.

142. Mahaffey KR: Factors modifying susceptibility to lead intoxication. In: Dietary and Environmental Lead: Human Health Effects, p 371, Mahaffey KR (ed.), Elsevier, Amsterdam, 1985.

143. Mahaffey KR, Annest JL: Association of erythrocyte protoporphyrin with blood lead level and iron status in the second National Health and Nutrition Survey, 1976–1980. Environ Res 41:327, 1986.

144. Mahaffey KR, Michaelson IA: The interaction between lead and nutrition. In: Low Level Lead Exposure, p 159, Needlemen HL (ed.), Raven Press, New York, 1980.

145. Mahaffey KR, Rader JI: Metabolic interactions: Lead, calcium and iron. Ann NY Acad Sci 355:285, 1980.

146. Mahaffey KR, Treloar S, Banis TA, et al: Differences in dietary intake of calcium and phosphorus in children having normal and elevated blood lead concentrations. J Nutr 107:, 1976.

147. Mahaffey KR, Annest JL, Roberts J, et al: National estimates of blood lead levels: United States, 1976–1980. Association with selected demographic and socioeconomic factors. N Engl J Med 307:573, 1982.

148. Maibach HI, Boisits EK (eds.): Neonatal Skin: Structure and Function, Marcel Dekker, New York, 1982.

149. Makinodan T, Hirokawa K: Normal aging of the immune system. In: Relations between Normal Aging and Disease, p 117, Johnson HA (ed.), Raven Press, New York, 1985.

150. Mallory TB, Gall EA, Brickley WJ: Chronic exposure to benzene (benzol) III. The pathologic results. J Ind Hyg Toxicol 21:355, 1939.

151. Martin-Bouyer G, Toga O, Lebreton R, et al: Outbreak of accidental hexachlorophene poisoning in France. Lancet 1:91, 1982.

152. Marzulli FN, Maibach H: Relevance of animal models: The hexachlorophene story. In: Animal Models in Dermatology, p 156, Maibach H (ed.), Churchill Livingstone, Edinburgh, 1975.

153. McLellan RK: Multiple chemical hypersensitivities. Ann Intern Med 111:953, 1989.

154. Mehta S: Drug disposition in children with protein energy malnutrition. J Pediatr Gastroenterol Nutr 2: 407, 1983.

155. Melia RJW, Florey C du V, Morris RW, et al: Child-

hood respiratory illness and home environment. II. Association between respiratory illness and nitrogen dioxide, temperature and relative humidity. Int J Epidemiol 11:164, 1982.

156. Menzel DB: Protection against environmental toxicants. In: Vitamin E: A Comprehensive Treatise, p 474, Machlin LJ (ed.), Marcel Dekker, New York, 1980.

157. Meredith PA, Moore MR, Goldberg A: The effect of calcium on lead absorption in rats. Biochem J 166:531, 1972.

158. Meydani M: Dietary effects on detoxification processes. In: Nutritional Toxicology, Vol II, p 1, Hathcock JN (ed.), Academic Press, Orlando, 1987.

159. Michaels R, Sigurdson M, Thurlbeck S, et al: Elastic recoil of the lung in cigarette smokers: The effect of nebulized bronchodilator and cessation of smoking. Am Rev Respir Dis 119:707, 1979.

160. Miller ON: Nutrition and drug metabolism. Fed Proc 35:2459, 1976.

161. Miller RW: How environmental effects on child health are recognized. Pediatrics 53:792, 1974.

162. Miyamoto R, Takafuji S, Suzuki S, et al: Environmental factors in the development of allergic reactions. In: Toxicological and Immunological Aspects of Drug Metabolism and Environmental Chemicals, p 553, Estabrook RW, Lindenlaub E, Oesch F, et al. (eds.), FK Schattauer Verlag, Stuttgart, 1988.

163. Mole RH: Irradiation of the embryo and fetus. Br J Radiol 60:17, 1987.

164. Moon RC, McCormick DL, Mehta RG: Inhibition of carcinogenesis by retinoids. Cancer Res 43 [Suppl]: 2469s, 1983.

165. Moore-Ede MC, Czeisler CA, Richardson GS: Circadian timekeeping in health and disease. Part 1: Basic properties of circadian pacemakers. N Engl J Med 309:469, 1983.

166. Moore-Ede MC, Czeisler CA, Richardson GS: Circadian timekeeping in health and disease. Part 2: Clinical implications of circadian rhythmicity. N Engl J Med 309:530, 1983.

167. Morselli PL, Garattini S, Sereni F: Basic and Therapeutic Aspects of Perinatal Pharmacology, Raven Press, New York, 1975.

168. Mossberg B, Afzelius BA, Ellasson R, et al: On the pathogenesis of obstructive lung disease: A study in the immotile-cilia syndrome. Scand J Respir Dis 59: 55, 1978.

169. Motulsky A: Pharmacogenetics. Prog Med Genet 3: 49, 1964.

170. Motulsky AG: Ecogenetics: Genetic variation in susceptibility to environmental agents. In: Human Genetics, Proceedings of the Fifth International Congress on Human Genetics, p 375, Excerpta Medica, Amsterdam, 1976.

171. Murray RF Jr: Tests of so-called genetic susceptibility. J Occup Med 28:1103, 1986.

172. Mustafa MG, Tierney DF: Biochemical and metabolic changes in the lungs with oxygen, ozone, and nitrogen dioxide toxicity. Am Rev Respir Dis 118:1061, 1978.

173. Nachman RI, Esterly NB: Increased skin permeability in preterm infants. J Pediatr 79:628, 1971.

174. Nebert DW: Genetic control of drug metabolism. In:

Pharmacologic Intervention in the Aging Process, p 55, Roberts J, Adelman R, Cristofalo VJ (eds.), Plenum Press, New York, 1977.

175. Nebert DW, Gonzalez FJ: P450 genes: Structure, evolution and regulation. Annu Rev Biochem 56:945, 1987.

176. Nebert DW, Levitt RC, Pelkonen O: Genetic variation in metabolism of chemical carcinogens associated with susceptibility to tumorigenesis. In: Carcinogens: Identification and Mechanisms of Actions, p 157, Griffin AC, Shaw CR (eds.), Raven Press, New York, 1979.

177. Needleman HL: The persistent threat of lead: A singular opportunity. Am J Public Health 79:643, 1989.

178. Neims AH, Warner M, Yang G, et al: Relative deficiency in the elimination of hexachlorophene by neonatal rodents. In: Basic and Therapeutic Aspects of Perinatal Pharmacology, p 177, Morselli PL, Garattini S, Sereni F (eds.), Raven Press, New York, 1975.

179. Netteshein P, Williams ML: The influence of vitamin A on the susceptibility of the rat lung to 3-methylcholanthrene. Int J Cancer 17:351, 1976.

180. Office of Technology Assessment, Congress of the United States: The Role of Genetic Testing in the Prevention of Occupational Disease, US Government Printing Office, Washington, 1983.

181. Ogston SA, Florey C du V, Walker CHM: The Tayside infant morbidity and mortality study: Effect on health of using gas for cooking. Br Med J 290:957, 1985.

182. Omenn GS: Predictive identification of hypersusceptible individuals. J Occup Med 24:369, 1982.

183. Omenn GS: Risk assessment, pharmacogenetic, and ecogenetics. In: Genetic Variability in Responses to Chemical Exposure, Banbury Report 16, p 3, Omenn GS, Gelboin HV (eds.), Cold Spring Harbor Laboratory, New York, 1984.

184. Omenn GS: Susceptibility to occupational and environmental exposures to chemicals. In: Ethnic Differences in Reactions to Drugs and Xenobiotics, p 527, Kalow W, Goedde HW, Agarwal DP (eds.), Alan R Liss, New York, 1986.

185. Omenn GS: Heredity and environmental interactions. Prog Clin Biol Res 241:323, 1987.

186. Omenn GS, Gelboin HV (eds.): Genetic Variability in Responses to Chemical Exposure, Banbury Report 16, Cold Spring Harbor Laboratory, New York, 1984.

187. Omenn GS, Motulsky AG: "Eco-genetics": Genetic variation in susceptibility to environmental agents. In: Genetic Issues in Public Health and Medicine, p 83, Cohen BH, Lilienfeld AM, Huang PC (eds.), Charles C Thomas, Springfield, IL, 1978.

188. Onishi S, Kawade N, Itoh S, et al: Postnatal development of uridine diphosphate glucuronyltransferase activity towards bilirubin and 2-aminophenol in human liver. Biochem J 184:705, 1979.

189. Owen G, Lippman G: Nutritional status of infants and young children. Pediatr Clin North Am 24:211, 1977.

190. Palmer S: Diet, nutrition, and cancer. Prog Food Nutr Sci 9:283, 1985.

191. Parke DV: Development of detoxication mechanisms in the newborn. In: Toxicology and the Newborn, p 1,

Kacew S, Reasor MJ (eds.), Elsevier, Amsterdam, 1984.

192. Parke DV, Ionnides C: The role of nutrition in toxicology. Annu Rev Nutr 1:207, 1981.

193. Proceedings of a Conference on the Susceptibility of the Fetus and Child to Chemical Pollutants: Pediatrics 53(Suppl):777, 1974.

194. Puchelle E, Zahm JM, Bertrand A: Influence of age on bronchial mucociliary transport. Scand J Respir Dis 60:307, 1979.

195. Randolph TC: Depressions caused by home exposure to gas and combustion products of gas, oil, and coal. J Lab Clin Med 46:942, 1955.

196. Randolph TC: The specific adaptation syndrome. J Lab Clin Med 48:934, 1956.

197. Randolph TC: Human Ecology and Susceptibility to the Chemical Environment. Charles C Thomas, Springfield, IL, 1962.

198. Randolph TC: Emergence of the specialty of clinical ecology. Clin Ecol 2:65, 1982.

199. Randolph TG, Moss RW: An Alternative Approach to Allergies, Lippincott & Cromwell, Philadelphia, 1980.

200. Rea WJ: Environmentally triggered small vessel vasculitis. Ann Allergy 38:245, 1977.

201. Rea WJ: Food and chemical susceptibility after environmental chemical overexposure: Case history. Ann Allergy 41:101, 1978.

202. Rea WJ: Environmentally triggered cardiac disease. Ann Allergy 40:243, 1978.

203. Rea WJ, Peters DW, Smiley RE, et al: Recurrent environmentally triggered thrombophlebitis: A five year followup. Ann Allergy 47:338, 1981.

204. Reinhardt CF: Chemical hypersusceptibility. J Occup Med 20:319, 1978.

205. Richey DP, Bender AD: Pharmacokinetic consequences of aging. Annu Rev Pharmacol Toxicol 17:49, 1977.

206. Roels HA, Balis-Jacques MN, Buchet JP, et al: The influence of sex and chelation therapy on erythrocyte protoporphyrin and U-ALA in lead exposed workers. J Occup Med 21:527, 1979.

207. Roskos KV, Guy RH, Maibach HI: Percutaneous absorption in the aged. In: The Aging Skin, p 455, Gilchrest BA (ed.), WB Saunders, Philadelphia, 1986.

208. Rowe L, Wills ED: The effect of dietary lipids and vitamin E on lipid peroxide formation, cytochrome P-450 and oxidative demethylation in the endoplasmic reticulum. Biochem Pharmacol 25:175, 1976.

209. Sato A, Nakajima T, Fujiwara Y, et al: Kinetic studies on sex differences in susceptibility to chronic benzene intoxication with special reference to body fat content. Br J Ind Med 32:321, 1975.

210. Schardein JL: Chemically Induced Birth Defects. Marcel Dekker, New York, 1985.

211. Schottenfeld D: Genetic and environmental factors in human carcinogenesis. J Chron Dis 39:1021, 1986.

212. Schottenfeld RS: Workers with multiple chemical sensitivities: A psychiatric approach to diagnosis and treatment. Occup Med 2:739, 1987.

213. Schottenfeld RS, Cullen MR: Recognition of occupation-induced posttraumatic stress disorders. J Occup Med 28:365, 1986.

214. Schrenk HH, Heimann H, Clayton GD, et al: Air pollution in Donora, PA. Epidemiology of the unusual smog episode of October, 1948. Public Health Bulletin 306, Federal Security Agency, Public Health Service, Division of Industrial Hygiene. US Government Printing Office, Washington, 1949.

215. Selikoff IJ, Hammond EC, Seldman H: Mortality experience of insulation workers in the United States and Canada, 1943–1976. Ann NY Acad Sci 330:91, 1979.

216. Shaikh RA, Warren AJ: Factors affecting susceptibility to neoplastic pulmonary disease. In: Variations in Susceptibility to Inhaled Pollutants, p 223, Brain JD, Beck BD, Warren AJ, et al. (eds.), The Johns Hopkins University Press, Baltimore, 1988.

217. Shakman RA: Nutritional influences on the toxicity of environmental pollutants. Arch Environ Health 28:105, 1974.

218. Sheppard D, Wong SC, Uehara CF, et al: Lower threshold and greater bronchomotor responsiveness of asthmatic subjects to sulfur dioxide. Am Rev Respir Dis 122:873, 1980.

219. Sheppard D, Salsho A, Nadel JA, et al: Exercise increases sulfur dioxide-induced bronchoconstriction in asthmatic subjects. Am Rev Respir Dis 123:486, 1981.

220. Shuman RM, Leech RW, Alvord EC Jr: Neurotoxicity of hexachlorophene in humans. II: A clinical pathological study of 46 premature infants. Arch Neurol 32:320, 1975.

221. Shusterman D, Balmes J, Cone J: Behavioral sensitization to irritants/odorants after acute overexposures. J Occup Med 30:66, 1988.

222. Shy CM, Goldsmith JR, Hackney JD, et al: Health effects of air pollution. American Thoracic Society, New York, 1978.

223. Sinclair D: Human Growth After Birth. 3rd ed., Oxford University Press, Oxford, 1978.

224. Singer EJ, Wegmann, PC, Lehman MD, et al: Barrier development, ultrastructure, and sulfhydryl content of the fetal epidermis. J Soc Cosmet Chem 22:119, 1971.

225. Smith LL: The response of the lung to foreign compounds that produce free radicals. Annu Rev Physiol 48:681, 1986.

226. Sorrell M, Rosen JF, Roginsky MR: Interactions of lead, calcium, vitamin D, and nutrition in lead-burdened children. Arch Environ Health 32:160, 1977.

227. Spatz L, Bloom AD, Paul NW (eds.): Detection of Cancer Predisposition: Laboratory Approaches, Monograph No. 3, March of Dimes Birth Defects Foundation, White Plains, New York, 1990.

228. Steel K, Gertman PM, Crescenze C, et al: Iatrogenic illness on a general medical service at a university hospital. N Engl J Med 304:638, 1981.

229. Stewart A, Kneale GW: Radiation dose effects in relation to obstetric x-rays and childhood cancer. Lancet 1:1185, 1970.

230. Stokinger HE, Mountain JT: Tests for hypersusceptibility to hemolytic chemicals. Arch Environ Health 6:495, 1963.

231. Stokinger HE, Mountain JT: Progress in detecting the worker hypersusceptible to industrial chemicals. J Occup Med 9:537, 1967.

232. Stokinger HE, Scheel LD: Hypersusceptibility and genetic problems in occupational medicine: A consensus report. J Occup Med 15:564, 1973.

233. Strope GL, Stempel DA: Risk factors associated with the development of chronic lung disease in children. Pediatr Clin North Am 31:757, 1984.

234. Szeinberg A, Adam A, Myers F, et al: A hematological survey of industrial workers with enzyme-deficient erythrocytes. Arch Ind Health 20:510, 1959.

235. Tager IB, Speizer FE: Risk estimates for chronic bronchitis in smokers: A study of male-female differences. Am J Respir Dis 113:619, 1976.

236. Terr AI: Environmental illness: A clinical review of 50 cases. Arch Intern Med 146:145, 1986.

237. Terr AI: Clinical ecology. J Allergy Clin Immunol 79:423, 1987.

238. Terr AI: "Multiple chemical sensitivities": Immunologic critique of clinical ecology theories and practice. Occup Med 2:683, 1987.

239. Terr AI: Clinical ecology in the workplace. J Occup Med 31:257, 1989.

240. Tokuhata GK, Lilienfeld AM: Familial aggregation of lung cancer in humans. J Natl Cancer Inst 30:289, 1963.

241. Tokuhata GK: Familial factors in human lung cancer and smoking. Am J Public Health 54:24, 1964.

242. Triggs EJ, Nation RI: Pharmacokinetics in the aged: A review. J Pharmacokinet Biopharm 3:387, 1975.

243. US Dept of Health and Human Services: The Health Consequences of Involuntary Smoking. A Report of the Surgeon General, Office of Smoking and Health, DHHS Publ No (CDC)87–8398, US Government Printing Office, Washington, 1986.

244. Vainio H, Hemminki K, Wilborn J: Data on the carcinogenicity of chemicals in the IARC Monographs program. Carcinogenesis 6:1653, 1985.

245. Vesell ES: Advances in pharmacogenetics. In: Progress in Medical Genetics IX, p 291, Steinberg AG, Bearn AG (eds.), Grune & Stratton, New York, 1973.

246. Vesell ES: Gene-environment interactions in drug metabolism. In: Clinical Pharmacology and Therapeutics, Proceedings of the First World Conference, London and Basingstoke, p 63, Macmillan, London, 1980.

247. Vesell ES: On the significance of host factors that affect drug disposition in man. Clin Pharmacol Ther 31:1, 1982.

248. Vesell ES: Effects of human physiologic and genetic variability on the development and expression of pollutant-related diseases. In: Environmental Impacts on Human Health: The Agenda for Long-term Research and Development, p 35, Draggan S, Cohrssen JJ, Morrison RE (eds.), Praeger, London, 1987.

249. Vesell ES: Pharmacogenetic perspectives on susceptibility to toxic industrial chemicals. Br J Ind Med 44: 505, 1987.

250. Vesell ES, Penno MB: Assessment of methods to identify sources of interindividual pharmacokinetic variations. Clin Pharmacokinet 8:378, 1983.

251. Vine MF, McFarland LT: Markers of susceptibility. In: Biological Markers in Epidemiology, p 196, Hulka BS, Wilcosky TC, Griffith, Oxford University Press, Oxford, 1990.

252. Vogel F: Modern problems of human genetics. Ergeb Inn Med Kinderheilkd 12:52, 1959.

253. Wanner A: State of the art: Clinical aspects of mucociliary transport. Annu Rev Respir Dis 116:73, 1977.

254. Ward E, Paigen B, Steenland K, et al: Aryl hydrocarbon hydroxylase in persons with lung or laryngeal cancer. Int J Cancer 22:384, 1978.

255. Wattenberg LW: Inhibition of carcinogenic effects of polycyclic hydrocarbons by benzyl isothiocyanate and related compounds. J Natl Cancer Inst 58:395, 1977.

256. Wattenberg LW: Inhibition of chemical carcinogenesis by antioxidants. In: Carcinogenesis. Vol 5: Modifiers of Chemical Carcinogenesis, p 85, Slage TJ (ed.), Raven Press, New York, 1980.

257. Wattenberg LW: Inhibitors of chemical carcinogens. J Environ Pathol Toxicol 3:35, 1980.

258. Wattenberg LW: Inhibitors of chemical carcinogens. In: Cancer: Achievements, Challenges, and Prospects for the 1980s, Vol 1, p 517, Burchenal JH, Oettgen HF (eds.), Grune & Stratton, Orlando, 1981.

259. Wattenberg LW: Chemoprevention of cancer. Cancer Res 45:1, 1985.

260. Wattenberg LW, Loub WD: Inhibition of polycyclic hydrocarbon-induced neoplasia by naturally occurring indoles. Cancer Res 38:1410, 1978.

261. Weinstock S, Beck BD: Age and nutrition. In: Variations in Susceptibility to Inhaled Pollutants, p 104, Brain JD, Beck BD, Warren AJ, et al. (eds.), The Johns Hopkins University Press, Baltimore, 1988.

262. Weksler ME: Biological basis and clinical significance of immune senescence. In: Clinical Geriatrics, 3rd ed., p 57, Rossman I (ed.), JB Lippincott, Philadelphia, 1986.

263. Wester RC, Maibach H: Comparative percutaneous absorption. In: Neonatal Skin, p 137, Maibach H, Boisits EK (eds.), Marcel Dekker, New York, 1982.

264. Whittmore AS, Korn EL: Asthma and air pollution in the Los Angeles area. Am J Public Health, 70:687, 1980.

265. Willett WC, MacMahon B: Diet and cancer: An overview. First of two parts. N Engl J Med 310:633, 1984.

266. Willett WC, MacMahon B: Diet and cancer: An overview. Second of two parts. N Engl J Med 310:697, 1984.

267. Wilson JF: Environment and Birth Defects. Academic Press, New York, 1973.

268. Wolff MS: Occupationally derived chemicals in breast milk. Am J Ind Med 4:259, 1983.

269. Woodhead AD, Bender MA, Leonard RC: Phenotypic Variations in Populations: Relevance to Risk Assessment, Plenum Press, New York, 1988.

270. Yamada DY, Kido T, Okada A, et al: Studies on the biological effects of low level lead exposures. Part 2: Biochemical responses and subjective symptoms in female lead workers. Jpn J Ind Health 23:383, 1981.

271. Zeidberg LD, Horton RJM, Landau E: The Nashville air pollution study V. Mortality from disease of the respiratory system in relation to air pollution. Arch Environ Health 15:214, 1967.

272. Ziegler EE, Edwards BB, Jensen RL, et al: Absorption and retention of lead by infants. Pediatr Res 12:29, 1978.

RECOMMENDED READINGS

Baker SR, Rogul M (eds.): Environmental Toxicity and the Aging Process, Alan R. Liss, New York, 1987.

Brain JD, Beck BD, Warren AJ, et al. (eds.): Variations in Susceptibility to Inhaled Pollutants. The Johns Hopkins University Press, Baltimore, 1988.

Calabrese EJ: Toxic Susceptibility: Male/Female Differences, John Wiley & Sons, New York, 1985.

Cooper RL, Goldman JM, Harbin TJ (eds.): Aging and Environmental Toxicology: Biological and Behavioral Perspectives, The Johns Hopkins University Press, Baltimore, 1991.

de Serres FJ, Pero RW (eds.): Individual Susceptibility to Genotoxic Agents in the Human Population, Plenum Press, New York, 1984.

Grandjean P, Idle Jr. J, Kello D (eds.): Ecogenetics: Genetic Predisposition to Toxic Effects of Chemicals, Routledge, Chapman & Hall, New York, 1991.

Kacew S, Reasor MJ (eds.): Toxicology and the Newborn. Elsevier, Amsterdam, 1984.

Kalow W, Goedde HW, Agarwal DP (eds.): Ethnic Differences in Reactions to Drugs and Xenobiotics, Alan R Liss, New York, 1986.

Omenn GS, Gelboin HV (eds.): Genetic Variability in Responses to Chemical Exposure. Banbury Report 16, Cold Spring Harbor Laboratory, New York, 1984.

Spatz L, Bloom AD, Paul NW (eds.): Detection of Cancer Predisposition: Laboratory Approaches, Monograph No. 3, March of Dimes Birth Defects Foundation, White Plains, New York, 1990.

Woodhead AV, Bender MA, Leonard RC (eds.): Phenotypic Variation in Populations: Relevance to Risk Assessment, Plenum Press, New York, 1988.

Part V

DISORDERS ASSOCIATED WITH EXPOSURE TO ENVIRONMENTAL CHEMICALS AND PHYSICAL AGENTS

13. DISORDERS OF THE NERVOUS SYSTEM

John R. Taylor

INTRODUCTION

The nervous system, in spite of its seemingly protected environment, is vulnerable to the effects of a host of toxins. Although the precise reasons for this vulnerability remain uncertain, the heterogeneity of cell types, the coatings required by many of the axons, and the rich blood supply needed by the metabolically active cells all present opportunities for many toxins to exert a noxious effect. Once attacked, the nervous system repairs itself poorly if at all, and the resulting dysfunction often endures. At times minor neural damage can create noticeable, even disabling, symptoms. Numerous authors have reviewed the effects of neurotoxic exposure (14,15,42,46,86,103,115).

The extent of neurological impairment from environmental toxins is difficult to know. The volitional toxic exposure to such "recreational" chemicals as ethanol, marijuana, and psychoactive drugs constitutes a problem of such magnitude that the effects of environmental toxins would seem to fade into obscurity. Yet the surreptitious and unwanted effects of environmental poisoning are seen as heinous and unacceptable. The extent of noxious environmental damage to the nervous system, as gauged by overt epidemics (e.g., the contamination of

flour by insecticides), seems small and confined. Unknown, however, is the extent of mild to moderate neurological disease, occurring in a deceptively sporadic pattern, that is caused by environmental pollution. Every neurologist, for example, has seen the patient with peripheral neuropathy, ataxia, or myelopathy with no identifiable cause and has pursued the matter no further than ordering the usual routine tests. Strident press reports of pollution crises add to the complexity of the problem and often cause the clinician to forget that environmental pollution, generally ubiquitous and in low concentration, may play a part in any patient's illness.

The physician trained to diagnose toxic illness clearly plays a critical role in the recognition of environmentally induced disease. Industrial engineers and hygienists can detect contamination, and toxicological animal studies can suggest potential human responses, but until the physician is trained and provided with the means to diagnose toxic illness, such illness will continue to flourish.

Chemical identification of toxic substances in the blood has achieved great accuracy in recent years; nevertheless, the "toxic screen" of blood or urine ordered by many physicians often does little more than provide a subterfuge from more thoughtful investigation. The matter is further complicated by the sensitivity of many chemical determinations. Such determinations often provide the physician with a number in a vacuum—a number with unknown significance. In all obscure cases, consultation with an experienced toxicologist may be far

Principles and Practice of Environmental Medicine, edited by Alyce Bezman Tarcher. Plenum Medical Book Company, New York, 1992.

more useful to the clinician than a battery of laboratory tests.

The discussion that follows focuses on the relationship between exposure to environmental chemicals and neurological disease. This issue is addressed with the realization that the number of neurotoxins that pose a significant health threat is largely unknown. Anger and Johnson recently listed more than 850 chemicals that have been reported to exert behavioral and neurotoxic effects (12). Of particular concern are the neurobehavioral effects of toxic exposure. Neurobehavioral changes may be the first indication of damage to the nervous system. This subject is discussed in Chapter 14.

ENVIRONMENTAL CHEMICALS ASSOCIATED WITH ADVERSE EFFECTS ON THE NERVOUS SYSTEM

From the wide range of chemicals known to cause neurological disease, the following groups are discussed: (1) the pesticides, (2) the halogenated industrial chemicals, including dioxin and the biphenyls, (3) the metals, including aluminum, arsenic, lead, and mercury, and (4) the solvents. Most neurotoxic events arise from exposure to pesticides, metals, and solvents. As seen in Table 13-1, neurotoxic exposures are encountered in both occupational and environmental settings. The ubiquitous

TABLE 13-1. Neurological Symptoms and Associated Toxic Substance Exposures[a]

Neurological effect	Neurotoxin	Major uses/sources of exposures[b]
Ataxia	Acrylamide	Polymer production, soil stabilization, gel chromatography, paper making, treatment of potable water and foods
	Chlordane	Agricultural industry, pesticide formulators and pest control workers
	Chlordecone (Kepone)	Processors or formulators of pesticides (use canceled by EPA in 1978)
	DDT	Herbicide for control of broad-leaf plants and plant growth regulator, workers engaged in manufacture, formulation, or application
	n-Hexane	Lacquers, printing inks, stains
	Manganese	Iron, steel industry, welding operations, metal operations of high manganese, fertilizers, manufacturers of fireworks, or matches, manufacturers using oxidation catalysts
	Mercury (especially methyl mercury)	Scientific instruments, amalgams, photography, taxidermy, pigments, electrical industry, felt making, textiles
	Methyl n-butyl ketone (MBK)	Paints, varnishes, quick-drying inks, lacquers, metal-cleaning compounds, paint removers
	Methyl chloride	Extractant for greases, oils, and resins. Solvent in synthetic rubber industry. Refrigerant, propellant in polystyrene foam production. Local anesthetic (freezing)
	Toluene	Manufacture of benzene, solvent for paints and coatings; component of automobile and aviation fuels; chemical fuel for manufacture of other chemical agents
Sacral neuropathy	Dimethylaminopropionitrile (DMAPN)	Manufacture of flexible polyurethane foams
Constricted visual fields	Mercury	*See Ataxia
Cranial neuropathy	Carbon disulfide	Manufacturers of viscose rayon; preservatives, rubber cement, electroplating industry, paints, textiles, varnishes
	Trichloroethylene	Degreasers; painting industry, paints, lacquers, varnishes; dry cleaning industry; rubber solvents, adhesive in shoe and boat industry; process of extraction of caffeine from coffee

TABLE 13-1. (*Continued*)

Neurological effect	Neurotoxin	Major uses/sources of exposures[b]
Headache	Lead	Solder, lead shot, illicit whiskey, insecticides, auto body shops, storage battery manufacturing plants, foundries, smelters, lead-based paints, lead stained glass, lead pipes
	Nickel	Electroplating industry, surgical and dental instruments, nickel–cadmium batteries, paints, inks, alloys, coinage
Impaired visual acuity	*n*-Hexane	*See Ataxia
	Mercury	*See Ataxia
	Methanol	Industrial solvent for inks, resins, adhesives, and dyes; ingredient in paints, varnishes, and plastics; starting material in syntheses of organic chemicals
Impaired psychomotor function	Carbon disulfide	*See Cranial neuropathy
	Lead	*See Headache
	Mercury	*See Ataxia
	Organophosphate	Agricultural industry, pesticide manufacturers, formulators and applicators
	Perchoroethylene and other solvents	Paint removers, degreasers, extraction agent for vegetable and mineral oils, dry cleaning industry, textile industry
Increased intracranial pressure	Lead	*See Headache
	Organotin compounds	Preservatives for wood, leather, paper, paints, textiles, additives
Memory impairment	Arsenic	Pesticides, pigments, antifouling paint, electroplating industry, seafood, smelting, semiconductors
	Carbon disulfide	*See Cranial neuropathy
	Lead	*See Headache
	Manganese	*See Ataxia
Myoclonus	Benzene hexachloride	Chemical intermediate, solvent for fats, oils, waxes, resins and certain synthetic rubbers, extractant of essential oils in perfume industry
Neurasthenia (preferably called organic-affective syndrome)	Mercury	*See Ataxia
	Acrylamide	*See Ataxia
	Arsenic	*See Memory impairment
	Lead	*See Headache
	Manganese	*See Ataxia
	Mercury	*See Ataxia
	Methyl *n*-butyl ketone (MBK)	*See Ataxia
	Methyl chloride	*See Ataxia
	Toluene	
Nystagmus	Mercury	*See Ataxia
Opsoclonus	Chlordecone (Kepone®)	*See Ataxia
Paraplegia	Organotin compounds	*See Increased intracranial pressure
Parkinson's syndrome	Carbon monoxide	Metallurgy, organic synthesis of petroleum products, manufacture of metal carbonyls
	Carbon disulfide	*See Cranial neuropathy
	Manganese	*See Ataxia
Psychosis or marked emotional instability (acute)	Carbon disulfide	*See Ataxia
	Manganese	*See Ataxia
	Toluene (rare)	*See Ataxia
Seizures	Lead	*See Headache
	Organic mercurials	Fungicide, preservative, disinfectant
	Organotin compounds	*See Paraplegia

[a]From Baker et al. (15).
[b]Sources of compounds mentioned elsewhere, marked with asterisk (*), are listed where cross-indexed.

nature of neurotoxic chemicals is illustrated by information derived from the toxic release inventory, which supplies data on toxic substances released into the environment from industrial sources in the United States. In 1987, 17 of the 25 chemicals released into the air in the greatest amounts have documented neurotoxic effects. Their release totaled 1.8 billion pounds (118).

Pesticides

Pesticide is a general term that includes insecticides, fungicides, rodenticides, and herbicides (53,82). The organophosphorus and carbamate insecticides comprise one of the most commonly encountered and most neurotoxic classes of pesticides used in the United States.

Organophosphorus Insecticides

The organophosphorus group of chemicals consists of approximately 50,000 different compounds. These compounds are all substituted esters of phosphoric acid, phosphonic acid, or phosphinic acid. Four such groups are recognized, based on the substituents.

About half of all the insecticides in the entire organic phosphorus family are included in the dimethoxy group. Malathion, first introduced in 1950, is the prototype chemical for this group. It is now marketed under a number of different trade names. The diethyl group of organophosphates includes parathion and diazinon. The triphenyl group includes triorthocresyl phosphate, which has no known insecticidal properties (29). In general, organic phosphorus compounds tend to hydrolyze in aqueous media and do not persist in the environment. Readers interested in a more detailed examination of the chemistry of these compounds are referred to the two references (53,82).

Carbamate Insecticides

Although the carbamates generally have a lower toxicity than the organophosphate insecticides, their range of toxicity is still quite broad. For example, aldicarb (Temik®) is extremely toxic by both the oral and dermal routes.

Distribution Pesticides are widely used throughout the world. More than a billion pounds are used each year in the United States alone. Their uses vary. The organophosphates such as malathion are distributed fairly evenly among agriculture, home and garden, and industry and commerce, whereas dichlorvos, with its appreciable vapor pressure, is used in flea collars. Monocrotophos is used almost exclusively in agriculture. Diazinon is

widely used around the home, in the vegetable garden, and on the lawn. The carbamates have a distribution similar to the organic phosphorus compounds but are generally used to a greater extent around the home.

The likelihood of exposure to pesticides varies with the compound and its use. Obviously, individuals living in proximity to sprayed field crops will experience some exposure. Some of the organophosphates find their way into ground water and nearby streams (76). Organophosphate and carbamate compounds may contaminate soils. Under these conditions, their disappearance depends, in part, on the particular characteristics of the soil. Because of their widespread use, pesticides are dispersed in low concentrations throughout the environment and are found, to some extent, in the nation's food and water supplies (119,120) (see Chapters 3 and 4).

Apart from agricultural workers, those engaged in the manufacture and transportation of pesticides are at increased risk of such exposure. Homeowners may also receive excessive pesticide exposure. A U.S. study reported that homeowners used from 5 to 10 lb of pesticides per acre per year (38). This use is often greater than that for agricultural purposes.

Toxicology The lipid-soluble organophosphorus compounds and the carbamates are absorbed by the skin, lung, and intestinal tract. Following absorption, the organophosphorus compounds are rapidly distributed throughout most of the body. These compounds are esters and readily react with numerous esterases within the body. Their toxicity depends on their ability to inhibit the activity of cholinesterase. Unlike the organophosphates, the carbamates do not form stable bonds with the cholinesterase enzyme. The biotransformation products of the organophosphorus compounds are excreted in the urine. Measuring their excretion is a means of assaying the degree of exposure (see Chapter 27).

Organochlorine Insecticides

Organochlorine insecticides have been widely used. These agents differ biologically from the lower-molecular-weight chlorinated hydrocarbons used as solvents. Spawned by the development of DDT by Muller in 1939, the organochlorine pesticides include such agents as chlordane, hexachlorocyclohexane (lindane), chlordecone (Kepone®), and toxaphene.

The entire group shares a number of common chemical properties. They are highly soluble in fats and oils and quite persistent in the environment and in biological systems. This persistence carries the potential for inadvertent exposure and chronic effects. The use of many of the organochlorine insecticides such as aldrin, chlordane, DDT, endrin, lindane, and toxaphene has been suspended or restricted in recent years (117).

Distribution The relatively low acute mammalian toxicity of the chlorinated hydrocarbons resulted in such widespread environmental use that most of the world's population has a body burden of these chemicals, particularly DDT. Two facts explain the continued presence of DDT and other organochlorine insecticides in humans and other animal forms. First, these stable, water-insoluble compounds have an environmental persistence that can be measured in years. Second, their bioaccumulation occurs through the food chain. Bioaccumulation results when an agent is persistent and displays no acute toxicity to the organisms involved. The material may then be concentrated directly from soil and water by plants and fish and then passed up the food chain by herbivores and carnivores. In this scheme man is the consumer at the top of the food chain.

Because of the ubiquitous environmental presence of the chlorinated hydrocarbon pesticides, farm workers and their families are at risk for excessive exposure to these agents, particularly if sanitary precautions are casual. Workers employed in factories that manufacture pesticides are also at risk. In the case of severe chlordecone (Kepone®) contamination that occurred in Hopewell, Virginia in 1975, the workers regularly arrived home with clothing heavily imbued with chlordecone dust (113). The level of chlordecone was higher in individuals living near the plant and decreased as the distance from the plant increased (28).

DDT, though banned for use in the United States in 1972, is still being produced for export. Substantial production of methoxychlor, chlordane, and some other organochlorine insecticides continues. Methoxychlor is widely used on cattle and other livestock. The use of chlordane has been banned except for subsurface ground insertion for termite control, and this has been sharply curtailed in the United States (117).

Toxicology Absorption of chlorinated hydrocarbon insecticides occurs by any route and is enhanced when the compounds are dissolved in lipid or organic solvent solutions. The lipid solubility of the compounds results in rapid compartmentalization into fat-rich organs such as brain, body fat, and liver. The half-life of these compounds in serum varies from hours for compounds like lindane to many months for compounds such as DDT, dieldrin, mirex, and chlordecone. The metabolism of chlordecone, a compound with a long half-life, has been well studied in man (52).

Herbicides

Herbicides, particularly 2,4-D and paraquat, have been widely disseminated in the environment. Herbicides are used in agriculture, in the control of plant growth along utility paths, and in the control of aquatic plants. Their use in agriculture is such that their purchase may often represent the farmer's greatest single expense. Herbicides are also applied to roadsides and paths to rid them of vegetation. They are used infrequently around the home or garden.

The chlorophenoxy herbicides 2,4-dichlorophenoxyacetic acid (2,4-D) and 2,4,5-trichlorophenoxyacetic acid (2,4,5-T) do not persist in the environment as do the organochlorine insecticides. Both 2,4-D and 2,4,5-T can be absorbed via the oral, dermal, and inhalation routes. Both are distributed widely, and both are excreted in the urine within a few days (49,63). In the past, substantial amounts of 2,4,5-T were used in the maintenance of highway, railroad, and power line rights of way in the United States, but its use has been abandoned. However, 2,4-D continues to be used for this purpose (117).

Halogenated Hydrocarbons

Polychlorinated Biphenyls

The polychlorinated biphenyls (PCBs), produced commercially since 1929, were formerly used as insulators in hydraulic fluids, plasticizers, lubricating fluids, and heat exchangers. Because of their chemical stability, these agents are ubiquitous in our environment. Because of their carcinogenic potential and their stability, the past use of PCBs is of some concern (34).

The PCBs are readily absorbed from the gastrointestinal tract. Their excretion is related to their metabolism. Those with increasing chlorine or bromine content are less readily metabolized and are deposited in adipose tissue. Some of the biphenyls may remain in the body for years (78).

Dioxins

The dioxins, which consist of two benzene rings interconnected by two oxygen atoms, have invaded the environment largely by accident. These compounds are unwanted byproducts formed in the manufacture of chlorophenyls and such related compounds as the herbicide 2,4,5-T. Dioxins were present in the herbicides used during the Vietnamese war, particularly in a substance labeled "Agent Orange," a mixture of 2,4-D and 2,4,5-T (see Chapter 26 for a further discussion of these agents).

The variation in toxicity of the dioxins, which

include 75 analogues, is greater than 150,000 (9,10). Because of its extreme toxicity to certain animals and its potential hazard to man, 2,3,7,8-tetrachloro-dibenzo-*p*-dioxin (TCDD) has been most completely studied. The term "dioxin" refers to this compound.

Tetrachlorodibenzodioxin (TCDD) is stable in storage and within the soil but quite sensitive to sunlight. The dioxins are readily absorbed from the gastrointestinal tract and stored in fat. The great differences in acute toxicity among species, particularly for TCDD, have not been explained. There is evidence that humans are not the most sensitive species. Reviews have summarized the industrial, toxicological, and clinical experience with TCDD and related compounds (10,58,61).

Metals

Aluminum

Aluminum is abundantly present. It is found in most foods and is widely used in food packaging and as a food additive. Aluminum is present in the average American diet in amounts between 5 and 50 mg/dy. Its absorption from the stomach is enhanced by the increased solubility of the aluminum salts in the acid environment. About 2% to 6% of the aluminum in antacid preparations are absorbed from the gastrointestinal tract (19,50).

Arsenic

The use of arsenic and its compounds in the United States exceeds 25,000 tons annually. Arsenic is used in the manufacture of pesticides, herbicides, and other agricultural products, with more than 80% of its yearly consumption going for this purpose (68). Arsenical rodenticides have been used for years. Arsenic is used in wood preservatives and in lead shot and is present as a contaminant in most smelting operations of other metals.

Human exposure to arsenic occurs through many food sources, particularly seafood. Arsenic also finds its way into drinking water in areas adjacent to mines containing arsenic-rich ores. Arsenic-laden dusts from smelters provide a source of community and occupational exposure. Workers are exposed to arsenic in the smelting, pesticide, chemical, and pharmaceutical industries.

The trivalent form of arsenic is usually the cause of toxicity. Arsenic in this form is readily absorbed by the gastrointestinal tract, the lungs, and the skin, especially if the skin is inflamed. Following absorption, arsenic is widely distributed, with highest concentrations in the liver, kidney, spleen, hair, and nails (21). Arsenic stored in the hair and nails remains for long periods of time. The remainder is excreted rapidly in the urine (79).

Lead

Lead has a wide distribution in the environment. Today, production exceeds 2.5 million tons annually worldwide. Storage batteries comprise over 40% of all use, followed by lead alkyls, other metallic uses, soldering cables and pipes, and lead-based paints (43).

The best-known organic compound is tetraethyl lead, an antiknock agent in gasoline. When burned, it is degraded into inorganic lead. Although exposure to tetraethyl lead occurs mainly in occupations involved with the production of gasoline, environmental exposure to lead also occurs from the use of lead-containing gasoline. The U.S. government restricted the use of lead in gasoline in 1975, but many motor vehicles still use leaded gasoline. Approximately 300,000 tons of organic lead compounds are produced annually.

The distribution of lead is so great that no geographic area escapes. The air in urban areas and near ore smelters has the highest concentrations of lead. Based on blood lead levels, urban dwellers show higher levels than do rural residents, with suburban citizens showing an intermediate level. The use of lead in interior paints led to a virtual epidemic of lead intoxication in the 1940s because of childhood pica. A small chip of paint containing 25% lead represents many times the acceptable daily lead intake. Paint produced today for household use in the United States, by federal regulation, can contain no more than 0.06% lead by dry weight. In some instances, paint manufactured before the 1940s contained more than 50% lead. Newsprint, decorated glassware, the glaze on some ceramics, and improperly manufactured food containers are other sources of lead exposure. High levels of lead may also be found in the dust and soil that collect lead from auto exhaust and from industrial emissions. Auto emissions near busy highways and streets provide another source of lead exposure.

A large number of occupations expose workers to lead intoxication. Among these are lead smelters and the battery and paint industries. Workers in small shops where lead is being heated are at particular risk. This includes automobile radiator repair and scrap metal smelting shops. Hobbyists engaged in making pottery, stained glass, and jewelry are also at risk.

The lungs are an important portal for the absorption of lead (43). It is estimated that workers who inhale lead oxide fumes absorb 40% of inhaled lead particles. Gastrointestinal absorption also occurs but is less efficient, as only 10% of the ingested lead is absorbed. The efficiency of absorption is much greater in children, with up to 50% being absorbed (3). Skin absorption occurs only with organic lead compounds.

After absorption, the lead is compartmentalized into blood, soft tissue, and bone. The lead in the blood and soft-tissue fractions is relatively labile, whereas the lead in bone, though stored in a mobilizable form, turns over very slowly. The half-life of lead in blood and soft tissue is 35 to 40 days, whereas the half-life of lead in bone is as long as 20 years (90,91). Blood lead levels represent recent exposure with an undefined input from past lead stores (83).

Mercury

Mercury exists in elemental, organic, and inorganic forms (50). Its use in industry and agriculture has burgeoned. Up to 5 to 10 million pounds are produced annually. Exposure to inorganic mercury is mostly occupational, whereas exposure to organic mercury takes place mainly through the food chain.

Mercury is used in agriculture as a fungicide, in the electrical industry, in paints, paper pulp manufacture, some synthetic processes, thermometers, jewelry, taxidermy, mercury vapor lights, and in a host of other applications. This extensive use results in a substantial environmental contamination, especially of water sources. Mercury tends to accumulate in fish swimming in contaminated waters. This problem is not limited to such well-known episodes of mercury contamination as that in the Minimata area of Japan. Fish in the American Great Lakes and other U.S. waters have been found to be contaminated with mercury (see Chapter 3). Worldwide it is common to have mercury-contaminated water that has received effluents from industry. Persons consuming fish regularly evidence an increased body burden of mercury (23). The consumption of grain treated with mercury has resulted in well-known episodes of intoxication. Dentists who utilize mercury amalgams have increased tissue levels of this agent.

Absorption of elemental mercury is probably limited to inhalation, since gastrointestinal absorption is extremely low. Absorption of inorganic mercury compounds readily occurs by any portal (20). Organic mercury compounds are absorbed efficiently by the respiratory and gastrointestinal tracts and rather slowly through the skin.

Inorganic mercury appears in higher concentrations in the kidney, and excretion is mainly in the urine. Its disappearance is rapid, in terms of days (59). Methyl mercury is excreted, in part, through the bile. It has a biological half-life of about 70 days in man (39).

Solvents

The list of liquids and gases that function as solvents is almost endless (11). Solvents in common use include n-hexane, kerosene, benzene, toluene, carbon tetrachloride, methyl bromide and chloride, trichloroethylene, trichloroethane, methyl and isopropyl alcohol, methyl-n-butyl ketone, acetone, formaldehyde, phenols, and cresols. All of these solvents are organic compounds with relatively low molecular weights.

Solvents are utilized by virtually every industry and invade the environment in abundance. Solvents such as n-hexane, toluene, and methyl-n-butyl ketone are used in glues and cements, paints, paint thinner, varnishes, and related substances. Agents such as Stoddard solvent, perchloroethylene, trichloroethylene, and methyl-n-butyl ketone are extensively employed as dry cleaning and degreasing agents. It is estimated that in the United States 222,000 workers are annually exposed to methyl-n-butyl ketone alone. Organic solvents are used in the production of other chemicals. For some, such as benzene, this accounts for the majority of their use.

Because of their volatility, solvent contamination of the environment may come about through improper storage, particularly indoors. Although this problem usually occurs in an occupational setting, it can also occur in the home through the use of such products as spot remover, paint, paint thinners, paint strippers, varnishes, and glues. Such products are often used in the home without adequate ventilation. Artists and hobbyists may be exposed to solvent concentrations as high as, if not higher than, those found in the workplace.

Although most of the solvents are readily absorbed when ingested, their physical nature makes inhalation and skin contact the most common routes of absorption. Following absorption, most solvents are quite rapidly eliminated.

Toxicological Assessment of Neurotoxicity

Assessing the neurotoxic effects of chemical exposure is assuming greater importance as regulatory agencies attempt to determine and predict the neurotoxic potentiation of toxic exposure. Several industrial and federal agencies have developed animal tests to evaluate the effects of known and potential neurotoxic substances. The interested reader is referred to several references for a review of this subject (115, 121).

EPIDEMIOLOGY

Implicating neurotoxic exposure in the development of neurological disease, particularly in an environmental setting, is extremely difficult. More often, exposure to neurotoxins goes unnoticed. This occurs, in part, because chronic low-level exposure may cause subclinical or asymptomatic disease that is detectable only if the exposed individual is required to function in a highly skilled job or at a complex intellectual level. The great reserve capacity of the nervous system often permits adequate function despite slowly progressive damage. By the time damage to the nervous system is apparent, evidence of toxic exposure may be unobtainable. Moreover, it has been postulated that the effects of early exposure to a neurotoxin may not be expressed until many years later, when natural aging depletes the functional reserve of the nervous system (26). In addition, few neurotoxins produce specific, easily recognizable symptoms. Exposure to the same substance at different concentrations may give rise to totally different clinical findings. Exposure to acute high levels of hexane, for example, results in narcosis, whereas low-level exposure is linked to distal axonopathy.

New Methodology for Studying the Effects of Neurotoxic Exposure

Assessment of the effects of neurotoxic exposure has depended primarily on a thorough neurological history, neurological examination, and electrophysiological testing. These costly and time-consuming methods cannot be applied to the study of large numbers of exposed individuals suffering from the subtle effects of low-dose pollutant exposure. With the development of new methodology, neuroepidemiologists may be able to more effectively evaluate the effects of neurotoxic exposure (121).

New tools, using sensitive automated devices, hold promise that a functional assessment of the nervous system can be applied to large populations. Advances in electrophysiological procedures, coupled with microcomputers, have resulted in the use of sensory evoked potentials, which allow a noninvasive objective and reliable evaluation of sensory pathways from the periphery to the cortex (31). Such testing can detect dysfunctions that are not clinically evident. Portable devices that quantitatively assess tactile and vibration thresholds from distalmost limb points have been used to screen for the presence of toxic neuropathy (13). Such measurements could assist in the early detection of such conditions (85). Tremometry, which measures slight changes in tremor frequency, distribution, and amplitude, has also been used to detect the early effects of neurotoxic exposure (40). Measuring conduction velocities in peripheral nerves has also been used for the detection of toxic neuropathies. If these technological advances are to be fully realized and applied to the discovery of neuro- and other toxins, reportable illnesses must be extended. Would the episode of chlordecone poisoning that occurred in Hopewell, Virginia in 1975 have been more quickly

identified if the unexplained tremor had been reported to a central agency? Speculation suggests an affirmative answer.

Environmental Factors in the Development of Certain Chronic Neurological Conditions

Concern about the neurotoxic effects of chemical exposure has mounted as epidemiologic studies contribute to the notion that environmental factors might increase the risk of such chronic neurological conditions as Parkinson's disease, Alzheimer's disease, amyotrophic lateral sclerosis (ALS), and brain cancer.

Research in Parkinson's disease was revolutionized in the early 1980s when Langston et al. reported irreversible parkinsonism induced by a contaminant of a "bad" batch of a synthetic narcotic. The toxic compound was identified as 1-methyl-4-phenyl-1,2,3,6-tetrahydropyridine (MPTP) (70,71, 122). This finding, which was reproduced in primates, alerted researchers to the possible role of environmental factors in the etiology of Parkinson's disease, particularly in younger individuals (17,65, 110). To date, a number of investigators have conducted epidemiologic studies searching for a link between environmental factors and Parkinson's disease. Many of these studies bolster the hypothesis that environmental factors may be involved in the etiology of some cases of Parkinson's disease (24, 27,48,54,57,111).

The studies by Spencer and his colleagues lend additional support to the concept that environmental factors may play a role in the development of Parkinson's disease, Alzheimer's disease, and motoneuron disease (105–107). Their research centered on a neurological disease formerly having a high incidence in the Chamorros, the indigenous people of Guam. These individuals suffered from amyotrophic lateral sclerosis, parkinsonism, and Alzheimer-type dementia (81,92). A decline in the high incidence of this disease, without evidence of a demonstable viral or inheritable cause, suggested the gradual disappearance of an environmental factor specifically linked to the Chamorros' mores. After much investigation, it was demonstrated the neurological events found in the Chamorros were related to the ingestion of a seed containing an unusual toxic amino acid called BMAA. The seed of the *Cycas circinalis* L. plant was traditionally used as a source of food and medicine for the Chamorros until after World War II. The epidemiologic data were further supported by animal studies. Feeding synthetic BMAA to macaques was followed by structural and functional neurological changes similar to those seen in motoneuron disease and parkinsonism (107).

Studies of the Guam ALS–Parkinson's dementia emphasize the potential importance of neurotoxic exposure that becomes clinically evident years after the initial exposure has occurred. Many Guamanians who left the island between the age of 20 and 30 developed their symptoms 30 years later. Thus, the effects of the neurotoxic exposure they received in their youth, before their departure from the island, became clinically apparent only with the steady loss of brain cells that accompanies advancing age.

Recent epidemiologic studies provide evidence that the incidence of motoneuron disease is increasing, particularly among the middle-aged (40 to 65 years). This increase appears to be present in the United States as well as in other countries (25,44,73). Without other explanations, it is reasonable to assume that exposure to some causative agent is also rising (73).

Studies have raised the question of a link between Alzheimer's disease and aluminum. Increased amounts of aluminum have been measured in the brains of patients dying with Alzheimer's disease. In addition, neurofibrillary tangles have been found in the brain in experimental aluminum toxicity studies and in Alzheimer's disease. Few epidemiologic studies have investigated this relationship. To date, however, there is no evidence that aluminum is a causal factor in the development of Alzheimer's disease (114).

Human exposure to extremely low levels of electromagnetic fields has recently come under scrutiny. Epidemiologic studies have noted some correlation between such exposure and an increase in the risk of cancer. The most consistent association is found in electrical workers and children, particularly for brain cancer and leukemia (2,33,97,98). Thus far the findings are inconclusive. Several large epidemiologic studies are now examining this question (1).

It is noteworthy that a review of cancer deaths in industrialized nations reveals an increase in brain tumor deaths in the elderly (37). It is unclear whether this increase merely reflects an improvement in diagnostic methods and increased longevity.

Neurotoxicity Associated with Episodes of Environmental and Occupational Contamination

Neurotoxicity in human populations has occurred with episodes of environmental and occupational contamination. A few selected examples are presented. For a more detailed listing of major neurotoxicity incidents the reader is referred to a government document (115).

Halogenated Hydrocarbon Pesticides

In the mid-1970s, a dramatic epidemic of neurological disease appeared in Hopewell, Virginia. Over half of the workers employed in a small chemical plant manufacturing chlordecone (Kepone®) became ill (112). Symptoms of neurotoxicity caused by exposure to this organochlorine pesticide included tremor, visual disturbances, mental changes, headache, and gait difficulties. Environmental contamination also occurred in connection with this widely publicized episode of chlordecone intoxication in the workplace. Persons exposed to this agent in nonoccupational settings were discovered to have chlordecone in their tissues. Overt neurotoxicity, however, was evident only in workers exposed to this agent.

Hexachlorophene

During the 1970s well-documented evidence of severe neurotoxicity was reported in newborn infants exposed to hexachlorophene (99,100). Because of its bactericidal qualities, this chlorinated phenolic compound gained wide use in newborn nurseries during the 1960s (47). Although hexachlorophene is no longer used for this purpose, the hexachlorophene episode clearly reflects the dangers of subjecting a susceptible population to an agent in relatively high concentrations before its toxicological features are adequately explored and before all the available toxicological data are reviewed and integrated. The details of this important episode are presented in Chapter 12.

Polyhalogenated Biphenyls

In Japan in 1968, an outbreak of an illness known as "Yusho" was caused by the ingestion of rice oil contaminated with Kanechlor 400, a commercial brand of polychlorinated biphenyls (PCBs). Over 1000 persons consumed the contaminated rice oil, which was used in cooking. The PCBs were originally thought to be the causal agents of Yusho. Recent studies, however, reveal that the rice oils also contained polychlorinated dibenzofurans (PCDFs) and polychlorinated quaterphenyls (PCQs). Because the PCDFs have greater toxicity than the PCBs, they are now considered the major causal agent in Yusho (77).

Apart from the characteristic acne-like skin eruptions, a considerable number of the Yusho victims complained of such neurological symptoms as headache and paresthesia in their extremities (66, 67). Evidence of peripheral neuropathy was also present in another outbreak of PCB poisoning that occurred in 1979 in Taiwan (95).

Herbicides and Dioxin

Episodes of occupational and environmental contamination from the herbicide 2,4,5-trichloro-dibenzo-*p*-dioxin (2,4,5-T) and from the contaminant 2,3,7,8-tetrachlorodibenzo-*p*-dioxin (TCDD) or dioxin have occurred. Neurotoxic effects have been reported in some instances but not in others (9,10).

In 1949 a discharge from an overheated reactor in a herbicide-producing factory in Nitro, West Virginia exposed a number of workers to 2,4,5-T contaminated with dioxin. A study to determine the long-term effects of this workplace exposure was reported by Suskind and Hertzberg in 1984 (108). Neurological examination and conduction velocity measurements performed on 204 exposed and 163 unexposed subjects revealed no differences between the exposed and unexposed groups. A 10-year follow-up of 55 workers in Czechoslovakia who were exposed to dioxin revealed that 17 workers had symptoms of neurological impairment, the most common being polyneuropathy (88).

In 1976 in Seveso, Italy, a short distance from Milan, there was an industrial accident that resulted in environmental contamination with dioxin. The accident, which occurred during the synthesis of trichlorophenol, released an estimated 650 to 1700 g of dioxin over an area about a mile long and half-mile wide, about 2.02 km^2 (35). About 37,000 people were estimated to have been exposed to varying amounts of TCDD. Many deaths occurred in rabbits and small farm animals, but no deaths in humans were recorded.

Studies evaluating the central and peripheral nervous system of inhabitants of the contaminated area were performed. Standard neurological tests were performed, and conduction velocity in the motor and sensory peripheral nervous system was measured. The results revealed no clear evidence of neurological abnormalities (93,94).

Metals

Arsenic Peripheral neuropathy has been reported in individuals chronically exposed to arsenic in well water (56). Individuals living near hazardous waste sites may be at increased risk. Arsenic present in stored chemicals is often sufficiently soluble, when wet, to seep into the ground water (41).

Lead The prevalence of acute lead poisoning is now quite low, with most urban medical centers in the United States seeing only a few cases annually. In contrast, the subtle behavioral changes that accompany childhood exposure to low levels of lead present a major public health threat. Numerous epidemiologic studies have addressed this important issue; they are reviewed in Chapter 14.

Studies evaluating the health effects of lead absorption among children living near a lead smelter revealed increased lead absorption associated with slowed nerve conduction and anemia (69). Fatal encephalopathy has also been reported from increased lead absorption in proximity to lead smelters (87).

The prevalence of symptomatic intoxication in workers in the lead industry is quite low. Asymptomatic intoxication, however, may be quite common. Using special techniques, Seppalainen and Hernberg performed motor nerve conduction measurements on 39 male lead workers. They found evidence of lead intoxication in 31. Twenty-four of these subjects displayed abnormalities on the standard electromyogram (101).

Mercury It was not until the outbreak of methyl mercury poisoning in Japan in the 1950s that the extreme toxicity of organic mercury compounds was appreciated. An industrial effluent containing large amounts of mercury contaminated the waters of the bay in Minamata, Japan. The mercury was converted to methyl mercury by marine biota. This accumulated in fish and shellfish, which were eventually consumed by the local residents. Ingestion of the contaminated fish resulted in widespread neurological disease (109). Although this episode of methyl mercury poisoning is one of the best known, its use as a fungicide in seed grain is the leading cause of mercury intoxication worldwide. The most severe episode occurred in Iraq in 1972. At this time 6530 persons were hospitalized, and 459 died, as a result of eating mercury-contaminated grain. Neurological sequelae were quite extensive, including disturbances in sensory, motor, and cognitive functions (16,96).

Solvents

The voluntary inhalation of solvents, particularly those commonly present in glue and paint thinner, by individuals desiring a "high" is a feature of recent decades. Toluene has been particularly abused. The offending products are readily available in hardware stores. In one epidemic, encephalopathy was noted in 19 children aged 14–18 years who engaged in the recreational use of toluene (72).

A particularly well-documented outbreak of neuropathy caused by solvent exposure occurred in the 1970s in a coated fabrics plant in Columbus, Ohio. The agent incriminated was methyl-*n*-butyl ketone. The interested reader is referred to reports of this classic study (6,7).

PATHOLOGY AND PATHOLOGICAL PHYSIOLOGY

An overview of neuropathology is of great help to the clinician. Such knowledge, when combined with information on the type and site of a toxic process and on the biochemistry of the offending agent, often helps the physician to predict the clinical manifestations of neurotoxicity and to proceed with clinical management.

Toxins adversely affect every aspect of neural function. Table 13-2 illustrates the pervasiveness of their damage. At a histopathological level the nervous system's ability to respond to an insult is restricted, whether the insult is toxic, infectious, degenerative, vascular, or metabolic. Neurons may be damaged, myelin may be lost, or axons may be injured. The sites of injury are influenced by such factors as the host, the agent, the dose, and the metabolic events within the host.

Spencer and Schaumburg have proposed a classification of neurotoxic responses based on cellular

TABLE 13-2. Patterns of Damage and Anatomic Areas of the Nervous System Affected by Various Agents[a]

Agent	Gray Matter type 1[b] — Anoxia					Prolonged anoxia				White Matter type 2[b]				Peripheral neuropathy types 3, 4, 5[b]			Local areas type 6[b]			
	Cortex IV	Cortex V	Hippocampus H_1	Caudate nucleus	Putamen	Hippocampus H_2	Fascia dentata	Globus pallidus	Subthalamus	Internal capsule	Corpus callosum	Optic chiasm	Schwann cells	Sensory n. thalamus	Anterior horn cells	Peripheral axons	Hippocampus H_3	Hypothalamus ventral n.	Mammillary body	Tegmentum
Acetylpyridine						+								+			+			
Acrylamide													+							
Azide	+		+	+	+				+	+	+	+								+
Barbiturate	+	+																		
Carbon disulfide	+		+	+										+		+				
Carbon monoxide							+	+		+	+	+								
Cyanide	+		+	+	+		+				+	+								+
DDT													+			+				
Glutamate														+				+		
Gold thioglucose								+										+		
Hexachlorophene										+	+									
Iminodipropionitrile											+				+					
Isoniazid										+	+	+			+					
Lead (inorganic)																				
Adults													+		+					
Children	+	+								+	+	+		+						
Malononitrile				+	+					+	+									
Manganese				+	+				++											
Mercury (organic)	+									+				+		+				
Methyl bromide	+						+									+				
Nitrogen trichloride	+	+	+	+	+		+													
Pyrithiamine																			+	+
Triethyl tin										+	+	+								
Triorthocresyl phosphate																+				
Vinca alkaloids													+		+					

[a] From Norton (86).

[b] Type 1, agents causing anoxia. Type 2, agents damaging myelin. Type 3, agents causing peripheral axonopathies. Type 4, agents causing primary damage to cell body of peripheral neurons. Type 5, agents damaging neuromuscular junction of motor nerve. Type 6, neurotoxicants causing localized CNS lesions.

targets of chemical agents (104). The scheme includes the following targets: neurons, glial cells and myelin, the neurotransmitter system, the nervous system vasculature, and muscles. The major limitations of this classification include the potential for certain agents to affect different sites in the nervous system, depending on the degree of exposure, and the lack of a valid experimental animal model for many neurotoxic substances. In many instances, however, the cellular target of the neurotoxic chemical is defined. In most cases the precise mechanism of injury is unknown.

A number of agents cause neuronal injury. Toluene and other solvents, for example, affect cortical neurons. Lead may affect both cortical neurons and anterior horn cells. At times, as with chlordecone, neurons in the mesencephalic reticular substance are preferentially affected. Organic mercurials attack neurons in the cerebellum and striate cortex. The clinical manifestation of neuronal loss is determined by the site of injury rather than by its pathological nature. Clinical evidence of neuronal loss will often be reflected in some combination of mental status change, seizures, visual loss, ataxia, and tremor or other involuntary movement.

Some agents damage conduction fibers by attacking the myelin or the axon. Triethyl tin affects the oligodendrocytes that create myelin in the central nervous system, whereas arsenic affects the myelin (and axons) of the peripheral nervous system. Methyl-n-butyl ketone causes an axonopathy in the peripheral nervous system. Peripheral nerve damage, whatever the cause, results in some combination of limb weakness, sensory loss, and areflexia. An injury to central nervous system myelin produces some combination of spasticity, incoordination of limb or ocular movement, poor motor control, and visual loss.

Other chemicals such as organic phosphorus and carbamate compounds, by inhibiting acetylcholinesterase, attack the neuromuscular junction. Such injury causes symptoms that are, in many respects, similar to myasthenia gravis. For an extensive review of the neuropathophysiology of toxins, the reader is referred to the book of Spencer and Schaumburg (103).

CLINICAL ASPECTS OF EXPOSURE TO ENVIRONMENTAL CHEMICALS ON THE NERVOUS SYSTEM

A high level of suspicion coupled with a careful exposure history are critical in establishing a relationship between toxic exposure and neurological disease. Toxic exposure produces a wide range of varied and complex neurological manifestations affecting both the central and peripheral nervous system (Tables 13-1 and 13-3). The clinical symptoms and laboratory findings often provide little help in identifying the offending agent. The task of discovery therefore resides primarily with the attending physician, who must collect, sort out, and integrate the data. Although the clinician frequently encounters numerous obstacles to establishing a diagnosis of neurotoxic disease, there are times when the diagnosis is freely available to the clinician who inquires about the patient's exposure pattern. Such was the case when an alert clinician uncovered the cause of the severe neurological problems linked to

TABLE 13-3.   Peripheral Nervous System Effects of Neurotoxic Chemicals

Effect	Toxin	Comments
Motor neuropathy	Lead	Primarily wrist extensors
		Wrist drop and ankle drop rare
Mixed sensorimotor neuropathy	Acrylamide	Ataxia common
		Desquamation of hands and soles
		Sweating of palms
	Arsenic	Distal paresthesias earliest symptom
		Painful limbs, especially in calves
		Hyperpathia of feet
		Weakness prominent in legs
	Carbon disulfide	Peripheral neuropathy rather mild
		CNS effects more important
	Carbon monoxide	Seen only after severe intoxication
	DDT	Seen only with ingestions
	n-Hexane and methyl n-butyl ketone (MBK)	Distal paresthesias and motor weakness
		Weight loss, fatigue, and muscle cramps common
	Mercury	Predominantly distal sensory involvement
		More common with alkyl mercury exposure

[a]From Baker et al. (15).

Kepone® exposure that took place in Hopewell, Virginia (28).

Neurotoxic agents causing structural damage almost always produce diffuse disease in the affected segment of the nervous system. The peripheral nerves, the long tracts of the spinal cord, the cerebellum, and the cerebrum are the segments of the nervous system most vulnerable to toxic assault. Such assault rarely produces focal or asymmetric injury of the nervous system.

Weakness, sensory loss, and encephalopathy are clinical evidence of nervous system injury incurred by exposure to neurotoxic chemicals. Weakness develops with neuromuscular blockade and neuropathy (Table 13-3). Sensory loss occurs with agents that produce a neuropathy. Encephalopathies are evidenced by seizures, ataxia, brainstem findings, movement disorders, and changes in mental status ranging from overstimulation to lethargy and coma (Table 13-1).

Neuromuscular blockade is produced by organic phosphorus compounds and by the carbamates. Neuropathy is produced by tri-ortho-cresyl phosphate, DDT, arsenic, n-hexane, trichloroethylene, methyl-n-butyl ketone, acrylamide, carbon disulfide, lead, dioxin, and halogenated biphenyls. Encephalopathy of one form or another is produced by mercury, arsenic, aluminum, toluene, carbon disulfide, methyl chloride, trichloroethylene, n-hexane, dinitrophenol, and the chlorinated hydrocarbons. There is some overlap between these groups because some chemicals, e.g., lead, have more than one manifestation. The reason for one manifestation occurring in lieu of another, as in the case of lead producing an encephalopathy in children and a neuropathy in adults, is incompletely understood.

The following section deals with the diagnosis and treatment of neurological disease caused by exposure to specific neurotoxins. It bears emphasis that all patients suffering from the acute or chronic effects of toxic exposure must be removed from the source of exposure. Adequate supportive treatment must also be given.

Organophosphate and Carbamate Insecticides

Ordinarily, the physician is able to elicit a clear history of exposure to insecticides, particularly if there is accidental exposure. Such exposure can occur in agricultural settings and with improper pest control in and around the home and in the garden.

Since both the organophosphates and carbamates inhibit cholinesterase activity, the rapidly developing symptoms are caused by the accumulation of endogenous acetylcholine. The symptoms involve both the central and autonomic nervous systems. The muscarinic effects of cholinergic activity consist of profound overstimulation of the parasympathetic nervous system. This results in such symptoms as pupillary constriction, increased salivation, excessive bronchial secretions, chest tightness, sweating, nausea, and vomiting. The nicotinic effects of cholinergic action at the neuromuscular junction produce muscular fibrillations and fasciculations. Muscle cramps may supervene and be quite severe. The accumulation of acetylcholine also afflicts the central nervous system. The earliest symptoms may be behavioral changes, which include anxiety and emotional lability. As exposure increases, headache, tremor, and drowsiness develop. Finally, ataxia, generalized seizures, coma, and death can occur (53,64).

Laboratory Findings

Depression of plasma and/or RBC cholinesterase is useful in detecting toxicity from organic phosphate and carbamate exposure. The rather marked variation in cholinesterase activity found among individuals often makes it difficult to interpret a single enzyme level. The best evidence of excessive exposure, therefore, lies in a comparison of the test results before and after exposure. A decrease of 25% of more in cholinesterase activity, when compared with a baseline figure, is evidence of excessive exposure (80) (for further discussion see Chapter 27).

Treatment and Prognosis

The specific treatment of organophosphorus intoxication is quite satisfactory if the diagnosis is made quickly and treatment is initiated early. The muscarinic side effects can be blocked with atropine. The maintenance of full atropinization may require repeated doses of atropine at intervals of 10 to 60 min for several hours. If the muscarinic symptoms reemerge, atropine should be reinstituted. The details of therapy for organophosphorus poisoning are found in several references (49,80).

The treatment of carbamate intoxication is similar to that caused by organophosphate insecticides except that the use of pralidoxime is contraindicated in carbaryl poisonings (49).

The prognosis of organophosphate and carbamate intoxication appears to be excellent if treatment is prompt and the individuals are otherwise in good health. The possible chronic behavioral sequelae of organophosphorus poisoning are discussed in Chapter 14.

Chlorinated Hydrocarbon Insecticides

The clinical characteristics of the neurotoxicity produced by the chlorinated hydrocarbon insecticides differ markedly from those produced by the cholinesterase inhibitors. In cases of chronic exposure, the patient's clinical history may not initially suggest toxicity from organochlorine exposure. This important clinical observation is well demonstrated in the patients who suffered from chlordecone intoxication. These individuals were seen for at least a year by numerous physicians without the nature of their illness being recognized. During this time their symptoms were attributed to "nerves," "flu," pneumonia, and psychiatric problems.

With acute intoxication with organochlorine insecticides, the history is often dramatic. Such agents as chlordane, dieldrin, toxaphene, and lindane may produce seizures soon after ingestion of an intoxicating dose. The potential for incorrect diagnosis still exists, since many of the intoxicated persons are children whose seizures could easily suggest other, more common causes. With acute toxicity, seizures begin from 20 min to a few hours after exposure to chlorinated hydrocarbons. Seizures resulting from chronic intoxication occur at variable periods after the onset of exposure. Seizures may be repeated for hours after their onset and may respond poorly to anticonvulsants.

Tremor, the other major manifestation of chlorinated hydrocarbon intoxication, has been extensively studied in chlordecone exposure. The tremor produced by chlordecone was not present at rest or in sleep. It was most evident with purposive movements, such as reaching for objects, and with static posture, as in holding the arms outstretched against gravity (112,113). With chronic chlordecone intoxication, the tremors were noted after only 6 weeks of exposure. There was a distinct cerebellar appearance to the tremor, which may lead to some difficulty with manual tasks. Incoordination was also noted.

Abnormal ocular motility has been noted with exposure to several of the organochlorine pesticides. Usually described as nystagmus, an ocular motility problem was a conspicuous feature of chlordecone intoxication. It was sufficiently severe to produce symptoms of blurred vision when the individual was reading or glanced quickly to the side. On examination these individuals were found to have a series of quick eye movements, small in amplitude and multidirectional, at the termination of a refixation saccade. These chaotic eye movements fit the definition of opsoclonus. Chlordecone was the first toxic agent known to induce opsoclonus in man. Patients suspected of suffering from neurotoxity should be carefully examined for this feature. Opsoclonus does not occur with slow-pursuit eye movements, which are used in routine examinations. Although neuropathy is an occasional feature of chlorinated hydrocarbon intoxication, it is seldom a severe or conspicuous manifestation.

Laboratory Findings

Chlorinated hydrocarbon insecticides rapidly appear in the blood and can be assayed chemically. Such analyses, however, are not readily available in most clinical laboratories. The blood level associated with acute poisoning has been determined for some of the organochlorine insecticides (113). In general, determinations of blood levels have limited usefulness in predicting health hazards, as dose–response relationships are unknown.

Treatment and Prognosis

The only specific treatment for chlorinated hydrocarbon intoxication is that employed by Cohn et al. in cases of chlordecone intoxication (32). These investigators demonstrated that the half-life of chlordecone was sharply reduced by oral administration of cholestyramine. This agent increased the fecal elimination of chlordecone by preventing its reabsorption from the gut. Cholestyramine, a nonabsorbable ion-exchange resin that binds bile acids, also binds chlordecone after its elimination in the bile. The oral administration of 16 g of cholestyramine per day increased the fecal concentration of chlordecone almost sevenfold. The half-life of chlordecone in the blood was reduced from 165 days to 80 days. Cholestyramine therapy resulted in a marked improvement in the signs and symptoms of chlordecone toxicity (32). To what extent cholestyramine therapy can be used in the treatment of toxicity produced by other chlorinated hydrocarbons is unknown. For recommendations regarding the treatment of acute poisoning with organochlorine insecticides, the reader is referred to several references (49,80).

Excessive exposure to the organochlorine insecticides may lead to prolonged symptomatology and disability. Seizures continuing for weeks following intoxication with the dieldrin group of chemicals have been reported (53). Although mental changes have been reported in association with the early clinical manifestations of intoxication with the organochlorines, dementia or other long-term mental changes have not been established.

Herbicides

With herbicide intoxication, a history of exposure may not be apparent immediately. The intoxicated patient may not be aware of his exposure, particularly exposure that occurs as a result of aerial spraying of herbicides. Symptoms of skin and mucous membrane irritation should raise the possibility of herbicide exposure, especially if accompanied by nausea. Most case reports have described complaints of skin burning rather than pruritus. This distinction can at times be useful in the diagnosis, as most inadvertent exposure to herbicides occurs outdoors.

Paraquat has caused hundreds of cases of human intoxication, often due to suicidal intentions. Ulceration of the mouth is common, along with hepatic, renal, and cardiac abnormalities. Pulmonary damage is prominent. Neurological involvement occurs in the form of an encephalopathy, but it is not usually paramount. The encephalopathy may be delayed for days following exposure (8). Survivors recover completely except for possible respiratory problems.

Neurological manifestations appear quickly in cases of 2,4-D and 2,4,5-T poisoning. Muscular twitching and weakness are noted, along with myalgia. Other manifestations include headache, flushed skin, abdominal pain, and cardiac arrhythmia. The phenoxy herbicides may induce a comatose state indistinguishable from other causes of toxic or metabolic coma (22,53).

Laboratory Findings

Although the concentration of herbicides can be determined in blood and urine, such determinations are not commonly performed in most clinical laboratories (see Chapter 27 for further discussion).

Treatment and Prognosis

There is no specific treatment for herbicide intoxication other than removal from exposure. The prognosis for recovery from herbicide intoxication is generally good. Some agents, especially paraquat, when taken in a large dose, as in a suicidal effort, carry a high mortality (80).

Aluminum

The only known neurological manifestation of aluminum toxicity in humans is a dementing disorder that occurs in patients undergoing long-term dialysis with nondeionized water. Such patients develop encephalopathy after being treated with hemodialysis from 3 to 7 years (4). The first symptom, characterized by a peculiar form of speech impairment, includes stuttering and misshapen word sounds. Some difficulty in finding words, in a manner not recognized as a variety of aphasia, is also present. The speech pattern is sufficiently unique that it is easily recognized by experienced neurologists and nephrologists. Seizures also occur. Within weeks to a few months after the onset of symptoms, all mental processes begin to deteriorate. The dementia progresses relentlessly until death ensues.

There is no specific treatment for dialysis encephalopathy. Chelation therapy has been employed in a few cases. The results are uncertain but promising. The incidence of dialysis encephalopathy has dropped markedly since deionized dialysates have become widely used.

Arsenic

Most significant arsenic exposure occurs in industrial settings in connection with smelting and metal and pesticide manufacture.

In acute arsenic poisoning the major symptoms are gastrointestinal. Those individuals surviving the acute phase and those chronically exposed to arsenic may develop symptoms involving a number of organ systems. The most common neurological manifestation of arsenic exposure is peripheral neuropathy. Over half of the patients with arsenical intoxication will develop this complication. The neuropathy may develop rapidly. In cases with repeated low-dose arsenic exposure, the neuropathy develops slowly over several years (60).

The neuropathy that occurs secondary to arsenic exposure is ordinarily symmetrical in distribution, involving both motor and sensory components. The initial symptoms of paresthesias of the feet and hands progress to sensory loss with substantial hyperpathia. Patients often cannot bear the discomfort of bed clothing or of walking. The motor involvement consists of distal limb weakness, more pronounced in the legs. Up to 50% of the patients have a foot drop. A lesser percentage develop a wrist drop as the upper limbs become involved (55).

Laboratory Findings

Arsenic toxicity can be difficult to evaluate. Because arsenic is rapidly distributed throughout the body, blood levels may not reflect recent exposure. Urine arsenic may be used as evidence of current or continuous exposure. The urinary concentration of arsenic in the general population ranges from 0 to 0.39 µg/mL. A 24-h excretion exceeding 0.1 mg is considered abnormal. Although it is possible for patients with arsenical neuropathy to have urine arsenic levels in the normal range, the levels are usually increased (55). Arsenic also enters hair, usually within 2 weeks following ingestion. Levels that exceed 0.1 mg per 100 g of hair are probably abnormal. Measuring arsenic in hair can be of help in evaluating environmental exposure. In the industrial setting, however, this determination has less value, as hair may be contaminated by the deposition of exogenous arsenic.

Treatment and Prognosis

The nature of the treatment of arsenic intoxication depends on whether the exposure has been acute or chronic. For specific treatment, dimercapto-propanol or British anti-Lewisite (BAL) is usually indicated in symptomatic arsenic poisoning. The details of treatment are found in two references (49,80).

In the chronic phase of arsenic intoxication, analgesics or carbamazepine may be required to ameliorate pain. The effectiveness of chelating agents such as BAL is open to considerable question. Recovery from the neuropathy is slow or may never occur.

Lead

Although the epidemics of lead poisoning seen in the United States in the 1940s in infants with a history of pica are now relatively rare, excessive environmental lead exposure remains the major environmental health hazard facing the nation's children (116). Young children, particularly those living in pre-World War II houses with peeling lead paint, are especially threatened by increased lead exposure. A detailed exposure history and careful evaluation are of the utmost importance in any child displaying neurotoxicity. Behavioral changes and learning impairments have been shown to be related to low-level lead exposure that occurs during fetal development and early childhood (84) (see Chapter 14 for a detailed discussion of the neurobehavioral effects of low-level lead exposure).

Acute lead poisoning is characterized by abdominal pain, fatigue, and hemolytic anemia. The abdominal pain may suggest the need of abdominal surgery. With high levels of lead exposure, the central nervous system is profoundly affected, as evidenced by seizures, delirium, and coma. Seizures may be focal or generalized and are relatively unresponsive to traditional anticonvulsants. In contrast, the early clinical manifestations of encephalopathy from chronic lead exposure are subtle and nonspecific. These include symptoms of listlessness, apathy, or bizarre behavior. At times irritability may be present (51).

Peripheral neuropathy associated with lead exposure is evidenced by distal motor weakness (102). Any motor neuropathy should be suspect, however. The neuropathy is often asymmetric. Sensory loss is a rarity.

Laboratory Findings

Blood lead determinations are the screening method of choice to identify elevated blood lead levels. Based on the evidence that some adverse health effects have been demonstrated in young children at blood lead levels as low as 10 μg/dL (0.5 μmol/L), the Centers for Disease Control (CDC) recommends that the surveillance of children begin at blood lead levels of 10 μg/dL (0.5 μmol/L). This level has been revised downward from the 1985

intervention level of 25 μg/dL (1.2 μmol/L) (30). Since it is impossible to select a single number to define lead poisoning in all groups of children, the CDC has outlined a series of steps to identify and prevent lead poisoning as the blood lead level increases (30).

A child with a blood lead level <μg/dL (<0.5 μmol/L) is not considered to be lead-poisoned. A blood lead level between 10 and 14 μg/dL (0.5–0.7 μmol/L) is considered to be in the border zone. The child should be tested again in about 3 months to make certain that the blood lead level does not increase. Blood lead levels between 10 and 14 μg/dL should trigger community-wide childhood lead-poisoning prevention activities. A child with a blood lead level between 15 and 19 μg/dL (0.7–0.9 μmol/L) should receive individual case management including nutritional and educational interventions and more frequent screening. A child with a blood lead level between 20 and 44 μg/dL (1–2.1 μmol/L) should receive environmental evaluation and remediation and a medical evaluation. This may include pharmacologic treatment. A child with lead levels between 45 and 69 μg/dL (2.2–3.3 μmol/L) needs medical and environmental intervention, including chelation therapy (30). A blood level of 70 μg/dL (3.4 μmol/L) is evidence of acute lead intoxication. This acute medical emergency should be managed by a physician experienced in treating children who are critically ill with lead poisoning (30).

In adults with blood lead levels betwen 40 and 80 μg/dL (1.9–3.8 μmol/L) clinical judgment tends to favor treating those who have symptoms or findings consonant with lead intoxication. According to regulations of the Occupational Safety and Health Administration, adult workers with blood lead levels averaging over 50 μg/dL (2.4 μmol/L) or above must be removed from occupational lead exposure until their blood levels fall below 40 μg/dL (1.9 μmol/L) (40). For a further discussion of the biological monitoring of lead exposure see Chapter 27.

Treatment and Prognosis

The specific treatment of choice for lead intoxication is chelation therapy. Three chelating agents, dimercaprol (British anti-Lewisite), d-penicillamine, and the calcium disodium salt of ethylene diamine tetraacetate (EDTA), are all effective chelating agents for lead. The details of therapy are given by Gosselin et al. (49). In 1991, the U.S. Food and Drug Administration approved succimer, an oral chelating agent for therapy of children with blood lead levels over 45 μg/dL (2.2 μmol/L) (30).

The prognosis in lead encephalopathy remains rather poor. Although the mortality in children is less than 5%, incidence of neurological sequelae including seizures or mental retardation is reportedly as high as 82% (89). Clearly the prevention of lead exposure is of the utmost importance, particularly in the young child. The prognosis of lead neuropathy, on the other hand, is quite good, particularly when it is discovered early and treated vigorously. Recovery requires several months.

Prevention

Lead poisoning is one of the most prevalent and preventable health problems in childhood. Since sufficient information on the pathways of lead exposure and the means of preventing such exposure is available, efforts can now be focused on eliminating childhood lead poisoning. The goal of lead-poisoning prevention activities should be to reduce children's blood lead levels below 10 μg/dL (0.5 μmol/L). In concert with community environmental programs and nutritional and education campaigns, physicians play a critical role in preventing childhood lead poisoning. This includes (1) teaching parents about major sources of lead exposure (e.g., peeling lead-based paint, lead-contaminated dust from paint that is disturbed in homes built before 1960—particularly during renovation); (2) assessing a child's risk for high-dose lead exposure; (3) screening children and interpreting blood lead test results; (4) making certain that lead poisoned children receive medical, environmental, and social service follow-ups; (5) emphasizing that strict precautions must be taken during the abatement of lead hazards in the home and such places as day-care centers; and (6) working with public health officials and others involved in the prevention of childhood lead poisoning (30). The Centers for Disease Control has recently published a booklet on the prevention of lead poisoning in young children; the reader is urged to review this important document (30) (see Chapters 14, 24, 27, and 28).

Organic Lead Compounds

The toxicity of organic lead is different from that of inorganic lead. The fat solubility of organic lead compounds encourages them to partition into the central nervous system, which has a high fat content. Most symptoms of neurotoxicity therefore stem from the central nervous system. Early symptoms include headache, insomnia, and central nervous system excitation. In cases of severe poisoning, hallucinations and seizures occur. The diagnosis of organic lead toxicity depends on a history of such exposure followed by the development of encephalopathy. The blood lead levels are elevated (19). In cases of organic lead intoxication, chelation therapy is of doubtful value.

Mercury

Exposure to inorganic and metallic forms of mercury is found primarily in an industrial setting. At times, however, children playing with droplets of metallic mercury receive excessive exposure to mercury vapor. The ingestion of contaminated fish is the major source of human exposure to organic mercury. The prenatal effects of mercury exposure are of major concern (see Chapter 24 for a discussion of this issue).

In cases of acute exposure to a large amount of inorganic mercury there is rapid development of gastrointestinal symptoms and shock, associated with renal tubular failure. In chronic mercury intoxication, the conspicuous neurological features reflect involvement of the central nervous system. This results from intoxication by either inorganic or organic mercury. Inorganic compounds tend to cause tremor, ataxia, and personality changes. Nervousness, irritability, and emotional lability occurring in workers in the hatting industry probably led to the phrase "mad as a hatter." Evidence of dermatitis, gingivitis, and stomatitis is also present.

Exposure to organic mercury compounds such as those used as pesticides and antifungal agents on seeds is primarily environmental. Exposure to methyl mercury almost always produces purely neurological illness. There is a characteristic hiatus between the onset of exposure and the onset of symptoms (75). Early symptoms are sensory, consisting of paresthesias of the extremities. The paresthesias begin distally in the limbs and spread proximally. The findings usually consist of mild sensory loss, which ultimately reaches the face, perioral areas, and tongue. Visual field constriction is a regular feature of organic mercury intoxication. The diagnosis is, in fact, in jeopardy if this feature is absent. Cerebellar ataxia of limbs, gait, and speech (dysarthria) is present in up to 95% of cases with organic mercury intoxication. Neurogenic deafness is another common feature. Other motor findings that may be seen include tremor, athetosis, and rigidity. Mental deterioration may also occur.

Laboratory Findings

Mercury is widely distributed in body tissues and fluids. Blood, urine, and tissue levels of mercury must be interpreted with considerable caution, however. Unexposed healthy persons have an average blood mercury concentration of 0.5 μg/100 mL, with most having a value below 3 μg/100 mL (45). Inorganic mercury compounds are excreted rapidly in the urine; hence, blood levels may not be significantly elevated in spite of serious illness. Urine levels may more accurately reflect recent exposure.

Nevertheless, there is often a poor correlation between urinary levels of mercury and toxicity (59). As a consequence, urinary excretion of mercury is more an index of recent exposure than proof that symptoms are related to mercury. Urine mercury concentrations in normal persons are usually less than 10 μg/mL. Blood levels are useful in evaluating organic mercury intoxication. Blood levels in unexposed workers should be less than 2 μg/L, whereas blood levels in asymptomatic workers exposed to organic mercury may be 10 μg/L (75).

Treatment and Prognosis

The therapy of mercury intoxication is not entirely satisfactory. With inorganic mercury intoxication, chelation therapy with BAL or d-penicillamine has proven quite useful (49). Specific therapy for organic mercury poisoning is not satisfactory: BAL may actually aggravate the poisoning by alkyl mercury compounds. This relates to the increased solubility of BAL–alkyl mercury complexes.

The prognosis of methyl mercury intoxication is partly determined by its concentration in the blood. In the epidemic of organic mercury poisoning that occurred in Iraq, only those individuals with moderate mercury toxicity improved (16). In cases of acute inorganic mercury poisoning, a high mortality rate prevails. In chronic inorganic mercury poisoning, the prognosis can be excellent, depending on the severity of the illness at the time the exposure ceases.

Solvents

Solvents are ubiquitous in the workplace and the environment. Their widespread use coupled with their ability to cause neurotoxicity give cause for concern. It is well established that the most common and serious consequence of overexposure to solvents is their adverse neurological effect. Solvents produce certain common nonspecific effects and other effects that are characteristic of exposure to specific solvents or classes of solvents. Solvents produce two forms of neurotoxicity: encephalopathy and peripheral neuropathy.

The acute toxic encephalopathy that follows exposure to organic solvents is characterized by euphoria, excitement, confusion, dizziness, headache, and motor incoordination. There is evidence that toxic encephalopathy can follow prolonged and repeated exposure to high concentrations of certain organic solvents. Whether repeated moderate exposure to these agents results in a chronic encephalopathy is controversial. A number of studies in the Scandinavian countries report a connection between chronic solvent exposure in the workplace and impaired function of the central nervous system. This subject is discussed in Chapter 14.

The best-known of the solvent encephalopathies is the chronic encephalopathy produced by toluene exposure. This agent is intentionally inhaled because it produces a euphoria or "high" (as in glue sniffing; paint sniffing). The "high," being rather brief, can be maintained by frequent inhalation of the fumes. The onset of the encephalopathy is insidious. It may begin with bizarre behavior, ataxia, or intellectual decline. Eventually all three manifestations are present (18,72).

The peripheral neuropathy produced by hexane can be used as an example of solvent-induced neuropathy. There are, however, important differences in the neuropathy caused by other agents. The neuropathy that develops secondary to hexane exposure in the workplace generally develops slowly. The initial symptom is sensory loss in the hands and feet (5). Facial numbness is rarely present with hexane neuropathy. In contrast, trichloroethylene exposure regularly produces involvement of the fifth cranial nerve (5). Acrylamide neuropathy differs from hexane neuropathy in that the loss of vibration and position sense is prominent, ataxia is common, and the Romberg sign is present. Although motor weakness is a feature of solvent neuropathy, it usually develops after the appearance of sensory symptoms. The motor weakness, though usually not severe, can become so if the exposure persists (5,36).

Laboratory Findings

In many instances, the biological monitoring of solvent exposure is unsatisfactory. In cases of toluene abuse the laboratory may be of help, as the whole-blood half-life of this agent ranges between 3 and 6 h. Since glue sniffers seldom go long without practicing their habit, toluene blood levels should be obtained if this syndrome is suspected. Blood levels of 1.0–2.5 mg/L are associated with symptoms, and death may occur with levels greater than 10 mg/L (74). The sweet, pungent odor of toluene often helps the clinician in making the diagnosis. Any young patient observed to have an encephalopathy and the distinctive odor on his breath, should immediately be tested for toluene intoxication (62). The chronic encephalopathy associated with toluene produces slowing in the EEG and evidence of brain atrophy with ventriculomegaly. The pathology of solvent neuropathy, particularly from hexane, is sufficiently unique that a sensory nerve biopsy showing such changes would strongly incriminate this agent.

Treatment and Prognosis

When exposure ceases, solvent neuropathy almost uniformly improves. Persons mildly affected will recover completely from exposure to hexane and most other solvents. The trigeminal nerve sensory loss inflicted by trichloroethylene exposure may endure for years. The acute encephalopathy seen with exposure to many solvents usually regresses, assuming that deep coma does not supervene. Some deaths linked to acute solvent exposure appear to be the consequence of cardiac arrhythmias (see Chapter 17 for a discussion of this problem).

The prognosis for recovery from toluene encephalopathy following cessation of exposure depends on the severity of the encephalopathy. In cases where serious encephalopathy has been present for months, minimal recovery occurs.

Differential Diagnosis of Neurotoxicity

The signs and symptoms of neurotoxic exposure are shared by many chemical agents and disease processes. The laboratory often provides little help in identifying the offending agent. Exposure to each of the chemical agents causing human illness may be accompanied by a number of abnormal laboratory findings that indicate nothing more specific than the disordered function of the affected organ(s). The clinician must be prepared to deal with this lack of specificity when evaluating the nervous system's response to chemical assault. Having a thorough grasp of the elements involved in the differential diagnosis of neurotoxic disease is therefore essential.

Weakness may result from exposure to many different chemicals. The following clinical features may be used in the differential diagnosis of this finding. With the organophosphate insecticides, the weakness is rapid in onset and not associated with sensory changes. Because pupillary miosis usually accompanies this weakness, vascular insults to the pons, particularly pontine hemorrhage, must be considered. The rapid onset of weakness is also suggestive of Guillain–Barré syndrome, and the distinction between these two may be quite difficult. If miosis is present, the diagnosis would favor an intoxication with organic phosphorus compounds. If gastrointestinal symptoms overshadow the weakness, the diagnosis of enteritis might be suggested. With the chest discomfort and respiratory stress that occur with toxicity with the organophosphates, a primary pulmonary or cardiac problem should be considered. Other entities that must be considered in a patient with weakness include poliomyelitis, myasthenia gravis, and botulism. Botulism can be a particular problem if it is not recollected that the pupil in botulism, if affected, is usually dilated rather than small. Involvement of bulbar musculature in botulism is also a distinguishing feature.

When considering the neurotoxic causes of peripheral neuropathy, which include exposure to such compounds as tri-ortho-cresyl phosphate, arsenic, lead, solvents, dioxin, and the halogenated biphenyls, other causes must also be remembered. Chief among these are diabetic and alcoholic neuropathy along with neuropathy from other toxic, metabolic, vascular, and inflammatory processes. Other factors may help to differentiate the neuropathy of toxic exposure from that of other conditions. The neuropathy of arsenic is usually painful and associated with skin changes that are different from those found with diabetic neuropathy. Arsenic often leads to gastrointestinal symptoms and may cause mental status changes as well. The neuropathy of lead intoxication, at times associated with lead colic, is primarily a motor neuropathy particularly affecting the radial nerve. This finding may be confused with a compressive radial neuropathy, often called "Saturday night palsy." Lead-induced wrist drop is ordinarily symmetrical, whereas "Saturday night palsy" is usually unilateral. The fact that arsenical neuropathy is principally a sensory neuropathy and lead neuropathy is principally a motor neuropathy should be of help in their clinical appraisal.

A neuropathy with a preponderant involvement of one or both fifth cranial nerves strongly suggests trichloroethylene intoxication. Although there are few other conditions that cause this problem, one must also consider multiple sclerosis, syringobulbia, brainstem and cerebellpontine angle neoplasm, or brainstem neurovascular disease.

The seizures associated with exposure to neurotoxins are no different from those arising from other causes. Seizures are a common feature of chlorinated hydrocarbon intoxication, and, if accompanied by tremor, their presence strongly suggests intoxication with these chemicals. Nevertheless, the same combination can be seen with alcohol abstinence syndrome. The seizures that accompany lead encephalopathy are not specific. The spinal fluid in such cases often exhibits some mild pleocytosis and increased protein. This finding often makes the clinician suspect encephalitis rather than lead intoxication. If papilledema and headache are present, a mass lesion in the brain must be considered.

Establishing the cause of the tremor of chlorinated hydrocarbon intoxication presents several pitfalls. If the history of toxic exposure is uncertain, benign essential tremor is a strong consideration. In such cases a good exposure history is of critical importance. Because the tremor induced by most toxic exposures, including the chlorinated hydrocarbons, is not a resting tremor, it is difficult to differentiate it from tremors caused by hyperthyroidism. On this basis, the resting tremor of parkinsonism should not be difficult to distinguish from that caused by toxic exposure.

The acute encephalopathy of solvent intoxication is not distinguishable from the acute encephalopathy seen with other psychoactive chemicals. The presence of an obvious "high" or of central nervous system stimulation might be more apt to suggest acute solvent encephalopathy than barbiturate intoxication, but there is overlap. The chronic encephalopathy associated with exposure to such solvents as toluene and with lead and arsenic intoxication is no different from that seen with a host of other causes. Some individuals with toluene encephalopathy have greater gait disturbances than might be expected with Alzheimer's disease. In addition, the young age of those afflicted with toxic encephalopathy serves to eliminate the presence of Alzheimer's disease. The presence of toluene in the blood, if the determination is performed soon after the patient is seen, can be of help in distinguishing toluene encephalopathy from other causes of encephalopathy.

The visual field changes in mercury intoxication are not often seen in encephalopathy caused by other processes. The constricted visual field must be separated from retinitis pigmentosa. This distinction is readily apparent because of the funduscopic differences. Constricted visual fields may resemble tunnel vision, suggestive of hysteria. Performance of careful visual fields at two separate distances usually makes the distinction between tunnel vision and funnel vision.

The encephalopathy seen with chronic dialysis is notable for its stuttering speech. This finding, however, could be mistaken for aphasia or for the language difficulty sometimes seen in Pick's disease. The opportunistic central nervous system infection, so commonly seen in patients receiving chronic dialysis, must always be excluded. The encephalopathy associated with mercury intoxication and the changes in mental status that occur with exposure to other chemical agents may resemble psychopathology from other causes, including schizophrenia.

In several of the neurological conditions described above, coexisting nonneurological manifestations may be of help in making the diagnosis. Lead toxicity, for example, may be associated with anemia, and mercury toxicity with renal failure.

To summarize: the clinical distinction between the various toxic states and other medical conditions is sometimes difficult. Certain rules are helpful. The rapid onset of weakness, particularly with muscle fasciculations, after exposure to a chemical should always raise the issue of organophosphate or carbamate intoxication. The presence of tremor and convulsions without an obvious alcoholic history compels the clinician to rule out chlorinated hydrocarbon intoxication. A neuropathic picture that is primarily wrist drop or is mainly a painful sensory neuropathy should suggest the possibility of lead or arsenic intoxication. A combination of paresthesias, concentric constriction of visual fields, and the insidious onset of ataxia suggests chronic organic mercury intoxication. A subacute encephalopathy in a young person requires the clinician to rule out toluene intoxication. The rapid development of a facial sensory loss with no other explanation suggests trichloroethylene intoxication.

In spite of these helpful clues, the correct diagnosis is established in toxic conditions by (1) obtaining a meticulous exposure history and scrupulously evaluating the patient, (2) maintaining a high level of suspicion of environmental factors in the etiology of disease, (3) using the laboratory judiciously, and (4) following the patient with perseverence. Physicians must be constantly vigilant because an accurate diagnosis of neurotoxic disease often results in specific therapy and always results in a reduction or avoidance of the toxic exposure.

SUMMARY

Exposure to neurotoxic agents is receiving increased attention, particularly as it is recognized that such agents pervade the environment. Neurotoxic chemicals target many levels of the nervous system and cause a variety of adverse effects. Clinicians must be constantly alert to the effects of neurotoxic exposure, even if that exposure occurred long before the onset of clinical symptoms.

REFERENCES

1. Ad Hoc Working Group, International Agency for Research on Cancer: Extremely low frequency electric and magnetic fields and risk of human cancer. Bioelectromagnetics 11:91, 1990.
2. Ahlbom A: A review of the epidemiologic literature on magnetic fields and cancer. Scand J Work Environ Health 14:337, 1988.
3. Alexander FW: The uptake of lead by children in differing environments. Environ Health Perspect 7: 155, 1974.
4. Alfrey AC, LeGendre GR, Kaethny WE: The dialysis encephalopathy syndrome: Possible aluminum intoxication. N Engl J Med 294:184, 1976.
5. Allen N: Solvents and other industrial organic compounds. In: Handbook of Clinical Neurology, Vol. 36, p 361, Vinken PJ, Bruyn GW (eds.), North-Holland, Amsterdam, 1979.
6. Allen N: Identification of methyl n-butyl ketone as the causative agent. In: Experimental and Clinical Neurotoxicology, p 834, Spencer PS, Schaumburg HH (eds.), Williams & Wilkins, Baltimore, 1980.
7. Allen N, Mendell JR, Billmair JD, et al: Toxic neuropathy due to methyl n-butyl ketone. Arch Neurol 32: 209, 1975.

8. Almog C, Tal E: Death from paraquat after subcutaneous injection. Br Med J 3:721, 1967.
9. American Medical Association: Health Effects of "Agent Orange" and Polychlorinated Dioxin Contaminants, AMA, Chicago, 1981.
10. American Medical Association: Health Effects of "Agent Orange" and Polychlorinated Dioxin Contaminants: An update, AMA, Chicago, 1984.
11. Andrews LS, Snyder R: Toxic effects of solvents and vapors. In: Casarett and Doull's Toxicology The Basic Science of Poisons, 3rd ed., p 636, Klaassen CD, Amdur MO, Doull J (eds.), Macmillan, New York, 1986.
12. Anger WK, Johnson BL: Chemicals affecting behavior. In: Neurotoxicity of Industrial and Commercial Chemicals, Vol. 1, O'Donoghue JL (ed.), CRC Press, Boca Raton, 1985.
13. Arezzo JC, Schaumburg NH, Peterson CA: Rapid screening for peripheral neuropathy: A field study with the optacon. Neurology 33:626, 1983.
14. Baker EL: Neurological and behavioral disorders. In: Occupational Health: Recognizing and Preventing Work-Related Disease, 2nd ed., p 399, Levy BS, Wegman DH (eds.), Little Brown, Boston, 1989.
15. Baker EL, Feldman RG, French JG: Environmentally related disorders of the nervous system. Med Clin North Am 74:325, 1990.
16. Bakir F, Damluji SF, Amin-Zaki L, et al: Methylmercury in Iraq. Science 181:230, 1973.
17. Barbeau A: Etiology of Parkinson's disease: A research strategy. Can J Neurosci 11:1457, 1983.
18. Barnes GE: Solvent abuse: A review. Int J Addict 14:1, 1979.
19. Baselt RC, Cravey RH: Disposition of Toxic Drugs and Chemicals in Man, 3rd ed., Year Book Medical Publishers, Chicago, 1990.
20. Batigelli MC: Mercury. In: Environmental and Occupational Medicine, p 449, Rom WN (ed.), Little, Brown, Boston, 1983.
21. Bennett DG Jr, Schwartz TE: Cumulative toxicity of lead arsenate in phenothiazine given to sheep. Am J Vet Res 32:727, 1971.
22. Berwick P: 2,4-Dichlorophenoxyacetic acid poisoning in man: Some interesting clinical and laboratory findings. JAMA 214:1114, 1970.
23. Birke G, Johenls AG, Plantin LO, et al: Studies on humans exposed to methylmercury through fish consumption. Arch Environ Health 25:77, 1972.
24. Bocchetta A, Bernardi F, Piccardi MP, et al: MPTP model: Renewed interest in environmental factors in Parkinson's disease. In: Neurodegenerative Disorders: The Role Played by Endotoxins and Xenobiotics, p 121, Nappi G, Hornykiewicz O, Fariello RG, et al. (eds.), Raven Press, New York, 1988.
25. Buckley J, Warlow C, Smith P, et al: Motor neuron disease in England and Wales, 1959–1979. J Neurol Neurosurg Psychiatry 46:197, 1983.
26. Calne DB, McGeer E, Eisen A, et al: Alzheimer's disease, Parkinson's disease and motoneuron disease: Abiotropic interaction between ageing and environment. Lancet 2:1067, 1986.
27. Caine S, Schoenberg B, Martin W, et al: Familial Parkinson's disease: Possible role of environmental factors. Can J Neurol Sci 14:303, 1987.
28. Cannon SB, Veazey JM Jr, Jackson RS, et al: Epidemic kepone poisoning in chemical workers. Am J Epidemiol 107:529, 1978.
29. Cavanaugh JB, Holler WC: Tri-ortho-cresyl phosphate poisoning. In: The Handbook of Clinical Neurology, Vol. 37, p 471, Vinken PJ, Bruyn GW (eds.), North-Holland, Amsterdam, 1979.
30. Centers for Disease Control: Preventing Lead Poisoning in Young Children, A Statement by the Centers for Disease Control, CDC, Atlanta, 1991.
31. Chiappa KH, Ropper AH: Evoked potentials in clinical medicine, I and II. N Engl J Med 306:1140–1150, 1205–1211, 1982.
32. Cohn NJ, Boylan JJ, Blanke RV: Treatment of chlordecone (Kepone) toxicity with cholestyramine. N Engl J Med 298:243, 1978.
33. Coleman M, Beral V: A review of epidemiological studies of the health effects of living near or working with electricity generation and transmission equipment. Int J Epidemiol 17:1, 1988.
34. Cordle R, Locke R, Springer J: Risk assessment in a federal regulatory agency: An assessment of risk associated with the human consumption of some species of fish contaminated with polychlorinated biphenyls (PCBs). Environ Health Perspect 45:171, 1982.
35. Coulston F, Pocchiari F (eds.): Accidental Exposure to Dioxins. Academic Press, Orlando, 1983.
36. Craft BF: Solvents and related compounds. In: Environmental and Occupational Medicine, p 511, Rom WN (ed.), Little, Brown, Boston, 1983.
37. Davis DL, Hoel D, Fox J, et al: International trends in cancer mortality in France, West Germany, Italy, Japan, England and Wales, and the USA. Lancet 2:474, 1990.
38. Environmental Studies Board, Commission on Natural Resources: Urban Pest Management, National Academy Press, Washington, 1980.
39. Falk RJO, Snihs L, Ekman U, et al: Whole body measurements of the distribution of mercury 203 in humans after oral intake of methylradiomercury nitrate. Acta Radiol 9:55, 1971.
40. Fawer RF, de Ribaupierre Y, Guillemen MP, et al: Hand tremor measurements: Methodology and application. In: Advances in the Biosciences, Vol 46, Neurobehavioral Methods in Occupational Health, p 137, Gilioli R (ed.), Pergamon Press, New York, 1983.
41. Feinglass M: Arsenic intoxication from well water in the United States. N Engl J Med 288:828, 1973.
42. Feldman R: Effects of toxins and physical agents on the nervous system. In: Neurology in Clinical Practice, p 1185, Bradley DM, Daroff R, Fenichil G, et al. (eds.), Butterworths, London, 1990.
43. Fischbein A: Environmental and occupational lead exposure. In: Environmental and Occupational Medicine, p 433, Rom WN (ed.), Little, Brown, Boston, 1983.
44. Flaten TP: Rising mortality from motoneuron disease. Lancet 1:1018, 1989.
45. Friberg L, Vostal J: Mercury in the Environment: An Epidemiologic and Toxicologic Appraisal. CRC Press, Boca Raton, 1972.
46. Gailli CL, Manzo L, Spencer PS (eds.): Recent Advances in Nervous System Toxicology, Plenum Press, New York, 1984.

47. Gluck L, Wood HR: Staphylococcal colonization in newborn infants with and without antiseptic skin care. N Engl J Med 268:1265, 1963.

48. Goldsmith JR, Herishanu Y, Agarbanel JM, et al: Clustering of Parkinson's disease points to environmental etiology. Arch Environ Health 45:89, 1990.

49. Gosselin RE, Smith RP, Hodge HC: Clinical Toxicology of Commercial Products, Williams & Wilkins, Baltimore, 1984.

50. Goyer RA: Toxic effects of metals. In: Casarett and Doull's Toxicology: The Basic Science of Poisons, 3rd ed., p 582, Klaassen CD, Amdur MO, Doull J (eds.), Macmillan, New York, 1986.

51. Graf JW: Clinical aspects of lead poisoning. In: Handbook of Clinical Neurology, Vol. 36, p 1, Vinken PJ, Bruyn CW (eds.), North-Holland, Amsterdam, 1979.

52. Guzelian PS: Comparative toxicology of chlordecone (Kepone) in humans and experimental animals. Annu Rev Pharmacol Toxicol 22:89, 1982.

53. Hayes WJ Jr: Pesticides Studied in Man. Williams & Wilkins, Baltimore, 1982.

54. Hertzman C, Wiens M, Bowering J, et al: Parkinson's disease: A case-control of occupational and environmental risk factors. Am J Ind Med. 17:349, 1990.

55. Heyman A, Pfeiffer JB Jr, Willett RW, et al: Peripheral neuropathy caused by arsenical intoxication: A study of 41 cases with observations on the effect of BAL (2,3-dimercapto-propanol). N Engl J Med 254:401, 1956.

56. Hindmarsh JT, McLetchie OR, Hefferman LPM, et al: Electromyographic abnormalities in chronic environmental arsenicism. J Anal Toxicol 1:270, 1977.

57. Ho SC, Woo J, Lee CM: Epidemiologic study of Parkinson's disease in Hong Kong. Neurology 39: 1314, 1989.

58. Huff JE, Moore JA, Aracci R, et al: Long term hazards of polychlorinated dibenzodioxins and polychlorinated dibenzofurans. Environ Health Perspect 36: 221, 1980.

59. Jacobs MB, Ladd AC, Goldwater LJ: Absorption and excretion of mercury in Man. VI: Significance of mercury in urine. Arch Environ Health 9:454, 1964.

60. Jenkins RB: Inorganic arsenic and the nervous system. Brain 89:479, 1966.

61. Kimbrough RD, Jensen AA (eds.): Halogenated Biphenyls, Terphenyls, Naphthalenes, Dibenzodioxins and Related Products, 2nd ed., Elsevier, Amsterdam, 1989.

62. King MD, Day RE, Oliver JS, et al: Solvent encephalopathy. Br Med J 283:664, 1981.

63. Kohli JD, Khanna RN, Gutta BN, et al: Absorption and excretion of 2,4-dichlorophenoxyacetic acid in man. Xenobiotica 4:97, 1974.

64. Koller WC, Klawans HL: Organophosphorus intoxication. In: Handbook of Clinical Neurology, Vol 37, p 541, Vinken PJ, Bruyn GS (eds.), North-Holland, Amsterdam, 1979.

65. Kopin IJ, Markey SP: MDTP toxicity implications for research in Parkinson's disease. Annu Rev Neurosci 11:81, 1988.

66. Kuratsune M: Yusho, with reference to Yu-Cheng. In: Halogenated Biphenyls, Terphenyls, Naphthalenes, Dibenzodioxins and Related Products, Kimbrough RD, Jensen AA (eds.), 2nd ed., p. 381, Elsevier, Amsterdam, 1989.

67. Kurolwa Y, Mural Y, Santa T: Neurological and nerve conduction velocity. Fukuoka Acta Med 60:462, 1969.

68. Landrigan PJ: Arsenic state of the art. Am J Ind Med 2:5, 1981.

69. Landrigan PJ, Baker EL, Feldman RG, et al: Increased lead absorption with anemia and slowed nerve conduction in children near a lead smelter. J Pediatr 89:904, 1976.

70. Langston JW, Ballard PA: Parkinson's disease in a chemist working with 1-methyl-4-phenyl-1,2,3,6-tetrahydropyridine. Lancet 1:747, 1985.

71. Langston JW, Ballard P, Tetrud JW, et al: Chronic parkinsonism in humans due to a product of merperidine-analogue synthesis Science 219:979, 1982.

72. Lewis JD, Moritz D, Mellis LP: Long term toluene abuse. Am J Psychiatry 138:368, 1981.

73. Lilienfeld DE, Chan E, Ehland J, et al: Rising mortality from motoneuron disease in the USA, 1962–84. Lancet 1:710, 1989.

74. Lush M, Oliver JS, Watson JM: The analysis of blood in cases of suspected solvent abuse with a review of results during the period October 1977 to July 1979. In: Forensic Toxicology: Proceedings of the European Meeting of the International Association of Forensic Toxicologists, p 301, Oliver JS (ed.), Croom Helm, London, 1980.

75. Marsh D: Organic mercury: methylmercury compounds. In: Handbook of Clinical Neurology, Vol 36, p 73, Vinken JP, Bruyn GS (eds.), North-Holland, Amsterdam, 1979.

76. Marshall E: The rise and decline of Temik. Science 229:1369, 1985.

77. Masuda Y, Yashimur H: Polychlorinated biphenyls and dibenzofurans in patients with Yusho and their toxicological significance. Am J Ind Med 5:31, 1984.

78. Mathews HB, Dedrick RL: Pharmokinetics of polychlorinated biphenyls. Annu Rev Pharmacol Toxicol 24:85, 1984.

79. Mealey J Jr, Brownwell GL, Sweet WH: Radiarsenile in plasma, urine, normal tissues and intracranial neoplasms. AMA Arch Neurol Psychiatry 81:310, 1959.

80. Morgan DP: Recognition and Management of Pesticide Poisoning, 4th ed, US Environmental Protection Agency, EPA 540/9-88-001, Washington, 1989.

81. Mulder DW, Kuland LT, Iriarte LLG: Neurologic diseases on the island of Guam, US. Armed Forces Med J 5:1724, 1954.

82. Murphy SD: Toxic effects of pesticides. In: Casarett and Doull's Toxicology: The Basic Science of Poisons, 3rd ed, p 519, Klaassen CD, Amdur MO, Doull J (eds.), Macmillan, New York, 1986.

83. Mushak P: Biological monitoring of lead exposure in children: Overview of selected biokinetic and toxicological issues. In: Lead Exposure and Child Development an International Assessment, p 129, Smith MA, Grant LD, Sors AI (eds.), Kluwer Academic, Dordrecht, 1988.

84. Mushak P, Davis MJ, Crocetti AF, et al: Prenatal and postnatal effects of low-level lead exposure: Integrated summary of a report to the U.S. Congress on childhood lead poisoning. Environ Res 50:11, 1989.

85. Neilson VK: The peripheral nerve function in chronic

renal failure: An analysis of the vibratory perception threshold. Acta Med Scand 191:287, 1972.

86. Norton S: Responses of the central nervous system. In: Casarett and Doull's Toxicology: The Basic Science of Poisons, 3rd ed, p 359, Klaassen CD, Amdur MO, Doull J (eds.), Macmillan, New York, 1986.

87. Oyangurem H, Perez E: Poisoning of industrial origin in the community. Arch Environ Health 13:185, 1966.

88. Pazderova-Vejlupkova J, Lukas E, Numcova M, et al: The development and prognosis of chronic intoxication by tetrachlordibenzo-*p*-dioxin in men. Arch Environ Health 36:5, 1981.

89. Perlstein MA, Attala R: Neurologic sequelae of plumbism in children. Clin Pediatr 5:292, 1966.

90. Rabinowitz MB, Wetherill GW, Kopple JD: Studies of human lead metabolism by use of stable isotope tracers. Environ Health Perspect 7:145, 1974.

91. Rabinowitz MB, Wetherill GW, Kopple JD: Kinetic analysis of lead metabolism in healthy humans. J Clin Invest 58:260, 1976.

92. Reed DM, Brody JA: Amyotrophic lateral sclerosis and parkinsonism dementia on Guam, 1945–1972. Am J Epidemiol 101:287, 1975.

93. Reggiani G: Estimation of the TCDD toxic potential in the light of the Seveso accident. Arch Toxicol Suppl 2:291, 1979.

94. Reggiani GM: The Seveso accident: Medical survey of a TCDD exposure. In: Halogenated Biphenyls, Terphenyls, Naphthalenes, Dibenzodioxins and Related Products, 2nd ed., p 45, Kimbrough RD, Jensen AA (eds.), Elsevier, Amsterdam, 1989.

95. Rogan WJ: Yu-Cheng. In: Halogenated Biphenyls, Terphenyls, Naphthalenes, Dibenzodioxins and Related Products, 2nd ed., p 401, Kimbrough RD, Jensen AA (eds.), Elsevier, Amsterdam, 1989.

96. Rustam H, Hamdi T: Methyl mercury poisoning in Iraq. Brain 97:499, 1974.

97. Savitz DA, Wachtel H, Barnes FA, et al: Case control study of childhood cancer and exposure to 60-Hz magnetic fields. Am J Epidemiol 128:21, 1988.

98. Savitz DA, John EM, Kleckner RC: Magnetic field exposure from electric appliances and childhood cancer. Am J Epidemiol 131:763, 1990.

99. Schuman RM, Leech RW, Alvord ED Jr: Neurotoxicity of hexachlorophene in the human. A clinicopathologic study of 248 children. Pediatrics 54:689, 1973.

100. Schuman RM, Leech RW, Alvord ED Jr: Neurotoxicity of hexachlorophene in the human. Arch Neurol 32:320, 1975.

101. Seppalainen AM, Hernberg S: Sensitive techniques for detecting subclinical lead neuropathy. Br J Ind Med 29:443, 1972.

102. Seto DYS, Freeman JM: Lead neuropathy in childhood. Am J Dis Child 107:337, 1964.

103. Spencer PS, Schaumburg HH (eds.): Experimental and Clinical Neurotoxicology, Williams & Wilkins, Baltimore, 1980.

104. Spencer PS, Schaumburg HH: An expanded classification of neurotoxic responses based on cellular targets of chemical agents. Acta Neurol Scand 70(Suppl 100):9, 1984.

105. Spencer PS, Nunn PB, Hugon J, et al: Motor neuron disease on Guam: Possible role of a food neurotoxin. Lancet 2:965, 1986.

106. Spencer PS, Roy DN, Ludolph A, et al: Lathyrism: Evidence for role of the neuroexcitatory BOAA. Lancet 2:1066, 1986.

107. Spencer PS, Nunn PB, Hugon J, et al: Guam amyotrophic lateral sclerosis–Parkinson–dementia linked to a plant excitant neurotoxin. Science 237:517, 1987.

108. Suskind RR, Hertzberg VS: Human health effects of 2,4,5-T and its toxic contaminants. JAMA 257:2372, 1984.

109. Takeuchi T, Eto N, Eto K: Neuropathology of childhood cases of methylmercury poisoning (Minamata disease) with prolonged symptoms with particular reference to the decortication syndrome. Neurotoxicology 1:1, 1979.

110. Tanner CM: The role of environmental toxins in the etiology of Parkinson's disease. Trends Neurosci 12:49, 1989.

111. Tanner CM, Chen B, Wang W, et al: Environmental factors and Parkinson's disease: A case-control study in China. Neurology 39:660, 1989.

112. Taylor JR, Selhorst JB, Houff SA, et al: Chlordecone intoxication in man: I: Clinical observations. Neurology 28:626, 1978.

113. Taylor JR, Selhorst JB, Calabrese VP: Chlordecone. In: Experimental and Clinical Neurotoxicology, p 407, Spencer PS, Schaumburg HH (eds.), Williams & Wilkins, Baltimore, 1980.

114. US Congress, Office of Technology Assessment: Losing a Million Minds: Confronting the Tragedy of Alzheimer's Disease and Other Dementias, US Government Printing Office, Washington, 1987.

115. US Congress, Office of Technology Assessment: Neurotoxicity: Identifying and Controlling Poisons of the Nervous System, Van Nostrand Reinhold, New York, 1990.

116. US Department of Health and Human Services, Public Health Service, Agency for Toxic Substances and Disease Registry: The Nature and Extent of Lead Poisoning in Children in the United States: A Report to Congress, Centers for Disease Control, Atlanta, 1988.

117. US Environmental Protection Agency: Suspended, Cancelled and Restricted Pesticides, 3rd revision, Washington, 1985.

118. US Environmental Protection Agency, Office of Pesticides and Toxic Substances: The Toxic Release Inventory: A National Perspective, 1987 EPA 560/4-89-006, Washington, 1989.

119. US Environmental Protection Agency, Office of Water, Office of Pesticides and Toxic Substances: National Pesticide Survey, Phase 1 Report: EPA's National Survey of Pesticides in Drinking Water Wells. EPA 570/9-90-015, Washington, 1990.

120. Winter CK, Seiber JN, Nuckton CF: Chemicals in the Human Food Chain, Van Nostrand Reinhold, New York, 1990.

121. World Health Organization: Principles and Methods for the Assessment of Neurotoxicity Associated with Exposure to Chemicals. Environmental Health Criteria 60, World Health Organization, Geneva, 1986.

122. Wright JM, Wall RA, Perry TL, et al: Chronic parkinsonism secondary to intranasal administration of a

product of meperidine-analogue synthesis. N Engl J Med 310:325, 1984.

RECOMMENDED READINGS

Baker EL, Feldman RG, French JG: Environmentally related disorders of the nervous system. Med Clin North Am 74:325, 1990.

Committee on Neurotoxicology and Models for Assessing Risk, National Research Council, National Academy Press, Washington, 1992.

Feldman R: Effects of toxins and physical agents on the nervous system. In: Neurology in Clinical Practice, Vol II, p 1185, Bradley WG, Daroff RB, Fenichel GM, et al. (eds.), Butterworth Heinemann, London, 1991.

Johnson BL (ed.): Preventing Neurotoxic Disease in Working Populations, John Wiley & Sons, New York, 1987.

Spencer PS, Schaumburg HH (eds.): Experimental and Clinical Neurotoxicology, Williams & Wilkins, Baltimore, 1980.

US Congress, Office of Technology Assessment: Neurotoxicity: Identifying and Controlling Poisons of the Nervous System, OTA-8A-436, US Government Printing Office, Washington, 1990.

14. NEUROBEHAVIORAL DISORDERS

David E. Hartman, Stephen Hessl, and Alyce Bezman Tarcher

INTRODUCTION

The nervous system is vulnerable to the harmful effects of many industrial and agricultural chemicals. Although it has long been recognized that toxic exposure affects the function of the brain and peripheral nerves, only recently has attention focused on behavioral changes as an indicator of toxic assault to the central nervous system.

Behavior can be thought of as the end product of the sensory, motor, affective, and integrative processes of the nervous system (102,105). Thus, any exposure that adversely affects behavior can impair our ability to function in our daily and working life. The importance of recognizing the link between toxic exposure and behavioral disorders stems in part from the impression that such changes may provide the earliest evidence of toxic injury to the central nervous system. In addition, many investigators suggest that the sensitivity of the brain to toxic substances provides an early barometer of their adverse effects. The toxic effects of exposure may be heralded by such subtle, insidious, and mild disturbances as depression, irritability, and fatigue long before more tangible effects appear (116,126, 131,147).

Early identification of toxic injury to the central nervous system is important because the prompt

Principles and Practice of Environmental Medicine, edited by Alyce Bezman Tarcher. Plenum Medical Book Company, New York, 1992.

removal of an individual from further hazardous exposure may prevent irreversible neurological injury. Early diagnosis obviously depends primarily on the alert physician. Too frequently, however, physicians have little awareness that exposure to toxic agents can lead to subtle changes in behavior, intellect, memory, and mood. Moreover, central nervous system toxicity induced by chronic exposure may go undetected because the symptoms are nonspecific and thus readily confused with other conditions. For example, behavioral changes in the elderly are usually attributed to the debilitating effects of advancing age, without consideration of the possibility that prolonged neurotoxic exposure may also be involved.

It was not generally recognized until recently that chemical exposure of the developing nervous system of the fetus and young child can lead to subtle long-lasting consequences. Past investigators were concerned primarily with the structural defects that resulted from prenatal exposure. However, in the 1960s, teratology expanded to include functional defects. This area of investigation, termed behavioral teratology, refers to the adverse behavioral effects of agents on developing organisms. It is one of the fastest growing and most challenging disciplines in neuroscience (11,119). The importance of behavioral teratology rests on the fact that the developing brain is particularly sensitive to toxic assault. Once brain injury is sustained, it remains for life (1,29). A number of agents are known to have adverse behavioral consequences on the neonate and on later development in both humans and animals. The effects of three environmental chemicals, i.e., lead, methyl mercury, and polychlorinated biphenyls, are discussed.

The advent of modern neuropsychological testing techniques has added immeasurably to our ability to assess functional disturbances of the central nervous system. Advances made in recent years have established that such testing affords sufficient sensitivity, reliability, and validity (69,143). Neuropsychological testing methods have been used to study the behavioral effects of exposure in groups of workers and in the individual.

This chapter focuses on the changes in mental functioning that may follow exposure to toxic chemicals. Particular attention is given to metals, solvents, and pesticides. The clinical implications of behavioral disorders induced by toxic exposure are discussed, as is neuropsychological testing: its rationale, uses, and limitations.

ENVIRONMENTAL CHEMICALS ASSOCIATED WITH NEUROBEHAVIORAL DISORDERS

Neurobehavioral disorders can arise from exposure to any of a wide range of toxic agents. Exposures to metals, solvents, and pesticides, however, are most commonly associated with these disorders (Table 14-1). A listing of agents having an adverse effect on behavior is far from complete. The magnitude of the problem is reflected in the fact that over 1000 new compounds are developed yearly. Approximately 70,000 chemicals and 2 million chemical mixtures are in common use.

In the United States alone, some 20 million workers are exposed to materials known to be neurotoxic. Solvents and pesticides, in particular, are widely used throughout the world. Solvents are used in industry in such agents as glues, paints, and degreasing agents. The problem of exposure to solvents and other neurotoxic agents is not confined to large industries. Nearly everyone at some time is exposed to solvents and especially solvent mixtures. Perhaps of greater concern is the potential for neurotoxic exposure of workers in small shops where hazards are often ignored. Pesticides pose a major neurotoxic hazard because of their vast global use in agriculture and in the home. Worldwide sales of pesticides increased from $2.7 billion in 1970 to $11.6 billion in 1980 and to an anticipated $18.5 billion in 1990 (94).

Neurotoxic hazards exist in the home, the school, and the community. Defective space heaters, lead-containing paint, and exposure to household pesticides have produced neurotoxic illness as severe as those arising from industrial exposure to carbon monoxide, lead, or organophosphates. Such neurotoxic agents as rubber cement, shellac, paint, paint thinner, and pesticides are often used in and around the home without adequate precaution and ventilation. Problems of exposure to neurotoxic agents may also exist for the artist and in schools where art is taught. Hobbyists and artists may also be at risk from lead exposure through such activities as stained glass work, jewelry making, and soldering of metal sculptures.

Lead is widely dispersed throughout our environment. Industrial exposure to lead may occur in foundries, smelters, auto body shops, and in the manufacture of electric storage batteries. Lead exposure also occurs in the general environment and in food, particularly food stored in cans sealed with lead solder. Drinking water may contain lead when it flows through lead pipes or pipes soldered with lead. Outdoor air contains lead, particularly in the vicinity of smelters or from the exhaust of autos using lead-containing gasoline.

Homes may also be contaminated with lead, particularly in old pre-World War II homes and apartments painted with lead-containing paint. Leaded paint continues to be the major source of environmental lead exposure. It is well documented that environmental lead contamination presents a major neurotoxic hazard for the fetus and young child (2,24,25,38,106). It is estimated that 17% of children (3–4 million) living in metropolitan areas in the United States are exposed to environmental sources of lead that place them at health risk. In addition, 400,000 fetuses are estimated to be at risk of excess absorption of lead as a result of maternal exposure (2).

Although adverse behavioral effects are now well recognized as a consequence of exposure to environmental and industrial agents, toxicity testing has only recently focused on the brain and its function. This attention follows the advances in neurobehavioral toxicology made over the past 10 to 20 years (10,138,143,147). Technical methods are now available for assessing a wide variety of central nervous system functions in the laboratory.

Well-developed animal models have emerged in the field of behavioral toxicology (138). Animal testing offers the promise of screening agents for neurotoxicity and ultimately providing regulatory agencies with data that may be of value in the process of risk assessment. Such testing, however, suffers from the problem of transposing behavioral endpoints observed in the laboratory to humans. Further, behavioral deficits have not been correlated with neuropathological or neurochemical changes (102,124,138). Neuroscientists actively continue to search for such correlates.

Human subjects have been used to investigate the neurobehavioral effects of chemical exposure. Human studies generally entail the assessment of neurobehavioral performance through the use of an

Table 14-1. Neurobehavioral Effects of Exposure to Common Neurotoxins[a]

Agent	Effect	Major uses/exposure sources
Arsenic	Memory impairment CNS symptoms (neurasthenia psychoorganic syndrome) Visual–motor impairment	Pesticides Pigments Antifouling paint Electroplating industry Seafood Smelters Semiconductor manufacturing
Lead	Memory impairment CNS symptoms (neurasthenia, psychoorganic syndrome) Visual–motor impairment Impaired neurobehavioral development in children	Solder Lead paint Illicit whiskey Insecticides Autobody shops Battery manufacturing plants Foundries, smelters Lead pipes Drinking water contaminated by lead pipes
Mercury	Memory impairment CNS symptoms (neurasthenia, psychoorganic syndrome) Visual–motor impairment	Scientific instruments (e.g., thermometers) Dental amalgams Electroplating industry Photography Feltmaking Textiles Pigments Taxidermy
Organic solvents	Memory impairment CNS symptoms (neurasthenia, psychoorganic syndrome) Visual–motor impairment	Dry cleaning fluid Degreasers Paint removers, glues Paints, lacquers Rubber solvents Adhesives in shoe and boot industry Auto and aviation fuels
Organophosphates	Memory impairment CNS symptoms (neurasthenia, psychoorganic syndrome Visual–motor impairment	Pesticides Agricultural industry
Carbon monoxide	Motor incoordination Impaired vigilance and attention ?CNS symptoms (neurasthenia, psychoorganic syndrome)	Exhaust fumes Acetylene welding Enclosed areas, mines, tunnels, and garages Emissions of cars and buses Poorly ventilated stoves, furnaces, and heaters

[a]From Anger and Johnson (9), Eskenazi and Maizlish (51), and Johnson (81).

exposure chamber in which a subject is exposed to a known concentration of a toxicant(s) for a prescribed period of time. Ethical and safety concerns severely restrict experimental research on humans. Moreover, human exposure studies are difficult and expensive to perform. Thus, relatively few human studies have been done thus far. The goal of human studies typically lies in the assessment of the acute neurobehavioral effects of chemical exposure and the identification of those effects that appear at low levels of exposure (39). One of the basic shortcomings of experimental studies is that exposure conditions rarely simulate those present in the real world (56).

To date, the guidelines for acute and subchronic toxicity testing issued by the Environmental Protection Agency refer only in passing to behavioral observations. With the exception of the organophosphate pesticides, the primary "evidence" of neurotoxic exposure is limited to neuropathological changes (8,125,141,146). Neurobehavioral toxicity has been incorporated into about 25% of workplace standards in the United States (9). This is in contrast to the Russians, who have used central nervous system function in setting workplace standards (44).

EPIDEMIOLOGY

In the past, epidemiologic studies revealed the link between toxic exposure and outbreaks of overt neurotoxic illness. Our present awareness that toxic exposures may be coupled with a subtle, less tangible form of neurotoxic illness reflected in behavioral changes stems primarily from epidemiologic studies initiated in the 1970s in Scandinavia. These studies report insidious behavioral changes in occupational groups chronically exposed to solvents (13,20,63,74).

Many epidemiologic studies have used neuropsychological test methods to identify the neurobehavioral effects of toxic exposure and to provide detailed objective evidence of such change. The functions assessed generally include memory, visuospatial skills, attention and cognitive tracking, motor abilities, verbal concept formation, personality, and mood. The benefits and limitations of neurobehavioral testing are discussed later in this chapter.

Prior to the availability of neuropsychological testing, clues to the behavioral effects of neurotoxic exposure depended on the gross description of exposed workers presented in case studies. Such studies described individuals with such problems as poor work performance, memory disturbances, confusion, and depression.

As a growing number of reports reveal a relationship between exposure and impaired central nervous system function, the importance of well-designed epidemiologic studies becomes apparent (14). Epidemiologic methods help to define the neurobehavioral effects of occupational/environmental exposure(s), the mode of onset, reversibility, dose-response relationships, populations at risk, maximal safe levels, and the efficacy of control measures. Unfortunately, epidemiologic studies encounter difficulty in characterizing toxic exposure. When studying the long-term effects of exposure, it is very difficult to reconstruct past exposure patterns. This problem is particularly troublesome in cases of solvent-induced dysfunction. In contrast to lead, biological monitoring provides no evidence of chronic exposure to solvents, since these agents are rapidly metabolized. A detailed discussion of biological monitoring is found in Chapter 27.

Most epidemiologic studies of behavioral neurotoxicity performed thus far have been cross-sectional studies of occupationally exposed groups; i.e., an exposed group of workers is compared with a group having less exposure or with a group with no exposure to the chemical(s) in question. Prospective studies are needed to provide insight into the pattern of neurobehavioral dysfunction that arises in relation to the duration and intensity of toxic exposure and its reversibility after exposure stops. Individual susceptibility in relation to age, gender, genetic factors, nutrition, medication, drugs, and ethanol use also needs to be explored. The question of neurotoxic exposure aggravating neuropsychiatric disorders also bears investigation.

Occupational Studies

Neurotoxicants were first identified in workplaces where toxic exposures are higher and more readily recognized. A review of clinical reports and epidemiologic studies describing neurobehavioral effects of workers exposed to lead, organic solvents, and organophosphate insecticides follows.

Lead

Symptoms of intoxication from inorganic lead exposure have been recognized for hundreds of years. As cases of severe acute lead encephalopathy become rarer, and as our methodology permits the assessment of less obvious behavioral dysfunction, attention is increasingly directed to the subtle central nervous system manifestations of lead exposure.

For example, workers chronically exposed to medium to low lead levels insidiously develop such symptoms as dizziness, headache, nausea, anorexia, nervousness, hyperirritability, sleeplessness, and fatigue (53). In some studies, blood lead levels or zinc protoporphyrin levels were correlated with the number of symptoms reported (17,90,158). Lead exposure generally appears to be linked to cognitive and psychomotor dysfunction and mood disturbances (18,61,117,123,142). Even though a precise threshold has not been found, several studies of lead-exposed workers reveal that subtle neurobehavioral changes can be detected even at very low levels of lead exposure (67,97,98). The importance of reducing lead exposure was shown by Baker et al., who noted an improvement in the behavioral performance of workers whose exposure to lead was reduced (21).

Solvents

The term "solvent" is used to describe individual substances as well as mixtures of organic solvents, which include gasoline, kerosene, thinners, glues, paints, and lacquers. From an epidemiologic perspective, the major health hazard arises not from exposure to isolated individual compounds but from exposure to solvent mixtures. Worldwide, it is thought that millions of individuals are exposed to solvent mixtures in the workplace and the general environment. The discussion thus focuses on the neurobehavioral effects of exposure to mixtures of organic solvents.

The neurobehavioral effects of acute exposure to high concentrations of organic solvents are well established. The euphoric, intoxicating central nervous system effects of sniffing solvent-containing spot remover, glues, and lacquer thinner have been widely observed (145). In contrast, defining the neurobehavioral effects of chronic exposure to relatively low levels of organic solvents has been a difficult and challenging task. The neurotoxic effects of exposure to organic solvents in the workplace have been amply reviewed (20,51,52,63,95).

Many cross-sectional epidemiologic studies done in Sweden, Finland, and Denmark indicate that workers, after years of exposure to organic solvent mixtures, display a variety of neurobehavioral deficits. The exposed groups consisted of printers; car, industrial, and house painters; wood workers; and workers exposed to jet fuels. Though the findings varied somewhat, disturbances in mood, impairment of motor coordination and speed, and reduction in short-term memory ability were noted. In addition, solvent-exposed workers were observed to complain more frequently of such symptoms as headache, irritability, fatigability, and insomnia (45,64,66,79,82,91,92). A study by Baker et al. in the United States revealed an increase in neurobehavioral symptoms in painters chronically exposed to organic solvents. The number of symptoms reported was proportional to an index of solvent exposure derived from work histories and other job information (22).

Research groups in Scandinavia studied the long-term effects of solvent exposure by examining the pension or disability records of workers who retired with neuropsychiatric illness (12,91,104,112). These investigators found that painters and some other solvent-exposed workers were roughly twice as likely to develop an incapacitating neuropsychiatric disorder than other workers. Workers with diagnoses of alcoholism were excluded from these studies. Psychiatric disorders associated with solvent exposures have been reviewed (133).

In many instances adverse behavioral effects were noted in workers who were exposed to mixed organic solvents at levels thought to be within a safe range. These findings may arise from inadequate safety levels and/or synergistic relationships among various solvent compounds that act to enhance their toxicity. The apparent persistence of central nervous system dysfunction observed in some cases, even after solvent exposure has stopped, is of concern.

Some investigators have not replicated the results of the Scandinavian studies (32,95). Moreover, there is a discrepancy between the number of patients reported to have toxic encephalopathy in Scandinavia and those reported for other industrialized European countries. To further investigate this problem, an International Working Group on the Epidemiology of the Chronic Neurobehavioral Effects of Organic Solvents was set up. Methodological guidelines related to such factors as study design, measurement of confounding variables, exposure data, and neurobehavioral and neurophysiological testing are being advanced to assure a consistent research approach that permits the comparability of data (139).

Although many epidemiologic studies provide evidence that central nervous system impairment is produced by prolonged exposure to low levels of organic solvents, this issue is unresolved. The uncertainty rests, in part, on the difficulty in characterizing the degree of exposure, the differences in neurobehavioral test methods used in the various studies, and the inability of most past studies to control adequately for such confounding factors as alcohol use that could lower test performance (62, 76,130). Despite the fact that a number of important questions remain unanswered, solvent-related toxicity affecting the central nervous system is rapidly becoming an important public health issue (15,16).

Pesticides: Organophosphorus Compounds

It has been estimated that the incidence of acute pesticide poisoning worldwide ranges between 500,000 and 2.9 million cases (80,153). Acute exposure to high concentrations of organophosphorus (OP) pesticides has a marked effect on the central nervous system. The onset and duration of symptoms in acute poisoning depend on the dose and duration of exposure, the route of entry, the intrinsic toxicity of the OP, and the susceptibility of the host (12,91,104,112). Symptoms of acute poisoning develop during exposure or within 4 to 12 h of exposure. There is usually a distinct constellation of central nervous system effects, which include anxiety, restlessness, emotional lability, headache, and impaired memory and concentration. Inhibition of plasma and/or RBC acetylcholinesterase enzyme activities is the most generally available and satisfactory biochemical index of excessive exposure to OP (see Chapter 27 for further discussion of this topic).

Many case reports note the presence of neurobehavioral sequelae following acute and chronic OP exposure. Common symptoms include impaired memory and concentration, confusion, agitation, depression, nervousness, irritability, insomnia, and forgetfulness (41,43,58,75,78,134,149).

Exposure to OP is reported to have delayed, persistent, or latent neuropsychological effects on the central nervous system (51). Evidence supporting the long-term neurobehavioral effects of OP exposure is derived from case reports, large case series, and cross-sectional epidemiologic studies of agricultural workers.

In some epidemiologic studies neuropsychological testing was performed on groups of workers who received varying degrees of exposure to OP for unspecified periods of time. The groups included farmers, agricultural workers, pest control workers, and industrial workers with accidental pesticide exposure. A limited range of neurobehavioral functions was evaluated in many studies, and only a few studies employed compatible test methods. Nonetheless, a number of investigators reported that exposed workers demonstrated impaired performance on psychometric testing (83,96,103).

The latent neurological sequelae of acute OP poisoning were studied by Savage et al. (121). In this epidemiologic study, differences in the results of neuropsychological testing were found between subjects with a history of acute pesticide poisoning and the controls. The median time elapsed from the last OP poisoning to the date of the neuropsychological examination was approximately 9 years. Some impairment of fine coordination and motor speed was found. However, major deficits were also encountered in cognitive performance. The findings were sufficiently subtle to be overlooked in the clinical neurological examination (121). Ensberg et al., studying workers with heavy exposure to a mixture of pesticides, noted that such complaints as recurring headache and abnormal fatigue were more frequent in workers with 4 years or more of exposure than among control subjects (46). Other researchers failed to note deficits in neurobehavioral function in workers exposed to OP (42,120).

The methodological shortcomings of epidemiologic studies lead to uncertainties about the long-term behavioral effects of OP exposure. Nonetheless, many investigators have described persistent symptoms and neurobehavioral deficits associated with acute and chronic OP exposure. These findings point the way for future studies.

Indoor Air Pollution: Sick Building Syndrome

The term "sick building syndrome" or "tight building syndrome" has been applied to symptoms experienced by a significant number of occupants of large office buildings. Over the past decade, building-related symptoms in nonindustrial settings have been widely reported (see Chapter 2). This problem is discussed in this chapter because many of the symptoms that form a part of the "sick building syndrome" are those found in a mild form of mood disturbance with a possible organic basis (16,60,144). Headache, fatigue, lethargy, irritability, and forgetfulness are commonly described in the sick building syndrome. Though these symptoms

are nonspecific, they are quite consistent with those described under conditions of low-level exposure to solvents and other agents. Other complaints include eye irritation, dry throat, burning mucous membranes, sinus congestion, skin irritation, cough, dyspnea, and dizziness. It is of interest that psychological symptoms in relation to indoor air pollution were described as early as 1955 (113).

From 1978 through 1985, the National Institute of Occupational Safety and Health (NIOSH) carried out 365 health hazard evaluations, primarily in government and private office buildings. In most instances air quality monitoring failed to identify concentrations of contaminants that were considered high enough to cause health problems. Nonetheless, chemical contaminants associated with building materials and pollutant sources within the building, such as carpeting, office furnishings, cleaning materials, paints and adhesives, and pollutants, accounted for about 30% of the air quality problems investigated. Inadequate ventilation and poor air quality were described as the primary cause of the symptoms in about 50% of the buildings investigated (60,144).

Environmental Studies

With the evolution of more sophisticated laboratory and epidemiologic methods, study of the effects of toxic exposure was extended from the workplace to the lower levels of exposure found in the general environment. Children were the logical subjects of such epidemiologic studies because they often encounter many of the toxic chemicals present in the workplace and because they are in many ways more susceptible than adults to toxic assault (107). Of all such epidemiologic studies, the effects of lead exposure on neuropsychological development in childhood have received the greatest attention (2,128).

Lead (Childhood Exposure)

Lead persists indefinitely and, as a consequence of industrialization, is widely dispersed throughout the environment. It is a health hazard especially for the fetus and young child. Because lead readily crosses the placenta during the entire period of gestation, the developing fetus is at risk for6lead exposure and toxicity. Young children are vulnerable to the effects of lead for a number of reasons. They ingest more lead than adults because of hand-to-mouth activity. They also absorb a larger amount of lead per unit body measure than do adults (157). Moreover, with greater movement of lead to bone, children retain a larger fraction of the absorbed lead than do adults (157). A number of studies reveal that the nutritional well-being of the child also plays a role in lead toxicity. A strong inverse correlation was found between iron status and blood lead levels (33). A similar relationship was observed between calcium intake and blood lead levels (129). Zinc deficiency also plays a role in enhanced lead absorption and toxicity risk (99).

Lead is associated with a broad range of toxicological effects. However, the developing central nervous system is a primary target organ for lead toxicity. Childhood lead toxicity was recognized in the United States in the earlier part of this century. Neurotoxicity was related to acute high-level lead exposure, which was often followed by severe encephalopathy. Though we are not free of such problems, particularly in urban ghettos, the attention of the medical and research community has shifted to analyzing the effects of low levels of lead exposure. Our efforts are directed to the neurotoxic effects of chronic, low-level lead exposure at concentrations that do not result in encephalopathic symptoms, miscarriages, or obvious neonatal deformities.

Epidemiologic studies are a primary means of identifying chronic injury to the developing central nervous system in relation to low levels of environmental lead exposure. Epidemiologic studies are of two general types: (1) cross-sectional or retrospective studies and (2) prospective or longitudinal studies. Prospective studies overcome some of the difficulties of retrospective studies by allowing investigators to follow exposed groups over a period of time during which lead exposure is measured in relation to changes in behavioral development.

Epidemiologic studies investigating the relationship between lead exposure and childhood development are bedeviled by many confounding factors and the methodological difficulties in dealing with these factors. For example, the course of child development may be affected by such forces as parental education and intelligence, the home environment, nutritional status, socioeconomic status, family size, and birth order. In addition, epidemiologic studies must face such issues as the adequacy of the marker used to indicate lead exposure, the use of insensitive or inappropriate measures to assess childhood development, and the lack of statistical power of studies in which small groups are sampled (108,140,155,156).

Cross-Sectional or Retrospective Studies Early epidemiologic research on lead exposure at low dose and childhood development conducted in the 1970s and 1980s consisted of cross-sectional or retrospective studies. Some studies revealed a lead effect, but others did not. An early and important study was performed in 1979 by Needleman and his co-workers. These investigators conducted a community-based study of children in the Boston area who had no known increased lead exposure. The deciduous teeth of the children were analyzed for lead content.

This measurement was used as an indicator of cumulative lead exposure. Based on the classroom teachers' rating scale of 2146 subjects, poorer behavior scores were recorded in direct relation to the child's dentine lead level. More detailed analyses were performed on 58 children with high dentine lead levels and 100 children with low dentine lead levels, taking into account various confounding variables. The children with high dentine lead had significantly lower scores on verbal IQ and other neurobehavioral tests (110).

A study of children in Edinburgh, Scotland performed by Fulton et al. revealed that blood lead levels below 25 μg/dL (1.2 μmol/L) were inversely related to cognitive ability and educational attainment (55). Hatzakis et al. in Lavrion, Greece also provided strong evidence of IQ deficits related to children's lead exposure at blood lead levels below 25 μg/dL (1.2 μmol/L) (73). Other investigators showed few if any apparent effects of low-level lead exposure on mental development after adjustment had been made for the confounding effects of the social environment and other factors (47,85, 127,152).

Prospective Studies The varied results noted above may in part be related to methodological issues, particularly those confounding variables that influence children's development. To overcome the methodological difficulties of the cross-sectional studies, a number of prospective studies were begun and are currently in progress in various parts of the world. These studies were designed to obtain a clearer definition of the interrelationship between low-level prenatal and postnatal lead exposure and neuropsychological development in childhood. Though the epidemiologic studies are being conducted independently, the investigators have exchanged information and ideas to strengthen the study design and analysis. Appropriate controls have been incorporated for many covariates and potentially confounding variables. The population under study is generally large enough to have the statistical power to detect subtle effects. The analytic methods for measuring blood lead levels are reliable. The consistent use of the Bayley Scales of Infant Development and other widely used test methods in the assessment of developmental effects permits the direct comparison of the results among the studies (2,38,140). The Bayley Scales of Infant Development comprise three indices of mental, motor, and emotional development for children from 2 to 30 months of age. The scales have a mean of 100 and a standard deviation of 16 (23).

Bellinger and co-workers, working in Boston, were the first to report the results of a prospective study assessing the relationship between prenatal lead exposure and postnatal development (24). In their cohort of 249 subjects, an inverse relationship was noted between infants' umbilical cord blood lead concentration and their scores at 6 months on the Bayley Mental Development Index. Cord blood lead levels were categorized as low (<3 μg/dL; <0.15 μmol/L), middle (6–7 μg/dL; 0.30–0.35 μmol/L), and high (10–24.9 μg/dL; 0.5–1.2 μmol/L). After adjustment for various covariates and confounders, the difference between the low- and high-lead groups was nearly 6 points on the the Mental Development Index. This pattern persisted with continued follow-up of these subjects at 12, 18, and 24 months of age (25,26). Lead levels in umbilical cord blood between 10 and 25μg/dL (0.5–1.2 μmol/L) were consistently associated with lower performance on tests of infant development administered at 6-month intervals through the second year of life. Up to 2 years of age the scores on the Mental Development Index were unrelated to the infants' postnatal blood lead levels.

Dietrich et al. studied 305 pregnant women residing in the inner city of Cincinnati. Lead was measured in the mother, from the umbilical cord, and from the newborn infants. All blood lead levels were less than 30 μg/dL (<1.4 μmol/L). Infant development, as measured at 6 months of age on the Bayley Mental Development Index, was inversely related to both prenatal and postnatal blood lead levels. Impaired performance was also related to reduced gestational age and reduced birth weight. Male infants and infants from the poorest families appeared to be especially sensitive (40).

Other workers also observed an effect of socioeconomic forces on the behavioral development of lead-exposed children (27,28). A study by Bellinger et al. revealed a class-dependent association between prenatal lead exposure and the Mental Development Index. The adverse effect on performance in children in lower socioeconomic strata was noted at the lower levels of prenatal exposure (blood lead levels of 6–7 μg/dL (0.30–0.35 μmol/L) (28). The influence of socioeconomic strata on lead toxicity is consistent with the results of other studies (72,84,152).

Another major prospective study is under way in Port Pirie, South Australia (101,150). A cohort of 537 children, living in a community situated near a lead smelter, are being studied to determine the effect of lead exposure on their mental development. The study thus far indicates that the blood lead concentration at each age, particularly at 2 and 3 years, and the integrated postnatal average concentration are inversely related to development at the age of 4. After adjustment for confounding factors, the children with an average postnatal blood lead level of 31 μg/dL (1.50 μmol/L) had a cognitive score 7.2 points lower than those with an average concentration of 10 μg/dL (0.50 μmol/L). Within the range of exposure studied, there was no evidence of a threshold dose for an effect of lead (101,150).

In Cleveland, prospective studies were conducted by Ernhart et al. Maternal and cord blood lead determinations were performed on 169 and 146 subjects, respectively. Of these samples, 132 were mother–infant pairs. Behavioral development was assessed at 6 months and at 2, 3, and 4 years of age. On the basis of this sampling, the authors concluded that their data showed no clear indication of an effect of low-level lead exposure on fetal and childhood development (48,49).

In 1988, Needleman and his co-workers reexamined 132 subjects who were first studied in 1979 and found that neurobehavioral dysfunction was still related to the lead content of teeth shed at the ages of 6 and 7. Thus, children with higher dentine lead levels were noted to have serious academic and socioeconomic problems as young adults. The problems were reflected in serious reading disabilities; deficits in vocabulary, fine motor skill, reaction time, and hand–eye coordination; and a dropout rate from high school seven times the national average (111). This 11-year follow-up study provides strong evidence that lead exposure during childhood has long-lasting effects.

In summary, a large and growing body of well-conducted epidemiologic studies demonstrate disturbances in early neurobehavioral development at blood lead levels that were formerly thought to be harmless (2,38). Blood lead levels as low as 10–15 μg/dL (0.5–0.7 μmol/L) and possibly lower constitute a level of concern for undesirable developmental outcomes in the fetus and young child (38,140). Evidence increasingly supports a link between low-level lead exposure during early development and later deficits in neurobehavioral performance (101, 111). Adverse developmental effects have been associated with both prenatal and postnatal exposure to low levels of lead (2,38). At present the developing central nervous system is considered to be the principal target organ for lead toxicity in children (2,38). Lead exposure during the prenatal period is particularly threatening. Indeed, it has been suggested that the behavioral teratogenic effects of lead may serve as a paradigm for transplacental toxicants (109). The magnitude of the problem is set forth by a policy statement from the American Academy of Pediatrics, which indicated that lead poisoning is one of the most significant health hazards facing young children in the United States (3); see also Chapters 13, 24, 27, and 28).

Mercury

The behavioral effect of prenatal exposure to methyl mercury in humans came to light after two episodes of environmental mercury contamination.

One episode occurred in Japan, the other in Iraq. In Japan in the 1950s, villagers living along Minamata Bay were exposed to methyl mercury through the ingestion of contaminated fish. The fish were contaminated with methyl mercury derived from factory waste dumped into the bay. It is noteworthy that exposed mothers generally displayed little evidence of toxicity, whereas fetal exposure resulted in striking evidence of toxicity. Children exposed prenatally evidenced severe neurological and psychological impairments. Cerebral palsy and mental retardation were widely reported, but congenital malformations were rare (50,118).

In Iraq in 1971, an outbreak of methyl mercury poisoning was caused by the accidental ingestion of seed grain treated with a methyl mercury fungicide. In contrast to the severe chronic exposure that occurred at Minamata Bay, the exposure in Iraq was shorter and more intense. Iraqi children exposed to methyl mercury prenatally were noted to have impaired mental development as well as problems with speech and motor function. Congenital malformations were rare (6,7).

Polychlorinated Biphenyls

Gladen et al. performed an epidemiologic study to determine whether exposure to polychlorinated biphenyls (PCBs) or dichlorodiphenyl dichloroethene (DDE), either prenatally or through breast feeding, affects the results on the Bayley Scales of Infant Development at 6 or 12 months of age. The subjects of the study were volunteer samples of 858 infants, of whom 802 had Bayley scores available at 6 months or 12 months or both. Chemical determinations and the assessment of infant development were performed independently. Higher transplacental exposure to PCBs was associated with lower psychomotor scores at both 6 and 12 months of age. In contrast, higher prenatal exposure to DDE was associated with higher mental scores at 6 months of age. No relationship was apparent at 12 months of age. No adverse effects were associated with breast feeding (59).

PATHOLOGY AND PATHOLOGICAL PHYSIOLOGY

Traditionally, the effect of toxic exposure on the nervous system was assessed by the changes seen on gross and microscopic examination. It is now generally appreciated that behavioral dysfunction supplies us with prime evidence of injury to the central nervous system and that any meaningful assessment of the effects of toxic exposure on the central nervous system must include behavioral observations in conjunction with analyses of the underlying structures and neurochemical processes (102). Such studies are complicated by the considerable reserve capacity of the central nervous system. It has been noted repeatedly on postmortem examinations that gross injury to the brain may be associated with surprisingly little apparent behavioral dysfunction. Conversely, alterations in behavior thus far have few obvious correlates with neuropathological or neurochemical changes.

Discovering the relationship between neurobehavioral deficits and underlying changes in the structure and function of the central nervous system is one of the major challenges facing behavioral scientists. The enormous structural heterogeneity of the nervous system in conjunction with its varied and complex biochemical reactions pose immense problems to investigators as they direct their attention to the neurochemical counterpart of behavioral dysfunction (29).

Clues to underlying neuropathology may be sought by comparing the patterns of functional deficits found in cases with defined central nervous system lesions with those produced by toxic exposure. In addition, combining the anatomic data obtained from such advanced techniques as positron emission tomography (PET) and magnetic resonance imaging (MRI) with neuropsychological testing methods should be of help in investigating structure–function correlations within the central nervous system (57).

CLINICAL ASPECTS OF NEUROBEHAVIORAL DISORDERS CAUSED BY TOXIC EXPOSURE

In recent years a number of studies have suggested that neurotoxic exposure in the workplace, at levels producing no obvious medical or neurological symptoms, produces measurable evidence of neurobehavioral dysfunction. Identifying the subtle changes in central nervous system performance that arise from toxic exposure(s) presents the clinician with a formidable task, particularly when the resulting dysfunction is nonspecific and thereby easily produced by a variety of conditions.

Medical History

To identify behavioral symptoms arising from toxic exposure, physicians must maintain a high index of suspicion. The early diagnosis of such problems almost uniformly rests with the clinician, who is in a unique position to detect changes in mental function and to consider toxic exposure as a potential cause. The clinical task generally begins with the identification of behavioral symptoms. This is followed by a detailed medical history designed to search for the conditions, including environmental/occupational exposure(s), that can produce such symptoms. The diagnostic steps used in evaluating patients with suspected neurotoxic behavioral disorders are outlined in Fig. 14-1.

The early effects of neurotoxic exposure on the central nervous system are typically insidious, heralded by such subtle subjective and nonspecific symptoms as dizziness, headache, depression, irritability, insomnia, fuzzy thinking, and memory impairment. Patients with such complaints need further scrutiny. Their ability to function in daily life should be queried. It may also be helpful to speak

with the patient's family and co-workers and to observe the patient's interactions with these individuals. Specific questions that may help in assessing neurobehavioral symptoms are found in Table 14-2.

It should be appreciated that patients of all ages may complain of "benign forgetfulness" that prevents them from recalling a name or a particular detail of a past event that in other respects is quite clear in their mind. In contrast, patients with actual dementia may not recall important events in their lives. In such cases, family members provide more accurate evidence of the patient's day-to-day dys-

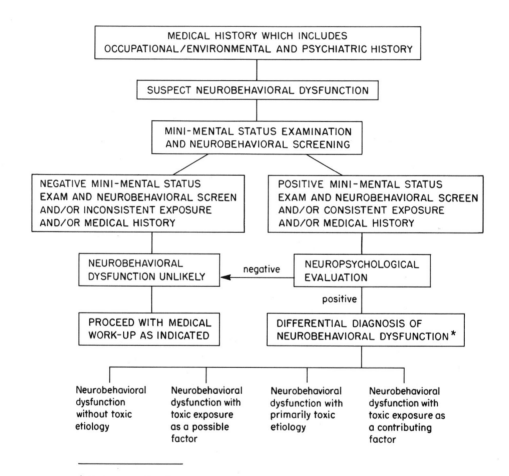

FIGURE 14-1. Diagnostic evaluation of neurobehavioral dysfunction with attention to neurotoxic etiology.

TABLE 14-2. Questions That Can Be Used to Screen for Neurobehavioral Symptoms[a]

Do you have a short memory? Is it getting worse?
Do you remember to deliver messages and keep appointments?
Do you often have problems concentrating?
Do you generally find it hard to get the meaning when reading newspapers and books?
Do you often feel irritable or depressed for no apparent reason?
Do you suffer from chronic severe fatigue?
Has your performance at work suffered?
Have your family relationships become difficult?

[a]Modified from Hogstedt et al. (77).

function than does the patient. In cases of true dementia, the patient no longer has the introspective capacity to recognize or remember cognitive deficits. The patient with "benign forgetfulness" usually needs reassurance, whereas the patient with suspected early dementia requires a thorough evaluation to define the cause and extent of the problem.

Identifying a link between the onset of behavioral symptoms and toxic exposure is often difficult, especially when the exposure is not well defined, chronic, or of low concentration. The diagnosis depends almost entirely on talking to patients and carefully piecing together their medical histories (see Chapter 11). Detailed information about current and past occupational/environmental exposures is essential. Exact information on the onset and progression of the behavioral symptoms in relation to exposure(s) is essential. Data on the duration and intensity of the exposure(s) are as important as information on the specific agent(s) involved. A job title generally does not provide sufficient exposure data. Query should be made into the precise nature of the exposure, the use of protective devices, and the degree of ventilation. For example, a painter should be asked if the paint is applied with a brush or as a spray and whether protective devices are used. Strong evidence for neurotoxic exposure is obtained when the patient's co-workers also complain of similar symptoms.

At times the physician may encounter a patient with a history of neurotoxic exposure and no apparent health problems. In such cases, evidence of neurobehavioral toxicity can be easily overlooked if the physician is not consistently vigilant to the possibility that neurobehavioral changes may be present. Since neurotoxic agents affecting behavior may also affect other elements of the nervous system, a general neurological survey of cranial nerve function and motor, sensory, and autonomic function is in order.

Toxic exposure in the home and community must be considered. Hobbies may be associated with significant solvent exposure. Pesticides may be heavily used in the home and garden. Workplace exposures may be carried into the home on contaminated clothing. Children are at high risk for the neurological effects of lead exposure. Physicians must therefore be aware of the potential avenues of lead exposure in and around the home. These sources include paint, soil, dust, food, water, air, and some folk medicines. Since it is well documented that behavioral dysfunction can arise from prenatal exposure to such agents as lead and mercury, physicians must be alert to toxic exposures occurring during pregnancy.

After the link between the neurological symptoms and exposure has been explored, information on medications and drug and alcohol abuse is obtained. A neurological review must include data on previous head injuries, infections, vascular accidents, neoplasms, dementia, and hereditary disorders. Nutritional factors and systemic disorders involving virtually all organs of the body must come under review (Fig. 14-1).

A psychiatric history is particularly important in patients with neurobehavioral dysfunction. Psychiatric disorders that occur in the presence of toxic exposure present the clinician with a diagnostic dilemma. Psychiatric disorders can mimic the symptoms of behavioral dysfunction found with neurotoxic exposure, and such exposure can give rise to psychiatric problems. At times, a detailed psychiatric history may suggest that a primary psychiatric disorder is less likely. For example, the absence of psychiatric problems before the onset of the exposure(s) in question and the relative absence of psychological, social, and economic problems that could trigger a psychiatric problem are of importance.

A social history provides an important insight into stressful conditions encountered by the patient. The patients' satisfaction with their work environment, their relationships with fellow workers, the degree of work stress, economic security, and fulfillment in family and social settings are all areas of inquiry. In cases of suspected neurotoxicity, patients should be queried about their plans to seek legal redress and monetary compensation. Such plans may play a role in the patient's symptomatology.

Physical Examination

A complete physical examination may offer clues to the diagnosis, especially by providing evidence of systemic disorders that may result in central nervous system dysfunction. The neurological examination, in addition to assessing sensory and motor function, should evaluate the patient's mental status.

Mental Status

If the patient's mental status (e.g., memory, personality, and intellect) appears to have changed, and/or the medical history corroborates the possibility of neurotoxic exposure, a simple, standardized mini-mental-status examination can be done in the office (54) (Table 14-3). This simple test can be invaluable in confirming the presence of *gross* cognitive deficits. To avoid offending or frightening patients or their families, considerable tact should be used when administering the mental status examination. The patient's schooling, previous accomplishments, and social background must be taken into account in interpreting the results. The physician should be aware of the rather loose relationship between the patient's subjective complaints and significant disruption of his or her mental status.

Laboratory Examination

Laboratory tests are often useful in searching for systemic disorders such as infections; metabolic,

liver, and kidney disorders; and structural abnormalities of the central nervous system that can cause alterations in central nervous system function. In some instances, evidence of excessive exposure to neurotoxic chemicals can be aided by biological monitoring of the patient's blood or urine (81). Such testing may be particularly helpful in cases of exposure to such agents as carbon monoxide, organophosphate pesticides, mercury, lead, and arsenic. Unfortunately, in the case of chronic exposure to organic solvents, such testing generally offers little help. These agents are usually metabolized quite rapidly, leaving no measurable evidence of past exposure. Documenting the nature and severity of past exposures is frequently one of the most difficult problems encountered by the physician and the epidemiologist. The reader is referred to Chapter 27 for a further discussion of this issue. Laboratory tests of use in assessing the etiology with neurobehavioral dysfunction are listed in Table 14-4.

NEUROPSYCHOLOGICAL TESTING

Rationale and Benefits

Neuropsychological testing is a relatively new methodology that provides an objective means of assessing, in depth, the functional impairment of the central nervous system (143). Such testing, designed to evaluate cognitive, behavioral, and psychomotor function, has proved useful in assessing patients with neurotoxic exposure. Neuropsychological tests are used to evaluate the mental function of working populations and individual patients exposed to neurotoxic agents. The tests are administered by a psychologist with specialized training (68,69). As it becomes more generally recognized that subtle central nervous system deterioration may arise from toxic exposure, neuropsychological testing will undoubtedly gain wider use.

It has been suggested that neuropsychological

TABLE 14-3. The Mini-Mental-Status Examination[a]

Test	Maximum Score[b]
Orientation	
What is the year, season, day, date, month?	5
Where are you? state, county, town, place, floor?	5
Registration	
Name three objects; state slowly and have patient repeat	3
(Repeat until patient learns all three.)	
Attention and calculation	5
Do reverse serial 7s (five steps) or spell "WORLD" backwards	
Recall	
Ask for the three unrelated objects noted above	3
Language	
Name from inspection a pencil, a watch	2
Have patient repeat "No ifs, ands, or buts"	1
Follow a three-stage command (Take a piece of paper, fold it, and put it on the floor)	3
Read and obey the following: Close your eyes; write a simple sentence; copy intersecting pentagons	1, 1, 1

[a] Adapted from Folstein et al. (54).
[b] Out of a possible score of 30, a mean score for dementia was between 9 and 10, that for depression with cognitive impairment was 19, and that for uncomplicated affective depression was between 27 and 28.

TABLE 14-4. Standard Laboratory Assessment in Cases of Neurobehavioral Dysfunction

1. Metabolic evaluation: electrolyte panel; calcium, phosphorus, magnesium, uric acid, creatinine, liver function tests
2. Complete blood count and sedimentation rate
3. Serologic test for syphilis
4. Thyroid function tests
5. Vitamin B^{12} and folic acid levels
6. Chest film
7. Computerized tomography or magnetic resonance imaging of the brain
8. Cerebrospinal fluid analysis

assessment offers the most sensitive means of examining the effects of toxic exposure (89). In a workplace setting, such testing may provide a means of monitoring industrial safety and thereby be useful in establishing exposure standards in the workplace. In the clinical setting, neuropsychological methods are helpful in detecting subtle neurotoxic states, in quantifying the degree of functional impairment, and in making a diagnosis. Progress made over the past 10 years indicates that neuropsychological test methods show a high degree of sensitivity and reliability within and across laboratories (81,143).

Limitations

A major limitation of neuropsychological testing is the nonspecific nature of the test results, which simply represent a set of performance scores that must be interpreted in the context of medical, occupational/environmental, educational, and psychological variables. To properly evaluate the influence of neurotoxic exposure on test performance, account must be taken of such confounding factors as age, sex, ethnic origin, educational experience, preexposure intellectual level, medication, drug and alcohol intake, nutrition, and disorders of the nervous system and other organs of the body. Other personal characteristics, which include motivation; emotional state; sleep deprivation; recent alcohol, drug, caffeine, or cigarette consumption; diurnal variation; and the degree of familiarity with the tests, may also affect the test results. These factors, by influencing test performance, may mask or mimic the effects of neurotoxic exposure. When referring patients to a neuropsychologist for evaluation, the physician must be assured that the examiner is properly experienced and attentive to possible confounding factors (71,81).

Certain conditions affecting neuropsychological performance pose problems that merit further discussion. A hypochondriacal response to environmental/occupational exposure leads some individuals to believe that they have suffered intellectual changes and memory deficits from toxic exposure. Neuropsychological test methods may not verify such a response, though including a personality assessment in the test battery may be helpful. Additional historical information may also provide clues in evaluating a hypochondriacal response.

In some cases patients malinger and use the neuropsychological examination in a search for secondary gain. This may occur particularly when toxic encephalopathy is a compensable disability. Solvent-induced encephalopathy associated with workplace exposure is currently a compensable disability in Scandinavia. Malingering may show up as a highly uneven and inconsistent test performance. Specific tests for malingering are available.

Differentiating cognitive deficits arising from toxic exposure from those arising from a psychiatric disorder, such as depressive reaction, often presents a problem. The difficulty arises because depression in itself may be associated with cognitive deficits, and neurotoxic exposure not uncommonly results in a depressive reaction (52,89). Because of this significant overlap, it is difficult to determine if the cognitive deficits observed on neuropsychological testing result entirely from neurotoxic exposure or the depression. In certain cases there may be no solution to this complex problem. It is often helpful, however, to evaluate more closely the deficit pattern observed on the tests of cognitive function and the nature of the depression.

Neuropsychological testing offers few clues to the underlying neuropathology. This is not surprising given the general lack of knowledge concerning neurotoxic influences on neuropathology. Moreover, the interpretation of neuropsychological tests in patients exposed to neurotoxic agents can be hampered, especially when their baseline performance prior to exposure is unavailable for comparison. In an epidemiologic setting, the impact of individual variability is somewhat compensated for by the number of subjects being studied. In the clinical setting, when patients are evaluated for diagnostic purposes, individual variability may obscure the analysis unless adequate population norms and/or educational, occupational, or service records are available (71,81).

The Neuropsychological Examination

It is generally accepted that neuropsychological test methods must be linked to three functional units of the central nervous system: the unit that maintains a sufficient state of arousal, the unit that transmits, elaborates, and stores information, and the unit that controls behavior. Thus, if neurotoxic effects are to be detected, even the most limited test battery should provide information about these important units (81).

The following criteria have been suggested for neuropsychological tests used to assess the effects of neurotoxic exposure. The test battery should include (1) tests known to measure functions that are affected by several neurotoxic agents; (2) tests that have been experimentally validated among groups of patients with neurotoxic disorders; (3) tests that are reliable; (4) tests that are psychometrically sound by virtue of measuring one or more well-defined functions; (5) tests that are relatively independent of such extraneous influences as the subject's cultural and educational backround; and (6) tests that have been considered in terms of costs (time, expertise, and equipment) and benefits (81).

In 1983, experts from the World Health Organization suggested a set of "core" neurobehavioral tests to be used in the evaluation of neurotoxicity. The short test battery emphasizes functions known to be affected by neurotoxic exposure (Table 14-5). A detailed description of the core tests is given by Johnson (81). As technology and knowledge advance, new and revised test methods will continue to be developed.

A recent testing approach uses a computer-administered neurobehavioral evaluation system specifically designed to assess neurotoxicity (19). Thus far, the neurobehavioral evaluation system (NES) has been used most extensively in the United States; however, translations of the system now exist in German, Italian, French, Dutch, and Finnish. The tests incorporated into the NES are, for the most part, computerized extensions of conventional neuropsychological procedures. There is a close relationship between the "core" tests recommended by the World Health Organization and the tests used in the NES system (86). Although the computerized neurobehavioral testing technique was developed to aid the epidemiologic study of populations exposed to neurotoxic agents, it has also been used in clinical and laboratory settings. The computerized testing system has many advantages for epidemiologic research, including portability, speed and accuracy of administration, and automatic data collection. However, there is concern that the computerized testing system could be administered poorly, used in inappropriate situations, and interpreted improperly (86).

At this writing, adequate norms are just beginning to be published for the NES. Until adequate normative data are available, the NES should not be used in individual clinical patients. With proper validation and adherence to ethical and methodological concerns, computerized neurobehavioral testing techniques promise to advance the assessment of neurobehavioral dysfunction and aid in the clinical diagnostic analysis of neurobehavioral toxicity (68,69,100).

CLASSIFICATION OF CENTRAL NERVOUS SYSTEM DISORDERS RELATED TO TOXIC EXPOSURE

Although central nervous system disturbances follow exposure to a wide variety of toxic chemicals, there is as yet no generally accepted system of classifying the resulting neurobehavioral dysfunctions. The classification presented in Table 14-6 has been suggested as a guide for clinical diagnosis and for characterizing subjects under epidemiologic investigation (15,154).

Acute Central Nervous System Conditions

A vast number of toxic agents, including solvents, pesticides, and metals, can give rise to acute confusional states. Patients exhibit a varied clinical picture. Acute exposure may result in mild, typically reversible, central nervous system dysfunction. With low levels of exposure, symptoms of headache, irritability, mild lethargy, and subtle alterations in alertness, attention, and concentration may be noted. Other symptoms of acute exposure include bizarre behavior, agitation, and hallucinations. In the absence of treatment or with higher levels of exposure, seizures, coma, and death may ensue. The intensity and duration of exposure as well as the nature of the toxic agent determine the degree of dysfunction and the probability that persistent impairment will remain (Table 14-6).

Chronic Central Nervous System Syndromes

The diagnostic criteria for chronic toxic encephalopathy have recently been more fully characterized. Efforts to provide a more detailed classification stemmed from reports that chronic exposure to organic solvents was associated with long-term central nervous system damage. Past researchers described solvent-associated "psychoorganic syndrome" or "neurasthenic" syndrome or "presenile dementia." Different interpretations were given to these terms by various research groups. In an effort to resolve the differences and provide a guide for clinical and epidemiologic studies, a classification scheme was developed at a World Health Organization workshop in 1985 and modified the same year at a workshop held in the United States (35,154).

The classification scheme identifies three chronic conditions affecting the central nervous system of solvent-exposed individuals: (1) central nervous system symptoms (type 1), (2) mild chronic toxic en-

TABLE 14-5. Neurobehavioral Test Methods[a]

Core tests	Functional domain
Aiming (pursuit aiming II)	Motor speed
	Motor steadiness
Simple reaction time	Attention/response speed
Digit symbol (WAIS-R[b])	Perceptual–motor speed
Santa Ana (Helsinki version)	Manual dexterity
Benton Visual Retention	Visual perception/ memory
Digit span (WAIS, WMS[c])	Auditory memory
POMS (Profile of Mood States)	Affect

[a]Modified from Johnson (81).
[b]Wechsler Adult Intelligence Scale—Revised.
[c]Wechsler Memory Scale.

TABLE 14-6. Clinical Manifestations and Causes of Central Nervous System Conditions[a]

Condition	Symptoms	Signs	Latency	Prognosis following exposure cessation	Major neurotoxic substances
Acute conditions					
1. Acute intoxication	Dizziness, lightheadedness, balance and gait impairment, incoordination, feeling "high"	Ataxia, slow psychomotor function	Minutes–hours	Reversible	Organic solvents, inhalation anesthetics
2. Acute toxic encephalopathy	Obtundation, coma, seizures, potentially fatal	Signs of diffuse central nervous system depression; reflex slowing, EEG slowing	Hours–days	Persistent deficits common	Solvents, lead, pesticides
Chronic syndromes					
1. Symptoms only	Mood changes (irritability, depression), sleep disorders; difficulty concentrating; memory complaints; symptoms are more noticeable to relatives than to patient	No objective signs	Weeks–months	Reversible	Carbon disulfide, lead, organic solvents
2. Mild chronic toxic encephalopathy					
A. Organic personality or mood disorders	Similar to those noted above; greater frequency and severity	Mood or personality inventories of potential value	Weeks–months	Incomplete reversibility possible but uncommon	Lead, organic solvents
B. Neurobehavioral impairment	Symptoms as above may be present	Reduced motor speed, reduced vigilance and reaction time, plus reduced performance on memory (short-term) testing and other tests of cognitive function (i.e., visuo-spatial ability)	Weeks–months	Potentially reversible, partial or complete	Carbon disulfide, lead, organic solvents, carbon monoxide (?)
3. Severe chronic toxic encephalopathy (dementia)	Significant loss of ability to perform activities of daily living: difficulty in comprehension, profound memory loss, reduced verbal fluency	Testing compatible with severe neurological damage and neuropsychological impairment as seen in dementia	Poorly reversible		Lead, organic solvents (e.g., toluene)

[a]From Johnson (81).

cephalopathy (types 2A and 2B), and (3) severe chronic toxic encephalopathy (type 3). Since the underlying pathophysiology is unclear in most cases, the central nervous system disorders may be thought of as syndromes rather than specific disease states (Table 14-6). Although the classification scheme deals with the chronic central nervous effects of long-standing solvent exposure, it may also apply to other agents. The chronic central nervous system syndromes linked to toxic exposure typically have an insidious onset. Mild cases have the potential for reversibility, whereas continued exposure to a toxic agent(s) increases the severity of the neurobehavioral dysfunction and results in irreversible injury to the central nervous system (81).

Central Nervous System Symptoms (Type 1)

The mildest form of chronic central nervous system dysfunction is reflected in nonspecific symptoms only (81). Typically, complaints include fatigue, irritability, sleep disturbances, loss of initiative, loss of sexual interest, loss of energy, difficulty in concentrating, and diminished mental efficiency (Table 14-6). These complaints occur prior to observable neuropsychological impairment. The WHO group described above applied the term "organic affective syndrome" to this category based on the diagnostic scheme developed by the American Psychiatric Association in 1980 (4). In 1987, the revised American Psychiatric Association nomenclature changed the category to "organic mood syndrome" (5).

Neurasthenia, a term used by psychiatrists in the past to define a neurosis characterized by such symptoms as chronic fatigue, insomnia, lack of energy, inability to concentrate, and moderate depression, has also been used to describe the early symptoms of toxic exposure.

Mild Chronic Toxic Encephalopathy (Types 2A and 2B)

This category, described as mild chronic toxic encephalopathy, is divided into two types, one characterized by a marked and sustained mood or personality disorder (2A) and the other by deficits in neurobehavioral function (2B) (81). The two categories may be separated for research purposes; however, it is not clear that separate clinical entities exist in exposed patients (Table 14-6).

Severe Chronic Toxic Encephalopathy (Type 3)

This category includes patients who suffer from global and severe deterioration of cognition and affect (81). Type 3 impairments can be characterized as a neurotoxicant-caused dementia (Table 14-6).

ESTABLISHING A DIAGNOSIS OF NEUROBEHAVIORAL DYSFUNCTION ARISING FROM TOXIC EXPOSURE

A diagnosis of behavioral dysfunction arising from toxic exposure largely depends on the old-fashioned method of talking to the patient and carefully piecing together his or her history. Establishing the diagnosis is frequently difficult because adequate data on the nature and degree of toxic exposure are often lacking and the effects of such exposure on the central nervous system are nonspecific.

In many cases central nervous system dysfunction cannot be attributed to a specific etiology unless there is acute toxic encephalopathy. Acute central nervous system dysfunction secondary to toxic exposure is frequently quite evident. In contrast, identifying chronic central nervous system dysfunction secondary to long-standing neurotoxic exposure is a formidable task. Typically, a multifactorial etiology is present. Under such conditions, the clinician must determine whether neurotoxic exposure constitutes a significant causal factor (Fig. 14-1). Despite the application of all available diagnostic methods, the final diagnosis usually depends on integrating the findings of a number of observers including family practitioners, internists, psychiatrists, nurses specializing in occupational medicine, neuropsychologists, and social workers.

The diagnosis of neurobehavioral dysfunction induced by toxic exposure depends on (1) identifying possible psychiatric causes; (2) identifying possible endogenous causes (i.e., disorders of the central nervous system and other organ systems; and (3) identifying possible exogenous causes (i.e., alcohol or drug abuse, medication, and occupational/environmental exposures (132).

Identifying Psychiatric Disorders

Distinguishing behavioral dysfunction induced by psychiatric disorders from that induced by toxic exposure often presents the physician with a diagnostic dilemma. Confusion arises because of the complex interrelationship between neurobehavioral dysfunction and neurotoxic exposure. At least five potential interrelationships exist (1) Behavioral dysfunction may be the direct effect of neurotoxic injury to the central nervous system. Mood disorders such as a depressive reaction arising from lead exposure or slowed, confused thinking secondary to pesticide exposure are examples. (2) Behavioral dysfunction may be secondary to the consequences of neurological impairment induced by toxic exposure. For example, a toxin-induced peripheral neuropathy resulting in the loss of fine motor control in a skilled worker can lead to a severe psychological response.

(3) Behavioral dysfunction may be secondary to the psychosocial stress of exposure or the fear of exposure. In some cases, under exposure conditions considered to be of very low risk, individuals develop bodily symptoms suggesting a physical disorder for which there is no known organic cause. The diagnosis of a somatoform disorder is based on the presence of psychological factors and the absence of organic findings. Some patients may develop a posttraumatic stress disorder characterized by physical, cognitive, and emotional complaints. This reaction, which may follow a single or repeated episodes of toxic exposure, involves reexperiencing the trauma or the symptoms associated with the exposure. (4) Behavioral dysfunction may be unrelated to the toxic exposure but linked to preexisting or predisposing psychological disturbances or to family, economic, or occupational problems. (5) Behavioral dysfunction may develop in an attempt to achieve secondary gain. Though malingering is probably overestimated, some patients consciously attempt to misrepresent their medical condition.

Psychiatric diagnostic criteria, as contained in the American Psychiatric Association Diagnostic and Statistical Manual of Mental Disorders (DSM-III-R), may help the clinician to determine if a psychiatric component is present (5). It should be remembered, however, that patients with a psychiatric disorder can also be exposed to neurotoxic agents. Therefore, a history or current evidence of a psychiatric disorder does not rule out the presence of toxic encephalopathy. At times, certain findings may suggest that a primary psychiatric disorder is unlikely. This includes the absence of previous psychiatric problems, an abrupt change in mood or behavior, rapid fluctuations of symptoms, a lack of response to standard psychiatric therapy, and the fact that the symptoms do not fit into one of the established psychiatric diagnostic categories.

Since a disorder of virtually any organ system of the body can give rise to impaired central nervous system function, all patients must receive a general medical evaluation along with appropriate laboratory studies. Specific disorders of the central nervous system such as infection, vascular accidents, hemorrhage, and tumors must be ruled out.

Identifying Neurotoxic Exposures

Identifying neurotoxic exposure as the source of behavioral dysfunction depends primarily on obtaining an appropriate history of occupational/environmental exposure and relating the symptomatology to such exposure. At times, biological monitoring may be helpful, particularly in cases of lead, arsenic, mercury, carbon monoxide, and or-

ganophosphate exposure. Alcohol and drug abuse, reactions to medications, and herbal remedies must always be considered.

Management

The cardinal principle of treating patients with neurobehavioral dysfunction from toxic exposure is stopping further exposure. In an occupational setting, the desired goal is the reduction of exposure concentrations to levels where neurobehavioral dysfunction does not occur. Reexposure to neurotoxins is to be avoided.

Multiple Chemical Sensitivity Syndrome

At times neurobehavioral problems may be difficult to classify. During recent years a number of observers, including physicians specializing in occupational medicine, have encountered patients who develop a recognizable constellation of symptoms in response to low levels of exposure to many different chemicals present in the workplace and general environment. Such patients become symptomatic at levels of exposure far less than those observed to cause disturbances in the general population (34,36, 123). Although the symptoms involve multiple organ systems, complaints of neurobehavioral dysfunction are usually quite prominent. Most patients complain of a form of mood disturbance characterized by depression, fatigue, irritability, mood swings, and an inability to think clearly or concentrate. A further discussion of this condition is found in Chapter 12.

Thus far, the constellation of symptoms presented by such patients has defied traditional diagnostic approaches. In the absence of explicable physical, pathological, and laboratory findings, considerable controversy surrounds this issue. To date, no uniform and appropriate nomenclature defines the clinical condition. Patients are often labeled by themselves or other observers by many different names, e.g., "hypersensitive," "hypersusceptible," or suffering from "environmental illness" or "20th century disease." Since the mechanism by which the exposures give rise to the patient's symptoms has not been defined, widely divergent theories are held involving psychiatric, immunologic, and toxicological causes (30,31,87,88,114,115,135–137).

Some observers believe that many, if not all, patients who complain of multiple chronic symptoms secondary to multiple low-level chemical exposures are in fact suffering from a psychiatric disorder and/or psychosocial disruptions (30,31,122). Many such patients meet the American Psychiatric Association DSM-III-R diagnostic criteria for a somatoform disorder or posttraumatic stress disorder.

What proportion of these individuals should be so classified remains unclear, however (37).

Other observers, taking careful note of the patient's clinical picture, have defined an acquired syndrome of multiple chemical sensitivities. (The term sensitivity is used by convention. No immunologic meaning is implied.) It is characterized by

recurrent symptoms referable to multiple organ systems, occurring in response to demonstrable exposure to many chemically unrelated compounds at doses well below those established in the general population to cause harmful effects. No single widely accepted test of physiologic function can be shown to correlate with symptoms (37).

This definition represents an early attempt to apply some diagnostic parameters to the complex clinical picture.

According to Cullen, the syndrome of multiple chemical sensitivities is characterized by the following major diagnostic features: (1) it is a chronic condition, acquired in relation to some documentable environmental exposure(s), insult(s), or illness(es); (2) the symptoms involve more than one organ system; (3) the symptoms recur and abate in response to predictable stimuli; (4) the symptoms are elicited by exposures to chemicals of diverse structural classes and toxicological modes of action; (5) the symptoms are elicited by exposures that are demonstrable (albeit at low level); (6) exposures that elicit symptoms are *very low*, for example, many standard deviations below "average" exposures known to cause adverse human responses; and (7) no single widely available test of organ system function can explain the symptoms (37).

Clearly, a diagnostic and therapeutic dilemma confronts the physician who encounters patients with untoward responses to multiple environmental pollutants and chemicals at low levels of exposure. This chronic clinical condition undoubtedly has many manifestations and multiple etiologies. Through the efforts of Cullen and the staff of the Yale–New Haven Occupational Medicine Program, an entire volume was devoted to the theories, data, and clinical observations of this complex clinical phenomenon. The interested reader is urged to consult this volume (36).

SUMMARY

This chapter has reviewed the changes in central nervous system function that arise from toxic exposure. The epidemiologic aspects of the problem are presented in some detail. The importance of neuropsychological test methods is emphasized. The complexity of the clinical picture and the difficulty in establishing the presence of neurobehav-

ioral dysfunction induced by toxic exposure are apparent throughout the discussion.

The pattern of neurobehavioral dysfunction induced by toxic exposure is nonspecific. The laboratory is generally of little help in identifying the offending occupational/environmental agent(s). The clinical diagnosis therefore depends primarily on an overall assessment of the general medical history, the occupational/environmental history, the psychiatric and social history, the physical and laboratory examination, the neurological and neuropsychological evaluation, and the role of all possible etiological factors. The final diagnosis is often based on the convergence of many disciplines, which include general, internal, and occupational medicine, neuropsychology, psychiatry, and the methodologies found in neuropsychological testing and biological monitoring. In many instances, a diagnostic dilemma can be resolved by close adherence to the disciplined approach outlined in this chapter.

REFERENCES

1. Abel EL: Behavioral Teratogenesis and Behavioral Mutagenesis, Plenum Press, New York, 1989.
2. Agency for Toxic Substances and Disease Registry: The Nature and Extent of Lead Poisoning in Children in the United States: A Report to Congress, United States Department of Health and Human Services, Public Health Service, Atlanta, 1988.
3. American Academy of Pediatrics: Statement on childhood lead poisoning. Pediatrics 79:457, 1987.
4. American Psychiatric Association: Diagnostic and Statistical Manual of Mental Disorders, 3rd ed., American Psychiatric Association, Washington, 1980.
5. American Psychiatric Association: Diagnostic and Statistical Manual of Mental Disorders, 3rd ed. rev., American Psychiatric Association, Washington, 1987.
6. Amin-Zaki L, Elhassani S, Majeed MA, et al: Intrauterine methylmercury poisoning in Iraq. Pediatrics 54:587, 1974.
7. Amin-Zaki L, Majeed MA, Elhassani SB: Prenatal methylmercury poisoning. Clinical observations over five years. Am J Dis Child 133:172, 1979.
8. Anger WK: Neurobehavioral testing of chemicals: Impact on recommended standards. Neurobehavioral Toxicol Teratol 6:147, 1984.
9. Anger WK, Johnson BL: Chemicals affecting behavior. In: Neurotoxicity of Industrial and Commercial Chemicals, p 51, O'Donoghue J (ed.), CRC Press, Boca Raton, 1985.
10. Annau Z (ed.): Neurobehavioral Toxicology. The Johns Hopkins University Press, Baltimore, 1986.
11. Annau Z, Eccles CU: Prenatal exposure. In: Neurobehavioral Toxicology, p 153, Annau Z (ed.), The Johns Hopkins University Press, Baltimore, 1986.
12. Axelson O, Hane M, Hogstedt C: A case-referent study on neuropsychiatric disorders among workers

exposed to solvents. Scand J Work Environ Health 2:14, 1976.

13. Axelson O, Hane M, Hogstedt C: Current aspects of solvent-related disorders. In: Developments in Occupational Medicine, p 237, Zenz C (ed.), Year Book Medical Publishers, Chicago, 1980.

14. Baker EL Jr: Epidemiologic issues in neurotoxicity research. Neurobehav Toxicol Teratol 7:293, 1985.

15. Baker EL: Organic solvent neurotoxicity. Annu Rev Public Health 9:233, 1988.

16. Baker EL, Fine LJ: Solvent neurotoxicity. J Occup Med 28:126, 1986.

17. Baker EL, Landrigan PJ, Barbour AG, et al: Occupational lead poisoning in the United States: Clinical and biochemical findings related to blood lead levels. Br J Ind Med 36:314, 1979.

18. Baker EL, Feldman RG, White RF, et al: Occupational lead neurotoxicity: A behavioral and electrophysiological evaluation. Study design and year one results. Br J Ind Med 41:352, 1984.

19. Baker EL, Letz R, Fidler A: A computer-administered neurobehavioral evaluation system for occupational and environmental epidemiology. J Occup Med 27:206, 1985.

20. Baker EL Jr, Smith TJ, Landrigan PJ: The neurotoxicity of industrial solvents: A review of the literature. Am J Ind Med 8:207, 1985.

21. Baker EL, White RF, Pothier LJ, et al: Occupational lead neurotoxicity: Improvement in behavioural effects after reduction in exposure. Br J Ind Med 42:507, 1985.

22. Baker EL, Letz RE, Eisen EA, et al: Neurobehavioral effects of solvents in construction painters. J Occup Med 30:116, 1988.

23. Bayley N: Bayley Scales of Infant Development, The Psychological Corporation, New York, 1969.

24. Bellinger D, Needleman HL, Leviton A, et al: Early sensory–motor development and prenatal exposure to lead. Neurobehav Toxicol Teratol 6:387, 1984.

25. Bellinger D, Leviton A, Needleman HL, et al: Low-level lead exposure and infant development in the first year. Neurobehav Toxicol Teratol 8:151, 1986.

26. Bellinger D, Leviton A, Waternaux C, et al: Longitudinal analyses of prenatal and postnatal lead exposure and early cognitive development. N Engl J Med 316:1037, 1987.

27. Bellinger D, Leviton A, Waternaux C, et al: Low-level lead exposure, social class, and infant development. Neurotoxicol Teratol 10:497, 1988.

28. Bellinger D, Leviton A, Waternaux C, et al: Lead, IQ, and social class. Int Epidemiology 18:180, 1989.

29. Boer GJ, Feenstra MGP, Mirmiran M, et al: Biochemical Basis of Functional Neuroteratology: Permanent Effects of Chemicals on the Developing Brain, Elsevier, Amsterdam, 1988.

30. Brodsky CM: "Allergic to everything": A medical subculture. Psychosomatics 24:731, 1983.

31. Brodsky CM: Multiple chemical sensitivities and other "environmental illness": A psychiatrist's view. Occup Med 2:695, 1987.

32. Cherry N, Hutchins H, Pace T, et al: Neurobehavioral effects of repeated occupational exposure to toluene and paint solvents. Br J Ind Med 42:291, 1985.

33. Chisolm JJ Jr: Dose–effect relationship for lead in young children: Evidence in children for interactions among lead, zinc and iron. In: Environmental Lead: Proceedings of the Second International Symposium on Environmental Lead Research, p 1, Lynam DR, Piantanida LG, Cole JF (eds.), Academic Press, Orlando, 1981.

34. Cone JE, Harrison R, Reiter R: Patients with multiple chemical sensitivities: Clinical diagnostic subsets among an occupational health clinic population. Occup Med 2:721, 1987.

35. Cranmer J, Goldberg L (eds.): Workshop on neurobehavioral effects of solvents. Neurotoxicology 7:1, 1986.

36. Cullen MR (ed.): Workers with multiple chemical sensitivities. Occup Med 2:655–805, 1987.

37. Cullen MR: The worker with multiple chemical sensitivities: An overview. Occup Med 2:655, 1987.

38. Davis JM, Svensgaard DJ: Lead and child development. Nature 329:297, 1987.

39. Dick RB, Johnson BL: Human experimental studies. In: Neurobehavioral Toxicology, p 348, Annau Z (ed.), The Johns Hopkins University Press, Baltimore, 1986.

40. Dietrich KN, Krafft KM, Bornschein RL, et al: Low-level fetal lead exposure effect on neurobehavioral development in early infancy. Pediatrics 80:721, 1987.

41. Dillie JR, Smith PW: Central nervous system effects of chronic exposure to organophosphate insecticide. Aerospace Med 35:475, 1964.

42. Durham WF, Wolfe HR, Quinby GE: Organophosphorus insecticides and mental alertness. Arch Environ Health 10:55, 1965.

43. Ecobichon DJ, Joy RM (eds.): Pesticides and Neurological Diseases, CRC Press, Boca Raton, 1982.

44. Elkins HB: Maximum acceptable concentrations, a comparison in Russia and the United States. Arch Environ Health 2:45, 1961.

45. Elofsson S, Gamberale F, Hindmarsh T, et al: Exposure to organic solvents. A cross-sectional epidemiologic investigation on occupationally exposed car and industrial spray painters with special reference to the nervous system. Scand J Work Environ Health 6:239, 1980.

46. Ensberg IFG, de Bruin A, Ziehuis RL: Health of workers exposed to a cocktail of pesticides. Int Arch Arbeitsmed 32:191, 1974.

47. Ernhart CB, Landa B, Wolf AW: Subclinical lead levels and developmental deficits: Reanalysis of data. J Learn Dis 18:475, 1985.

48. Ernhart CB, Morrow-Tlucak M, Marier M, et al: Low level lead exposure in the prenatal and early preschool periods: Early preschool development. Neurotoxicol Teratol 9:259, 1987.

49. Ernhart CB, Morrow-Tlucak M, Wolf AW, et al: Low level lead exposure in the prenatal and early preschool periods: intelligence prior to school entry. Neurotoxicol Teratol 11:161, 1989.

50. Eskenazi B: Behavioral teratology. In: Perinatal Epidemiology, p 216, Bracken MB (ed.), Oxford University Press, Oxford, 1984.

51. Eskenazi B, Maizlish NA: Effects of occupational exposure to chemicals on neurobehavioral function-

ing. In: Medical Neuropsychology: The Impact of Disease on Behavior, p 223, Tarter RE, Van Thiel DH, Edwards KL (eds.), Plenum Press, New York, 1988.

52. Feldman RG, Ricks NL, Baker EL: Neuropsychological effects of industrial toxins: A review. Am J Ind Med 1:211, 1980.

53. Fischbein A, Thornton JC, Lilis R, et al: Zinc protoporphyrin, blood lead and clinical symptoms in two occupational groups with low-level exposure to lead. Am J Ind Med 1:391, 1980.

54. Folstein MF, Folstein SE, McHugh PR: Minimental State: A practical method for grading the cognitive state for the clinician. J Psychiatr Res 12:189, 1975.

55. Fulton M, Thomson G, Hunter R, et al: Influence of blood lead on the ability and attainment of children in Edinburgh. Lancet 1:1221, 1987.

56. Gamberale F: Use of behavioral performance tests in the assessment of solvent toxicity. Scand J Work Environ Health 11(Suppl 1):65, 1985.

57. Gazzaniga MS: Organization of the human brain. Science 245:947, 1989.

58. Gershon S, Shaw FB: Psychiatric sequelae of chronic exposure to organophosphorus insecticides. Lancet 1:1371, 1971.

59. Gladen BC, Rogan WJ, Hardy P, et al: Development after exposure to polychlorinated biphenyls and dichlorodiphenyl dichloroethene transplacentally and through human milk. J Pediatr 113:991, 1988.

60. Godish T: Indoor Air Pollution Control, Lewis Publishers, Chelsea, Michigan, 1989.

61. Grandjean P, Arnvig E, Beckmann J: Psychological dysfunction in lead-exposed workers: Relation to biological parameters of exposure. Scand J Work Environ Health 4:295, 1978.

62. Grasso P: Neurotoxic and neurobehavioral effects of organic solvents on the nervous system. Occup Med 3:525, 1988.

63. Grasso P, Sharratt M, Davies DM, et al: Neurophysiological and psychological disorders and occupational exposure to organic solvents. Food Chem Toxicol 22:819, 1984.

64. Gregersen P, Angelsø B, Nielsen TE, et al: Neurotoxic effects of organic solvents in exposed workers: An occupational neuropsychological and neurological investigation. Am J Ind Med 5:201, 1984.

65. Hane M, Axelson O, Blume J, et al: Psychological function changes among house painters. Scand J Work Environ Health 3:91, 1977.

66. Hänninen H, Eskelinen L, Husman K, et al: Behavioral effects of long-term exposure to a mixture of organic solvents. Scand J Work Environ Health 2:240, 1976.

67. Hänninen H, Hernberg S, Mantere P, et al: Psychological performance of subjects with low exposure to lead. J Occup Med 20:683, 1978.

68. Hartman DE: On the use of clinical psychology software: Practical, legal, and ethical concerns. Prof Psychol Res Pract 17:462, 1986.

69. Hartman DE: Artificial intelligence or artificial psychologist? Conceptual issues in clinical microcomputer use. Prof Psychol Res Pract 17:528, 1986.

70. Hartman DE: Neuropsychological toxicology: Identification and assessment of neurotoxic syndromes. Arch Clin Neuropsychol 2:45, 1987.

71. Hartman DE: Neuropsychological Toxicology: Identification and Assessment of Human Neurotoxic Syndromes. Pergamon Press, New York, 1988.

72. Harvey P, Hamlin M, Kumar R: Blood lead, behavior and intelligence test performance in preschool children. Sci Total Environ 40:45, 1984.

73. Hatzakis A, Kokkevi A, Maravelias C, et al: Psychometric intelligence deficits in lead-exposed children. In: Lead Exposure and Child Development: An International Assessment, p 211, Smith MA, Grant LD, Sors AI (eds.), Kluwer Academic Publishers, Dordrecht, 1989.

74. Hernberg S: Neurotoxic effects of long-term exposure to organic hydrocarbon solvents: Epidemiologic aspects. In: Mechanisms of Toxicity and Hazard Evaluation, Holmstedt B, Lauwerys R, Mercier M, et al. (eds.), p 937, Elsevier, Amsterdam, 1980.

75. Hirshberg A, Lerman Y: Clinical problems in organophosphorus insecticide poisoning. The use of a computerized information system. Fundam Appl Toxicol 4:5209, 1984.

76. Hogstedt C, Axelson O: Long-term health effects of industrial solvents: A critical review of the epidemiologic research. Med Lav 77:11, 1986.

77. Hogstedt C, Hane M, Axelson O: Diagnostic and health care aspects of workers exposed to solvents. In: Developments in Occupational Medicine, p 249, Zenz C (ed.), Year Book Medical Publishers, Chicago, 1980.

78. Holmes JH, Gaon MD: Observations on acute and multiple exposure to anticholinesterase agents. Trans Am Clin Climatol Assoc 68:86, 1956.

79. Husman K, Karli P: Clinical neurological findings among car painters exposed to a mixture of organic solvents. Scand J Work Environ Health 6:33, 1980.

80. Jeyaratnam J: Health problems of pesticide usage in the Third World. Br J Ind Med 42:505, 1985.

81. Johnson BL (ed.): Prevention of Neurotoxic Disease in Working Populations. John Wiley & Sons, New York, 1987.

82. Knave B, Olson BA, Elofsson S, et al: Long-term exposure to jet fuel. II. A cross-sectional epidemiologic investigation on occupationally exposed workers with special reference to the nervous system. Scand J Work Environ Health 4:19, 1978.

83. Korsak RJ, Sato MM: Effects of chronic organophosphate pesticide exposure on the central nervous system. Clin Toxicol 11:83, 1977.

84. Landrigan PJ, Kreiss K, Xintarus C, et al: Clinical epidemiology of occupational neurotoxic disease. Neurobehav Toxicol 2:43, 1980.

85. Lansdown R, Yule M, Urbanowicz MA, et al: The relationships between blood-lead concentrations, intelligence, attainment and behavior in a school population: The second London study. Int Arch Occup Environ Health 57:225, 1986.

86. Letz R, Baker EL: Computer-administered neurobehavioral testing in occupational health. Semin Occup Med 1:197, 1986.

87. Levin AS, Byers VS: Environmental illness: A disorder of immune regulation. Occup Med 2:669, 1987.

88. Levine SA, Reinhardt JH: Biochemical-pathology initiated by free radicals, oxidant chemicals, and thera-

peutic drugs in the etiology of chemical hypersensitivity disease. Orthomol Psychiatry 12:166, 1983.

89. Lezak MD: Neuropsychological assessment in behavioral toxicology—developing techniques and interpretive issues. Scand J Work Environ Health 10 (Suppl 1):25, 1984.

90. Lilis R, Valciukas JA, Malkin J, et al: Effects of low-level lead and arsenic exposure on copper smelter workers. Arch Environ Health 40:38, 1985.

91. Linström K: Changes in psychological performance of solvent-poisoned and solvent-exposed workers. Am J Ind Med 1:69, 1980.

92. Linström K, Wickström G: Psychological function changes among maintenance house painters exposed to low levels of organic solvent mixtures. Acta Psychiatr Scand 67(Suppl 303):81, 1983.

93. Linström K, Riihimäki H, Hänninen K: Occupational solvent exposure and neuropsychiatric disorders. Scand J Work Environ Health 10:321, 1984.

94. Lotti M: Production and use of pesticides. In: Toxicology of Pesticides: Experimental, Clinical and Regulatory Perspectives, p 15, Costa LG, Galli CL, Murphy SD (eds.), Spring-Verlag, Berlin, 1987.

95. Maizlish NA, Langolf GD, Whitehead LW, et al: Behavioural evaluation of workers exposed to mixtures of organic solvents. Br J Ind Med 42:579, 1985.

96. Maizlish NA, Schenker M, Weisskopf C, et al: A behavioral evaluation of pest control workers with short-term low-level exposure to the organophosphate diazinon. Am J Ind Med 12:153, 1987.

97. Mantere P, Hänninen H, Hernberg S: Subclinical neurotoxic lead effects: Two-year follow-up studies with psychological test methods. Neurobehav Toxicol Teratol 4:725, 1982.

98. Mantere P, Hänninen H, Hernberg S, et al: A prospective follow-up study on psychological effects in workers exposed to low levels of lead. Scand J Work Environ Health 10:43, 1984.

99. Markowitz ME, Rosen JF: Zinc (Zn) and copper (Cu) metabolism in CaNa$_2$EDTA-treated children with plumbism. Pediatr Res 15:635, 1981.

100. Matarazzo JD, Matarazzo RG: Clinical psychological test interpretations by computer: Hardware outpaces software. Comput Human Behav 1:235, 1986.

101. McMichael AJ, Baghurst PA, Wigg NR, et al: Port Pirie cohort study: Environmental exposure to lead and children's abilities at the age of four years. N Engl J Med 319:408, 1989.

102. Mello NK: Behavioral toxicology: A developing discipline. Fed Proc 34:1832, 1975.

103. Metcalf DR, Holmes JH: EEG, psychological and neurological alterations in humans with organophosphate exposure. Ann NY Acad Sci 160:357, 1969.

104. Mikkelsen S: A cohort study of disability pension and death among painters with special regard to disabling presenile dementia as an occupational disease. Scand J Soc Med 16(Suppl):34, 1980.

105. Mitchell CL, Tilson HA, Cabe PA: Screening for neurobehavioral toxicity: Factors to consider. In: Nervous System Toxicology, p 229, Mitchell C (ed.), Raven Press, New York, 1982.

106. Needleman HL (ed.): Low Level Lead Exposure: The Clinical Implications of Current Research, Raven Press, New York, 1980.

107. Needleman HL: Epidemiological studies. In: Neurobehavioral Toxicology, p 279, Annau Z (ed.), The Johns Hopkins University Press, Baltimore, 1986.

108. Needleman HL: Low level lead exposure in the fetus and young child. Neurotoxicology 8:389, 1987.

109. Needleman HL: The neurotoxic, teratogenic, and behavioral teratogenic effects of lead at low doses: A paradigm for transplacental toxicants. In: Transplacental Effects of Fetal Health, p 279, Scarpelli DG, Magaki G (eds.), Alan R Liss, New York, 1988.

110. Needleman HL, Gunnoe C, Leviton A, et al: Deficits in psychologic and classroom performance of children with elevated dentine lead levels. N Engl J Med 300:689, 1979.

111. Needleman HL, Schell A, Bellinger D: The long-term effects of exposure to low doses of lead in childhood: An 11-year follow-up report. N Engl J Med 322:83, 1990.

112. Olsen J, Sabroe S: A case-reference study of neuropsychiatric disorders among workers exposed to solvents in the Danish wood and furniture industry. Scand J Soc Med 16(Suppl):44, 1980.

113. Randolph TC: Depression caused by home exposures to gas and combustion products of gas, oil, and coal. J Lab Clin Med 46:942, 1955.

114. Randolph TC: Human Ecology and Susceptibility to the Chemical Environment, Charles C. Thomas, Springfield, IL, 1962.

115. Randolph TC: Emergence of the specialty of clinical ecology. Clin Ecol 2:65, 1982.

116. Reiter L: Use of activity measures in behavioral toxicology. Environ Health Perspect 26:9, 1978.

117. Repko JD, Corum CR, Jones PD, et al: The effects of inorganic lead on behavioral and neurologic function, National Institute for Occupational Safety and Health, Publication no. 78–128, Washington, 1978.

118. Reuhl KR, Chang LW: Effects of methylmercury on the development of the nervous system: A review. Neurotoxicology 1:21, 1979.

119. Riley EP, Vorhees CV (eds.): Handbook of Behavioral Teratology, Plenum Press, New York, 1986.

120. Rodnitzky RL, Levin HS, Mick DL: Occupational exposure to organophosphate pesticides: A neurobehavioral study. Arch Environ Health 30:98, 1975.

121. Savage EP, Keefe TJ, Mounce LM, et al: Chronic neurological sequelae of acute organophosphate pesticide poisoning. Arch Environ Health 43:38, 1988.

122. Schottenfeld RS: Workers with multiple chemical sensitivities: A psychiatric approach to diagnosis and treatment. Occup Med 2:739, 1987.

123. Schottenfeld RS, Cullen MR: Organic affective illness associated with lead intoxication. Am J Psychiatry 141:1423, 1984.

124. Sette WF: Complexity of neurotoxicological assessment. Neurotoxicol Teratol 9:411, 1987.

125. Sette WF, Levine TE: Behavior as a regulatory endpoint. In: Neurobehavioral Toxicology, p 391, Annau Z (ed.), The Johns Hopkins University Press, Baltimore, 1986.

126. Silbergeld EK: Indirectly acting neurotoxins. Acta Psychiatr Scand 67(Suppl 303):16, 1983.

127. Smith M, Delves T, Lansdown R, et al: The effects of lead exposure on urban children: The Institute of Child Health/Southhampton study. Dev Med Child Neurol 47 [Suppl]:1, 1983.

128. Smith MA, Grant LD, Sors AI (eds.): Lead Exposure and Child Development: An International Assessment, Kluwer Academic, Dordrecht, 1989.

129. Sorrell M, Rosen JF, Roginsky M: Interactions of lead, calcium, vitamin D and nutrition in lead-burdened children. Arch Environ Health 32:160, 1977.

130. Spencer PS, Schaumburg HH: Organic solvent neurotoxicity. Scand J Work Environ Health 11(Suppl 1): 53, 1985.

131. Spyker JM: Assessing the impact of low level chemicals on development: Behavioral and latent effects. Fed Proc 34:1836, 1975.

132. Strub RL, Black FW: Neurobehavioral Disorders: A Clinical Approach, 2nd ed., FA Davis, Philadelphia, 1989.

133. Struwe G, Wennberg A: Psychiatric and neurological symptoms in workers occupationally exposed to organic solvents. In: Biology Psychiatry, p 253, Perris C, Struwe G, Jannson B (eds.), Elsevier/North-Holland, Amsterdam, 1981.

134. Tabershaw IR, Cooper WC: Sequelae of acute organic phosphate poisoning. J Occup Med 8:5, 1966.

135. Terr AI: Environmental illness: A critical review of 50 cases. Arch Intern Med 146:145, 1986.

136. Terr AI: "Multiple chemical sensitivities": Immunologic critique of clinical ecology theories and practice. Occup Med 2:683, 1987.

137. Terr AI: Clinical ecology in the workplace. J Occup Med 31:257, 1989.

138. Tilson HA, Mitchell CL: Neurobehavioral techniques to assess the effects of chemicals on the nervous system. Annu Rev Pharmacol Toxicol 24:425, 1984.

139. Triebig G, Bleecker M, Giliole R, et al: International working group on the epidemiology of the chronic neurobehavioral effects of organic solvents. Int Arch Occup Environ Health 61:423, 1989.

140. US Environmental Protection Agency: Air Quality Criteria for Lead (EPA report no.EPA/600/8-83/028aF–dF), Office of Health and Environmental Assessment, Research Triangle Park, 1986.

141. US Environmental Protection Agency: Health Effects Test Guidelines (EPA 560.6-83-001, PB 83-257691), National Technical Information Services, Alexandria, VA, 1989.

142. Valciukas JA, Lilis R, Eisinger J, et al: Behavioral indicators of lead neurotoxicity: Results of a clinical field survey. Int Arch Occup Environ Health 41:217, 1978.

143. Vorhees CV: Reliability, sensitivity, and validity of behavioral indices of neurotoxicity. Neurotoxicol Teratol 9:445, 1987.

144. Wallingford KM, Carpenter J: Field experience overview: Investigating sources of indoor air quality problems in office buildings. In: Proceedings of IAQ '86: Managing Indoor Air for Health and Energy Conservation, p 448, American Society of Heating, Refrigerating and Air-Conditioning Engineers, Atlanta, 1986.

145. Watson JM: Solvent abuse by children and young adults: A review. Br J Addict 75:27, 1980.

146. Weiss B: Behavior as an early indicator of pesticide toxicity. Toxicol Ind Health 4:351, 1988.

147. Weiss B, Laties VG (eds.): Behavioral Toxicology, Plenum Press, New York, 1975.

148. White R, Feldman RG: Neuropsychological assessment of toxic encephalopathy. Am J Ind Med 11:395, 1987.

149. Whorton MD, Obrinsky DL: Persistence of symptoms after mild to moderate acute organophosphate poisoning among 19 farm field workers. J Toxicol Environ Health 11:347, 1983.

150. Wigg NR, Vimpani GV, McMichael AJ, et al: Port Pirie cohort study: Childhood blood lead and neuropsychological development at age two years. J Epidemiol Commun Health 42:213, 1988.

151. Winneke G, Kraemer U: Neuropsychological effects of lead in children: Interactions with social background variable. Neuropsychobiology 11:195, 1984.

152. Winneke G, Kraemer U, Brockhaus U, et al: Neuropsychological studies in children with elevated tooth-lead concentration. II: Extended study. Int Arch Occup Environ Health 108:231, 1983.

153. World Health Organization: Safe Use of Pesticides, Technical Report Series No. 9, World Health Organization, Geneva, 1973.

154. World Health Organization: Chronic Effects of Organic Solvents on the Central Nervous System and Diagnostic Criteria, World Health Organization and Nordic Council of Ministers, Copenhagen, 1985.

155. Yule W: Methological and statistical issues. In: The Lead Debate: The Environment, Toxicology and Child Health, p 193, Lansdown R, Yule W (eds.), Croom Helm, London, 1986.

156. Yule W, Rutter M: Effect of lead on children's behavior and cognitive performance: A critical review. In: Dietary and Environmental Lead: Human Health Effects, p 211, Mahaffey K (ed.), Elsevier, Amsterdam, 1985.

157. Ziegler EE, Edwards BB, Jensen RL, et al: Absorption and retention of lead by infants. Pediatr Res 12:29, 1978.

158. Zimmerman-Tansella C, Campara P, D'Andrea F, et al: Psychological and physical complaints of subjects with low exposure to lead. Hum Toxicol 2:615, 1983.

RECOMMENDED READINGS

Annau Z (ed.): Neurobehavioral Toxicology, The Johns Hopkins University Press, Baltimore, 1986.

Hartman DE: Neuropsychological Toxicology: Identification and Assessment of Human Neurotoxic Syndromes. Pergamon Press, London, 1988.

Johnson BL (ed.): Prevention of Neurotoxic Illness in Working Populations, John Wiley & Sons, New York, 1987.

Riley EP, Vorhees CV (eds.): Handbook of Behavioral Teratology, Plenum Press, New York, 1985.

Smith MA, Grant LD, Sors AL (eds.): Lead Exposure and Child Development: An International Assessment, Kluwer Academic, Dordrecht, 1989.

Weiss B, Laties VG (eds.): Behavioral Toxicology, Plenum Press, New York, 1975.

15.   DISORDERS OF THE SKIN

Ronald C. Wester and Howard I. Maibach

INTRODUCTION

By providing a barrier between the body and its physical, chemical, and biological environment, the skin functions as one of the protective organs of the body. Although its barrier properties are impressive, the skin provides a portal of entry and a vulnerable target for many environmental chemicals. There can be, for example, sufficient percutaneous absorption of such substances as aniline dye, cyanide salts, numerous solvents, organophosphates, and other insecticides to produce toxic symptoms (55). Direct exposure of the skin to the vast number of environmental chemicals can result in a wide range of adverse responses. This chapter discusses the adverse effects of such exposure on the skin.

ENVIRONMENTAL CHEMICALS AND PHYSICAL AGENTS ASSOCIATED WITH ADVERSE EFFECTS ON THE SKIN

Chemical Agents

The number of man-made chemicals entering the environment has increased dramatically over the past 50 years. Exposure to these agents in the workplace and general environment can be associated with such adverse dermal effects as contact dermatitis, photosensitivity, acne and chloracne, pigmen-

tary disturbances, urticaria, and cancer. Atmospheric conditions such as changes in the ozone layer also contribute to the development of skin disease, particularly skin cancer (25,30,31,47,53, 57,60,62,105).

All varieties of chemical agents have been incriminated in the etiology of skin disease. Included are such agents as solvents, nonsolvent petroleum products, metals, pesticides, plastics, resins, soaps, detergents, cleaning agents, glues, pastes, adhesives, cement, mortar, and wet plaster. The dermatologic effects of pollutant exposure in the general environment have been less dramatic and less documented than those encountered in the workplace. Nonetheless, there is increasing recognition that the vast array of environmental chemicals coming in direct contact with the skin provides this organ with a ready source of hazardous exposure.

The home and its environs are an important source of toxic exposure. Such consumer products as paints, solvents, cleansers, adhesives, and pesticides are regularly used in the home environment, often with less attention to their hazards and with fewer protective devices than are found in industry. Cosmetics, soaps, detergents, dyes, fire retardants, and perma-press agents are sources of exposure in the home. Many of the materials used in hobbies and by artists adversely affect the skin and other organs. Yet a large number of these materials are inadequately labeled as to their hazard and chemical content. Pesticides, in high concentration, are often used in the home environment (33). Exposure to organic chemicals in water used for drinking and bathing may occur through dermal absorption (100). Proximity to industry and hazardous waste sites

Principles and Practice of Environmental Medicine, edited by Alyce Bezman Tarcher. Plenum Medical Book Company, New York, 1992.

provides a source of pollutant exposure in the community and in and around the home (3,10). Finally, workers may bring home from their workplace such hazardous chemicals as asbestos, lead, beryllium, arsenic, and polycyclic compounds (48).

Depletion of the Ozone Layer

Changes in atmospheric conditions, particularly ozone depletion in the stratosphere, are cause for concern. This concern arises from the fact that ozone, formed in the atmosphere, limits the amount of harmful solar ultraviolet (UV) radiation reaching the earth. Only a fraction of the UV radiation emitted by the sun reaches the surface of the earth. Ultraviolet radiation with a wavelength from 240 to 290 nm (UVC) is almost totally screened by the ozone layer, and only a portion with a wavelength from 290 to 320 nm (UVB) penetrates the ozone layer. The UVB spans the absorption spectra of DNA. Therefore, the ozone layer provides crucial protection against the carcinogenic impact of sunlight on humans. Chronic UV exposure has been linked to the development of basal-cell and squamous-cell carcinoma. These neoplasms are found with increased frequency in fair-skinned individuals who spend time outdoors (52,94). It has been calculated that for each 1% decrease in the ozone layer, at least a 4% increase in nonmelanoma skin cancer can be expected (86). The ozone that acts as a protective shield in the stratosphere is the same substance that acts as a hazardous pollutant at ground level.

Concern about the depletion of the ozone layer first emerged in the 1970s and focused on the chlorofluorocarbons (CFCs). These man-made compounds are widely used throughout the world as propellants in aerosol spray cans, as coolants in refrigerators, freezers, and air conditioners, in the manufacture of polystyrene foam, and as solvents. They are not broken down when emitted into the atmosphere. The CFCs slowly move upward to reach the stratosphere, where their projected half-life is 75 years or more. Models of stratospheric ozone indicate that CFCs are capable of destroying hugh numbers of ozone molecules (21). A report issued in 1988 by an international group of scientists indicated that the ozone layer around the earth was being reduced much faster than the models had predicted (67). These findings, when coupled with the fact that the chlorofluorocarbons now present in the stratosphere will continue to react with ozone molecules for years to come, caused a number of nations take steps necessary to reduce the production of chlorofluorocarbons (46). In 1990, 93 nations agreed that by the end of the century they would halt the production of chemicals that destroy the atmosphere's ozone shield.

Toxicology

The dermal and systemic toxicity of exposure to many chemicals depends on the degree to which they penetrate the skin. Factors affecting percutaneous absorption have therefore received a great deal of attention (13,81–83).

Factors Influencing Percutaneous Absorption

Stratum Corneum The main factor governing percutaneous absorption is the permeability barrier of the skin. The skin is composed of two layers known as epidermis and dermis. The epidermis is the thinner outer layer composed of epithelial tissue; the dermis is the thicker inner layer consisting mainly of connective tissue (Fig. 15-1). The permeability barrier resides principally in the stratum corneum, the outmost layer of the epidermis.

The differences noted in the percutaneous absorption in various parts of the body are partially correlated with the thickness of the stratum corneum. Its thickness varies with location. The skin on the palms and soles has a much thicker epidermis than that in other areas. Lowest absorption is noted on skin of the hands and soles, whereas greatest absorption is noted on the skin of the genitalia (36). Skin with damage to the stratum corneum is more permeable than is normal skin (81).

Apart from the barrier defenses provided by the stratum corneum, percutaneous absorption is influenced by a number of other factors such as the dose, the surface area, the character of the agent, the vehicle in which the agent is carried, and the location and condition of the skin itself (Table 15-1).

Concentration and Surface Area Dermal absorption is dependent on the concentration of the applied dose and on the surface area of application. As the applied dose is increased, the total amount absorbed into the body increases (97). Increasing the surface area of the applied dose also increases absorption (70).

Substance and Vehicle In general, lipids and lipid-soluble compounds and small molecules having both lipid and water solubility penetrate the skin quite easily. Ionization reduces skin absorption. Water penetrates the skin with extreme difficulty. The percutaneous absorption of any compound, however, can be profoundly affected by the vehicle in which it is carried. The partition coefficient of a compound between the vehicle and the skin in large part determines its absorption. Low solubility of a compound in the vehicle will tend to drive the compound into the skin, whereas high solubility will have the opposite effect. Some vehicles may damage the stratum corneum and thereby increase ab-

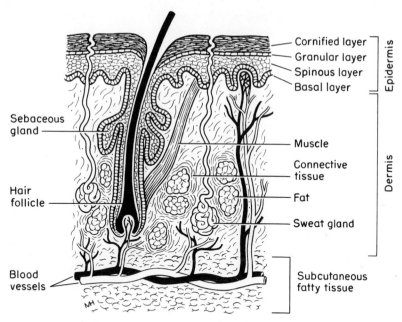

FIGURE 15-1. Diagram of a cross-section of human skin.

TABLE 15-1.   Conditions Affecting Percutaneous Absorption

Dose, concentration, and surface area
Vehicle used for agent being absorbed
Multiple dose application
Skin site of application
Condition of the skin
Occlusion of the skin
Skin metabolism

sorption. Other vehicles may enhance absorption or contain an agent(s) that enhances absorption (81–83).

Anatomic Site The extent of absorption depends on the anatomic site to which the compound is applied. This is true for humans and animals. High total absorption occurs through the skin of head, neck, and axilla—all areas that receive significant cosmetic and environmental exposure. The female genitalia show greater absorption than does the skin of the forearm. The site of greatest absorption, however, is the scrotum (35). The general pattern of regional variation in skin absorption holds for a variety of chemical moieties examined (steroids, pesticides, and antimicrobials) (54,102). The potential for systemic toxicity is therefore increased

when toxic exposure occurs at skin sites having enhanced absorption.

Occlusive Covering When a compound applied to the skin is covered—either intentionally, as with bandaging, or unintentionally, by the donning of clothing—percutaneous absorption is usually increased. Such occlusive covering increases the hydration and temperature of the skin, which in turn increases absorption. Occlusion also prevents an applied compound from being wiped off or from evaporating. Occlusion is the most practical clinical means of enhancing percutaneous absorption.

The reservoir effect is an example of the skin's ability to hold agents in the stratum corneum and to subsequently release them slowly into the body. This phenomenon is evident when the absorption of a drug applied to the skin is increased by hydrating the skin through the use of an occlusive dressing. The reservoir effect is also strikingly evident after cutaneous exposure to solvents, when, long after skin exposure has ceased, solvents continue to appear in blood and exhaled air (95,100).

Skin Metabolism

Skin is far more than a passive barrier that restricts the entrance of chemical agents into the body. The skin is a viable membrane that can metabolize an assortment of drugs, chemicals, and steroid hormones and thereby modify their effects. Although the dermis constitutes approximately 95% of the mass of human skin, the smaller epidermal layer accounts for the major portion of the biochemical transformations occurring in the skin. The skin appendages, such as sweat glands, hair follicles, and sebaceous glands, which extend into the dermal layer, are also metabolically active (6,7,9,71,72).

The skin utilizes many of the metabolic pathways found in other tissues and contains many of the same drug-metabolizing enzymes found in the liver. In vitro studies indicate that the activity of the cutaneous enzymes is about 2% of that found in the liver (71,72). The action of enzymes present in the microsomal portion of the cell generally leads to the detoxication and excretion of foreign chemicals. However, in some cases microsomal enzymes activate chemicals to form metabolites that are more toxic than the parent compound from which they are derived. The skin is capable of transforming nontoxic foreign chemicals into toxic compounds. The metabolism of the polycyclic aromatic hydrocarbon benzo[a]pyrene provides an excellent example of this process. Benzo[a]pyrene, a ubiquitous environmental pollutant found in tar, automobile exhaust, and some charcoal-broiled foods, is not carcinogenic. After undergoing metabolism by the microsomal enzyme system, benzo[a]pyrene is transformed into a diol-epoxide, a potent carcinogen (39,72). (See Chapter 9 for a discussion of the metabolism of foreign substances.)

Since the skin receives a major part of the body's exposure to environmental pollutants, its metabolic activity has important implications. Any toxic or potentially toxic chemical that penetrates the skin must go through the metabolically active epidermis before entering the systemic circulation. A chemical can thus be activated or detoxified by cutaneous enzymes before entering the body. It is possible that certain chemicals may be more toxic after topical application than when taken orally. The skin's metabolism can thus be an important factor in the pattern of dermal and systemic toxicity that follows exposure to foreign chemicals.

When there is little or no skin metabolism of a topically applied chemical, the chemical is introduced unchanged into the systemic circulation. Under these conditions the skin's defense against toxic exposure depends primarily on its barrier function.

Dermal Toxicity Testing

A number of tests, including animal assays, have been used to make predictions of dermal toxicity in humans. The complex aspects of dermal toxicity testing have been reviewed (37,68,98). New techniques for assessing dermal toxicity are increasingly dependent on in vitro methods such as tissue culture. These methods, which have been widely used to establish the safety of plastics in medical devices implanted in the human body, are being used to screen new skin products for safety.

Methods for Measuring Percutaneous Absorption

Ideally, information on the dermal absorption of a particular compound in humans is best obtained through studies performed in humans. However, since many compounds are potentially too toxic to test in man, studies must be performed utilizing other techniques. Percutaneous absorption has been measured by two major methods: (1) in vitro diffusion cell technique and (2) in vivo determinations, which generally utilize radiolabeled compounds (98). To insure their applicability to the clinical situation, the relevance of the studies using these techniques must constantly be challenged.

In vitro techniques involve placing a piece of animal or human skin in a diffusion chamber containing physiological saline. The compound under investigation is applied to one side of the skin. The compound is then assayed at regular intervals on the other side of the skin (91). Artificial membranes may also be used. The skin may be intact or separated into epidermis and dermis. The advantages of the in vitro techniques are that the methodology is easy to use and results are obtained quickly. The major disadvantage is the limited relevance of the conditions present in the in vitro system to those found in humans.

Percutaneous absorption in vivo is usually determined by the indirect method of measuring radioactivity in excreta following the topical application of a labeled compound. In human studies, the plasma level of a topically applied compound is usually extremely low, often below assay detection. For this reason tracer methodology is used. After the topical application of the carbon-14- or tritium-labeled compound, the total amount of radioactivity excreted in urine or in urine plus feces is determined. The amount of radioactivity retained in the body or excreted by a route not assayed (CO_2) is corrected for by determining the amount of radioactivity excreted following parenteral administration. Absorption represents the amount of radioactivity excreted, expressed as a percentage of the applied dose (99). Percutaneous absorption can also be assessed by the ratio of the areas under the concentration-versus-time curves following the topical and intravenous administration of a radiolabeled compound. The metabolism of a compound by the skin as it is absorbed will not be detected by this method (101). A biological response, such as vasoconstriction after the topical application of steroids, has also been used to assess dermal absorption in vivo.

EPIDEMIOLOGY

The association between the development of skin disease and exposure to toxic chemicals has long been recognized. Contamination of the workplace is an obvious source of toxic exposure to the skin. Less obvious is the toxic exposure that occurs through contamination of the general environment. Although many cutaneous disorders arise from exposure to toxic chemicals in the environment, information on incidence of skin disease related to chemical exposure is derived from occupational sources. These data depend on statistical compilations of occupational disease reports, clinical studies of epidemics, clinical case reports, and a few epidemiologic studies (29,43,61,65,73,89). The validity of such data may be seriously compromised by such problems as underreporting, inadequate exposure data, and improper diagnoses.

After the exclusion of accidental injuries, which account for about 97% of cases, skin disease accounts for over one-third of all occupationally related illnesses (61). Of all the occupational categories, agricultural activities and manufacturing have the highest incidence of occupationally related skin disease. In agriculture, nearly two-thirds of occupational illnesses were based on skin disease. The most recent compilation of occupational skin diseases obtained from the U.S. Bureau of Statistics Survey indicates that the rate and number of cases declined from 1973 through 1983. Although this decline may be attributed to such factors as worker education, increasing automation, and enclosure of automated processes, it is generally accepted that the true incidence of occupational skin disease may be 10 to 50 times that reported (92). Information on occupational skin disease reflects the incidence of skin disease that follows immediately on an exposure. The role of occupational exposure in the development of chronic skin disease is unknown.

Contact dermatitis constitutes about 80% to 90% of occupational skin disease. Over three-quarters of the cases of contact dermatitis arise from irritation rather than allergy. Based on data from California, soaps, detergents, cleaning agents, and solvents are most often cited as causal agents. The solvents most frequently involved are acetone, chlorinated hydrocarbons, toluene, xylene, petroleum distillate, and alcohols (16).

Although allergic contact dermatitis is much less prevalent than irritant contact dermatitis, a number of sensitizing agents are present in the home as well as the workplace. Because exposure to even minute concentrations of a sensitizing agent is followed by an adverse dermal response in the sensitized individual, many ordinary measures to reduce such exposure are often ineffective.

Epidemiologic studies have been helpful in identifying certain environmental factors associated with skin cancer. Foremost in importance are the epidemiological studies that link UV radiation from the sun to the development of skin cancer. There is a vast literature to support this relationship. Population studies done in the 1960s and 1970s revealed that fair-skinned people living near the equator have an increased incidence of skin cancer (24,42). Additional studies showed that basal-cell carcinoma and squamous-cell carcinoma occur primarily on the light-exposed areas of the skin. Moreover, these tumors are more prevalent in lightly pigmented people who spend time outdoors and who sunburn easily (85,94).

The relationship between UV exposure and melanoma is more complex than that present in the case of basal-cell and squamous-cell carcinoma of the skin. Numerous studies indicate that the incidence of melanoma in Caucasian populations has been increasing over the past 30 years. A consistent inverse relationship between the incidence of melanoma and latitude has been observed. Of interest are studies that indicate that melanoma risks are increased in individuals exposed to high doses of UV radiation for short periods of time but not in populations having more gradual exposure (26,47, 51,90). Of the four main types of melanomas, the lentigo maligna, which arises on sun-exposed skin, seems related to cumulative UV exposure (63).

Epidemiologic studies have incriminated environmental arsenic contamination as a cause of skin cancer. Studies in Taiwan reveal that individuals exposed to inorganic arsenic through contaminated well water have an incidence of skin cancer many times higher than that of the general population (104). These findings have been confirmed (4).

Susceptibility and Cutaneous Toxicity

A number of specific environmental and host factors can affect the development of dermatologic disease following toxic exposure (20). Environmental factors are exogenous agents to which an individual is exposed, whereas host factors are those factors present in the exposed individual. Host factors may be inherited or acquired.

Specific environmental factors that may alter the risk of environmental/occupational skin disease include exposure to chemical, physical, and biological agents in air, food, and water in the workplace and in the home. Other factors include personal hygiene, protective devices, ambient temperature and humidity, general cleanliness of the workplace and the home, and the life style of an individual as reflected in the use of medications and drugs.

Host factors that can alter the risk of toxic skin disorders include such genetically determined features as surface oils, skin thickness, pigmentation, hairiness, sweat gland activity, scar formation, vascular response, healing characteristics, metabolic status, and immunologic condition (20,103). An individual's age, nutritional status, and the presence of certain chronic skin conditions are other host factors that may determine an individual's predisposition to develop skin disease secondary to toxic exposure.

Age is especially important in affecting the prevalence and pattern of toxic dermatoses of large numbers of individuals. Age-dependent conditions function at each end of the life cycle to increase susceptibility to toxic exposure. The infant, particularly the premature one, because of its immature development, large surface area in relationship to body weight, and reduced dermal barrier, has shown the greatest toxicological response to topical agents not ordinarily considered to be highly toxic.

Numerous well-documented episodes of infantile poisoning from the dermal absorption of topically applied agents have been reported (99). The most striking example of this phenomenon occurred with the use of hexachlorophene, an antibacterial agent that formerly was added to soaps and baby powders. In France, a sudden outbreak of hexachlorophene poisoning occurred in infants who were exposed to talcum powder containing hexachlorophene. Premature infants also suffered brain damage from repeated bathing with soap containing hexachlorophene (56,87).

The aged, whose numbers are increasing significantly in many highly industrialized societies, are also more susceptible to toxic exposure. The skin, along with other organs, is compromised by age. Among the well-documented changes in the aged skin are increased dryness and diminished lipid content, both of which exert influence over the barrier function of the skin. The proliferative capacity of the epidermis is also reduced with age (11,77).

Although relatively few epidemiologic studies have investigated the factors that predispose individuals to develop environmental/occupational skin disease, two major conclusions can be drawn from the work done thus far. (1) The skin of atopic individuals and those with atopic dermatitis is generally more susceptible to irritants, dusts, and sharp changes in heat and/or humidity. (2) Fair-skinned individuals are more susceptible to the adverse effects of UV radiation (43,79,85,94).

PATHOLOGY AND PATHOLOGICAL PHYSIOLOGY

The skin responds to toxic exposure in a variety of ways (1,31,53). Toxic responses of the skin have been described and classified primarily on the basis of morphological changes (Table 15-2). These responses for the most part are nonspecific in that widely different toxic agents can cause similar pathological responses. The biochemical and physiological events underlying most toxic skin responses are poorly understood. Notable exceptions are the advances that have been made in explaining the events underlying cutaneous carcinogenesis and radiation- and immune-induced skin injury (18,19, 41,80).

Contact Dermatitis

Contact dermatitis is the most commonly observed dermal response to chemical exposure. The term refers to an inflammatory condition induced by exposure of the skin to an offending agent. Contact dermatitis may arise as an irritant or allergic skin response (1,38).

Irritant Contact Dermatitis

Irritant contact dermatitis develops as a direct, local, and toxic effect and does not involve immunologic mechanisms. Irritant dermatitis is usually limited to the areas of exposure. It is manifest by dermal reactions, which range from mild erythema, edema, scale formation, and thickening to vesiculation, necrosis, and ulceration. Chemicals with strong irritant qualities can adversely affect the skin after one brief exposure. Most chemicals found in the workplace and in the home, however, are relatively weak irritants requiring repeated, prolonged skin contact before visible changes are induced. Virtually any substance may have a direct irritant

TABLE 15-2. Adverse Skin Reactions to Environmental and Occupational Agents

Contact dermatitis
Irritant
Allergic
Acneiform disorders
Oil acne
Chloracne
Pigmentary disorders
Hyperpigmentation
Hypopigmentation
Photosensitivity
Phototoxic reactions including actinic changes and porphyria cutanea tarda
Photoallergic reactions
Contact urticaria
Radiodermatitis
Skin cancer
Squamous-cell carcinoma
Basal-cell carcinoma
Certain types of melanoma

effect on the skin. The most commonly encountered irritants are acids, alkalis, solvents, soaps, and detergents (Table 15-3). Many individuals, particularly those in the workplace, are exposed to multiple skin irritants. The irritation that ensues may be the cumulative result of multiple exposures. Once skin inflammation has taken place, the barrier function of the skin is compromised, and the skin thereby becomes even more susceptible to irritation.

Allergic Contact Dermatitis

Allergic contact dermatitis has clinical and pathological features similar to contact dermatitis caused by irritants. It develops as an immunologic reaction to a chemical agent and is an expression of cell-mediated delayed hypersensitivity. The pathogenic events leading to allergic contact dermatitis require a number of steps that are well characterized. The sensitization process begins when simple low-molecular-weight chemicals, termed haptens, combine with skin proteins to form a full antigen. The antigen then interacts with the epidermal Langerhans cells or macrophages. After processing by the Langerhans cells, the antigen interacts with thymus-derived or T lymphocytes. Langerhans cells or T lymphocytes migrate from the skin to the paracortical area of the regional lymph nodes. At this point two populations of sensitized T lymphocytes are formed. One set is termed effector T lymphocytes; the second set is called memory cells. The effector T lymphocytes circulate in the peripheral blood, travel to the skin surface, and release the substances that mediate the inflammatory skin reaction associated with further antigen contact. The memory cells, on contact with the same or a closely related antigen, proliferate and produce new populations of sensitized lymphocytes (80).

The development of allergic contact dermatitis proceeds according to the following time sequence. First, there is the interval during which contact with the potential allergen occurs without evidence of sensitization. This interval, termed the refractory period, may last only a few days or a long interval. The refractory period is followed by an incubation or latent period during which the actual development of sensitization takes place. This process may take from 4 days to several weeks. After dermal sensitization is complete, reexposure to the sensitizing antigen, even in minute concentrations, gives rise to fulminant contact dermatitis within 48 to 72 h (1). This interval, known as the eliciting phase (reaction time), is the basis of the diagnostic "patch test" for allergic contact dermatitis.

The causes of contact allergic dermatitis are varied, and there are great differences in antigenic potency. Although the workplace is a major source of antigenic exposure, a large number of antigenic agents such as perfumes, hair dyes, cosmetic colorants, and resins and dyes in clothing are found in the home and in products made for personal use. Some common important allergens are shown in Table 15-3.

Oil Acne and Chloracne

Contact with lubricating oils and greases may cause comedonal plugging or pustular folliculitis having microscopic features resembling acne vulgaris. Acneiform eruptions are most often encountered in machinists and other workers coming in contact with petroleum derivatives (23).

Chloracne is a distinct and more serious and persistent form of acne. It is caused by exposure to various chlorinated or brominated aromatic compounds having a particular molecular structure. Exposure to halogenated naphthalenes, diphenyls, azoxybenzenes, dibenzofurans, and dioxin has been

TABLE 15-3. Chemical Agents Commonly Associated
with Irritant and Allergic Dermatitis

Irritant dermatitis agent	Allergic dermatitis agent
Acids	Metals
Inorganic and organic	Nickel and nickel salts
Alkalis	Chromium salts
Inorganic and organic	Cobalt salts
Metal salts	Organomercurials
Solvents	Rubber additives
Alcohols	Methyl methacrylate and other acrylic monomers
Ketones	Pentaerythritol triacrylate and other multifunctional
Chlorinated	acrylates
Others	Ethylenediamine, hexamethylenetetramine, and other
Soaps	aliphatic amines
Detergents	Formaldehyde

associated with chloracne. Lesions may appear after exposure has ceased (88). Cases of chloracne have been reported following occupational exposure or accidental environmental contamination. Notable episodes of environmental contamination associated with outbreaks of chloracne occurred in Seveso, Italy in 1976, when an industrial accident resulted in widespread exposure to tetrachlorodibenzo-*p*-dioxin (TCDD or "dioxin"), in Japan in 1968, and in Taiwan in 1979, when cooking oil was accidently contaminated with polychlorinated diphenyls (PCBs), polychlorinated dibenzofurans, and polychlorinated quaterphenyls (17,50,58,75).

Chloracne is characterized by multiple closed comedones and straw-colored cysts. The lesions are commonly found on the cheeks, temples, ears, and behind the ears. In severe cases, inflammatory changes occur, and involvement spreads to the shoulders, trunk, buttocks, and scrotum. Histological changes are typified by a keratinization of the sebaceous gland ducts followed by the disappearance of the sebaceous gland and the formation of keratin-filled cysts (88).

Pigmentary Disorders

Chemical agents can modify skin color by staining and discoloration or by affecting melanization. Staining of the skin occurs when dyes bind to keratin in the stratum corneum. Most staining is encountered at the site of exposure to such agents as aniline dye, nitric acid, trinitrotoluene, and copper. The systemic absorption of such heavy metals as silver, mercury, or arsenic may produce a diffuse discoloration of skin.

Hyperpigmentation, the most commonly encountered pigment problem, may follow an episode of chemical or thermal injury to the skin. Hyperpigmentation may also result from contact, ingestion, or injection of substances that are photosensitizers (see below). Such agents may cause inflammatory reactions, followed by hyperpigmentation, in sun-exposed areas. The loss of cutaneous pigmentation can arise after chemical injury that is severe enough to destroy melanocytes. It can also be caused by a variety of phenolic or catecholic derivatives in connection with exposure to such agents as rubber, photographic developing solutions, and lubricating oils.

Photosensitivity

Photosensitivity is used to describe an unusual vulnerability to the effects of ultraviolet and/or visible radiation. This condition becomes clinically apparent as an acute sunburn or eczema on sun-exposed skin surfaces. Photosensitivity commonly arises from the presence of certain exogenous chemicals in the skin that respond to ultraviolet radiation by initiating events that are broadly similar to contact dermatitis. Photosensitivity reactions may arise through phototoxicity or photoallergy. These reactions are analogous to irritant and allergic contact dermatitis except for the added requirement of ultraviolet radiation. Phototoxicity does not involve immunologic mechanisms, whereas photoallergy requires involvement of the immune system. Exogenous chemicals associated with phototoxicity and photoallergy are shown in Table 15-4 (28,30,32).

Porphyria Cutanea Tarda

Porphyria cutanea tarda is characterized by bullous eruptions, photosensitivity, hyperpigmentation, and excessive hair growth. Porphyria cutanea tarda may appear after exposure to organochlorine compounds, the most important being hexachlorobenzene and dioxin. Exposure to these agents may interfere with porphyrin metabolism by reducing hepatic uroporphyrinogen decarboxylase activity. Excessive amounts of uroporphyrins are thereby formed and deposited in the skin. The photochemical action spectrum for skin photosensitivity corresponds closely with the absorption spectrum of uroporphyrin (8,69). An epidemic of porphyria cutanea tarda occurred in Turkey in the 1950s when seed grain treated with hexachlorobenzene was introduced into the food supply. Hexachlorobenzene was formerly widely used as a fungicide (84).

Contact Urticaria

Generalized and localized urticaria can be caused by the absorption of a variety of foreign agents. Generalized urticaria, when related to occupational/environmental exposure, usually results from inhalation of allergenic material and is accompanied by symptoms of inhalant allergy. Localized urticarial reactions (both immunologic and nonimmunologic) may occur from the dermal absorption

TABLE 15-4. Chemical Agents Associated with Phototoxicity and Photoallergy

Phototoxic reactions
  Polyaromatic hydrocarbons
  Pitch, asphalt, coal tars, oils, anthracene, acridine, phenanthrene
  Painting and photographic chemicals
    Amyl-*o*-dimethylaminobenzoic acid
  Furocoumarins (psoralens)
Photoallergic reactions
  Halogenated salicyanilides and related agents
  4,6-Dichlorophenylphenol

of foreign agents. Contact urticaria may be associated with delayed dermatitis, bronchial asthma, and symptoms of itching and burning.

Radiodermatitis

About 2 to 3 weeks after the skin is exposed to relatively high doses of ionizing radiation, an acute reaction takes place. This reaction is similar to that noted with ultraviolet radiation. Erythema is followed by blistering, erosions, and epilation. With increasing exposure necrosis may also occur. Some months or years following radiation injury of the skin, atrophy, telangiectasia, fibrosis, and depigmentation develop.

Skin Cancer

Because of its external location, more is known about the etiology and pathogenesis of skin cancer in relation to exposure than is known about any other malignancy. It is well established that human skin is susceptible to carcinogenesis by exposure to chemical carcinogens and radiation (105) (Table 15-5). The rodent skin has been used extensively to study the pathogenesis of such important environmental carcinogens as polycyclic aromatic hydrocarbons, ultraviolet, and ionizing radiation.

Chemical Carcinogenesis

The basic experimental protocol by which many of the essential concepts in carcinogenesis were established evolved from studies of mouse skin. Mouse skin provided the earliest experimental model for the study of chemical carcinogenesis. Evidence collected over the past decade indicates that the processes observed in mouse skin are analogous to the malignant transformations that occur in other

organs (74,105). For a further discussion of this process, the reader is referred to Chapters 9 and 26.

Early studies of chemical carcinogenesis using the skin of the mouse revealed a latency period in the development of cancer. From these observations, it was possible to identify two distinct stages, initiation and promotion, in the process of chemical carcinogenesis (12,78). Additional studies revealed that the chemical agents that induce skin cancer bind covalently to DNA in mouse skin. The extent of DNA binding, in general, was proportional to the carcinogenic potency of the agent (7,14,105). Further investigation revealed that the carcinogenic potential of a number of chemical agents is realized only after they are metabolized to active intermediates capable of binding covalently with cellular macromolecules (66).

Much attention has been focused on benzo[a]-pyrene, a polycyclic aromatic hydrocarbon that produces skin cancer. The metabolites of benzo[a]-pyrene generally fall into three classes: phenols, quinones, and dihydrodiols. It is the dihydrodiols that, when metabolized to diol-epoxides, become potent carcinogens. The diol-epoxides are the metabolic intermediates of benzo[a]pyrene that react with cellular DNA, RNA, and proteins (96). Other polycyclic aromatic hydrocarbons such as 3-methylcholanthrene and benz[a]anthracene derivatives also induce skin tumors through the formation of reactive metabolites. Knowledge of the active metabolites of specific polycyclic aromatic hydrocarbons and their binding to cellular macromolecules has reached a high level of sophistication (7,40, 45,105). Apart from the polycyclic aromatic hydrocarbons, nitrosamines, nitrosamides, aromatic amines, and alkylating agents have been shown to induce skin cancer in the rodent.

Radiation (Ultraviolet and Ionizing) Carcinogenesis

Ultraviolet Radiation Chronic repeated exposure to ultraviolet radiation after a latent period of varying length is closely associated with human skin cancer, particularly basal-cell and squamous-cell cancers. Those individuals who sunburn easily and have considerable exposure to solar ultraviolet radiation are particularly susceptible. The clinical and epidemiologic evidence to support this observation has been amply reviewed (27,93).

The mouse skin, so effectively used in the study of chemical carcinogenesis, has also provided insight into ultraviolet carcinogenesis. Experimental studies have established that ultraviolet radiation between 290 and 320 nm (UVB) induces skin cancer. In mouse skin, most experimentally induced cancers are squamous-cell carcinomas. Ultraviolet radiation has demonstrated cancer-initiating and -promoting properties. The short-wave length UVB

TABLE 15-5. Chemical and Physical Factors Associated with the Development of Human Skin Cancer

Agent	Type of cancer
Ultraviolet light 280–320 nm (UVB)	Basal-cell carcinoma Squamous-cell carcinoma Certain melanomas
Ionizing radiation	Basal-cell carcinoma Squamous-cell carcinoma
Arsenic	Basal-cell carcinoma Squamous-cell carcinoma
Soot, coal tar, pitch, petroleum products, creosote, coke, greases	Squamous-cell carcinoma

produces direct photochemical damage as evidenced by a variety of DNA lesions, which include pyrimidine dimers, pyrimidine adducts, and DNA strand breaks (44). A number of mechanisms function to repair the DNA damaged by ultraviolet light (19).

Certain individuals have an inherited susceptibility to the carcinogenic effects of solar radiation based on their diminished ability to repair light-induced DNA damage (18). Such individuals, with an autosomal recessive genetic disease termed xeroderma pigmentosum, have a high incidence of skin cancer at a young age (49).

Based primarily on evidence derived from animal studies, there appears to be an additive and/or synergistic effect between environmental chemicals and radiation in the induction of skin cancer. This phenomenon may be linked to (1) chemical photosensitization that leads to toxic injury, (2) additive effects of dermal exposure to chemical and physical carcinogens, and (3) cancer-promoting effects of certain chemicals on ultraviolet-initiated skin cancer. To date, these relationships have not been demonstrated in humans (34). Examining the relationship of sun-induced skin cancer in humans to chemical exposure gains importance as new compounds are introduced into the environment.

Ionizing Radiation A few years after Roentgen's discovery of x rays in the early 20th century, ionizing radiation was incriminated in the development of skin cancer. At this time individuals exposed to low doses of x rays were noted to develop skin cancer.

The rat skin has provided an excellent model for studying radiation carcinogenesis. In this model, dose-response and time-response characteristics and the cellular and biochemical effects of radiation-induced carcinogenesis have been investigated (15).

In general, higher doses of radiation produce squamous-cell carcinomas, whereas lower doses of radiation produce more basal-cell carcinomas (2). The dose-response relationship of radiation-induced carcinogenesis typically rises to a peak and then declines at higher doses.

A variety of cellular and biochemical changes are induced by ionizing radiation. One of the most readily observed effects of ionizing radiation is the appearance of aberrant chromosomes. This picture may be the result of simple breakage of the chromosomes or the interaction of the broken ends to form rearrangements. X-ray-induced ionizations break one or both strands of DNA, damage many sites in the purine and pyrimidine rings, and produce DNA-protein cross-links. The damage incurred by ionizing radiation is linked to the ionization of cellular water and biological molecules. Free radicals derived from the ionization of water are highly unstable and chemically reactive. The biological effects of radiation-induced free radical reactions are intensified in the presence of oxygen. The radiation energy deposited produces molecular excitations, largely dissipated as heat, and is of little importance (5, 19,59).

The interaction of ionizing radiation with chemical carcinogens has received limited attention. Using the skin of experimental animals, McGregor demonstrated that the number of tumors induced by ionizing radiation increased when cigarette smoke condensate was subsequently applied to the skin (64). The interrelationship between ionizing radiation and the myriad chemical agents and physical agents present in the workplace and general environment promises to be an important area of future investigation.

CLINICAL ASPECTS OF EXPOSURE TO ENVIRONMENTAL CHEMICALS AND PHYSICAL AGENTS ON THE SKIN

Establishing the Diagnosis

Establishing the diagnosis of occupational and/or environmental skin disease is largely dependent on a thorough medical history and a carefully performed physical examination. A skilled history and physical examination establish a diagnosis by searching for answers to the following key questions: (1) Are the appearance and distribution of the skin lesions compatible with a reaction to a chemical, physical, or biological agent? (2) Is there a history of exposure to a toxic agent(s) in the workplace or general environment that could cause such lesions? (3) Did the exposure occur before the onset of the skin disease? (4) Does removal of the suspected causal exposure improve the skin disease? It should be appreciated, however, that chronic dermatosis may not improve rapidly even when the inciting agent is removed.

The medical history should include a detailed description of the skin lesions, their localization, spread, progression, and improvement. Information on events, activities, and exposures surrounding the onset and the change of the skin disease should be noted. By relating external events to the onset and modification of the patient's skin disease, the physician may discover its cause. Work activities, for example, at the onset of the skin disease offer a means of isolating offending agents. A clear understanding of present and past working conditions and exposures is of critical importance. Environmental exposures from personal products and from agents used in the home must be considered. Since host factors play a role in the development of environmental and occupational skin disease, the patient's ethnic makeup and family history of skin problems must be considered. A history of atopy, excessive sun exposure, or previous skin reactions to topical medication, cosmetics, and jewelry must be determined. The components of the history are shown in Table 15-6.

A physical examination, performed under good lighting, should note the general appearance, distribution, and character of the skin lesions. The distribution of the skin lesions often helps to determine the etiological agent. Dermatitis from liquids usually occurs on the dorsal aspects of the hands, on the lateral surfaces of the fingers, and on the arms. The face and neck are commonly affected by fumes and airborne agents. Dusts frequently cause problems at the collar line and belt region.

At times the presence of occupational/environmental skin disease will be quickly apparent. Many times the appearance of the skin lesions belies their toxic origin. Thus, such endogenous conditions as atopic dermatitis, nummular eczema, chronic hand eczema, and psoriasis must be considered in the diagnosis. The physician must also be aware that skin disease can be worsened by exposure to chemical agents.

The patch test is one of the most useful diagnostic procedures for identifying occupational/environmental skin disease. The test is performed if allergic contact dermatitis is suspected and if the inciting agent is unknown. Patch testing is usually performed using common test substances, which are marketed for this purpose. Unfortunately, many allergens encountered in the workplace and generally environment have not been commercially prepared for testing. Unless specifically tested, these allergens may be overlooked.

The chemicals to be tested are dissolved in a vehicle in nonirritating concentrations and applied to an impervious adhesive tape, which is then fixed to the skin. The patch tests are applied to the upper or lower back or occasionally to the lateral side of the upper arm. The test units are generally removed after 2 or 3 days. The appearance of an eczematous lesion under the patch within 2 to 4 days provides evidence of a delayed hypersensitivity reaction to the applied agent. This response presumes a prior skin sensitization to the test substance that developed very recently or in years past. As with all assays, there are false-positive and false-negative reactions with patch testing. The most common cause of a false-positive reaction is the use of irritant substances as test materials. A false-negative reaction often stems from using too low a concentration of the test agent or from a failure to duplicate the conditions present during the dermatitis i.e., sweating, friction, etc. The relevance of a positive patch test in detecting the cause of dermatitis depends on the clinician's awareness and on the importance of the allergen in the patient's environment. Details of the methodology used in diagnostic patch testing are found in the following references (1,22).

Treatment and Prevention

The cause of a toxic skin response should be identified as precisely and promptly as possible, for the prompt removal of the causal agent often improves the prognosis. Once the causal agent(s) has been identified, the patient must be informed and instructed in its avoidance. The treatment program must be individualized. The stage of disease, the patient's age, and the factors that enhance the patient's susceptibility to skin disease must be considered in a treatment program. Patients with healed dermatitis should be aware that even though their skin appears normal, it is more vulnerable to environmental insult. Patients with allergic dermatitis must be informed that their skin lesions will recur on reexposure to the offending agent. The details of treating occupational/environmental skin disease are found in several references (1,60).

Preventing environmental and occupational skin disease depends on eliminating or minimizing the patient's contact with irritating, sensitizing, carcinogenic, and depigmenting agents. Exposure to ultraviolet must be minimized, particularly in the case of susceptible individuals. This goal is ap-

---

TABLE 15-6. Pertinent Medical History in the Diagnosis of Environmental and Occupational Skin Disease

Present illness
  The skin lesion, its nature, and distribution
  Progression and regression as related to occupational and environmental exposures and activities
  Effects of weekends, vacations, sick leave
  Response to therapy
  Evaluation of patient's susceptibility to skin problems
Past medical history
  Previous skin problems including atopy
  History of allergies
Medications
  Prescribed and over-the-counter
Family history
  Skin disease, atopy, and allergy
Environmental and occupational history
  Environmental history
    Exposure in the home and its vicinity
      Cleaning products, etc.
      Jobs around the house, etc.
    Hobbies
    Personal habits
    Recreational habits
  Occupational history
    Nature and conditions of work(s), materials used, protective devices, skin-cleaning methods

proached in part through a program of education. As the stratospheric ozone shield continues to deteriorate, protecting the skin from ultraviolet radiation assumes far greater importance.

Workers should be aware of the composition of chemicals used on the job, their potential hazards, the importance of protective measures, and personal hygiene. A similar awareness is necessary for chemicals found in personal products and in the home environment. Emphasis must be placed on properly using, storing, and disposing of hazardous chemicals present in the home and workplace. Skin contact with hazardous agents should be avoided, and when contact occurs the skin should be washed as soon as possible.

Other methods of prevention are dependent on forces beyond the control of the individual. These include replacing offending irritants, allergens, or carcinogens with a suitable alternative and modifying manufacturing practices so that automatic equipment and closed processes isolate the worker from hazardous exposures.

SUMMARY

The skin, by providing a barrier between the body and the environment, bears the brunt of the body's exposure to environmental chemicals and physical agents. Since the skin's response to environmental assault is apparent, it has received considerable attention. Exposure to environmental chemicals and physical agents can be associated with such diverse reactions as contact dermatitis, photosensitivity, acne and chloracne, pigmentary disturbances, urticaria, and cancer. All varieties of environmental chemicals have been incriminated in the etiology of skin disease. Most recently, the continued depletion of the ozone layer, which provides protection against the carcinogenic impact of sunlight, has added a new dimension of concern.

REFERENCES

1. Adams RM (ed): Occupational Skin Disease, 2nd ed., WB Saunders, Philadelphia, 1990.
2. Albert RE, Phillips ME, Bennett P, et al: The morphology and growth characteristics of radiation-induced epithelial skin tumors in the rat. Cancer Res 29:658, 1969.
3. Andelman JB, Underhill DW (eds.): Health Effects from Hazardous Waste Sites. Lewis Publishers, Chelsea, Michigan, 1987.
4. Armondo VI, Angel AO: Chronical arsenicism. Bol Med Hosp Infant 36:849, 1979.
5. Baxendale JH: Effects of oxygen and pH in radiation chemistry of aqueous solutions. Radiat Res 4 (Suppl): 114, 1964.

6. Bickers DR: The skin as a site of drug and chemical metabolism. In: Current Concepts in Cutaneous Toxicity, p 95, Drill VA, Lazar P (eds.), Academic Press, Orlando, 1980.
7. Bickers DR: Drug, carcinogen, and steroid hormone metabolism in the skin. In: Biochemistry and Physiology of the Skin, p 1169, Goldsmith LA (ed.), Oxford University Press, New York, 1983.
8. Bickers DR: Photosensitization by porphyrins. In: Biochemistry and Physiology of the Skin, p 755, Goldsmith LA (ed.), Oxford University Press, New York, 1983.
9. Bickers DR, Das M, Mukhtar H: Pharmacological modification of epidermal detoxification systems. Br J Dermatol 115(Suppl 31):9, 1986.
10. Binder S, Forney D, Kaye W, et al: Arsenic exposure in children living near a former copper smelter. Bull Environ Contam Toxicol 39:114, 1987.
11. Blank IH: The effect of hydration on the permeability of the skin. In: Percutaneous Absorption, p. 97, Bronaugh RL, Maibach HI (eds.), Marcel Dekker, New York, 1985.
12. Boutwell RK: Some biological aspects of skin carcinogenesis. Prog Exp Tumor Res 4:207, 1964.
13. Bronaugh RL, Maibach HI (eds.): Percutaneous Absorption: Mechanisms-Methodology-Drug Delivery, 2nd ed., Marcel Dekker, New York, 1989.
14. Brooks P, Lawley PD: Evidence for the binding of polynuclear aromatic hydrocarbons to the nucleic acids of mouse skin: Relation between carcinogenic hydrocarbons and their binding to deoxyribonucleic acid. Nature 202:781, 1964.
15. Burns FJ, Albert RE: Radiation carcinogenesis in rat skin. In: Radiation Carcinogenesis, p 198, Upton AC, Albert RE, Burns FJ, et al. (eds.), Elsevier, Amsterdam, 1986.
16. California Department of Industrial Relations, Division of Labor Statistics and Research: Occupational Skin Disease in California (with Special Reference to 1977), California Department of Industrial Relations, San Francisco, 1982.
17. Caramaschi F, DelCorno G, Favaretti C, et al: Chloracne following environmental contamination by TCDD in Seveso, Italy. Int J Epidemiol 10:135, 1981.
18. Cleaver JE: DNA damage and repair in light sensitive human skin disease. J Invest Dermatol 54:181, 1970.
19. Cleaver JE: DNA damage and repair. In: Radiation Carcinogenesis, p 43, Upton AC, Albert RE, Burns FJ, et al. (eds.), Elsevier, Amsterdam, 1986.
20. Cohen SR: Risk factors in occupational skin disease. In: Occupational and Industrial Dermatology, 2nd ed, p 6, Maibach HI (ed.), Year Book Medical Publisher, Chicago, 1987.
21. Committee on Causes and Effects of Changes in Stratospheric Ozone, National Research Council: Causes and Effects of Stratospheric Ozone Reduction: An Update, 1983, National Academy Press, Washington, 1983.
22. Cronin E: Contact Dermatitis, Churchill Livingston, Edinburgh, 1980.
23. Crow KD: Chloracne and its potential clinical implications. Clin Exp Dermatol 6:243, 1981.
24. Davis NC: Sunlight and melanomas. Lancet 1:803, 1971.

25. Drill VA, Lazar P (eds.): Current Concepts in Cutaneous Toxicity, Academic Press, Orlando, 1980.
26. Elwood J, Gallagher R, Davison J, et al: Sunburn, suntan and the risk of cutaneous malignant melanoma: The Western Canada Melanoma Study. Br J Cancer 53:543, 1985.
27. Emmett EA: Ultraviolet radiation as a cause of skin tumors. CRC Crit Rev Toxicol 2:211, 1974.
28. Emmett EA: Phototoxicity from exogenous agents. Photochem Photobiol 30:429, 1979.
29. Emmett EA: The skin and occupational diseases. Arch Environ Health 39:344, 1984.
30. Emmett EA: Toxic responses of the skin. In: Casarett and Doull's Toxicology, 3rd ed., p 412, Klaassen CD, Amdur MO, Doull J (eds.), Macmillan, New York, 1986.
31. Emmett EA: Occupational dermatosis. In: Dermatology in General Medicine, 3rd ed., p 1567, Fitzpatrick TB, Eisen AZ, Wolff K, et al. (eds.), McGraw-Hill, New York, 1987.
32. Emmett EA: Photobiologic effects. In: Occupational and Industrial Dermatology, 2nd ed., p 94, Maibach HI (ed.), Year Book Medical Publishers, Chicago, 1987.
33. Environmental Studies Board, Commission on Natural Resources: Urban Pest Management, National Academy Press, Washington, 1980.
34. Epstein JH: Cutaneous cancer and environmental chemicals. In: Occupational and Industrial Dermatology, 2nd ed., p 121, Maibach HI (ed.), Year Book Medical Publisher, Chicago, 1987.
35. Feldmann RJ, Maibach HI: Regional variation in percutaneous penetration of ^{14}C cortisone in man. J Invest Dermatol 48:181, 1967.
36. Feldmann RJ, Maibach HI: Absorption of some organic compounds through the skin in man. J Invest Dermatol 54:339, 1969.
37. Fischer T, Maibach HI: Patch testing in allergic contact dermatitis: An update. In: Occupational and Industrial Dermatology, 2nd ed., p 190, Maibach HI (ed.), Year Book Medical Publisher, Chicago, 1987.
38. Fisher AA: Contact Dermatitis, 3rd ed., Lea & Febiger, Philadelphia, 1986.
39. Gelboin HV: Benzo(a)pyrene metabolism, activation and carcinogenesis. Role and regulation of mixed function oxidases and related enzymes. Physiol Rev 60:1107, 1980.
40. Gelboin HV, T'so POP (eds.): Polycyclic Hydrocarbons and Cancer, Vols 1 and 2, Academic Press, Orlando, 1978.
41. Goldsmith LA (ed.): Biochemistry and Physiology of the Skin, Oxford University Press, New York, 1983.
42. Haenszel W: Variations in skin cancer incidence within the United States. Natl Cancer Inst Monogr 10:225, 1963.
43. Hanifin JM: Epidemiology of atopic dermatitis. In: Epidemiology of Allergic Diseases, p 116, Schlumberger HD (ed.), Karger, Basel, 1987.
44. Harm W: Biological Effects of Ultraviolet Radiation. Cambridge University Press, Cambridge, 1980.
45. Jeffrey AM, Kinoshita T, Santella RM, et al: The chemistry of polycyclic aromatic hydrocarbons-DNA adducts. In: Carcinogenesis: Fundamental Mechanisms and Environmental Effects, p 565, Pullman B, T'so POP, Gelboin H (eds.), Reidel Publishing, Dordrecht, 1980.
46. Johnston K: First steps in ozone protection agreed. Nature 329:189, 1987.
47. Jones RR: Ozone depletion and cancer risk. Lancet 2:443, 1987.
48. Knishkowy B, Baker EL: Transmission of occupational disease to family contracts. Am J Ind Med 9:543, 1986.
49. Kraemer KH: Xeroderma pigmentosum. In: Clinical Dermatology, p 1, Demis DJ, Dobson R, McGuire J (eds.), Harper & Row, New York, 1981.
50. Kuratsume M, Shapiro RE (eds.): PCB Poisoning in Japan and Taiwan, Alan R Liss, New York, 1984.
51. Lancaster H: Some geographical aspects of the mortality from melanoma in Europeans. Med J Aust 1:1092, 1956.
52. MacKie RM, Rycroft MJ: Health and the ozone layer. Br Med J 297:369, 1988.
53. Maibach HI (ed.): Occupational and Industrial Dermatology, 2nd ed., Year Book Medical Publishers, Chicago, 1987.
54. Maibach HI, Feldmann RJ, Milby TH, et al: Regional variation in percutaneous penetration in man: Pesticides. Arch Environ Health 23:208, 1960.
55. Malkinson FD: Percutaneous absorption of toxic substances in industry. Arch Ind Health 21:87, 1960.
56. Martin-Bouyer G, Toga O, Lebreton R, et al: Outbreak of accidental hexachlorophene poisoning in France. Lancet 1:91, 1982.
57. Marzulli FN, Maibach HI (eds.): Dermatotoxicology, 4th ed., Hemisphere Publishing, New York, 1991.
58. Masuda Y, Kuroki H, Karaguchi K, et al: PCB and PCDF congeners in the blood and tissues of Yusho and Yu-Chen patients. Environ Health Perspect 59:53, 1985.
59. Matheson MS: Formation and detection of intermediates in water radiotypes. Radiat Res 4(Suppl):1, 1964.
60. Mathias CGT: Occupational dermatoses. In: Occupational Medicine, 2nd ed., p 132, Zenz C (ed.), Year Book Medical Publishers, Chicago, 1988.
61. Mathias CGT: Occupational skin diseases, United States. Arch Dermatol 124:1519, 1988.
62. Mathias CGT, Maibach HI: Perspectives in occupational dermatology. West J Med 137:191, 1982.
63. McGovern V, Shaw H, Milton G, et al: Is malignant melanoma arising in a Hutchinson's melanotic freckle a separate disease entity? Histopathology 4:235, 1980.
64. McGregor JF: Enhancement of skin tumorigenesis by cigarette smoke condensate following β-irradiation in rats. J Natl Cancer Inst 68:605, 1982.
65. Mennè T, Christophersen J, Maibach HI: Epidemiology of allergic contact sensitization. In: Epidemiology of Allergic Diseases, p 132, Schlumberger HD (ed.), Karger, Basel, 1987.
66. Miller EC: Some current perspective on chemical carcinogenesis in humans and experimental animals. Cancer Res 38:1479, 1978.
67. National Aeronautics and Space Administration (NASA): Executive Summary of the Ozone Trends Panel, NASA, Washington, 1988.
68. National Research Council: Principles and Procedures for Evaluating the Toxicity of Household Substances, National Academy of Sciences, Washington, 1977.
69. Nichol AW, Collins AG: Porphyria cutanea tarda. In:

Dermatotoxicology, 3rd ed., p 607, Marzulli FN, Maibach HI (eds.), Hemisphere Publishing, Washington, 1987.

70. Noonan PK, Wester RC: Percutaneous absorption of nitroglycerin. J Pharm Sci 69:365, 1980.

71. Noonan PK, Wester RC: Cutaneous biotransformation and some pharmacological and toxicological implications. In: Dermatotoxicology, 3rd ed., p 71, Marzulli FN, Maibach HI (eds.), Hemisphere Publishing, Washington, 1987.

72. Pannatier A, Jenner P, Testa B, et al: The skin as a drug-metabolizing organ. Drug Metab Rev 8:319, 1978.

73. Paul E, Greilich RC, Dominante G: Epidemiology of urticaria. In: Epidemiology of Allergic Diseases, p 87, Schlumberger HD (ed.), Karger, Basel, 1987.

74. Pitot HC: Fundamentals of Oncology, 3rd ed., Marcel Dekker, New York, 1986.

75. Pocchiari F, Silano V, Samplieri A: Human health effects from accidental release of tetrachlorodibenzo-p-dioxin (TCDD) at Seveso, Italy. Proc NY Acad Sci 320:300, 1979.

76. Pohl RJ, Philpot RN, Fouts JR: Cytochrome P-450 content and mixed function oxidase activity in microsomes isolated from mouse skin. Drug Metab Disp 4:442, 1976.

77. Roskos KV, Guy RH, Maibach HI: Percutaneous absorption in the aged. Dermatol Clin 4:455, 1986.

78. Rous P, Kidd JG: Conditional neoplasms and subthreshold neoplastic states. J Exp Med. 73:365, 1941.

79. Rystedt I: Work-related hand eczema in atopics. Contact Derm 12:164, 1985.

80. Safai B, Good RA (eds.): Immunodermatology, Plenum Press, New York, 1981.

81. Scheuplein RJ: Permeability of the skin: A review of major concepts. Curr Prob Dermatol 7:172, 1978.

82. Scheuplein RJ, Blank IH: Permeability of the skin. Physiol Rev 51:702, 1971.

83. Scheuplein RJ, Bronaugh RL: Percutaneous absorption. In: Biochemistry and Physiology of the Skin, p 1255, Goldsmith LA (ed.), Oxford University Press, Oxford, 1983.

84. Schmid R: Cutaneous porphyria in Turkey. N Engl J Med 263:367, 1960.

85. Scotto J, Fraumeni JF Jr: Skin (Other Than Melanoma). In: Cancer Epidemiology and Prevention, p 996, Schottenfeld D, Fraumeni JF Jr (eds.), WB Saunders, Philadelphia, 1982.

86. Scotto J, Fears TR, Fraumeni JF Jr: Solar radiation. In: Cancer Epidemiology and Prevention, p 254, Schottenfeld D, Fraumeni JF Jr (eds.), WB Saunders, Philadelphia, 1982.

87. Shuman RM, Leech RW, Alvord EC Jr: Neurotoxicity of hexachlorophene in humans. II. A clinical pathological study of 46 premature infants. Arch Neurol 32:320, 1975.

88. Taylor JS: Environmental acne: Update and overview. Ann NY Acad Sci 320:295, 1979.

89. Taylor JS: Occupational disease statistics. Arch Dermatol 124:1557, 1988.

90. Teppo L, Pakkanen M, Hakulinen T: Sunlight as a risk factor of malignant melanoma of the skin. Cancer 41:2018, 1978.

91. Tregear RT: Physical Properties of Skin. Academic Press, New York, 1966.

92. United States Occupational Safety and Health Administration: Report of the Advisory Committee on Cutaneous Hazards, NIOSH, Washington, 1978.

93. Urbach F: Geographic pathology of the skin cancer. In: The Biologic Effects of Ultraviolet radiation, p 635, Urbach F (ed.), Oxford University Press, Oxford, 1969.

94. Urbach F, Epstein JH, Forbes PD: Ultraviolet carcinogenesis: Experimental, global and genetic aspects. In: Sunlight and Man: Normal and Abnormal Photobiological Responses, p 259, Fitzpatrick TB, Madhukar A (eds.), University of Tokyo Press, Tokyo, 1974.

95. Vickers CFH: Reservoir effect of human skin: Pharmacological speculation. In: Percutaneous Absorption of Steroids, p 19, Mauvais-Jarvis P, Vickers CFH, Wepierre J (eds.), Academic Press, Orlando, 1980.

96. Weinstein IB, Jeffrey AN, Jennette KW, et al: Benzo-(a)pyrene diol-epoxides as intermediates in nucleic acid binding in vitro and in vivo. Science 193:592, 1976.

97. Wester RC, Maibach HI: Relationship of topical dose and percutaneous absorption in rhesus monkey and man. J Invest Dermatol 67:518, 1976.

98. Wester RC, Maibach HI: Percutaneous absorption relative to occupational dermatology. In: Occupational and Industrial Dermatology, p 241, Maibach HI (ed.), Year Book Medical Publisher, Chicago, 1987.

99. Wester RC, Maibach HI: In Vivo Percutaneous Absorption. In: Dermatotoxicology, 3rd ed., p 135, Marzulli FN, Maibach HI (eds.), Hemisphere Publishing, Washington, 1987.

100. Wester RC, Maibach HI: Percutaneous absorption of organic solvents. In: Occupational and Industrial Dermatology, 2nd ed., p 213, Maibach HI (ed.), Year Book Medical Publisher, Chicago, 1987.

101. Wester RC, Noonan PK: Topical bioavailability of potential anti-acne agent (SC-23110) as determined by cumulative excretion and areas under plasma concentration time curves. J Invest Dermatol 70:92, 1978.

102. Wester RC, Noonan PK, Maibach HI: Variations in percutaneous absorption of testosterone in the rhesus monkey due to anatomic site of application and frequency of application. Arch Dermatol Res 267:229, 1980.

103. Worobec SM, DiBeneditto JP: Perspectives on occupational dermatoses. In: Cutaneous Toxicity, p 253, Drill VA, Lazar P (eds.), Raven Press, New York, 1984.

104. Yeh S: Relative incidence of skin cancer in Chinese in Taiwan with special reference to arsenical cancer. Natl Cancer Inst Monogr 10:81, 1963.

105. Yuspa SH: Cutaneous carcinogenesis: Natural and experimental. In: Biochemistry and Physiology of the Skin, p 1115, Goldsmith LA (ed.), Oxford University Press, New York, 1983.

RECOMMENDED READINGS

Adams RM (ed.): Occupational Skin Disease, 2nd ed, WB Saunders, Philadelphia, 1990.

Fisher AA: Contact Dermatitis, 3rd ed., Lea & Febiger, Philadelphia, 1986.

Maibach HI (ed.): Occupational and Industrial Dermatology, 2nd ed., Year Book Medical Publisher, Chicago, 1987.

16. DISORDERS OF THE LUNGS

Dean Sheppard

INTRODUCTION

The lung has a far greater external surface area (almost 70 m^2) and encounters more of the external environment (about 9000 L of air daily) than any other organ. As a result, the lung is both a common target for environmental disease and an important point of entry for pollutants that cause toxicity to other organs. The significance of adverse effects of air pollution on the lung became apparent in the aftermath of several episodes of severe air pollution that occurred in the middle part of this century. The worst of these episodes occurred in the Meuse Valley, Belgium in 1930, in Donora, Pennsylvania in 1948, and in London, England in 1952. They were all associated with clear-cut acute increases in mortality (90). The excess deaths attributable to air pollution during these episodes were generally clustered among patients with pulmonary diseases. Following the Donora episode there was one report of exacerbation in 88% of asthma patients surveyed (80).

As a result of the recognition that air pollution can cause respiratory mortality as well as morbidity, increasing attention has been focused on the adverse respiratory effects of exposure to pollutants (100). Three methods have been employed to identify the adverse effects of specific constituents of polluted air and to estimate the likelihood that these

effects would occur in people under various conditions of exposure. These methods are epidemiologic studies, controlled acute human exposure studies, and exposure studies in experimental animals. Each method has important strengths and weaknesses.

Methods of Determining the Effect of Pollutant Exposure

Epidemiologic Studies

The major advantage of epidemiologic studies in estimating the adverse effects of pollution on the lung is that they allow investigation of large numbers of people exposed to pollution under real-life conditions (17). Demonstrations of an adverse response in association with air pollution in an epidemiologic study thus provides the strongest evidence that such a response will actually take place under naturally occurring conditions of exposure. Failure to find an adverse effect in epidemiologic studies, however, cannot be taken as definitive evidence that such a response will not occur. The use of epidemiologic studies to search for causative relationships between specific pollutants and specific adverse health effects has been hampered by a number of methodological problems (17).

At the time of the previously described episodes of severe pollution in London in 1952, in the Meuse Valley, Belgium in 1930, and in Donora, Pennsylvania in 1948, only crude methods were available to measure the constituents of polluted air. As a result the adverse effects of these episodes were related to smoke density or sulfate concentrations.

Principles and Practice of Environmental Medicine, edited by Alyce Bezman Tarcher. Plenum Medical Book Company, New York, 1992.

The roles of other pollutants could not be assessed (90). Since air pollution is a complex mixture of many different gases and particulates, the failure to measure individual constituents made meaningful comparisons between air pollution episodes difficult. Recently methods have been developed to measure many of the constituents of polluted air. These measurements have demonstrated that some pollutants are present in significantly higher concentrations in indoor air than in outdoor air (18,94). On this basis, any attempt to relate adverse health effects to the concentrations of pollutants measured outdoors may be hampered by the confounding effects of widely different concentrations of indoor pollutants (94).

Another major limitation of epidemiologic studies for estimating the health effects of a given pollutant is the difficulty in estimating the relevant lung dose of various pollutants actually received by individuals living in a polluted area (17). For instance, most studies attempt to relate observed effects to the average concentration of a pollutant occurring over some period of time—generally longer than one hour and often as long as 1 year. Some of the adverse effects of pollutants, however, are primarily determined by the highest concentration encountered over a very short period of time. Although sulfur dioxide, for example, can cause severe bronchoconstriction in subjects with asthma after 3–5 min of exposure, such short-term peak concentrations of sulfur dioxide may not be reflected in the long-term average concentrations (85,87).

Finally, epidemiologic studies are hampered by the fact that most of the adverse effects potentially caused by air pollution are also commonly attributable to numerous other factors. Tuberculosis, for example, does not occur in the absence of the causative organism; but exacerbations of asthma, recurrent upper respiratory infections and even lung cancer clearly occur quite commonly in the absence of air pollution.

Human Exposure Studies

Controlled human exposure studies provide the opportunity to quantify the effects of various doses of a single pollutant or pollutant mix on pulmonary function. This is accomplished in the absence of many of the confounding factors present in the general environment. By the appropriate selection of subjects, segments of the population predicted to be at increased risk for adverse effects can be studied, and a range of exposure conditions (e.g., rest, vigorous exercise, oral breathing, and nasal breathing) can be examined. Although these studies are ideally suited for studying acute effects of pollutants, they cannot be easily applied to investigate chronic effects.

Exposure Studies in Experimental Animals

Exposure studies in experimental animals provide the opportunity to determine the mechanisms of acute and chronic response to constituents of polluted air. A broader range of pollutant concentrations can be employed than would be acceptable in human studies. In addition, the effects of exposure to high pollutant concentrations can be identified. Such exposure would ordinarily occur only rarely or over long intervals at lower exposure concentrations. The major limitation of animal studies predicting human dose-response relationships is the large variation in response to exposure between species. For example, dogs, a species commonly used for studying effects of pollutants, can often tolerate more than 200 ppm of sulfur dioxide without developing significant bronchoconstriction. People with asthma can develop marked bronchoconstriction from inhaling 0.5 ppm or less (8,9, 50,87,88).

The chapter now focuses on agents that adversely affect the lung and then proceeds with a discussion of epidemiology and pathological physiology. It concludes with a presentation of the clinical implications of pollutant exposure on the lung.

ENVIRONMENTAL CHEMICALS ASSOCIATED WITH ADVERSE EFFECTS ON THE LUNG

The overwhelming majority of environmental chemicals that potentially injure the lung are encountered by inhalation of polluted air. The few exceptions, such as the herbicide paraquat, which causes lung injury after absorption through the gastrointestinal tract, is not discussed in this section. As noted in Chapter 2, the constituents of polluted indoor air are somewhat different from those of polluted outdoor air, though some pollutants such as nitrogen dioxide and carbon monoxide are commonly found in both locations. Many pollutants may be found in higher concentrations in indoor air than outdoor air (18,34,94) (see Chapter 2). A list of some of the commonly encountered pollutants associated with adverse pulmonary effects is presented in Table 16-1 (11).

Sulfur oxides, ozone, and nitrogen dioxide are the three most widely encountered pollutants that cause well-documented adverse pulmonary effects. Sulfur dioxide, one of the major pollutants, is produced by the combustion of such sulfur-containing fossil fuels as coal and oil. The major sources of environmental pollution with sulfur dioxide are power plants and oil refineries. Until recently indoor concentrations have generally been lower than outdoor concentrations. Kerosene space heaters, however, have introduced a new source of sulfur dioxide

TABLE 16-1. Major Pollutants Associated with Adverse Pulmonary Effects[a]

Pollutant	Outdoor sources	Indoor sources	Adverse effects
Sulfur oxides	Power plants, oil refineries, smelters	Kerosene space heaters	Bronchoconstriction
Oxides of nitrogen	Automobile exhaust, power plants, oil refineries	Gas stoves and furnaces, kerosene space heaters	Airway injury, impaired lung defenses (pulmonary edema, bronchiolitis)
Ozone	Automobile exhaust	Aircraft cabins, electrical appliances, ozone generators	Airway injury, impaired lung defenses (pulmonary edema, bronchiolitis)
Polycyclic hydrocarbons	Diesel exhaust	Cigarette smoke	Lung cancer
Asbestos	Asbestos-processing plants	Insulation, building materials, workers' clothing	Mesothelioma (lung cancer, pulmonary fibrosis)
Ionizing radiation	—	Building materials	Lung cancer
Arsenic	Smelters	Cigarette smoke	Lung cancer
Allergens	Pollen	Animal dander, house dust mites	Exacerbations of asthma

[a]From Boushey and Sheppard (11).

in indoor air. Since commercially available kerosene contains varying amounts of sulfur, the use of kerosene heaters can, under some operating conditions, produce indoor atmospheres containing up to 5 ppm sulfur dioxide. This is more than 30 times higher than the present primary air quality standard of 0.14 ppm (72,94).

Sulfur dioxide is also widely used and produced in industry, particularly in smelters, paper pulp mills, and wineries. These industrial sources can lead to the exposure of workers and of neighboring residential areas. Once released into the atmosphere, sulfur dioxide combines with other pollutants to form a variety of particulate aerosols. These will vary from place to place in particle size distribution and chemical species. Nearly all of the particles that remain suspended in air are less than 10 μm in diameter, with the numerical majority in the submicrometer fractions. Commonly encountered sulfur-containing compounds, in addition to sulfur dioxide, include sulfuric acid, sulfites, and various metallic, acidic, and ammonium sulfates.

The instruments generally used to monitor these pollutants do not separate such particles by specific particle size or chemical composition. They give information only about SO_2, total suspended particulates, and sometimes total suspended sulfates. Since sulfur dioxide is a highly water-soluble gas, it is primarily deposited and absorbed from the upper airways. Very little inhaled SO_2 reaches the distal regions of the lung (33). This is in contrast to inhaled sulfate particles. The major sites of deposition of such inhaled particles are determined by their size. Thus, submicrometer aerosols may be deposited primarily in the lung periphery.

Ozone, another important cause of adverse effects on the lung, is predominantly an outdoor pollutant. It is produced from a complex interaction between emissions of volatile organic compounds and nitrogen oxides in the presence of sunlight. Ozone is encountered in high concentrations in areas with large numbers of automobiles and frequent sunlight, such as the Los Angeles basin. Ozone is also found as an indoor pollutant in the cabins of high-altitude commercial aircraft, especially during trans-Pacific flights, which pass through a low-lying section of the ozone layer in the earth's atmosphere (6). Since ozone is considerably less soluble in water than is sulfur dioxide, a high percentage of inhaled ozone reaches peripheral regions of the lung. As a result, ozone can cause lung injury at any point from the upper airways to the alveoli (29,35,49,58).

Nitrogen dioxide is an oxidation product of nitric oxide. Nitric oxide is in turn produced by fixation of atmospheric nitrogen with oxygen under conditions of high-temperature combustion. Nitrogen dioxide is thus an important byproduct of all high-temperature combustion. Outdoors it emanates from power plants and automobile exhaust. Indoors it comes from the combustion of natural gas (or kerosene) in home heaters and stoves. Indoor concentrations can be many times higher than outdoor concentrations. Peak hourly concentrations between 200 and 700 mg/m³ have been measured in kitchens and other rooms of homes during conventional gas cooking (94). (The National Ambient Air Quality Standard is 100 mg/m³.) Because nitrogen dioxide is relatively insoluble in water, it can have effects in any region of the lung.

In outdoor air another major group of pollutants of concern are carcinogens (91). These include arsenic, which is generally present in the vicinity of smelters, and polycyclic hydrocarbons, which are emitted from diesel engines and petroleum refineries. Since these carcinogens are also present in tobacco smoke, they can be found in considerably higher concentrations in indoor than in outdoor air (94). Indoor air also contains radon daughters released from construction materials and soil below and around buildings, formaldehyde released from synthetic fabrics, cigarette smoke, urea-formaldehyde foam insulation, and such building materials as plywood and particle board (21,73). Indoor air may also contain asbestos, which can be found in ceiling and floor tiles, in sprayed-on insulation, and on the outside and inside of boilers and heating ducts (19). All of these pollutants, except formaldehyde, have been shown to increase the risk for lung cancer in workers exposed to high concentrations (108). Formaldehyde has been shown to be a carcinogen in animal studies. Much attention is directed to investigating the contribution of formaldehyde exposure to respiratory and other forms of cancer in humans (48,67).

None of the aforementioned carcinogens, except tobacco smoke, has been shown to cause lung cancer in concentrations that may be found in indoor or outdoor air. Large epidemiologic studies in Japan demonstrated a significantly greater incidence of lung cancer in nonsmoking spouses of smokers than in nonsmoking spouses of nonsmokers (43,44). These results, along with numerous other studies showing an increased risk of lung cancer among nonsmokers exposed to environmental tobacco smoke, support the conclusion that involuntary smoke inhalation is a cause of lung cancer (20,43,44,99).

Reports indicate that other indoor air pollutants increase the risk for lung cancer. Household exposure to asbestos has been associated with the development of mesothelioma in family members of asbestos workers, who presumably brought home asbestos fibers on their workclothes (5,103). A report from China reveals that lung cancer mortality is among the highest in Xuan Wei County, Yunnan Province. Lung cancer, found especially in women, was more closely associated with indoor burning of "smoky" coal than with tobacco smoking (65).

Several materials present in polluted air have been shown to produce adverse effects on the lung, but generally at concentrations considerably higher than those found in ambient air. Most notable among these is formaldehyde, which can be an important component of indoor air (21). Formaldehyde can cause eye, nose, and throat irritation at concentrations below the highest level recorded inside residences (0.1–2.4 ppm) (21,106). High concentrations of formaldehyde have been recorded in mobile homes.

The lung is also an important point of entry for pollutants that cause adverse effects on other organs and may also affect the lung (60,71). The effects of these pollutants, which include lead, carbon monoxide, nitrosamines, polyaromatic hydrocarbons, pesticides, and volatile organics (e.g., toluene, xylene, benzene, chloroform, gasoline) are discussed in Part V.

EPIDEMIOLOGY

Epidemiology studies have identified four major types of adverse pulmonary effects that can be attributed to ambient air pollution. These are increases in respiratory mortality, exacerbations of asthma, an increased incidence of acute respiratory illnesses, and increased disability in patients with chronic obstructive lung disease. Several other possible effects, including an increased incidence of lung cancer and an increased prevalence of asthma, have been suggested but not proven.

Mortality

A clear-cut acute increase in mortality was noted in association with several episodes of urban air pollution that resulted from the combined effects of uncontrolled industrial effluents and several days of severe air stagnation. During the worst of these episodes, the London fog of 1952, excess deaths were observed on the first day and continued for several weeks (59). The total excess number of deaths attributable to pollution (above the number expected for the same time period) was 4000. These deaths, occurring primarily among patients with preexisting heart and lung disease and persons over 45 years of age, were mainly from bronchitis, pneumonia, and other acute respiratory and cardiac disorders (59). Precise measurements of the concentrations of specific pollutants are not available from these episodes. Acute increases in mortality from pollution have not recurred in these locations since control measures were instituted. These measures were designed primarily to reduce ground-level concentrations of sulfur dioxide and of total suspended particulates.

The episodes of acute increases in mortality have led several investigators to examine the relationship between air pollution of lesser magnitude and variations in mortality. Overall, these studies have suggested a positive association between pollution and daily mortality (55,94,112). It has not been possible to define a relationship between a given pollutant concentration and an expected number of deaths because other forces such as influenza epidemics, temperature extremes, and holiday weekend accidents also have strong effects on variation in daily mortality.

Exacerbations of Asthma

Extreme sensitivity of the airways to a wide variety of exogenous stimuli is a characteristic feature of asthma. It is therefore not surprising that patients with asthma constitute a segment of the population that is at particularly high risk for the adverse effects of environmental pollution. Since asthma is a common disease, affecting 3–8% of the U.S. population, the effects of air pollution on this group contribute significantly to the respiratory morbidity attributable to environmental factors (27). Several studies have reported an increase in symptomatic exacerbations of asthma and/or an increase in clinic or emergency room visits by patients with asthma in association with increases in air pollution (15,90,109,111).

In addition to the adverse effects of urban air pollution from industrial effluents, "environmental asthma" occasionally results from residential exposure to specific point-source emissions. Rural residents living near grain elevators may develop symptomatic asthma from exposure to grain dust. Residents near a castor bean plant have been reported to develop asthma attacks from exposure to bean dust effluents (23). Patients with asthma have been reported to develop bronchoconstriction from the inhalation of tobacco smoke, allergens, and other components of indoor air (2,12,76). It is therefore possible that some energy conservation measures that decrease indoor ventilation exacerbate asthma.

Acute Respiratory Illness

Several epidemiologic studies have noted an increased incidence of acute respiratory illnesses associated with increases in air pollution (3,28,30, 56,105,107). Since many of these studies have been based on questionnaire responses from residents and physicians in polluted areas, the precise etiological agents responsible for these respiratory illnesses generally have not been defined. It appears likely, however, that air pollution can increase the incidence of both viral upper respiratory infections and pneumonia. There is evidence suggesting that several different patterns of air pollution can lead to increased acute respiratory illnesses. The pulmonary effects of locally released toxic air pollutants have received scant attention except for the disastrous industrial leak of methyl isocyanate in Bhopal, India in 1984 (61).

The pollutant mix that results from the combustion of sulfur-containing fossil fuels, and which predominates in urban areas of the eastern and midwestern United States, is composed primarily of sulfur oxides, suspended particles, and oxides of nitrogen. Studies from several cities in these regions have shown an association between the intensity of air pollution and the incidence of upper respiratory infections and pneumonia (3,28,56). This suggests that sulfates, particulates, and/or oxides of nitrogen, either alone or in combination, contribute to the development of such infections. They do so, presumably, by impairing local host defense mechanisms (3,28,102). Other studies from the Los Angeles basin, where high concentrations of ozone are produced as a result of heavy use of automobiles in a sunny climate, have demonstrated a similar association between ozone concentrations and acute respiratory illnesses (30,105).

Clinical studies have investigated the effects of ozone in ambient air on respiratory function in children (42,93). Respiratory function was measured over a 4-week period on a daily basis in 91 children in a summer camp in northwestern New Jersey. After 2 weeks, spirometric indices decreased in one-third of the children. It was not possible to demonstrate the specific effects of other environmental factors, which included heat stress and acid aerosol concentration, on the ozone-associated response. The ozone levels during the study never exceeded the current federal ambient air standard of 0.12 ppm (93). An additional study of the effects of ambient ozone on respiratory function was performed on 43 children attending a summer camp in the San Bernardino mountains in California. This study also revealed that lung function changed in a negative fashion in relation to ambient ozone levels. These changes were reversed as ambient ozone decreased (42). The effects of ozone exposure on respiratory function have been reviewed (47,58).

Chronic Lung Disease

Studies conducted in various cities around the world have suggested an association between the prevalence of chronic respiratory symptoms (e.g., cough, sputum production, shortness of breath) and combined sulfate and particulate pollution (52,64,110). One such study of nearly 10,000 British adults found that cigarette smokers have a higher rate of cough, phlegm, and chronic bronchitis than do nonsmokers. The difference between smokers and nonsmokers increased with increasing pollution, suggesting that there was synergism between the effects of pollution and cigarette smoking. The study also found significant differences in symptoms between residents of urban and rural areas, differences that could not be explained by cigarette smoking alone (52). Prevalence rates for these respiratory symptoms increased with increasing air pollution, independently of cigarette smoking. A significant weakness in this study was the failure to consider the effects of occupation or social class. Industrial workers, for example, are more likely to have a greater occupational exposure to pollutants and to live in areas of high air pollution than are professionals. It is therefore difficult to be certain that the observed effects were not caused in part by exposure to higher concentrations of pollutants in the workplace. Thus, methodological problems, especially the problem of eliminating the effects of cigarette smoking and occupational exposure, make it difficult to determine either the importance of air pollution to the overall incidence of chronic bronchitis or the concentrations of pollutants required to produce this effect.

Several studies have demonstrated an association between increased symptoms or disability in patients with preexisting chronic obstructive lung disease and ambient levels of pollution. This is especially the case when there are relatively high concentrations of sulfates and particulates (72,110). In Britain, where there have been improvements in air quality over the past 25 years, the relationship between daily fluctuations in air pollution and exacerbations of chronic obstructive lung disease is no longer apparent (90,109).

Indoor Air Pollution

Epidemiologic research on the health effects of indoor air pollution has increased steadily in recent years (2,76,77,99). Some epidemiologic studies have investigated the carcinogenic effects of passive exposure to tobacco smoke, and others have examined the effects of exposure to such common indoor contaminants as combustion products, formaldehyde and other aldehydes, volatile organic compounds, and radon (7,10,17,22,28,34,46,63,68,73, 76,77). Research in this area was prompted by the concern that energy-saving measures that result in reduced ventilation could increase pollutant levels and thereby adversely affect health. Some of the commonly encountered indoor air pollutants associated with adverse pulmonary effects are found in Table 16-1.

Some studies report a higher incidence of acute respiratory illnesses among children living in homes with gas stoves, but other studies do not confirm these effects (62,63,68,92,100). It is noteworthy, however, that the nitrogen dioxide concentrations can be up to seven times higher in homes using gas stoves than in those using electric stoves (92). Although the respiratory effects of residential exposure to NO_2 appear to be small, it has become increasingly evident that passive exposure to tobacco smoke imposes a significant hazard to the respiratory tract, especially for the young (13,14,31, 76,98,100). Young children passively exposed to cigarette smoke show a higher incidence of acute respiratory illnesses. Their frequency increases with the amount of parental smoking, particularly in the

mother (16,96). The link between involuntary smoking and the incidence of respiratory illness is evident primarily during the first 1–2 years of life (70,96). Respiratory symptoms, particularly wheezing, appear more often in the children of smokers than of nonsmokers (107). Longitudinal studies of children whose parents smoke reveal that the rate of increase in FEV_1 during their growth is less than expected (16,96).

Host Factors

On the basis of the epidemiologic studies discussed above, it is possible to identify a number of host factors that are associated with an increased risk of suffering the adverse respiratory effects of air pollution. Clearly, patients with asthma and chronic obstructive lung disease are at increased risk. Such patients may develop increased symptoms, disability, and—in extreme cases—death as a result of pollutant exposure. Older individuals, perhaps because of their increased baseline susceptibility to respiratory infections, also constitute a high-risk group. Children, too, may be at increased risk of developing acute respiratory illnesses from outdoor and indoor air pollution (15,62,63,79,90, 92,101,104,107). Passive smoking poses a particular risk for children below the age of 2 years. The children of smokers have an increased incidence of acute respiratory illnesses, chronic cough, and phlegm (16,70,96,99,107).

Although there are, as yet, no supporting data, it is possible that other groups are also at increased risk of experiencing the adverse respiratory effects of air pollution. One such group includes immunocompromised patients who have increased susceptibility to respiratory infections. Once respiratory infections are established in such patients, their morbidity and mortality rates are sharply increased. Patients with abnormalities in local pulmonary defense mechanisms compose another group at risk for sustaining adverse respiratory effects of pollutant exposure. This includes individuals with α_1-antitrypsin deficiency. Such individuals are certainly at risk from the effects of the high concentrations of pollutants present in mainstream cigarette smoke; they might also be at increased risk from cigarette smoke found in indoor air. Finally, patients with a deficiency of such vitamins as C and E, which play a role in antioxidant defense, might suffer the adverse effects of oxidant pollutants.

PATHOLOGY AND PATHOLOGICAL PHYSIOLOGY

The lung has a limited number of possible responses to injury. Most patterns of pulmonary pathology can therefore be produced by many dissimilar initial insults. One such insult is exposure to environmental pollutants (11,36,45,54,90). It is possible to produce airway disease, interstitial fibrosis, pulmonary edema, lung cancer, or increased susceptibility to pulmonary infections in experimental animals by exposing them to various environmental pollutants. Although extrapolating the results of animal experiments to predict a dose-response relationship between a pollutant and an adverse effect in people is fraught with difficulties, much important information can be obtained from animal experimentation. First, it is possible to identify the specific adverse responses most likely to occur from exposure to a specific pollutant at several different intensities of exposure. By illustration, exposure to low concentrations of sulfur dioxide can cause an increase in mucus secretion or bronchoconstriction, whereas exposure to high concentrations can cause fatal pulmonary edema. Second, by performing studies in several different species, investigators increase the power of such experiments to predict effects in humans. Third, by studying a group of animals under well-controlled conditions over long periods of time, it may be possible to identify effects of a given pollutant that would be impossible to identify under the complex and continually changing conditions of natural exposure.

In the following sections, the most common patterns of environmentally induced lung injury are discussed. The discussion is based on human and animal studies in which toxic agents have clearly been shown to be injurious to the lung.

Airway Dysfunction

The airways are the point of entry of environmental agents into the lung. They are also the major site of deposition of water-soluble gases and many inhaled particles. It is therefore not surprising that the airways are a common site of environmentally induced injury. The airways respond to injury in two ways: first, by contraction of airway smooth muscle (bronchoconstriction), and second, by alterations in mucus secretion. Both of these responses can be elicited in experimental animals and in human subjects by inhalation of environmental pollutants.

There are two distinctly different mechanisms by which environmental pollutants can lead to bronchoconstriction. The first mechanism involves activation of airway smooth muscle contraction without histological evidence of airway injury or inflammation. The second mechanism involves a local inflammatory response that is the result of direct injury to the airway epithelium (82,84).

The first mechanism is best exemplified by the effects of sulfur dioxide. Inhaling sulfur dioxide in concentrations as low as 0.1 ppm can cause bronchoconstriction in human subjects with asthma (87). This is in contrast to the concentrations of 100 ppm or more that may be required to cause histological evidence of airway injury in experimental animals (87,88). The precise mechanism by which sulfur dioxide ultimately leads to smooth muscle contraction is presently under investigation. It appears, however, that more than one mechanism is involved. Activation of the vagus nerve is clearly important. Cutting or cooling the vagus nerves in cats abolishes the bronchoconstriction produced by high concentrations of sulfur dioxide (>10 ppm). If the vagus nerve is intact, as when a laryngeal pouch is anatomically separated from the lower airway, instillation of sulfur dioxide produces bronchoconstriction (66). The bronchoconstriction caused by inhalation of low concentrations of sulfur dioxide (<2 ppm) in subjects with asthma is partially, but not entirely, a result of a vagal reflex. This is supported by the observation that bronchoconstriction can be partially inhibited by prior administration of muscarinic antagonist drugs (85,97). The bronchoconstriction associated with exposure to low concentrations of sulfur dioxide may also involve the nonimmunologic release of mediators from airway mast cells. It can be inhibited by treatment with disodium cromoglycate, a drug thought to work by inhibition of mast cell activation (86).

Other sulfur-containing pollutants, notably sulfuric acid, are also capable of activating airway smooth muscle contraction at concentrations far lower than those that produce histological abnormalities. The ability to induce bronchoconstriction, however, does not appear to be merely a function of the "irritating" nature of specific pollutants. Some pollutants such as formaldehyde, although irritating, cause little or no bronchoconstriction (89). Sulfur dioxide, in concentrations as low as 0.1 ppm, produces bronchoconstriction, even though at this dose there is very little evidence of irritation (87).

Direct injury to the airway epithelium, producing an inflammatory response, is the second mechanism by which environmental pollutants can lead to bronchoconstriction. Although airway injury that induces a local inflammatory response may cause little if any immediate bronchoconstriction, it can lead to a dramatic increase in the bronchoconstrictor response to such agents as histamine or cholinergic agonists. This pattern of exaggerated bronchoconstrictor response, called airway hyperresponsiveness, is a central feature of asthma.

Ozone is an example of the pollutants that can cause this type of airway response (45,84). Unlike sulfur dioxide, ozone in concentrations close to that encountered in ambient air causes disruption of airway epithelial cells and recruitment of inflammatory cells to the airway epithelium (29,49). Although the inhalation of ozone in concentrations of 0.4–2.0 ppm may not in itself produce bronchoconstriction, it does enhance the bronchoconstriction produced by histamine and by cholinergic agonists. This effect has been observed in humans and in animals (37,45,54). In dogs, this response has been shown to be caused by recruitment of neutrophils to the epithelium. It does not occur in the absence of neutrophil recruitment and can be abolished by depleting the animals of neutrophils before ozone exposure (45). The gradient of neutrophil concentrations across the airway wall (highest in the epithelium, lowest in the lamina propria) suggests that this recruitment results from ozone-induced release of a chemotactic factor from airway epithelial cells (45).

Nitrogen dioxide is the other important air pollutant that can induce airway injury and airway hyperresponsiveness in concentrations close to those encountered in polluted air (4,69).

The effects of air pollutants on mucus secretion have been more difficult to study than the effects on smooth muscle contraction. Various pollutants have been shown to increase or decrease mucociliary clearance both in people and in animals (25). Clearance, the process by which foreign particles are removed from the airway surface, is affected by ciliary beating, airway caliber, and mucus secretion. Relatively high concentrations of sulfur dioxide (>25 ppm) have been shown to increase acutely the output from individual submucosal glands in dogs (H. L. Hahn, personal communication). The chronic administration of even higher concentrations (200–500 ppm) has led to hypertrophy of submucosal glands (as occurs in chronic bronchitis) in the same species (78). The relationship of these findings to possible effects of exposure to the much lower concentrations (generally < 0.5 ppm) that occur in polluted urban air is unclear.

Impairment of Lung Defense Mechanisms

Exposure to air pollutants at concentrations close to those encountered in urban air has been shown to increase susceptibility to a variety of respiratory infections in a number of species (35). These findings are of special interest in light of the epidemiologic evidence (discussed earlier) that air pollution increases the frequency of acute respiratory illnesses, and that pneumonia was an important cause of death during the severe episodes of air pollution.

Susceptibility to infections is commonly studied by inoculating experimental animals with a specific concentration of organisms of known virulence either before, during, or after exposure to clean air or to the pollutant under investigation. Using this method, investigators have demonstrated increased mortality rates from respiratory infections in animals exposed to nitrogen dioxide, ozone, sulfate aerosols, and heavy metals such as cadmium, nickel, and manganese. The observed effects are particularly important with regard to ozone and nitrogen dioxide. These agents, in concentrations less than those observed in polluted air, have been shown repeatedly to increase susceptibility to infection (35,90). Although the causes of impaired defense against pulmonary infections have not been definitively established, one mechanism may be the inhibition of alveolar macrophage function. Such inhibition has been demonstrated after exposure to both ozone and nitrogen dioxide (35,90).

Interstitial Fibrosis

Inhalation of a variety of inorganic dusts, most notably asbestos and free silica, can cause interstitial pulmonary fibrosis. The mechanism by which these dusts produce lung injury appears to involve the activation of alveolar macrophages with or without the subsequent recruitment of neutrophils to the interstitium and air spaces (24,26). These activated macrophages (and neutrophils) release oxygen-derived free radicals and protelytic enzymes, leading to tissue injury and collagen production (24,26). In addition, products released by these inflammatory cells, and perhaps chemical components of the dusts themselves, may also directly stimulate increased collagen production (24, 26). Although the development of interstitial fibrosis generally requires long-term high-dose exposure to the offending dust, there is clearly marked variability among individuals in susceptibility to this effect. It is therefore impossible to determine a "no-effect" dose with certainty. Asbestos, in particular, being extremely inert, persists in the lung for many years after inhalation; it can continue to induce an inflammatory response for many years after exposure ceases. Therefore, the calculated dose of asbestos to any individual must take into account the individual's calculated life expectancy as well as the number of fibers inhaled (5,19). Interstitial fibrosis from inhaled asbestos is generally thought of as an occupational disease; whether it can result from nonoccupational exposure that occurs when asbestos-laden dust is carried home on work clothing is unknown. Whether asbestos-induced fibrosis can result from the chronic low-dose exposure encountered in buildings with asbestos insulation is as yet unknown.

Pulmonary Edema and Bronchiolitis Obliterans

High concentrations of several pollutants have been found to produce injury to the epithelium lining the alveoli or to the terminal and respiratory bronchioles in humans and in animals (78). The likelihood that a particular pollutant will cause such injury is determined by its ability to injure cells and by its solubility in water. Since the oropharynx, nasopharynx, and tracheobronchial tree are lined by an aqueous layer, gases with high water solubility, such as sulfur dioxide or ammonia, dissolve in this lining layer. The distal regions of the lung are reached only when these gases are present at extremely high initial concentrations. Gases such as ozone or nitrogen dioxide, which are less water soluble, are much more likely to get to the smallest bronchioles and alveoli. Pollutant gases with relatively low water solubility are generally not present in sufficient concentrations in polluted air to cause injury to the bronchioles and alveoli. Bystanders or workers exposed to toxic spills or industrial accidents have evidenced alveolar and terminal airway injury after inhalation of chlorine, ammonia, nitrogen dioxide, or ozone (95).

The pathology of alveolar injury involves damage to type I alveolar cells and capillary endothelial cells. Such injury results in increased alveolar endothelial and epithelial permeability and alveolar flooding with protein-rich fluid. This type of pulmonary edema is indistinguishable from other forms of the adult respiratory distress syndrome. Patients who can be supported through the initial episode of pulmonary edema usually recover completely and regain normal pulmonary function. Terminal airway injury, on the other hand, can initiate a continuous inflammatory response that leads to fibrosis and complete obliteration of peripheral airways (called bronchiolitis obliterans). This lesion, associated with irreversible airflow obstruction on pulmonary function testing, can cause progressive respiratory failure and death (32).

Neoplasms

Certain environmental pollutants have been shown to act as carcinogens both in experimental animals and in heavily exposed people. Since the lung filters particles and gases out of inhaled air, these carcinogens can be concentrated in the respiratory tract and, as in the case of asbestos, may remain there for many years.

In heavily exposed workers, inhaled carcinogens have been shown to increase the incidence of all cell types of carcinoma of the lung. Whereas some agents appear to cause only a single type of tumor (e.g., chloromethyl ether causes primarily small-cell carcinoma), other agents (e.g., asbestos) appear to increase the incidence of all major cell types (Table 16-2).

Mesothelioma is a rare tumor, usually associated with exposure to asbestos (1). Along with lung cancer and pulmonary fibrosis, asbestos causes mesothelioma in a dose-dependent fashion. Mesothelioma may occur after exposure to doses lower than those required to produce the other pulmonary complications. The fact that wives and children of asbestos insulation workers have developed mesothelioma suggests that high-dose nonoccupational exposure can lead to the development of mesothelioma (5,103).

Ambient air contains a number of known carcinogens. Polycyclic aromatic hydrocarbons are present in low concentrations, and agents such as arsenic and vinyl chloride are concentrated near point sources of pollution. Although some studies have reported an association between air pollution and the geographic distribution of lung cancer, this association has been weak and inconsistent and could be explained by such factors as cigarette smoking or occupational exposure (90).

Indoor air can also contain such known carcinogens as radon daughters, asbestos fibers, formaldehyde, and cigarette smoke. Radon enters indoor air from soil adjacent to buildings, from the water supply, and from building materials. A colorless, odorless, radioactive gas, it is a decay product of uranium that is present in the earth's crust (73). Since the radioactivity of soil and rock vary greatly, the radon concentration in indoor air can vary by several orders of magnitude. The increased incidence of lung cancer observed in uranium miners is the basis of the concern about exposure to radon in indoor air (73). Exposure to α radiation from radon decay products is one of the best-documented hazards from ionizing radiation. The indoor levels of radon are manyfold lower than those encountered in an occupational setting. However, there is wide agree-

TABLE 16-2.   Potential Environmental Lung Carcinogens

Agent	Source of exposure	Cell type
Ionizing radiation	Building materials	Oat cell
Asbestos	Insulation, floor and ceiling tiles, work clothes (indoors)	All
Polycyclic hydrocarbons	Sidestream smoke (indoors)	All
Metals (nickel, arsenic, chromium, cadmium)	Near point-source emissions (outdoors)	?

ment that risk is proportional to the exposure. The greater the exposure to radon, the higher is the risk for lung cancer. Although there are no studies that link radon contamination indoors to lung cancer, this problem represents an important public health issue (39,74). Scientific uncertainty exists, however, in assessing the risk associated with exposure to indoor radon (75).

Asbestos fibers can invade indoor air from adjacent milling or mining operations and from asbestos insulation used around or inside heating ducts, furnaces, and water pipes. Other important sources include asbestos-containing floor and ceiling tiles, especially when these materials deteriorate or are being replaced during building renovations. Whether the low concentrations of asbestos that are present in some indoor air conditioners will increase the incidence of lung cancer remains to be seen (19).

As previously mentioned, the evidence of an increased incidence of lung cancer in some populations exposed to environmental tobacco smoke supports the conclusion that involuntary smoking is a cause of lung cancer (20,43,44).

All known lung carcinogens exhibit a long latency period between the onset of exposure and the development of visible tumors. Although this latency period may be somewhat shorter in the case of extremely high-dose exposure, tumors rarely develop in less than 15 years from the onset of exposure to the carcinogenic agent. As a result, identification of an association between exposure to a particular agent and human lung cancer cannot be made until the agent has been present in the environment for a number of years. The most important lung carcinogen by far is cigarette smoke, which plays a role in the production of approximately 90% of all lung cancers. This fact tends to obscure the role of other agents, which may have additive or synergistic effects with cigarette smoke (45,60,67, 71,91).

CLINICAL ASPECTS OF POLLUTANT EXPOSURE ON THE LUNGS

Obviously the most effective way to deal with the adverse effects of pollutants on the lung is first to identify the responsible agents and then to decrease their concentrations in the environment. This goal is best accomplished by governmental regulation, judicial action, and public education. The diagnosis and treatment of individual patients with environmentally induced pulmonary disorders represent small parts of the response to this problem, but ones that are the unique responsibility of health practitioners. Recognizing a possible association between a patient's disorder and an environmental exposure serves two important functions. First, it allows the practitioner to incorporate envi-

ronmental control measures into patient management. Second, it may provide the data base for identifying as-yet-undocumented adverse effects of pollutants on the lung.

Asthma

Pollutants can have two distinct effects on asthma. First, patients with preexisting asthma may frequently develop symptomatic exacerbations from exposure to environmental agents such as air pollutants (82). Second, previously healthy individuals may develop asthma from pollutant exposure.

Exacerbation of Preexisting Asthma

Sulfur dioxide, in concentrations that are sometimes greater than in polluted outdoor air (>0.25 ppm), is a potent stimulus to bronchoconstriction in subjects with asthma (87). This gas is found in highest concentrations (occasionally exceeding 2 ppm) in close proximity to such point sources of emission as coal- and oil-fired power plants, oil refineries, and smelters. Even higher concentrations (up to 5 ppm) can be produced indoors by the use of high-sulfur kerosene in kerosene space heaters (53).

Several factors have been shown to increase an individual patient's risk of developing sulfur-dioxide-induced bronchoconstriction. The first is the patient's degree of underlying airway responsiveness. Subjects with asthma who uniformly have increased airway responsiveness have been shown to be extremely sensitive to the bronchoconstrictive effects of sulfur dioxide (51,57,83,85). The second important factor is an individual's minute ventilation during exposure.

The magnitude of bronchoconstriction increases as ventilation is increased during exercise and voluntary hyperpnea (9,87). This effect results not merely from the increased amount of sulfur dioxide inhaled through the mouth during hyperpnea but also from the increased percentage of inhaled gas that bypasses the upper airway scrubbing mechanisms during conditions of rapid air flow (33). On this basis sulfur dioxide, in concentrations (0.5 ppm) that generally have no effect on lung function when inhaled at rest, will often cause severe symptomatic bronchoconstriction when inhaled during moderate or heavy exercise. As might be expected, exercising subjects with even mild asthma are much more sensitive. These subjects routinely develop asthma when inhaling levels of sulfur dioxide of 0.4 ppm and higher, and this effect occurs with exposures as brief as 2 min (84). Noteworthy is the fact that sulfur dioxide concentrations at or above 0.4 ppm can be found near point sources of sulfur dioxide emissions and in homes heated with kerosene space heaters (83).

The third factor is the oronasal distribution of ventilation. Since sulfur dioxide is a highly water-soluble gas, its dispersion in the airway is heavily dependent on the mode of breathing. During nasal breathing most of it is taken up by the moist nasal mucosa. During oral breathing considerably more sulfur dioxide reaches the lungs (33). Conditions such as exercise and nasal obstruction, which are associated with oral breathing, tend to increase the magnitude of sulfur-dioxide-induced bronchoconstriction (38).

Finally, the temperature and humidity of inspired air are important factors. Sulfur dioxide causes considerably more bronchoconstriction when inhaled in cold or dry air than when inhaled in warm, humid air (8,88). It is possible to gauge roughly the effects of a given concentration of sulfur dioxide in a given individual on the basis of his or her degree of airway responsiveness, activity during exposure, degree of nasal patency, and the ambient temperature and humidity.

A number of other environmental agents can cause bronchoconstriction either by direct or by immunologic mechanisms. Animal dander and house dust mites are important components of indoor air that can cause bronchoconstriction by immunologic mechanisms. As with other indoor pollutants, concentrations of these materials may increase as air turnover rates are decreased. Recognition of these pollutants as potential causes of exacerbations of asthma is important, since specific control measures may lead to dramatic clinical improvement.

Medical History In all patients with asthma, attention to possible environmental causes of exacerbations is an essential part of the medical history. Determining the pollutant exposure of patients with asthma is important for two reasons. The first is the well-established relationship between exposure and bronchoconstriction. The second is that the most commonly identified cause of exacerbation of asthma, namely a recent upper respiratory infection, may be affected by environmental pollutants.

Since the workplace is the most common site of intense exposure to chemical agents, particular attention should be paid to the patient's occupation and its specific exposures. Information should also be obtained about the location of the patient's home, particularly in relation to nearby point sources of sulfur dioxide or other industrial emissions. If the patient complains of bronchoconstriction during exercise, it is important to determine whether this problem occurs in association with increased ambient pollutant concentrations in proximity to point sources of emission. Since exercise is an important factor in potentiating pollutant-induced asthma, the considerations noted above are clinically important.

Information about indoor air quality in the patient's place of residence is especially valuable in evaluating exacerbations of asthma. As previously mentioned, kerosene space heaters can produce high concentrations of sulfur dioxide and nitrogen dioxide. For this reason they should never be used by patients with asthma. Cigarette smoke is also a potent bronchoconstrictor. It is therefore important to determine whether the patient lives or works with smokers. The presence of specific common antigens such as animal dander, wool, goose down, and excessive amounts of house dust should be determined. Also important is the method(s) used for home heating and cooking and whether adequate furnace filters and kitchen ventilation are present and in use. The age and construction of the building, the type of insulation material used, and the pattern of indoor ventilation should be determined. Hobbies—such as carpentry, furniture refinishing, and soldering and the use of cleaning agents and insecticides—that might increase indoor pollution should be queried. Finally, evidence of response to other known stimuli to bronchoconstriction, such as fog, cold air, outdoor allergens, and emotional stress should be sought.

Differential Diagnosis Although exacerbations of asthma are thought to be responses to exogenous stimuli, the specific stimuli responsible for a given exacerbation are often difficult to identify with certainty. For specific allergens such as house dust mite or animal dander, skin prick tests can often confirm an immediate hypersensitivity response. However, a positive skin test does not prove that the provocative allergen is responsible for the patient's symptoms of asthma. Repeated symptomatic exacerbations in close temporal association with specific pollutant exposure (e.g., dyspnea and wheezing that occur whenever a roommate is smoking a cigarette) provides the strongest available evidence of a causative role for that pollutant. Even this type of evidence, however, must be tempered by the knowledge that many other concurrent stimuli might be responsible for the observed effect.

Management Despite frequent uncertainty about the role of a particular pollutant in exacerbating a given patient's asthma, it is reasonable to suggest environmental measures aimed at minimizing the adverse effect of pollutants. To minimize the effects of outdoor pollution, patients with asthma should not reside or perform vigorous physical exercise near point-source emitters of sulfur dioxide (e.g., coal- or oil-fired power plants, smelters, and oil refineries). In addition, such patients should decrease their level of physical exertion during episodes of significant outdoor pollution with sulfates, ozone, or nitrogen dioxide.

Since urban populations generally spend more than 90% of the time indoors, patients with asthma should minimize the effects of indoor pollution. They should, for example, not use kerosene space heaters and should, if at all possible, avoid living or working in close proximity to cigarette smoke. If they live in homes with gas stoves, the stoves should be equipped with properly functioning exhaust fans. The fans should always be turned on when the stove or oven is in use. Forced-air heaters should be equipped with filters that are replaced regularly. Bare floors are preferred to carpets, which trap and retain dust-borne allergens. Since wool, goose down, and animal dander are common allergens, asthmatics should avoid exposure to these materials, especially if they demonstrate positive skin-prick test responses. Some patients with hypersensitivity to house dust mites may benefit from putting coverings over pillows and mattresses, which are the common breeding areas for house dust mites. Finally, since the nose is an important filter for pollutants, treatment of any nasal obstruction that is so commonly present in the asthmatic may significantly diminish pollutant exposure.

Pollutants as a Cause of Asthma in Previously Healthy People

Over 100 separate agents found in the workplace are known to cause asthma in previously healthy workers (81). Many of these materials may also be inhaled in high concentrations when they are used inside the home. Some agents (e.g., toluene diisocyanate released from polyurethane varnishes) have been associated with the onset of asthma in this nonoccupational setting. In addition, rare "outbreaks" of asthma have been described among residents living near a castor-bean-processing plant or grain-processing and storage facilities. Such "outbreaks" are presumably caused by exposure to effluents from these plants (23). Exposure to high concentrations of formaldehyde over a period of years has been reported to cause asthma in two previously healthy dialysis nurses (40,41). Whether chronic exposure to the lower concentrations (generally less than 1 ppm) released into indoor air from new construction materials, fabrics, and urea-formaldehyde foam insulation is also capable of causing asthma remains to be determined. There is at present no evidence that links chronic or repeated exposure to ozone or nitrogen dioxide with persistent asthma. Acute exposure to these pollutants, however, can cause short-lived increases in airway responsiveness suggestive of asthma.

Diagnosis The first step in establishing a diagnosis of environmentally induced asthma is establishing a diagnosis of asthma. This diagnosis requires a history of episodic cough, dyspnea, or wheezing. Such symptoms are usually made worse by one or more of the commonly recognized stimuli to bronchoconstriction, such as exercise, viral upper respiratory infections, and fog. It is important to keep in mind that in mild asthma, coughing is frequently the only symptom.

The medical history should include inquiry into the nature of the patient's workplace exposure as well as into known causes of asthma in the home. This includes information about the hobbies of all household members. The nature of any industry in the vicinity of the patient's home should also be determined. In seeking a temporal relationship between exposure to specific materials and symptoms of asthma, the practitioner should keep in mind that delayed bronchoconstrictor responses, occurring 4–12 h after exposure, are quite common (81). It should also be remembered that the longer the patient has had symptoms of asthma, the less likely he or she is to improve when away from exposure to the responsible agent.

A history of atopy, including hay fever and eczema, neither supports nor detracts from a diagnosis of occupationally or environmentally induced asthma. Depending on the responsible agent, the incidence of atopy in individuals with asthma may not differ from that found in the general population (81).

The physical examination is frequently normal in patients with asthma. During symptomatic episodes, scattered wheezes, prolonged expiration, and lung hyperinflation may be present. Although measurements of forced expired volume in 1 s (FEV_1) and forced vital capacity (FVC) are frequently normal between symptomatic episodes, there may be a reduction in FEV_1, FVC, and in the ratio of FEV_1 : FVC. These abnormalities in pulmonary function, if present, usually improve after inhalation of a β-adrenergic agonist drug such as isoproterenol. Failure to improve after bronchodilator therapy does not rule out a diagnosis of asthma.

If screening pulmonary function tests are normal, the diagnosis of asthma can be confirmed by demonstrating exaggerated sensitivity to an inhaled bronchoconstrictor drug such as histamine or methacholine. Evidence that the asthma is caused by exposure to a particular agent can then be sought by frequently measuring the peak expiratory flow with a portable peak-flow meter. A diary of symptoms and detailed recording of activities and exposure should be kept concurrently. Demonstration of repeated drops in peak flow of more than 20% below base line in a temporal relationship to specific exposures strongly implicates those exposures as an important factor contributing to the patient's asthma.

More definitive evidence can be obtained by specific inhalation challenge studies. These studies should include exposure to several doses of the suspected agent and to a placebo on different days in a blinded fashion. Since late responses are frequent, inhalation challenge studies should be continued for at least 12–24 h. Such studies are complex and should be done only in centers with appropriate facilities to safely generate and monitor the challenge conditions.

Management If the causative link between a particular pollutant and the development of asthma is firmly established, the most important approach to treatment is avoidance of that pollutant. When asthma is associated with outdoor pollution emanating from a particular source, the responsibility of reducing the emissions rests with the polluting facility. When asthma is the result of an exposure in the home, further use of the offending agent should be avoided. When asthma is related to an agent(s) present in the workplace, the patient should be counseled to avoid such exposure.

Acute Massive Exposure to Toxic Gases

As previously discussed, acute massive exposure to toxic gases can cause diffuse severe lung injury. The first symptoms of exposed individuals may be upper airway obstruction or bronchospasm. Progressive respiratory failure associated with pulmonary edema and bronchiolitis may develop over several hours or days. These deep lung effects are most likely to occur after exposure to gases (such as phosgene or nitrogen dioxide) that are relatively insoluble. Although a history of exposure to a toxic spill is usually obvious, there are a few exceptions to this rule. For example, the degradation products of Teflon® produced when empty Teflon-coated pans are inadvertently heated can produce this pattern of diffuse lung injury. Teflon®-caused lung injury often appears many hours after the period of exposure. The inhalation of nitrogen dioxide can occur when individuals enter unvented grain silos. Such exposure takes place under these circumstances because nitrogen dioxide, produced from decomposing grain, is denser than air and settles to the ground.

When first seen, the patient may appear relatively well with only mild tachypnea. Early on, the physical examination frequently reveals wheezes or rhonchi, which reflect airway injury and reflex bronchoconstriction. The presence of conjuctival and pharyngeal erythema may be an important clue to mucosal injury. The presence of stridor implies life-threatening upper airway obstruction. It indicates a need for immediate admission to an intensive care unit. Although the initial chest radiograph is usually normal, arterial blood gases often show a mild to moderate hypoxemia. Blood gases are therefore a very important index of lung injury.

During the next 12–72 h hypoxemia may progress, and diffuse parenchymal infiltrates, indicative of pulmonary edema, may appear on the chest x-ray. Over the same period of time, increasing airway obstruction may develop and be associated with a dramatic increase in mucus secretion and sloughing of large areas of the tracheobronchial epithelium. The sloughed epithelial "casts" can occlude major airways, leading to segmental, lobar, or even whole-lung atelectasis. Three to 7 days after the initial injury, bacterial pneumonia frequently develops as a result of impaired pulmonary defenses.

Management

Early assessment of the likelihood of severe lung injury is based on estimated exposure dose, signs of mucosal injury, pulmonary auscultatory findings, and the degree of arterial hypoxemia. Upper airway obstruction may require endotracheal intubation. Bronchoconstriction should be treated with inhaled β-adrenergic agonists and systemic theophylline. Although corticosteroids should be considered in patients with severe airway obstruction unresponsive to conventional therapy, they should not be used routinely.

Therapy should be primarily supportive. Patients who develop severe hypoxemia or ventilatory failure will require endotracheal intubation and mechanical ventilation. Antibiotics should not be used unless the patient develops a bacterial pneumonia, which frequently occurs between the third and seventh days. Bronchoscopy can confirm the presence of diffuse airway injury. It is probably unnecessary, however, unless lobar atelectasis develops. In this case it can be helpful in removing the airway epithelial "casts."

Prognosis

Most patients with acute lung injury from toxic gas inhalation recover completely over a period of weeks to months. Some patients, however, go on to develop progressively severe distal airway obstruction (bronchiolitis obliterans). There have been scattered published reports of previously healthy people who have developed long-standing airway hyperresponsiveness and clinically significant asthma after a single episode of acute inhalation injury.

Respiratory Infections

As previously mentioned, epidemiologic evidence suggests an association between pollutant exposure and acute respiratory illnesses (3,16,28, 30,46,56,62,92,102,104,105,107). This association is strengthened by the finding that pollutant exposure increases susceptibility to infections in animals. Information about exposure to pollutants is therefore important in evaluating patients with recurrent respiratory infections. Exposure to sources of indoor pollution appears to be especially undesirable for young children. Children have been shown to develop an increased incidence of acute respiratory illnesses in association with parental smoking (16,70, 104,107). The presence of indoor air pollution from gas stoves may also pose a respiratory hazard to the young (62,92). In evaluating children with recurrent acute respiratory illnesses, information about parental smoking, cooking fuels, home heating, and home and kitchen ventilation should be sought. If patients with recurrent respiratory infections are found to have significant exposure to pollutants, appropriate control measures should be instituted.

SUMMARY

The recognition that air pollution poses a health hazard became apparent as an aftermath of several air pollution episodes that occurred in the middle part of this century. A large body of literature now describes the properties, sources, and distribution of pollutants found in both indoor and ambient air. The respiratory effects of such agents as sulfur dioxide, nitrogen dioxide, ozone, and environmental cigarette smoke have been investigated in epidemiologic studies, in short-term clinical studies, and by acute and chronic exposures of laboratory animals. These studies have identified certain adverse respiratory effects linked to pollutant exposure. It is therefore incumbent on physicians to explore a possible relationship between a patient's respiratory disorder and pollutant exposure. A recognition of this relationship provides the physician with an opportunity to incorporate environmental control measures in the care of the patient.

REFERENCES

1. Aisner J, Wiernik PH: Malignant mesothelioma. Chest 74:438, 1978.
2. American Thoracic Society: Environmental controls and lung disease. Am Rev Respir Dis 142:913, 1990.
3. Angel JH, Fletcher CM, Hill ID, et al: Respiratory illness in factory and office workers. A study of minor respiratory illnesses in relation to changes in ventilatory capacity, sputum characteristics, and atmospheric pollution. Br J Dis Chest 59:66, 1965.
4. Bauer MA, Utell MJ, Morrow PE, et al: Inhalation of 0.30 ppm nitrogen dioxide potentiates exercise-induced bronchospasm in asthmatics. Am Rev Respir Dis 134:1203, 1986.
5. Becklake MR: Asbestos-related diseases of lung and other organs: Their epidemiology and implications for clinical practice. Am Rev Respir Dis 114:187, 1976.
6. Bennett G: Ozone contamination of high altitude aircraft cabins. Aerospace Med 33:969, 1962.
7. Berkey CS, Ware JH, Dockery DW, et al: Indoor air pollution and pulmonary function growth in preadolescent children. Am J Epidemiol 123:250, 1986.
8. Bethel RA, Epstein J, Sheppard D, et al: Potentiation of sulfur dioxide-induced bronchoconstriction by airway cooling. Am Rev Respir Dis 127:161, 1983.
9. Bethel RA, Erle DJ, Epstein J, et al: Effect of exercise rate and route of inhalation on sulfur dioxide induced bronchoconstriction in asthmatic subjects. Am Rev Respir Dis 128:592, 1983.
10. Blot MJ, Yu Z-Y, Boice JD Jr, et al: Indoor radon and lung cancer in China. J Natl Cancer Inst 82:1025, 1990.
11. Boushey HA, Sheppard D: Air pollution. In: Textbook of Respiratory Medicine, p 1617, Murray JF, Nadel JA (eds.), WB Saunders, Philadelphia, 1988.
12. Boushey HA, Holtzman MJ, Sheller JR, et al: State of the art: Bronchial hyperreactivity. Am Rev Respir Dis 121:389, 1980.
13. Burchfield CM, Higgins MW, Keller JB, et al: Passive smoking in childhood. Respiratory conditions and pulmonary function in Tecumseh, Michigan. Am Rev Respir Dis 133:966, 1986.
14. Charlton A: Children's cough related to parental smoking. Br Med J 288:1646, 1984.
15. Chiaramonte LT, Bongiorno JR, Brown R, et al: Air pollution and obstructive respiratory disease in children. NY State J Med 70:394, 1970.
16. Committee on Environmental Hazards: Involuntary smoking—a hazard to children. Pediatrics 77:755, 1986.
17. Committee on Epidemiology of Air Pollutants, National Research Council: Epidemiology and Air Pollution, National Academy Press, Washington, 1985.
18. Committee on Indoor Pollutants, National Research Council: Indoor Pollutants, National Academy Press, Washington, 1981.
19. Committee on Nonoccupational Health Risks of Asbestiform Fibers, National Research Council: Asbestiform Fibers: Nonoccupational Health Risks. National Academy Press, Washington, 1984.
20. Committee on Passive Smoking, National Research Council: Environmental Tobacco Smoke, Monitoring Exposures and Assessing Health Effects, National Academy Press, Washington, 1986.
21. Committee on Toxicology, National Research Council: Formaldehyde—An Assessment of Health Effects, National Academy Press, Washington, 1980.
22. Cone JE, Hodgson MJ (eds.): Problem buildings: Building-associated illness and the sick building syndrome. Occup Med 4:575–797, 1989.
23. Cowan DW, Thompson HS, Paulus HJ, et al: Bronchial asthma associated with air pollutants from the grain industry. J Air Pollut Control Assoc 13:546, 1963.
24. Craighead JE, Mossman BT: The pathogenesis of asbestos-associated diseases. N Engl J Med 306:1446, 1982.
25. Dalhamm T: Mucous flow and ciliary activity in the trachea of healthy rats exposed to respiratory irritant gases (SO$_2$, NH$_3$, NCHO). Acta Physiol Scand 36:1, 1956.

26. deShazo, RD: Current concepts about the pathogenesis of silicosis and asbestos. J Allergy Clin Immunol 70:41, 1982.

27. Dodge RR, Burrows B: The prevalence and incidence of asthma and asthma-like symptoms in a general population sample. Am Rev Respir Dis 122:567, 1980.

28. Dohan FC: Air pollutants and incidence of respiratory disease. Arch Environ Health 3:387, 1961.

29. Dungworth D, Goldstein E, Ricci PF: Photochemical air pollution—Part II. Specialty conference. West J Med 142:523, 1985.

30. Durham WH: Air pollution and student health. Arch Environ Health 28:241, 1974.

31. Ekwo EE, Weinberger MW, Lachengruch PA, et al: Relationship of parental smoking and gas cooking to respiratory disease in children. Chest 84:662, 1983.

32. Epler GR: The spectrum of bronchiolitis obliterans. Chest 83:161, 1983.

33. Frank NR, Yoder RE, Brain JD, et al: SO$_2$(^{35}S labeled) absorption by the nose and mouth under conditions of varying concentration and flow. Arch Environ Health 18:315, 1969.

34. Gammage RB, Kaye SV (eds.): Indoor Air and Human Health. Lewis Publishers, Chelsea, Michigan, 1985.

35. Gardner DE: Effects of environmental chemicals on host defense response of the lung. In: Biological Relevance of Immune Suppression as Induced by Genetic Therapeutic and Environmental Factors, p 275, Dean JH, Padrathsingh M (eds.), Van Nostrand, New York, 1981.

36. Gardner DE, Crapo JD, Massaro EJ (eds.): Toxicology of the Lung, Raven Press, New York, 1988.

37. Golden JA, Nadel JA, Boushey HA: Bronchial hyperirritability in health subjects after exposure to ozone. Am Rev Respir Dis 118:287, 1978.

38. Goldstein E, Hackney JD, Rokaw SN: Photochemical air pollution—Part I. Specialty conferences. West J Med 142:369, 1985.

39. Harley N, Samet JM, Cross FT, et al: Contribution of radon and radon daughters to respiratory cancer. Environ Health Perspect 70:17, 1986.

40. Hendrick DJ, Lane DJ: Formalin asthma in hospital staff. Br J Ind Med 34:607, 1975.

41. Hendrick DJ, Lane DJ: Occupational formalin asthma. Br J Ind Med 34:11, 1977.

42. Higgins ITT, D'Arcy JB, Gibbons DI, et al: Effects of exposure to ambient ozone on ventilatory lung function in children. Am Rev Respir Dis 141:1136, 1990.

43. Hirayama T: Nonsmoking wives of heavy smokers have higher risk of lung cancer: A study from Japan. Br Med J 282:183, 1981.

44. Hirayama T: Cancer mortality in nonsmoking women with smoking husbands based on a large-scale cohort study in Japan. Prev Med 13:680, 1984.

45. Holtzman MJ, Fabbri LM, O'Byrne PM, et al: Importance of airway inflammation for hyperresponsiveness induced by ozone. Am Rev Respir Dis 127:686, 1983.

46. Honicky RE, Osborne JS III, Akpom CA: Symptoms of respiratory illness in young children and the use of wood-burning stoves for indoor heating. Pediatrics 75:567, 1985.

47. Horstman D, McDonnell W, Abdul-Salaam S, et al: Changes in pulmonary function and airway reactivity due to prolonged exposure to typical ambient ozone levels. In: Atmospheric Ozone Research and Its Policy Implications, p 755, Schneider T, Lee SD, Wolters GJR, et al. (eds.), Elsevier, Amsterdam, 1989.

48. International Agency for Research on Cancer: Some industrial chemicals and dyestuffs. In: Formaldehyde, Vol 29, IARC Monographs on the evaluation of the carcinogenic risk of Chemical in Humans, p 345, IARC, Lyon, 1982.

49. Kerhl HR, Vincent LM, Kowalsky RJ, et al: Ozone exposure increases respiratory epithelial permeability in humans. Am Rev Respir Dis 135:1124, 1987.

50. Kirkpatrick MB, Sheppard D, Nadel JA, et al: Effect of the oronasal breathing route on sulfur dioxide-induced bronchoconstriction in exercising asthmatic subjects. Am Rev Respir Dis 125:627, 1982.

51. Koenig JQ, Pierson WE, Horike M, et al: Effects of SO$_2$ plus NaCl aerosol combined with moderate exercise on pulmonary function in asthmatic adolescents. Environ Res 25:340, 1981.

52. Lambert PM, Reid DD: Smoking, air pollution, and bronchitis in Britain. Lancet 1:853, 1970.

53. Leaderer BP: Air pollution emissions from kerosene space heaters. Science 218:1113, 1982.

54. Lee LY, Bleecker ER, Nadel JA: Effect of ozone on the bronchomotor response to inhaled histamine aerosol in dogs. J Appl Physiol 43:626, 1977.

55. Lepper MH, Shioura N, Carnow B, et al: Respiratory disease in an urban environment. Arch Ind Med 38:36, 1969.

56. Levy D, Gent M, Newhouse MT: Relationship between acute respiratory illness and air pollution levels in an industrial city. Am Rev Respir Dis 116:167, 1977.

57. Linn WS, Venet TG, Shamoo DA, et al: Respiratory effects of sulfur dioxide in heavily exercising asthmatics: A dose response study. Am Rev Respir Dis 127:278, 1983.

58. Lippmann M: Effects of ozone on respiratory function and structure. Annu Rev Public Health 10:49, 1989.

59. Logan WPD: Mortality in London fog incident. Lancet 1:336, 1953.

60. Matanoski G, Fishbein L, Redmond C, et al: Contributions of organic particulates to respiratory cancer. Environ Health Perspect 70:37, 1986.

61. Mehta PS, Mehta AS, Mehta SJ, et al: Bhopal tragedy's health effects. JAMA 264:2781, 1990.

62. Melia RJW, Florey C, Altman DG, et al: Association between gas cooking and respiratory disease in children. Br Med J 2:149, 1977.

63. Melia RJW, Florey C, Morris RW, et al: Childhood respiratory illness and home environment. II: Association between respiratory illness and nitrogen dioxide, temperature, and relative humidity. Int J Epidemiol 11:164, 1982.

64. Mork T: A comparative study of respiratory disease in England and Wales and Norway, Norwegian University Press, Oslo, 1962.

65. Mumford JL, He XZ, Chapman RS, et al: Lung cancer and indoor air pollution in Xuan Wei China. Science 235:217, 1987.

66. Nadel JA, Salem H, Tamplin B, et al: Mechanism of

bronchoconstriction during inhalation of sulfur dioxide. J Appl Physiol 20:164, 1965.

67. Nelson N, Levine RJ, Albert RE, et al: Contribution of formaldehyde to respiratory cancer. Environ Health Perspect 70:23, 1986.

68. Ogston SA, Florey C, Walker CHM: The Tayside infant morbidity and mortality study: Effect on health of using gas for cooking. Br Med J 290:957, 1985.

69. Orehek J, Massari JP, Gayrard P, et al: Effect of short-term low-level nitrogen dioxide exposure on bronchial sensitivity of asthmatic patients. J Clin Invest 57:301, 1976.

70. Pedreira FA, Guandolo VL, Feroli EJ, et al: Involuntary smoking and incidence of respiratory illness during the first year of life. Pediatrics 75:594, 1985.

71. Peters JM, Thomas D, Falk H, et al: Contributions of metals to respiratory cancer. Environ Health Perspect 70:71, 1986.

72. Petrilli FL, Agnese G, Kanitz S: Epidemiological studies of air pollution effects in Genoa, Italy. Arch Environ Health 12:733, 1966.

73. Radford EP: Potential health effects of indoor radon exposure. Environ Health Perspect 62:281, 1985.

74. Samet JM: Radon and lung cancer. J Natl Cancer Inst 81:745, 1989.

75. Samet JM, Nero AV Jr: Indoor radon and lung cancer. N Engl J Med 320:591, 1989.

76. Samet JM, Marbury MC, Spengler JD: Health effects and sources of indoor air pollution. I. Am Rev Respir Dis 136:1486, 1987.

77. Samet JM, Marbury MC, Spengler JD: Health effects and sources of indoor air pollution. II. Am Rev Respir Dis 137:221, 1988.

78. Scanlon PD, Seltzer J, Drazen JM: Chronic sulfur dioxide exposure. Physiologic and histologic correlation. Am Rev Respir Dis 129:A236, 1984.

79. Schenker MB, Samet JM, Speizer FE: Risk factors for childhood respiratory disease: The effects of host factors and home environmental exposures. Am Rev Respir Dis 128:1035, 1983.

80. Schrenk HH, Heiman H, Clayton GD, et al: Air Pollution in Donora, Pennsylvania. Epidemiology of the Unusual Smog Episode of October 1948, Public Health Bulletin 306, US Government Printing Office, Washington, 1949.

81. Sheppard D: Occupational asthma. West J Med 137:480, 1982.

82. Sheppard D: Mechanisms of bronchoconstruction from nonimmunologic environmental stimuli. Chest 90:585, 1986.

83. Sheppard D: Sulfur dioxide and asthma—a double-edged sword? J Allergy Clin Immunol 82:961, 1988.

84. Sheppard D: Mechanisms of acute increases in airway responsiveness caused by environmental chemicals. J Allergy Clin Immunol 81:128, 1988.

85. Sheppard D, Wong SC, Uehara CF, et al: Lower threshold and greater bronchomotor responsiveness of asthmatic subjects to sulfur dioxide. Am Rev Respir Dis 122:873, 1980.

86. Sheppard D, Nadel JA, Boushey HA: Inhibition of sulfur dioxide-induced bronchoconstriction by disodium cromoglycate in asthmatic subjects. Am Rev Respir Dis 124:257, 1981.

87. Sheppard D, Saisho A, Nadel JA, et al: Exercise increases sulfur dioxide-induced bronchoconstriction in asthmatic subjects. Am Rev Respir Dis 123:486, 1981.

88. Sheppard D, Eschenbacher WL, Boushey HA, et al: Magnitude of the interaction between the bronchomotor effects of sulfur dioxide and those of dry (cold) air. Physiology 26:A-23, 1983.

89. Sheppard D, Eschenbacher WL, Epstein J: Absence of bronchomotor response to up to 3 ppm formaldehyde in subjects with asthma. Environ Res 35:133, 1984.

90. Shy CM, Goldsmith JR, Hackney JD, et al: Health Effects of Air Pollution. American Thoracic Society, New York, 1978.

91. Speizer FE: Overview of the risk of respiratory cancer from airborne contaminants. Environ Health Perspect 70:9, 1986.

92. Speizer FE, Fermis B, Bishop Y, et al: Respiratory disease rates and pulmonary function in children associated with NO_2 exposure. Am Rev Respir Dis 121:3, 1980.

93. Spektor DM, Lippmann M, Loiy PJ, et al: Effects of ambient ozone on respiratory function in active normal children. Am Rev Respir Dis 137:313, 1988.

94. Spengler JD, Sexton K: Indoor air pollution: A public health perspective. Science 221:9, 1983.

95. Sumner W, Haponik E: Inhalation of irritant gases. Clin Chest Med 2:273, 1981.

96. Tager IB, Weiss ST, Munoz A, et al: Longitudinal study of the effects of maternal smoking on pulmonary function studies in children. N Engl J Med 309:699, 1983.

97. Tam E, Sheppard D, Epstein J, et al: Lack of dose dependency for ipratropium bromide's inhibitory effect on sulfur dioxide-induced bronchospasm in asthmatic subjects. Am Rev Respir Dis 127:257, 1983.

98. Taskin DP, Clark VA, Simmons M, et al: The UCLA population studies of chronic obstructive respiratory disease. Relationship between paternal smoking and children's lung function. Am Rev Respir Dis 129:891, 1984.

99. US Department of Health and Human Services: The Health Consequences of Involuntary Smoking, A Report of the Surgeon General. US Dept Health and Human Services, Public Health Services, Office of Smoking and Health, DHHS Pub No. (CDC)87-8398, Washington, 1986.

100. Utell MJ, Samet JM: Environmentally mediated disorders of the respiratory tract. Med Clin North Am 74:291, 1990.

101. Vedal S, Schenker MB, Samet JM, et al: Risk factors for childhood respiratory disease. Am Rev Respir Dis 130:187, 1984.

102. Verma MP, Schilling FJ, Becker WH: Epidemiological study of illness absences in relation to air pollution. Arch Environ Health 18:536, 1969.

103. Viana NJ, Polan AK: Non-occupational exposure to asbestos and malignant mesothelioma in females. Lancet 2:1061, 1978.

104. Ware JH, Dockery DW, Spiro A III, et al: Passive smoking, gas cooking and respiratory health of children living in six cities. Am Rev Respir Dis 129:366, 1984.

105. Wayne WS, Wehrle PF: Oxidant air pollution and school absenteeism. Arch Environ Health 19:315, 1969.

106. Weber-Tschopp A, Fischer T, Grandjean E: Irritating effects of formaldehyde on men. Int Arch Occup Environ Health 39:207, 1977.
107. Weiss ST, Tager IB, Speizer FE, et al: Persistent wheeze: Its relation to respiratory illness, cigarette smoking, and levels of pulmonary function in a population sample of children. Am Rev Respir Dis 122: 697, 1980.
108. Weiss W: Lung cancer and occupational lung disease. Clin Chest Med 2:289, 1981.
109. Whittmore AS, Korn EL: Asthma and air pollution in the Los Angeles area. Am J Public Health 70:687, 1980.
110. Yashizo T: Air pollution and chronic bronchitis. Osaka Univ Med J 20:10, 1968.
111. Zeidberg LD, Prindle RA, Landau E: The Nashville air pollution study. I. Sulfur dioxide and bronchial asthma. A preliminary report. Am Rev Respir Dis 84: 489, 1961.
112. Zeidberg LD, Horton RJM, Landau E: The Nashville air pollution study. V. Mortality from diseases of the respiratory system in relation to air pollution. Arch Environ Health 15:214, 1967.

RECOMMENDED READINGS

Committee on the Epidemiology of Air Pollutants, National Research Council: Epidemiology and Air Pollution. National Academy Press, Washington, 1985.

Gardner DE, Crapo JD, Massaro EJ (eds.): Toxicology of the Lung, Raven Press, Washington, 1988.

Samet JM, Marbury MC, Spengler JD: Health effects and sources of indoor air pollution I. Am Rev Respir Dis 136:1486, 1987.

Samet JM, Marbury MC, Spengler JD: Health effects and sources of indoor air pollution. II. Am Rev Respir Dis 137:221, 1988.

Samet JM, Spengler JD (eds.): Indoor Air Pollution: A Health Perspective, Johns Hopkins University Press, 1991.

Utell MJ, Samet JM: Environmentally mediated disorders of the respiratory tract. Med Clin North Am 74:291, 1990.

Watson AY, Bates RR, Kennedy D (eds.): Air Pollution, the Automobile, and Public Health, National Academy Press, Washington, 1988.

17. DISORDERS OF THE HEART AND BLOOD VESSELS

Kenneth D. Rosenman

INTRODUCTION

Chemical exposure can cause acute injury to the myocardium and precipitate a cardiovascular crisis when there is preexisting myocardial disease. When there is no clinical evidence of an immediate cardiovascular reaction to a toxic exposure, our knowledge about the relationship is limited. Thus, the risks that chemical exposure impose on the development of cardiovascular disease are unknown.

It is vital to gain this understanding. Cardiovascular disease, in particular coronary artery disease (CAD), is the major cause of death in the United States. Approximately 500,000 or 40% of all deaths each year are attributed to this cause. It is estimated that 1.2 million individuals have an acute myocardial infarction each year. An additional 6 million individuals are estimated to have ischemic heart disease. Hypertension affects 20–30% of the population, depending on race and age. Another 9% of all deaths are attributed to cerebrovascular disease.

The underlying process in the majority of patients with coronary artery disease is atherosclerosis. Although a great deal is known about such risk factors as hypertension, family history, serum lipoprotein patterns, cigarette smoking, and dia-

betes, surprisingly few investigators have focused on the relationship between cardiovascular disease and environmental exposure. Only a few reviews of this subject are available (36,46,56,62,63).

Epidemiologists in search of a link between CAD and exposure to environmental chemicals are hampered by a number of methodological problems: (1) Techniques for measuring an individual's exposure to ambient pollution have only recently been developed. These measurements are not yet as simple as asking a patient if he or she smokes. Thus, most studies depend on a sampling obtained from fixed locations in neighborhoods. (2) There are no reliable noninvasive tests for measuring the development of atherosclerosis in asymptomatic populations exposed to various noxious agents. (3) There are few distinctive laboratory or pathological features of chemically induced cardiovascular disease. (4) The development of CAD, in particular, is known to be related to numerous risk factors. Thus, if pollutant exposure is a risk factor, it can easily be obscured by other causal factors. (5) The cardiovascular risk of low-dose environmental exposure is probably low and therefore difficult to assess. This assumption is related to the fact that smokers, despite their high exposure to carbon monoxide, increase their risk of CAD less than twofold (37).

Because of these factors, the known associations between CAD and environmental pollution are scarce. Even in the workplace, where exposures are higher and more easily quantified, information on the association between chemical exposures and

Principles and Practice of Environmental Medicine, edited by Alyce Bezman Tarcher. Plenum Medical Book Company, New York, 1992.

cardiovascular disease is limited (46,62,63). In this connection, it should be appreciated that indoor air pollution from hobbies or chemical use at home can cause equivalent or even greater levels of exposure than those found in the workplace. Food and water contamination have also been associated with significant levels of pollutant exposure (2,60,78).

Not unexpectedly environmental factors currently recognized as most important in the etiology of CAD are personal life-style habits. The reason for this is twofold. First, life-style factors are frequently the ones to which there is highest exposure. Second, it is often possible to measure such factors at the individual level. Smoking provides an excellent example of toxic exposure on a personal level that can be determined quite easily.

Traditionally the astute physician has frequently been the first to recognize chemically related diseases, especially in the occupational setting. For the reasons cited above, however, this ability is limited in relation to cardiovascular disease—in particular to CAD. Despite these limitations, physicians must consider a link between exposure and cardiovascular disease. All patients must be questioned about past and present exposures and their intensity and relationship to the onset of illness. A list should be made of any symptoms that recur in relation to activity as well as to exposure(s).

The importance of obtaining such data is well illustrated in the following case report (76). A retired executive sustained an acute myocardial infarction shortly after stripping wood in a poorly ventilated area. After being admitted to the hospital the patient told his physician about the paint stripping. The physician noted that the product contained 80% methylene chloride. The label cautioned that the product be used only with adequate ventilation. The physician saw no causal relationship between the patient's recent exposure to the paint remover and his acute myocardial infarction. After his recovery from his first myocardial infarction, the patient went on to have two more myocardial infarctions. On each occasion he had used the product containing 80% methylene chloride. The last episode was fatal. Had the clinician been more alert, an investigation of the toxic properties of methylene chloride would have revealed it to be rapidly metabolized to carbon monoxide, an agent that can be associated with myocardial ischemia.

This chapter focuses on the link between exposure to environmental chemicals and cardiovascular disease. It begins by citing the agents that adversely affect the cardiovascular system and then continues with a discussion of epidemiology and pathological physiology. It concludes with a discussion of the clinical implications of such exposure on the cardiovascular system.

ENVIRONMENTAL CHEMICALS ASSOCIATED WITH ADVERSE EFFECTS ON THE HEART AND BLOOD VESSELS

The agents listed in Table 17-1 are associated, to varying degrees of certainty, with the development of cardiovascular disease. Those associations that are well documented involve acute effects and cardiomyopathy. For the adverse effects noted with a question mark, no firm association is established. Individuals with preexisting underlying CAD are at increased risk of developing the acute effects noted in Table 17-1 (34,39,51,89). At the levels of carbon monoxide, sulfur dioxide, and particulates found in ambient air or during severe pollution episodes, individuals with underlying heart or lung disease are more vulnerable than the general adult population (51). Most documented adverse cardiovascular effects outside of the workplace involve exposures in the home or to contaminated food or water.

Carbon Monoxide

Carbon monoxide is a ubiquitous pollutant that adversely affects the cardiovascular system. It is a fairly stable, odorless, and colorless gas. It mixes with air at all temperatures. Its affinity for hemoglobin is about 200 times greater than oxygen; myoglobin has an affinity for carbon monoxide 50 times that of oxygen. Carbon monoxide displaces oxygen from hemoglobin by binding with the more labile oxygen sites on the hemoglobin molecule. This decreases the oxygen-carrying capacity of the blood and causes the oxygen dissociation curve to shift to the left. For this reason an individual with 50% reduction in hemoglobin as a result of anemia may be less impaired than one whose hemoglobin is 50% saturated with carbon monoxide (24,34). The individual with anemia may have few symptoms, whereas the individual with excess carbon monoxide exposure may be severely impaired.

Carbon monoxide is produced whenever fuel is incompletely burned. Vehicle exhaust is the major outdoor source. Carbon monoxide is widely present in indoor air. Clinicians must be alert to the possibility of carbon monoxide exposure. Proximity to combustion sources, particularly in a confined space (running a car in a garage, for example), must be considered a potential indicator for carbon monoxide exposure. Improperly vented wood stoves, space heaters, and gas stoves can produce high levels of carbon monoxide (82). Emissions from kerosene and gas space heaters can, in a small room with only moderate ventilation, increase the concentration of carbon monoxide (65). Elevated levels of carbon monoxide in the patient compartment of ambulances have been reported (40).

It is well documented that ambient concentra-

TABLE 17-1. Factors Associated with Environmental (Nonwork-Related) Cardiovascular Disease

Substance	Mode of exposure	Cardiovascular abnormalities or disease	
		Acute	Chronic
Arsenic	Ingestion: food, water		Cardiomyopathy, peripheral vascular disease
Cadmium	Inhalation: ambient atmosphere		Increased mortality from CAD[a]? Hypertension?
Carbon monoxide	Inhalation: ambient atmosphere, home	Myocardial infarction Angina Arrhythmias Sudden death	Increased atherosclerosis?
Cobalt	Ingestion: food		Cardiomyopathy
Fluorocarbons	Inhalation: home	Arrhythmias? Sudden death	
Hydrocarbons	Inhalation: home	Arrhythmias? Sudden death?	
Lead	Ingestion: paint chips		Cardiomyopathy Hypertension?
Methylene chloride	Inhalation: home		(Metabolized to Carbon monoxide in body; see "carbon monoxide" above)
Soft water	Ingestion: water		Increased mortality from cardiovascular diseases
Episodes of high urban air pollution	Inhalation: ambient atmosphere	Increased mortality from cardiac disease	

[a]Coronary artery disease.

tions of carbon monoxide in specific locations can become very high. Wright et al. demonstrated that, depending on such conditions as traffic density and location (i.e., in an underpass), pedestrians may be exposed to concentrations up to 100 ppm (91).

Table 17-2 shows the percentage of the United States population with carboxyhemoglobins greater than 2% (68). Individuals with atherosclerotic disease may become symptomatic with a carboxyhemoglobin greater than 2% (3,6,47,72). There is a trend for carboxyhemoglobin levels to be higher in winter than in summer and higher in urban than in rural areas. These findings suggest that furnaces,

fireplaces, unvented gas stoves, and space heaters are indoor sources of carbon monoxide. They also indicate that ambient carbon monoxide levels are higher in winter than in summer.

The actual exposure and subsequent effect will depend on the length of time an individual spends in any one spot. Carboxyhemoglobin levels will increase with continued exposure. The time it takes to reach equilibrium between air levels of carbon monoxide and serum carboxyhemoglobin is dependent on the pulmonary ventilation. When an individual is at rest, equilibrium is reached within 8 h. With increased physical activity, equilibrium is

TABLE 17-2. Percentage of Individuals with Carboxyhemoglobin Greater Than 2.0% for Nonsmokers by Age, Season, and Urbanization Status[a]

Age (years)	Season	Population standard metropolitan statistical area			
		≥1,000,000 central city	≥1,000,000 not central city	<1,000,000	Rural
12–74	Winter	8.5%	5.0%	4.9%	4.5%
	Summer	0	4.4%	0.2%	0.9%
3–11	Winter	3.3%	0.3%	4.9%	2.6%
	Summer	0	0	0.1%	0

[a]From Rosenman (63). Data derived from Radford and Drizd (58), based on 8411 carboxyhemoglobin results.

reached sooner (20). The following equation can be used to estimate approximate carboxyhemoglobin levels with shorter periods of exposure:

$$\% \text{ carboxyhemoglobin} = \% \text{ carbon monoxide in air} \times \text{ time (in minutes)} \times k$$

where 10,000 ppm carbon monoxide = 1% and k is a constant with a value of 3 at rest, 5 for light physical work, 8 for moderate physical work, and 11 for heavy physical work (50). The period of time used in the equation cannot be greater than the time it takes to reach equilibrium. Table 17-3 shows carboxyhemoglobin levels found at equilibrium with different ambient levels of carbon monoxide.

Hydrocarbons and Aerosol Propellants

Halogenated hydrocarbons, particularly the low-molecular-weight chlorinated alkanes and/or fluorinated methane or ethane derivatives, are widely used as fire extinguishing agents, solvents, and refrigerants (52).

Exposure to these halogenated hydrocarbons has been associated with sudden death, presumably from cardiac arrhythmia. Fluorocarbons were formally used as propellants in aerosol cans. Although these agents are no longer present in aerosol cans, they may be found in coin-operated dry cleaning machines. Aerosol sniffing has been a source of high exposure to halogenated hydrocarbons. The hydrocarbons currently used in household products are less arrhythmogenic than the agents used previously, as tested in one experimental animal system

(59). All such agents, however, have not been tested for their arrhythmogenic potential. Ambient levels of hydrocarbons, even around industrial sites (i.e., refineries), have not been reported to cause arrhythmias.

Metals

Low levels of arsenic, cadmium, mercury, and cobalt are found naturally in water and soil. Industrial contamination of air, water, food, and soil increases human exposure to these heavy metals.

Environmental exposure to arsenic has occurred through use of arsenical pesticides, air pollution from smelters, and from contaminated food and water. The highest ambient air levels of arsenic are found around smelters of nonferrous metal ores such as copper. In some locations it also occurs in relatively high concentrations in well water. Arsenic is present in many foods. Seafood contains the highest concentration of arsenic in the United States food supply (23).

Cadmium is produced in the process of smelting zinc and lead. Such smelters contribute to environmental cadmium pollution. Increasing amounts of cadmium are being released into the environment from such sources as disposal of sewage sludge and the burning of waste and fossil fuels. Cadmium is also present in cigarette smoke. Food is the major nonindustrial source of cadmium exposure (64).

The sources of human exposure to lead include food, drinking water, paint chips, contaminated soil, and the inhalation of indoor and ambient air.

TABLE 17-3. Carboxyhemoglobin (COHb) at Equilibrium for Varying Concentrations of Carbon Monoxide[a]

Concentration of carbon monoxide (ppm)		COHb (%)	Comments
0		0.36–0.9; average 0.5	Endogenous production increases with hemolysis, pregnancy, and administration of phenobarbital and diphenylhydantoin
9	Environmental Protection Agency average ambient air standard	1.7	
35	Environmental Protection Agency peak ambient air standard for 1 h National Institute of Occupational Safety and Health recommended average for 10-h work day	5.4	
50[b]	Occupational Safety and Health standard average allowed for 8-h work day	7.36	
400	Average concentration in cigarette smoke during inhalation and dilution with air	1–10; average 4 (varies with number of cigarettes smoked)	

[a]Data derived from Coburn et al. (20) and Radford and Drizd (58). From Rosenman (63).
[b]Recently lowered to 35 ppm.

Exposure to leaded paint chips and the inhalation of dust containing lead has been the major source of lead exposure for children. The major source of lead exposure for the general population in the United States has been emissions from the use of leaded gasoline in automobiles. Following restrictions on the use of lead in gasoline in the United States, the lead emission from automobiles has decreased by almost 75% from 1975 to 1984. Leaching from lead pipes or lead solder or from underground rock formations by soft water can also increase lead exposures. Reports of lead exposure on this basis have come from parts of Scotland and England. Individuals living near smelters and in houses with flaking lead paint manufactured before 1978 are subject to increased lead exposure. Young children are particularly susceptible to excess lead exposure and are more likely to be exposed, given their tendency to put things in their mouths.

Ingestion of fish is a major route of environmental exposure to organic mercury. This occurs because mercury, discharged into the waterways from industrial sources and transformed into organic mercury by microorganisms, bioaccumulates in fish. It has been reported that mercury-containing paints used in homes are a source of exposure (1). Mercury is used in a variety of industrial processes. These include the production of chlorine and caustic soda, electrical apparatus, and special antifouling and mildew-proofing of paints (64). The issue of mercury leaching from amalgams in dental fillings has been raised (19).

With increased exposure all the metals accumulate in the body. They have varied rates of absorption depending on the mode of exposure and the specific form of the metal compound. They are preferentially stored in specific tissues in the body. The heart is generally not the preferential site of accumulation. Rather, the metals are concentrated in such organs as bone, brain, liver, and kidney. All of the toxic metals are excreted, to some extent, in the urine.

EPIDEMIOLOGY

Episodes of Air Pollution

Acute exposure to high levels of air pollutants has been associated with increased mortality. Such episodes have been described in the Meuse Valley in Belgium in 1931, in Donora, Pennsylvania in 1948, and in London in 1952 (39). In retrospect, similar episodes were noted to have taken place in London in 1873, 1880, 1882, 1891, 1892, and 1948. In the 1952 episode, 4000 deaths in excess of those that would normally have occurred were noted. In all these episodes meteorological conditions caused stagnation of the air and the buildup of pollutants. The in-

creased death rate was attributed to chronic heart or lung disease (39) and bronchitis or pneumonia (51).

The most extensively studied acute air pollution episode occurred in October 1948 in Donora, Pennsylvania (67). The town, located in the valley of the Monongahela River, south of Pittsburgh, was the site of a zinc and steel plant. Twenty excess deaths were noted in a 4½-day period. Most of the deaths (17 of them) occurred on the third day. A household survey of approximately 15,000 individuals showed that 42.7% had various respiratory and gastrointestinal symptoms. The ages of those dying were between 52 and 84. Twice as many men as women died. The mortality rate among blacks was four times that found in the white population. There was no elevation of viral titers or other evidence of an influenza epidemic. Most deaths were attributed to chronic heart disease or bronchial asthma.

Since measurements of the concentration of specific pollutants were not made during the episode, the excess deaths was presumed to be linked to increased levels of sulfur dioxide and particulates.

Carbon Monoxide

Epidemiologic studies of carbon monoxide in the ambient air have examined the effect of acute and chronic exposures. A study of the about 9000 patients encountered at an emergency room in Denver in the mid-1970s found a statistically significant increase in patients with cardiorespiratory complaints. This occurred on the same day or the day after the ambient level of carbon monoxide was increased (49). The excess cardiorespiratory complaints were attributed to elevated levels of ambient carbon monoxide. The mean 1-h peak ambient air levels of carbon monoxide from "high-carbon-monoxide days" was 27.2 ± 4.3 ppm, compared to the "low-carbon-monoxide days" level of 12.1 ± 1.8 ppm. The 24-h average levels were 9.3 ± 1.4 ppm versus 5.9 ± 0.8 ppm. Similar findings have not been reported from other locations. The possibility that Denver's lower atmospheric oxygen pressure may accentuate the carbon monoxide effect has not been assessed (49).

A study done in the late 1960s in Los Angeles, and another in the early 1970s in Baltimore, failed to find a relationship between ambient carbon monoxide levels and the incidence of myocardial infarction and/or sudden death (47,48). In 1958, one study reported a link between case fatality rates of patients hospitalized with myocardial infarction and atmospheric carbon monoxide pollution in Los Angeles. The carbon monoxide level ranged between 5.4 and 14.5 ppm (21). Further analysis of these data suggests that there were methodological problems and/or the possibility of an influenza epidemic.

A series of case reports shows that carboxyhemoglobin levels 20% and greater are associated with acute myocardial infarctions (89). DeBias and co-workers demonstrated that monkeys with acute myocardial infarction are more susceptible to ventricular fibrillation when their carboxyhemoglobin levels range between 8.4% and 10.2% (27).

A syndrome called "Shinshu myocardosis," related to chronic carbon monoxide exposure, was described in 1955 in Japan (33). The population at risk spent the winter months in their homes manufacturing mats in enclosed rooms heated by charcoal fires. Carboxyhemoglobin levels reached 20–30%. One thousand twenty-two individuals were examined. Thirty-five percent had abnormal heart findings. With other known causes excluded, 18% were thought to have the syndrome. Symptoms varied with the severity of the disease. Less seriously affected individuals had stiffness of the shoulders, backache, fatigue, vertigo, and facial edema. More severe symptoms included dyspnea on exertion, substernal tightness and pain, numbness of the upper extremities, paroxysmal nocturnal dyspnea, and anginal attacks. Cardiac enlargement was found on chest x ray. Electrocardiographic abnormalities included arrhythmias, low voltage, depressed ST segments, and prolongation of QRS complexes. Under treatment, the condition persisted as long as 3 to 5 years. Remodeling of the rooms to allow for more ventilation markedly reduced morbidity.

Several clinical studies have investigated the effects of low levels of carbon monoxide exposure on cardiovascular function in individuals with coronary artery disease (4,6–8).

Anderson et al. exposed subjects with angina pectoris to low levels of carbon monoxide that resulted in mean carboxyhemoglobin levels of 2.9% and 4.5%. These subjects had significantly decreased exercise capacity as evidenced by a shortened duration of exercise before the onset of chest pain (4).

Aronow noted that low-level carbon monoxide exposure (50–100 ppm) over 2–4 h decreases exercise tolerance and increases the duration of ischemic pain in individuals with preexisting angina, chronic obstructive lung disease, or claudication (6). Carboxyhemoglobin levels averaged between 2.8% and 4.5% in patients included in these studies. Patients with angina showed a decreased exercise tolerance. Subjects with angina were also observed to develop increased ischemic symptoms after driving on the Los Angeles freeways for 90 min with the car windows open (8). Carboxyhemoglobin levels of 3.2–5.0% were measured after the 90-min freeway drive. Neither the increase in carboxyhemoglobin nor the decrease in exercise tolerance was seen when the subjects received compressed purified air during the 90-min freeway drive. Healthy middle-aged volunteers who raised their mean carboxyhemoglobin level from 1.67% to 3.95% by breathing 100 ppm carbon monoxide for 1 h had a 5% reduction in exercise tolerance without chest pain or EKG changes (7).

Allred et al. demonstrated a decreased exercise capacity in patients with known coronary artery disease who were exposed to carbon monoxide (3). The study was designed to evaluate the effects of blood carboxyhemoglobin levels of 2% and 4% on the development of myocardial ischemia during graded exercise in a population of patients with documented coronary artery disease. With exposure to carbon monoxide, the length of time to the onset of angina was decreased, and the presence of myocardial ischemia was confirmed by electrocardiographic changes. The results of this study confirm previous findings and indicate that carboxyhemoglobin blood levels of 2–3% exacerbate myocardial ischemia in subjects with coronary artery disease.

Forty-one nonsmokers with documented coronary artery disease were exposed to carbon monoxide levels that raised their carboxyhemoglobin to either 4% or 6%. At 6% the number and complexity of ventricular arrhythmias increased significantly during exercise (72).

The levels of carboxyhemoglobin noted above are found in individuals who smoke one to two packs of cigarettes per day, in passive smokers in an unventilated room, in the workplace where ambient air standards allow workers to have up to 5.4% carboxyhemoglobin, and in firemen who do not use respiratory protection.

The relationship between cigarette smoking and increased risk of myocardial infarction is well documented (81). Although the actual etiological agent is not agreed on, nicotine and carbon monoxide are considered the two most likely causal agents (80).

Halogenated Hydrocarbons

Of four reports that assessed a possible association between blood pressure and serum levels of polychlorinated biphenyls (PCBs), only one found an association. This study of 458 persons demonstrated a link between serum polychlorinated biphenyl (PCB) blood levels and an elevated diastolic, but not systolic, blood pressure (45). No relationship was found between the metabolites of dichlorodiphenyltrichloroethane (DDT) and blood pressure. These findings contrasted with an earlier report that showed an association between DDT metabolites and systolic and diastolic blood pressure (66).

A positive association is also reported between serum levels of PCBs and serum levels of triglycerides or cholesterol. For the most part such findings are reported in occupationally exposed groups. This association, however, has also been described when there was excessive exposure to PCBs in the community or in food (45,83). The association may be secondary to the solubility of PCBs in serum lipids.

Exposure to halogenated hydrocarbons has been linked to sudden deaths among asthmatics and also among individuals who abuse household products for their intoxicant effect (30). The abused substances include fluorocarbons, chlorinated hydrocarbons, and such agents as benzene, gasoline, and toluene. Acute dysrhythmias appear to be the cause of death in individuals who abuse these agents (12).

In one study, autopsies done on six young individuals revealed no anatomic cause of death. Suffocation was not the cause of death, as the victims were usually found at varying distances from the plastic bags filled with the substances they had been inhaling. Arrhythmias have also been reported when certain halogenated hydrocarbons were used as anesthetic gases. In an occupational setting, arrhythmias were reported in pathologists who used monofluoromethane in the preparation of frozen sections (75).

Although deaths among asthmatics may have been related to a delay in seeking medical attention, other hypotheses have included the high dose of isoproterenol (allowed in over-the-counter inhalants in certain countries) or a combined effect of fluorocarbon propellant and the hypoxemia of an asthma attack (92).

Ten male subjects between the ages of 20 and 24 recreated the use of consumer products containing fluorocarbon propellants in a laboratory setting (84). Pulmonary function studies and electrocardiograms were performed after 15 s, 45 s, and 60 s of exposure on different days. After a 15-s exposure, one subject had intermittent first-degree A-V block. Exposure for 60 s produced negative T waves in two subjects, atrioventricular block in one, and bradycardia and increased variability of heart rate in the majority of the other seven subjects.

Water Hardness and Cardiovascular Disease

In 1957 a Japanese researcher correlated the acidity of drinking water, as reflected in the sulfate-carbonate ratio, with elevated stroke mortality (25). Subsequent work in the United States showed a similar inverse relationship between cardiovascular mortality and the hardness of the water (25,28, 68,69,85). Studies within regions or states, however, do not consistently support such a relationship (71). The metals dissolved in soft water may vary from one region to another. Numerous reports identify different metals and trace elements in drinking water with an increased incidence of cardiovascular disease (71). Therefore, no clear association exists between the individual components of drinking water and cardiovascular disease. Despite the inconsistencies found with individual components, corrosiveness of water was consistently correlated with deaths from atherosclerotic heart disease (70).

Trace elements or metals contained in most public water supplies make up a very small percentage of an individual's total intake (71). The one exception to this is magnesium. Hard water probably contributes 10–20% of this element to the diet (71). It has therefore been suggested that greater attention be given to magnesium—its dietary sources, requirements, and metabolism (71).

A few studies done thus far show a low myocardial magnesium in patients dying suddenly from myocardial infarction. Such findings lend support to the theory that magnesium deficiency is a factor in CAD (5,16). They do not, however, eliminate the possibility that low myocardial magnesium is the consequence, not a cause, of sudden death. Studies from Great Britain that consistently show a relationship between soft water and cardiovascular disease show little or no correlation with the magnesium content of water (29,54).

Metals

Arsenic

Contamination of drinking water, beer, and food with various heavy metals has been associated with cardiomyopathy or peripheral vascular disease.

Arsenic was first noted to have an effect on the heart in 1900, when Reynolds reported his clinical observations of patients who, for many months, had been drinking beer contaminated with arsenic (60,61). Arsenic contamination of beer was traced to one supplier of invert sugar for breweries, who used sulfuric acid contaminated with arsenic to make the invert sugar from cane. Beers from 100 breweries in northern England were affected. The concentration of arsenic in beer was 2–4 ppm. Thousands of cases of illness were reported. Although the fatality rate is unknown, deaths occurred from congestive heart failure. The basis of cardiomyopathy found with arsenic contamination of beer has not been discovered. Subsequent reports of arsenic poisoning describe peripheral vascular disease rather than congestive heart failure.

In the 1960s in Antofagosta, Chile, a number of children were found to have chronic arsenic poisoning. The source of the arsenic exposure was traced to the water supply, which contained arsenic from natural sources in a concentration of 0.8 ppm (normal < 0.01 ppm). A part of the clinical picture included peripheral vascular disease as evidenced by Raynaud's syndrome, ischemia of the tongue, and hemiplegia with partial occlusion of the carotid artery (17). Other symptoms and signs included chronic diarrhea, abdominal pain, rhinitis, chronic cough, herpes of the lip, acrocyanosis, abnormal skin pigmentation, and hyperkeratosis. Except for the absence of neurological changes and congestive heart failure, the clinical findings were similar to those seen with the ingestion of arsenic-contaminated beer.

Increased peripheral vascular disease was also reported in individuals living in southwest Taiwan. These individuals had ingested well water that had been contaminated with arsenic for as long as 45 years (78). The concentration of arsenic in the well water ranged from 0.01 to 1.82 ppm. In a survey of 40,421 of the 44,519 exposed individuals, 7418 had hyperpigmentation, 2868 had keratosis, 428 had skin cancer, and 360 had "blackfoot disease." The "blackfoot disease," caused by severe arteriosclerosis, was associated with gangrene in approximately 70% of the individuals who were affected. Similar vascular changes were reported in German vinedressers and cellarmen who drank wine contaminated with arsenic and who were also exposed in the workplace (23). Chronic arsenic exposure in the copper smelters is associated with an increased mortality from CAD rather than from cardiomyopathy or peripheral vascular disease (10).

Cadmium

Although cadmium is nephrotoxic and a strong inducer of hypertension in animals, its role in the etiology of hypertension is unclear. Carroll reported a correlation between ambient levels of cadmium and death rates from hypertension and arteriosclerotic disease (18). Voors et al., in an autopsy study of 75 individuals, showed a correlation between increased levels of liver and aortic cadmium and heart-related deaths (86). Glauser and associates have reported a link between serum cadmium levels and the prevalence of hypertension (32). A study by Beever et al., however, does not support the link between blood cadmium and hypertension (15).

A study in rats demonstrates that as cadmium is added to the drinking water, the maximal increase in blood pressure occurs at the low-dose range. This response occurs when the cadmium intake is 10 to 20 μg/kg of body weight per day (44). It is of interest that this intake of cadmium approaches that of the average American adult. These findings may help to explain why the cardiovascular effects of cadmium are noted with exposure to the low environmental levels rather than at the relatively high levels present in the workplace.

Lead

The cardiovascular effects of lead exposure have received attention for many decades. Most of the early clinical observations of lead-related cardiovascular effects lack epidemiologic support. Chest pain, myocarditis, and conduction abnormalities, however, have been reported in children and adults with lead poisoning (31,43,56). The adults had all been exposed occupationally. The children had been exposed through the ingestion of paint chips. In a series of 30 children with blood lead greater than 60 μg/100 dL, 70% had abnormal electrocardiograms (74).

More recently epidemiologic studies have investigated the relationship between hypertension and lead exposure. A survey of newly diagnosed hypertensives in Great Britain reported a statistically significant increase in serum lead in males with hypertension (14). A positive correlation between lead levels in the liver and aorta of autopsied individuals and heart-related deaths has also been reported (86). Blood lead levels in younger men and women (aged 21–55 years) were associated with increased blood pressure. These findings were noted in a study done on about 20,000 individuals who were selected as a representative sample of the civilian, noninstitutionalized population in the United States. Individuals with diastolic blood pressures greater than or equal to 90 mm Hg had a significant increase in blood lead levels (17.9 μg/dL versus 16.9 μg/dL). Such levels are typically found among individuals without work exposure or other unusual exposure to lead (38).

Newly diagnosed male hypertensives with a serum creatinine greater than 1.5 mg/dL excreted increased lead when given a chelating agent. In contrast, newly diagnosed hypertensives with serum creatinines less than 1.5 mg/dL and individuals without hypertension but with renal disease did not excrete increased amounts of lead when given a chelating agent (13). Similar findings were noted in patients with gout. These findings suggest an association between environmental lead exposure and hypertension, particularly in individuals who also have renal impairment or gout.

Additional epidemiologic studies also lend support to the presence of a relationship between low levels of lead exposure and increases in blood pressure (35,57,77). Pirkle et al., in an analysis of NHANES II data for white males between the ages of 40 and 59, showed an association between blood lead and both systolic and diastolic blood pressures. This relationship remained even after adjustment for all factors known to be correlated with an elevation in blood pressure. The relationship between blood lead and blood pressure was characterized by large initial increments in blood pressure at relatively low blood lead levels, followed by a leveling off of blood pressure increments at high blood levels (57). This response in humans is in keeping with the biphasic increases in blood pressure observed in rodents exposed to lead (77).

Mercury

During the early part of the 1960s, in Iraq, hundreds of individuals became ill after ingesting bread contaminated with mercury. The most common symptoms involved the neurological system (insomnia, tremor of the hands, dysarthria, and ataxia). Electrocardiographic changes were reported in one case in a group of 42 patients (26).

Cobalt

An important episode of food contamination occurred in the early 1960s. Brewers in Canada began to add cobalt to beer to stabilize the foam. This increased the cobalt concentration in beer to 1.2 ppm from the usual concentration of 0.075 ppm. Within 1 month, cases of cardiomyopathy were noted in heavy beer drinkers (53). In a series of 49 cases reported from Quebec the mortality rate was 21.6%. Other series were reported from Nebraska and Minnesota and from Belgium. Only one such case has been reported in an industrial setting (11).

PATHOLOGY AND PATHOLOGICAL PHYSIOLOGY

Carbon Monoxide

Adverse health effects of carbon monoxide can be divided into those occurring acutely and those that appear only after years of chronic exposure. Chronic effects are not well documented, although it has been reported that smokers with a carboxyhemoglobin greater than 5% were 21 times more likely than those with a level less than 3% to develop myocardial infarctions, angina pectoris, and intermittent claudication (87,88). Acute exposure to carbon monoxide causes a reduction in cardiac output, a reduction in the amount of oxygen that can be transported by hemoglobin to myocardial tissues and other organs, and an inhibition of mitochondrial enzymes such as cytochrome oxidase. Carbon monoxide also binds to myoglobin. Oxygen transport to muscle mitochondria is also inhibited (79).

The possibility that atherosclerosis develops after long-term exposure to carbon monoxide is suggested by animal studies. These show increased vascular permeability, increased potential for lipid deposition in vessels, and increased platelet adhesiveness (79).

Hydrocarbons

Exposure to sufficient levels of halogenated hydrocarbons may cause a dysrhythmia. The presence of heart disease probably enhances the susceptibility to this effect. In addition to sensitizing the heart to the arrhythmogenic effect of catecholamines, halogenated hydrocarbons have a negative inotropic effect on the heart. There are numerous mechanisms that may explain the arrhythmogenic effect of the halogenated hydrocarbons. Evidence supports such mechanisms as a direct effect on the cardiac conduction system, an effect on the adrenergic and/or cholinergic receptors, and/or an effect through a change in potassium levels. A number of mechanisms have been suggested to explain the depressant effect of the halogenated hydrocarbons on the heart. These include interference with the autonomic nervous control of the heart, metabolic processes for energy production and/or utilization, and the process of excitation-contraction coupling (92).

Animal models have been used to assess the cardiotoxicity of these halogenated hydrocarbons. The following conclusions are drawn from animal testing: (1) the threshold concentration for initiation of an arrhythmia is independent of the duration of exposure; (2) sensitization of the myocardium to epinephrine after exposure to a halogenated hydrocarbon ceases once the hydrocarbon is eliminated from the bloodstream; (3) the arrhythmogenic effect varies between animal species; (4) halogenated derivatives of aliphatic hydrocarbons are more active than the corresponding unsubstituted hydrocarbons (i.e., tetrachloroethane versus ethane) (92). One classification scheme, using dogs, rated the strength of various hydrocarbons for their sensitizing properties. In this system benzene, chloroform, heptane, and trichlorethylene were the most active (59). All the fluorocarbons have some arrhythmogenic effect. Combined exposure to noise and a fluorocarbon is more sensitizing than exposure to the fluorocarbon alone (59).

Metals

Arsenic, cadmium, and mercury have a high affinity for protein sulfhydryl groups and would react with enzymes in the heart. However, the heart may be protected from the toxic effects of these heavy metals because they are preferentially concentrated in other organs (52).

Chronic arsenic ingestion is associated with "blackfoot disease." Histological studies demonstrate that this condition is secondary to arteriosclerosis obliterans or thromboangitis obliterans (78).

Myocardial involvement has been reported in cases of lead poisoning. Kline presented autopsy findings in five patients with chronic lead poisoning. Myocardial changes were described in all cases. There were cloudy swellings of the myocardial fibers, interstitial edema, and foci of inflammatory cells (43). Lead myocarditis has also been reported by other workers (31).

An increase in the urinary excretion of catecholamine metabolites is reported in children and experimental animals with lead exposure (73). Increased vagal tone has been suggested as the mechanism of atrioventricular conduction defects (55). In rats lead increases the arrhythmogenic potential of epinephrine even after a lead-free period of 4 months (90).

Cobalt

The pathology of the cobalt cardiomyopathy found in beer drinkers in the early 1960s is well described. The myocardium of all victims showed similar tissue destruction and thrombi in the heart and major arteries. Polycythemia, pericardial effusions, and thyroid hyperplasia were also found (2). Why the comparatively low doses of cobalt found in beer caused such a toxic effect has never been adequately explained. For example, an individual drinking 24 pints of beer ingested about 8 mg of cobalt. In cases of anemia, physicians have prescribed as much as 150 mg of cobalt per day. The synergistic effect of alcohol, cobalt, and a protein-poor diet has been suggested as the basis of this unique cardiomyopathy. This assumption is supported by the observation that well-nourished individuals who drank the cobalt-containing beer in amounts equal to those who developed cardiomyopathy escaped without harm (41).

CLINICAL ASPECTS OF EXPOSURE TO ENVIRONMENTAL CHEMICALS ON THE HEART AND BLOOD VESSELS

Heart disease related to environmental exposure generally does not have a unique clinical or pathological picture. For this reason a thorough history is the most important element linking heart disease to noxious exposure. The case history presented in the introduction to this chapter vividly illustrates the importance of determining a patient's activity, location, and exposure at the time symptoms occur.

Coronary Artery Disease and Peripheral Vascular Disease

The effect of carbon monoxide on the heart is linked to the duration and degree of anoxia and the condition of the myocardium. Thus, a patient with CAD will be more susceptible to carbon monoxide exposure than one with good coronary circulation. On this basis all patients complaining of myocardial ischemic pain should be asked about their exposure to chemicals. The clinician must search for an environmental cause when assessing the frequency of symptoms and their relationship to activity and location. In addition to ischemic pain, carbon-monoxide-exposed individuals may complain of headache, dizziness, drowsiness, or nausea. It is well to remember that ischemic symptoms can appear long before the "classic" picture of carbon monoxide poisoning occurs. Thus, the cherry red color of the skin or mucous membranes is rarely seen (89).

Intermittent claudication, a symptom caused by circulatory insufficiency, may be increased with exposure to carbon monoxide (9). As a result, an exposure history must be obtained in all patients with symptoms of intermittent claudication.

The laboratory is very helpful in cases of excessive carbon monoxide exposure. Carboxyhemoglobin is easily measured: an arterial blood gas is not necessary; venous blood collected in a heparinized tube can be used. This determination is most important, as the likelihood of developing symptoms from exposure to carbon monoxide increases with the level of blood carboxyhemoglobin. Environmental measurement of carbon monoxide can discover the source of the exposure. An instantaneous monitor with a probe is the best method for finding the source of the carbon monoxide.

Dysrhythmias

Dysrhythmias may be produced with exposure to halogenated hydrocarbons or carbon monoxide. Additional symptoms may include recurrent dizziness, headaches, lightheadedness, and nausea. Individuals with chronic exposure to halogenated hydrocarbons may also have eye or noise irritation, reddened pharyngeal mucosa, tearing, or a runny nose.

Depending on the particular solvent, abnormalities in blood, kidney, or liver function may be found. Renal tubular acidosis, for example, is described in individuals who sniff toluene. Actual measurement of the chemical in serum, exhaled air, or as a metabolite in the urine is sometimes possible. Dysrhythmias from chemical exposure have no distinguishing characteristics. They can be supraventricular or ventricular in origin. Continuous EKG monitoring accompanied by a diary of activity can document the relationship between exposure and dysrhythmia. Air sampling performed at the location where the patient is symptomatic is also useful in confirming the diagnosis.

Cardiomyopathy

Many agents have an adverse effect on the myocardium and may cause cardiomyopathy. Included in this list are alcohol, hormones, and such drugs as antibiotics, antineoplastic, and psychotherapeutic agents. Of the agents encountered in the workplace and general environment, the metallic compounds have a direct toxic effect on the myocardium and peripheral vasculature.

The cardiovascular findings associated with chronic arsenic exposure may include Raynaud's syndrome, acrocyanosis, and hypertension. Peripheral vascular disease with keratosis, hyperpigmentation, and/or skin cancer in non-sun-exposed areas suggest arsenic exposure (23).

Changes in the electrocardiogram may appear with lead and mercury exposures. For lead, the abnormalities reported include tachycardia, atrial arrhythmias, both shortening and prolongation of PR intervals, prolongation of QT intervals, inversion of T waves over the lateral precordium, and wide QRS-T angles. Severe abnormalities may be found among children with a marked elevation in blood lead. For mercury, the predominant findings may include ST segment depression, prolongation of the QT interval, and multifocal and multiple ventricular ectopic beats.

To confirm exposure, biological measurements of the appropriate heavy metal can be made. Prolonged subacute exposure, giving rise to the findings described above, would undoubtedly be associated with abnormal levels. For arsenic, determinations are done in urine. Hair may also be used, as it is a good reflection of the amount of inorganic arsenic absorbed during its growth. Care is needed in interpreting urinary arsenic levels because values up to 200 μg/L may be found, depending on dietary intake (50). Blood lead and erythrocytic protoporphyrin levels are commonly done to evaluate lead exposure. Urinary and serum levels are usually performed for evaluating mercury exposure (50).

Hypertension

Although the link between hypertension and toxic exposure is not well established, clinicians should obtain an exposure history in all patients with hypertension. A history of heavy metal exposure is particularly important in individuals with renal disease, since some human studies have reported an association between cadmium and lead exposure and hypertension (13,32,38,57). The fact that most cases of hypertension occur without known cause lends further support to a search for exogenous factors that increase the risk of this common disease.

Clinical Management

The clinical management of heart disease related to chemical exposure is similar to that for heart disease caused by other factors. In addition, however, it is important to eliminate or lower the exposure.

Governmental authorities currently monitor air quality and recommend that the elderly and the chronically ill stay indoors and reduce strenuous activities during air pollution alerts. Individual practitioners can lend their support to this recommendation.

In some instances it is possible to provide specific therapy along with eliminating the exposure. For example, with excessive exposure to carbon monoxide, oxygen is administered. Inhaled carbon monoxide is generally excreted in 4 to 5 h. With oxygen administration this time is reduced. Oxygen replaces the carbon monoxide in the hemoglobin molecule and also provides additional oxygen dissolved in the blood. With severe intoxication hyperbaric oxygen can further increase the excretion of carbon monoxide (42).

Chelating agents such as EDTA and BAL are indicated for heavy metal intoxication in situations where symptoms or organ damage requires an immediate reduction in heavy metal body burdens. Under these conditions removing the patient from the source of exposure is not enough to give a rapid therapeutic response. For lead, a reversal in the cardiac findings is seen with chelation therapy. In one series, only four of 30 (13%) electrocardiograms remained abnormal after chelation therapy (74). In another report, a child's congestive heart failure and encephalopathy were reversed after treatment with a chelating agent (31).

SUMMARY

Although we have relatively little understanding of the risks that chemical exposure imposes on the cardiovascular system, there is increasing evidence that carbon monoxide, at levels present in the general environment, has the potential to exacerbate myocardial ischemia in patients with coronary artery disease. Adverse cardiovascular effects may also occur with exposure to metals, chemicals, and other gases. It is therefore necessary that clinicians consider such exposure when evaluating patients with cardiovascular disease.

REFERENCES

1. Agocs MM, Etzel RA, Parrish RG, et al: Mercury exposure from interior latex paint. N Engl J Med 323: 1096, 1990.

2. Alexander CS: Cobalt and the heart. Ann Intern Med 70:411, 1969.
3. Allred EN, Bleecker ER, Chaitman BR, et al: Short-term effects of carbon monoxide exposure on the exercise performance of subjects with coronary artery disease. N Engl J Med 321:1426, 1989.
4. Anderson EW, Andelman RJ, Strauch JM, et al: Effects of low-level carbon monoxide exposure on onset and duration of angina pectoris: A study on 10 patients with ischemic heart disease. Ann Intern Med 79:46, 1970.
5. Anderson TW, Neri LC, Shreiber GB, et al: Ischemic heart disease, water hardness and myocardial magnesium. Can Med Assoc J 113:199, 1975.
6. Aronow WS: Effect of ambient level of carbon monoxide on cardiopulmonary disease. Chest 74:1, 1978.
7. Aronow WS, Cassidy J: Effect of carbon monoxide on maximal treadmill exercise: A study of normal persons. Ann Intern Med 83:496, 1975.
8. Aronow WS, Harris CN, Isbell MW, et al: Effect of freeway travel on angina pectoris. Ann Intern Med 72:669, 1972.
9. Aronow WS, Stemmer EA, Isbell MW: Effect of carbon monoxide exposure on intermittent claudication. Circulation 49:415, 1974.
10. Axelson O, Dahlgreen E, Jonsson CD, et al: Arsenic exposure and mortality: A case referent study from a Swedish copper smelter. Br J Ind Med 35:360, 1978.
11. Barborik JM, Dusek J: Cardiomyopathy accompanying industrial cobalt exposure. Br Heart J 34:113, 1972.
12. Bass M: Sudden sniffing death. JAMA 21:2075, 1970.
13. Batuman V, Landy E, Maesaka JK, et al: Contribution of lead to hypertension with renal impairment. N Engl J Med 309:17, 1983.
14. Beevers DG, Erskine E, Robertson M: Blood lead and hypertension. Lancet 2:1, 1976.
15. Beevers DG, Goldberg A, Campbell BC, et al: Blood cadmium in hypertensives and normotensives. Lancet 2:1222, 1976.
16. Behr G, Burton P: Heart-muscle magnesium. Lancet 2:450, 1973.
17. Borgono JM, Greiber R: Epidemiological study of arsenicism in the city of Antofagosta. In: Proceedings of the University of Missouri's 5th Annual Conference on Trace Substances in Environmental Health, p 13, Hemphill DD (ed.), University of Missouri, Columbia, 1972.
18. Carroll RE: The relationship of cadmium in the air to cardiovascular disease death rates. JAMA 198:177, 1966.
19. Clarkson TW: Mercury—an element of mystery. N Engl J Med 323:1137, 1990.
20. Coburn RF, Forster RE, Kane PB: Consideration of the physiological variables that determine the blood carboxyhemoglobin in man. J Clin Invest 44:1899, 1965.
21. Cohen RI, Deane M, Goldsmith JR: CO and survival from myocardial infarction. Arch Environ Health 19:510, 1969.
22. Committee on Lead in the Human Environment, National Research Council: Lead in the Human Environment, National Academy Press, Washington, 1980.
23. Committee on Medical and Biologic Effects of Environmental Pollutants, National Research Council: Arsenic, National Academy Press, Washington, 1977.
24. Committee on Medical and Biological Effects of Environmental Pollutants, National Research Council: Carbon Monoxide, National Academy Press, Washington, 1977.
25. Comstock GWG: Water hardness and cardiovascular disease. Am J Epidemiol 110:375, 1979.
26. Dahhan SS, Orfaly H: Electrocardiographic changes in mercury poisoning. Am J Cardiol 14:178, 1964.
27. DeBias DA, Banerjee CM, Birkhead NC, et al: Effects of CO inhalation on ventricular fibrillation. Arch Environ Health 31:42, 1976.
28. Dudley EF, Beldin RA, Johnson BC: Climate water hardness and coronary artery disease. J Chron Dis 22:25, 1969.
29. Elwood PC, St. Leger AS, Morton M: Mortality and the concentration of elements in tap water in county boroughs in England and Wales. Br J Prev Soc Med 31:178, 1977.
30. Frank R: Are aerosol sprays hazardous? Am Rev Respir Dis 112:485, 1975.
31. Freeman R: Reversible myocarditis due to chronic lead poisoning in childhood. Arch Dis Child 40:389, 1965.
32. Glauser SC, Bello CT, Glauser EM: Blood-cadmium levels in normotensive and untreated hypertensive humans. Lancet 1:717, 1976.
33. Goldsmith JR: CO research—recent and remote. Arch Environ Health 21:118, 1970.
34. Goldsmith JR, Aronow WS: Carbon monoxide and coronary heart disease: A review. Environ Res 10:236, 1975.
35. Goyer RA: Lead toxicity: From overt to subclinical to subtle health effects. Environ Health Perspect 86:177, 1990.
36. Hackney JD: Relationship between air pollution and cardiovascular disease: A review. In: Clinical Implication of Air Pollution Research, p 89, Finkel AJ, Duel WC (eds.), Publishing Sciences Group, Acton, MA, 1974.
37. Hammond EC: Smoking in relation to death rates of one million men and women. In: Epidemiological Approaches to the Study of Cancer and Other Diseases, p 1, Hanzel W (ed.), US Public Health Service, National Cancer Institute, Monograph 19, Bethesda, 1966.
38. Harlan WR, Landis JR, Schmouder RL, et al: Blood lead and blood pressure relationship in the adolescent and adult US population. JAMA 253:530, 1985.
39. Heimann H: Effects of air pollution on human health. In: Air Pollution, p 159, Columbia University Press, World Health Organization, New York, 1961.
40. Iglewicz R, Rosenman KD, Iglewicz B, et al: Elevated levels of carbon monoxide in the patient compartment of ambulances. Am J Public Health 74:511, 1984.
41. Kesteloot H, Roelandt J, Williams J, et al: Enquiry into the role of cobalt in the heart of disease of chronic drinkers. Circulation 37:854, 1968.
42. Kindwall EP: Carbon monoxide. In: Occupational Medicine: Principles and Practical Applications, 2nd ed., p 563, Zenz C (ed.), CRC Press, Boca Raton, 1990.
43. Kline TS: Myocardial changes in lead poisoning. AMA J Dis Child 99:48, 1960.
44. Kopp SJ, Gloner J, Parry HM, et al: Cardiovascular actions of cadmium at environmental exposure levels. Science 217:837, 1982.

45. Kreiss K, Zack MM, Kimbrough RD, et al: Association of blood pressure and polychlorinated biphenyl levels. JAMA 245:2505, 1981.

46. Kristensen TS: Cardiovascular diseases and the work environment. A critical review of the epidemiologic literature on chemical factors. Scand J Work Environ Health 15:245, 1989.

47. Kuller LH, Cooper M, Perper J: Epidemiology of sudden death. Arch Intern Med: 129:714, 1972.

48. Kuller LH, Radford EP, Swift D, et al: Carbon monoxide and heart attacks. Arch Environ Health 30:477, 1975.

49. Kurt TL, Moglielnicki RP, Chandler JE: Association of the frequency of acute cardiorespiratory complaints with ambient levels of carbon monoxide. Chest 74:10, 1978.

50. Lauwerys RR: Industrial Chemical Exposure: Guidelines for Biological Monitoring, Biomedical Publications, Davis, CA, 1983.

51. Logan WPD: Mortality in the London fog incident, 1952. Lancet 1:336, 1953.

52. Magos L: The effects of industrial chemicals on the heart. In: Cardiac Toxicology, Vol II, p 203, Balazs T (ed.), CRC Press, Boca Raton, 1981.

53. Morin YL, Foley AR, Martineau G, et al: Quebec beer-drinkers' cardiomyopathy. Can Med Assoc J 97:881, 1967.

54. Morris JN, Crawford MD, Heady JA: Hardness of local water supplies and mortality from vascular disease. Lancet 1:869, 1961.

55. Myerson RM, Eisenhaver JH: Atrioventricular conduction defects in lead poisoning. Am J Cardiol 11:409, 1963.

56. Petronio L: Chemical and physical agents of work-related cardiovascular disease. Eur Heart J 9(Suppl): 26, 1988.

57. Pirkle JL, Schwartz J, Landis JR, et al: The relationship between blood lead levels and blood pressure and its cardiovascular risks. Am J Epidemiol 121:246, 1985.

58. Radford EP, Drizd TA: Blood Carbon Monoxide Levels in Persons 3–74 Years of Age: United States, 1976–1980. Advanced Data from Vital and Health Statistics of the National Center for Health Statistics, DHHS (PHS)82-1250 76:24, 1982.

59. Reinhardt CF, Azar A, Maxfield ME, et al: Cardiac arrhythmias and aerosol "sniffing." Arch Environ Health 22:265, 1971.

60. Reynolds ES: Epidemic of arsenical poisoning in beer-drinkers in the north of England during the year 1900. Lancet 1:98, 1901.

61. Reynolds ES: An account of the epidemic outbreak of arsenical poisoning occurring in beer drinkers in the north of England and midland countries in 1900. Lancet 1:166, 1901.

62. Rosenman KD: Cardiovascular disease and environmental exposure. Br J Ind Med 36:85, 1979.

63. Rosenman KD: Environmentally related disorders of the cardiovascular system. Med Clin North Am 74: 361, 1990.

64. Safe Drinking Water Committee, National Research Council: Drinking Water and Health, National Academy Press, Washington, 1977.

65. Samet JM, Marbury MC, Spengler JD: Health effects and sources of indoor air pollution. Am Rev Respir Dis 136:1486, 1987.

66. Sandifer SH, Keil JE: Pesticide exposure: Association with cardiovascular risk factors. In: Proceeding of the University of Missouri's 5th Annual Conference on Trace Substances in Environmental Health, p 329, Hemphill DD (ed.), University of Missouri, Columbia, 1972.

67. Schrenk H, Heinmann H, Clayton GD, et al: Air pollution in Donora, Pennsylvania. Epidemiology of the unusual smog episode of October 1948. Public Health Bull 306, U.S. Government Printing Office, Washington, 1949.

68. Schroeder HA: Relation between mortality from cardiovascular disease and treated water supplies. JAMA 172:1902, 1960.

69. Schroeder HA: Municipal drinking water and cardiovascular death rates. JAMA 195:81, 1966.

70. Schroeder HA, Kraemer LA: Cardiovascular mortality, municipal water and corrosion. Arch Environ Health 28:303, 1974.

71. Sharret AR: Water hardness and cardiovascular disease. Americal Heart Association Task Force Report. Circulation 63:247A, 1981.

72. Sheps DS, Herbst MC, Hinderliter AL, et al: Production of arrhythmias by elevated carboxyhemoglobin in patients with coronary artery disease. Ann Intern Med 113:343, 1990.

73. Silbergeld EK, Chisolm JJ Jr: Lead poisoning: Altered urinary catecholamine metabolites as indicators of intoxication in mice and children. Science 192:153, 1976.

74. Silver W, Rodrigues-Torres R: Electrocardiographic studies in children with lead poisoning. Pediatrics 41: 1124, 1968.

75. Speizer FE, Wegman DH, Ramirez A: Palpitation rate associated with fluorocarbon exposure in a hospital setting. N Engl J Med 292:624, 1975.

76. Stewart RD, Hake CL: Paint remover hazard. JAMA 235:398, 1976.

77. Symposium on Lead-Blood Pressure Relationships: Environ Health Perspect 78:139, 1988.

78. Tseng WP, Chu HM, How SW, et al: Prevalence of skin cancer in an endemic area of chronic arsenicism in Taiwan. J Natl Cancer Inst 40:453, 1964.

79. Turino GM: Effect of carbon monoxide on the cardiorespiratory system. Carbon monoxide toxicity: Physiology and biochemistry. American Health Association Task Force Report. Circulation 63:253A, 1981.

80. US Department of Health Education and Welfare: The Health Consequences of Smoking, NIH 76-1221:230, USDHEW, 1975.

81. US Department of Health Education and Welfare: Smoking and Health: A Report of the Surgeon General, Publication #79-50066, USDHEW, Washington, 1979.

82. US Environmental Protection Agency: Proceedings Conference on Wood Combustion Emissions Assessment, EPA-600/9-81029, USEPA, Washington, 1981.

83. Urabe H, Kada H, Asahi M: Present state of Yusho patients. Ann NY Acad Sci 120:273, 1979.

84. Valic F, Skuric Z, Bantic A, et al: Effects of fluorocarbon propellants on respiratory flow and ECG. Br J Ind Med 34:130, 1977.

85. Voors AW: Minerals in the municipal water and atherosclerotic heart disease. Am J Epidemiol 93:259, 1971.

86. Voors AW, Johnson WD, Shuman MS: Additive statis-

tical effect of cadmium and lead on heart-related disease in a North Carolina autopsy series. Arch Environ Health 37:98, 1982.

87. Wald M, Howard S, Smith PE, et al: Association between atherosclerotic disease and carboxyhemoglobin levels in tobacco smokers. Br Med J 1:761, 1973.

88. Weir FW, Fabiano UL: Reevaluation of the role of carbon monoxide in production of aggravation of cardiovascular disease processes. J Occup Med 24:519, 1982.

89. Whorton MD: Carbon monoxide intoxication: A review of 14 patients. J Am Coll Emerg Physicians 5:505, 1976.

90. Williams BJ, Griffith WH, Albrecht CM, et al: Effects of chronic lead treatment on some cardiovascular responses to norepinephrine in the rate. Toxicol Appl Pharmacol 40:407, 1977.

91. Wright GR, Jewczyk S, Onrot J, et al: Carbon monoxide in the urban atmosphere hazards to the pedestrian and the street-worker. Arch Environ Health 30:123, 1975.

92. Zakhari S, Alviado DM: Cardiovascular toxicology of aerosol propellants, refrigerants, and related solvents. In: Cardiovascular Toxicology, p 281, Van Stee EW (ed.), Raven Press, New York, 1982.

RECOMMENDED READINGS

Kristensen TS: Cardiovascular diseases and the work environment: A critical review of the epidemiologic literature on chemical factors. Scand J Work Environ Health 15:245, 1989.

Rosenman KD: Cardiovascular disease and environmental exposure. Br J Ind Med 36:85, 1979.

Rosenman KD: Environmentally related disorders of the cardiovascular system. Med Clin North Am 74:361, 1990.

18.   DISORDERS OF THE DIGESTIVE SYSTEM

John G. Banwell and Peter Yang

INTRODUCTION

The major function of the digestive system is to provide for the nutrient requirements of the host in the form of water, electrolytes, protein, carbohydrate, fat, vitamins, and macro- and micronutrients. In carrying out this function, the gastrointestinal tract is inevitably exposed to a variety of foreign chemical compounds that may have a deleterious action on intestinal functions. This chapter is concerned with the adverse effects of environmental chemicals entering the gastrointestinal tract.

Since very early times, it has been recognized that many naturally occurring toxic materials are found in foodstuffs (9,38). In today's environment, however, food and water contain an important source of new and potentially toxic compounds. These compounds include complex inorganic and organic chemicals, heavy metals, plasticizers, food additives, such agricultural chemicals as pesticides and fertilizers, and many other industrial agents (6,12,18,40,42,44,70). Unlike food additives, environmental contaminants enter the food supply inadvertently. Although such contamination is generally long-term and in low concentration, many well-documented incidences of high-level contamination have been recorded (1,42).

Physicians have traditionally developed skills to identify certain diseases of occupational origin and illnesses caused by the ingestion of poisons. However, specialized new skills and knowledge are now required if physicians are to identify the adverse health effects of environmental contamination by the wide variety of chemical agents used in industry and in the home. The physician's task is particularly difficult because environmental chemicals are generally present in low concentrations over long periods of time (12,40–42, 44). In addition, knowledge of biological processes gained during the last 20 years emphasizes the delayed effects of exposure exerted through genetic influences, the transplacental passage of chemicals, and the initiation and promotion of carcinogenesis (26,47).

Physicians must play a much wider and more complex role, which varies from identifying the characteristic clinical features of acute poisoning to defining new diseases caused by exposure to environmental chemicals. They must be aware that some adverse reactions to chemical agents occur only in particularly susceptible individuals (39,43). The reader is referred to Chapter 12 for a detailed discussion of this issue. Clinicians have the added responsibility of advising patients on methods of reducing exposure to environmental chemicals and devising strategies to be observed once exposure has occurred.

ENVIRONMENTAL CHEMICALS ASSOCIATED WITH ADVERSE EFFECTS ON THE DIGESTIVE SYSTEM

The number and quantity of chemical substances entering the environment have increased steadily since the Industrial Revolution. Initially, clinical concern for certain contaminants was raised by epidemiologists who observed that exposure to

Principles and Practice of Environmental Medicine, edited by Alyce Bezman Tarcher. Plenum Medical Book Company, New York, 1992.

particular compounds (lead poisoning in paint workers, scrotal cancer in chimney sweeps, and leukemia in fluorescent dye workers are examples) could lead to specific disabilities. Gradually, the risk to health from chemically contaminated water and food was recognized.

In the past, man-made chemicals caused much less illness than did naturally occurring toxic agents. However, recent episodes of food contamination, particularly with agricultural chemicals, indicate that constant control must be exercised to avoid adverse health effects (1,42). In a survey of the 50 states requested by the U.S. Congress, the Office of Technology Assessment reported 243 episodes of environmental contamination of food between 1968 and 1978 (42). Inadvertent or accidental contamination of food may result from agricultural, mining, and industrial activities (42) (see Chapter 3). Table 18-1 lists some of the environmental chemicals that commonly enter the digestive system.

Direct exposure of the digestive system to environmental chemicals occurs via the mouth, through swallowing of contaminated material, or through swallowing mucus that contains inhaled materials. Indirect exposure may occur from agents introduced via the skin, through parenteral administration, and from materials entering from the biliary tract. The adverse effects of environmental chemicals on the digestive system depend on whether their action causes direct injury to the intestinal cell surface, affects the metabolism of the intestinal cell, affects the host's immune system, or affects the intestinal microbial flora. Table 18-2 presents a summary of the potential adverse gastrointestinal reactions to various foreign chemicals.

EPIDEMIOLOGY

Epidemiologic studies of gastrointestinal diseases have implicated environmental factors, primarily in the etiology of gastrointestinal cancer. By comparing the type and incidence of cancer in populations with different eating habits, life styles, and occupations and noting the changes that occur with migration, epidemiologists have determined that the development of certain types of cancer depends more on environmental factors than on genetic makeup (24,47,59).

Epidemiologic studies have implicated environmental factors in the development of esophageal, gastric, and colon cancer. Data thus far indict smoking, alcohol consumption, nutrition, genetic susceptibility, and low socioeconomic status in the pathogenesis of gastrointestinal cancer, rather than variations in exposure to chemical carcinogens (59). Studies reveal that nutritional factors, in particular, may play an important role in the development of stomach and colon cancer (59). The identification and quantitation of the dietary determinants of cancer are of major interest (8,59).

Asbestos Exposure and Gastrointestinal Cancer

Although chemical agents have not been implicated in the etiology of gastrointestinal cancer, asbestos exposure may play a role in the development of esophageal, gastric, and colorectal cancers (11, 53). This relationship, however, is much less clear than the well-established correlation between asbestos exposure in the workplace and the development

TABLE 18-1. Environmental Chemicals Entering the Digestive System through the Contamination of Food[a]

Source	Chemical	Foods contaminated
Agriculture	Pesticides	Meats, fish, poultry, dairy products
	Organochlorine	
	DDT and related compounds	
	Organophosphates and carbamates	Grains and cereals
	Diazinon, carbaryl, and related compounds	Fruits and vegetables
Industry		
Electrical	Polychlorinated biphenyls (PCBs)	Fish, human milk
Wood preservative	Pentachlorophenol	Various foods
Impurities in chlorophenols	Dioxin	Fish, cow's milk, beef fat
Smelters	Arsenic	Seafood
Smelters, sewer sludge	Cadmium	Grains, vegetables, meat, fish
Auto exhaust, canning industry	Lead	Grains, vegetables, canned foods
Electrical apparatus, control equipment	Mercury	Fish, seafood

[a]Derived from references 12, 41, 42, 44, and 70.

TABLE 18-2. Potential Adverse Gastrointestinal Reactions to Chemical Exposure

Chemical agent	Gastrointestinal reaction
Carcinogens	
Asbestos	Gastrointestinal cancer
Acrylonitrile	Gastric, duodenal ulcers
Butylated hydroxytoluene	Stomach hyperplasia and cancer
Polycyclic hydrocarbons	Stomach cancer
Corrosive poisons	
Strong alkali/acid	Esophagus, gastric necrosis
Organic compounds	
Phenol/Lysol	Esophagus, gastric necrosis
Volatile agents (ethyl alcohol)	Gastritis
Nitrosoguanidines	Gastritis
Inorganic compounds	
Nonmetallic	
Phosphorus	Mucosal erosions: stomach and intestine
Metallic	
Arsenic, bismuth, copper, gold, manganese, nickel, vanadium	Gastritis, vascular congestion, mucosal sloughing of intestine

of lung cancer and mesothelioma. The incidence of gastrointestinal cancer in relation to asbestos exposure has been studied in two different groups: populations ingesting contaminated water supplies and individuals exposed in the workplace.

A number of epidemiologic studies have investigated populations whose municipal water supplies are contaminated with asbestos from natural mineral deposits, industry, or water pipes (34). The incidence of gastrointestinal cancers was studied in six geographic areas (San Francisco, Duluth, Quebec, Connecticut, Florida, and western Washington) in the United States and Canada (34). Although some studies suggest an increased risk, no consistent increase in the incidence of gastrointestinal cancer was noted. A review of the reports on 21 cohorts of workers exposed to asbestos failed to show evidence of increased risk for colorectal cancer (69). All of these epidemiologic studies were limited, particularly by the inability to determine the degree of asbestos exposure (11,30).

Studies reveal that peritoneal mesotheliomas are clearly linked to asbestos exposure in the workplace (11). In contrast, studies of various groups of asbestos workers reveal an increased incidence of gastrointestinal cancer in some but not all of the occupational groups (11,37,53). In many cases, epidemiologic studies examining the risk of gastrointestinal cancer in asbestos workers were hampered by possible diagnostic inaccuracy and by a failure to specify where within the gastrointestinal tract the cancer occurred (30,37). To date, many attempts to induce gastrointestinal tumor in animals by administering oral doses of asbestos have yielded negative results (11).

A number of reports point to excessive gastrointestinal disease and cancer in textile workers, metal workers, and chemical workers (2,46,50,62, 66). These findings may warrant further epidemiologic investigation.

Nitrosamines and Gastric Cancer

Nitrates and related compounds present in such dietary sources as drinking water, cured meats, and cereals have been implicated in the etiology of stomach cancer (19,21,63). Armijo and Coulson reported a strong correlation between the use of nitrate fertilizer in Chile and the death rate from gastric cancer (4). Other studies in Colombia, Japan, Iran, China, England, and the United States (Hawaii) reveal a relationship between the intake of food and water with high levels of nitrate or nitrite and an increased incidence of gastric cancer (5,13, 14,19,23).

Although these studies suggest an association between nitrates and related compounds and stomach cancer, they do not provide clear evidence of such a relationship (10).

PATHOLOGY AND PATHOLOGICAL PHYSIOLOGY

As a portal of entry, the gastrointestinal mucosa may be exposed to high concentrations of many xenobiotics in food (42). No other organ can be challenged by such a variety of harmful chemicals as the intestinal mucosa. It is a source of astonishment that the gut mucosa has evolved mechanisms that seem to deal so effectively with toxic agents. The mechanisms for this resistance reside in certain physiological and biochemical characteristics of the gastrointestinal tract. In particular, they reside in (1) the integrated response of nausea and vomiting, which results in the rejection of materials entering the stomach (61); (2) the denaturation and inactivation of some toxic materials by the acid-peptic environment of the stomach; (3) the secretion of intestinal fluids that dilute toxic agents in the bowel lumen (56); (4) the intraluminal and intracellular biodegradation of toxic agents (7,20,45); (5) the presence of a mucus layer, which reduces the access of foreign materials to the intestinal cells (17,35); (6) the rapid turnover and shedding of epithelial cells, which help rid the body of ingested toxins (16); (7) the presence of plasma membranes and glycoproteins, which may affect the absorption of toxic agents (29); (8) the degradation of certain foreign agents by the gut microflora (55); and (9) the excretion of toxic agents in fecal waste, which may be facilitated by increased bowel motility and the induction of diarrhea. Chapter 8 presents a detailed discussion of gastrointestinal defenses against exposure to environmental chemicals.

A variety of different experimental methods may be used to assess the effects of exposure to environmental chemicals on: (1) the histology of the mucosal surface, (2) mucosal cell proliferation, (3) nutrient absorption by the intestine, and (4) intestinal motility (67).

Many of the studies that assess the effects of toxic agents exposure have been performed on animals. The results of using animals to define toxicity for man and the mechanisms of injury caused by xenobiotics and other chemicals may be difficult to interpret because of interspecies variability. Such differences include anatomic variations (e.g., ruminant versus monogastric), the distribution and composition of the intestinal microflora, and functional differences in the small bowel mucosa. In this context, correlation of carcinogens causing gastrointestinal tumors in animals with the human disease counterpart may be limited. Examples would include dimethylhydrazine for induction of colon carcinoma and the induction of duodenal ulcer in rats by acetonitrile.

In general, the effects of chronic low-dose exposure to environmental chemicals on intestinal function have not been examined in any detail in man or in animals (54). Few studies have investigated the specific effects of various environmental contaminants on the gastrointestinal tract. Little is known, for example, about the effect of such exposure on active or facilitated transport or passive diffusion in the gut.

Effects of Foreign Chemicals on Cell Membranes

The brush border membrane of the intestinal cell is the site at which cell contents are separated from the luminal environment. Toxic chemicals may affect transport processes in the cell membrane (48). Changes in passive cation permeability occur when red blood cells are exposed to heavy metals and when p-chloromercury phenylsulfonate alters anionic permeability channels (51). The Na^+, K^+-ATPase pump is sensitive to organochlorine compounds: DDT may act as a noncompetitive inhibitor through its interaction with the hydrophobic regions of the protein or lipid membrane (27). Sodium-coupled intestinal sugar transport has been studied by utilizing intestinal membrane vesicles. Mercury has been shown to impair the carrier function in this system (48).

Other Toxic Actions on Mucosal Cells

Rats treated with malathion show reduced glucose and glycine absorption associated with a depression of brush border membrane disaccharide activity. In contrast, dieldrin augments glucose uptake and is associated with increased disaccharidase activity (57). Lipid assimilation is augmented in rats exposed to 2,3,7,8-tetrachlorodibenzo-p-dioxin (TCDD or "dioxin"). However, no specific physiological effect was observed on monosaccharide or amino transport absorption sites (58).

Mucosal Metabolism of Foreign Compounds

Once absorbed into the intestinal mucosa, xenobiotics may undergo biotransformation before they pass into the general circulation. Xenobiotic metabolism is catalyzed by the cytochrome P-450-dependent mixed-function oxidases (monooxygenases). This microsomal system, which modifies foreign chemicals so that they can be excreted by the kidney, may also generate highly cytotoxic reactive metabolites. The digestive system has been shown to be well supplied with the biochemical pathways necessary for the biotransformation of foreign chemicals (71). Chapter 8 discusses the mechanisms by which the gastrointestinal tract guards against exposure to environmental chemicals, including their metabolism by the intestinal mucosa. Chapter 9 discusses in detail the biotransformation of foreign chemicals.

Nitrosamines and Gastric Cancer

Specific chemical carcinogens have not been clearly identified in the pathogenesis of gastrointestinal cancer in humans. However, a link between gastric cancer and a broad class of compounds containing the N-nitroso group is provided by the epidemiologic finding previously mentioned and by the evidence that these compounds are potent carcinogens in experimental animals (31,33).

Interest in the association between the dietary

nitrates and cancer of the stomach stems from the recognition that nitrates and nitrites, though not in themselves carcinogenic, can lead to the formation of carcinogenic nitrosamines. This reaction is known to occur within the human intestine through the action of the gastrointestinal microflora (49). N-Nitroso compounds (nitrosamines and nitrosamides) are formed when amines and amides react with nitrite (31). Although preformed nitrosamines may be present in such foods as nitrite-cured meats, some cheeses, fish, and beer, their formation within the body is quantitatively more important (63,64).

Studies show that nitrosamines are formed in saliva and gastric juice by the combination of nitrite with secondary and tertiary amines (32,60). The secondary and tertiary amines are derived from dietary sources. The nitrites are formed, largely from ingested nitrates, through the action of nitrite-reducing bacteria present in saliva and gastric juice (52,65). Nitrite concentrations in gastric juice therefore depend on the level of dietary nitrate and on bacterial populations having nitrate-reducing activity. Dietary nitrate is widely distributed in drinking water, in such foods as cured meats and some cheeses, and in foods contaminated by nitrate fertilizers (63). It is of interest that increased concentrations of nitrate are being found in rivers and ground water throughout the world. Most of the nitrate is derived from inorganic and organic nitrogen fertilizers, which leach from the soil. The nitrate contamination of ground water is of particular concern because, in many regions, it is the source of drinking water (see Chapter 4).

It has been postulated that gastric cancer may be related to the endogenous formation of nitrosamines in the stomach (25,68). This hypothesis is supported by the following evidence. Low gastric acidity is found in conditions associated with atrophic gastritis or following peptic ulcer operations. These conditions are known to have a predisposition to gastric cancer. An increased number of nitrite-forming bacteria are found in the stomachs of individuals with reduced gastric acidity (49). Bacterial proliferation in the stomach is noted to be a function of gastric acidity. Reduced gastric acidity appears to allow the proliferation of nitrate-reducing bacteria within the stomach (the stomachs of normal persons are relatively sterile except immediately after eating).

An inverse relationship between gastric nitrite concentration and hydrogen ion concentration is reported, with hypochlorhydric subjects having a significant increase in gastric juice nitrite concentration (52). A positive correlation is noted in humans between gastric pH and nitrosamine concentration and between gastric pH and an increase in the concentration of nitrites (49,52). A significant relationship is also reported between raised nitro-

samine and nitrite levels in gastric juice and the growth of nitrate-reducing bacteria. Increased levels of nitrosamine are reported in patients with gastric cancer and in conditions associated with or conducive to gastric cancer (49). Patients with pernicious anemia, atrophic gastritis, partial gastrectomy, and vagotomy had nitrosamine levels similar to those measured in patients with gastric carcinoma (49).

It has been postulated that the marked decrease in the incidence of gastric cancer in the United States over the past four decades may be related to the widespread use of refrigeration, which inhibits the conversion of nitrate to nitrite, and to lowering the amount of nitrate that is used in food additives. In addition, there is evidence that the formation of N-nitroso compounds in chemical systems, in nitrite-preserved meat, in humans, and in experimental animals is inhibited by the presence of vitamins C and E (36).

CLINICAL ASPECTS OF EXPOSURE TO ENVIRONMENTAL CHEMICALS ON THE DIGESTIVE SYSTEM

Except for cases of acute poisoning, there is little evidence of a link between exposure to environmental chemicals and gastrointestinal disease. Nevertheless, physicians should be alert to the possibility of such a relationship. Information on past and present toxic exposure should be obtained from all patients suffering from gastrointestinal disease. The onset of such acute symptoms as nausea, vomiting, colicky pain, and diarrhea, in particular, should elicit questions about recent changes in occupational and environmental exposures. Even in cases in which the gastrointestinal symptoms are unrelated to toxic exposure, the questions may be of value. They may, by alerting the patient to the dangers of toxic exposure, help in the early recognition and control of such exposure.

Gastrointestinal Injury Caused by Caustic Agents

Ingestion of a variety of caustic agents may cause a wide range of injuries to the gastrointestinal mucosal surfaces. The severity and frequency of such injuries have increased since the introduction of concentrated liquid alkaline and acid cleaners in the 1960s. Accidental intake characteristically occurs in children when such agents are mistaken for other solutions (e.g., milk). Psychotic and suicidal persons and those suffering from alcoholism are also at risk for such exposure.

Caustic injury to the gastrointestinal tract is usually produced by the ingestion of strong alkali or strong acids. Sodium and potassium hydroxides in liquid or granular form are used as drain cleaners, washing powders, soaps, and in Clinitest® tablets. Their concentration may range from 9% in liquid form to 100% in the solids. Acids are commonly used in toilet bowl cleansers, antirust compounds, battery fluid, and swimming pool cleaners. Other fluids used to clean drains may contain sodium or ammonium hypochlorite.

Alkaline agents are often tasteless and odorless. They rapidly penetrate into tissues and cause solubilization of the lipid components of cell membranes. This produces liquefactive necrosis accompanied by an intense inflammatory reaction and saponification of all layers of the viscus (mucous membrane, submucosa, and muscular wall). Ingestion of granular materials causes focal injuries. Liquid alkali may cause generalized diffuse damage to nasopharynx, esophagus, and stomach.

Acid substances produce a coagulative necrosis that causes the formation of a protective eschar, which delays further injury. Although esophageal injury may occur, major damage usually involves the stomach. The severity of caustic injury to the gastrointestinal tract is classified as follows. First-degree lesions, producing erythema and edema, involve the mucosa and submucosa. No scarring or stricture follows healing. Second-degree lesions penetrate the submucosa and the muscular walls. The sloughing of tissue that occurs 1–2 weeks after injury results in deep ulceration and the production of granulation tissue. Over the weeks or months after exposure, scarring and stricture formation may cause such complications as esophageal and antral stenosis. Third-degree lesions cause perforations with resultant mediastinitis and peritonitis.

Clinical Features

Many patients who do not have oropharyngeal involvement may have few complaints. Other patients may have salivation along with edema and ulceration of the palate and pharynx. Dysphagia and odynophagia may herald esophageal injury; however, the degree of esophageal injury correlates poorly with oropharyngeal findings. Gastric injury is reflected by epigastric pain and the vomiting of blood or coffee-ground materials. Perforation of a viscus is marked by increased pain and the presence of fever and abdominal rigidity. The development of an esophageal and antral stricture, which may be delayed up to 2 to 6 weeks after exposure, is characteristically associated with dysphagia and weight loss. Vomiting may indicate a gastric obstruction.

Diagnosis

The extent and severity of injury are defined by upper gastrointestinal endoscopy. Chest and abdominal roentgenograms may reveal evidence of perforation. Barium contrast radiography, though less sensitive in the acute phase of injury, may be useful in defining such delayed complications as strictures, ulcerations, thickened gastric folds associated with atony, and dilatation of the duodenal bulb. Stenotic lesions may resemble carcinomatous changes. The differential diagnosis is usually evident from the medical history. However, if the patient is seen long after the initial injury, peptic lesions, carcinoma, and unusual inflammatory disorders of the gastrointestinal tract (syphilis or Crohn's disease) must be considered.

Treatment

Alkaline neutralization and dilution with water are unlikely to be of help in the emergency treatment of alkali ingestion. Tissue damage occurs early and rapidly after alkali ingestion, and the heat produced by the neutralization reaction may further increase tissue injury. Ingested acid may be diluted advantageously with water and milk. The induction of emesis is to be discouraged. Hemodynamic and respiratory support and surgical intervention for perforation may be necessary. Few if any clues accurately predict which patients will experience a delayed perforation of the esophagus or stomach.

In well-controlled animal studies, steroid therapy has been of help in inhibiting fibroblastic reaction and the growth of granulation tissue during the healing of injured tissue. A controlled trial, however, failed to show any efficiency of corticosteroids in preventing stricture formation (3). Animal studies indicate that antibiotics may be used to prevent secondary infection. The use of an H_2-receptor antagonist to reduce gastric acidity and volume and total parenteral nutrition are additional approaches to management.

Esophageal stricture, once established, is treated with esophageal dilatation by bouginage. A strong association has been reported between caustic injury to the esophagus and the development of squamous carcinoma at this site years after the initial injury. An incidence 6–10% higher than normal is cited.

Gastrointestinal Injury Caused by Chemical Agents

Chemical compounds foreign to the human body and without a physiological or nutritional role on entry into the GI tract are all potentially toxic (7). These agents, derived from a myriad of sources, range from such synthetic chemicals as pesticides and chlorinated hydrocarbons to such heavy metals as lead, cadmium, and mercury. Unfortunately, at this time, the intestinal effect of exposure to most of these environmental contaminants, particularly at low concentrations, is for the most part unknown.

A recent epidemic of poisoning from contamination of foodstuffs by toxic oil emphasizes the potential danger of chemical pollution (28). The epidemic occurred in Spain and resulted in over 300 deaths. Evidence favored the notion that ingestion of rapeseed oil contaminated with aniline was the cause. The disease syndrome that followed the exposure was unique and unlike any acute poisoning previously encountered.

The illness began with complaints of nonproductive cough, dyspnea, pleuritic chest pain, headache, and fever. A marked eosinophilia accompanied by gastrointestinal symptoms of nausea, vomiting, diarrhea, and abdominal pain became prominent after about 1 month. The disease was self-limited in most instances. However, some patients developed myalgia and muscle atrophy. A few went on to develop scleroderma-like skin thickening, pulmonary hypertension, Raynaud phenomenon, sicca syndrome, and dysphagia. Histopathological features of a vasculitis were associated with abdominal pain and mesenteric vein thrombosis. These observations suggest that involvement of the immune system is partially responsible for the toxic-oil syndrome. A similar presentation was described in individuals exposed to a single batch of L-tryptophan. Although gastrointestinal complaints were minimal, eosinophilic infiltration of the gastrointestinal tract was present (22). These syndromes provide an excellent example of the wide range of tissue damage that may occur after pollutant ingestion. It also indicates the importance of careful clinical observation and epidemiologic and laboratory analyses in episodes of environmental contamination.

Gastrointestinal Cancer

Despite comparative epidemiologic data that implicate environmental factors in the pathogenesis of esophageal, gastric, and colon cancer, specific chemicals have not been clearly linked to the development of gastrointestinal cancer in humans. To date, limited studies suggest that certain occupational groups (e.g., chemical workers, textile workers, and possibly asbestos workers) face a greater risk of gastrointestinal cancer. Since almost all known human carcinogens were first recognized by alert physicians or patients themselves (15), physicians must be attentive to the hazards of toxic exposure.

SUMMARY

There is evidence that many hundreds of chemical substances ranging from pesticides and poly-chlorinated biphenyls to heavy metals, such as lead, cadmium, and mercury, contaminate the environment and enter the intestinal tract. For the most part their effects on the intestine are unknown. However, an episode of contamination of foodstuffs by toxic oil resulted in gastrointestinal symptoms along with a wide range of tissue damage. The occurrence of the toxic-oil syndrome serves to alert physicians to the potential adverse effects of ingesting environmental chemicals.

REFERENCES

1. Aldicarb food poisoning from contaminated melons—California. Leads from the MMWR. JAMA 256:175, 1986.
2. American Occupational Medical Association: NIOSH Advises Handling Acrylonitrile as Though a Human Carcinogen, AOMA Report, Arlington Heights, Illinois, 1977.
3. Anderson KD, Rouse TM, Randolph JG: A controlled trial of corticosteroids in children with corrosive injury of the esophagus. N Engl J Med 323:637, 1990.
4. Armijo R, Coulson AH: Epidemiology of stomach cancers in Chile: The role of nitrogen fertilizer. Int J Epidemiol 4:301, 1975.
5. Armijo R, Gonzalez M, Orellana AH, et al: Epidemiology of gastric cancer in Chile: II. Nitrate exposures and stomach cancer frequency. Int J Epidemiol 10:57, 1981.
6. Banwell JG; Environmental contaminant effects on human intestinal function. In: Intestinal Toxicology, p 193, Schiller CJ (ed.), Raven Press, New York, 1984.
7. Chambra RS: Intestinal absorption and metabolism of xenobiotics. Environ Health Perspect 33:61, 1979.
8. Committee on Diet, Nutrition and Cancer, National Research Council: Diet, Nutrition and Cancer, National Academy Press, Washington, 1982.
9. Committee on Food Protection, National Research Council: Toxicants Occurring Naturally in Foods, National Academy of Sciences, Washington, 1973.
10. Committee on Nitrite and Alternative Curing Agents in Food, National Research Council: The Health Effects of Nitrate, Nitrite, and N-Nitroso Compounds, National Academy Press, Washington, 1981.
11. Committee on Nonoccupational Risks of Asbestos Fibers, National Research Council: Asbestiform Fibers: Nonoccupational Health Risks. National Academy Press, Washington, 1984.
12. Committee on Scientific and Regulatory Issues Underlying Pesticide Use Patterns and Agricultural Innovation, National Research Council: Regulating Pesticides in Food; The Delaney Paradox, National Academy Press, Washington, 1987.
13. Correa P, Haenszel W, Cuello S, et al: A model for gastric cancer epidemiology. Lancet 2:58, 1975.
14. Cuello C, Correa P, Haenszel W, et al: Gastric cancer in Columbia 1. Cancer risk and suspect environmental agents. J Natl Cancer Inst 57:1015, 1976.
15. Doll R: Pott and the prospects for prevention. Br J Cancer 321:263, 1975.

16. Eastwood GL: Gastrointestinal epithelial renewal. Gastroenterology 72:962, 1977.

17. Forstner G, Wesley A, Forstner J: Clinical aspects of gastrointestinal mucus. In: Mucus in Health and Disease II, p 189, Chantler EN, Elder JB, Elstein M (eds.), Plenum Press, New York, 1982.

18. Gartrell MJ, Cran JC, Podrebarac DS, et al: Pesticides, selected elements and other chemicals in adult total diet samples Oct 1980–Mar 1982. J Assoc Off Anal Chem 69:146, 1986.

19. Haenszel W, Kurihara M, Segi M, et al: Stomach cancer among Japanese in Hawaii. J Natl Cancer Inst 49:969, 1972.

20. Hartiala K: Metabolism of hormones, drugs and other substances by the gut. Physiol Rev 53:496, 1973.

21. Hartman PE: Putative mutagens and carcinogens in food, 1. Nitrate/nitrite ingestion and gastric cancer mortality. Environ Mutagen 5:111, 1983.

22. Hertzman PA, Blevins WL, Mayer J, et al: Association of the eosinophilia myalgia syndrome with the ingestion of tryptophan. N Engl J Med 322:869, 1990.

23. Higginson J: Etiological factors in gastrointestinal cancer in man. J Natl Cancer Inst 37:527, 1966.

24. Higginson J, Jenson OM, Muir CS: Environmental carcinogenesis: A global problem. Curr Prob Cancer 5:1, 1981.

25. Hill MJ, Hawksworth G, Tattersall G: Bacteria, nitrosamines and cancer of the stomach. Br J Cancer 28:562, 1973.

26. Interdisciplinary Panel on Carcinogenicity. Criteria for evidence of chemical carcinogenicity. Science 225:682, 1984.

27. Janicki RH, Kinter WB: DDT inhibits Na,K,Mg- ATPase in the intestinal mucosae and gills of marine teleosts. Nature 233:148, 1971.

28. Kilbourne EM, Rigau-Perez JG, Heath CW, et al: Clinical epidemiology of toxic-oil syndrome. N Engl J Med 309:1408, 1983.

29. Lamont JT, Ventola A: Synthesis and secretion of colonic glycoproteins: Evidence for shedding in vivo of low molecular weight membrane components. Biochim Biophys Acta 629:553, 1980.

30. Levine DS: Does asbestos exposure cause gastrointestinal cancer? Dig Dis Sci 30:1189, 1985.

31. Lijinsky W, Taylor HW: Nitrosamines and their precursors in food. In: Origins of Human Cancer. Cold Spring Harbor Conferences on Cell Proliferation, Vol 4, p 1579, Hiatt W, Watson JD, Winsten JA (eds.), Cold Spring Harbor Laboratory, New York, 1977.

32. Lijinsky W, Taylor HW, Snyder C, et al: Malignant tumours of liver and lung in rats fed aminopyrine or heptamethyleneimine together with nitrite. Nature 244:176, 1973.

33. Magee PN: Nitrosamines and Human Cancer. Banbury Report 12, Cold Spring Harbor Laboratory, New York, 1982.

34. March GM: Review of epidemiological studies related to ingested asbestos. Environ Health Perspect 53:49, 1983.

35. McNabb PC: Host defense mechanisms at mucosal surfaces. Annu Rev Microbiol 35:477, 1981.

36. Mirvish SS: Effects of vitamins C and E on N-nitroso compound formation, carcinogenesis, and cancer. Cancer 58(8 Suppl):1842, 1986.

37. Morgan RW, Foliart DE, Wong O: Asbestos and gastrointestinal cancer: A review of the literature. West J Med 143:60, 1985.

38. Morton ID: Naturally occurring toxins in foods. Proc Nutr Soc 36:101, 1977.

39. Motulsky A: Ecogenetics: Genetic variation in susceptibility to environmental agents. In: Human Genetics: Proceedings of Fifth International Congress in Human Genetics, p 375, Excerpta Medica, Amsterdam, 1976.

40. Munro IC, Charbonneau SM: Environmental contaminants. In: Food Safety, p 141, Robert HR (ed.), John Wiley & Sons, New York, 1981.

41. Newberne PM, Conner MW: Food additives and contaminants: An update. Cancer 58:1851, 1986.

42. Office of Technology Assessment: Environmental Contaminants in Food, US Government Printing Office, Washington, 1979.

43. Omenn GS, Gelboin HV (eds.): Genetic Variability in Responses to Chemical Exposures. Banbury Report 16, Cold Spring Harbor Laboratory, New York, 1984.

44. Palmer S, Mathews RA: The role of non-nutritive dietary constituents in carcinogenesis. Surg Clin North Am 66:891, 1986.

45. Pantuck EJ, Hsiao KC, Kuntzman R, et al: Intestinal metabolism of phenacetin in the rat: Effects of charcoal-broiled beef and raw chow. Science 187:744, 1975.

46. Pickle LW, Gottlieb MS: Pancreatic cancer mortality in Louisiana. Am J Public Health 70:256, 1980.

47. Pitot HC: Fundamentals of Oncology, Marcel Dekker, New York, 1986.

48. Pritchard JB: Toxic substances and membrane function. Fed Proc 38:2220, 1979.

49. Reed PI, Haines K, Smith PLR, et al: Gastric juice N-nitrosamines in health and gastroduodenal disease. Lancet 2:550, 1981.

50. Ross R, Nichols P, Wright W, et al: Asbestos exposure and lymphomas of the gastrointestinal tract and oral cavity. Lancet 2:1118, 1982.

51. Rothstein A, Takeshita M, Knauf PA: Chemical modification of proteins involved in the permeability of the erythrocyte membrane ions. Biomembranes 3:393, 1972.

52. Ruddell WSG, Bone ES, Hill MJ, et al: Gastric-juice nitrite. A risk factor for cancer in the hypochlorhydric stomach. Lancet 2:1037, 1976.

53. Safe Drinking Water Committee, National Research Council: Drinking Water and Health, Vol 5, National Academy Press, Washington, 1983.

54. Schedl HP: Environmental agents and intestinal disease in man. In: Intestinal Toxicology, p 209, Schiller CM (ed.), Raven Press, New York, 1984.

55. Scheline RR: Metabolism of foreign compounds by gastrointestinal microorganisms. Pharmacol Rev 25:451, 1973.

56. Schiller CM (ed.): Intestinal Toxicology, Raven Press, New York, 1984.

57. Schiller CM, Walden R, Shoaf CR: Studies on the mechanism of 2,3,7,8-tetrachloro-dibenzo-p-dioxin toxicity: Nutrient assimilation. Fed Proc 41:1426, 1982.

58. Schiller CM, Shoaf CR, Chapman DE: Alterations of intestinal function by chemical exposure: Animal model. In: Intestinal Toxicology, p 133, Schiller CM (ed.), Raven Press, New York, 1984.

59. Schottenfeld D, Fraumeni JF (eds.): Cancer Epidemiol-

ogy and Prevention, WB Saunders, Philadelphia, 1982.

60. Sen NP, Smith DC, Schwinghamer L: Formation of N-nitrosamines from secondary amines and nitrite in human and animal gastric juice. Food Cosmet Toxicol 7:301, 1969.

61. Sleisenger MH, Fordtran JS (eds.): Gastrointestinal Disease: Pathophysiology, Diagnosis and Management, 4th ed., WB Saunders, Philadelphia, 1989.

62. Suskind RR, Hertzberg VS: Human health effects of 2,4,5-T and its toxic contaminants. JAMA 251:2372, 1984.

63. Tannenbaum SR: N-Nitroso compounds: A perspective on human exposure. Lancet 1:629, 1983.

64. Tannenbaum SR, Fett D, Young VR, et al: Nitrite and nitrate are formed by endogenous synthesis in the human intestine. Science 200:487, 1978.

65. Tannenbaum SR, Moran D, Rand W, et al: Gastric cancer in Colombia IV. Nitrite and other ions in gastric contents of residents from a high risk region. J Natl Cancer Inst 62:9, 1979.

66. Vobecky J, Devroede G, Lacaille J, et al: An occupational group with a high risk of large bowel cancer. Gastroenterology 75:221, 1978.

67. Walsh J: Methods in gastrointestinal toxicology. In: Principles and Methods of Toxicology, p 475, Hayes AW (ed.), Raven Press, New York, 1982.

68. Weisburger JH, Raineri R: Dietary factors and the etiology of gastric cancer. Cancer Res 35:3269, 1975.

69. Weiss W: Asbestos and colorectal cancer. Gastroenterology 99:876, 1990.

70. Winter CK, Seiber JN, Nuckton CF (eds.): Chemicals in the Human Food Chain, Van Nostrand Reinhold, New York, 1990.

71. Wollenberg P, Ullrich V: The drug monooxygenase system in the small intestine. In: Extrahepatic Metabolism of Drugs and Other Foreign Compounds, p 267, Gram TC (ed.), SP Medical & Scientific Books, New York, 1980.

RECOMMENDED READINGS

Schiller CJ (ed.): Intestinal Toxicology, Raven Press, New York, 1984.

Winter CK, Seiber JN, Nuckton CF (eds.): Chemicals in the Human Food Chain, Van Nostrand Reinhold, New York, 1990.

19. DISORDERS OF THE LIVER

Philip S. Guzelian

INTRODUCTION

Very little is known about the clinical aspects of "environmental hepatology," especially when compared to the extensive experimental investigations of the hepatotoxic effects of environmental agents. The very advantages that have made the liver popular as an organ for general studies of cell biology, biochemistry, and physiology also make the liver attractive for studies of the effects of potentially toxic substances.

The liver carries out a diverse array of specialized biochemical and physiological functions. These include the synthesis and release of numerous plasma proteins; maintenance of carbohydrate, glycerolipid, sterol, and amino acid homeostasis; and biotransformation of potentially toxic exogenous substances. Furthermore, the liver can be readily sampled in experimental animals, can be maintained as an isolated perfused organ, or can be examined under conditions of cell culture for many days in vitro. Of the many compounds examined in one of these systems, few fail to affect at least one liver function. Yet, authoritative reviews conclude that there is scant evidence for clinically significant liver disease resulting from exposure to small amounts of toxic substances in the environment and that where such disease exists, it is usually subtle and clinically inconspicuous (76,97).

Principles and Practice of Environmental Medicine, edited by Alyce Bezman Tarcher. Plenum Medical Book Company, New York, 1992.

Definitions of Environmental Hepatotoxicity

A major source of confusion is the lack of consensually validated definitions for "toxicity" in general or, more specifically, for "hepatotoxicity." The least-restrictive definition of toxicity is "any deviation from the normal state." For the isolated hepatocyte this definition would encompass any change in the amount or activity of a given enzyme (increase or decrease), in the structure or composition of a membrane or organelle, in the ultrastructural appearance of the cell, or in the overall integrated activity of the cell. Extended to the intact liver, this definition would also include any changes relevant to the integrated tissue such as blood flow and distribution, bile production and flow, or metabolic interactions with other organs. Finally, in clinical medicine any perceived (or perceivable) alteration in liver structure, physiological function, or biochemical characteristics would be defined as "hepatotoxicity."

An obvious difficulty with this broad definition is that changes that are beneficial would be termed "toxic." For example, infants with physiological jaundice of the newborn are treated with phenobarbital to stimulate the capacity of the liver to eliminate bilirubin. It seems inappropriate to regard this change evoked by phenobarbital as hepatotoxic. Therefore, use of "toxicity" is usually confined to changes that are not beneficial (often expressed with the use of vague modifiers such as "adverse" liver effects, liver "injury," liver "damage," "impaired" liver function, etc.). Coupling modifiers such as "potential" or "possible" add to the lack of precision. Moreover, there are substantial disagreements on what changes are beneficial, indifferent, or injurious.

Difficulties in defining toxicity might be circumvented by employing the concept of a biological or, in clinical practice, a clinical threshold for toxicity. Continuing advances in technology increase the sensitivity of detecting structural, biochemical, or physiological changes, even though it may be uncertain whether such changes are significant for the cell, the organ, or the individual.

It is theoretically possible that some changes are biologically insignificant, falling beneath the threshold for biological importance. Such endpoints for the individual hepatocyte might include survival or the ability to carry out functions characteristic of the liver. For example, a compound that damaged the plasma membrane of the hepatocyte, leading to loss of maintenance of transmembrane ion concentration and cell death, would be hepatotoxic. On the other hand, an agent that appeared only to decrease an enzyme in a biosynthetic pathway would not be termed hepatotoxic unless (or until) it could be demonstrated that endpoints of biological significance were affected.

Endpoints relevant to the integrated tissue might include normal growth and development, ability to reproduce, life span, etc. Additional endpoints for human effects include a sense of well-being, ability to carry out regular activities of daily living, and the maintenance of sufficient reserve liver function to resist the effects of diseases of the liver or of other organs.

The concept of clinical thresholds is well known to physicians, who must often decide whether a particular physical or laboratory finding is clinically meaningful. For example, treatment with the drug isoniazid transiently and asymptomatically increases the serum transaminase in 5–20% of patients. Only in 1–2% will there be progressive morphological and biochemical changes resulting in morbidity, permanent loss of liver function, or death (65). Should the mild, self-limited elevations of transaminase be considered hepatotoxic, or does this change fall beneath the clinical threshold for significant liver damage? The answer may depend on individual value judgments. Similar disagreements over the effects of environmental chemicals on human health may be directly traceable to the failure to distinguish between a demonstrable effect and the clinical or biological relevance of that effect.

ENVIRONMENTAL CHEMICALS ASSOCIATED WITH ADVERSE EFFECTS ON THE LIVER

Several lists of environmental agents incriminated in injury to the liver have been compiled (76,97,98). These are summarized in Table 19-1. In many instances evidence for hepatotoxicity may be scant, reflecting no more than one or two case reports. In other cases exposure to the agent resulted from an accident or suicidal ingestion involving extremely high doses far exceeding those encountered in the environment.

Distribution

It may be seen from the list of potential or established hepatotoxic substances (Table 19-1) that this array of compounds defies simple classification

TABLE 19-1. Agents in the Environment Incriminated in Injury to the Liver

Adulterated cooking oil	Dimethyl nitrosamine	Pentachlorophenol
Amanita phalloides	Dinitrophenol	Perchlorothylene
Aminotriazole	Diphenyl oxide	Phenobarbital
Anabolic steroids	Epichlorohydrin	Phenytoin
Antimony	Ethionine	Phosphorus
Arsenicals	Ethylene dibromide	Ponceau-MX
Benzene	Galactosamine	Pyrethins
Beryllium	Halogenated aromatics	Safrole
Bismuth	Halides	Senecio alkaloids
Boranes	Halogenated paraffins	Styrene
Bush tea	Heliotropium	Talune
Carbonates	Herbal remedies	Thallium
Carbon tetrachloride	Hexachlorobenzene	Tetrachlorethylene
Chromium	Hydrazines	Tetrachlorodibenzo-*p*-dioxin
Crotalaria	Hypoglycin	Tetrachlorethane
Cyanide	Lead methylene chloride	Thorotrast
Cycasin	Methylenedianiline	Toluene diisocyanate
Cymene	Mycotoxins (aflatoxin)	Trichlorethylene
DDT	Naphthalene	Trinitrotoluene
4,4'-Diaminodiphenylmethane	Organochlorine pesticides	Xylene
Dieldrin	Paraquat	Vinyl chloride
Diethyl nitrosamine		

according to physical properties, chemical characteristics, or distribution. Pollutants may be found in the air, either out of doors or inside, in urban or rural settings, or as contaminants in food and water. The home, school, areas of recreation, and workplace usually contain products incorporating chemicals that are potentially toxic. Examples of household products in this category would be antifreeze, cleaning agents, polishes and waxes, mothballs, paint products, pesticides, and inks. The presence of these agents within easy access of children or suicidal patients can lead to either accidental or intentional ingestion of toxic doses. This need not be acute. Persistent consumption of ethanol in large amounts might be regarded as chronic intentional poisoning of the liver.

Food represents a common source of ingestion of contaminants. These need not be artificial. There are a number of naturally occurring substances (for example, poisonous mushrooms) that are known to be hepatotoxic. Ingestion of mushrooms from the *Amanita* genus containing amatoxins or phallotoxins produces massive hepatic necrosis, often resulting in liver failure, hemorrhage, and death. Pyrrolidizine alkaloids are produced by more than 200 species of plants commonly found in tropical climates that may be found in "bush teas" or in wheat and other grain products (64). These agents damage the hepatic vasculature, leading to occlusive disease of the hepatic veins.

Other examples of naturally occurring toxic substances include hypoglycin A, a fruit product that causes acute fatty liver in "Jamaican vomiting sickness," which resembles Reye's syndrome. Safrol and isosafrol were consumed by the public at large prior to recognition that these agents are hepatotoxic and carcinogenic in experimental animals. Mycotoxins (e.g., aflatoxin), which commonly contaminate grain or peanuts, are known to produce liver cytotoxicity and carcinogenesis in experimental animals and may do the same in humans.

Other sources of food contamination are exemplified by unusual mass contaminations such as the "Epping jaundice" caused by bread baked from flour contaminated with 4,4'-diaminodiphenylmethane (54); the toxic porphyria among Turks who ate wheat contaminated with hexachlorobenzene (82); "Yusho," the epidemic among Japanese who ate rice oil containing polychlorinated biphenyls (34); and almost all the residents of the state of Michigan who were exposed to polybrominated biphenyls (4) (a mixture of hepatotoxic chemicals) spread through the food chain from contamination of cow feed. A final example that could be included as a continuing mass contamination is the appearance in seafood of numerous potentially hepatotoxic substances bioaccumulated by the marine life living in polluted streams, lakes, rivers, and oceans. Finally, it should

be noted that manufacturers add thousands of different substances to processed food including artificial flavoring, coloring agents, or preservatives such as nitrites, which may directly or indirectly carry the risk of developing injury to the liver. Food may also contain residues of insecticides, herbicides, fumigants, and other chemicals used in its growth or processing.

Toxicology

Dose is the dominant factor determining the potential toxic outcome of an exposure to an environmental agent. For many toxic substances a sufficient dose, regardless of other factors, will lead to predictable toxic outcome in all exposed individuals. However, for lesser doses there are other important modifying factors. The route of administration or contact (dermal, inhalation, or ingestion) may be important depending on the physical and chemical properties of the toxic agent. Differences in absorption ("bioavailability") or distribution may be important. Inhaled toxic substances may never reach the liver, whereas the liver represents the first organ of postabsorption contact for most ingested substances. As discussed later, metabolism, and especially interindividual differences in metabolism, may be key in determining the outcome of exposure to an agent. Since the liver clears toxic substances from the blood and excretes them into bile, the liver may be exposed to these substances longer and in higher concentrations than are other organs.

EPIDEMIOLOGY

Most of the agents established as hepatotoxic for man have been related to single incidents involving exposure to large amounts of the agent, as an accidental or intentional exposure, often in the workplace. Occupational toxicity was responsible for the recognition of chlorinated biphenyls, trinitrotoluene, tetrachlorethane, and dimethylnitrosamine as hepatotoxic substances. With better industrial hygiene, incidents of toxicity in the workplace have decreased. Investigators are now performing epidemiological studies of populations exposed to these industrial chemicals in small amounts.

Because clinical chemistry tests relevant to the liver are inexpensive and readily obtained, an assessment of "hepatotoxicity" is often included in population studies. There are, in addition to the inherent nonspecificity of liver tests used as the endpoint in such studies, severe limitations in the usefulness of such epidemiologic approaches. A comprehensive survey of a large industrial work force showed that age, sex, and diurnal and seasonal variations could exert important influences on liver tests, making it imperative to select control groups carefully for meaningful interpretation (27). Unfortunately, there are few population studies of "normal" liver chemistry tests other than in hospital or clinic groups.

When the disease is rare—such as angiosarcoma of the liver in workers exposed to vinyl chloride—the cause-and-effect relationship is often evident and does not require complicated epidemiologic studies. On the other hand, with common diseases such as hepatocellular carcinoma, the most common tumor in man worldwide (50), the insensitivity of classical epidemiology presents a problem. There is a strong association between hepatitis B virus infection and hepatocellular carcinoma. However, epidemiologists still have difficulty in agreeing whether or not aflatoxin, a potent experimental liver carcinogen, is a proven carcinogenic or cocarcinogenic agent for the liver in humans.

Consider a less potent hepatocarcinogenic agent that might increase human cancer risk by only a few percent but would affect thousands of people. Conclusive risk assessment for such an agent in man (if obtainable at all) would require leviathan epidemiologic studies. Hence, establishing whether or not a particular agent is toxic to the liver in humans is an extremely difficult problem that in most instances transcends current scientific methodology. To circumvent this problem, a new approach combining traditional clinical and epidemiologic studies with the use of highly advanced biotechnology is currently being developed (40,72). This approach, which incorporates biological markers into analytical epidemiologic research, is termed molecular epidemiology (40). Its purpose is to evaluate directly in humans the biologically relevant dose of a compound, the potential genetic susceptibility to exposure to that dose, and the early events that may presage a toxic outcome (see Chapters 1 and 27).

PATHOLOGY AND PATHOLOGICAL PHYSIOLOGY

Classification of Adverse Effects

Table 19-2 summarizes the syndromes of hepatotoxicity that may be caused by environmental agents. For most of the examples listed a cause-and-effect relationship seems well established. The pathological patterns produced by environmental agents encompass the entire repertoire of the responses of the liver to injury. Some industrial chemicals or household agents are known to produce hepatic necrosis. Carbon tetrachloride or trichlorethane, when given in repeated exposures, can lead to continuing necrosis, fibrosis, subacute hepatic necrosis, and possible cirrhosis. Whether or not exposures to smaller amounts of these substances over a lifetime are responsible for "cryptogenic cirrhosis" remains speculative. It is unusual to find cholestasis as the sole manifestation of liver injury. Fatty metamorphosis, established only by liver biopsy, can be produced by the agents listed in Table 19-2 but also accompanies excessive alcohol ingestion, obesity, diabetes, and many other disease states.

Hypertrophy of the endoplasmic reticulum (microsomal enzyme induction) has clearly been demonstrated in human beings exposed to toxic substances in the environment. However, considering the definitions discussed in the introduction of this chapter, it is open to question whether this response represents hepatotoxicity per se, or is rather an adaptive response of the liver (see paragraph be-

TABLE 19-2. Summary of Syndromes of Hepatotoxicity
Caused by Environmental Agents

Toxic manifestations	Examples of environmental toxins reported in man
1. Hepatic necrosis	Chlorinated aliphatics in high doses (CCl_4, tetrachloroethane); mushroom toxins; phosphorus; mycotoxins; high doses of polychlorinated biphenyls (PCBs)
2. Cholestasis	Methylenediamine (Epping jaundice); dinitrophenol; chromium
3. Fatty metamorphosis	Small doses of chlorinated aliphatics; some organochlorine pesticides; 2,3,7,8-tetrachlorodibenzodioxin
4. Hypertrophy of endoplasmic reticulum	Polychlorinated biphenyls; some organochlorine pesticides
5. Venoocclusive disease	Plant toxins (pyrrolidizine alkaloids); therapeutic liver irradiation
6. Granuloma	Beryllium
7. Hepatoportal fibrosis	Vinyl chloride; arsenic
8. Cirrhosis	Chlorinated aliphatics; aromatics; aflatoxin; arsenic; plant toxins
9. Hepatocellular carcinoma	Aflatoxin; ethanol
10. Angiosarcoma	Vinyl chloride; arsenic

low). Hypertrophy of the endoplasmic reticulum is accompanied by an increase (or decrease) in the concentration of drug-metabolizing enzymes in the liver. Changes in the levels of these enzymes may increase or decrease the rate of metabolism of many exogenous or endogenous compounds and may also alter the pharmacological profile of the metabolites produced.

Since metabolites may be more toxic or less toxic than the parent drug, and since the amount and type of metabolites produced may depend critically on the profile of drug-metabolizing enzymes, induction of this system carries the potential of enhancing toxic chemical interactions. It also may serve as a protective response. An important aspect of this manifestation is that for most chemicals, even those that are potent inducers of liver microsomal enzymes, relatively high doses are required to produce this response. Hence, proliferation of the smooth endoplasmic reticulum usually indicates a relatively large exposure to an inducer, often a lipophilic chemical that is slowly eliminated from the liver (see Chapter 9).

Venocclusive disease, granulomas, hepatoportal fibrosis, and cirrhosis. There are only limited examples in the United States of venocclusive disease, granulomas, or hepatoportal fibrosis caused by environmental agents. Cirrhosis has been identified as an outcome of a single or repeated exposure to an environmental agent. However, it is also an extremely common disease in the general public, making it difficult to use cirrhosis as an epidemiologic endpoint for incriminating other toxic agents. The most commonly established causes of cirrhosis in the United States are ethanol ingestion, viral hepatitis, infections with either hepatitis B virus or non-A, non-B viruses.

Hepatocellular carcinoma is commonly found in geographic regions endemic for hepatitis B virus (50). In these regions the food is heavily contaminated with the experimental liver carcinogen, aflatoxin. In the Western world, hepatocellular carcinoma and ethanol consumption are commonly associated (almost always occurring in the setting of preexisting cirrhosis). It is uncertain whether ethanol is a direct carcinogen or whether it alters liver architecture and regenerative patterns, leading to cirrhosis, which secondarily fosters liver malignancy. A key, as yet unanswered, question is whether the risk of human hepatocellular carcinoma is increased by exposure to any of the numerous chemicals that, when fed at high doses for the lifetime of rats or mice, produce hepatocellular carcinoma.

With new emphasis on chemical testing and regulations and increased vigilance regarding pollution of the environment from industrial sources, it seems likely that future exposure to substances known to be liver carcinogens in rodents will be reduced. Nevertheless, many of these compounds are ubiquitous in the environment (primarily the halogenated, aliphatic, or aromatic hydrocarbon chemicals). For example, most residents of Michigan carry body burdens of polybrominated biphenyls, and almost all adults have detectable residues of DDE in their bodies. Yet the available epidemiologic studies have failed to show evidence of DDT or its metabolites causing liver carcinogenesis in humans. It may be argued that these studies have insufficient power to detect an increase in hepatocellular carcinoma or that the latent period for expression of malignancy is longer than the almost 50 years since widespread use of DDT began. The same argument may also be raised to explain the lack of excess liver cancer in humans receiving phenobarbital, a drug that promotes liver cancer in rodents. Answers to these questions would significantly advance our understanding of the relevance of extrapolating to man the results of toxicity testing in animals.

Angiosarcoma is a rare tumor that arises from the epithelial cells lining the liver sinusoid (7,61,92). This was an extraordinarily rare tumor prior to its appearance in vinyl chloride workers or in people exposed to arsenic or the radioactive contrast agent thorotrast.

Pathophysiology of Hepatocellular Toxicity

It is clear that biochemical or morphological evidence of hepatotoxicity in animals cannot be extrapolated to man with certainty. However, there have been important advances in understanding the mechanisms of hepatotoxicity and hepatocarcinogenesis. This body of knowledge, derived largely from animal experimentation, stemmed from the recognition that liver microsomal enzymes are capable of metabolizing drugs, carcinogens, and other foreign compounds. An entire field of research has developed focusing on the role of these enzymes as an important biochemical locus for interaction between humans and their chemical environment (9,17,69,87) (see Chapter 9).

A simplified schematic representation of the pathways for the disposition of foreign substances in the liver is presented in Fig. 19-1. Most often, environmental agents are lipophilic and, hence, are not readily excreted in aqueous media such as urine or bile. Hepatic metabolism converts these substances to more polar, readily excretable forms. The reactions are carried out largely in the endoplasmic reticulum of the hepatocyte or "microsomes" (as these membranes are called when extracted and isolated by differential centrifugation).

A key component of the microsomes is cytochrome P-450. This group of hemoprotein isoenzymes binds the chemical and also binds oxygen and cata-

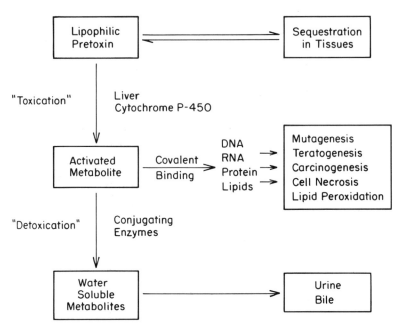

FIGURE 19-1. Generalized pathways for the disposition of some environmental hepatotoxins. From Guzelian (28).

lyzes the oxidation of many foreign substances (9,69). In some instances, biooxidation of foreign compounds renders them not only more water soluble but also pharmacologically inactive. However, most potentially toxic compounds require similar biooxidation reactions to be converted into toxic forms (metabolic activation). Unless promptly disposed of, these oxygenated metabolites may chemically interact with nucleic acids or other macromolecules in the hepatocyte, initiating a chain of events leading to cytotoxicity or malignancy. Prompt removal of metabolically activated toxic substances is carried out by a series of conjugating enzymes capable of converting these metabolites to water-soluble derivatives that are inactive pharmacologically (detoxication) (see Chapter 9).

There are several examples of enzymes that serve to detoxify the activated metabolites formed by the cytochrome P-450 enzymes. Liver cytosol contains a series of glutathione-S-transferases that catalyze the combination of oxygenated species with glutathione, a sulfur-containing tripeptide present in high concentrations in many cells including the hepatocyte. Glutathione likely serves as an important buffer, preventing interactions between oxygenated metabolites and the sulfhydryl groups of important macromolecules. Another conjugating enzyme is microsomal epoxide hydratase, which catalyzes the conversion of potentially reactive epoxides or arene

oxides (products of cytochrome P-450 reactions) to water-soluble dialcohols (see Chapter 9).

It may be reasoned that the metabolic disposition of a foreign compound in the liver will depend not only on the dose but also on differences between the rates of enzymatic activation of the compound and the availability of pathways for inactivation of its reactive metabolites. Hence, factors that alter the profile of the many isozyme forms of activating or detoxifying enzymes in the liver may be important determinants of the development of toxicity.

It is well recognized that cytochrome P-450 is inducible by many environmental compounds, including lipophilic drugs, some natural agents, carcinogens, and environmental pollutants (69,87). For example, when any of a large number of organochlorine pesticides or polycyclic aromatic hydrocarbons are administered, there are increases in the concentration of hepatic cytochrome P-450, the xenobiotic-metabolizing activity of the microsomes, and the rate of clearance of test compounds by the liver. These appear to be adaptive responses of the liver, since the cytochrome concentration promptly falls once the concentrations of these inducing chemicals in the liver have been sufficiently reduced through metabolism or redistribution to other tissues. There is substantial evidence that the amounts and types of cytochromes P-450 and their inducibility are under genetic control (69). Contrasting with the effects of inducers are the decreases in cytochrome P-450 found in many physiological or pathophysiological states (49). The recent availability of advanced techniques in recombinant DNA and molecular genetics should facilitate progress in understanding interindividual variations in sensitivity to toxic substances.

An important category of compounds commonly found in the environment are those extremely hydrophobic chemicals (e.g., halogenated biphenyls, organochlorine pesticides) that undergo little, if any, metabolism and elimination by the liver (Fig. 19-1). Chronic exposure to small amounts of these chemicals leads to their accumulation in tissues and membrane lipids. We know little regarding the biochemical and biophysical aspects of this sequestration or of the basic forces that establish distribution of these chemicals in the body. Many of these compounds are toxic or carcinogenic in rodent liver. This prompts concern that these chemicals may also foster malignancies in human tissue by acting as "promoters" of biochemically initiated premalignant hepatocytes (see below) or by inducing cytochrome P-450 and, hence, rendering the individual more susceptible to other procarcinogens. (See Chapter 27 for a discussion of the role of environmental chemicals in human cancer causation.)

Concepts in the Pathophysiology of Hepatocellular Carcinoma

The problems of extrapolation from experimental animals to humans is perhaps nowhere better illustrated than in the subject of hepatocellular carcinoma. Despite the fact that many persistent chemicals in the environment cause liver tumors when administered at high doses to experimental animals, it is as yet unknown whether organochlorine pesticides, polyhalogenated biphenyls, etc. also produce cancer in humans exposed chronically to small amounts of these substances. Investigation of this problem by classic epidemiology in human populations is difficult because of the long latent period for emergence of human malignancy.

An advance in the pathophysiology of experimental chemical carcinogenesis has been the establishment of a multistage model of liver cancer, analogous to that previously established for the skin (23, 24,73,74). For example, Farber and his associates have developed a multistep model for liver carcinogenesis that can be divided into two stages (Fig. 19-2). The first stage, initiation, can be produced by exposing rats to known chemical procarcinogens that, when metabolically activated, interact with DNA and produce mutations. These short-term biochemical changes, however, will resolve immediately unless there is prompt application of a second stimulus capable of evoking hepatocyte replication (e.g., partial hepatectomy). Thus, the initiating process results in conversion of some normal hepatocytes into "preneoplastic" hepatocytes. These postulated cells (presently unrecognizable) are irrevocably committed to retain the potential for developing into hepatocellular carcinomas, and yet, they will remain dormant for the life of the animal unless a second series of manipulations, termed promotion, is applied.

Although there are many "promotion" protocols, all have in common the simultaneous exposure of the liver to a stimulus for hepatocyte replication combined with an antimitogenic stimulus. Farber (24) has proposed that such opposing forces for replication offer a selective advantage for survival of the preneoplastic hepatocytes. These cells proliferate, forming foci or nodules of phenotypically altered hyperplastic cells. These hyperplastic foci will revert to latent, preneoplastic hepatocytes if the promoting stimuli are stopped. However, if selection pressures are maintained, overt hepatocellular carcinomas will develop.

It may be inferred from these models that carcinogenesis involves sequential exposure to a number of stimuli producing a series of rare events that infrequently lead to cancer. For cancers to be produced the individual must be exposed to both initiating and promoting influences in sufficient amounts and in the correct sequence (73). It is obvious that models such as these should be most useful for future attempts to investigate the mechanisms of carcinogenesis and also to establish dose dependency, quantitatively as a rational means of fixing permissible amounts of initiators or promoters in the environment.

Sirica et al. tested chlordecone (Kepone®) in a two-stage rat model of hepatocarcinogenesis (84). In these studies, in both males and females, chlordecone acted largely as a liver tumor promoter rather than as a complete hepatic carcinogen. Dose-response experiments revealed that the hepatocarcinogenic effects of long-term chlordecone administration became undetectable in noninitiated rat liver at concentrations in the same range as those measured in human biopsies taken from exposed workers who exhibited no liver abnormalities.

Of interest was the marked gender difference in the incidence of malignant liver tumors caused by chlordecone promotion in rats. Hepatocellular cancer was seen in up to 63% of female rats whose livers had previously been initiated with a subcarcinogenic dose of diethylnitrosamine given 24 h after partial hepatectomey and then promoted by 27 weeks of chlordecone administration. In contrast, none of comparably treated males had malignant liver tumors, even after 44 weeks of chlordecone administration. Although the toxicity of chlordecone in women has never been studied, it is of interest that increased risk for primary liver cancer was noted among women exposed to solvents (33).

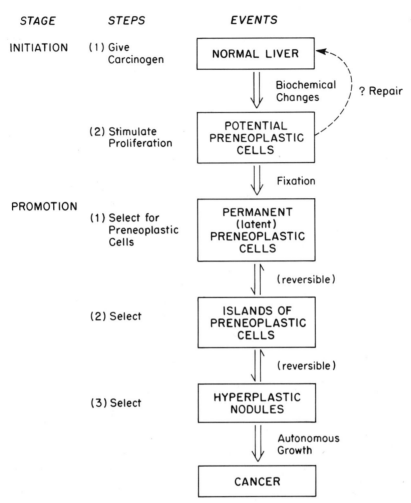

FIGURE 19-2. Multistep model of chemical carcinogenesis. From Guzelian (28).

CLINICAL ASPECTS OF EXPOSURE OF THE LIVER TO ENVIRONMENTAL CHEMICALS

Clinical Characteristics

Clinically overt liver failure manifested by jaundice, hepatic encephalopathy, or portal hypertension is readily diagnosed on clinical grounds but is a rare complication of exposure to environmental chemicals. When liver failure is related to exposure it generally is due to either accidental or intentional contact with large amounts of hepatotoxin. A far more common but difficult problem is the evaluation of mild, asymptomatic, clinically inconspicuous evidence of liver effects of exposure to a potential hepatotoxic substance. Often this is discovered by routine laboratory tests in a medical surveillance

program. Mild injury to the liver may accompany clinically overt toxicity to other organ systems. In these instances the challenge to the physician is to establish a cause-and-effect relationship between exposure and abnormalities on liver tests. Establishing this relationship in an individual patient may be impossible because standard clinical tests of liver structure and function, including liver biopsy, although often quite sensitive, reveal only nonspecific changes. The following examples serve to illustrate this point.

Polychlorinated biphenyls. Several studies of groups of electrical workers whose average serum or blood concentrations of polychlorinated biphenyls (PCBs) were in the range of 33.4 to 524 ng/mL revealed statistically significant changes in liver tests, summarized in Table 19-3. The findings were not entirely

TABLE 19-3. Effects of Some Environmental Chemicals on Clinical Tests of the Liver

Agent	Liver tests					References
	Hepatomegaly	BR[a]	AST[b]/ALT[c]	GTP[d]	Enzyme induction	
PCB[e]	+	↓	↑	↑	+	14, 25, 62, 85
"Yusho"[f]	+	↑|↓	–	N.R.	N.R.	36, 58, 68
PBB[g]	N.R.*	–	↑	↑	N.R.	4, 55
DDT[h]	N.R.	↓	–	↑	+	56, 67, 75
HCH[i]	+	–	–	–	+	37
Chlordecone (Kepone®)	+	–	–	–	+	15, 28
Chlorinated dioxins	+	–	↑	N.R.	+	45, 51
Vinyl chloride	+	–	↑	↑	–	7, 8, 61, 63, 86, 92, 96
Solvents	–	–	↑	N.R.	–	21, 88

[a]Bilirubin.
[b]Aspartate amino transferase (SGOT).
[c]Alanine amino transferase (SGPT).
[d]γ-Glutamyl transpeptidase.
[e]Polychlorinated biphenyls.
[f]"Rice oil disease" due to the ingestion of rice cooking oil contaminated with PCBs, polychlorinated dibenzofurans, and dibenzodioxins. The episode occurred in Japan in 1968.
[g]Polybrominated biphenyls.
[h]2,2-Bis-(p-chlorophenyl)-1,1,1-trichloroethane).
[i]Hexachlorocyclohexane.
*N.R., not reported.

uniform among these studies. A significant number of the workers, on physical examination, were found to have liver enlargement. The serum bilirubin tended to be in the lower range of normal, whereas serum transaminase activity tended to be in the high-normal range or slightly elevated. The serum γ-glutamyl transpeptidase (GTP) activity was positively correlated with the serum level of PCBs. The latter result was also reported in people exposed to sludge contaminated with PCBs (6) and in residents of Triana, Alabama, who were exposed to PCBs (57).

The lack of consistency in demonstrating the effects of PCBs on common liver tests is unexplained. PCBs may cause induction of the liver microsomal drug metabolizing enzyme systems in man as is the case for experimental animals (3). "Yusho" (Table 19-3) refers to the outbreak of poisonings in Japan in people who consumed rice oil that contained PCBs (34) plus polychlorinated dibenzofurans and dibenzodioxins. Initially, many of the patients presented with hepatomegaly, and in one series 11% were said to show jaundice (58). A subsequent study 7 years after the outbreak showed that there was a statistically significant reduction in serum bilirubin that correlated inversely with residual serum levels of poorly excreted PCB isomers (36). Transaminase levels were said to be normal. Studies of two large cohorts exposed to polybrominated biphenyls (PBBs) revealed no significant change in bilirubin, slight elevations in transaminase and GTP, and an elevation in urinary porphyrins that positively correlated with serum levels of PBBs (4,55) (Table 19-3).

Dichlorodiphenyltrichloroethane (DDT). Cross-sectional studies of groups with different serum DDT levels revealed hypobilirubinemia but no consistent relationship with transaminase (66). A positive correlation was found between the GTP and the levels of serum DDT and its isomers in residents of Triana, Alabama (56). Evidence for induction of liver drug-metabolizing enzymes was found in one study of DDT workers (75) (Table 19-3).

Hexachlorocyclohexane (HCH). In studies of workers occupationally exposed to HCH for up to 18 years, there was still evidence of induction of liver enzymes 7 years after the last exposure. However, their physical examinations, standard liver chemistry tests, and rates of elimination of indocyanine green and galactose were all normal (37) (Table 19-3). Hexachlorocyclohexane (a component of lindane) is an insecticide ingredient that, like PCBs, is highly lipophilic and is slowly excreted from the body.

Chlorodecane (Kepone®). Among the most complete data on the effects of exposure to an environmental agent of the class of lipophilic organochlorine chemicals in humans are the results of studies of 32 workers exposed to high concentrations of chlordecone (30). Despite the fact that these workers had high concentrations of chlordecone in their serum, adipose tissue, and liver (15), standard liver screening tests were in each case repeatedly negative (30). However, there was liver enlargement, and tests for liver microsomal enzyme induction were positive (Table 19-3). Clearance of sulfobromophthalein (BSP) was normal in all of these patients, and liver biopsies revealed only nonspecific alterations (30).

Workers exposed to chlorinated phenols and to contaminants (including 2,3,7,8-tetrachlorodibenzodioxin or dioxin) had hepatomegaly and mild abnormalities of liver tests (51). Evidence of liver microsomal enzyme induction was reported in children exposed to dioxin as a result of an explosion in a factory in Seveso, Italy (45). Liver biopsies of workers in a plant producing chlorinated phenols showed only mild "reactive" (or nonspecific) hepatitis, Kupffer cell hyperplasia, mild fatty infiltration, and slight periportal fibrosis (71).

Vinyl chloride. Exposure to vinyl chloride over a prolonged period of time clearly increases the risk of developing angiosarcoma of the liver, noncirrhotic portal hypertension, peliosis hepatitis (localized areas of sinusoidal dilatation with dropout of hepatocytes), hepatic fibrosis, or cirrhosis (7,8,63,86).

There are several prospective screening programs for detecting those individuals exposed to vinyl chloride who may be developing liver disease (61,90). Available algorithms for screening begin in general with standard chemistry tests, including the GTP, and progress to the clearance of an organic anion dye and then to liver biopsy, angiography, or other invasive diagnostic tests.

Some experts have concluded that best results were obtained with the use of GTP, as the least specific but most sensitive test, plus the alkaline phosphatase, as the test with highest specificity, particularly when compared with clearance of indocyanine green (90). None of the federally recommended tests for screening vinyl chloride workers proved to be of added benefit.

Other investigators have concluded that ultrasonographic evaluation of the liver, spleen, and abdomen offers greater specificity and sensitivity as a screening technique for workers exposed to vinyl chloride (96). They point out that 35% of their control subjects had liver test abnormalities when examined by standard chemistry tests. This illustrates a problem associated with the use of sensitive liver tests in mass screening endeavors, namely, the lack of appropriate control values on the incidence of abnormalities of liver chemistries in unexposed populations.

Organic solvents. Interest in subtle liver injury was prompted by two studies of subjects exposed to organic solvents (21,88). These studies of selected workers revealed mild increases in transaminase, liver biopsy findings of mild fatty metamorphosis, focal hepatocellular necrosis, and mild portal fibrosis. These provocative reports of possibly overlooked liver injury from exposure to common chemicals in the environment have been the subject of stern editorial disapproval (5,46,59). Nevertheless, the possibility of liver injury caused by exposure to organic solvents should be regarded as a hypothesis worthy of further investigation.

Hepatic porphyria. Hepatic porphyria (porphyria cutanea tarda) has been reported in humans exposed to hexachlorobenzene (89), PCBs, PBBs, or chlorinated dibenzodioxins, but not in chlordecone-poisoned workers. This likely relates to the failure of chlordecone to bind to the liver cytosolic "Ah receptor," which is believed to mediate effects of the other chemicals on the liver (and other tissues) (69). The porphyria results from partial inhibition of the heme biosynthetic pathway at the step of decarboxylation of uroporphyrin (89).

Diagnostic Tests

Liver biopsy. Liver biopsy remains an indispensable tool for establishing the diagnosis and prognosis of possible liver injury in patients who are seen because of abnormalities in nonspecific screening liver tests. It is surprising, however, to realize how little information is available on human liver histopathology in people exposed to ubiquitous environmental pollutants. Some of the most complete information comes from 12 needle liver biopsy specimens in chlordecone-exposed workers (Table 19-4). Light microscopic examination of specimens from these patients revealed only nonspecific changes, including minimal steatosis, hyperglycogenation of nuclei, and focal proliferation of reticuloendothelial cells. Similarly, ultrastructural changes in these liver biopsies showed residual bodies, branched mitochondria, paracrystalline inclusions, plasma membrane blebs, and proliferation of the endoplasmic reticulum.

The mitochondrial changes are nonspecific and

TABLE 19-4. Liver Histology in 12 Patients with Chlordecone Poisoning[a]

Finding	No. of patients
Light microscopy	
Vacuolated nuclei	3
Increased cytoplasmic pigment (lipofuscin)	11
Fatty infiltration	3
Portal inflammatory cells (mild)	5
Portal fibrosis (mild)	3
Focal areas of proliferated reticuloendothelial cells	3
Electron microscopy	
Proliferated smooth endoplasmic reticulum	11
Dilated, vesiculated rough endoplasmic reticulum	6
Lipid vacuoles	8
Branched mitochondria with paracrystalline inclusions	4
Blebs in hepatocyte sinusoidal membrane	4

[a]From Guzelian et al. (30).

have been noted in a wide variety of pathological conditions of the liver. One reported human liver biopsy in a patient exposed to polychlorinated biphenyls also revealed mitochondrial abnormalities (35). As indicated in the preceding section, many mild chemical exposures lead only to nonspecific reactive hepatitis on liver biopsies. However, in the case of vinyl chloride exposure, characteristic morphological features may be present.

It is unfortunate that so little histological information is available. Presumably, this is because of the belief that liver biopsy is unwarranted on clinical grounds. Nevertheless, when performed by an experienced hepatologist, liver biopsy carries only a small risk, and, as illustrated in the case of the chlordecone-poisoned workers, the information gained may be essential for diagnosis, for management, and ultimately for designing a rational approach to treatment.

Induction of microsomal enzymes. A prominent effect of lipophilic environmental agents, especially the halogenated hydrocarbon chemicals, is to induce both in animals and in man the enzymes in the smooth endoplasmic reticulum responsible for xenobiotic biotransformation. The clinical consequences of this effect are unknown. But concern is raised because induction of liver microsomal enzymes may alter the pathways or rates of metabolism of other xenobiotics or of endogenous substances such as lipoproteins (2). Another concern is that many compounds that induce drug-metabolizing enzymes also are classified as tumor promoters in experimental carcinogenesis systems. Hence, it would be desirable to have simple, specific, and clinically practical tests that would recognize liver microsomal enzyme induction in humans (Table 19-5).

One approach is measuring the clearance of model drugs that rely on liver metabolism for their elimination. Clearance can be assessed from the rate of disappearance from plasma or saliva (for example, antipyrine or tolbutamide) or from the rate of appearance in the breath of metabolites derived from radioactively labeled drug substrates [for example, aminopyrine (32), caffeine (78), or phenacetin (10)]. Accelerated metabolism of these drugs in subjects exposed to agents that induce microsomal

enzymes presumably reflects accumulation in the microsomes of cytochromes P-450, which may be rate limiting for the oxidative metabolism and elimination of many foreign and endogenous compounds. Urinary excretion of steroid metabolites may also serve as a reflection of the cytochrome-P-450-mediated drug-oxidizing activity, since steroids serve as substrates for these versatile hemoproteins. Many of the compounds that induce the cytochromes P-450 in the liver also induce microsomal enzymes involved in the metabolism of glucuronic acid (43). Therefore, increased urinary excretion of glucaric acid, a breakdown product of glucuronic acid, may signify enzyme induction and proliferation of the smooth endoplasmic reticulum in the liver (18,41,42).

Microsomal enzyme induction in the liver may be associated with elevated γ-glutamyl transpeptidase (GTP) activity in the serum (see below). Finally, it has been suggested that leukocyte δ-aminolevulinic acid synthetase activity may serve as a convenient, noninvasive way to monitor induction of liver microsomal enzymes (77).

It is of interest that the frequently noted generalities about induction of human liver microsomal enzymes by lipophilic chemicals such as organochlorine pesticides, polyhalogenated biphenyls, and related compounds are based on surprisingly few studies (Table 19-6). These studies show the half-life of antipyrine plasma was significantly reduced in people exposed to polychlorinated biphenyls (3), to a mixture of chlorinated hydrocarbons (primarily DDT but also including chlordane and lindane) (53), to a skin cream containing lindane (38), or to HCH (37). Accelerated clearance of antipyrine from saliva was found in persons exposed to pesticides (20). Unfortunately, none of these studies compared the concentrations of the environmental chemical inducer in plasma or liver to the effect on liver drug-metabolizing activity. It is therefore uncertain whether there is a threshold concentration of these environmental agents required to achieve induction in human liver. It has been established, however, that antipyrine half-life was shortened in chlordecone-poisoned workers (Table 19-6) at a time when the concentration of this pesticide in the plasma was no less than 1000 ng/mL. Workers exposed to DDT exhibited accelerated clearance of phenylbutazone and increased urinary excretion of 6 β-hydroxycorticosterol with a possible threshold for this effect being associated with a serum concentration of DDT of 300–500 ng/mL (75).

Excretion of urinary glucaric acid has received little attention as a way to test for microsomal enzyme induction in the liver by environmental chemicals. Slight elevations of urinary glucaric acid were found in workers making the pesticide Endrin (93). One study of workers exposed to DDT failed to

TABLE 19-5. Methods of Recognizing Liver Microsomal Enzyme Induction in Humans

1. Clearance of drugs (e.g., antipyrine, tolbutamide)
2. Breath tests (aminopyrine, caffeine, diazepam)
3. Urinary steroid metabolites
4. Urinary glucaric acid
5. Serum glutamyl transpeptidase activity
6. Leukocyte δ-aminolevulinic acid synthase activity

TABLE 19-6. Effect of Lipophilic Chlorinated Hydrocarbons on Clearance of Antipyrine in Humans

	Antipyrine half-life		
Agent	Control (n)	Exposed (n)	Reference
1. PCB[a]	15.6 (5)	10.8 (5)	9
2. DDT[b] (and others)	13.1 (33)	7.7 (26)	26
3. Lindane	12.9 (3)	11.7 (9)	27
4. HCH[c]	14.7 (4)	7.4 (6)	19
5. Chlordecone (Kepone®)	14.8 (3)	7.5 (10)	20

[a]Polychlorinated biphenyls.
[b]2,2-bis-(p-chlorophenyl)-1,1,1-trichloroethane.
[c]Hexachlorocyclohexane.

reveal elevated excretion of urinary glucaric acid (66). However, the highest serum DDT concentration in this group (167 ng/mL) was less than the apparent threshold associated with liver enzyme induction in another group of DDT workers as based on the measurements of drug clearance or excretion of steroid metabolites (75). Hence, it remains uncertain whether DDT (even in higher doses) affects urinary excretion of glucaric acid.

Definitive evidence that an organochlorine chemical can increase urinary excretion of glucaric acid comes from studies of chlordecone-poisoned workers (30). After these workers had been placed on cholestyramine, an orally administered anionic binding resin that stimulates the elimination of chlordecone from the body (15), chlordecone concentrations in the plasma fell to low or undetectable values, and the excretion of glucaric acid fell into the normal range. From these results, the estimated serum level of chlordecone associated with enzyme induction in the liver is in the range of 100–500 ng/ml.

Epidemiologists have come to rely on GTP as a marker not just for liver disease but also for induction of liver microsomal enzymes. However, data indicate that the enzyme is not found in the liver exclusively but is present in most tissues of the body (bone being a notable exception), with significant amounts in kidney, pancreas, spleen, and intestine (70). A second important point is that GTP is not primarily a microsomal enzyme, as it has been localized to the hepatocyte plasma membrane (13,44, 91). It is also found in the apical portions of some human bile duct cells and possibly in nonparenchymal liver cells (13,26).

Enthusiasm for using the GTP test, especially as a marker for induction of liver microsomal enzymes, is tempered because GTP activity in human serum is increased in association with numerous physiological or pathological conditions (83). Patients receiving drugs, particularly antiepileptic drugs such as barbiturates and phenytoin, have significantly increased GTP activity (80,95). The enzyme is increased in almost every form of hepatobiliary disease, including subtle forms of liver injury (12,19,38,48,83,94). GTP is also elevated in diabetes or other pancreatic diseases (47,70), in kidney diseases (60), in congestive heart failure (81), in angina (31), in myocardial infarction (1), and in many other conditions (22). The consumption of alcohol, even in moderate amounts, may elevate the GTP activity (79). The GTP is elevated in children and also appears to be higher in adult males than in females (52). Indeed, birth control pills appear to decrease GTP, at least under conditions where the enzyme is elevated in viral hepatitis (16).

In addition to false-positive results for liver enzyme induction, the GTP can give false-negative results as well. For example, administration of rifampicin to normal subjects increased clearance of hexobarbital and urinary glucaric acid, and yet GTP activity remained normal (11). Moreover, despite the strong evidence for induction of liver microsomal enzymes in chlordecone-poisoned workers, GTP activity remained normal (30). Thus, an elevated GTP activity, particularly when taken out of clinical context, as in an epidemiologic study, need not indicate liver involvement, let alone induction of drug-metabolizing enzymes in the liver.

In summary, the induction of microsomal enzymes is a prominent effect of exposure to lipophilic environmental agents. Although the clinical implications of such enzymatic changes are unclear, they would be expected to alter the hepatic metabolism of a number of exogenous and endogenous substances. For this reason the various clinical methods of evaluating the induction of hepatic drug-metabolizing enzymes were discussed in detail.

Treatment

There are no specific treatments for hepatotoxicity caused by environmental agents apart from those generally applicable to liver disease from drugs or other causes. In the case of acute liver failure, intensive supportive care is indicated. With chronic liver diseases, particularly those resulting in chronic liver failure, treatment of hepatic encephalopathy or portal hypertension becomes the major focus of medical attention. A general principle of drug-induced liver disease is that cessation of drug administration often results in resolution of the signs and symptoms of liver injury. It seems likely that this would also be true for environmental agents, provided that, like drugs, these agents have a short biological half-life in man.

A troublesome problem is the potential hepatic effects of lipophilic environmental chemicals that are excreted at very slow rates (if at all) from the body. These agents may persist in the tissues for many years. Only minimal amounts of these chemicals (e.g., organochlorine pesticides, polyhalogenated biphenyls) are excreted in urine or in bile, through the skin, or in the breath. Until recently there was no remedy for this problem.

However, as a result of intensive investigations of the chlordecone-poisoned workers, it has been discovered that there exists in humans a nonbiliary pathway for translocation of chlordecone from the blood into the intestinal lumen, probably representing transmucosal transport by the gut itself [reviewed by Guzelian (29)]. This pathway appears to account for the minimal amounts of chlordecone appearing in the stool. Furthermore, it was discovered that this pathway is inhibited by bile normally flowing into the intestine.

When the bile is removed from the intestine, either surgically by diversion of the bile duct or medically by oral administration of cholestyramine (a nonabsorbable agent that binds bile acids), increased amounts of chlordecone appeared in the stool, accompanied by the accelerated disappearance of the compound from the body. This stimulated chemical detoxification by treatment with cholestyramine was accompanied by almost complete amelioration of the signs and symptoms of chlordecone toxicity. Based on preliminary data from a number of laboratories, it appears that the transmucosal pathway can be manipulated pharmacologically to stimulate the excretion not only of chlordecone but of many other slowly excreted lipophilic substances. If so, this development offers promise as a means for safe and effective treatment for people exposed to these ubiquitous and persistent environmental agents.

SUMMARY

In past years, before there was intense concern about health consequences of toxic chemicals in the environment, and before modern industrial hygiene was widely instituted, clinically overt (and often fatal) liver injury resulted from exposure to many kinds of environmental hepatotoxins. Presently, a more common occurrence is clinically inconspicuous liver effects that carry an uncertain cause-and-effect relationship with possible etiological agents. Important advances have been made in understanding the pathogenesis of cytotoxicity, mutagenesis, and carcinogenesis in experimental animals and the important role that the liver plays in these toxic disease processes. With the blending of talents of clinical hepatologists and toxicologists, it may be possible to develop noninvasive methods for examining host genetic or acquired factors that determine the metabolic outcome of exposure to potentially toxic substances in the environment. Undoubtedly, future research will be directed to discover whether environmental agents are causative or provocative factors in such diseases as cryptogenic cirrhosis, immunologic liver diseases, or hepatocellular carcinomas.

REFERENCES

1. Agostini A, Ideo G, Stabilini R: Serum gamma-glutamyl transpeptidase activity in myocardial infarction. Br Heart J 27:688, 1965.
2. Alcohol, HDL cholesterol and liver microsomal induction. Lancet 1:8367, 1984.
3. Alvares AP, Fischbein A, Anderson MD, et al: Alterations in drug metabolism in workers exposed to polychlorinated biphenyls. Clin Pharmacol Ther 22:140, 1977.
4. Anderson HA, Wolff MS, Lilis R, et al: Symptoms and clinical abnormalities following ingestion of polybrominated-biphenyl contaminated food products. Ann NY Acad Sci 320:684, 1979.
5. Axelson O: Solvents and the liver. Eur J Clin Invest 13:109, 1983.
6. Baker EL, Landrigan PJ, Glueck CJ, et al: Metabolic consequences of exposure to polychlorinated biphenyls (PCB) in sewage sludge. Am J Epidemiol 112:553, 1980.
7. Berk PD: Vinyl chloride-associated liver disease. Ann NY Acad Sci 84:717, 1976.
8. Blendis LM, Smith PM, Lawrie BW, et al: Portal hypertension in vinyl chloride monomer workers: A hemodynamic study. Gastroenterology 75:206, 1978.
9. Blumberg WE: Enzymic modification of environmental intoxicants: The role of cytochrome P-450. Q Rev Biophys 2:481, 1978.
10. Breen KJ, Bury RW, Calder IV, et al: A [14C]phenacetin breath test to measure hepatic function in man. Hepatology 4:47, 1984.
11. Breimer DD, Zilly W, Richter W: Influence of rifampicin on drug metabolism: Differences between hexobarbital and anti-pyrine. Clin Pharmacol Ther 21:470, 1977.
12. Burrows S, Feldman W, McBride F: Serum gamma glutamyl transpeptidase. Am J Clin Pathol 64:311, 1975.

13. Busachi C, Mebis J, Broeckaert L, et al: Histochemistry of γ-glutamyl transpeptidase in human liver biopsies. Pathol Res Pract 172:99, 1981.

14. Chase K, Wong D, Thomas D, et al: Clinical and metabolic abnormalities associated with occupational exposure to polychlorinated biphenyls (PCBs). J Occup Med 24:109, 1982.

15. Cohn WJ, Boylan JJ, Clanke RV, et al: Treatment of chlordecone (Kepone) toxicity with cholestyramine. N Engl J Med 298:243, 1978.

16. Combes B, Shore GM, Cunningham FG, et al: Serum gamma-glutamyl transpeptidase activity in viral hepatitis suppression in pregnancy and by birth control pills. Gastroenterology 72:271, 1977.

17. Conney AH, Burns JJ: Metabolic interactions among environmental chemicals and drugs. Science 178:576, 1972.

18. Cunningham JL, Evans DAP: Urinary D-glucaric acid excretion and acetanilide pharmacokinetics before and during diphenylhydantoin administration. Eur J Clin Pharmacol 7:387, 1974.

19. Cushcieri A, Baker PR: Gamma-glutamyl-transpeptidase in hepatobiliary disease—value as an enzymatic liver function test. Br J Exp Pathol 55:110, 1974.

20. Dossing M: Changes in hepatic microsomal enzyme function in workers exposed to mixtures of chemicals. Clin Pharmacol Ther 32:340, 1982.

21. Dossing M, Arlien-Soborg P, Petersen LM, et al: Liver damage associated with occupational exposure to organic solvents in house painters. Eur J Clin Invest 13:151, 1983.

22. Ellis G, Worthy E, Goldberg DM: Lack of value of serum gamma-glutamyl transferase in the diagnosis of hepatobiliary disease. Clin Biochem 12:142, 1979.

23. Emmelot P, Scherer E: The first relevant cell stage in rat liver carcinogenesis: A quantitative approach. Biochim Biophys Acta 605:247, 1980.

24. Farber E, Cameron R: The sequential analysis of cancer development. Adv Cancer Res 31:125, 1980.

25. Fischbein AL, Wolff MS, Lilis R, et al: Clinical findings among PCB-exposed capacitor manufacturing workers. Ann NY Acad Sci 320:703, 1979.

26. Galteau MM, Siest G, Ratansavanh D: Effect of phenobarbital on the distribution of gamma-glutamyltransferase between hepatocytes and nonparenchymal cells in the rat. Cell Mol Biol 26:267, 1979.

27. Gidlow DA, Church JF, Clayton BE: Haematological and biochemical parameters in an industrial workforce. Ann Clin Biochem. 20:341, 1983.

28. Guzelian PS: Environmental toxins and the liver. Pract Gastroenterol 5:26, 1981.

29. Guzelian PS: Comparative toxicology of chlordecone (Kepone) in humans and experimental animals. Annu Rev Pharmacol Toxicol 22:89, 1982.

30. Guzelian PS, Vranian G, Boylan JJ, et al: Liver structure and function in patients poisoned with chlordecone (Kepone). Gastroenterology 78:206, 1980.

31. Hedworth-Whitty RB, Whitfield JB, Richardson RW: Serum gamma-glutamyl transpeptidase activity in myocardial ischemia. Br Heart J 29:432, 1967.

32. Hepner GW, Vesell ES: Assessment of aminopyrine metabolism in man by breath analysis after oral administration of ¹⁴C-aminopyrine: Effects of phenobarbital, disulfiram and portal cirrhosis. N Engl J Med 291:1384, 1974.

33. Hernberg S, Kauppinen T, Riala R, et al: Increased risk for primary liver cancer among women exposed to solvents. Scand J Work Environ Health 14:356, 1988.

34. Higuchi K (ed): PCB Poisoning and Pollution. Academic Press, New York, 1976.

35. Hirayama C, Irisa T, Tamamoto T: Fine structural changes of the liver in a patient with chloribiphenyls intoxication. Fukuoka Acta Med 60:455, 1969.

36. Hirayama C, Okumura M, Nagai J, et al: Hypobilirubinemia in patients with polychlorinated biphenyls poisoning. Clin Chim Acta 55:97, 1974.

37. Hoensch H, Andre M, Gruner J: Inducing effect of B-hexachlorocyclohexane (B-HCH) on human hepatic drug metabolism. Liver Metab Dis 76:15, 1982.

38. Horwitz CA, Burke MD, Henie W, et al: Late persistence of serum gamma-glutamyl transpeptidase activity after mononucleosis. Gastroenterology 72:1322, 1977.

39. Hosler J, Tschanz C, Hignite CE, et al: Topical application of lindane cream (Kwell) and antipyrine metabolism. J Invest Dermatol 74:51, 1979.

40. Hulka BS, Wilcosky TC, Griffith JD: Biological Markers in Epidemiology, Oxford University Press, Oxford, 1990.

41. Hunter J, Maxwell JD, Carrella M, et al: Urinary D-glucaric-acid excretion as a test for hepatic enzyme induction in man. Lancet 1:572, 1971.

42. Hunter J, Maxwell JD, Stewart DA, et al: Increased hepatic microsomal enzyme activity from occupational exposure to certain organochlorine pesticides. Nature 237:399, 1972.

43. Hunter J, Maxwell JD, Stewart DA, et al: Urinary D-glucaric acid excretion and total liver content of cytochrome P-450 in guinea pigs: Relationship during enzyme induction and following inhibition of protein synthesis. Biochem Pharmacol 22:743, 1973.

44. Huseby NE: Subcellular localization of gamma-glutamyltransferase activity in guinea pig liver. Effect of phenobarbital on the enzyme activity levels. Clin Chim Acta 94:163, 1979.

45. Ideo G, Bellati G, Bellobuono A, et al: Increased urinary D-glucaric acid excretion by children living in an area polluted with tetrachlorodibenzoparadioxin (TCDD). Clin Chim Acta 120:273, 1982.

46. Industrial solvents and the liver. Lancet 1:8316, 1983.

47. Jacobs WLW: Gamma-glutamyl-transpeptidase in diseases of the liver, cardiovascular system and diabetes mellitus. Clin Chim Acta 38:419, 1972.

48. Kampa IS, Jarzabek J, Clain J: The use of gamma-glutamyl transpeptidase in differentiating liver from bone isoenzymes of alkaline phosphatase. Clin Biochem 9:234, 1976.

49. Kato R: Drug metabolism under pathological and abnormal physiological states in animals and man. Xenobiotica 7:25, 1977.

50. Kew MC: The hepatitis-B virus and hepatocellular carcinoma. Semin Liver Dis 1:31, 1981.

51. Kimbrough RD, Grandjean P: Occupational exposure. In: Halogenated Biphenyls, Terphenyls, Naphthalenes, Dibenzodioxins and Related Products, 2nd ed., p 485, Kimbrough RD, Jensen AA (eds.), Elsevier, Amsterdam, 1989.

52. Knight JA, Haymond RE: Gamma-glutamyltransferase and alkaline phosphatase activities compared in

serum of normal children and children with liver disease. Clin Chem 27:48, 1981.

53. Kolmodin B, Azarnoff DL, Sjoqvist F: Effects of environmental factors on drug metabolism: Decreased plasma half-life of antipyrine in workers exposed to chlorinated hydrocarbon insecticides. Clin Pharmacol Ther 10:638, 1969.

54. Kopelman H, Scheuer P, Williams R: The liver lesion in Epping jaundice. Q J Med 35:553, 1966.

55. Kreiss K, Roberts C: Serial PBB levels, PCB levels, and clinical chemistries in Michigan's PBB cohort. Arch Environ Health 37:141, 1982.

56. Kreiss K, Zack MM, Kimbrough RD, et al: Cross-sectional study of a community with exceptional exposure to DDT. JAMA 245:1926, 1981.

57. Kreiss K, Zack MM, Kimbrough RD, et al: Association of blood pressure and polychlorinated biphenyl levels. JAMA 245:2505, 1981.

58. Kuratsune M, Shapiro RE (eds.): PCB Poisoning in Japan and Taiwan, Alan R Liss, New York, 1984.

59. Kurppa K, Vainio H: Study design, liver disease and house painters' exposure to organic solvents. Eur J Clin Invest 13:113, 1983.

60. Lehmann D, Prentice M, Rosalki SB: Plasma gamma-glutamyltranspeptidase activity following renal transplantation. Am J Clin Invest 7:148, 1970.

61. Makk L, Creech JL, Whelan JG, et al: Liver damage and angiosarcoma in vinyl chloride workers. JAMA 230:64, 1974.

62. Maroni M, Colombi A, Arbosti G, et al: Occupational exposure to polychlorinated biphenyls in electrical workers. II. Health effects. Br J Ind Med 38:55, 1981.

63. Marsteller HJ, Lelbach WK, Muler R, et al: Unusual splenomegalic liver disease as evidenced by peritoneoscopy and guided liver biopsy among polyvinyl chloride production workers. Ann NY Acad Sci 246:95, 1975.

64. McLean EK, Mattocks AR: Environmental liver injury: Plant toxins. In: Toxic Injury of the Liver (Part B), p 517, Farber E, Fisher M (eds.), Marcel Dekker, New York, 1980.

65. Mitchell JR, Zimmerman HJ, Ishak KG, et al: Isoniazid liver injury: Clinical spectrum, pathology and probable pathogenesis. Ann Intern Med 84:181, 1976.

66. Morgan DP, Lin LI: Blood organochlorine pesticide concentrations, clinical hematology and biochemistry in workers occupationally exposed to pesticides. Arch Environ Contam Toxicol 7:423, 1978.

67. Morgan DP, Roan CC: Liver function in workers having high tissue stores of chlorinated hydrocarbon pesticides. Arch Environ Health 21:14, 1974.

68. Nagayama J, Masuda Y, Kuratsune M: Chlorinated dibenzofurans in Kanechlor and rice oil used by patients with "Yusho." Fukuoka Acta Med 66:593, 1975.

69. Nebert DW, Eisen HJ, Hegishi M, et al: Genetic mechanisms controlling the induction of polysubstrate monooxygenase (P-450) activities. Annu Rev Pharmacol Toxicol 21:431, 1981.

70. Orlowski M: The role of gamma-glutamyl transpeptidase in the internal diseases clinic. Arch Immunol Ther Exp 11:1, 1963.

71. Pazderova-Vejlupkova J, Lukas E, Nemcova M, et al: The development and prognosis of chronic intoxication by tetrachlordibenzo-p-dioxin in men. Arch Environ Health 36:5, 1981.

72. Perera FP, Weinstein IB: Molecular epidemiology and carcinogen DNA adduct detection: New approaches to studies of human cancer causation. J Chron Dis 35:581, 1982.

73. Pitot HC: Fundamentals of Oncology, 3rd ed., Marcel Dekker, New York, 1986.

74. Pitot HC, Sirica AE: The stages of initiation and promotion in hepatocarcinogenesis. Biochim Biophys Acta 605:191, 1980.

75. Poland A, Smith D, Kuntzman R, et al: Effect of intensive occupational exposure to DDT on phenylbutazone and cortisol metabolism in human subjects. Clin Pharmacol Ther 11:724, 1970.

76. Popper H, Gerber MA, Schaffner F, et al: Environmental hepatic injury in man. Prog Liver Dis 6:605, 1979.

77. Rapeport WG, McInnes GT, Thompson GG, et al: Hepatic enzyme induction and leucocyte delta-aminolaevulinic acid synthase activity: Studies with carbamazepine. Br J Clin Pharmacol 16:133, 1983.

78. Renner E, Wietholtz H, Huguenin P, et al: Caffeine: A model compound for measuring liver function. Hepatology 4:38, 1984.

79. Rosalki SB, Rau D: Serum gamma-glutamyl transpeptidase activity in alcoholism. Clin Chim Acta 39:41, 1972.

80. Rosalki SB, Tarlow D, Rau D: Plasma gamma-glutamyl transpeptidase elevation in patients receiving enzyme-inducing drugs. Lancet 2:376, 1971.

81. Rutenberg AM, Goldbarg JA, Peneda FP: Plasma gamma-glutamyl transpeptidase. Clin Chem 15:124, 1969.

82. Schmid R: Cutaneous porphyria in Turkey. N Engl J Med 263:397, 1960.

83. Selinger MJ, Matloff DS, Kaplan MM: γ-Glutamyl transpeptidase activity in liver disease: Serum elevation is independent of hepatic GGTP activity. Clin Chim Acta 125:283, 1982.

84. Sirica AE, Wilkerson CS, Wu LL, et al: Evaluation of chlordecone in a two-stage model of hepatocarcinogenesis: A significant sex difference in the hepatocellular carcinoma incidence. Carcinogenesis 10:1047, 1989.

85. Smith AB, Schloemer J, Lowry LK, et al: Metabolic and health consequences of occupational exposure to polychlorinated biphenyls. Br J Ind Med 39:361, 1982.

86. Smith PM, Crossley IR, Williams DMJ: Portal hypertension in vinyl-chloride production workers. Lancet 2:602, 1976.

87. Snyder R, Remmer H: Classes of hepatic microsomal mixed function oxidase inducers. Pharmacol Ther 7:203, 1979.

88. Sotaniemi EA, Sutinen S, Sutinen S, et al: Liver injury in subjects occupationally exposed to chemicals in low doses. Acta Med Scand 212:207, 1982.

89. Strik JJTWA, Koeman JH (eds.): Chemical Porphyria in Man, Elsevier, Amsterdam, 1979.

90. Tamburro CH, Greenberg R: Effectiveness of federally required medical laboratory screening in the detection of chemical liver injury. Environ Health Perspect 41:117, 1981.

91. Tazi A, Ratansavanh D, Galteau MM, et al: Hepatic membrane gamma-glutamyltransferase solubilization facilitated after administration of phenobarbital. Pharmacol Res Commun 11:211, 1979.

92. Thomas LB; Vinyl-chloride-induced liver disease: From idiopathic portal hypertension (Banti's syndrome) to angiosarcomas. N Engl J Med 292:17, 1975.

93. Vrij-Standhardt WG, Strik JJTWA, Ottevanger CF, et al: Urinary D-glucaric acid and urinary total porphyrin excretion in workers exposed to endrin. In: Chemical Porphyria in Man, p 113, Strik JJTWA, Koeman JE (eds.), Elsevier/North-Holland, Amsterdam, 1979.

94. Whitfield JB, Pounder RE, Neale G, et al: Serum γ-glutamyl transpeptidase activity in liver disease. Gut 13:702, 1972.

95. Whitfield JB, Moss DW, Neale S, et al: Changes in plasma γ-glutamyl transpeptidase activity associated with alterations in drug metabolism in man. Br Med J 1:316, 1973.

96. Williams DMJ, Smith DPM, Taylor KJ, et al: Monitoring liver disorders in vinyl chloride monomer workers using greyscale ultrasonography. Br J Ind Med 33:152, 1976.

97. Zimmerman HJ: Syndromes of environmental hepatoxicity. In: Hepatotoxicity, The Adverse Effects of Drugs and Other Chemicals on the Liver, p 279, Appleton-Century Crofts, New York, 1978.

98. Zimmerman HJ, Maddrey WC: Toxic and drug-induced hepatitis. In: Diseases of the Liver, p 591, Schiff L, Schiff ER (eds.), JB Lippincott, Philadelphia, 1987.

RECOMMENDED READINGS

Plaa GL, Hewitt WR (eds.): Toxicology of the Liver, Raven Press, New York, 1982.

Zimmerman HJ, Maddrey WC: Toxic and drug-induced hepatitis. In: Diseases of the Liver, p 591, Schiff L, Schiff ER (eds.), JB Lippincott, Philadelphia, 1987.

20.   DISORDERS OF THE KIDNEY AND URINARY TRACT

William F. Finn

INTRODUCTION

There is evidence that many environmental chemicals produce acute and chronic renal damage (3,13, 17,60,61,124). The extent to which these agents cause clinically significant renal disease, however, has not been determined. Nor has the population at risk been clearly defined. The occurrence of many forms of acute and chronic renal failure without known cause and the presence of marked racial and regional differences in the incidence of chronic end-stage renal disease raise the question of the health hazard presented by environmental nephrotoxins.

There are several obstacles to identifying agents with nephrotoxic potential. These include a constantly changing environmental millieu, the presence of multiple exposures, the lack of simple and reliable tests to identify early renal injury, and the fact that renal failure can occur many years after the initial exposure to environmental nephrotoxins, when all evidence of exposure has disappeared. In addition, end-stage renal disease has many common characteristics regardless of its cause. These factors explain the virtual absence of epidemiologic data on the number of people who develop end-stage renal disease as a result of acute or chronic exposure to environmental nephrotoxins.

In the sections that follow, the relationship between exposure to environmental chemicals and renal injury is discussed. It will be obvious that more information is needed to delineate the role of environmental nephrotoxins in the development of acute and chronic renal impairment.

ENVIRONMENTAL CHEMICALS ASSOCIATED WITH ADVERSE EFFECTS ON THE KIDNEY

The list of environmental chemicals associated with toxic renal damage is shown in Table 20-1. Renal injury, associated with toxic exposure, may be acute or chronic and involve tubular, glomerular, or interstitial structures. The specific nature of the injury will depend on the properties of the substances involved, the intensity of exposure, and various host factors.

Acute Injury

When renal disease occurs immediately after toxic exposure, the relationship is apparent (82). Environmental chemicals producing acute renal injury can be separated into the following categories: organic solvents; heavy metals; various insecticides, herbicides, and fungicides; and miscellaneous agents. Some may trigger severe hemolytic reactions, causing hemoglobinuria. Others may lead to the destruction of striated muscle, and myoglobinuria will result. The consequent "pigment nephropathy" is not an uncommon form of acute renal failure.

Principles and Practice of Environmental Medicine, edited by Alyce Bezman Tarcher. Plenum Medical Book Company, New York, 1992.

TABLE 20-1.   Environmental Chemicals Associated with Renal Disease

Acute renal failure	Pigment nephropathy	Interstitial nephritis
Organic solvents	Hemoglobinuria	Cadmium
Carbon tetrachloride	Aniline	Lead
Chloroform	Arsine	Radiation
Ethylene dichloride	Cresol	Aflatoxins?
Toluene	Naphthalene	Glomerulonephritis
Trichloroethylene	Nitrobenzene	Hydrocarbons?
Heavy metals	Phenol	Silicon
Arsenic	Sodium chlorate	Nephrotic syndrome
Cadmium	Toluene	Mercury
Chromium	Myoglobinuria	Hydrocarbons?
Lead	Carbon monoxide	
Mercury	Mercuric chlorate	
Uranium		
Pesticides		
Chlorinated hydrocarbons		
Organophosphorus compounds		
Bipyridinium compounds		
Pentachlorophenol		

Chronic Injury

Many environmental nephrotoxins may cause subtle changes in renal structure and function. Such changes are difficult to detect and may only later be manifested as chronic indolent renal disease. Although the list of agents thought to be associated with chronic renal failure is shorter than the list of agents causing acute disease, the net effect may be greater (102). Injury may take the form of chronic interstital nephritis, chronic glomerulonephritis, or some forms of the nephrotic syndrome.

Heavy Metals

Arsenic

Arsenic is used in insecticides, ant poisons, weed killers, wallpaper, antifouling paint, ceramics, wood preservatives, and glass (5,56). The inorganic arsenicals such as arsenic trioxide are more toxic than are the organic compounds (95). Absorption occurs following inhalation or ingestion. The soluble compounds are readily absorbed via skin and mucous membranes and excreted primarily in the urine. Repeated doses are cumulative. Toxicity results when arsenic combines with sulfhydryl enzymes and interferes with cellular oxidative processes. Arsine is an extremely toxic gas produced by the action of acid on metal in the presence of arsenic. It is a hazard to workers in metallurgic industries who deal with ores contaminated by arsenic. Exposure to concentration as low as 10 ppm can cause death.

Cadmium

Cadmium is a major byproduct of zinc production (55,89,92). It is used industrially as a component in nickel–cadmium batteries; in the manufacture of alloys, paints, and glass; in electroplating and soldering; and as a stabilizer in plastics. Cadmium is found in cigarette smoke, seafood, and drinking water. As a result of wide exposure and a half-life that may exceed 30 years, the body content of cadmium slowly accumulates and may eventually reach about 30 mg. There is a wide consensus that the cadmium content of food is the major source of cadmium for the general population. Following absorption, cadmium tends to accumulate in the liver and kidney. It is bound to metallothionein, a low-molecular-weight cysteine-rich apoprotein.

Accumulation within the kidney continues even as other tissue concentrations fall. It appears that a certain level of cadmium must accumulate within the kidney before overt damage is produced. Urinary cadmium excretion increases when defects occur in the tubular reabsorption of metallothionein. Later, as tubular injury progresses to the point of death, there is a decrease in the renal cortical concentration of cadmium. Thereafter, renal cadmium levels may fall despite the fact that liver concentrations continue to rise. Blood values greater than 0.7 μg/dL, urine values above 20 μg/L, and renal cortical concentrations exceeding 200 μg/g wet kidney weight are thought to be associated with toxicity.

Lead

Occupational exposure to lead occurs in smelters, in lead paint removal, and in the manufacture of storage batteries, paint, pottery, and pewter. Environmental lead exposure can occur through the use of inadequately glazed pottery and the ingestion of lead-containing food or water. The addition of lead to gasoline and paint provides another source of lead exposure (122).

There are three forms of lead intoxication: acute inorganic lead poisoning from the inhalation of lead oxide; lead poisoning caused by the inhalation or absorption through the skin of tetraethyl lead; and chronic inorganic lead poisoning from inorganic lead in the form of lead oxide, lead carbonate, or similar compounds (41). Initially, the highest concentrations can be found in the kidney. Here its concentration is 50 times greater in the cortex than in the medulla. From the kidney, lead is excreted in the urine and redistributed to other tissues, most notably bone. The rate of urinary excretion of lead depends on the duration of exposure as well as on the absolute body burden.

It appears that a major toxic effect of lead involves the inhibition of cellular respiration. This results from the tendency for lead to accumulate in mitochondria and from the defects in mitochondrial structure and function that follow.

Mercury

Mercury exists in the form of inorganic salts, gases, and organic mercury compounds (7,62). In the inorganic form, mercury is present either as the free metal or in an ionic form such as mercurous or mercuric salt. In the organic form, the mercury is bound covalently to at least one carbon atom. The phenol and methoxymethyl compounds degrade to inorganic mercury, whereas alkyl mercury compounds remain as organic compounds.

The free metallic form is found in thermometers and barometers. It is not absorbed from the gastrointestinal tract, and toxicity occurs only with inhalation of the vapor. Inorganic salts, such as mercuric chloride used as an antiseptic, are highly nephrotoxic, as are organic salts such as phenyl mercuric proprionate, used as a fungicide. Chronic exposure to alkyl compounds such as methyl mercury have been associated primarily with neurological rather than renal injury. Renal lesions have resulted from organic mercury poisoning, however (41). These compounds are absorbed from the gastrointestinal tract and are bound to plasma proteins and hemoglobin. They are distributed mainly in the liver and kidney. In the kidney, mercury is preferentially accumulated in proximal tubular epithelial cells. Renal excretion occurs by tubular secretion rather than by glomerular filtration. Some mercury is also excreted in the feces. The urine concentration of mercury is normally less than 20 μg/L. Mercury tends to form highly undissociated linkages to sulfhydryl groups, evokes changes in membrane potentials, and blocks a number of enzymatic reactions.

Epidemics of mercury poisoning have occurred in Japan and Iraq. In Japan fish were contaminated by industrial waste containing methyl mercury (78). In Iraq alkyl-mercury fungicides contaminated grain used for bread (40). In the latter case, 6000 people were affected, and 500 deaths occurred. In both epidemics, poisoning with alkyl mercury primarily affected the nervous system rather than the kidney.

Silicon

Silicon is a major constituent of the earth's crust. Its toxicity arises from the production of free silica as found in quartz and flint. Granite, sandstone, and slate are also sources of free silica. Individuals working in mines, quarries, potteries, and foundries are exposed to particles 1 to 5 μm in size. These particles cause adverse effects when inhaled. Sandblasters are likely to be at risk. Silicon is partially eliminated by the kidney. It is partially reabsorbed by the epithelial cell of the proximal tubule. This results in cytoplasmic vacuoles and structural changes in mitochondria and lysosomes. Silicon may also affect enzyme systems within the kidney and alter the molecular integrity of the glomerular basement membrane. Silicon does not inhibit Na^+,K^+-ATPase activity as do such heavy metals as cadmium, lead, mercury, and copper (100).

Uranium

Exposure to uranium is limited to its use in the nuclear industry. Soluble compounds, particularly those complexed with bicarbonate, are readily absorbed from the gastrointestinal tract, with over 50% excreted by the kidneys within the first 24 h. Toxicity is related to severe effects on mitochondrial function of proximal tubular epithelial cells (64).

Organic Solvents

Carbon Tetrachloride

Carbon tetrachloride is widely used as an industrial solvent (4). At one time it was a common household cleaning agent. Carbon tetrachloride continues to be used in insecticide sprays and in fire extinguishers. It is a volatile, heavier-than-air liquid that is toxic in concentrations greater than 100 ppm. Absorption occurs through the gastrointestinal tract following ingestion and through the lungs during exposure to vapor. Toxicity is more likely to occur when the agent is used in confined or poorly ventilated areas. Carbon tetrachloride is hepatotoxic and nephrotoxic. It accumulates in the highest concentration in adipose tissue, liver, bone marrow, blood, brain, and kidney. Over 50% is exhaled in unaltered form, and the remainder is eliminated by the liver and kidneys. Hepatic and renal toxicity increase when ethyl alcohol or isopropyl alcohol is consumed during the period of exposure. Carbon tetrachloride is thought to be converted to toxic metabolites via microsomal metabolism.

Chloroform

Chloroform is a volatile, sweet-smelling, nonflammable liquid. It is used chiefly as a refrigerant, an aerosol propellant, and in the synthesis of fluorinated resins. It is also produced during the chlorination of water. Although chloroform exerts its primary toxic effects on the central nervous system and liver, it is also nephrotoxic. It is absorbed through the lungs or gastrointestinal tract and is eventually metabolized by the microsomal enzymes. Chloroform is thought to be transformed into a toxic product by microsomal metabolism. On this basis the ingestion of polybrominated biphenyls, known to be inducers of microsomal enzyme activity, enhances chloroform nephrotoxicity. The degree of enhancement is proportional to the concentration of polychlorinated biphenyl in the diet (68).

Trichloroethylene

Trichloroethylene is a nonflammable liquid that is used as an industrial solvent and household cleaning agent. Its vapor is readily absorbed, with rapid accumulation in adipose tissue. The maximal allowable concentration is 200 ppm. Trichloroethylene undergoes biotransformation to produce a number of metabolites, which are slowly eliminated. It is insoluble in water but soluble with ether or chloroform. A portion of the observed toxicity may be a result of the interaction with these solvents (57).

Pesticides

The term "pesticide" is a generic name that includes insecticides, herbicides, and fungicides. Nephrotoxicity has been associated with the use of two major categories of insecticides—the organophosphorus compounds and the chlorinated hydrocarbons (85) and the bipyridyl group of herbicides, particularly paraquat (85).

Insecticides

Organophosphorus compounds such as parathion are powerful inhibitors of carboxylic esterase enzymes, including acetylcholinesterase (true cholinesterase) and pseudocholinesterase. Although the predominant pharmacological and toxicological effects of organophosphates result from inhibition of acetylcholinesterase of the nervous system (86), there is some evidence that absorption of organophosphorus compounds may result in a variety of renal tubular disorders (130). Abnormalities in the absorption of glucose, amino acids, and phosphate have been observed, along with the inability to concentrate urine properly. It has been suggested that these abnormalities are caused by organophosphate metabolites such as p-nitrophenols.

Chlorinated hydrocarbons such as chlordane, in contrast to the organophosphorus compounds, accumulate in human and animal tissue. They enter the body by way of the skin or lungs. There have been cases of acute oliguric renal failure associated with their use (32).

Acute renal failure may be a component of systemic toxicity with other insecticides. Fluoride, used in roach powder, is a general protoplasmic poison because of its ability to inactivate proteolytic and glycolytic enzymes. Phosphorus is used in insect and rodent poisons, in fireworks, and in the manufacture of fertilizer. In the form of a yellow or white powder phosphorus is highly poisonous. Boric acid is a white crystalline powder used as an antiseptic, as a food preservative, and as a buffering and fungistatic agent in talcum powder. Sodium borate is used as an antiseptic, as a cleaning agent, and as an insecticide spray and dust. These substances are toxic to all cells.

Herbicides

Paraquat is a widely used herbicide that is marketed as an aerosol, as a granule, or as a 20% to 40% concentrated aqueous solution. Severe systemic toxicity has been reported from the latter form. Once absorbed, paraquat is promptly eliminated by the kidney. When renal insufficiency occurs, its accumulation in the body may lead to additional pulmonary injury.

The mechanism of toxicity is thought to be related to the generation of a free radical, the superoxide ion (O_2^{-}), and to the peroxidation of lipid cellular membranes. It has been suggested that high concentrations of oxygen used in the therapy of paraquat toxicity may increase the production of O_2^{-} and hydrogen peroxide. As a result, oxygen therapy given before paraquat is completely removed from the body may carry increased risk of lung injury.

EPIDEMIOLOGY

The overall incidence of acute renal failure from toxic exposure has recently been estimated to be as high as 27% with antibiotics emerging as the most important cause (1,3,111). At one time exposure to substances such as heavy metals or organic solvents accounted for approximately 10% of the total cases of acute renal failure (96). With the decreased use of heavy metals as medicinal agents and the employment of less toxic solvents, this figure has decreased. Several studies support a link between exposure to such substances as cadmium and lead and the appearance of renal insufficiency (76,105, 125,132). The incidence of idiopathic chronic interstitial nephritis is increasing. Whether this finding represents the effects of prolonged exposure to new chemical agents or simply reflects changing diagnostic criteria is uncertain.

Defining the role of toxic exposure in the development of end-stage renal disease is a singularly important task (27). To date all such estimates depend on inferences drawn from surveys of patients entering dialysis or transplantation programs. Table 20-2 summarizes the results of several such surveys performed in the United States to identify the abnormality associated with end-stage renal disease (23,34,97). Conditions such as glomerulonephritis, hypertension, and interstitial nephritis account for approximately 60% of the cases. Illnesses such as diabetes mellitus, polycystic kidney disease, and other hereditary and nonhereditary diseases account for another 25% of the cases. This leaves about 15% of the cases of end-stage renal disease without known cause.

The decision to include an individual patient in a particular category is often arbitrary. Little if any consideration is given to the possibility that exposure to environmental pollutants has influenced the development of glomerulonephritis, interstitial nephritis, or hypertension. Occupational or environmental histories that might implicate toxic exposure in the etiology of the patient's end-stage renal disease are rarely available.

Social and demographic data reveal that the incidence of end-stage renal disease in the United States is substantially higher in blacks than whites. Indeed, the yearly incidence in blacks is more than three times that found in whites. On this basis blacks compose about 30% of the patients undergoing dialysis in the United States. Blacks are found to have a much higher incidence of renal failure from glomerulonephritis, hypertension, interstitial nephritis, diabetes mellitus, and unknown causes. Notably, blacks have a 17-fold higher incidence of kidney failure related to hypertension. Only polycystic renal disease and miscellaneous forms of renal failure are higher in whites than in blacks (Table 20-3).

Studies also indicate that end-stage renal disease is more prevalent among the poor. In 1976, 36% of the patients had a total household income below the poverty level and 72% had incomes below the median family range (39). In these patients accurate occupational profiles are particularly difficult to obtain because their employment patterns have often been erratic.

The dramatic impact of end-stage renal failure can be more fully understood when it is realized that, worldwide each year, more than 500,000 patients are added to this group. There is little data available on the incidence of end-stage renal failure in developing countries. However, some European countries treat over 70 new patients per million population per year. In Japan and the United States over 100 new patients per million population are treated per year (27).

In the United States in 1987, approximately

TABLE 20-2. Classification of Renal Disease in Patients on Maintenance Dialysis[a]

Diagnosis	Percentage of total patients			
	1977	1979	1982	Combined
Glomerulonephritis	31.6	29.6	13.3	30.0
Hypertension	25.3	13.0	25.6	18.9
Unknown	5.5	19.4	22.6	15.2
Interstitial nephritis	11.8	8.4	23.3	11.5
Diabetes	12.5	7.2	8.8	9.2
Polycystic kidney disease	5.8	11.6	3.7	8.5
Other	7.5	10.8	3.7	8.6
Total	100	100	100	100
Number of patients	296	1111	721	2128

[a]Compiled from data reported by Easterling (34), Burton and Hirschman (23), and Rostand et al. (97).

TABLE 20-3.   Risks of Diseases Causing Renal Failure According to Race[a]

Diagnosis	Percentage of total patients		Yearly incidence per 100,000 population	
	Black	White	Black	White
Glomerulonephritis	20.4	31.8	2.79	0.96
Hypertension	41.2	9.7	6.17	0.36
Unknown	10.8	10.2	2.60	0.90
Interstitial nephritis	11.2	18.6	2.24	0.89
Diabetes	10.2	12.6	1.50	0.46
Polycystic kidney disease	1.6	8.7	0.24	0.34
Other	4.6	8.2	0.26	0.57
Total	100	100	15.8	4.48

[a]Compiled from data reported by Easterling (34) and Rostand et al. (97).

158,000 people with irreversible renal failure were kept alive by dialysis therapy. An estimated 9000 renal transplants were performed in 1988. The annual cost for these forms of treatment was about $3.4 billion in 1987. In view of the limited rehabilitation achieved by dialysis, the complications associated with transplantation, and the tremendous costs involved, efforts should be directed toward identifying the specific causes of renal disease. Factors that result in progression and the irreversible decline in renal function must also be identified.

The fact that a substantial number of patients develop end-stage renal disease for unknown reasons, and that the incidence is skewed in favor of blacks and those with marginal incomes, deserves scrutiny. The influence of chemical exposure on the development of end-stage renal disease merits investigation.

PATHOLOGY AND PATHOLOGICAL PHYSIOLOGY

The susceptibility of the kidney to toxic damage is related to several aspects of normal renal function. First, the blood flow to the kidney per gram of tissue weight is greater than that to any other organ. On this basis the total amount of toxin delivered to the kidney may be disproportionately high. Second, even if toxic agents arrive at the kidney in low concentration, the processes of glomerular filtration, tubular reabsorption and secretion make it likely that high renal concentrations will develop. Third, the high metabolic activity of tubular epithelial cells make the kidney particularly vulnerable to the actions of metabolic inhibitors. Fourth, the kidney's metabolic capacity, which generally detoxifies compounds, may transform some nontoxic agents into ones with significant nephrotoxicity (69,98) (see Chapter 9).

Mechanisms of Toxicity

Renal injury may be the result of a direct toxic effect or an immunologic response. Toxicity may also be produced by indirect means—when, for example, renal metabolism of environmental contaminants potentiates the action of nephrotoxic agents.

Direct Toxic Effects

The toxicity of environmental pollutants is determined by their chemical properties, the duration and extent of exposure, and the nature of the host response. Evidence of renal toxicity is related to the site of action, the degree of damage, and the ability of the kidney to compensate for the loss of function. The renal vasculature, the glomerlar capillary membrane, and the tubular epithelial cell may all be subjected to direct toxic injury.

Involvement of the renal vasculature leads to changes in renal vascular resistance with either a redistribution of blood flow within the kidney, a decrease in the total blood flow, or both. Changes in renal vascular resistance, by affecting glomerular filtration, may decrease the clearance of a number of substances.

Toxicity directed to the glomular capillary membrane may change the ultrafiltration coefficient, a product of the glomerular capillary surface area and hydraulic conductivity. A decrease in either figure results in a proportional decrease in the filtration rate. Changes in pore size or configuration or neutralization of the fixed negative charges are also of importance. They may affect the ability of various substances to pass the glomerular barrier.

Toxicity can occur within tubular epithelial cells, in particular those of the proximal tubule. Indeed, toxicity may be limited to a specific cell type or to a particular organelle within the cell, depending on their particular functional characteristics. Some compounds may have a major effect on tubular epithelial cell membranes. Others selectively alter the function of lysosomes, mitochondria, nuclei, or the endoplasmic reticulum (47). Disruption of intracellular organelles, particularly those providing energy for cellular respiration, may lead to cell death and loss of the integrity of the tubular epithelium. If such damage takes place, renal filtrate may passively move into the renal interstitium.

Immunopathological Mechanisms

There is evidence that the toxicity of certain environmental agents may be mediated, in part, by immunologic mechanisms (see Chapters 10 and 23 for a discussion of immune mechanisms). Such injury may cause glomerular or tubulointerstitial disease (33,129).

In general, based on their pathogenesis, there are four categories of adverse immunologic reactions. Type I, the anaphylactic or immediate hypersensitivity reaction, involves the binding of antigen or preformed IgE antibodies attached to mast cells and basophils. Type II, the cytotoxic reaction, results from the reaction of antibody with cell-bound antigen and leads to activation of the complement cascade and cell death. Type III, the immune complex reaction, causes tissue damage through the formation of immune complexes in situ or in the circulation. Type IV, the delayed hypersensitivity reaction, is mediated primarily by T lymphocytes (see Chapters 10 and 23).

At the present time, there is little to suggest that the type I response mediates the nephrotoxic effects of environmental pollutants. It appears, however, that a type II response may follow nephrotoxic exposure. Toxic agents may so alter glomerular or tubular membranes that autoantigens are produced. With the subsequent formation of autoantibodies, a type II response ensues. The type III response is likely to be most important because a nephrotoxin may act as a full antigen or as a hapten. This response may involve the deposition of immune complexes formed in the vascular compartment. The type IV response, once thought to be of little significance in renal injury, may play a role in some forms of interstitial disease.

Xenobiotic Metabolism

In general, foreign compounds (xenobiotics), once absorbed, are distributed to various tissues where they undergo biotransformation into nontoxic metabolites, which are then excreted. At times, however, the process of biotransformation produces metabolites that are more toxic than the parent compound. The enzymes responsible for the metabolism of xenobiotics include mixed-function oxidases located in the microsomes (see Chapter 9). Although these enzymes are generally much less active in the kidney than in the liver, certain specific cell types—particularly those in the last third of the proximal tubule—show considerable activity. Several environmental pollutants—most notably the polybrominated biphenyls (PBBs), the polychlorinated biphenyls (PCBs), some halogenated dibenzodioxins, and hexachlorobenzene—have the capacity to increase the activity of the mixed-function oxidases. Under these conditions the toxicity of those xenobiotics that are converted to toxic products via microsomal metabolism is enhanced (see Chapter 9). The enhancement of chloroform nephrotoxicity after the ingestion of PBBs is an example of this process.

Host Factors

Host factors may alter renal toxicity by influencing the metabolism of xenobiotics, the renal concentration of toxic agents, or the susceptibility to cell injury. Patients with glucose-6-phosphate dehydrogenase deficiency, for example, may be at increased risk to chemical exposure. Because of the increased susceptibility of their red blood cells, exposure to such chemicals as naphthalene, toluidine blue, and trinitrotoluene increases the potential for hemolysis (18). The hemoglobinuria that may follow increases the risk of secondary renal injury.

Changes with Renal Growth and Aging

Renal susceptibility to toxic damage increases with age. This phenomenon may in part be related to the anatomic and functional changes that occur with growth, maturation, and aging (30,38,50,107). At birth, the human kidney contains a full complement of nephrons. During the first year, the glomeruli and tubular structures mature and increase in size. The increase in mass is reflected by a marked increase in kidney weight. After the first year, growth slows. By the age of 18 to 20 years, maturity is reached. A plateau in structural and functional development persists until the third or fourth decade. Thereafter, regressive changes take place, most marked within the renal vasculature and glomeruli. Renal blood flow decreases about 10%, with a greater reduction appearing after the age of 60 years. Since the glomerular filtration rate, muscle mass, and creatinine production also decrease with age, the serum creatinine concentration remains constant. The susceptibility to injury from nephrotoxic agents increases with age. When injury does occur, it is likely to be more severe and to result in more permanent damage (50).

Factors Determining Progression to Chronicity

The early detection of renal injury is most important since, once established, there is a propensity for many forms of renal disease to progress on their own accord. A critical event separating self-limited from progressive renal failure may be the stimuli producing compensatory hypertrophy or the effects of this process.

With the initial injury it is assumed that a certain proportion of the nephrons are irreversibly damaged. Adaptive changes occurring in the remaining nephrons, while the renal filtration rate remains near normal, may ultimately cause the premature death of those nephrons that have undergone the greatest hypertrophy. Since the number of sclerotic glomeruli is increased in the markedly hypertrophic kidney, it has been proposed that the hyperperfusion associated with compensatory hypertrophy is deleterious (22,101). An increase in the glomerular capillary hydrostatic pressure or a change in the glomerular capillary membrane may also contribute to the progressive glomerular damage and subsequent tubular atrophy. Whatever the cause, the loss of the hypertrophied nephrons contributes to a progressive decrease in the renal filtration rate. It also stimulates other less-involved nephrons to undergo hypertrophy, repeating a vicious cycle. Eventually, the compensatory processes in some nephrons are unable to keep up with the progressive loss of other nephrons. Renal function then deteriorates. The extent to which environmental agents stimulate or even retard the process of compensatory hypertrophy is largely unexplored.

Changes with Diet

Although malnutrition does not appear to be linked to an increased incidence of parenchymal renal disease, it may cause developmental abnormalities in the very young and physiological defects in adults. For example, if a caloric deficiency occurs early in the growth phase, when rapid cell multiplication is taking place, the kidneys may not reach their proper weight or number of cells. Unlike some animals in which cell multiplication continues after birth, the newborn human kidney has its full complement of cells. Malnutrition following birth would not be expected to adversely affect kidney size. There have been reports, however, that the kidneys of infants dying from protein–calorie malnutrition are smaller than normal and show signs of chronic contraction and scarring.

In adults malnutrition is associated primarily with physiological defects in renal function. Fasting, for example, is associated with a naturesis that is abolished by carbohydrate refeeding. The naturesis is related to changes in glucagon levels (106) and

to the need to excrete metabolically generated anions (103). With prolonged malnutrition, although renal blood flow and glomerular filtration rate are thought to be normal, other physiological parameters may be adversely affected. In particular, the responses to salt and water loads are abnormal. This is reflected in the propensity for edema formation when excess salt is available.

When the kidney is stimulated to undergo compensatory hypertrophy, dietary protein restriction retards this response. In experimental animals and humans with chronic renal disease, limiting phosphorus intakes slows the progressive decline in renal function (119).

CLINICAL ASPECTS OF EXPOSURE TO ENVIRONMENTAL CHEMICALS AND PHYSICAL AGENTS ON THE KIDNEY

When a medical history is taken from a patient suffering from renal disease, specific information on present and past exposures to noxious agents should be obtained. Such inquiry may uncover vital clues to the cause of the patient's illness (126). Familiarity with the agents linked to acute and chronic renal disease will facilitate the search for such exposure (Table 20-1).

Acute Renal Failure

Acute renal failure is marked by a progressive rise in the concentration of serum creatinine and other nitrogenous compounds. There are a number of causes of acute renal failure. Of particular concern are those cases caused by ischemic insults and nephrotoxic agents. Such forms of acute renal failure are frequently accompanied by a reduction in urine output to less than 500 mL per day. Even if urine flow rates are unaltered, parenchymal injury is reflected by changes in the composition of the urine. These changes tend to separate postischemic and nephrotoxic acute renal failure from situations in which reduced renal function results from changes in systemic hemodynamics. The inability to form a concentrated urine is a prominent abnormality in acute renal failure.

When acute renal failure occurs in association with drugs and toxins, the overall mortality rate is approximately 37%. In those who survive, renal function generally returns to life-sustaining levels, but in only a few is recovery complete. In a small percentage of patients various degrees of structural and functional impairment persist indefinitely (43).

In all patients with acute renal failure, the possibility of exposure to an environmental nephrotoxin must be considered. Frequently, particular elements of the clinical presentation suggest a specific etiologic agent.

Environmental agents that have received the widest attention in connection with acute renal failure include organic solvents, heavy metals, and various pesticides (Table 20-1).

Organic Solvents

Carbon Tetrachloride The toxic manifestations of carbon tetrachloride may include central nervous system depression, vomiting, abdominal pain, constipation, diarrhea, and fever. More severe exposure results in centrilobular liver necrosis and/or acute renal failure (109). In general, the renal injury follows hepatic impairment when renal excretion of the toxic agent takes place. Symptoms occur following both inhalation and ingestion of carbon tetrachloride. Hepatic and renal toxicity is increased if ethyl alcohol is consumed during the period of exposure (88). A similar potentiation has been described with isopropyl alcohol (46). A reduction in urine volume may not be apparent for 48 h or longer. Jaundice may not be apparent until the fourth day. The oliguria can be expected to persist for 1 to 2 weeks, with gradual recovery thereafter. Unlike other forms of nephrotoxic acute renal failure, the urine sediment may contain an impressive number of red blood cells, leading to an erroneous diagnosis of acute glomerulonephritis. When acute renal failure occurs in association with hepatitis, the diagnosis of organic solvent toxicity should be considered. Treatment, largely supportive, may involve the use of peritoneal dialysis or hemodialysis until recovery occurs.

Toluene Glue sniffing and other forms of solvent abuse are not uncommon (128). The typical solvent sniffer is a boy, 13 to 15 years of age, from a middle- or low-income family, who inhales the vapors of model glues placed in plastic bags (72). Adults often tend to inhale vapors from a rag saturated with spray paints. Other psychoactive substances may be used as well (110). The patient may present with abdominal pain, nausea and vomiting, mild fever, and generalized weakness. In addition, signs of adhesive on the face may be revealed by a "glue-sniffers rash." This develops from repeated application of a plastic bag to the nose (121). At levels greater than 200 ppm, toluene causes transient euphoria, excitement, exhilaration, and tinnitus. At concentrations higher than 600–800 ppm, confusion, auditory and visual hallucinations, and nausea and vomiting are prominent symptoms. Liver and kidney damage may occur simultaneously or as independent manifestations of toluene toxicity.

The most common renal abnormalities are tubular acidification defects. These appear to be of the type 1 or distal tubular variety. This injury results in a hyperchloremic metabolic acidosis and an inappropriately alkaline urine. At times, damage to the proximal tubules may predominate and lead to the appearance of Fanconi's syndrome, i.e., phosphaturia, glycosuria, amino-aciduria, and type 2 hypercholeremic acidosis. If distal tubular function is intact, the urine pH may be acidic. Profound muscle weakness, with or without rhabdomyolysis, may occur in association with severe hypokalemia. Reversible acute renal failure has been reported, as has the development of recurrent urinary calculi (114). Proteinuria and hematuria may be found in some instances.

Heavy Metals

Arsenic When arsenic is ingested in large amounts, the initial symptoms include a dry, burning sensation in the mouth and throat. This is followed by crampy abdominal pain, severe vomiting, and diarrhea. Vertigo, delirium, and coma are quite obvious manifestations of central nervous system involvement. Death may occur with circulatory collapse and liver and renal failure. Hemodialysis has been found to be effective treatment for renal failure in some studies (51) but not others (104). BAL (2,3,-dimercapto-1-propanol or dimercaprol) is of value in acute arsenic poisoning (53,84).

Mercury Poisoning with inorganic mercury such as mercury bichloride (sublimate) was once a common identifiable cause of acute renal failure. The initial manifestations of acute mercury poisoning arise primarily from the gastrointestinal tract and include a severe burning sensation and vomiting. As excretion occurs, additional gastrointestinal tract symptoms such as pain, vomiting, colic, and diarrhea develop. In the kidney, the terminal portions of all proximal tubules are involved. Gastrointestinal bleeding is a common complication of acute mercury-induced renal failure. The toxic dose of $HgCl_2$ is from 0.5 to 2.5 g with a mean of approximately 1.5 g. Recovery is expected if the patient survives. The initial stage can be treated with dialysis. Chronic renal failure following chronic inorganic mercury poisoning has been described (120).

Herbicides

Paraquat The ingestion of large amounts of paraquat results in a severe burning sensation in the mouth and pharynx, repeated vomiting, and the rapid onset of pulmonary edema and hemorrhage. The mortality associated with the concentrated solution approaches 50%, with death usually from progressive respiratory failure. Smaller doses are associated with an asymptomatic period of several days, followed by the development of pulmonary infiltrates. Hypoxemia, decreased lung volumes, low lung compliance, and an impaired diffusing capacity for carbon monoxide occur. Renal insufficiency may be noted during this time (44,118).

Histological examination of the kidneys reveals lesions of the tubular epithelial cells. There are a range of proximal tubular dysfunctions, including renal glycosuria, amino-aciduria, and impaired phosphorus, uric acid, and sodium transport. Recovery from paraquat poisoning may occur despite acute renal failure.

If paraquat has been ingested, immediate administration of an absorbent is the one theurapeutic measure most likely to favorably affect the outcome. Additional therapeutic measures are presented by Gosselin et al. (53) and Morgan (84).

Pigment Nephropathy

Myoglobinuria and hemoglobinuria can be produced by exposure to chemical agents (Table 20-1). When hemoglobinuria and myoglobinuria accompany acute renal failure, it is difficult to define their role in the development of renal damage. Such coexistent factors as abnormalities in blood pressure and the adverse effects of toxic agents tend to obscure the role of hemoglobinuria and myoglobinuria on renal function (15,45,48,113). In conditions associated with hemoglobinuria or myoglobinuria, an osmotic diuresis should be induced.

Tubulointerstitial Nephritis

Acute tubulointerstitial nephritis is marked by interstitial edema and infiltration with inflammatory cells, some of which appear in the urine. Both morphological and functional evidence of tubular epithelial cell injury is present. Chronic tubulointerstitial nephritis is distinguished by the presence of interstitial fibrosis and tubular atrophy. The manifestations of tubulointerstitial nephritis depend on the extent of injury, the tubular segment(s) most severely involved, and the degree of compensation achieved by the less severely involved nephrons. When the proximal tubule is damaged, such substances as sodium, glucose, amino acids, and low-molecular-weight proteins, ordinarily reabsorbed or metabolized at this site, appear in the urine. Damage to more distal structures including the loop of Henle, the distal convoluted tubule, and the collecting duct is accompanied by an inability to maximally concentrate and dilute the urine. Since the former effect is more pronounced than the latter, polyuria may result. Acidification of the urine also occurs at the distal sites. Thus, damage in this area may lead to metabolic acidosis.

Up to one-third of biopsy-confirmed cases of acute tubulointerstitial nephritis cannot be ascribed to either an infectious or a drug-related process. This finding raises the possibility that environmental agents may play a role. Exposure to cadmium, lead, and radiation is associated with tabulointerstitial nephrites (Table 20-1).

Cadmium

The kidneys are involved in both acute and chronic cadmium intoxication (76). The kidney is considered to be the critical target organ involved in long-term occupational or environmental exposure to cadmium. The earliest observable effect of chronic cadmium poisoning is the development of proteinuria, which is tubular in origin. An analysis of the urine protein shows the presence of β_2-microglobulin, retinol-binding protein, and α_1-microglobulin.

Determination of specific low-molecular-weight proteins in the urine is used as a method to detect proximal tubular impairment in populations with occupational or environmental exposure to cadmium (17). Injury to proximal tubular epithelial cells also results in the presence of amino-aciduria, enzymuria, and glycosuria. In patients with chronic interstitial nephritis associated with cadmium exposure, the diagnosis is aided by a marked increase in the urinary concentration of β_2-microglobulin, which can be confirmed by determining the renal concentration of cadmium (36). More recently, however, the measurement of β_2-microglobulin has been replaced with the measurement of retinol-binding protein. This substance also reflects tubular proteinuria and is much more stable in acidic urine (17).

With low exposure, cadmium concentration in the urine may provide an index of the cadmium level in the body and the kidney. With increased cadmium exposure, a time lag exists before cadmium in the urine correlates with exposure. When renal dysfunction occurs, the loss of cadmium increases (55,74).

It is noteworthy that 100,000 workers are exposed to cadmium or cadmium compounds. In workers with a high level of exposure, urinary cadmium concentrations averaged 45.7 μg/L, whereas office workers with a low level of exposure had urinary cadmium concentrations that averaged 13.1 μg/L. Significant differences in renal function were noted in the two groups (105). In Japan, the ingestion of cadmium in contaminated rice and water led to the development of a painful bone disease associated with the Fanconi syndrome. This condition, referred to a "itai-itai" or "ouch-ouch disease," was more common in postmenopausal women (116).

Lead

At least two types of renal impairment may be found in association with lead poisoning. In the first and more acute form, generalized defects in proximal tubular function result in the Fanconi syndrome with amino-aciduria, glycosuria, and phosphaturia. Serum uric acid levels are generally elevated because of a defect in the tubular secretion of uric acid. Occasionally, the urine contains cells with eosinophilic intranuclear incisions composed of lead and protein (54). These abnormalities most often occur in children following several months of heavy lead ingestion. Although this impairment is generally rapidly reversible, it is likely that some cases go on to develop chronic lead nephropathy (115). Various factors, such as the amount of calcium in the diet, the presence of iron deficiency, and exposure to sunlight and vitamin D, may influence the amount of lead absorbed and the severity of the disease.

Chronic lead nephropathy, the second type of renal impairment associated with lead poisoning, is qualitatively different from the Fanconi syndrome. It is an indolent disease difficult to separate from other forms of chronic, slowly progressive renal insufficiency. In the absence of a history of acute lead nephropathy, the diagnosis may be suspected when the course of the renal disease is protracted, without definable cause, and associated with symmetrical contraction of both kidneys. Evidence of excessive lead absorption is supplied by determining urinary lead excretion using the calcium disodium salt of ethylenediaminetetraacetic acid (EDTA) lead mobilization test (see below).

The incidence of chronic lead nephropathy is difficult to determine, as studies of the long-term effects of acute plumbism have yielded somewhat different results (59,115). Nevertheless, long-term effects of chronic lead exposure have been described in three groups: those with occupational exposure, with gout, and with hypertension (16,125).

The first group includes workers with an established history of occupational lead exposure (125). In a survey of 158 lead workers with 3 to 10 years of exposure, 17% were hypertensive, and 18% had impaired renal function (79). In another study of 140 asymptomatic workers, 113 had abnormal total lead burdens as determined by the EDTA lead mobilization test. A reduction in the glomerular filtration rate was present in nearly 40% of the subjects. Of particular interest was the finding that the glomerular filtration rate improved by as much as 20% with chronic EDTA therapy (126).

The second group includes patients with gout (123,132). It is well established that chronic lead toxicity is associated with saturnine gout. Numerous studies have shown that 40–50% of patients with chronic lead nephropathy are so afflicted (9,37,131). In patients with gout, the severity of the renal failure was directly related to the amount of lead mobilized (10). Viewed in a different fashion, it may be presumed that in patients with gout, but

without overt evidence of lead toxicity, a certain number will have saturnine gout.

The third group includes patients thought to have essential hypertension (112). A study of two groups of hypertensive patients showed that in patients with a serum creatinine level above 1.5 mg/dL, the mean excretion of lead was 680 μg per 3 days. In contrast, those patients with a normal serum creatinine level had a mean excretion rate of lead of 340 μg per 3 days (11). These data suggest that a certain percentage of patients thought to have primary or essential gout may actually be afflicted with chronic lead intoxication. The question also arises whether the renal insufficiency commonly thought to be a consequence of gouty nephropathy or nephrosclerosis may be times be a manifestation of lead nephropathy.

In cases with chronic low-level lead exposure, a lead mobilization test may provide evidence of excessive lead absorption. The test is performed by measuring the urinary lead excretion following the administration of EDTA. One gram of EDTA is given twice, 8 to 12 h apart. During this time, a 24-h urine specimen is collected. An excessive body lead burden is indicated by excretion of more than 1000 μg of lead per day. Alternatively, 1 g of EDTA in 250 mL of 5% glucose solution may be given intravenously over the course of 1 h. Urine is collected at 24-hr intervals for 3 consecutive days. Excretion of more than 600 μg per 3 days is indicative of excess body lead. Weeden et al. found no evidence of EDTA nephrotoxicity in patients with renal insufficiency when the test was done as described above (127). EDTA is used in the treatment of acute and chronic lead poisoning. The dose is dependent on the severity of the illness (53).

Radiation Nephritis

The dose of radiation required to produce renal damage is thought to be in excess of 2300 R delivered to both kidneys within a 5-week period (73). It is difficult to define an exact dose inasmuch as there are a number of variables that determine the renal response to radiation. Age is an important determinant. Children, because of their pattern of organ growth, may be unusually susceptible to radiation. Adults can be at increased risk if they suffer from renal disease. The area and technique of irradiation, the extent of perirenal fat, and the concomitant administration of chemotherapeutic agents such as vincristine or actinomycin D may also modify the effects of radiation (6). It is possible that radiation from a variety of sources such as diagnostic x rays, the use of radioactive isotopes, or radiation from atomic explosions could lead to the development of clinical nephritis. But to date no such cases have been reported. In most instances radiation injury to the kidneys occurred during or after a course of deep x-ray treatment for pelvic carcinoma.

Radiation nephritis has been separated into five clinical categories: acute radiation nephritis, chronic radiation nephritis, asymptomatic proteinuria, benign essential hypertension, and late malignant hypertension (8,80,81). Acute radiation nephritis is associated with a variable degree of proteinuria, hypertension, and uremia. It may occur prior to or without the development of other symptoms. After a lag period of 3 to 9 months in children or 6 to 13 months in adults, cells and casts appear in the urine, and there are edema, hypertension, and nocturia. Of those who recover from the effects of acute radiation nephritis, a significant proportion will develop evidence of chronic renal impairment.

Chronic radiation nephritis may develop insidiously or as a complication of acute radiation nephritis. In contrast to the widespread vascular damage seen in acute radiation nephritis, chronic radiation nephritis is associated with tubular degeneration and interstitial nephritis. At times, asymptomatic proteinuria may be the only abnormality found. Mild elevation of the arterial blood pressure may also be an isolated finding. On occasion chronic radiation nephritis is associated with proteinuria and progresses to malignant hypertension. The development of malignant hypertension is the most severe complication. In contrast to those patients who develop malignant hypertension as a complication of acute radiation nephritis, there exists a group who may develop malignant hypertension months to years after exposure to radiation. It is particularly important to remember that when the irradiation of one kidney is followed by malignant hypertension, nephrectomy may provide the cure.

Chronic Glomerulonephritis

Chronic glomerular disease is an insidious process generally accompanied by albuminuria and microscopic hematuria. Its onset is often impossible to date, and its diagnosis is usually delayed until a secondary complications such as hypertension, anemia, or metabolic bone disease develops. In some instances the diagnosis may be suspected only after an abnormal urine sediment is found during a routine examination. In patients with chronic renal failure, the progressive decline in the glomerular filtration rate is too slow, and the deviation from the steady-state condition too small, to result in day-to-day changes in the serum creatinine or blood urea nitrogen concentrations. When found, a decrease in kidney size supports the chronic and irreversible nature of the condition. Examination of tissue obtained by percutaneous renal biopsy may confirm that the primary process involved glomerular structures. Frequently, such a distinction is clouded by a number of nonspecific changes that occur in all forms of chronic renal failure.

Occasionally, a more aggressive form of glomerular disease occurs in which renal function is lost over a period of weeks or months. This rapidly progressive glomerulonephritis can be identified by the presence of glomerular epithelial crescents in renal biopsy specimens. At times the kidney may be the only organ affected. On other occasions, the renal abnormalities may be part of a systemic disease that is often a result of a severe vasculitis. The agents associated with this process are discussed below (Table 20-1).

Solvents

There is concern that prolonged, excessive exposure to hydrocarbons, interacting with as yet unidentified host factors, predispose the kidney to glomerular injury or aggravate injury from other causes. The evidence supporting this position, though suggestive, is incomplete (26,29,42,75,83, 87,93,94).

The marked male predominance in patients with glomerulonephritis may indicate that occupational or environmental factors peculiar to males are contributory factors (133). An apparent association of Goodpasture's syndrome, a form of rapidly progressive glomerulonephritis, with exposure to petroleum products has also been reported (66). It has been reported that previous exposure to hydrocarbon solvents is a common feature among some groups of patients with crescentic glomerulonephritis or proliferative glomerulonephritis (12). Remissions and exacerbations of the nephrotic syndrome are noted to follow removal from and reexposure to solvents (24). A historical relationship between glomerulonephritis and exposure to hydrocarbons has also been described (43). Chronic exposure to gasoline vapors is claimed by some workers (66) to produce glomerulonephritis in rats. These findings have not been confirmed by other workers (129).

Silicon Nephropathy

Silicon, partly eliminated by the kidney, produces a dose-related nephropathy with chronic glomerular and tubulointerstitial disease. Glomerular lesions show a mild focal and segmental proliferative glomerulonephritis. Tubular changes consist of areas of hypertrophy and degeneration (19,52, 58,99). During the course of the illness, there are no functional tubular abnormalities, as may occur with cadmium. The urinary sediment tends to be normal, although protein of glomerular origin is present. Hypertension is commonly present. The diagnosis can be established by determining the silicon content of the kidney, which may be as high as 150 to

264 ppm dry weight (52,58,99). This contrasts with values of 14.2 ± 13.3 ppm dry weight in normal kidneys and 23.8 ± 25.1 ppm dry weight in kidneys with other forms of chronic disease (52).

In a series of 20 patients with chronic silicosis, 40% had renal insufficiency, and 20% had proteinuria (70). In another series of 45 patients who died with advanced silicosis, 51% had glomerular and tubular lesions. Occasionally, the renal disease may progress rapidly and be a part of a multisystem involvement (19).

Nephrotic Syndrome

Definition

The nephrotic syndrome is associated with heavy proteinuria (generally in excess of 3 g per 24 h), hypoalbuminemia, and edema. Abnormalities in lipid metabolism with hypercholesterolemia and hypertrigliceridemia are frequently present along with lipiduria. At the onset, the glomerular filtration rate need not be depressed and is occasionally elevated. The nephrotic syndrome may occur in conjunction with a variety of systemic diseases. It may also be a manifestation of primary glomerular injury, which occurs without a known cause. Under such conditions, the nephrotic syndrome is termed "idiopathic" and is classified according to the light and electron microscopic appearance of the glomeruli and their immunofluorescent patterns. It is noteworthy that chronic occupational exposure to mercury salts produces lesions similar to those found in some forms of idiopathic nephrotic syndrome.

Mercury

Exposure to both organic and inorganic mercury may produce nephrosis. The intensity and duration of the mercury exposure most likely determine whether acute tubular necrosis or proteinuria will appear. Large intravenous doses of mercury, given experimentally, produce selective necrosis of the proximal tubules. Smaller subcutaneous doses of mercury compounds given over a long period of time produce an immune-complex nephropathy manifested as mesangiopathic proliferative glomerulonephritis or as membranous glomerulonephritis. Nephrosis caused by mercury exposure has been reported in chemical plant workers and following the use of teething powders, skin-lightening creams, and ammoniated mercury ointments for psoriasis. The nephrotic syndrome has also been reported in two children after exposure to mercury-containing tuna fish (41).

Glomerular abnormalities on light microscopy are generally absent. Immunofluorescence may show diffuse generalized finely granular deposition of IgG and C3 along the glomerular basement membrane in an epimembranous distribution. The vessels and interstitium are normal. Within the proximal tubular cell cytoplasm there are heterogeneous electron-dense phagolysosomes. These contain finely granular electron-opaque material having the typical x-ray dispersion spectrum of mercury. Various mechanisms have been proposed to account for the immunopathological findings in mercury nephropathy (117).

Apart from the proteinuria, large quantities of mercury may be found in the urine. The mercury content of the hair may be increased. Once exposure to mercury is eliminated, recovery generally follows.

Toxic Exposure during Hemodialysis

Patients with renal insufficiency and, in particular, those receiving chronic hemodialysis are vulnerable to changes in their environment. The decreased excretory and metabolic capacity of the kidneys allows substances ordinarily excreted to accumulate in the body. In addition, noxious compounds usually detoxified by the kidney may have adverse effects on other organ systems. Hemodialysis itself provides another source of exposure to a number of potentially toxic substances (Table 20-4).

A progressive neurological disease, the so-called dialysis encephalopathy syndrome, occurs in some patients with chronic renal failure (2). This condition, which may be fatal, has been correlated with increased levels of aluminum in the central nervous system. This finding may be linked to the use of aluminum-containing antacids and/or high aluminum levels in the water used for hemodialysis.

Contamination of the water supply may also be responsible for a number of acute toxic reactions. Most notable are those associated with oxidative damage to red blood cells. Toxic methemoglobinemia has occurred when well water contaminated with nitrate was used to make the dialysate (25). Hemolysis has followed exposure to dialysates containing copper (67), chloramine (35), and formaldehyde (91). Untoward reactions in patients receiving hemodialysis have also been related to dialysate water containing excessive amounts of calcium, magnesium (49), and possibly fluoride (108).

Interactions between the blood and plastic tubing used during hemodialysis can also pose problems. Necrotizing dermatitis has followed the direct exposure of blood to the polyvinyl chloride tubing (20). These symptoms, thought to be an immunologic response, may be prevented by using polyvinyl tubing coated with polyurethane. The spallation and migration of silicone from the blood pump tubing have resulted in hypersplenism, pancytopenia (21), and, occasionally, granulomatous hepa-

TABLE 20-4. Toxic Exposure during Hemodialysis

Source	Agent	Reaction
Dietary supplementation	Aluminum	Neurological abnormalities
Water supply	Nitrates	Toxic methemoglobinemia
	Copper, chloramine, formaldehyde	Hemolysis
	Aluminum	Neurological abnormalities
	Calcium, magnesium	Hard-water syndrome
	Fluoride	Bone disease
Plastic tubing	Polyvinyl chloride	Necrotizing dermatitis
	Silicone	Hypersplenism
		Granulomatous hepatitis
Dialyzers	Plasticizers	Respiratory distress
	Particulates	
	Sterilant residuals	
	Reaction products	

titis (77). A syndrome characterized by respiratory distress, with or without wheezing, may occur when dialyzers contain various particulates, plasticizers, sterilant residuals, or reaction products (90).

The examples cited above are illnesses produced by exposure to toxin in a therapeutic setting and affecting a particularly susceptible patient population. Clinicians should remain alert to the possibility of toxic exposure in other therapeutic situations.

Carcinogenesis

Exposure to chemical agents has been implicated in the development of neoplasms of the renal parenchyma, renal pelvis and ureter, and urinary bladder (14,31,63,71) (Table 20-5). Such exposure is not implicated in the development of nephroblastomas or renal sarcomas. Renal adenomas and adenocarcinomas account for approximately 85% of all renal neoplasms and about 2% of all cancer deaths in men and women. Commonly referred to as hypernephromas, these tumors arise from cells of the proximal convoluted tubule. Squamous cell carcinomas, being much less common, account for 5–6% of renal neoplasms.

In the late 19th century it was first reported that men working in the aniline dye industry had an increased incidence of bladder cancer. Later it was appreciated that bladder cancer was linked to employment in the rubber and electric cable industries and that its development was associated with exposure to a number of aromatic amines (28,65). Exposure to 2-naphthylamine, 4-aminodiphenyl (xenylamine), and 4,4'-diaminodiphenyl (benzidine) have been linked to bladder carcinoma (65).

Transitional-cell carcinomas of the renal pelvis and ureter may be induced by the same exogenous carcinogens that produce bladder tumors. Workers in aniline dye, rubber, textile, and plastic industries have a higher incidence of these tumors, which account for 7–8% of renal neoplasms.

Smokers appear to develop bladder cancer at about twice the rate of nonsmokers. This may reflect increased exposure to such agents as polycyclic aromatic hydrocarbons, dialkylnitrosamines, and aromatic amines, all of which are present in cigarette smoke.

TABLE 20-5. Chemical Agents Associated with Cancer of the Urinary Tract

Renal parenchyma
  Renal adenoma and adenocarcinoma
    Aromatic amines
    Nitroso compounds
    Hydrazines
    Alkylating agents
    Anticancer agents
    Cadmium and lead
  Squamous cell carcinoma
    Various chemical carcinogens
Renal pelvis, ureter, bladder, and urethra
  Transitional cell carcinoma
    Aromatic amines
      2-Naphthylamine
      Xenylamine
      Benzidine
    Cigarette smoke

SUMMARY

Although a variety of chemicals have been identified as nephrotoxic agents, it is very difficult to define the extent of nephrotoxicity associated with chronic exposure to environmental agents. The problem relates, in part, to the kidney's ability to compensate for the effects of nephrotoxicity and its continuing deterioration even after the nephrotoxic exposure has ceased. The importance of focusing on this complex issue becomes apparent when it is realized that worldwide each year more than 500,000 patients develop end-stage renal failure, in most cases without known cause.

REFERENCES

1. Abuelo JG: Renal failure caused by chemicals, foods, plants, animal venoms, and misuse of drugs. Arch Intern Med 150:505, 1990.
2. Alfrey AC, LeGendre GR, Keahny WD: Dialysis encephalopathy Syndrome: Possible aluminum intoxication. N Engl J Med 293:184, 1976.
3. Anderson RJ, Linas SL, Henrich WL, et al: Nonoliguric acute renal failure. N Engl J Med 296:1134, 1977.
4. Andrews LS, Snyder R: Toxic effects of solvents and vapors. In: Casarett and Doull's Toxicology: The Basic Science of Poisons, 3rd ed., p 636, Klaassen CD, Amdur MO, Doull J (eds.), Macmillan, New York, 1986.
5. Arena JM, Drew RH (eds.): Poisoning: Toxicology, Symptoms, Treatments, 5th ed., Charles C. Thomas, Springfield, IL, 1986.
6. Arneil GC, Emmanuel IG, Slatman GE, et al: Nephritis in two children after irradiation and chemotherapy for nephroblastoma. Lancet 1:960, 1974.
7. Arnow R: Mercury. In: Clinical Management of Poisoning and Drug Overdose, p 637, Haddad LM, Winchester JF (eds.), WB Saunders, Philadelphia, 1983.
8. Arruda JAL: Radiation nephritis. In: Tubulointerstitial Nephropathies, p 275, Cotran R (ed.), Churchill Livingstone, Edinburgh, 1983.
9. Ball GV, Morgan JM: Chronic lead ingestion and gout. South Med J 61:21, 1961.
10. Batuman V, Maesaka JK, Haddad B, et al: The role of lead in gout nephropathy. N Engl J Med 304:520, 1981.
11. Batuman V, Landy E, Maesaka JK, et al: Contribution of lead to hypertension with renal impairment. N Engl J Med 309:17, 1983.
12. Beirne GJ, Brennan JT: Glomerulonephritis associated with hydrocarbon solvents. Arch Environ Health 24:365, 1972.
13. Bennett WM, Elzinger LW, Porter GA: Tubulointerstitial disease and toxic nephropathy. In: The Kidney, 4th ed., Vol. 2, p 1430, Brenner BM, Rector FC Jr (eds.), WB Saunders, Philadelphia, 1991.
14. Bennington JL, Laubscher FA: Epidemiologic studies on carcinoma of the kidney—association of renal adenocarcinoma with smoking. Cancer 21:1069, 1968.
15. Berlin R: Haff disease in Sweden. Acta Med Scand 129:560, 1948.
16. Bernard BP, Becker CE: Environmental lead exposure and the kidney. Clin Toxicol 26:1, 1988.
17. Bernard A, Lauwerys R: Epidemiological application of early markers of nephrotoxicity. Toxicol Lett 46:293, 1989.
18. Beutler E: Hemolytic Anemia in Disorders of Red Cell Metabolism. Plenum Press, New York, 1978.
19. Bolton WK, Suratt PM, Sturgill BC: Rapidly progressive silicon nephropathy. Am J Med 71:823, 1981.
20. Bommer J, Ritz E, Konrad A: Necrotizing dermatitis resulting from hemodialysis with polyvinyl chloride tubing. Ann Intern Med 91:869, 1979.
21. Bommer J, Ritz E, Waldherer R: Silicon-induced splenomegaly in a patient on hemodialysis. N Engl J Med 395, 1977, 1981.
22. Brenner BM, Meyer TW, Hostetter TH: Dietary protein intake and the progressive nature of kidney disease. N Engl J Med 307:652, 1982.
23. Burton BT, Hirschman GH: Demographic analysis: End-stage renal disease and its treatment in the United States. Clin Nephrol 11:47, 1979.
24. Cagnoli L, Casanova S, Pasquali S, et al: Relation between hydrocarbon exposure and the nephrotic syndrome. Br Med J 280:1068, 1980.
25. Carlson DJ, Shapiro FL: Methemoglobinemia from well water nitrates: A complication of home dialysis. Ann Intern Med 73:757, 1970.
26. Churchill DN, Fine A, Gault MH: Association between hydrocarbon exposure and glomerulonephritis. An appraisal of the evidence. Nephron 33:169, 1983.
27. Commission of the European Communities and the International Programme on Chemical Safety, United Nations/World Health Programme, World Health Organization: Consensus statement on the health significance of nephrotoxicity. Toxicol Lett 46:1, 1989.
28. Connoly JG (ed.): Carcinoma of the Bladder, Raven Press, New York, 1981.
29. Daniell WE, Couser WG, Rosenstock L: Occupational solvent exposure and glomerulonephritis. JAMA 259:2278, 1988.
30. Darmady EM, Offer J, Woodhouse MA: The parameters of the aging kidney. J Pathol 109:195, 1973.
31. Davin T, Casio F, Kjellstrand CM: Association of cancer with primary renal disease and/or uremia. In: Cancer and the Kidney, p 857, Riselbach RE, Garnick MB (eds.), Lea & Febiger, Philadelphia, 1982.
32. Derbes VJ, Dent JH, Forrest WW, et al: Fatal chlordane poisoning, JAMA 158:1367, 1955.
33. Druet P, Bernard A, Hirsch F: Immunologically mediated glomerulonephritis induced by heavy metals. Arch Toxicol 50:187, 1982.
34. Easterling RE: Racial factors in the incidence and causation of end-stage renal disease (ESRD). Trans Am Soc Artif Intern Organs 23:28, 1977.
35. Eaton JW, Kolpin CF, Swofford HS, et al: Chlorinated urban water: A cause of dialysis-induced hemolytic anemia. Science 181:463, 1973.
36. Ellis KJ, Morgan WD, Zanzi I, et al: In vivo measurement of critical level of kidney cadmium: Dose effect studies in cadmium smelter workers. Am J Ind Med 1:339, 1980.
37. Emmerson BT: Chronic lead nephropathy. The diagnostic use of calcium EDTA and the association with gout. Aust Ann Med 12:310, 1963.
38. Epstein M: Effects of aging on the kidney. Fed Proc 38:168, 1979.

39. Evans RW, Blagg CR, Bryan FA: Implications for health care policy: A social and demographic profile of hemodialysis patients in the United States. JAMA 345:487, 1981.

40. Eyl TB: Organic mercury food poisoning. N Engl J Med 284:706, 1971.

41. Felton JS, Kahn E, Salick B, et al: Heavy metal poisoning: Mercury and lead. Ann Intern Med 76:779, 1972.

42. Finn R, Fennerty RG, Ahmad R: Hydrocarbon exposure and glomerulonephritis. Clin Nephrol 14:173, 1980.

43. Finn WF: Recovery from acute renal failure. In: Acute Renal Failure, p 753, Brenner BM, Lazarus JM (eds.), WB Saunders, Philadelphia, 1983.

44. Fisher HK, Humphries M, Bails R: Paraquat poisoning: Recovery from renal and pulmonary damage. Ann Intern Med 75:731, 1971.

45. Flamenbaum W, Gehr M, Gross M, et al: Acute renal failure associated with myoglobinuria and hemoglobinuria. In: Acute Renal Failure, p 269, Brenner BM, Lazarus JM (eds.), WB Saunders, Philadelphia, 1983.

46. Folland DS, Schaffner W, Ginn HE, et al: Carbon tetrachloride toxicity potentiated by isopropyl alcohol. JAMA 236:1853, 1976.

47. Fowler BA: Ultrastructural and biochemical localization of organelle damage from nephrotoxic agents. In: Nephrotoxic Mechanisms of Drugs and Environmental Toxins, p 315, Porter GA (ed.), Plenum Press, New York, 1982.

48. Fowler BA, Weissberg JB: Arsine poisoning, N Engl J Med 291:1171, 1974.

49. Freeman RM, Lawton RL, Chamberlain MA: Hardwater syndrome. N Engl J Med 275:1113, 1967.

50. Friedman SA, Raizner AE, Rasen H, et al: Functional defects in the aging kidney. Ann Intern Med 76:41, 1972.

51. Giberson A, Vaziri D, Mirahamadi K, et al: Hemodialysis of acute arsenic intoxication with transient renal failure. Arch Intern Med 136:1303, 1976.

52. Giles RD, Sturgill BC, Suratt PM, et al: Massive proteinuria and acute renal failure in a patient with acute silicoproteinosis. Am J Med 64:336, 1978.

53. Gosselin RE, Smith RP, Hodge HC: Clinical Toxicology of Commercial Products, 5th ed., Williams & Wilkins, Baltimore, 1984.

54. Goyer RA: Effects of toxic, chemical and environmental factors on the kidney. In: Monographs in Pathology 20, p 202, Chung J, Spargo BH, Mostofi FK, et al. (eds.), Williams & Wilkins, Baltimore, 1979.

55. Goyer, RA: Cadmium nephropathy. In: Nephrotoxic Mechanisms of Drugs and Environmental Toxins, p 305, Porter GA (ed.), Plenum Press, New York, 1982.

56. Goyer RA: Toxic effects of metals. In: Casarett and Doull's Toxicology: The Basic Science of Poisons, 3rd ed., p 582, Klaassen CD, Amdur MO, Doull J (eds.), Macmillan, New York, 1986.

57. Haug E: Trichloroethylene poisoning: Acute renal failure caused by trichloroethylene inhalation treated with peritoneal dialysis. Tidsskr Nor Laegeforen 90:288, 1970.

58. Hauglustaine D, Van Damme B, Daenens P, et al: Silicon nephropathy: A possible occupational hazard. Nephron 26:219, 1980.

59. Henderson DA: A follow-up of cases of plumbism in children. Aust Ann Med 3:219, 1954.

60. Hook JB (ed.): Toxicology of the Kidney, Raven Press, New York, 1981.

61. Hook JB, Hewitt WR: Toxic responses of the kidney. In: Casarett and Doull's Toxicology: The Basic Science of Poisons, p 310, Klaassen CD, Amdur MO, Doull A (eds.), Macmillan, New York, 1986.

62. Joselow MM, Louria DB, Browder AA: Mercurialism: Environmental and occupational aspects. Ann Intern Med 76:119, 1972.

63. Kadamani S, Nabih AR, Nelson RY: Occupational exposure and risk of renal cell carcinoma. Am J Ind Med 15:131, 1989.

64. Kazantis G: Heavy metals and renal damage. Eur J Clin Invest 9:3, 1979.

65. King CM: The origins of urinary bladder cancer. In: Bladder Cancer, p 13, Bonney WW, Prout GR (eds.), Williams & Wilkins, Baltimore, 1980.

66. Klavis G, Drommer W: Goodpasture's syndrome and the effect of benzene. Arch Toxicol 26:40, 1970.

67. Klein WJ Jr, Metz EN, Price AR: Acute copper intoxication: A hazard of hemodialysis. Arch Intern Med 129:463, 1973.

68. Kluwe WM: The nephrotoxicity of low molecular weight halogenated alkane solvents, pesticides, and chemical intermediates. In: Toxicology of the Kidney, p 179, Hook JB (ed.), Raven Press, New York, 1981.

69. Kluwe WM, Hook JB: Effects of environmental chemicals on kidney metabolism and function. Kidney Int 18:648, 1980.

70. Kolev K, Doitschinov D, Todorov D: Morphologic alteration in the kidneys by silicosis. Medna Lav 61:205, 1970.

71. Kolonel LN: Association of cadmium with renal cancer. Cancer 37:1782, 1976.

72. Kroeger RM, Moore RJ, Lehman TH, et al: Recurrent urinary calculi associated with toluene sniffing. J Urol 123:89, 1980.

73. Kunkler PB, Farr RF, Luxton RF: Limit of renal tolerances to x-rays. Investigation into renal damage occurring following treatment of tumors of testis by abdominal baths. Br J Radiol 25:190, 1952.

74. Lauwerys RR: Industrial Chemical Exposure: Guidelines for Biological Monitoring, Biomedical Publications, Daris, California, 1983.

75. Lauwerys R, Bernard A, Vian C, et al: Kidney disorders and heme toxicity from organic solvent exposure. Scand J Work Environ Health 11(Suppl 1):83, 1985.

76. Lee JS, White KL: A review of the health effects of cadmium. Am J Ind Med 1:307, 1980.

77. Leong AS-Y, Dianey APS, Gove DW: Spallation and migration of silicone from blood-pump tubing in patients on hemodialysis. N Engl J Med 306:135, 1982.

78. Lesato K, Wakashin M, Wakashin Y, et al: Renal tubular dysfunction in Minamata disease: Detection of renal tubular antigen and beta-2-microglobulin in the urine. Ann Intern Med 86:731, 1977.

79. Lilis R, Fischbein A, Eisenger J, et al: Prevalence of lead disease among secondary lead smelter workers and biological indications of lead exposure. Environ Res 14:255, 1977.

80. Luxton RW: Radiation nephritis. Lancet 2:1221, 1961.

81. Madrazo A, Schwarz G, Churg J: Radiation nephritis: A review. J Urol 114:822, 1975.
82. Maher JF: Renal considerations: A. Acute renal failure complicating intoxication. In: Clinical Management of Poisoning and Drug Overdose, p 170, Haddad LM, Winchester JF (eds.), WB Saunders, Philadelphia, 1983.
83. Mehlman MA, Henistreet CP III, Thorpe JJ, et al; (eds.): Renal Effects of Petroleum Hydrocarbons, Princeton Scientific, Princeton, NJ, 1984.
84. Morgan DP: Recognition and Management of Pesticide Poisonings, 4th ed., US Environmental Protection Agency, EPA 54/9-88-001, Washington, 1989.
85. Murphy JD: Toxic effects of pesticides. In: Casarett and Doull's Toxicology: The Basic Science of Poisons, 3rd ed., p 519, Klaassen CD, Amdur MO, Doull J (eds.), Macmillan, New York, 1986.
86. Namba T, Nolte CT, Jackrel J, et al: Poisoning due to organophosphate insecticides. Am J Med 50:475, 1971.
87. Nelson NA, Robins TG, Port FR: Solvent nephrotoxicity in humans and experimental animals. Am J Nephrol 10:10, 1990.
88. New PS, Lubash GD, Scherr L, et al: Acute renal failure associated with carbon tetrachloride intoxication. JAMA 181:903, 1962.
89. Nordberg GF: Metabolism of cadmium. In: Nephrotoxic Mechanisms of Drugs and Environmental Toxins, p 285, Porter GA (ed.), Plenum Press, New York, 1982.
90. Odgen MA: New-dialyzer syndrome. N Engl J Med 301:1262, 1980.
91. Orringer EP, Mattern WD: Formaldehyde-induced hemolysis during chronic hemodialysis. N Engl J Med 294:1416, 1976.
92. Perry HM, Thind GS, Perry EF: The biology of cadmium. Med Clin North Am 60:759, 1976.
93. Ravnskov U: Possible mechanisms of hydrocarbon-associated glomerulonephritis. Clin Nephrol 23:294, 1985.
94. Ravnskov U, Forsberg B, Skerfving S: Glomerulonephritis and exposure to organic solvents. Acta Med Scand 105:575, 1979.
95. Robertson WD: Arsenic and other heavy metals. In: Clinical Management of Poisoning and Drug Overdose, p 656, Haddad LM, Winchester JF (eds.), WB Saunders, Philadelphia, 1983.
96. Rosa RM, Brown RS: Acute renal failure associated with heavy metals and organic solvents. In: Acute Renal Failure, p 321, Brenner BM, Lazarus JM (eds.), WB Saunders, Philadelphia, 1983.
97. Rostand SG, Kirk KA, Rutsky EA, et al: Racial differences in the incidence of treatment for end-stage renal disease. N Engl J Med 306:1276, 1982.
98. Rush FG, Smith JH, Newton JF, et al: Chemically induced nephrotoxicity: Role of metabolic activation. CRC Crit Rev Toxicol 13:99, 1984.
99. Saita B, Zavaglia O: La funzionalita renale nei silicotici. Medna Lav 42:41, 1951.
100. Saldanha LF, Rosen VJ, Gonick HG: Silicon nephropathy. Am J Med 59:95, 1975.
101. Schimamuria T, Morris AB: A progressive glomerulosclerosis occurring in partial five-sixths nephrectomy. Am J Pathol 79:95, 1975.
102. Schreiner GE: Renal considerations: Chronic drug nephrotoxicity. In: Clinical Management of Poisoning and Drug Overdose, p 185, Haddad LM, Winchester JF (eds.), WB Saunders, Philadelphia, 1983.
103. Sigler MH: The mechanism of the natriuresis of fasting. J Clin Invest 55:377, 1975.
104. Smith SB, Wombolt DG, Venkatesan R: Results of hemodialysis and hemoperfusion in the treatment of acute arsenic ingestion. Clin Exp Dialysis Apheresis 5:399, 1981.
105. Smith TJ, Anderson RJ, Reading JC: Chronic cadmium exposures associated with kidney function effects. Am J Ind Med 1:319, 1980.
106. Spark RF: Renin, aldosterone and glucogen in the natriuresis of fasting. N Engl J Med 292:1335, 1975.
107. Spitzer A (ed.): The Kidney during Development: Morphology and Function. Masson, Paris, 1982.
108. Spreepado Rao TK, Friedman EA: Fluoride and bone disease in uremia. Kidney Int 7:125, 1975.
109. Stewart RD, Boettner EA, Southworth RR, et al: Acute carbon tetrachloride intoxication. JAMA 183:994, 1963.
110. Streicher HZ, Gabow PA, Moss AH, et al: Syndromes of toluene sniffing in adults. Ann Intern Med 94:758, 1981.
111. Suki WN, Minuth AN, Terrell JB: Acute renal failure: A study of etiology, prognosis and the role of furosemide. Clin Dial Transplant Forum 5:123, 1975.
112. Symposium on Lead–Blood Pressure Relationships: Environ Health Perspect 78:3–139, 1988.
113. Symvoulidis A, Voudiclaris S, Mountokalakis T, et al: Acute renal failure in G-6 PD deficiency. Lancet 2:819, 1972.
114. Taher SM, Anderson RJ, McCartney R, et al: Renal tubular acidosis associated with toluene "sniffing." N Engl J Med 290:765, 1974.
115. Tepper LB: Renal function subsequent to childhood plumbism. Arch Environ Health 7:82, 1963.
116. Tsuchiya K: Proteinuria of workers exposed to cadmium fumes. Arch Environ Health 14:875, 1967.
117. Tubbs RR, Gephardt GN, McMahon JT, et al: Membranous glomerulonephritis associated with industrial mercury exposure. Study of pathogenic mechanisms. Am J Clin Pathol 77:409, 1982.
118. Vaziri ND, Ness RL, Fairshter RD, et al: Nephrotoxicity of paraquat in man. Arch Intern Med 139:172, 1979.
119. Walzer M: Delay of progression of renal failure. In: Prevention of Kidney Disease and Long-Term Survival, p 23, Avram MM (ed.), Plenum Press, New York, 1982.
120. Wands JR, Weiss SW, Yardley JH, et al: Chronic inorganic mercury poisoning due to laxative abuse. Am J Med 57:92, 1974.
121. Watson JM: Clinical and laboratory investigations in 132 cases of solvent abuse. Med Sci Law 18:40, 1978.
122. Wedeen RP: Lead nephropathy. In: Nephrotoxic Mechanisms of Drugs and Environmental Toxins, p 255, Porter GA (ed.), Plenum Press, New York, 1982.
123. Wedeen RP: Lead and the gouty kidney. Am J Kidney Dis 5:559, 1983.
124. Wedeen RP: Occupational renal disease: In-depth review. Am J Kidney Dis 3:241, 1984.

125. Wedeen RP, Maesaka JK, Weiner B, et al: Occupational lead nephropathy. Am J Med 59:630, 1975.
126. Wedeen RP, Mallik DK, Batuman V: Detection and treatment of occupational lead nephropathy. Arch Intern Med 139:53, 1979.
127. Weeden RP, Batuman V, Landy E: The safety of the EDTA lead mobilization test. Environ Res 30:58, 1983.
128. Will AM, McLaren EH: Reversible renal damage due to glue sniffing. Br Med J 283:525, 1981.
129. Wilson CB: Drug- and toxin-induced nephritides: Anti-kidney antibody and immune complex mediation. In: Nepthrotoxic Mechanisms of Drugs and Environmental Toxins, p 383, Porter GA (ed.), Plenum Press, New York, 1982.
130. Wyckoff DW: Diagnostic and therapeutic problems of parathion poisoning, Ann Intern Med 68:875, 1968.
131. Wyngaarden J, Kelley WM: Gout and Hyperuricemia, Grune & Stratton, New York, 1976.
132. Yu T: Lead nephropathy and gout. Am J Kidney Dis 5:555, 1983.
133. Zimmerman SW, Groehler K, Beirne GJ: Hydrocarbon exposure and chronic glomerulonephritis. Lancet 2:119, 1975.

RECOMMENDED READINGS

Bach PH, Lock EA (eds.): Nephrotoxicity In Vitro to In Vivo, Animals to Man. Plenum Press, New York, 1989.
Bennett WM, Elzinger LW, Porter GA: Tubulointerstitial Disease and Toxic Nephropathy. In: The Kidney, p 1430, Vol 2, Brenner BM, Rector FC Jr (eds.), WB Saunders, Philadelphia, 1991.
Porter GA (ed.): Nephrotoxic Mechanisms of Drugs and Environmental Toxins, Plenum Press, New York, 1982.

21. DISORDERS OF THE HEMATOPOIETIC SYSTEM

William A. Newton, Jr., and Alyce Bezman Tarcher

INTRODUCTION

This chapter focuses on the relationship between exposure to environmental chemicals and physical agents and disorders of the hematopoietic system. The hematopoietic system includes the formed elements of the blood as well as the bone marrow, spleen, lymph nodes, and reticuloendothelial tissue. It is uniquely constructed to provide the body with a vast capacity for cell renewal. To balance the loss of mature cells and to provide for rapid expansion in response to bodily insults, cellular renewal must be maintained throughout life. The relative accessibility of the blood and bone marrow creates the potential for providing early clues to the effects of toxic exposure. A wide range of hematological disorders may follow exposure to such environmental agents as solvents, heavy metals, insecticides, nitrates, nitrites, and ionizing radiation (45,77,106, 126,199,211). This information, plus the fact that many hematological disorders develop without known cause, should alert the physician to environmental exposure as a potential hematological hazard.

ENVIRONMENTAL CHEMICALS AND PHYSICAL AGENTS ASSOCIATED WITH ADVERSE EFFECTS ON THE HEMATOPOIETIC SYSTEM

It is well established that exposure to such agents as benzene, lead, carbon monoxide, nitrates, and ionizing radiation may be responsible for a wide range of hematological disorders (1,6,7,44,50,77, 136,156,179,202). Exposure to a variety of other chemicals, including metals, solvents, chlorophenoxy herbicides, pesticides such as γ-benzene hexachloride (lindane), chlordane, heptachlor, dieldrin, DDT, pentachlorophenol, and mothproofing chemicals has been linked, with varying degrees of certainty, to hematological toxicity (Table 21-1) (7,13,26, 30,32,38,57,60–62,67,85,90,92,105,112,115,117,118, 120,139,150,166,172,175,202,208,222).

Benzene

Of all known human carcinogens, benzene is commercially the most important and has the greatest potential for exposure in the workplace and general environment. Benzene is produced by petroleum refining and coal tar distillation. It has been used in large volumes by industry for many years. Benzene was originally used as a volatile solvent and later used in the synthesis of organic chemicals. Benzene is extensively used in the petroleum, explosive, plastics, pesticide, and rubber industries and as an octane booster in lead-free gasoline. It constitutes about 1% of U.S. gasoline and 5% of European gasoline.

It has been estimated that as many as 2 million U.S. workers may be exposed to benzene. Since it is

Principles and Practice of Environmental Medicine, edited by Alyce Bezman Tarcher. Plenum Medical Book Company, New York, 1992.

TABLE 21-1. Lymphohematological Disorders Associated
with Environmental and Occupational Exposures[a]

Lymphohematological disorder	Exposure(s)
Hemolytic anemia	Arsine, lead, copper, formaldehyde, aniline, napthalene, paradichlorobenzene
Hypoproliferative anemia	Arsenic, lead, benzene, aluminum
Thrombycytopenia	Benzene, ionizing radiation, organochlorine pesticides
Neutropenia	Arsenic, benzene, organochlorine pesticides
Aplastic anemia	Arsenic, benzene, ionizing radiation, organochlorine pesticides, trinitroglycerine
Leukemia	Electromagnetic radiation
Acute nonlymphocytic leukemia	Benzene, ionizing radiation
Acute lymphocytic leukemia	Benzene, ionizing radiation
Chronic myelogenous leukemia	Benzene, ionizing radiation
Chronic lymphocytic leukemia	Benzene
Hodgkin disease	Chlorophenoxyacetic acid herbicides
Non-Hodgkin lymphoma	Chlorophenoxyacetic acid herbicides, ionizing radiation
Multiple myeloma	Benzene, ionizing radiation
Methemoglobinemia	Nitrates, nitrites, aromatic nitro and amino compounds
Carboxyhemoglobinemia	Carbon monoxide

[a]Data from references 44, 55, 77, 101, 128, 165, 190, 194, 214, 227, and 237.

a common component of gasoline, benzene is also present in ambient air, particularly in urban areas where gasoline consumption is high (205). Benzene has not been used in consumer products in the United States since 1978. It may, however, be a contaminant in products containing petroleum distillates, with higher levels being present in such agents as stove and lantern fuels, brush cleaners, and rubber cements. The most important source of benzene exposure for smokers is mainstream smoke from their cigarettes (205).

Lead

Repeated ingestion of lead-pigment paint accounts for most symptomatic cases of lead intoxication. Household dust in old houses accounts for increased lead absorption in many young children (42). It is estimated, for example, that 27 million homes in the United States are contamined by lead paint (130). Unfortunately, hazards are also associated with the "deleading" of homes of children suffering from lead poisoning (9). Young children who live close to lead smelters may also show some evidence of increased lead absorption (123; see also Chapters 13, 14, and 28).

Since 1977, paint produced for household use in the United States must, by regulation, contain no more than 0.06% (600 ppm) lead by dry weight. In contrast, some paints manufactured in the 1940s for indoor use contained more than 50% (500,000 ppm) lead by dry weight. It should be understood that laws that effectively ban lead from household paints do not extend to artist's paints. Artists, teachers, and parents should therefore be aware of the sources of lead in such art supplies as oil paints, ceramic glazes, and copper enamels. Lead exposure may also occur during soldering operations and the firing of lead-containing ceramic glazes and copper enamels (see Chapters 13, 14, and 28).

The widespread nature of lead pollution accounts for chronic exposure to this element. Although lead in food generally provides a source of low-level exposure, foods can at times be an important source of exposure. This occurs if crops are grown near heavily traveled roads or near stationary industrial sources of lead contamination. Canned foods may contain high concentrations of lead when lead solder is used in the seams of the can. Under these conditions, the leaching of lead occurs particularly in the presence of acidic foods. Lead contamination of acidic foods and beverages through storage in improperly lead-glazed ceramicware also occurs. Water may be an important source of lead exposure when lead pipes and soldered points are used. The availability of lead-free gasoline removes an important source of lead pollution. Tetraethyl lead, a volatile organic liquid, is still present in some gasolines in concentrations of 0.1% or less. This compound slowly decomposes in the atmosphere, and from 25% to 75% of the lead in combusted automotive fuel is discharged into the atmosphere as inorganic lead salts (see Chapters 2–4).

Carbon Monoxide

Carbon monoxide, a product of incomplete combustion, is a ubiquitous pollutant. It is found in auto exhausts, furnaces, boilers, and fires. High concentrations are present in urban areas in conjunction with heavy auto and truck traffic. Carbon monoxide is also commonly present indoors. Unvented heating and cooking sources and cigarette smoke produce carbon monoxide. Elevated levels of carbon monoxide are found in underground garages. Garages attached to homes are also common sources of carbon monoxide in indoor air.

Nitrates and Nitrites

The presence of large quantities of nitrates in the water supply poses a threat of methemoglobinemia, particularly for the infant (114,136). In the past, nitrate contamination in rural wells or cisterns came primarily from feed lots, home sewage, or surface water runoff. At present, much of the nitrate contamination of rural wells and public water supplies in agricultural areas is derived from the excessive use of chemical fertilizers. Over the past 25 years, the use of chemical fertilizer throughout the world has grown dramatically. Ground and surface waters worldwide have thus become increasingly contaminated with nitrates from nitrogen-fertilized cropland (83,171; see also Chapter 4).

Pesticides

Pesticide is a general term used to include chemicals that control insects (insecticide), weeds (herbicide), plant diseases (fungicide), rodents (rodenticide), etc. Initially, farmers were the primary users of pesticides. However, as new chemicals were produced and new uses were developed, new types of users were found. Today, pesticides are still a major part of agriculture's production tools, but they are also used by industry, governments, municipalities, commercial pesticide applicators, and the public, including homeowners and backyard gardeners. The percentage used by agriculture has declined to approximately 50% of the total pesticide production. About 20% of all pesticides sold is used in the towns and cities. In developed countries, demand is leveling off or decreasing as pesticides with more specific activity and lower required dosages are developed and used. Consumption of pesticides in the United States declined 20% between 1973 and 1983 to 1.1 billion pounds (134). In contrast, herbicide use has grown substantially, and it now occupies about 40% of the world's agrochemical market (134). In the United States approximately 480 million pounds of herbicides are used annually (168).

The organochlorine pesticides, which include DDT, aldrin, dieldrin, chlordane, hepatochlor, lindane, and toxaphene, were widely used between the mid-1940s and the mid-1960s. These compounds have come under increasing disfavor because of their persistence in the environment, their concentration in the food chain, their ecotoxicity, and the fact that many are carcinogenic in animal assays (103). Agricultural use of many of the organochlorine insec-

ticides was banned in the United States in the 1970s. In 1987, the use of chlordane and heptachlor as a treatment for termites in U.S. homes was stopped. Human monitoring programs reveal the persistence of organochlorine residues in adipose tissue and blood (203).

The chlorophenoxy herbicides have been widely used in vast amounts since the late 1940s. The compounds 2,4,5-trichlorophenoxyacetic acid (2,4,5-T) and 2,4-dichlorophenoxyacetic acid (2,4-D) have been used in farming, in forest management, in backyard gardens, and for weed control along roadsides (226). The use of 2,4,5-T, which formerly was contaminated with varying amounts of dioxin, was suspended by the Environmental Protection Agency in 1979. Vast amounts of 2,4-D continue to be used, however, There is no evidence that 2,4-D is contaminated with dioxin.

Ionizing Radiation

Exposure of the population to ionizing radiation stems from a number of sources. These include natural radiation, medical radiation, consumer products, occupational and industrial operations, nuclear power generation, fallout from nuclear weapons testing, accidents from nuclear power plants, and environmental contamination from nuclear weapons plants (167,169). Of particular concern is a report released by the Department of Energy that reveals very serious radioactive pollution problems involving a number of weapons factories in the United States. Not only have radioactive and toxic wastes been discharged into the atmosphere, but soil and surface and ground water contamination has occurred as well (215).

Toxicology

Our understanding of normal hematopoiesis and of the adverse effects of toxic exposure on this process has depended on the development of increasingly sophisticated methodology. In the past, the toxic effects on the blood and bone marrow were monitored primarily by analyzing hemograms and then assessing the number of circulating blood cells. Newer methods for assessing bone marrow injury include in vivo and in vitro stem-cell assays, flow cytofluorometry, and cytogenetic techniques. The interested reader is encouraged to consult other references for a detailed discussion of this technology and its application (52,108,231).

EPIDEMIOLOGY

Despite the fact that primary hematological diseases and malignancies of the lymphoid and hematopoietic systems are relatively uncommon, these conditions have received the attention of many investigators. Aplastic anemia and leukemia, in particular, have been the focus of many studies (8,14, 28,29,74,80,81,97,100,127,128,144,193,204,206,208).

A number of epidemiologic studies have searched for an association between disorders of the lymphohematopoietic system and exposure to toxic agents. The effectiveness of such an investigation is limited, however, in part by the rarity of these disorders (62,194,211). Moreover, it is apparent that large individual differences exist in the susceptibility of the lymphohematopoietic system to toxic exposure. Genetic variability and other factors such as age, coexisting exposures, the presence of disease, and nutritional and physiological status undoubtedly influence host susceptibility.

Aplastic Anemia

Aplastic anemia is characterized by a bone marrow deficiency that results in inadequate production of erythrocytes, granulocytes, and platelets. Epidemiologic studies reveal that aplastic anemia is more prevalent in the Orient than in other parts of the world. This disease is rare before 1 year of age, remains at an intermediate level until the age of 50, and then increases in incidence with old age (37). In both the East and the West, chloramphenicol appears to be the agent most commonly incriminated in the genesis of aplastic anemia (37,99, 100,229).

The rarity of aplastic anemia has limited its study by epidemiologic methods. The only viable means of assessing its epidemiologic characteristics and associations depends on a large population-based, case–control study. A recent international cooperative study of this type was performed to investigate the relationship between analgesic use and agranulocytosis and aplastic anemia (207). The rarity of aplastic anemia suggests that its appearance after toxic exposure depends on unique individual susceptibility.

Investigation of the relationship between aplastic anemia and exposure to toxic agents has relied primarily on the observations of alert clinicians and on epidemiologic studies of occupational groups. Exposure to a variety of environmental agents has been reported to be associated with aplastic anemia. These include benzene, trinitrotoluene, arsenic, DDT, lindane, chlordane, heptachlor, and ionizing radiation (37,72,77,180–182,187,193).

A large series of case reports beginning more than 50 years ago noted a relationship between benzene exposure and aplastic anemia (58,145). These clinical observations have been supported by a number of epidemiologic studies (78,104,124,178, 219). Of note are the observations of Aksoy et al.,

who studied Turkish workers in the handicraft leather industry. These studies showed that exposure to benzene-containing glue was followed by cases of aplastic anemia that often was a forerunner of acute myelogenous leukemia. When the benzene-containing glue was replaced by another agent, the incidence of these blood disorders decreased dramatically (3–5).

Many clinical case reports have described the appearance of aplastic anemia after an individual was exposed to one of a number of different pesticides, primarily organochlorines. In many instances these reports depict individuals who received relatively high levels of exposure (151,173,177,180–182, 184,187,229).

An epidemiologic study by Wang and Gufferman explored the relationship between aplastic anemia and exposure to organochlorine pesticides (224). Using the occupation stated on the death certificate as an indicator of possible exposure to an organochlorine pesticide, these investigators failed to find an association between aplastic anemia and occupational pesticide exposure. Such a relationship cannot be excluded because of the limitations involved in using the occupation recorded on the death certificate as an index of exposure.

Radiation injury to the bone marrow can lead to aplastic anemia (59,206). This effect is secondary to destruction of the stem cells in the bone marrow (51). The rate and degree of damage to the formed elements of the blood can often serve as a crude reflection of radiation injury. In cases of acute radiation injury, the hematopoietic system is the system most likely to sustain injury. The complications that develop are secondary to a nonfunctioning bone marrow. Injury to the hematopoietic system occurs after exposure to doses of irradiation between 2 and 10 Gy (200 and 1000 rad) (59,163).

Leukemia

The leukemias comprise a varied group of malignancies that arise primarily from the bone marrow. As immunologic, chromosomal, and biochemical advances are made, the classification of the leukemias will continue to change. Epidemiologic studies have perceived differences among four basic forms of leukemia: acute lymphocytic leukemia (ALL), acute nonlymphocytic leukemia (ANLL), chronic granulocytic leukemia (CGL), and chronic lymphocytic leukemia (CLL) (128). In many epidemiologic studies of leukemia, however, the diagnosis has been used without further definition of the type of leukemia.

Descriptive epidemiologic studies of leukemia reveal that the geographic variation in its incidence is generally less than that seen in other cancers. The major exception to this observation is CLL, which is rare in Oriental countries. This difference persists in persons of Oriental ancestry living outside the Orient (96). The incidence of leukemia varies with age. There are about five cases per 100,000 between the ages of 2 and 4 years; one to two cases per 100,000 in young adults; and over 30 cases per 100,000 in those over 50. In general, ALL occurs in children; CLL arises in the elderly; and ANLL appears chiefly in adults. Males are more subject to CLL, and Caucasians have a higher incidence of leukemia than blacks. Host susceptibility is observed in a number of studies. Apart from the racial variation previously noted, certain hereditary conditions such as Down syndrome and ataxia telangiectasia carry an increased risk of leukemia or lymphoma (97,155).

Environmental Agents

Epidemiologists have studied various occupational groups to discover chemicals that pose a potential hematological hazard. Such studies have identified certain occupations associated with an increased risk of leukemia or lymphoma. These include rubber workers, metal workers, refinery workers, painters, chemical production workers, chemists, farmers, shoe-manufacturing production workers, chemists, farmers, and workers in the health care professions (24–26,30,101,128,144,170,211).

Epidemiologic studies have alerted the medical community to a potential link between leukemia in children and chemical exposure received by their parents. Several reports have noted an increased risk for leukemia in children whose parents were exposed to hydrocarbons and chlorinated solvents in the workplace and whose parents used pesticides in the home (64,82,98,135,217,218). Other studies, however, failed to confirm these findings (89,188, 195). Solvent-contaminated drinking water has been cited as a potential risk factor in the excess number of cases of childhood leukemia discovered in the residents of Woburn, Massachusetts (121). The validity of this relationship has been questioned (143). Immunologic abnormalities have also been described in a population chronically exposed to solvent-contaminated drinking water (35). These findings have not been confirmed. It is anticipated that future studies will address the role of exposure to hydrocarbons, chlorinated solvents, and pesticides in the etiology of childhood leukemia. The documentation and timing of such exposure in relation to the inception of pregnancy and fetal development are of importance.

Benzene

With the exception of benzene, specific chemicals have not been incriminated in the etiology of leukemia. The causal relationship between benzene exposure and the development of myelomonocytic leukemia, acute promyelocytic leukemia, and erythroleukemia is now amply demonstrated (23,78,79, 124,179). A series of case reports, beginning in 1928, were critical in focusing the attention of epidemiologists on the relationship between benzene and leukemia (6,32,58,145,219). Subsequent epidemiologic and animal studies supported these clinical observations (23,104,146,178,205,219).

Pesticides

Over the past 30 years, a variety of pesticides, particularly organochlorines, have been reported to be associated with a range of hematological disorders. These include anemia, aplastic anemia, leukemia, neutropenia, thrombocytopenia, and hemolytic anemia (Table 21-1). The association is based almost exclusively on clinical case reports describing adverse hematological reactions generally occurring after exposure to relatively high pesticide levels (60, 62,86,92,105,110,111,117,132,133,149,162,164,166,173, 176,177,180–182,187,192,193,221,228,233,235). Clinical case reports have obvious limitations in establishing environmental agents as health hazards; nonetheless, such observations are often essential in alerting the scientific community to an environmental hazard, which can then be studied epidemiologically and in the experimental laboratory (93,154).

Few epidemiologic studies have examined cancer risk associated with a specific pesticide exposure, as it is difficult to identify exposed groups of adequate size who are not also exposed to other chemicals (197). Wang and MacMahon performed a retrospective mortality study of 1403 workers employed in the manufacture of chlordane and heptachlor (225). No excess in hematological or more common malignancies was noted. However, the populations studied were small, and the period of follow-up was limited. A population-based case-referent study in Kansas performed by Zahm et al. examined the relationship among soft-tissue sarcoma, Hodgkin disease, and insecticide use. Soft-tissue sarcoma was found to be higher among farmers who mixed or applied insecticides. Farmers who failed to use any protective equipment to reduce insecticide exposure were at a significantly increased risk for soft-tissue sarcoma. The risk appeared to be limited to exposures occurring prior to the mid-1950s, primarily to chlorinated hydrocarbon insecticides (237).

Herbicides

Concern for the long-term health effects of pesticide exposure prompted a number of epidemiologic studies to see if farmers, because of their agricultural exposures, are at increased risk for certain cancers. Farmers have had potentially large exposure to pesticides (including herbicides) since the 1960s. In addition, they frequently come in contact with a number of other toxic chemicals, which include solvents, paints, welding fumes, fuels, and oils. Over the years a number of studies have suggested that farmers are at increased risk for such malignancies as Hodgkin disease, leukemia, non-Hodgkin lymphoma, multiple myeloma, and cancers of the lip, stomach, prostate, skin, and connective tissue (2,13,24–26,33,34,39,40,49,131,147,174,186,194).

Epidemiologic studies from Scandinavia, Italy, and the United States suggest that individuals exposed to chlorophenoxy herbicides are at increased risk of developing Hodgkin disease, non-Hodgkin lymphoma, and soft tissue sarcoma (46,63,87–89, 101,137,220,237).

Of the studies done thus far, the population-based case–control study of Kansas farmers performed by Hoar et al. offers the greatest statistical power (101). This study was performed to determine the effect of the agricultural use of herbicides and insecticides on the incidence of soft-tissue sarcoma, Hodgkin disease, and non-Hodgkin lymphoma. A sixfold increase of non-Hodgkin lymphoma was observed among farmers exposed to herbicides. The excesses were associated with the use of phenoxyacetic acid herbicides, specifically 2,4-D (101). To date, however, the International Agency for Research in Cancer has found limited evidence for carcinogenicity of chlorophenoxy herbicides in humans (103).

The epidemiologic studies noted above raise the issue of pesticide exposure as a risk factor for certain cancers among farmers. Identifying specific etiologic agents promises to be particularly difficult because farmers are exposed, in varying degrees, to a wide range of hazardous agents, including pesticides, fertilizers, solvents, ultraviolet light, and dusts.

Ionizing Radiation

The carcinogenic risks from exposure to ionizing radiation have been studied more extensively than have other environmental carcinogens (44,213). An important advantage of studying the effects of radiation exposure lies in the fact that the dose can be easily measured or reasonably well estimated retrospectively. Moreover, for many populations, particularly those exposed for medical reasons, fairly accurate and complete records are available.

As with other carcinogens, there is a latent period between irradiation and the clinical appearance of cancer. The latent period is inversely related to the level of radiation exposure. Latent periods ranging from a few years to as long as 20 years or

more have been observed. The latent period varies among species and with the type of cancer induced, usually being shorter for leukemia than for solid tumors (27,156,214). A recent report from the National Research Council on the effects of exposure to low levels of ionizing radiation provides no new data to contradict the theory that the carcinogenic effect of radiation exposure is directly related to the dose (44).

Clinical case reports first alerted the scientific community to the appearance of leukemia in workers who had received excessive radiation exposure (69). Excessive mortality from leukemia was also observed in radiologists and patients treated with x–ray for ankylosing spondylitis (50,56,212). Two radioisotopes used for diagnostic and therapeutic purposes are also known to induce leukemia in humans. These include thorotrast, a radioactive material formerly used in radiology as a contrast medium, and phosphorus-32, used in the treatment of polycythemia (158,159).

Epidemiologic studies of Japanese atomic bomb survivors show an excess of all types of leukemia except chronic lymphatic leukemia (17). The earliest cases of leukemia appeared about 2 years after the bombing. The latent period, generally between 5 and 10 years, was shorter in young survivors. The incidence of leukemia in individuals exposed to the atomic bomb was still somewhat greater than expected 30 years after exposure (44,128,153,156,157).

Multiple myeloma increases in frequency after irradiation (44,55). This relationship is observed in atomic bomb survivors, in patients after radiation therapy for ankylosing spondylitis, and in nuclear plant workers (44,55,56,209). Some observers have noted an increase in non-Hodgkin lymphoma after irradiation in humans (44,55). No increase in Hodgkin disease has been noted (44).

The catastrophic accident that occurred in April 1986 at the Chernobyl nuclear power plant in the USSR once again alerted the medical community to the health problems that can arise from radiation exposure. It has been estimated that because of the accident up to 28,000 extra cancer deaths may arise in the entire Northern Hemisphere (75,76). Since analysis of atomic-bomb survivors revealed that granulocytic leukemia occurred after a short latent period of 2 to 5 years after exposure, it will be important to observe its incidence in the 24,000 Soviets who are estimated to have received a collective dose of about 10,000 Gy (1 million person-rads, averaging about 43 rads per person) (75).

Numerous epidemiologic studies have investigated the carcinogenic effects of the fallout from nuclear weapons tests in the United States over southern and eastern Utah in the 1950s. An initial study by Lyon et al. revealed increased mortality from leukemia among children that then declined when surface testing stopped (138). A reanalysis by Land et al. concluded that the relationship noted by Lyon et al. was based on an anomalously low rate of childhood leukemia in southern Utah during the 1944–1949 period that was used as the baseline rate in the Lyon study (122).

In 1984, Johnson reported an excess incidence of leukemia as well as other cancers related to the fallout from nuclear testing. The large excess of leukemia noted in this study, which according to currently accepted risk estimates would require an exposure of 100 rad (1 Gy) or more, has raised the question of recall bias (113). A reanalysis by Machado et al. using slightly different time periods and geographic boundaries revealed a significant excess of deaths from leukemia associated with radioactive fallout in southwestern Utah (140).

Cancer risk associated with residence near a nuclear power facility or a nuclear weapons plant has recently come under investigation. A number of observers have noted an excess number of cases of childhood leukemia in proximity to nuclear power facilities in Britain and the United States (15,19,43, 47,70,71,94,95,102,183,216). To date, a general increase in the incidence of cancer has not been observed in individuals living in the vicinity of nuclear installations (47,48,65). The public health implications of these observations are unresolved. The growing number of positive findings merits further investigation.

Radiation exposure prenatally or during childhood is of concern since it may be followed by cancer. An excess in leukemia was noted in children who had survived the A bomb (31,155). Thus far two cases of childhood cancer were observed among in-utero-exposed survivors of the atomic bomb (236). However, the incidence of childhood leukemia was not increased in such survivors (236). Increased susceptibility to malignant disease, including leukemia, following prenatal radiation from diagnostic x–rays was first noted by Stewart et al. (201). Additional studies, including studies of twins, generally support these initial observations (91,141). A report from the National Research Council tentatively concluded that susceptibility to the carcinogenic effects of irradiation is high during prenatal life (44). This interpretation is complicated by the fact that little increase in susceptibility has been observed among prenatally exposed experimental animals, and there is no biological explanation for such an increase in susceptibility (142,157,160,161). The interested reader is referred to a comprehensive review of the health effects of ionizing radiation (44).

Electromagnetic Radiation

Over the past decade a number of epidemiologic studies have examined the relationship between cancer and exposure to electromagnetic fields (165,234). The question was first raised in 1979, when Wertheimer and Leeper reported that children who lived in homes near electrical power lines were two to three times more likely to develop cancer, particularly leukemia, lymphomas, and nervous system tumors, than children who live in homes a greater distance from these high current configurations (227). These results were generally confirmed by a subsequent case–control study performed by Savitz et al. (190). A risk ratio calculated by Savitz et al., of about 1.5, was lower than that reported by Wertheimer and Leeper. Other studies looking for such a correlation have produced mixed results (68,210). Investigation of workers exposed to electromagnetic fields reveal a general pattern of low increased risk of leukemia (36,152,189,196,198,234). Currently, no conclusions can be drawn regarding the carcinogenic effect of electromagnetic field exposure. Several large epidemiologic studies are now in progress to investigate this question.

In 1989, a background paper containing a comprehensive review and analysis of the pertinent literature and policy recommendations related to the biological effects of electromagnetic fields was issued by the U.S. Office of Technology Assessment (165). A key finding of this report indicates that 60-Hertz and other low-frequency electromagnetic fields can interact with individual cells and organs to produce biological changes. The public health implications of such exposure remain unclear.

PATHOLOGY AND PATHOLOGICAL PHYSIOLOGY

Toxic assault on the hematopoietic system may be reflected in a wide variety of adverse responses. These include (1) a general or partial suppression of hematopoiesis, (2) abnormal hematopoiesis, (3) interference with the functional capacity of the blood without a decrease in cell numbers, (4) increased demand for formation of blood elements, and (5) malignant transformation (126).

Suppression of Hematopoiesis

The suppressive effect of chemical exposure on hematopoiesis occurs in the case of chronic benzene exposure. At the turn of the century investigators first observed that benzene-exposed workers developed aplastic anemia. Subsequent studies revealed that the severity of bone marrow failure was a direct function of the degree of benzene exposure. Thus, the effects of benzene on hematopoiesis can range from a mild cytopenia to complete destruction of the bone marrow. Dose patterns are observed in humans and animals (77,124).

Chronic benzene exposure suppresses hematopoiesis by destroying the pluripotential stem cell responsible for red blood cells, granulocytic white blood cells, and platelets. Although it is apparent that a metabolite(s) of benzene rather than benzene itself is responsible for its hematological toxicity, the precise nature of this interaction is unclear. There are a number of metabolites of benzene that are capable of damaging critical bone marrow constituents. These include oxygenated derivatives of benzene such as benzene epoxide, open-ring metabolites of benzene such as muconaldehyde, and polyhydroxylated metabolites of benzene such as benzoquinone (107,124,125,191,200,205). Benzene-induced suppression of hematopoiesis is generally a reversible phenomenon, providing the exposed individual does not quickly succumb to aplastic anemia.

Abnormalities in Hematopoiesis

Under some circumstances, toxic exposure can have a predominant effect on a specific cellular element. The interaction of lead with the heme biosynthetic pathway illustrates how toxic exposure can adversely affect hematopoiesis. The effect of lead on heme synthesis takes place on bone marrow erythroblasts, which contain mitochondria. The vulnerability of red blood cell maturation in bone marrow may in part be linked to the preferential deposition of lead at this site (148).

The following metabolic effects are characteristic of lead toxicity on heme biosynthesis (Fig. 21-1). There is an inhibition of porphobilinogen synthase (formerly δ-aminolevulinic acid dehydratase), coproporphyrinogen oxidase (coprogenase), and ferrochelatase (heme synthetase), with a resultant increased urinary excretion of δ-aminolevulinic acid and coproporphyrin and the accumulation of protophorphyrin in red blood cells. Lead toxicity also results in a compensatory increase in the activity of the enzyme aminolevulinic acid synthetase. This effect is caused by a depletion of heme, the end product of the heme biosynthetic pathway, which exerts a primary control on the activity of this enzyme.

Alterations in the heme biosynthetic pathway provide an index of lead toxicity, notably, the presence of increased erythrocyte protophorphyrin. Red blood cell protoporphyrin begins to increase with

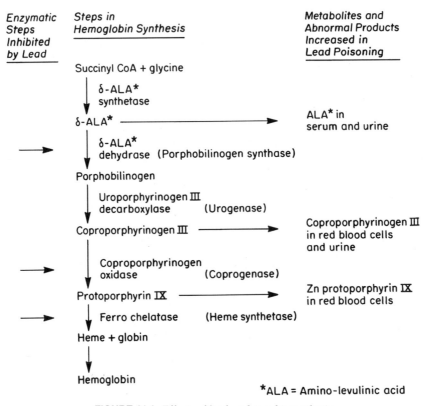

FIGURE 21-1. Effects of lead on heme biosynthesis.

blood lead levels of about 20 µg/dL (1 µmol/L). It persists for the life span of the red cell, thus reflecting the average inhibition of heme synthesis over the preceding 3 months (42). Erthrocyte protophorphyrin is also elevated in iron deficiency; blood lead levels must therefore be measured to provide evidence of lead toxicity. Since erythrocyte protophorphyrin concentration is not sensitive enough to identify children with blood lead levels below about 25 µg/dL (1.2 µmol/L), it is no longer the screening test of choice for lead poisoning (41).

Interference with the Functional Capacity of Normally Formed Cells

Certain environmental chemicals may impair the optimal function of various cellular elements of the hematopoietic system. Most notable are those agents that interfere with the oxygen delivery system of the red blood cell. Future studies will undoubtedly incriminate a range of toxic chemicals that impair the function of the formed elements of the hematopoietic system. For example, immunologic dysfunction of peripheral blood lymphocytes has been noted after exposure to certain chemicals (18,73). The subject of immunotoxicology and its clinical implications are discussed in Chapter 23.

Carboxyhemoglobinemia

Carbon monoxide interferes with the normal oxygen-carrying capacity of the blood by combining with hemoglobin to form carboxyhemoglobin (COHb). Carbon monoxide in ambient and indoor air diffuses through the lungs into the blood. Hemoglobin has approximately 220 times greater affinity for carbon monoxide than for oxygen, and the high affinity of carbon monoxide for hemoglobin prevents the uptake of oxygen from the lungs. Small elevations of carbon monoxide in ambient air can result in a relatively large displacement of oxygen from hemoglobin (202). The CO binds reversibly with hemoglobin; thus, when an acute exposure ceases, oxyhemoglobin is formed once again.

The primary mechanism of CO toxicity is the formation of COHb, which disrupts the normal transport of oxygen to the tissues. This occurs in two ways: (1) CO displaces oxygen on the hemoglobin carrier so that the hemoglobin has a reduced capacity to carry oxygen; (2) CO makes it more difficult for the oxygen that is still transported by hemoglobin to be released at the tissue level.

Methemoglobinemia

Methemoglobin is formed when the heme iron of hemoglobin is changed from the ferrous to the ferric state. Under these conditions, the red blood cell is incapable of delivering oxygen to the tissues. Of the chemicals capable of mediating the oxidation of hemoglobin, organic and inorganic nitrites and nitrates are the best known and of major importance. Environmental exposure to nitrates stems increasingly from the use of chemical fertilizers. During the last decade, ground water and drinking water in many major agricultural areas of the world have both evidenced rising levels of nitrate. Synthetic nitrogen is the fertilizer nutrient of primary concern in ground-water contamination (84). Although the ingested nitrates are relatively nontoxic, their conversion to nitrites by intestinal bacterial is linked to the formation of methemoglobin (136).

The oxidation of heme iron to produce methemoglobin occurs continuously under ordinary conditions. The major system responsible for the reduction of ferric iron to ferrous iron is an NADH-dependent methemoglobin reductase.

Infants during the first 4 months of life are at high risk of methemoglobin formation. At this age, the NADH-reductase system is not completely developed, and the relatively low acidity of the stomach provides an excellent environment for bacteria that convert nitrate to nitrite. Nitrate-contaminated well water is a common cause of methemoglobinemia in infants (114). Methemoglobin levels generally decline spontaneously once exposure ceases. Severely afflicted patients have been treated with methylene blue (114).

Increased Production of Blood Elements

Hemolytic Processes

A hemolytic process results in the premature destruction of red blood cells, which normally survive in the circulation about 120 days. A number of agents such as lead, copper, formaldehyde, aniline, and arsine can produce hemolysis by nonimmune mechanisms (21). Arsine, a toxic gas now widely used in the microelectronics industry, is particularly noted for its ability to produce severe hemolysis. The hemolytic process presumably is in part related to arsine's role in the formation of irreversible complexes with sulfhydryl groups of the red blood cell membrane (21,223).

Lead poisoning may be associated with a modest reduction in red blood cell survival. Although the mechanism of this shortened life span is not totally understood, the fact that lead inhibits pyrimidine 5'-nucleotidase is of interest. A congenital deficiency of this enzyme is characterized by a hemolytic anemia with basophilic stippling morphologically similar to that found in lead poisoning (22). The normochromic, microcytic or normochromic, normocytic anemia found with lead toxicity is thus the result of hemolysis as well as of decreased red blood cell production. Anemia is not an early index of lead toxicity. It is associated with high blood lead levels and chronic exposure (11,42).

Hemolytic anemia associated with exposure to certain oxidant chemicals is more likely to occur when the oxidant defense mechanisms of the red blood cell are compromised. A prime example of this problem is the hereditary deficiency of glucose-6-phosphate dehydrogenase (G-6-PD). In its mild and more common form, this enzyme deficiency is found in about 12% of black males in the United States. Glucose-6-phosphate dehydrogenase deficiency, the most common enzyme abnormality of the pentose phosphate pathway, reduces the capacity of the red blood cell to maintain glutathione in the reduced state. Because of this, the red blood cell is susceptible to damage by oxidant agents. Most notable is the predisposition of such individuals to develop hemolytic anemia following the ingestion of such oxidant drugs as primaquine, nalidixic acid, nitrofurantoin, sulfanilamide, and sulfamethoxazole. Individuals with G-6-PD deficiency appear to be at little risk from the inhalation of oxidant gases but may be susceptible to the oxidizing chemical trinitrotoluene, found in the workplace (10,20,21).

Malignant Changes

As previously noted, of all known human carcinogens, benzene has the greatest potential for exposure in the workplace and general environment. The extensive use of benzene has led to a number of studies investigating the mechanism of its leukemogenesis. Although the mechanism by which benzene acts as a chemical carcinogen is not resolved, studies during the past decade have provided a range of important information. Benzene toxicity is reflected primarily on the pluripotential stem cells of the bone marrow and on lymphocytic cells (12,54,107,109). There is evidence that benzene exposure produces cytogenetic effects. A significant increase in sister chromatid exchanges in bone marrow has been observed in mice after benzene exposure (53,66,79).

Studies of benzene metabolism reveal that, as with many other chemical carcinogens, the expression of benzene toxicity requires that it be metabolized to an active metabolite(s) (53,116,191). Bone marrow cells contain the enzymes necessary for converting benzene to its active metabolite(s). Additional evidence suggests that DNA is a likely target, as the covalent binding of benzene and its metabolites to DNA has been demonstrated (185,191). For further discussion of the mechanisms involved in chemical carcinogenesis, and benzene leukemogenesis in particular, the reader is referred to Chapter 26 and other reviews (53,116,205).

CLINICAL ASPECTS OF EXPOSURE TO ENVIRONMENTAL CHEMICALS AND PHYSICAL AGENTS ON THE HEMATOPOIETIC SYSTEM

Toxic exposure has been incriminated in the etiology of such hematological disorders as anemia, aplastic anemia, acute and chronic myelogenous leukemia, acute lymphocytic leukemia, and cyanotic states (Table 21-1). These responses are nonspecific. Only in the case of hypoxia from carboxyhemoglobinemia does the hematological response reflect exposure to a specific agent. The basis for linking a hematological disorder to toxic exposure therefore depends primarily on the medical history. In light of the variety of hematological disorders that may arise from toxic exposure, a thorough exposure history must be obtained in almost every patient with a hematological disturbance.

The identification of toxic exposure in the workplace and general environment has classically been the role of the alert clinician. When confronted with a patient with a hematological disorder, the physician must investigate the patient's present and past occupational exposures. Inquiry must be made into exposures within and surrounding the home. The jobs of family members may also be important, as contaminants in the workplace may be brought into the home (119). In most instances patients do not provide exposure information spontaneously. Physicians must therefore ask the patient directly about exposure to fumes, dusts, gases, chemicals, radiation, etc. and have sufficient background knowledge to inquire about specific agents that have been incriminated in the etiology of hematological disorders (Table 21-1).

Physicians are obligated to be aware of pollutant problems found in their community and of the associated health risks. For example, the risk of methemoglobinemia in infants is increased in farming communities where drinking water may be contaminated with nitrates from chemical fertilizers, manure, and septic tanks (114). Pesticide contamination of drinking water from contaminated wells is also a health hazard. The risk of lead poisoning is increased for poor children living in dilapidated pre-World War II inner-city housing (129). Pollutant exposure linked to hematological disorders may be increased in communities surrounding a smelter (123).

Since the manifestations of hematological disease caused by toxic exposure cannot be differentiated from those caused by drugs, internal derangements of the body, or unknown causes, standard clinical tools are used to assess the presence and the type of hematological dysfunction.

The medical history reveals the presence of a hematological disorder in a number of ways. Anemia may be uncovered by direct questions related to a previous diagnosis of anemia or "low blood." A history of excessive acute and/or chronic blood loss is obviously important, as are symptoms of weakness, fatigue, angina, and exertional dyspnea. A history of jaundice and pigmented urine may indicate a hemolytic process, whereas a history of easy bruising and cutaneous and mucosal petechiae may signal a problem with hemostasis. Excessive bacterial, fungal, or viral infections may herald the presence of neutropenic or lymphopenic disorders. The above findings are manifestations of an underlying disease process, which in turn must be considered in terms of environmental and occupational exposure to such agents as heavy metals, solvents, pesticides, nitrites, nitrates, carbon monoxide, and ionizing radiation (Table 21-1).

The physical examination may confirm the presence of a hematological disorder by revealing pallor of the skin and mucous membrane secondary to anemia. The presence of cyanosis alerts the clinician to a possible defect in oxygen transport. Lymphadenopathy, localized or generalized, raises the possibility of a disorder affecting lymphoid tissue and alerts the clinician to consider such neoplastic diseases as Hodgkin disease, non-Hodgkin lymphoma, and acute and chronic lymphocytic leukemia. Abnormal bleeding or the presence of petechiae may reflect an inadequate number of platelets and/or their impaired function.

Laboratory methods of evaluating the various hematological disorders can be found in standard hematological texts (230,232). As previously noted, the laboratory examination rarely reveals that a hematological disorder stems from toxic exposure and even more rarely from a specific exposure. Nonetheless, the laboratory at times can be helpful in the diagnosis of environmental and occupational hematological disease.

In some cases exposure to toxic agents linked to hematological disorders can be assessed through laboratory testing, i.e., lead, arsenic, aniline derivatives, or certain pesticides. In other instances, the products of toxic exposure, i.e., carboxyhemoglobin and methemoglobin can, can be measured in the circulating red blood cell (16,226). At times a hereditary susceptibility to hematological toxins, i.e., G-6-PD, can be identified.

The primary treatment of occupational and environmental hematological disorders depends on removing the patient from the source of exposure and/or removing the exposure itself. Detailed descriptions of additional modes of therapy for hematological disorders are found in standard hematological texts and current publications (230,232).

SUMMARY

The hematopoietic system, which includes the formed elements of the blood as well as the bone marrow, spleen, lymph nodes, and reticuloendo- thelial system, has a vast capacity for cellular renewal. The relative accessibility of the blood and bone marrow for examination may provide early evidence of toxic exposure. It is well established that a wide range of hematological disorders may follow exposure to such agents as benzene, lead, carbon monoxide, nitrates, and ionizing radiation. A variety of other chemicals have also been linked, with varying degrees of certainty, to hematological toxicity. In light of this information and the fact that many hematological disorders develop without apparent etiology, it is essential that environmental exposure(s) be considered in all such disorders.

REFERENCES

1. Adamson RH, Seiber SM: Chemically induced leukemia in humans. Environ Health Perspect 39:93, 1981.
2. Agu AU, Christensen BL, Buffler PA: Geographic patterns of multiple myeloma: Racial and industrial correlates, state of Texas, 1969–71. J Natl Cancer Inst 65:735, 1980.
3. Aksoy M: Malignancies due to occupational exposure to benzene. Haematologica 65:370, 1980.
4. Aksoy M: Different types of malignancies due to occupational exposure to benzene: A review of recent observations in Turkey. Environ Res 23:181, 1980.
5. Aksoy M, Erdem S: Follow-up study on the mortality and the development of leukemia in 44 pancytopenic patients with chronic exposure to benzene. Blood 52:285, 1978.
6. Aksoy M, Erdem S, DinCol G: Leukemia in shoeworkers exposed chronically to benzene. Blood 44:837, 1974.
7. Albahary C, Dubrisay J, Guerin J: Pancytopenie rebelle au lindane (isomere α de l'hexachlorocyclohexane). Arch Mal Prof 18:687, 1957.
8. Alderson M: The epidemiology of leukemia. In: Advances in Cancer Research, p 2, Klein G, Weinhouse S (eds.), Academic Press, Orlando, 1980.
9. Amital Y, Graef JW, Brown MJ, et al: Hazards of "deleading" homes of children with lead poisoning. Am J Dis Child 141:8, 1987.
10. Amoruso MA, Ryer J, Easton D, et al: Estimating of risk of glucose 6-phosphate dehydrogenase-deficient red cells to ozone and nitrogen dioxide. J Occup Med 28:473, 1986.
11. Angle CR, McIntire MS: Children, the barometer of environmental lead. In: Pediatrics, p 3, Barness LA (ed.), Year Book Medical Publishers, Chicago, 1982.
12. Aoyama K: Effects of benzene inhalation on lymphocyte subpopulations and immune response in mice. Toxicol Appl Pharmacol 85:92, 1986.
13. Axelson O: Pesticides and cancer risks in agriculture. Med Oncol Tumor Pharmacother 4:207, 1987.
14. Bader JL: Epidemiology of leukemia and related diseases—Summary. In: Advances in Comparative Leukemia Research, p 439, Yohn DS, Lapin A, Blakeslee JR (eds.), Elsevier/North-Holland, Amsterdam, 1979.
15. Barton CJ, Roman E, Ryder HM, et al: Childhood leukaemia in west Berkshire. Lancet 2:1248, 1985.

16. Baselt RC, Cravey RH: Disposition of Toxic Drugs and Chemicals in Man, 3rd Ed., Year Book Medical Publishers, Chicago, 1989.

17. Beebe GW, Kato H, Land CE: Studies of the mortality of A-bomb survivors: Mortality and radiation dose 1950–74. Radiat Res 75:138, 1978.

18. Bekesi JG, Roboz JP, Fischbein A, et al: Immunotoxicology: Environmental contamination by polybrominated biphenyls and immune dysfunction among residents of the State of Michigan. Cancer Detect Prev 1 (Suppl):29, 1987.

19. Beral V: Cancer near nuclear installations. Lancet 1: 556, 1987.

20. Beutler E: Hemolytic Anemia in Disorders of Red Cell Metabolism, Plenum Press, New York, 1978.

21. Beutler E: Chemical toxicity of the erythrocyte. In: Toxicology of the Blood and Bone Marrow, p 39, Iron RD (ed.), Raven Press, New York, 1985.

22. Beutler E, Baranki PV, Geagler J, et al: Hemolytic anemia due to pyrimidine-5'-nucleotidase deficiency: Report of eight cases in six families. Blood 56: 251, 1980.

23. Bigliani EC: Leukemia associated with benzene exposure. Ann NY Acad Sci 271:143, 1976.

24. Blair A, Thomas TL: Leukemia among Nebraska farmers: A death certificate study. Am J Epidemiol 110:264, 1979.

25. Blair A, White DW: Death certificate study of leukemia among farmers from Wisconsin. J Natl Cancer Inst 66:1027, 1981.

26. Blair A, Malker H, Cantor KP, et al: Cancer among farmers: A review. Scand J Work Environ Health 11: 397, 1985.

27. Boice JD, Fraumeni JF Jr: Radiation Carcinogenesis: Epidemiology and Biological Significance, Raven Press, New York, 1984.

28. Böttiger LE: Epidemiology and aetiology of aplastic anemia. Hamatol Bluttransfus 24:27, 1979.

29. Böttiger LE, Böttiger B: Incidence and cause of aplastic anemia, hemolytic anemia, agranulocytosis and thrombocytopenia. Acta Med Scand 210:475, 1981.

30. Brandt L: Environmental factors and leukaemia. Med Oncol Tumor Pharmacother 2:7, 1985.

31. Brill AB, Tomonaga M, Heyssel RM: Leukemia in man following exposure to ionizing radiation. A summary of the findings in Hiroshima and Nagasaki, and comparison with other human experience. Ann Intern Med 56:590, 1962.

32. Browning E: Toxicity and Metabolism of Industrial Solvents. Elsevier, Amsterdam, 1965.

33. Burmeister LF: Cancer mortality in Iowa farmers, 1971–1978. J Natl Cancer Inst 66:461, 1981.

34. Burmeister LF, Everett GD, VanLier SF, et al: Selected cancer mortality and farm practices in Iowa. Am J Epidemiol 118:72, 1983.

35. Byers VS, Levin AS, Ozonoff DM, et al: Association between clinical symptoms and lymphocyte abnormalities in a population with chronic domestic exposure to industrial solvent-contaminated domestic water supply and a high incidence of leukaemia. Cancer Immunol Immunother 27:77, 1988.

36. Calle E, Savitz DA: Leukaemia in occupational groups with presumed exposure to electrical and magnetic fields. N Engl J Med 313:1476, 1985.

37. Camitta BM, Storb R, Thomas ED: Aplastic anemia pathogenesis, diagnosis, treatment and prognosis. N Engl J Med 306:645, 1982.

38. Campbell DM, Davidson RJL: Toxic hemolytic anemia in pregnancy due to a pica for paradichlorobenzene. Br J Obstet Gynaecol 77:657, 1970.

39. Cantor KP: Farming and mortality from non-Hodgkin's lymphoma: A case–control study. Int J Cancer 29:239, 1982.

40. Cantor KP, Blair A: Farming and mortality from multiple myeloma: A case–control study with the use of death certificates. J Natl Cancer Inst 72:251, 1984.

41. Centers for Disease Control: Preventing Lead Poisoning in Young Children, US Department of Health and Human Services, Atlanta, 1991.

42. Chisolm JJ Jr: Lead poisoning. In: Pediatrics, 18th ed., p 732, Rudolph AM (ed.), Hoffman JIE (co-ed.), Axelrod S (assist ed.), Appleton & Lange, Norwalk, Connecticut, 1987.

43. Clapp RW, Cobb S, Chan CK, et al: Leukemia near Massachusetts nuclear power plant. Lancet 2:1324, 1987.

44. Committee on the Biological Effects of Ionizing Radiation, National Research Council: Health Effects of Exposure to Low Levels of Ionizing Radiation, BIER V, National Academy Press, Washington, 1990.

45. Conference on Target Organ Toxicity: Blood. Environ Health Perspect 39:1–105, 1981.

46. Cook RR: Dioxin, chloracne and soft-tissue sarcoma. Lancet 1:618, 1981.

47. Cook-Mozaffari P: Cancer near nuclear installations. Lancet 1:855, 1987.

48. Cook-Mozaffari P, Ashwood FL, Vincent T, et al: Cancer Incidence and Mortality in the Vicinity of Nuclear Installations. England and Wales, 1950–1980. Studies on Medical and Population Subjects, No. 51, Her Majesty's Stationery Office, London, 1987.

49. Council on Scientific Affairs: Cancer risk of pesticides in agricultural workers. JAMA 260:959, 1988.

50. Court Brown WM, Doll R: Mortality from cancer and other causes after radiotherapy for ankylosing spondylitis. Br Med J 2:1327, 1965.

51. Cronkite EP: Radiation-induced aplastic anemia. Semin Hematol 4:273, 1967.

52. Cronkite EP: Regulation and structure of hemopoiesis: Its application in toxicology. In: Toxicology of the Blood and Bone Marrow, p 17, Irons RD (ed.), Raven Press, New York, 1985.

53. Cronkite EP: Chemical leukemogenesis: Benzene as a model. Semin Hematol 24:2, 1987.

54. Cronkite EP, Inoue T, Carsten AL, et al: Effects of benzene inhalation on murine pluripotent stem cells. J Toxicol Environ Health 9:411, 1982.

55. Cuzick J: Radiation-induced myelomatosis. N Engl J Med 304:204, 1981.

56. Darby SC, Doll R, Gill SK, et al: Long term mortality after a single treatment course with X-rays in patients treated for ankylosing spondylitis. Br J Cancer 55: 179, 1987.

57. Dawson JP, Thayer WW, Desforges JF: Acute hemolytic anemia in the newborn infant due to naphthalene poisoning. Report of two cases with investigation into the mechanism of the disease. Blood 13:1113, 1958.

58. Delore P, Borgomano C: Leucémie aiguë au cours de l'intoxication benzénique: sur l'origine toxique de certaines leucémies aiguës et leurs relations avec les anémies graves. J Med Lyon 9:227, 1928.

59. Donati RM, Gantner GE: Hematological aspects of radiation exposure. In: Blood Disorders Due to Drugs and Other Agents, p 241, Girdwood RH (ed.), Excerpta Medica, Amsterdam, 1973.

60. Duell PB, Morton WE: Henoch–Schonlein purpura following thiram exposure. Arch Intern Med 147:778, 1987.

61. Enterline PE, Marsh GM: Mortality studies of smelter workers. Am J Ind Med 1:251, 1980.

62. Epstein SS, Ozonoff D: Leukemias and blood dyscrasias following exposure to chlordane and heptachlor. Teratogen Carcinogen Mutagen 7:527, 1987.

63. Eriksson M, Hardell L, Berg NO, et al: Soft-tissue sarcoma and exposure to chemical substances: A case-referent study. Br J Ind Med 38:27, 1981.

64. Fabia J, Thuy TO: Occupation of the father at time of birth of children dying of malignant disease. Br J Prev Soc Med 28:98, 1974.

65. Forman D, Cook-Mozaffari P, Darby S, et al: Cancer near nuclear installations. Nature 329:499, 1987.

66. Forni A: Chromosomal aberrations in monitoring exposure to mutagens–carcinogens. In: Monitoring Human Exposure to Carcinogenic and Mutagenic Agents, p 325, Berlin A, Draper M, Hemminki K, et al. (eds.), IARC Scientific Publications No. 59, International Agency for Research on Cancer, Lyon, 1984.

67. Friberg L, Martensson J: Case of panmyelophthisis after exposure to chlorophenothane and benzene hexachloride. AMA Arch Ind Hyg 8:166, 1953.

68. Fulton JP, Cobbs C, Preble L, et al: Electrical wiring configurations and childhood leukemia in Rhode Island. Am J Epidemiol 113:292, 1980.

69. Furth J, Lorenz E: Carcinogenesis by ionizing radiation. In: Radiation Biology, Vol 1, p 1145, Hollaender A (ed.), McGraw–Hill, New York, 1954.

70. Gardner MJ, Hall AJ, Downes S, et al: Follow up study of children born to mothers resident in Seascale, West Cumbria (birth cohort). Br Med J 295:822, 1987.

71. Gardner MJ, Hall AJ, Downes S, et al: Follow up study of children born elsewhere but attending schools in Seascale, West Cumbria (school cohort). Br Med J 295:819, 1987.

72. Gewin HM: Benzene hydrochloride and aplastic anemia. JAMA 296:1624, 1959.

73. Gibson GG, Hubbard R, Parke DV (eds.): Immunotoxicology, Academic Press, Orlando, 1983.

74. Girdwood RH (ed.): Blood Disorders Due to Drugs and Other Agents, Excerpta Medica, Amsterdam, 1974.

75. Goldman M: Chernobyl: A radiobiological perspective. Science 238:622, 1987.

76. Goldman M, Chairman: Health and Environmental Consequences of the Chernobyl Nuclear Power Plant Accident (Report DOE/ER-0332), Department of Energy, Washington, 1987.

77. Goldstein BD: Hematotoxicity in humans. In: Benzene Toxicity: A Critical Evaluation. J Toxicol Environ Health 2 (Suppl):69, 1977.

78. Goldstein BD: Risk assessment and risk management of benzene by the Environmental Protection Agency. Banbury Rep 19:293, 1985.

79. Goldstein BD, Snyder CA: Benzene leukemogenesis. In: Genotoxic Effects of Airborne Agents, p 277, Tice RR, Costa DL, Schaich KM (eds.), Plenum Press, New York, 1982.

80. Greene MH: Non-Hodgkin's lymphoma and mycosis fungoides. In: Cancer Epidemiology and Prevention, p 754, Schottenfeld D, Fraumeni JF (eds.), WB Saunders, Philadelphia, 1982.

81. Grufferman S: Hodgkin's disease. In: Cancer Epidemiology and Prevention, p 739, Schottenfeld D, Fraumeni JF Jr (eds.), WB Saunders, Philadelphia, 1982.

82. Hakulinen T, Salomen T, Teppo L: Cancer in the offspring of fathers in hydrocarbon related occupations. Br J Prev Soc Med 30:138, 1976.

83. Halberg GR: Agricultural chemicals in ground water: Extent and implications. Am J Alt Agric 2:3, 1987.

84. Halberg GR: The impact of agricultural chemicals on ground water quality. Geo-J 15:283, 1987.

85. Hallowell M: Acute hemolytic anemia following the ingestion of paradichlorobenzene. Arch Dis Child 34:74, 1959.

86. Hamilton HE, Morgan DP, Simmons A: A pesticide (dieldrin)-induced immunohemolytic anemia. Environ Res 17:155, 1978.

87. Hardell L, Eriksson M: The association between soft-tissue sarcomas and exposure to phenoxyacetic acids: A new case-referent study. Cancer 62:652, 1988.

88. Hardell L, Sandstrom A: Case–control study: Soft-tissue sarcomas and exposure to phenoxy-acetic acids or chlorophenols. Br J Cancer 39:711, 1979.

89. Hardell L, Eriksson M, Lenner P, et al: Malignant lymphoma and exposure to chemicals, especially organic solvents, chlorophenols and phenoxyacids or chlorophenols. Br J Cancer 43:169, 1981.

90. Harden RA, Baetjer AM: Aplastic anemia following exposure to paradichlorobenzene and naphthalene. J Occup Med 20:820, 1978.

91. Harvey EB, Boice JD Jr, Honeyman M, et al: Prenatal x-ray exposure and childhood cancer in twins. N Engl J Med 312:541, 1985.

92. Hassan AB, Seligmann H, Bassan HM: Intravascular haemolysis induced by pentachlorophenol. Br Med J 291:22, 1985.

93. Hatch MC, Stein ZA: The role of epidemiology in assessing chemical-induced disease. In: Mechanisms of Cell Injury: Implications for Human Health, p 303, Fowler BA (ed.), John Wiley & Sons, New York, 1987.

94. Heasman MA, Kemp IW, Macharen AM, et al: Incidence of leukaemia in young people in west of Scotland. Lancet 1:118, 1984.

95. Heasman MA, Kemp IW, Urquhart JD, et al: Childhood leukaemia in Northern Scotland. Lancet 1:266, 1986.

96. Heath CM Jr: Hereditary factors in leukemia and lymphomas. In: Cancer Genetics, p 233, Lynch HT (ed.), Charles C Thomas, Springfield, IL, 1976.

97. Heath CM Jr: The leukemias. In: Cancer Epidemiology and Prevention, p 728, Schottenfeld D, Fraumeni JF Jr. (eds.), WB Saunders, Philadelphia, 1982.

98. Hemminki K, Saloniemi I, Salonen T, et al: Child-

hood cancer and parental occupation in Finland. J Epidemiol Commun Health 35:11, 1981.

99. Hibino S: Aplastic anemia. Rinsho Ketsueki 16:299, 1975.

100. Hibino S, Takaku F, Shahidi N (eds.): Aplastic Anemia, University Park Press, Baltimore, 1978.

101. Hoar SK, Blair A, Holmes FF, et al: Agricultural herbicide use and risk of lymphoma and soft-tissue sarcoma. JAMA 256:1141, 1986.

102. Hole DJ, Gillis CR: Childhood leukemia in the west of Scotland. Lancet 2:525, 1986.

103. IARC: IARC Monographs on the Evaluation of Carcinogenic Risk to Humans, Supplement 7, International Agency for Research on Cancer, Lyon, 1987.

104. Infante PF, Rinsky RA, Wagoner JK, et al: Leukaemia in benzene workers. Lancet 2:76, 1977.

105. Infante PF, Epstein SS, Newton WA: Blood dyscrasias and childhood tumors and exposure to chlordane and heptachlor. Scand J Work Environ Health 4:137, 1978.

106. Irons RD (ed.): Toxicology of the Blood and Bone Marrow, Raven Press, New York, 1985.

107. Irons RD, Neptun DA: Effects of the principal hydroxy-metabolites of benzene on microtubule polymerization. Arch Toxicol 45:297, 1980.

108. Irons RD, Stillman WS: Flow cytofluorometric analysis of blood and bone marrow. In: Toxicology of the Blood and Bone Marrow, p 101, Irons RD (ed.), Raven Press, New York, 1985.

109. Irons RD, Heck HD, Moore RJ, et al: Effects of short-term benzene administration on bone marrow cell cycle kinetics in the rat. Toxicol Appl Pharmacol 51:339, 1979.

110. Jedlicka VL, Hermanska Z, Smida I, et al: Paramyeloblastic leukaemia appearing simultaneously in two blood cousins after simultaneous contact with gamma-xane (hexachlorocyclohexane). Acta Medica Scand 161:447, 1958.

111. Jenkyn LR, Budd RC, Fein SH, et al: Insecticide/herbicide exposure, aplastic anemia and pseudotumor cerebri. Lancet 2:368, 1979.

112. Jennings GH, Gower ND: Thrombocytopenic purpura in toluene di-isocyanate workers. Lancet 1:406, 1963.

113. Johnson CJ: Cancer incidence in an area of radioactive fallout downwind from the Nevada test site. JAMA 251:230, 1984.

114. Johnson CJ, Bonrud PA, Dosch TL, et al: Fatal outcome of methemoglobinemia in an infant. JAMA 257:2796, 1987.

115. Kaiser L, Schwartz KA: Aluminum-induced anemia. Am J Kidney Dis 6:348, 1985.

116. Kalf GF, Post GB, Snyder R: Solvent toxicology: Recent advances in the toxicology of benzene, the glycol ethers, and carbon tetrachloride. Annu Rev Pharmacol Toxicol 27:399, 1987.

117. Karpinski RE: Purpura following exposure to DDT. J Pediatr 37:373, 1950.

118. Kjeldsberg CR, Ward HP: Leukemia in arsenic poisoning. Ann Intern Med 77:935, 1972.

119. Knishkowy B, Baker EL: Transmission of occupational disease to family contacts. Am J Ind Med 9:543, 1986.

120. Kulis JC: Chemically induced, selective thrombocytopenic purpura. Arch Intern Med 116:559, 1965.

121. Lagakos SW, Wessen BJ, Zelen M: An analysis of contaminated well water and health effects in Woburn, Massachusetts. J Am Statist Assoc 81:583, 1986.

122. Land CE, McKay FW, Machado SG: Childhood leukemia and fallout from the Nevada nuclear tests. Science 223:139, 1984.

123. Landrigan PJ, Baker EL, Feldman RG, et al: Increased lead absorption with anemia and slowed nerve conduction in children near a lead smelter. J Pediatr 89:904, 1976.

124. Laskin S, Goldstein BD (eds.): Benzene toxicity, a critical evaluation. J Toxicol Environ Health 2 (Suppl):1, 1977.

125. Latriano L, Goldstein BD, Witz G: Formation of muconaldehyde, an open-ring metabolite of benzene in mouse liver microsomes: An additional pathway for toxic metabolites. Proc Natl Acad Sci USA 83:8356, 1986.

126. Leventhal BG, Khan AB: Hematopoietic system. In: Environmental Pathology, p 344, Mottet NK (ed.), Oxford University Press, Oxford, 1985.

127. Lilienfeld AM (ed.): Review in Cancer Epidemiology, Vol 1, Elsevier/North-Holland, Amsterdam, 1980.

128. Linet MS: The Leukemias: Epidemiologic Aspects, Oxford University Press, New York, 1985.

129. Lin-Fu JS: Vulnerability of children to lead exposure and toxicity. N Engl J Med 289:1229, 1973.

130. Lin-Fu JS: Children and lead: New finding and concerns. N Engl J Med 307:615, 1982.

131. Linos A, Kyle RA, Elveback LR, et al: Leukemia in Olmsted County, Minnesota, 1965–1974. Mayo Clin Proc 53:714, 1978.

132. Loge JP: Aplastic anemia following exposure to benzene hexachloride (lindane). JAMA 193:110, 1965.

133. Lorand IC, Souza CA, Costa FF: Haematological toxicity associated with agricultural chemicals in Brazil. Lancet 1:404, 1984.

134. Lotti M: Production and use of pesticides. In: Toxicology of Pesticides: Experimental, Clinical and Regulatory Perspectives, p 15, Costa LG, Galli CL, Murphy SD (eds.), Springer-Verlag, Berlin, 1987.

135. Lowengart RA, Peters JM, Cicioni C, et al: Childhood leukemia and parents' occupational and home exposures. J Natl Cancer Inst 79:39, 1987.

136. Lukens JN: The legacy of well-water methemoglobinemia. JAMA 257:2793, 1987.

137. Lynge E: A follow-up study of cancer incidence among workers in manufacture of phenoxy herbicides in Denmark. Br J Cancer 52:259, 1985.

138. Lyon JL, Klauber MR, Gardnes JW, et al: Childhood leukemias associated with fallout from nuclear testing. N Engl J Med 300:397, 1979.

139. Mabuchi K, Lilienfeld AM, Snell LM: Cancer and occupational exposure to arsenic: A study of pesticide workers. Prev Med 9:51, 1980.

140. Machado SG, Land CE, MacKay FW: Cancer mortality and radioactive fallout in southwestern Utah. Am J Epidemiol 125:44, 1987.

141. MacMahon B: Prenatal exposure and childhood cancer. J Natl Cancer Inst 28:1173, 1962.

142. MacMahon B: Some recent issues in low-exposure radiation epidemiology. Environ Health Perspect 81:131, 1989.

143. MacMahon B, Prentice RL, Rogan WJ, et al: An

analysis of contaminated well water and health effects in Woburn, Massachusetts. Comments. J Am Statist Assoc 81:597, 1986.

144. Magrath I, O'Conor GT, Ramot B (eds.): Pathogenesis of Leukemias and Lymphomas: Environmental influences, Raven Press, New York, 1984.

145. Mallory TB, Gall EA, Brickley WJ: Chronic exposure to benzene (benzol). III. The pathologic results. J Ind Hyg Toxicol 21:355, 1939.

146. Maltoni C, Scarnato C: First experimental demonstration of the carcinogenic effects of benzene: Long-term bioassays on Sprague–Dawley rats by oral administration. Med Lav 70:352, 1979.

147. Markovitz A, Crosby WH: Chemical carcinogenesis: A soil fumigant, 1,3-dichloropropene, as possible cause of hematologic malignancies. Arch Intern Med 144:1409, 1984.

148. Marks GS: Exposure to toxic agents: The heme biosynthetic pathway and hemoproteins as indicators. CRC Crit Rev Toxicol 15:151, 1985.

149. Mastromatteo E: Hematological disorders following exposure to insecticides. Can Med Assoc J 90:1166, 1964.

150. McMillan R: Environmental thrombocytopenic purpura, JAMA 242:2434, 1979.

151. Mendeloff AI, Smith DE (ed.): Exposure to insecticides, bone marrow failure, gastrointestinal bleeding and uncontrollable infections. Clinico-pathologic conference. Am J Med 19:274, 1955.

152. Milham S: Mortality from leukemia in workers exposed to electrical and magnetic fields. N Engl J Med 307:249, 1982.

153. Miller RW: Delayed effects occurring within the first decade after exposure of young individuals to the Hiroshima atomic bomb. Pediatrics 18:1, 1956.

154. Miller RW: Pollutants and children: Lessons from case histories. In: Guidelines for Studies of Human Populations Exposed to Mutagenic and Reproductive Hazards, p 155, Bloom AD (ed.), March of Dimes Birth Defects Foundation, White Plains, New York, 1981.

155. Miller RW: Some persons at high risk of lymphoproliferative diseases. In: Pathogenesis of Leukemias and Lymphomas: Environmental Influences, p 201, Magrath IT, O'Conor GT, Ramot B (eds.), Raven Press, New York, 1984.

156. Miller RW, Beebe GW: Leukemia, lymphoma, and multiple myeloma. In: Radiation Carcinogenesis, p 245, Upton AC, Albert RE, Burns FJ, et al. (eds.), Elsevier, Amsterdam, 1986.

157. Miller RW, Boice JD Jr: Radiogenic cancer after prenatal or childhood exposure. In: Radiation Carcinogenesis, p 379, Upton AC, Albert RE, Burns FJ, et al. (eds.), Elsevier, Amsterdam, 1986.

158. Modan B, Lilienfeld AM: Polycythemia vera and leukemia—the role of radiation treatment. A study of 1222 patients. Medicine 44:305, 1965.

159. Mole RH: The radiobiological significance of the studies with 224-Ra and thorotrast. Health Phys 35:167, 1978.

160. Mole RH: Irradiation of the embryo and fetus. Br J Radiol 60:17, 1987.

161. Monson RR, MacMahon B: Prenatal x-ray exposure and cancer in children. In: Radiation Carcinogenesis:

Epidemiology and Biological Significance, p 97, Boice JD, Fraumeni JF Jr (eds.), Raven Press, New York, 1984.

162. Morgan DP, Stockdale EM, Roberts RJ, et al: Anemia associated with exposure to lindane. Arch Environ Health 35:307, 1980.

163. Morgan KZ, Turner JE: Principles of Radiation Protection, John Wiley & Sons, New York, 1967.

164. Muirhead EE, Groves M, Guy R, et al: Acquired hemolytic anemia, exposure to insecticides and positive Coombs test dependent on insecticide preparations. Vox Sang 4:277, 1959.

165. Nair I, Morgan MG, Florig HK: Biological Effects of Power Frequency Electric and Magnetic Fields, US Congress, Office of Technology Assessment, Washington, 1989.

166. Nalbandian RM, Pearce JF: Allergic purpura induced by exposure to p-dichlorobenzene. JAMA 194:238, 1965.

167. National Council on Radiation Protection and Measurements: Ionizing Radiation Exposure of the Population of the United States, NCRP Report No. 93, NCRP, Washington, 1987.

168. National Research Council: Regulating Pesticides in Food. The Delaney Paradox, National Academy Press, Washington, 1987.

169. Nuclear Energy Agency: The Radiological Impact of the Chernobyl Accident in OECD Countries, Organisation for Economic Co-operation and Development, Paris, 1987.

170. Olsson H, Brandt L: Risk of non-Hodgkin's lymphoma among men occupationally exposed to organic solvents. Scand J Work Environ Health 14:246, 1988.

171. Organisation for Economic Co-operation and Development: Water Pollution by Fertilizers and Pesticides, OECD, Paris, 1986.

172. Orringer EP, Mattern WD: Formaldehyde-induced hemolysis during chronic hemodialysis. N Engl J Med 294:1416, 1976.

173. Palva HLA, Kolvisto O, Palva IP: Aplastic anemia after exposure to a weed killer, 2-methyl-4-chlorphenoxyacetic acid. Acta Haematol 53:105, 1975.

174. Pearce NE, Smith AH, Fisher DO: Malignant lymphoma and multiple myeloma linked with agricultural occupation in a New Zealand Cancer registry-based study. Am J Epidemiol 121:225, 1985.

175. Pozzi C, Marai P, Ponti R, et al: Toxicity in man due to stain removers containing 1,2-dichloropropane. Br J Ind Med 42:770, 1985.

176. Rankin AM: A review of 20 cases of aplastic anemia. Med J Aust 2:95, 1961.

177. Reeves JD, Driggers DA, Kiley VA: Household insecticide associated aplastic anaemia and acute leukaemia in children. Lancet 2:300, 1981.

178. Rinsky RA, Young RJ, Smith AB: Leukemia in benzene workers. Am J Ind Med 2:217, 1981.

179. Rinsky RA, Smith AB, Hornung R, et al: Benzene and leukemia. N Engl J Med 316:1044, 1987.

180. Roberts HJ: Aplastic anemia due to pentachlorophenol and tetrachlorophenol. South Med J 56:632, 1963.

181. Roberts HJ: Aplastic anemia due to pentachlorophenol. N Engl J Med 305:1650, 1981.

182. Roberts HJ: Aplastic anemia and red cell aplasia due to pentachlorophenol. South Med J 76:45, 1983.

183. Roman E, Beral V, Carpenter L, et al: Childhood leukaemia in the West Berkshire and Basingstoke and North Hampshire District Health Authorities in relation to nuclear establishments in the vicinity. Br Med J 294:597, 1987.

184. Roodman GD, Reese EP Jr, Cardamone JM: Aplastic anemia associated with rubber cement used by a marathon runner. Arch Intern Med 140:703, 1980.

185. Rushmore T, Snyder R, Kalf G: Covalent binding of benzene and its metabolites to DNA in rabbit bone marrow mitochondria in vitro. Chem Biol Interact 49:133, 1984.

186. Saftias AF, Blair A, Cantor K, et al: Cancer and other causes of death among Wisconsin farmers. Am J Ind Med 11:119, 1987.

187. Sanchez-Medal L, Gastanedo JP, Garcia-Rojas F: Insecticides and aplastic anemia. N Engl J Med 269:1365, 1963.

188. Sanders BM, White GC, Draper GJ: Occupations of fathers of children dying of neoplasms. J Epidemiol Commun Health 35:245, 1981.

189. Savitz D, Calle E: Leukemia and occupational exposure to electromagnetic fields: Review of epidemiologic surveys. J Occup Med 29:47, 1987.

190. Savitz DA, Wachtel H, Barnes FA, et al: Case–control study of childhood cancer and exposure to 60-Hz magnetic fields. Am J Epidemiol 128:21, 1988.

191. Sawahata T, Rickert DE, Greenlee WF: Metabolism of benzene and its metabolites in bone marrow. In: Toxicology of the Blood and Bone Marrow, p 141, Irons RD (ed.), Raven Press, New York, 1985.

192. Schmid JR, Kiely JM, Pease GL, et al: Acquired pure red cell agenesis: Report of 16 cases and review of the literature. Acta Haematol 30:255, 1963.

193. Scott JL, Cartwright GE, Wintrobe MM: Acquired aplastic anemia: An analysis of thirty-nine cases and review of the pertinent literature. Medicine 38:119, 1959.

194. Sharp DS, Eskenazi B: Delayed health hazards of pesticide exposure. Annu Rev Public Health 7:441, 1986.

195. Shaw G, Lavey R, Jackson R, et al: Association of childhood leukemia with maternal age, birth order and paternal occupation. Am J Epidemiol 119:788, 1984.

196. Sheikh K: Exposure to electromagnetic fields and the risk of leukemia. Arch Environ Health 41:56, 1986.

197. Shindell S, Ulrich S, Glefer EE: Epidemiology and chlorinated hydrocarbon insecticides. In: Toxicology of Halogenated Hydrocarbons, p 50, Khan MAQ, Stanton RH (eds.), Pergamon Press, New York, 1981.

198. Shore RE: Electromagnetic radiations and cancer. Cancer 62:(Suppl):1747, 1988.

199. Smith RP: Toxic responses of the blood. In: Casarett and Doull's Toxicology: The Basic Science of Poisons, 3rd ed., p 223, Klaassen CD, Amdur MO, Doull J (eds.), Macmillan, New York, 1986.

200. Snyder R, Longacre SL, Witmer CM, et al: Biochemical toxicology of benzene. In: Review in Biochemical Toxicology, Vol 3, p 123, Hodgson E, Bend JR, Philpot RM (eds.), Elsevier/North-Holland, Amsterdam, 1981.

201. Stewart A, Webb J, Giles D, et al: Malignant disease in childhood and diagnostic irradiation in utero. Lancet 2:447, 1956.

202. Stewart RD: The effect of carbon monoxide on humans. Annu Rev Pharmacol 15:409, 1975.

203. Strassman SC, Kutz FW: Trends of organochlorine pesticide residues in human tissues. In: Toxicology of Halogenated Hydrocarbons, p 38, Khan MAQ, Stanton RH (eds.), Pergamon Press, New York, 1981.

204. Swanson M, Cook R: Drugs, Chemicals and Blood Dyscrasias, Drug Intelligence, Hamilton, Illinois, 1977.

205. Symposium on Benzene Metabolism, Toxicity and carcinogenesis: March 14–16, Research Triangle Park, NC. Environ Health Perspect 82:1–344, 1989.

206. Szklo M: Aplastic anemia. In: Review of Cancer Epidemiology, Vol 1, p 219, Lilienfeld AM (ed.), Elsevier/North-Holland, Amsterdam, 1980.

207. The International Agranulocytosis and Aplastic Anemia Study: Risks of agranulocytosis and aplastic anemia. A first report of their relation to drug use with special reference to analgesics. JAMA 256:1749, 1986.

208. Timonen TTT, Ilvonen M: Contact with hospital, drugs and chemicals as aetiological factors in leukaemia. Lancet 1:350, 1978.

209. Tolley HD, Marks S, Buchanan JA, et al: A further update of the analysis of mortality of workers in a nuclear facility. Radiat Res 95:41, 1983.

210. Tomenius L: 50-Hz electromagnetic environment and the incidence of tumors in Stockholm county. Bioelectromagnetics 7:191, 1986.

211. Tsongas TA: Occupational factors in the epidemiology of chemically induced lymphoid and hemopoietic cancers. In: Toxicology of the Blood and Bone Marrow, p 149, Irons RD (ed.), Raven Press, New York, 1985.

212. Ulrich H: The incidence of leukemia in radiologists. N Engl J Med 234:45, 1946.

213. United Nations Scientific Committee on the Effects of Atomic Radiation: Sources, Effects and Risk of Ionizing Radiation, United Nations, New York, 1988.

214. Upton AC, Albert RE, Burns RJ, et al: Radiation Carcinogenesis, Elsevier, Amsterdam, 1986.

215. US Department of Energy, Environment, Safety and Health, Office of Environmental Audit: Environmental Survey—Preliminary Summary Report of the Defense Production Facilities, DOE, Washington, 1988.

216. Urquhart J, Cutler J, Burke M: Leukaemia and lymphatic cancer in young people near nuclear installations. Lancet 1:384, 1986.

217. Van Steensel-Moll HA, Valkenburg HA, Van Zanen GE: Childhood leukemia and parental occupation. Am J Epidemiol 121:216, 1985.

218. Vianna NJ, Kovasznay B, Polan A, et al: Infant leukemia and parental exposure to motor vehicle exhaust fumes. J Occup Med 26:679, 1984.

219. Vigiliani EC, Saita G: Benzene and leukemia. N Engl J Med 271:872, 1964.

220. Vineis P, Terracini B, Ciccone G, et al: Phenoxy herbicides and soft-tissue sarcomas in female rice weeders: A population-based case-referent study. Scand J Work Environ Health 13:9, 1987.

221. Vodopick H: Cherchez la chienne. Erythropoietic hypoplasia after exposure to α benzene hexachloride. JAMA 234:850, 1975.

222. Wahlberg P, Nyman D: Turpentine and thrombocytopenic purpura. Lancet 2:215, 1969.

223. Wald PH, Becker CE: Toxic gases used in the micro-electronics industry. Occup Med 1:105, 1986.
224. Wang HH, Grufferman S: Aplastic anemia and occupational pesticide exposure: A case–control study. J Occup Med 23:364, 1981.
225. Wang HH, MacMahon B: Mortality of workers employed in the manufacture of chlordane and heptachlor. J Occup Med 21:745, 1979.
226. Wang RGM, Franklin CA, Honeycutt RC, et al. (eds.): Biological Monitoring for Pesticide Exposure. ACS Symposium Series 382, American Chemical Society, Washington, 1989.
227. Wertheimer N, Leeper E: Electrical wiring configuration and childhood cancer. Am J Epidemiol 109:273, 1979.
228. West I: Lindane and hematologic reactions. Arch Environ Health 15:97, 1967.
229. Williams DM, Lynch RE, Cartwright GE: Drug-induced aplastic anemia. Semin Hematol 10:195, 1973.
230. Williams WJ, Beutler E, Erslev AJ, et al: Hematology, 4th ed., McGraw-Hill, New York, 1990.
231. Wilson FD: Clonogenic stem and progenitor cell assays for the evaluation of chemically induced myelotoxicity. In: Toxicology of the Blood and Bone Marrow, p 65, Irons RD (ed.), Raven Press, New York, 1985.
232. Wintrobe MM, Lee GR, Boggs DR, et al: Clinical Hematology, Lea & Febiger, Philadelphia, 1981.
233. Woodliff HJ, Connor PM, Scopa J: Aplastic anemia associated with pesticides. Med J Aust 1:628, 1966.
234. World Health Organization: Magnetic Fields, Environmental Health Criteria 69, World Health Organization, Geneva, 1987.
235. Wright C-S, Doan CA, Haynie HC: Agranulocytosis occurring after exposure to D.D.T. pyrethrum aerosol. Am J Med 1:562, 1946.
236. Yoshimoto Y, Kato H, Schull WJ: Risk of cancer among children exposed in utero to A-bomb radiation, 1950–84. Lancet 2:665, 1988.
237. Zahm HS, Blair A, Holmes FF, et al: A case-referent study of soft-tissue sarcoma and Hodgkin's disease. Scand J Work Environ Health 14:224, 1988.

RECOMMENDED READINGS

Irons RD (ed.): Toxicology of the Blood and Bone Marrow, Raven Press, New York, 1985.
Scott JL, Cartwright GE, Wintrobe MM: Acquired aplastic anemia: An analysis of thirty-nine cases and a review of the pertinent literature. Medicine 38:119, 1959.
Sharp DS, Eskenazi B: Delayed health hazards of pesticide exposure. Annu Rev Public Health 7:441, 1986.
Symposium on Benzene Metabolism, Toxicity and Carcinogenesis: Environ Health Perspect 82:1–344, 1989.
Tsongas TA: Occupational factors in the epidemiology of chemically induced lymphoid and hemopoietic cancers. In: Toxicology of the Blood and Bone Marrow, p 149, Irons RD (ed.), Raven Press, New York, 1985.

22. DISORDERS OF THE THYROID

Eduardo Gaitan

INTRODUCTION

A large variety of naturally occurring and man-made compounds pose the danger of thyroid disease by interfering with thyroid function. These compounds can alter thyroid structure and function by acting directly on the gland or by affecting its regulatory mechanisms. The gland may increase in size to become a goiter. Thyroid hormone secretion may remain adequate or become insufficient, depending on dietary iodine intake or the presence of underlying thyroid disease.

No fewer than 5% of the world's population have goiters, which in many cases are associated with other disorders. This condition constitutes a major public health problem. Three hundred million individuals with goiter live in developing countries where iodine deficiency is prevalent, and despite iodine prophylaxis, 100 million individuals with goiter are found in industrialized nations.

Endemic goiter and iodine deficiency are commonly associated with cretinism, congenital hypothyroidism, and various degrees of impairment of growth and mental development (conditions grouped under the name of iodine deficiency disorders). In contrast, iodine-sufficient goiters are associated with

autoimmune thyroiditis, hypothyroidism, hyperthyroidism, and probably thyroid carcinoma (46).

Of the countless theories that have been proposed to explain the cause of endemic goiter, only a few are supported by experimental evidence: the presence of nutritional iodine deficiency, the presence of goitrogens in foodstuffs, and factors relating to the quality of the drinking water (44,117).

The importance of iodine deficiency in goitrogenesis and the prevention and treatment of endemic goiter by iodine supplementation are firmly established. However, epidemiologic and experimental evidence indicates that certain environmental pollutants may be responsible for many goiters. Several categories of naturally occurring and man-made antithyroid agents may enter the water, air, and food and thereby become important environmental goitrogenic factors in man and other animals. Their effects may be additive to those of iodine deficiency, making the manifestations of iodine deficiency disorders more severe (46).

Environmental chemicals that cause goiter—also known as environmental goitrogens—are the focus of this chapter. The study of environmental goitrogens requires the understanding, interest, and collaboration of multiple disciplines, some outside the confines of the biological sciences. The difficulty in complying with this requirement has fragmented our knowledge and prevented the effective investigation of many questions that surround this important and controversial issue. The public health and socioeconomic impact of environmental goitrogens is practically unknown.

Principles and Practice of Environmental Medicine, edited by Alyce Bezman Tarcher. Plenum Medical Book Company, New York, 1992.

ENVIRONMENTAL CHEMICALS AND PHYSICAL AGENTS ASSOCIATED WITH ADVERSE EFFECTS ON THE THYROID

Agents known to have goitrogenic and/or antithyroid effects on humans and other animal species are listed in Table 22-1.

Environmental antithyroid and goitrogenic compounds are naturally occurring or man made. They can be airborne or present in foodstuffs, in contaminated water supplies, in waste-water effluents, and as waste products of industrial processes (44,46).

Polyhydroxyphenols and Phenol Derivatives

Phenolics are the major organic pollutants in waste-water effluents from various types of coal-treatment processes (44,59,70,94). Resorcinol, substituted resorcinols, and other antithyroid phenolic pollutants are present in concentrations as high as 5 g/L in coal-derived effluents. Resorcinol and a substituted resorcinol, m-dihydroxyacetophenone, have been identified as contaminants in the water supply of endemic goiter districts in the coal-rich Appalachian area of eastern Kentucky and in western Colombia (41,42,44,66).

Resorcinol (1,3-dihydroxybenzene) is discussed here as a prototype of this group of compounds. Apart from their general chemical characteristics, these compounds share common sources, antithyroid properties, and pharmacokinetics. Because it is markedly different from the other compounds in this group, 2,4-dinitrophenol is discussed separately.

Resorcinol

Resorcinol (m-dihydroxybenzene) (Fig. 22-1) is a colorless crystalline substance freely soluble in water, alcohol, and other organic solvents (53,135). It is used industrially in the production of dyes, plasticizers, textiles, resins, pharmaceuticals, and adhesives for wood, plastics, and rubber products. In 1974, the production of resorcinol in the United States was 16 million kilograms. Typically, industrially produced resorcinol has a purity greater than 99.5%. The threshold limit value for occupational exposure to resorcinol was set in 1976 as 45 mg/m^3 (10 ppm) (110,135).

As early as the 1950s, the goitrogenic effect of resorcinol was demonstrated when patients applying resorcinol ointments for the treatment of varicose ulcers developed goiters (14,99). In the years that followed several investigators demonstrated, both in vitro and in vivo, the antithyroid effect of resorcinol and several other parent phenolic and phenolic–carboxylic compounds (3,21,30,31,73,106,

119,136). In 1964, Burges, Hurst, and Walkden from the Botanical Laboratories in Liverpool demonstrated that resorcinol and the phenolic and phenolic–carboxylic compounds that possess antithyroid activity are in fact degradation monomeric products of humic substances. This finding was subsequently confirmed by other investigators (11, 15,17,18,54,103,105,109). The chemical structures of these compounds are shown in Fig. 22-1.

Formerly, only geochemists and agronomists knew of the existence of humic substances. Now, water scientists, environmentalists, biologists, and chemists are coming to realize that these substances participate in and often control many reactions that occur in soils and water. Humic substances are currently considered the principal organic components of soil and waters.

Humic substances are high-molecular-weight complex polymeric organic compounds present in soils and water. They account for more than 90% of total organic matter in water. These substances are also important constituents of coal, shale, and other carbonaceous sedimentary rocks. At the heart of the process of humification is the production and polymerization of phenolic and carboxylic benzene rings. Up to 70% of flavonoid humic substances may be made up of these subunits (17,55,115). The vast distribution of the phenolic derivatives of humic substances provides sufficient reason to question and investigate their relationship to thyroid disease (21).

Resorcinol is readily absorbed from the gastrointestinal tract and excreted primarily in the urine (110). About half is excreted as the monoglucuronide, 15% as monosulfate, and 10% in free form (50). Pharmacokinetic data obtained from the rat following subcutaneous administration of [^{14}C]resorcinol show rapid plasma clearance. About 94% of radioactivity appears in the urine within 24 h. Most of the agent (about 80%) is excreted as a glucuronide conjugate. Only a small fraction (10%) appears as the free compound (82).

Resorcinol is irritating to skin and mucous membranes. The compound resembles phenol in its systemic actions. Ingestion may produce hypothermia, hypotension, decreased respiratory rate, cyanosis, metahemoglobinemia, hemoglobinuria, tremors, convulsions, and death. Central stimulation is more prominent than with phenol (53,110,135). Long-term oral or inhalation studies are required to assess the chronic effects of resorcinol exposure (110).

Coal-Conversion Processes Phenols are the major organic pollutants in aqueous effluents from coal-conversion processes. Coal-conversion waste waters contain, in addition to phenolics, thiocyanate and disulfides, which are also known to possess antithyroid and goitrogenic properties. Typical coal

TABLE 22-1. Environmental Agents Producing Goitrogenic and/or Antithyroid Effects[a]

Compounds	In vivo[b] Humans	In vivo[b] Animals	In vitro systems[b]
Sulfurated organics			
Thiocyanate (SCN⁻)	+	+	+
Isothiocyanates	NT	+	+
L-5-Vinyl-2-thiooxazolidone (goitrin)	+	+	+
Disulfides (R-S-S-R)	NT	+	0,+(?)[c]
Flavonoids (polyphenols)			
Glycosides	NT	+	+
Aglycones	NT	+	+
C-ring fission metabolites (i.e., phloroglucinol, phenolic acids)	NT	+	+
Polyhydroxyphenols and phenol derivatives			
Phenol	NT	NT	+
Catechol (1,2-dihydroxybenzene)	NT	NT	+
Resorcinol (1,3-dihydroxybenzene)	+	+	+
Hydroquinone (1,4-dihydroxybenzene)	NT	NT	+
m-Dihydroxyacetophenones	NT	NT	+
2-Methylresorcinol	NT	+	+
5-Methylresorcinol (orcinol)	NT	+	+
4-Methylcatechol	NT	NT	+
Pyrogallol (1,2,3-trithydroxybenzene)	NT	+	+
Phloroglucinol (1,3,5-trihydroxybenzene)	NT	+	+
4-Chlororesorcinol	NT	+	+
3-Chloro-4-hydroxybenzoic acid	NT	NT	+
2,4-Dinitrophenol	+	+	0
Pyridines			
3-Hydroxypyridine	NT	NT	+
Dihydroxypyridines	NT	+	+
Phthalate esters and metabolites			
Diisobutyl phthalate	NT	NT	0
Dioctyl phthalate	NT	NT	0
o-Phthalic acid	NT	NT	0
m-Phthalic acid	NT	NT	0
3,4-Dihydroxybenzoic acid (DHBA)	NT	NT	+
3,5-Dihydroxybenzoic acid	NT	NT	+
Polychlorinated (PCB) and polybrominated (PBB) biphenyls			
PCBs (Aroclor)	NT	+	NT
PBBs and PBB oxides	+	+	NT
Other organochlorines			
Dichlorodiphenyltrichloroethane (p,p'-DDT)	NT	+	NT
Dichlorodiphenyldichloroethane (p,p'-DDE) and dieldrin	NT	+	NT
2,3,7,8-Tetrachlorodibenzo-p-dioxin (TCDD)	NT	+	NT
Polycyclic aromatic hydrocarbons (PAH)			
Benzo[a]pyrene (BaP)	NT	+(?)	NT
3-Methylcolanthrene (MCA)	NT	+	NT
7,12-Dimethylbenzanthracene (DMBA)	NT	+	NT
Inorganics			
Excess iodine	+	+	+
Lithium	+	+	+

[a]From Gaitan (44).
[b]Symbols used: +, active; 0, inactive; NT, nontested.
[c]Inactive in thyroid peroxidase assay; active (?) in thyroid slices assay.

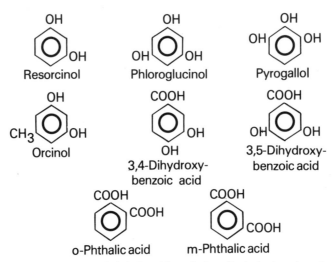

FIGURE 22-1. Chemical structures of phthalic acids and phenolic derivatives from humic substances.

gasification waste water, tons of which must be disposed of, has the following composition: phenolics, 2 g/L; thiocyanate, 1 g/L; S^{2-}, 0.2 g/L; cyanide, 0.1 g/l, and ammonia, 5 g/L (59,70). Resorcinol and other antithyroid phenolic pollutants (2-methyl- and 5-methyl resorcinol or orcinol) comprise as much as 5 g/L in the aqueous effluent from a bench-scale coal-liquefaction unit (94). In addition to the other toxic effects of phenols, their potential for a deleterious effect on the thyroid must be considered. This consideration reinforces the need for their removal if coal-conversion processes are to be environmentally acceptable.

Current methods for removing phenolics from industrial waste include solvent extraction, microbial degradation, absorption on activated carbon, and chemical oxidation (59,70,78). Although these methods may be effective, they suffer from such shortcomings as high cost, incompleteness of purification, formation of hazardous byproducts, and limited applicability to wide ranges of concentration (70,78).

The limited supply of natural gas and petroleum in the United States has focused increased attention on the development and expansion of processes for the conversion of coal to liquid and gaseous fuels (93,125). The expansion of coal-conversion technology points out the urgent need to develop cost-effective techniques for removing phenolics from coal-conversion waste waters. It also means that there must be quantitative assessment and monitoring procedures for the coal-conversion processes (87) as well as epidemiologic studies to investigate the relationship between thyroid disease and exposure to phenolic derivatives.

Chlorination Treatment of Waters The presence of halogenated organic compounds with known or potential harmful effects has awakened public health and environmental concerns (65). These compounds are produced by the chlorination of water supplies and are found in sewage and power plant cooling waters (64,65).

Compounds such as 4-chlororesorcinol and 3-chloro-4-hydroxybenzoic acid, present at microgram per liter concentrations (parts per billion) in treated domestic sewage and cooling waters, possess antithyroid activities (39). Whether these pollutants exert additive or synergistic antithyroid effects and/or act as "triggers" of autoimmune thyroiditis requires investigation, particularly because more than 60 soluble chloroorganics have been identified in the primary and secondary effluents of typical domestic sewage treatment plants (64).

2,4-Dinitrophenol

2,4-Dinitrophenol (DNP) is formed of yellow crystals that are very sparingly soluble in cold water but readily soluble as a crystalline sodium salt. It is soluble in alcohol and various organic solvents (135).

Derivatives of DNP are widely used in agriculture and industry. 2,4-Dinitrophenol is an insecticide, herbicide, and fungicide. It is used in the manufacture of dyes, in the preservation of timber, and as an indicator (135).

2,4-Dinitrophenol is readily absorbed through intact skin and the respiratory tract (135). Poisoning may thus occur after crop spraying with DNP (75). The compound causes toxicity by the uncoupling of oxidative phosphorylation in the mitochondria of cells throughout the body. Exposure to this agent can result in a syndrome characterized by lassitude, malaise, headache, increased perspiration, thirst, and dyspnea. It may produce malignant hyperthermia, profound weight loss, respiratory failure, and death (75,135). Because DNP compounds are widely used, it is possible that some patients with fever of unknown origin have unrecognized DNP poisoning. Animal studies have shown that the lethal dose (LD50) of DNP is the same for several species when expressed per kilogram body weight. Major factors in determining toxicity appear to be ambient temperature and oxygen concentration (75).

The administration of 2,4-DNP causes a marked reduction in circulating thyroid hormones (16,89). The effects of exposure to DNP compounds on the thyroid gland have not yet been investigated.

Phthalate Esters and Phthalic Acid Derivatives

This section focuses on di(2-ethylhexyl)phthalate (DEHP), also known as dioctyl phthalate (DOP), and dibutyl phthalate (DBP). The *ortho-*, *meta-*, and *para*-phthalic acids are also discussed. These substances are found as impurities of the phthalate industrial process, biodegradation products of phthalate esters, and monomeric derivatives of humic substances. Phthalic acid is so named because the standard source has always been oxidation of the abundant coal tar constituent naphthalene. The most abundant of these compounds is DEHP. It has been isolated, along with DBP, from the water supply of a district in Colombia known to have a high incidence of endemic goiter.

Structurally, phthalic acid esters, or phthalate esters, consist of paired ester groups on a dicarboxylic benzene ring. Phthalate esters are synthesized commercially by condensation of appropriate alcohols with phthalic anhydride. Specific phthalate esters with short alkyl groups such as dimethyl and dibutyl phthalates are quite soluble in water. Because of their lipophilic structures, long-chain dialkylphthalates such as DEHP are relatively insoluble in aqueous media. At standard temperature and pressure the volatility of these agents is low. This is true particularly of such branched- and long-chain compounds as DEHP (88,90,96,135). Phthalic acid decomposes at 200–230°C and is best identified by conversion to phthalic anhydride, the industrial substrate of phthalate esters (88,90).

Phthalate esters are commonly used as plasticizers to impart flexibility to plastics, particularly polyvinyl chloride polymers (PVC). Phthalate esters in the United States have been used mainly as plasticizers for substances used in building and construction, home furnishings, cars, wearing apparel, food wrappings, medical tubing, and intravenous bags (90,96,135). Phthalates may be present in con-

centrations up to 40% of the weight of the plastic. DEHP is the most widely used plasticizer. The annual production of phthalate esters in the United States alone was estimated in 1972 to be 1 to 2 billion pounds. Worldwide production reached about 4 billion pounds (79,81,83,96,100).

Phthalate esters, ubiquitous in their distribution, are among the priority pollutants listed by the U.S. Environmental Protection Agency. They have been frequently identified as water pollutants (12, 36,45,47,79,81,83,96). Although they are most commonly the result of industrial pollution, they also appear naturally in shale, crude oil, petroleum, plants, and as fungal metabolites (90).

Phthalate esters are well absorbed from the gastrointestinal tract. Phthalates are widely distributed in the body, the liver being the major initial repository organ. Clearance from the body is rapid. Short-chain phthalates can be excreted unchanged or following complete hydrolysis to phthalic acid. Prior to excretion most longer-chain compounds are converted, by oxidative metabolism, to polar derivatives of the monoesters. Marked differences in metabolism of phthalates exist between primates and rats. The major route of phthalate ester elimination from the body is urinary excretion (25,74,79,90,96).

Both DEHP and other phthalates have been shown in various animal species to exert hepatotoxic, cytotoxic, teratogenic, and mutagenic effects (25,74,79,90,96). Animal studies indicate that phthalate esters can cause significant perturbation of metabolism in liver, heart, testes, adrenals, and brain (25,74,79,90,96).

Phthalate esters leach out of finished PVC products into blood and physiological solutions. The entry of these plasticizers into the patient's bloodstream during blood transfusion, intravenous fluid administration, or hemodialysis has been a matter of concern among public health officials and the medical community (35,74,79,90,96).

Patients undergoing maintenance hemodialysis receive a yearly dose of 16 to 23 g of DEHP, which is 10 to 20 times that producing hepatotoxicity in the transfused rhesus monkey (96). Except for necrotizing cutaneous vasculitis and nonspecific, nonfatal hepatitis (35), the toxic effects of this chronic exposure are still unknown. A high incidence of goiter in patients receiving maintenance hemodialysis has been reported (76,101). Whether phthalate ester metabolites and/or contaminants in the water entering the patient's bloodstream are responsible for this condition remains to be determined.

Although phthalate esters and phthalic acids do not possess intrinsic antithyroid activity, they undergo degradation by gram-negative bacteria to form dihydroxybenzoic acid (DHBA) (32,67,103). This agent is known to possess antithyroid properties (21,45,136) (Table 22-1; Fig. 22-2). Phthalates are

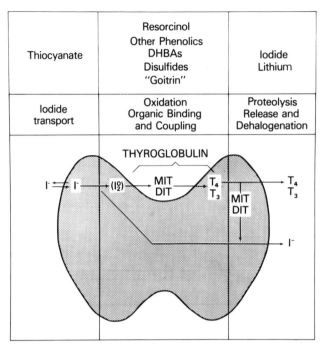

FIGURE 22-2. Environmental goitrogens and their sites of action in the thyroid gland. DHBAs, dihydroxybenzoic acids; I, iodide; I⁻, inorganic iodide; (I$_2^O$), oxidized iodide; MIT, monoiodotyrosine; DIT, diiodotyrosine; T_4, thyroxine; T_3, triiodothyronine. From Gaitan (44).

also actively concentrated and metabolized by several species of fish (25,79,81,83). Whether these widely distributed pollutants exert deleterious effects on the thyroid of humans and other animal species has not been investigated.

Polychlorinated and Polybrominated Biphenyls

Polychlorinated (PCB) and polybrominated biphenyls (PBB) are aromatic compounds containing two benzene nuclei with two or more substituent chlorine or bromine atoms. The PCBs are a mixture of chlorinated biphenyls that have been produced commercially by chlorination of biphenyl. Commercially prepared PCBs, identified by the trade name "Aroclors," are complex mixtures of different chlorobiphenyls and isomers. The PCBs are chemically very inert, resistant to corrosive chemicals, insoluble in water (0.04–0.2 ppm), and have a low vapor pressure. Their extreme stability contributes to their commercial usefulness and long-term deleterious environmental and health effects (22,69,110,135). The PBBs are analogous complex mixtures of different bromobiphenyls having physicochemical properties similar to PCBs (135).

The PCBs had a wide variety of industrial ap-

plications that steadily increased until 1977. At that time their use in the United States was restricted to such closed systems as electric transformers, capacitors, and heat transformers (13,22). The PBBs have been used commercially as flame retardants.

Worldwide, the population is subjected to low-level PCB exposure in air, water, and food (22). There is growing evidence that atmospheric transport is the primary means by which PCBs have global distribution from their sites of use and disposal. Plant foliage accumulates the vapor of PCBs from the atmosphere (13). In addition to their occurrence in surface water (rivers, lakes, etc.), PCBs have also been detected in U.S. drinking water, their concentration being limited by their solubility (3 μg/L; 3 ppb) (110). The most significant human exposures occur primarily in an industrial setting and during the consumption of contaminated fresh-water fish. The high PCB levels found in several species of fish (5 mg/kg in lake fish) have prompted reassessment of the PCB action levels (5,22,95). Polychlorinated biphenyls are also found in the milk of nursing mothers (mean 2 mg/L; 2 ppm) (104,110). The American Academy of Pediatrics recommends testing for PCBs in women who have eaten large amounts of sport fish or who have been occupationally exposed (104).

Polybrominated biphenyl contamination of the food chain occurred in Michigan in 1973 when PBB was accidently mixed in with cattle feed. This event resulted in widespread destruction of contaminated animals and raised concern over toxic effects of this exposure in humans (71). In a recent study in Michigan, breast milk of lactating women contained detectable levels of PBBs (104).

In general, PCBs and PBBs have high lipid solubility and resistance to physical degradation. They are slowly metabolized, and their excretion is limited. Long-term low-level exposure to the organohalides results in their gradual accumulation in fat, including the fat of breast milk. PCBs have been found in the adipose tissue of 30 to 45% of the general population (5,95,104,110).

The biological and toxicological properties of PCB mixtures may vary depending on their isomeric composition. Oral administration of PCBs to various mammals results in rapid and almost complete (90%) intestinal absorption. The degradation and elimination of PCBs depend on the hepatic microsomal enzyme system (110). The excretion of PCBs is related to the extent of their metabolism. Those with greater chlorine content have a correspondingly longer biological half-life in mammals. This resistance to metabolism is reflected in their deposition in adipose tissue. The PCBs, however, have very low acute toxicity in all animal species tested, and PBBs have biological properties similar to PCBs.

Both PCBs and PBBs are strong inducers of hepatic microsomal mixed-function oxidase enzymes. They can modify the toxicity of other agents and alter the peripheral metabolism of various hormones. It has been shown, for example, that PCB-exposed rats have increased excretion of circulating T_4 (6). They also develop goiter after such exposure. The PCBs are hepatotoxins and induce liver hypertrophy, hepatocellular adenomas, and carcinomas in Sherman rats (1,8,110). Because of their carcinogenic potential and widespread distribution, PCBs are among the priority pollutants listed by the EPA (22,110).

"Yusho disease" has been attributed to accidental contamination of rice bran oil with PCBs in Japan in 1968. Thyroid structure and function were not evaluated in the Yusho studies. Recent studies have revealed that polychlorodibenzofurans (PCDFs), highly toxic contaminants of the PCB preparation, are the main causative agent in the pathogenesis of Yusho disease (72).

Recent evidence suggests that some individuals exposed to PBB during the contamination episode in Michigan in 1973 may have a persistent immunologic dysfunction (10). A negative nonsignificant correlation between serum PBB and T_4 concentration was observed in 1978–1979 among Michigan residents exposed to PBBs in 1973 (71). Serum total thyroxine (T_4), a relatively insensitive parameter of thyroid function, was the only measure of thyroid function performed in the PBB-exposed population.

Other Organochlorines

DDT [2,2-bis-(p-chlorophenyl)-1,1,1-trichloroethane], a polychlorinated nondegradable heavily used pesticide, is produced by condensing chlorobenzene with chloral. DDT is practically insoluble in water and highly soluble in fat. It is resistant to destruction by light and oxidation (108,135). Dieldrin is one of the cyclodiene insecticides. Like DDT and DDE it is very stable, both environmentally and biologically (108, 135).

At the height of DDT use in the United States in 1963, production was about 176 million pounds. It was registered for use in 334 agriculture commodities. DDT has been used very extensively all over the world, both in malaria control and in agriculture. Its use was banned in the United States in 1972.

Because of its persistence in the environment, DDT and its breakdown products, DDE and DDD, are ubiquitous contaminants of water and of virtually every food product. Fish from Lake Michigan may contain DDT residues in excess of the 7 ppm, the FDA "safe limit." The low acute toxicity of DDT, coupled with its stability and pervasiveness, permits DDT to be biomagnified through the food chain. The overall magnification of DDT from water to fish may exceed a factor of 3×10^6. Humans reside at the top of this food chain. Human milk is contaminated: DDT residues averaging 0.08 ppm have appeared in United States samples.

Similar conditions prevail for dieldrin and the cyclodienes. Perhaps 600 million pounds of these highly chlorinated cyclic organic insecticides have been dispersed into the soil, air, water, and food in the United States during the last 30 years. Dieldrin is heavily bioconcentrated in the lipids of terrestrial and aquatic wildlife, humans, and foods, especially in animal fats and milk. Residues in milk can be particularly high because of the ingestion of these insecticides with forage. Dieldrin was banned in the United States in 1974.

DDT is reductively dechlorinated in biological systems to form DDE and DDD. DDE, the predominant residue stored in tissues, reaching about 70% in humans, is much less toxic than DDT. DDE is slowly eliminated from the body; little is known about its degradation pathway. DDT is also slowly eliminated from the human body through reduction to DDD and other more water-soluble derivatives (108,135).

DDT is of moderate acute toxicity to man and most other organisms. Poisoning may occur by ingestion or by absorption through the skin or respiratory tract. The estimated oral fatal dose is 500 mg/kg body weight. The major concern of low-level DDT exposure relates to the chronic effects of such exposure. These include liver damage and carcinogenesis.

The cyclodiene insecticides, particularly the persistent epoxide dieldrin, present the greatest hazards of all residual pesticides. At low dosages, they produce malignant hepatomas. Dieldrin, like DDT and DDE, is among the priority pollutants listed by the EPA.

DDT, DDE, and dieldrin are known to cause marked alterations in thyroid gland structure and function in birds (6,60–62). Since all these compounds induce microsomal enzyme activity, they may affect thyroid hormone metabolism in a way that is similar to the polyhalogenated biphenyls. The impact of these widely dispersed pollutants on the human thyroid is unknown.

Sulfurated Organics

The sulfurated organic goitrogens, though primarily naturally occurring, may also be man made.

Thiocyanate, Isothiocyanates, Thioglycosides, and Goitrin

Thiocyanate and isothiocyanates have been demonstrated as the goitrogenic principles in *Cruciferae*, i.e., cabbage, broccoli, and cauliflower; the potent antithyroid compound "goitrin" has been isolated from yellow turnips and from *Brassica* seeds (28,38,73). Cyanogenic glucosides (thiocyanate precursors) have also been found in several staple foods (cassava, maize, bamboo shoots, sweet potatoes, lima beans) used in the Third World. After ingestion, these glucosides can readily undergo enzymatic conversion to SCN.

It has also been shown that isothiocyanates react spontaneously with amino groups to form disubstituted thiourea derivatives, which produce a thiorurea-like antithyroid effect. Thioglucosides may also be transformed to isothiocyanate derivatives and in some instances to thiocyanate. A mustard oil glucoside yields SCN through the action of "myrosinase," a thioglucosidase enzyme contained in plants.

Ingestion of pure progoitrin, a naturally occurring thioglucoside, elicits antithyroid activity in rats and man in the absence of myrosinase. The antithyroid activity of progotrin results from its partial conversion in the animal into the more potent goitrogen, 1,5-vinyl-2-thiooxazolidone or "goitrin." This ability of plants and animals to readily convert inactive precursors into goitrogenic agents must be considered when investigating the possible etiological role of dietary elements in sporadic or endemic goiter. Specifically, it should be appreciated that the actual concentration of thiocyanates or isothiocya-

nates in a given foodstuff may not represent its true goitrogenic potential. Similarly the absence of these compounds does not negate a possible antithyroid effect. Man-made thiocyanate is found in high concentrations (1 g/L) in waste-water effluents of coal-conversion processes (59,70). It is also found in body fluids as a metabolite of hydrogen cyanide gas inhaled while smoking (73,97,98).

Aliphatic Disulfides

The major volatile components of onions and garlic have been identified as small aliphatic disulfides. These compounds have marked antithyroid activity in rats (23,112,113). Organic sulfide pollutants are present in high concentration in waste-water effluents of coal-treatment plants (59,70). Organic disulfides have been identified as water contaminants in the United States (12). They have also been found in the water supply of a Colombian district having a high incidence of endemic goiter (36,47). Methyl, diethyl, and diphenyl disulfides are the compounds most frequently isolated in the United States. However, dimethyl trisulfide, dimethyl sulfoxide, and diphenylene sulfide have also been isolated.

Irradiation

In the event of a nuclear reactor accident as occurred in 1986 in Chernobyl, USSR, radioisotopes of iodine would be released into the environment. After the Chernobyl accident, ^{131}I was readily measured in the atmosphere. The radioisotopes of iodine enter the body and are concentrated in the thyroid gland, where they remain for varying lengths of time. Although it is known that radioactive iodine can induce thyroid neoplasms, the precise level that may be tumorigenic is unknown. High levels of radioactive iodine are ablative to the thyroid gland (9).

EPIDEMIOLOGY

Goiter

Most goitrogens exert greater activity in the presence of such environmental conditions as iodine deficiency, poor sanitation, and malnutrition. The disease that results under these circumstances is called "endemic goiter" (26,117). Environmental goitrogens may also act on the thyroid in the presence of adequate iodine intake. When the disease is associated with an adequate iodine intake (75–300 μg per day), it is called "sporadic or nontoxic goiter." A prevalence rate of 10% or more is arbitrarily defined as goiter endemia. In the case of endemic goiter and iodine deficiency, the socioeconomic impact is dreadful. Endemic cretinism and various degrees of impaired growth and mental development occur in a large segment of the population.

In the case of sporadic or nontoxic goiter in the United States, there is an association with hyperthyroidism and probably with thyroid carcinoma. These possibilities provide the impetus for exhaustive studies, which are done to furnish appropriate diagnosis and treatment. Clearly, this takes a huge toll in the cost of medical and surgical care (127).

Currently more than 400 million individuals throughout the world are thought to be affected by endemic and nontoxic goiter. In Idjwi Island (Kivu Lake) and the Ubangi area in central Africa as much as 60% of the population are affected by goiter. Thiocyanate from a cyanogenic glucoside (linamarin) in cassava, a staple food, acting in the presence of extreme iodine deficiency, is thought to be the cause of most of these goiters (28).

In iodine-sufficient areas such as western Colombia, South America, pollution of the water supplies with shale- and coal-derived organic compounds (resorcinol, disulfides, phthalic acid ester metabolites) are thought to be the cause of most goiters. About 15% of the population is so afflicted in these areas (28,36,38,40–42,45,66,84).

Similar conditions are found in some areas of the United States. As many as 9 to 30% of the children living in the coal- and shale-rich areas of eastern Kentucky develop goiter despite an adequate iodine intake (41,57,77,117,121,122,129). These figures, far in excess of goiter prevalence in other areas of the United States, suggest that region-specific environmental factors are at the cause of this condition.

A high incidence of goiter has been documented among patients with advanced renal failure undergoing maintenance hemodialysis. The prevalence of goiter was reported to be 58% in Salt Lake City, Utah (101) and 37% in Chicago, Illinois (76). These rates are much higher than those expected in a matched control population. Although the cause of these goiters is unknown, the plasticizers (i.e., DEHP) leaching from the dialysis equipment and/or the organic pollutants present in the 100 to 240 L of dialysate to which such patients are exposed constitute potential sources of goitrogenicity.

Hypothyroidism

In the early 1950s sporadic goiter and hypothyroidism were observed in patients applying resorcinol ointments for the treatment of varicose ulcers (14,99). Similar situations were documented in patients receiving long-term thiocyanate treatment for hypertension (26,58,73). This goitrogenic effect of SCN is more evident in the presence of iodine deficiency.

Several observations suggest that resorcinol and SCN cross the human placenta and may cause both goiter and neonatal hypothyroidism (107,131). It has been further postulated that SCN acting in conjunction with iodine deficiency may be the cause of endemic cretinism in central Africa (28).

An increased prevalence of primary hypothyroidism (11%) was documented among workers in a plant that manufactured PBBs and PBB oxides (4). These subjects had elevated titers of antithyroid microsomal antibodies, indicating that hypothyroidism was probably a manifestation of lymphocytic thyroiditis. This response was perhaps a PBB-induced pathogenic autoimmune response or exacerbation of underlying subclinical disease. The association between environmental pollutant exposure and autoimmune thyroiditis has not been investigated, even though the incidence of this disorder has steadily increased in the United States during the past five decades (37).

The administration of 2,4-DNP to human volunteers resulted in a rapid and pronounced decline of circulating thyroid hormones (16,89). The biological significance of this observation and the public health impact of this pollutant on the thyroid are still unknown.

Autoimmune Thyroiditis

A study conducted in Olmsted County, Minnesota, in which all diagnosed cases of lymphocytic or autoimmune (Hashimoto) thyroiditis from 1935 to 1967 were reevaluated, indicates a rise in incidence from 7/100,000 to 69/100,000 population over the 32-year period. A similar upward trend was observed at the University of Michigan Hospital. Based on the examination of 2642 thyroid glands removed from 1915 to 1963, the frequency of autoimmune thyroiditis rose from 0.4% between 1915 and 1925, before iodine was introduced, to 9.3% some 35 years after the iodine prophylaxis program was established.

In Breathitt County, a coal-rich area of eastern Kentucky, antithyroid microsomal antibodies were elevated in 20% of the children with goiters but in only 6% of controls (57). Recent studies demonstrate a continued high incidence of goiter, autoimmune thyroiditis, and subclinical hypothyroidism in eastern Kentucky and show that iodine deficiency is not the cause of these goiters (41). The question thus arises: do the same region-specific environmental factors that cause goiter operate in genetically predisposed individuals to trigger the pathogenic mechanism leading to autoimmune thyroiditis?

Goitrous lymphocytic thyroiditis has been observed after administration of the carcinogens methylcholanthrene and dimethylbenzanthracene (polycyclic aromatic hydrocarbons) and carbon tetrachloride to the BUF inbred strain of rats (134). Similarly, injection of mouse thyroglobulin with bacterial lipopolysaccharide or with complete Freund's adjuvant containing mycobacteria induces lymphocytic thyroiditis in "good-responder" mice, whereas "poor-responder" strains develop little pathological response. "Good" and "poor" responders differ in their H-2 haplotype (134).

Polynuclear aromatic hydrocarbons (PAH) (2, 6,65,91,108), many of which are known to be carcinogenic to animals and to induce autoimmune thyroiditis in the BUF rat (134), have been found repeatedly in domestic water supplies. The PAH are present in industrial and municipal waste effluents. They also occur naturally in soils, ground water, and surface water and in their sediments and biota. A potent carcinogenic PAH compound, benzo[a]-pyrene, is widely distributed. It has been detected in water after conventional water treatment processes (108).

Thyroid Nodules

About 4% of adults in the United States have palpable thyroid nodules, and of those autopsied as many as 30% were found to have thyroid nodules. Some 8 million Americans are currently thought to have clinically significant thyroid nodules (26,33, 126,127).

Little has been done to elucidate the cause of this very common thyroid disorder. Most nodules correspond histologically to follicular adenomas. Follicular adenomas in the United States are histologically identical to the adenomas of multinodular goiters in endemic areas of other parts of the world. The association of hyperthyroidism with follicular adenomas is well recognized (37,48,92,128).

Thyroid Cancer

Investigations on morbidity and geographic pathology of thyroid carcinomas (24,37,56,117,130) demonstrate that the incidence of thyroid cancer in the endemic goiter area of western Colombia is as much as ten times that observed in nonendemic areas such as Puerto Rico, New York, and Connecticut. Follicular and anaplastic types of thyroid cancer are found in the endemic goiter areas, but the incidence of papillary carcinoma is similar to that in nonendemic regions. Follicular adenomas were associated with follicular and anaplastic carcinomas in 78% and 97% of the cases, respectively. Similar observations were made in endemic goiter areas of Finland.

One of the best methods of experimentally inducing follicular adenomas in rats, even in the presence of adequate iodine intake, is the administration of antithyroid goitrogenic compounds. The addi-tion of small amounts of a carcinogen (acetylaminofluorene or benzo[a]pyrene) results in the development of thyroid carcinomas. There are invasion of blood vessels and metastasis to the lungs, characteristic of the follicular type of carcinoma. If given alone, the carcinogen will not act on the thyroid. It appears that the antithyroid agent behaves as a "tumor promoter" to the action of the carcinogen on the thyroid gland. Although sustained and prolonged administration of a goitrogen by itself in the rat eventually results in development of thyroid carcinomas, it takes much longer than when the goitrogen is administered in the presence of a carcinogen (19,29). It is of interest that 60 years ago Twort and Twort (124) produced goiter in a high percentage of animals by painting shale oil on the skin of mice. These "petrol goiters" harbored carcinoma in a few mice.

The full relevance of the above observations in the pathogenesis of thyroid nodules and cancer and autoimmune thyroiditis in man remains to be determined.

Effect of Exposure to Radiation

Radiation exposure to the head and neck in childhood and adolescence has been related to the subsequent appearance of thyroid cancer (9,19,20, 26,27,80,114). The frequency of thyroid cancer increased as much as 100-fold after significant x-ray radiation was given to children and adolescents for thymus enlargement, hypertrophy of the tonsils and adenoids, and for the treatment of acne. Doses ranging between 200 and 700 rads were used. The prevalence of thyroid carcinomas in this population reached 2% to 7%. The average latency period is 20 years. Fortunately, most of these neoplasms are well-differentiated papillary carcinomas with a low degree of malignancy and a good prognosis. Benign thyroid nodules also occur after radiation with a higher frequency than do carcinomas. In large series of patients undergoing thyroid surgery, one out of three single nodules found at physical examination was histologically diagnosed as carcinoma. The development of thyroid nodules and cancer has also been observed in rats experimentally exposed to radiation.

The tumorigenic potential is different depending on the source of radiation. For instance, there is evidence indicating that iodine-131 is less tumorigenic than x rays. Some estimates show that ^{131}I is 5 to 20 times less tumorigenic. Since a nuclear reactor accident could release radioisotopes of iodine into the environment, the Environmental Hazards Committee of the American Thyroid Association has addressed the issue of using stable iodine as a thyroidal blocking agent (9).

Based on the continuing study of atomic bomb

survivors and other irradiated populations, the following generalizations appear to apply: (1) There is greater susceptibility to radiation-induced thyroid cancer during early childhood. The tumors do not become apparent until after puberty. (2) Women are two to three times more susceptible than men to spontaneous and radiation-induced thyroid cancer. (3) Radiogenic thyroid cancer is often preceded or accompanied by the presence of benign thyroid nodules. The frequency of hypothyroidism and simple goiter is higher in individuals who were exposed to large doses of radiation in their youth. (4) Radiogenic thyroid cancer is generally papillary as opposed to follicular or mixed histopathology, and (5) the development of overt thyroid cancer is related to hormonal stimulation such that a sustained elevation of thyroid-stimulating hormone levels increases the risk of thyroid cancer (20).

Host Factors

In both endemic and sporadic goiter, diffusely enlarged thyroid glands are more common in young individuals, and nodular glands are mainly seen in the female adult population (117,123). Autoimmune thyroid disease also occurs more frequently in women.

A relationship between loci in the major histocompatibility complex (MHC) and susceptibility to autoimmune thyroid disease has been demonstrated in man. For instance, the histocompatibility (HLA)-DR5 antigen is seen with increased frequency in patients with goitrous thyroiditis, whereas atrophic thyroiditis is associated with the HLA-DR3 (134).

Individuals with underlying or subclinical thyroid disease, such as lymphocytic thyroiditis, are more susceptible to the action of goitrogenic materials (i.e., excess iodine, lithium salts, resorcinol, and possibly PBBs). Some diffuse and nodular goiters or thyroid nodules correspond to entities other than those related to environmental goitrogens. For this reason, careful clinical examination, special laboratory tests, and diagnostic procedures must be conducted to provide an adequate diagnosis and treatment.

Other Animal Species

Goiters related to environmental pollutants also occur in animal species other than man (mammals, birds, and fish). For example, PCBs, DDT, DDE, and dieldrin have been shown to cause marked alterations in the thyroid gland of gulls and pigeons (60–63). Coho salmon in Lake Erie and Lake Ontario have a high incidence of goiter, whereas those in Lake Michigan do not. Since these findings cannot be explained on the basis of low levels of iodine, it is probable that contamination of the water with natural and man-made goitrogens is the cause (85,86,116,132).

PHYSIOLOGY AND PATHOPHYSIOLOGY

To understand the involvement of environmental chemicals in the pathogenesis of thyroid disease, a brief review of thyroid gland physiology is necessary. This review, by identifying the site of action and the physiological mechanisms disrupted by environmental chemicals, provides the basis for understanding how such exposure can lead to goitrogenesis, with or without hypothyroidism.

Figure 22-2 illustrates the three main steps in thyroid gland function. It also lists some environmental pollutants that act directly in the gland by interfering with the process of hormonal synthesis.

The first step involves the active uptake or concentration of inorganic iodide by the thyroid. Environmental goitrogens such as thiocyanate (SCN) interfere with this process. Since SCN has a molecular volume and a charge similar to those of iodide, it competes with iodide for transport in the thyroid cell. The goitrogenic effect of SCN, however, is overcome by iodine administration.

The second step entails the incorporation of oxidized iodine into the amino acid tyrosine—within the peptide sequence of thyroglobulin—to form monoiodotyrosine (MIT) and diiodotyrosine (DIT). These compounds are precursors of the active thyroid hormones triiodothyronine (T_3) and thyroxine (T_4). This process of organification is mediated by the action of the thyroidal peroxidase enzyme. Resorcinol and its phenolic and phenolic–carboxylic (DHBAs) parent compounds, aliphatic disulfides, and "goitrin" inhibit the process of organification.

The third step consists of the release of the active thyroid hormones, T_3 and T_4, into the circulation. Excess iodide and lithium salts block this step.

Because of their antithyroid effects, the administration of any of the substances affecting the three steps of thyroid hormone synthesis eventually results in goiter formation. In some instances hypothyroidism may also develop. For this reason such agents are called antithyroid or goitrogenic compounds. It becomes apparent that an absolute lack of dietary iodine or a decrease in iodine utilization because of environmental pollutants or both can result in "sporadic" or "endemic" goiter (26,38,58).

Thyrotropin (TSH) from the anterior pituitary regulates the rate of synthesis and secretion of thyroid hormones. In turn, T_4 and T_3 act directly on the pituitary to inhibit thyrotropin secretion (102). Since TSH also exerts a morphogenetic effect on the gland, any increase in thyrotropin secretion that follows exposure to antithyroid compounds would be expected to cause thyroid enlargement. The mechanism that induces the trophic changes leading to goiter formation is not well understood. Conversely, a decrease in thyrotropin secretion results in decreased synthesis and release of T_4 and T_3 and involution of the thyroid gland. The antithyroid effect of 2,4-dinitrophenol (DNP) results in part from an inhibition of the pituitary TSH mechanism (52).

Once T_4 and T_3 are released into the circulation, they are instantaneously bound to serum carrier proteins (26,58); DNP interferes with T_4 binding (51,133,137), further decreasing serum T_4 concentration. The PCBs exert a similar effect (7,8).

All circulating T_4 and 20% of T_3 are derived from the thyroid gland. The rest of T_3 is produced by outer ring monodeiodination of T_4 in peripheral tissues. Although deiodination is most important, there are two other major pathways for the metabolism and excretion of thyroid hormones. These include the oxidative deamination or transamination of the amino acid residue and the sulfate and glucuronide conjugation of the phenolic ring (26,58).

In addition to inhibiting the TSH mechanism and interfering with T_4 binding, DNP also accelerates the disappearance of T_4 from the circulation, thereby lowering the serum T_4 concentration even more (51). It is well known that DNP uncouples oxidative phosphorylation and stimulates the activity of the enzyme ATPase, but the mechanism by which DNP alters T_4 metabolism is unknown.

The thyroid hormones, in both free and conjugated forms, are excreted into the intestine along with small amounts of their deiodinated metabolites (26,58). Glucuronide conjugation, through the action of a UDP-glucuronyltransferase, occurs primarily in the liver; sulfate conjugation takes place mainly in the kidney through the action of a sulfate transferase. Under normal circumstances, however, little T_4 and T_3 are excreted in the conjugated form.

Polychlorinated biphenyls (PCBs) are potent hepatic microsomal enzyme inducers (8,110). Investigators have demonstrated that rats exposed to PCBs exhibit a greatly enhanced biliary excretion of circulating T_4. The T_4 is excreted as a glucuronide, which is then lost in the feces (6,7). This response is probably secondary to induction of hepatic microsomal T_4-UDP-glucuronyltransferase. The enhanced peripheral metabolism and reduced binding of T_4 to serum proteins in PCB-treated animals result in markedly decreased serum T_4 concentrations. These low levels stimulate the pituitary–thyrotropin–thyroid axis, and this eventually results in goiter formation (6,7).

Although PCB-treated animals exhibit decreased serum T_4, their T_3 levels are unchanged. This observation may be explained by the following considerations. The relative iodine deficiency brought about by the accelerated metabolism of T_4 may induce increased thyroidal T_3 secretion as well as increased peripheral deiodination of T_4 to T_3 (6,7). Polybrominated biphenyls (PBBs) appear to act similarly to PCBs. There is, however, some indication that they may also interfere directly with the process of hormonal synthesis in the thyroid gland (1).

In conclusion, environmental chemicals may cause goiter and/or hypothyroidism directly by acting on the thyroid gland or indirectly by altering its regulatory mechanisms and/or the peripheral metabolism and excretion of thyroid hormones. Environmental chemicals, operating in genetically predisposed individuals, may trigger the pathogenic mechanisms that lead to goiter formation and autoimmune thyroiditis. Although this process has been induced experimentally in the BUF rat (68,134), it has not yet been demonstrated in man.

The antithyroid and goitrogenic activities of compounds or materials having potential goitrogenicity can be determined by in vitro and in vivo assays (44). These methods can be of great help in evaluating the effect of chemical exposure on the thyroid gland. In vitro assays include (1) inhibition of thyroid peroxidase activity and (2) inhibition of uptake and/or organification of radioactive iodine in thyroid slices, lobes, or cell suspensions (bovine, porcine, rat, etc.). In vivo assays include measuring the following: (1) suppression of thyroid gland activities (uptake, organification, hormone release) by acute administration of test material (rats and mice); (2) goitrogenicity (increase in thyroid weight) by chronic administration of test material (usually in the rat); (3) other parameters related to goitrogenesis, i.e., gastrointestinal absorption of iodide, gastrointestinal loss of T_4, serum concentrations and peripheral metabolism of thyroid hormones; and (4) induction of autoimmune thyroiditis (positive circulating antithyroid antibodies, thyroid immunofluorescence, and lymphocytic infiltration) by administration of test material in susceptible strains of rats and mice.

CLINICAL ASPECTS OF EXPOSURE TO ENVIRONMENTAL CHEMICALS AND PHYSICAL AGENTS ON THE THYROID

Epidemiologic and experimental evidence indicates that environmental chemicals may be responsible for many goiters (43–46,111). Until these environmental factors are better defined, effective prevention and treatment cannot be implemented. The clinician is therefore restricted to the conventional and current forms of treatment—observation, administration of thyroid hormones, and surgery. As part of the clinical history, however, the physician should inquire about the intake of excessive iodine, lithium salts, and resorcinol-containing drugs. Exposure to PCBs, PBBs, and DNP should also be determined. A history of radiation to the face and neck in childhood and adolescence should not be overlooked.

Diffuse Goiters

Clinical and Laboratory Characteristics

Diffuse goiter is defined as an enlargement of the thyroid gland, which maintains its anatomic configuration. Most patients with diffuse goiters related to environmental goitrogens in iodine-sufficient areas are clinically and chemically euthyroid. Careful inspection and palpation of the neck are the only examinations needed to determine the presence or absence of a goiter. Hypothyroidism in the early stages is difficult to diagnose clinically. The finding of raised serum TSH levels with low normal T_4 but normal T_3 levels in persons with no clinical evidence of thyroid deficiency has been termed subclinical hypothyroidism. Thus, serum TSH measurement is the most sensitive indicator of impending thyroid failure (118,123). Once T_4 and T_3 levels are below normal, typical clinical manifestations of hypothyroidism become apparent (cold intolerance, slow relaxation of deep tendon reflexes, dry skin, puffiness, etc.).

Differential Diagnosis

Lymphocytic or autoimmune thyroiditis with or without hypothyroidism must be considered. High serum TSH is present when there is clinical or subclinical thyroid deficiency. High titers of antithyroid peroxidase microsomal and thyroglobulin antibodies are usually found. Histologically, there is lymphocytic infiltration of the thyroid.

Diffuse goiters with hyperthyroidism (Graves' disease) must be considered. This condition is rarely seen below 18 years of age. This diagnosis is usually established by the characteristic clinical and laboratory findings.

Treatment

Euthyroid diffuse goiters most commonly need observation only or suppression with oral thyroid hormone (l-thyroxine, 0.2 mg daily). Hypothyroidism with or without goiter requires thyroid supplementation (l-thyroxine, 0.1–0.15 mg daily).

Nodular Goiters and Thyroid Nodules

Clinical Characteristics

Nodular goiter is defined as an enlargement of the thyroid distorting its normal anatomic configuration. Careful clinical, laboratory, and special test evaluations are necessary (127).

Differential Diagnosis

Thyroid carcinomas, colloid nodules, cysts, and other conditions such as focal thyroiditis and parathyroid adenoma must be considered in differential diagnosis of thyroid nodules.

Treatment

Depending on the findings, treatment consists of observation, suppression with thyroid hormone, or surgery. Costs for diagnosis and treatment of a thyroid nodule currently may be very high.

Prevention and Control

As discussed in this chapter, environmental pollutants may be responsible for many goiters. However, it is clear that a number of studies must be done before a causal relationship between pollutant exposure and thyroid disease is established and before the risk of such exposure is understood. It must be shown that people with goiter were exposed to a suspected environmental goitrogen(s) and that the degree of exposure was greater than that of a control, nongoitrous population. A dose–response assessment that characterizes the relationship between the intensity of exposure and the incidence of thyroid disease is also important.

At this time, with the exception of dietary iodine deficiency, the public health and socioeconomic impact of environmental antithyroid and goitrogenic agents is practically unknown. At present, when available, medical or surgical treatments for individuals are being applied in iodine-sufficient goiter areas, but not measures for prevention and control.

SUMMARY

Epidemiologic and experimental evidence emphasizes the complex and multifactorial etiology of endemic goiter. The important role of iodine deficiency as an etiologic factor in endemic goiter is firmly established, but there is evidence that other environmental factors can play equally important roles in the pathogenesis of this condition. A large number of agents in the environment are known to interfere with thyroid gland function. Antithyroid compounds, either naturally occurring or man made, may enter the air, water, and food and thereby become important environmental goitrogenic factors in man and other animals.

Environmental chemicals that cause goiter are known as environmental goitrogens. These agents may act directly on the thyroid gland or indirectly by altering regulatory mechanisms, the peripheral metabolism, or excretion of thyroid hormones. In the presence of dietary iodine deficiency, the action of environmental goitrogens may be enhanced. The mechanisms that induce the trophic changes leading to goiter formation, and in some instances to hypothyroidism, are not well understood.

REFERENCES

1. Allen-Rowlands CR, Castracane VD, Hamilton MF, et al: Effect of polybrominated biphenyls (PBB) on the pituitary–thyroid axis of the rat. Proc Soc Exp Biol Med 166:506, 1981.
2. Andelman JB, Sness MJ: Polynuclear aromatic hydrocarbons in the water environment. Bull WHO 43:479, 1970.
3. Arnott DG, Doniach I: The effects of compound allied to resorcinol upon the uptake of radioactive iodine (^{131}I) by the thyroid of the rat. Biochem J 50:473, 1952.
4. Bahn AK, Mills JL, Synder PJ, et al: Hypothyroidism in workers exposed to polybrominated biphenyls. N Engl J Med 302:31, 1980.
5. Barsano CP: Environmental factors altering thyroid function and their assessment. Environ Health Perspect 38:71, 1981.
6. Barsano CP: Polyhalogenated and polycyclic aromatic hydrocarbons. In: Environmental Goitrogenesis, p 115, Gaitan E (ed.), CRC Press, Boca Raton, 1989.
7. Bastomsky CH: Goiters in rats fed polychlorinated biphenyls. Can J Physiol Pharmacol 55:288, 1977.
8. Bastomsky CH, Murphy PVN, Banovac K: Alterations in thyroxine metabolism produced by cutaneous application of microscope immersion oil. Effects due to polychlorinated biphenyls. Endocrinology 98:1309, 1976.
9. Becker DV, Braverman LE, Dunn JT, et al: The use of iodine as a thyroidal blocking agent in the event of a reactor accident. Report of the Environmental Hazards Committee of the American Thyroid Association. JAMA 252:659, 1984.
10. Bekesi JG, Roboz JP, Solomon S, et al: Altered immune function in Michigan residents exposed to polybrominated biphenyls. In: Immunotoxicology, p 182, Gibson GG, Hubbard R, Parke DV (eds.), Academic Press, Orlando, 1983.
11. Black AP, Christman RF: Chemical characteristics of fulvic acids. J Am Water Works Assoc 55:897, 1963.
12. Brass HJ, Feige MA, Halloran T, et al: The national organic monitoring survey: A sampling and analysis for purgeable organic compounds. In: Drinking Water Quality Enhancement through Source Protection, p 393, Pojasek RB (ed.), Ann Arbor Science, Ann Arbor, 1977.
13. Buckley EH: Accumulation of airborne polychlorinated biphenyls in foliage. Science 216:520, 1982.
14. Bull GM, Fraser R: Myxoedema from resorcinol ointment applied to leg ulcers. Lancet 1:851, 1950.
15. Burges NA, Hurst HM, Walkden B: The phenolic constituents of humic acid and their relationship to the lignin of the plant cover. Geochem Cosmol Acta 28:1547, 1964.
16. Castor CM, Beierwaltes WH: Depression of serum protein-bound iodine levels in man with dinitrophenol. J Clin Endocrinol Metab 15:862, 1955.
17. Choudry GG: Humic substances: Part 1: Structural aspects. Toxicol Environ Chem 4:209, 1981.
18. Christman RF, Chassemi N: Chemical nature of organic color in water. J Am Water Works Assoc 58:723, 1966.
19. Christov K, Raichev R: Experimental thyroid carcinogenesis. Curr Top Pathol 56:79, 1973.
20. Committee on the Biological Effects of Ionizing Radiations, National Research Council: Health Effects of Exposure to Low Levels of Ionizing Radiation. BIER V, National Academy Press, Washington, 1990.
21. Cooksey RC, Gaitan E, Lindsay RH, et al: Humic substances, a possible source of environmental goitrogens. Org Geochem 8:77, 1985.
22. Cordle F, Locke R, Springer J: Risk assessment in a federal regulatory agency: An assessment of risk associated with the human consumption of some species of fish contaminated with polychlorinated biphenyls (PCBs). Environ Health Perspect 45:171, 1982.
23. Cowan JW, Saghir AR, Salji JP: Antithyroid activity of onion volatiles. Aust J Biol Sci 20:683, 1967.
24. Cuello C, Correa P, Eisenberg H: Geographic pathology of thyroid carcinoma. Cancer 23:230, 1969.
25. Daniel JW: Toxicity and metabolism of phthalate esters. Clin Toxicol 13:257, 1978.
26. DeGroot LJ: Thyroid gland. In: Endocrinology, Vol I, p 305, DeGroot LJ, Cahill GH Jr, Martini L, et al. (eds.), Grune & Stratton, New York, 1979.
27. DeGroot LJ, Reilly M, Pinnameneni K, et al: Retrospective and prospective study of radiation-induced thyroid disease. Am J Med 74:852, 1983.
28. Delange F, Ahluwalia R (eds.): Cassava Toxicity and Thyroid: Research and Public Health Issues. International Development Research Centre (IDRC-207e), Ottawa, 1983.
29. Doniach I: Experimental thyroid tumors. In: Tumours of the Thyroid Gland. Neoplastic Diseases at Various Sites, Vol VI, p 73, Smither DW (ed.), Livinstone, Edinburgh, 1970.
30. Doniach I, Fraser R: Effects of resorcinol in the thyroid uptake of ^{131}I in rats. Lancet 1:855, 1950.
31. Doniach I, Logothetopoulos J: The goitrogenic action of resorcinol in rats. Br J Exp Pathol 34:146, 1953.
32. Engelhardt G, Wallnofer PR, Hutzinger O: The microbial metabolism of di-n-butyl phthalate and related dialkyl phthalates. Bull Environ Contam Toxicol 13:342, 1975.
33. Farook MA: Observations on the epidemiology, histology and classification of thyroidal nodules and adenomas. Int Surg 50:540, 1968.
34. Fishbein L: Toxicity of chlorinated biphenyls. Annu Rev Pharmacol 14:139, 1974.
35. Friedman EA, Lundin AP: Environmental and iatrogenic obstacles to long life on hemodialysis. N Engl J Med 306:167, 1982.
36. Gaitan E: Water-borne goitrogens and their role in the etiology of endemic goiter. World Rev Nutr Diet 17:53, 1973.
37. Gaitan E: Iodine deficiency and toxicity. In: Proceedings Western Hemisphere Nutrition Congress IV, p

56, White PL, Selvey N (eds.), Publishing Sciences Group, Acton, Mass., 1975.

38. Gaitan E: Goitrogens in the etiology of endemic goiter. In: Endemic Goiter and Endemic Cretinism, p 219, Stanbury JB, Hetzel B (eds.), John Wiley & Sons, New York, 1980.

39. Gaitan E, Lindsay RH, Cooksey RC, et al: Antithyroid activities of resorcinol and its methyl and chloro derivatives present in effluents from coal liquefaction and chlorinated domestic sewage plants. In: Proceedings American Thyroid Association, ATA, Quebec, 1982.

40. Gaitan E: Endemic goiter in western Colombia. Ecol Dis 2:295, 1984.

41. Gaitan E: Iodine-sufficient goiter and autoimmune thyroiditis: The Kentucky and Colombian experience. In: Frontiers in Thyroidology, p 19, Medeiros-Neto G, Gaitan E (eds.), Plenum Press, New York, 1986.

42. Gaitan E: Symposium on thyroid disorders: Possible role of environmental pollutants and naturally-occurring agents. Am Chem Soc Div Environ Chem 26:58–85, 1986.

43. Gaitan E: Goitrogens. Bailliere Clin Endocrinol Metab 2:683, 1988.

44. Gaitan E: Environmental Goitrogenesis, CRC Press, Boca Raton, 1989.

45. Gaitan E: Phthalate esters and phthalic acid derivatives. In: Environmental Goitrogenesis, p 107, Gaitan E (ed.), CRC Press, Boca Raton, 1989.

46. Gaitan E: Goitrogens in food and water. Annu Rev Nutr 10:21, 1990.

47. Gaitan E, Island DP, Liddle GW: Identification of a naturally occurring goitrogen in water. Trans Assoc Am Physicians 82:141, 1969.

48. Gaitan E, Wahner HW, Cuello C, et al: Endemic goiter in the Cauca Valley, II. Studies of thyroid pathophysiology. J Clin Endocrinol 29:675, 1969.

49. Gaitan E, Merino H, Rodriquez G, et al: Epidemiology of endemic goiter in western Colombia. Bull WHO 56:403, 1978.

50. Garton GA, Williams RT: Studies in detoxication. 21. The fates of quinol and resorcinol in the rabbit in relation to the metabolism of benzene. Biochem J 44:234, 1949.

51. Goldberg RC, Wolff J, Greep RO: The mechanism of depression of plasma protein bound iodine by 2,4-dinitrophenol. Endocrinology 56:560, 1955.

52. Goldberg RC, Wolff J, Greep RO: Studies on the nature of the thyroid–pituitary interrelationship. Endocrinology 60:38, 1957.

53. Goodman LS, Gilman A, Gilman AG (eds.): Goodman and Gilman's The Pharmacological Basis of Therapeutics, 7th ed., Macmillan, New York, 1985.

54. Greene G, Steelink C: Structure of soil humic acid II. Some copper oxide oxidation products. J Org Chem 27:170, 1962.

55. Hartenstein R: Sludge decomposition and stabilization. Science 212:743, 1981.

56. Hedinger CE (ed.): Thyroid Cancer, Vol 12, UICC Monograph Series. Springer-Verlag, Berlin, 1969.

57. Hollingsworth DR, Butcher LK, White SD: Kentucky Appalachian goiter without iodine deficiency. Am J Dis Child 131:866, 1977.

58. Ingbar SH, Braverman LE (eds.): Werner's The Thyroid, 5th ed., JB Lippincott, Philadelphia, 1986.

59. Jahnig CE, Bertrand RR: Aqueous effluents from coal-conversion processes. Chem Eng Prog 72:51, 1976.

60. Jefferies DJ, French MC: Avian thyroid: Effects of pp'DDT on size and activity. Science 166:1278, 1969.

61. Jefferies DJ, French MC: Hyper- and hypo-thyroidism in pigeons fed DDT: An explanation for the "thin eggshell" phenomenon. Environ Pollut 1:235, 1971.

62. Jefferies DJ, French MC: Changes induced in the pigeon thyroid by pp'DDT and dieldrin. J Wildl Mgmt 36:24, 1972.

63. Jefferies DJ, Parslow JLF: Effect of one polychlorinated biphenyl on size and activity of gull thyroid. Bull Environ Contam Toxicol 8:306, 1972.

64. Jolley RL, Gorchev H, Hamilton DH Jr: Analysis of organic constituents in natural and process waters by high-pressure liquid chromatography. In: Trace Substances in Environmental Health—XI, p 247, Hemphill DD (ed.), The University of Missouri, Columbia, 1975.

65. Jolley RL, Gorchev H, Hamilton DH Jr (eds.): Water Chlorination: Environmental Impact and Health Effects, Vol 2, Ann Arbor Science, Ann Arbor, 1978.

66. Jolley RL, Gaitan E, Lee NE, et al: Resorcinol, a potent antithyroid compound, detected in the water supply of a Colombian district with endemic goiter. Am Chem Soc Div Environ Chem 23:179, 1983.

67. Keyser P, Basayya GP, Eaton RW, et al: Biodegradation of the phthalates and their esters by bacteria. Environ Health Perspect 18:159, 1976.

68. Kieffer JD, Vickery AL Jr, Ridgway EC, et al: Induction of breast cancer by nitrosomethylurea in rats of the Buffalo strain: Frequent association with thyroid disease. Endocrinology 107:1218, 1980.

69. Kimbrough RD: The toxicity of polychlorinated compounds and related chemicals. CRC Crit Rev Toxicol 2:445, 1974.

70. Klibanov AM, Tu TM, Scott KP: Peroxidase-catalyzed removal or phenols from coal-conversion waste waters. Science 221:259, 1983.

71. Kreiss K, Roberts C, Humphrey HEB: Serial PBB levels, PCB levels, and clinical chemistries in Michigan's PBB cohort. Arch Environ Health 37:141, 1982.

72. Kuratsune M, Shapiro RE (eds.): PCB Poisoning in Japan and Taiwan. Progress in Clinical and Biological Research, Vol 137, Alan R Liss, New York, 1984.

73. Langer P, Greer MA (eds.): Antithyroid Substances and Naturally Occurring Goitrogens. S Karger, Basel, 1977.

74. Lawrence WH, Tuell SF: Phthalate esters: The question of safety—an update. Clin Toxicol 15:447, 1979.

75. Leftwich RB, Floro JF, Neal RA, et al: Dinitrophenol poisoning: A diagnosis to consider in undiagnosed fever. South Med J 75:182, 1982.

76. Lim VS, Fang VS, Katz AL, et al: Thyroid dysfunction in chronic renal failure. J Clin Invest 60:522, 1977.

77. London WT, Koutras DA, Pressman A, et al: Epidemiology and metabolic studies of a goiter endemic in eastern Kentucky. J Clin Endocrinol Metab 25:1091, 1965.

78. Luthy RD, Tallon JT: Biological treatment of coal

gasification process waste water. Water Res 14:1269, 1980.

79. Marx JL: Phthalic acid esters: Biological impact uncertain. Science 178:46, 1972.

80. Maxon HR, Thomas SR, Saenger EL, et al: Ionizing irradiation and the induction of clinically significant disease in the human thyroid gland. Am J Med 63:967, 1977.

81. Mayer FL, Stalling DL, Johnson JL: Phthalate esters as environmental contaminants. Nature 238:411, 1972.

82. Merker PC, Young D, Doughty D, et al: Pharmacokinetics of resorcinol in the rat. Res Commun Chem Pathol Pharmacol 38:367, 1982.

83. Metcalf RL, Booth GM, Schuth CK, et al: Uptake and fate of di-2-ethylhexyl phthalate in aquatic organisms and in a model ecosystem. Environ Health Perspect 4:27, 1973.

84. Meyer JD, Gaitan E, Merino H, et al: Geologic implications on the distribution of goiter in Colombia, SA. Int J Epidemiol 7:25, 1978.

85. Moccia RD, Leatherland JF, Sonstegard RA: Increasing frequency of thyroid goiters in Coho salmon (Oncorhynchus kisutch) in the Great Lakes. Science 198:425, 1977.

86. Moccia RD, Leatherland JF, Sonstegard RA: Quantitative interlake comparison of thyroid pathology in Great Lakes Coho (Oncorhychus kisutch) and chinook (Oncorhynchus tschawytscha) salmon. Cancer Res 41:2200, 1981.

87. Morris SC, Moskowitz PD, Sevian WA, et al: Coal-conversion technologies: Some health and environmental effects. Science 206:654, 1979.

88. Morrison RT, Boyd RM (eds.): Organic Chemistry, 3rd ed., Allyn and Bacon, Boston, 1978.

89. Nemeth S: Short-term decrease of serum protein-bound iodine concentration after administration of 2,4-dinitro-phenol in man. J Clin Endocrinol Metab 18:225, 1958.

90. Peakall DB: Phthalate esters: Occurrence and biological effects. Residue Rev 54:1, 1975.

91. Pelkonen O, Nebert DW: Metabolism of polycyclic aromatic hydrocarbons: Etiologic role in carcinogenesis. Pharmacol Rev 34:189, 1982.

92. Pendergrast WT, Milmore BK, Marcus SC: Thyroid cancer and thyrotoxicosis in the United States. Their relationship to endemic goiter. J Chron Dis 13:22, 1961.

93. Perry H: Coal in the United States: A status report. Science 222:377, 1983.

94. Pitt WW, Jolley RL, Jones G: Characterization of organics in aqueous effluents of coal-conversion plants. Environ Int 2:167, 1979.

95. Proceedings of the Conference on PCBs: Environ Health Perspect 45:1, 1982.

96. Proceedings of the Conference on Phthalates: Environ Health Perspect 45:1, 1982.

97. Prue DM, Martin JE, Hume AS: A critical evaluation of thiocyanate as a biochemical index of smoking exposure. Behav Ther 11:368, 1980.

98. Prue DM, Martin JE, Hume AS, et al: The reliability of thiocyanate measurement of smoking exposure. Addict Behav 6:99, 1981.

99. Quentin JG, Hobson BM: Varicose ulceration of the legs and myxoedema and goiter following application of resorcinol ointment. Proc R Soc Med 44:164, 1951.

100. Rall DP: The invisible pollution. N Engl J Med 287:1146, 1972.

101. Ramirez G, Jubiz W, Gutch CF, et al: Thyroid abnormalities in renal failure: A study of 53 patients on chronic hemodialysis. Ann Intern Med 79:500, 1973.

102. Reed-Larsen P: Thyroid–pituitary interaction. N Engl J Med 306:23, 1982.

103. Ribbons WW, Evans WC: Oxidative metabolism of phthalic acid by soil pseudomonads. J Biochem 76:310, 1960.

104. Rogan WJ, Bagniewska A, Damstra T: Pollutants in breast milk. N Engl J Med 30:1450, 1980.

105. Rook JJ: Chlorination reaction of fulvic acids in natural waters. Environ Sci Tech 11:478, 1977.

106. Rosenberg N: The antithyroid activity of some compounds that inhibit peroxidase. Science 115:503, 1952.

107. Roti E, Grundi A, Braverman LE: The placental transport, synthesis and metabolism of hormones and drugs which affect thyroid function. Endocr Rev 4:11, 1983.

108. Safe Drinking Water Committee, National Research Council: Drinking Water and Health, Vol 1, National Academy Press, Washington, 1977.

109. Safe Drinking Water Committee, National Research Council: Drinking Water and Health, Vol 2, National Academy Press, Washington, 1980.

110. Safe Drinking Water Committee, National Research Council: Drinking Water and Health, Vol 3, National Academy Press, Washington, 1980.

111. Safran M, Paul TL, Roti E, et al: Environmental factors affecting autoimmune thyroid disease. Endocrinology Metab Clin North Am 16:327, 1987.

112. Saghir AR, Cowan JW, Salji JP: Goitrogenic activity of onion volatiles. Nature 211:87, 1966.

113. Saghir AR, Cowan JW, Salji JP: The molecular structure of sulphides in relation to antithyroid activity. Eur J Pharmacol 2:399, 1968.

114. Schneider AB, Favus MJ, Stachura ME, et al: Incidence, prevalence and characteristics of radiation-induced thyroid tumors. Am J Med 64:243, 1978.

115. Schnitzer M, Khan S (eds.): Humic Substances in the Environment, Marcel Dekker, New York, 1972.

116. Sonstegard R, Leatherland JF: The epizootiology and pathogenesis of thyroid hyperplasia in Coho salmon (Oncorchynchus kisutch) in Lake Ontario. Cancer Res 36:4467, 1976.

117. Stanbury JB, Hetzel B (eds.): Endemic Goiter and Endemic Cretinism, John Wiley & Son, New York, 1980.

118. Surks MI: Laboratory aids in the diagnosis of hypothyroidism. Thyroid Today 1:4, 1977.

119. Taurog A: Biosynthesis of iodoamino acids. In: Handbook of Physiology, Section 7, Vol 3, p 101, Greer MA, Solomon DH (eds.), Williams & Wilkins, Baltimore, 1974.

120. Train RE: The environment today. Science 201:320, 1978.

121. Trowbridge FL, Hand KE, Nichaman MZ: Findings relating to goiter and iodine in the ten-state nutrition survey. Am J Clin Nutr 28:712, 1975.

122. Trowbridge FL, Matovinovic J, McLaren GD, et al:

Iodine and goiter in children. Pediatrics 56:82, 1975.

123. Tunbridge WG: Screening for thyroid disease in the community. Thyroid Today 5:5, 1982.

124. Twort JM, Twort CC: Disease in relation to carcinogenic agents among 60,000 experimental mice. J Pathol Bacteriol 35:219, 1932.

125. US Committee for Energy Awareness: Energy options. C310/100, P.O. Box 37012, Washington, DC 20013, 1983.

126. Vander JB, Gaston EA, Dawber TR: The significance of nontoxic thyroid nodules. A final report of a 15-year study of the incidence of thyroid malignancy. Ann Intern Med 69:537, 1968.

127. Van Herle AJ (Moderator), Rich P, Ljung B-M E, Ashcraft MW, et al. (discussants): The thyroid nodule. Ann Intern Med 96:221, 1982.

128. Vidor GI, Stewart JC, Wall JR, et al: Pathogenesis of iodine-induced thyrotoxicosis. Studies in northern Tasmania. J Clin Endocrinol 37:901, 1973.

129. Vought RL, London WT, Stebbing GE: Endemic goiter in northern Virginia. J Clin Endocrinol Metab 27:1381, 1967.

130. Wahner HW, Cuello C, Correa P, et al: Thyroid carcinoma in an endemic goiter area, Cali Colombia. Am J Med 49:58, 1966.

131. Walfish PG: Drug and environmentally induced neonatal hypothyroidism. In: Congenital Hypothyroidism, p 303, Dussault JH, Walter P (eds.), Marcel Dekker, New York, 1983.

132. Walker CR: Pre-1972 knowledge on nonhuman effects of polychlorinated biphenyls. In: Proceedings of the National Conference on Polychlorinated Biphenyls, p 268, Environmental Protection Agency, Publ 560-6-75-004, USEPA, Washington, 1976.

133. Wayne EJ, Koutras DA, Alexander WD (eds.): Clinical Aspects of Iodine Metabolism, Blackwell Scientific, London, 1964.

134. Weetman AP, McGregor AM: Autoimmune thyroid disease: Developments in our understanding. Endocr Rev 5:309, 1984.

135. Windholz M (ed.), Budavari S (co-ed.), Blumetti RF, et al. (assoc. eds.): The Merck Index, 10th ed., E. Merck & Co., Rahway, NJ, 1983.

136. Woeber K, Ingbar SH: Antithyroid effects of noncalorigenic congeners of salicylate, with observations on the influence of serum proteins on the potency of antithyroid agents. Endocrinology 76:584, 1965.

137. Wolff J, Standaert ME, Rall J: Thyroxine displacement from the serum and depression of serum protein-bound iodine by certain drugs. J Clin Invest 40:1373, 1961.

RECOMMENDED READINGS

Gaitan E: Goitrogens. Bailliere Clin Endocrinol Metab 2:683, 1988.

Gaitan E (ed.): Environmental Goitrogenesis, CRC Press, Boca Raton, 1989.

Gaitan E: Goitrogens in food and water. Annu Rev Nutr 10:21, 1990.

23. DISORDERS OF THE IMMUNE SYSTEM

Alf Fischbein and Alyce Bezman Tarcher

INTRODUCTION

In recent years much attention has been focused on the immune system. Remarkable advances have been made in our understanding of the mechanism of action and the control of immune responses. Basic research in immunology is proceeding so rapidly that it is difficult for even the most dedicated student to keep up to date with all of the developments in the field. Coincident with this burgeoning knowledge has been an increased concern about the possible health effects of pollution.

During the past decade, a substantial number of animal studies have shown that a variety of chemicals commonly encountered in the workplace and widely distributed in the general environment are capable of inducing changes in immune function (17,26,39,46,56,68,138,160,161,178). The overall consequences of immune modulation can be categorized into two types of reactions, namely, immunosuppression and immunopotentiation (41,70,170) (Fig. 23-1). The consequences of immunosuppression range from various forms of infections to malignant diseases, whereas immunopotentiation may be associated with the development of allergic or autoimmune diseases (41,144,169).

Allergic reactions (i.e., hypersensitivity responses) are presently the most widely recognized chemically induced immunotoxic events observed clinically in humans. A large number of foreign chemicals are known to induce allergic reactions in human populations (18,71,74,118,123,125,145). In occupational settings alone, large numbers of workers develop immunologic illnesses especially affecting the lungs and skin. Such sequelae are recognized to be among the most frequent and costly health problems encountered (118). A chemically induced hypersensitivity response is not to be confused with the terms "chemical hypersensitivity syndrome," "multiple chemical sensitivities," or "total allergic syndrome." This syndrome, which is discussed in Chapters 11 and 14, is poorly defined and understood. There is no definitive evidence to date to suggest that it is immunologically mediated (38).

Except for chemically induced allergic reactions and immune dysfunction observed in a few studies of populations inadvertently exposed to environmental chemicals, there are relatively few studies that have addressed the question of whether environmental chemicals produce immunotoxic effects in humans. In light of the importance of the immune system in maintaining health, the prospect that agents inducing immune dysfunction in animals may also have insidious immunotoxic effects in humans is cause for concern. Given the release of foreign chemicals into the environment with potential for exposure to humans, immunotoxic chemicals may play a greater role in disease causation than is currently appreciated. The lack of immunotoxicity studies in man indicates a pressing need to develop strategies to assess the effects of chemical exposure

Principles and Practice of Environmental Medicine, edited by Alyce Bezman Tarcher. Plenum Medical Book Company, New York, 1992.

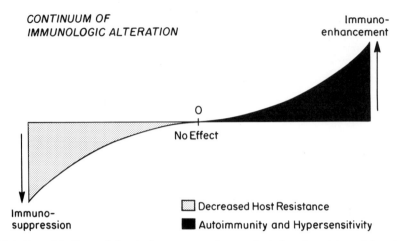

FIGURE 23-1. Potential effects of chemical exposure on immunologic function. Adapted from Bick (20).

on immune function in human populations and to extend the study of immunotoxicology from the research laboratory to the epidemiologic and clinical arenas.

This chapter is designed to provide the reader with an overview of the relationship between xenobiotic exposure and immune function and to draw attention to its potential clinical importance.

ENVIRONMENTAL AND INDUSTRIAL CHEMICALS ASSOCIATED WITH ADVERSE EFFECTS ON THE IMMUNE SYSTEM

During the past decade a growing list of diverse environmental and industrial chemicals have been reported to alter immune function (17,26,41,44,46,

68,138,161,184,187). In most instances, information on immunotoxicity in humans is incomplete and derived from studies in animals, primarily rodents. As noted previously, with the exception of agents producing allergic reactions, very few foreign chemicals have been studied for their immunotoxic potential in humans. Table 23-1 lists a few of the agents that have been reported to affect the immune system adversely in animals or in humans. It is apparent that agents with immunotoxic potential are of diverse origin and structure and are widely dispersed in the environment. A complete catalogue of drugs and chemicals reported to influence immune function can be found in a volume by Descotes (46).

The realization that many environmental chemicals can affect immune function adversely prompted the emergence of the discipline of immunotoxicol-

TABLE 23-1. Some Environmental and Industrial Agents Reported to Produce Immune Dysfunction in Animals or in Humans[a]

Agents	Examples
Metals	Arsenic, beryllium, lead, mercury, cadmium, chromium, selenium, zinc
Pesticides	Organochlorines: aldrin, DDT, mirex, lindane
	Organophosphates: parathion, methylparathion
	Carbamates: carbaryl
Halogenated aromatic hydrocarbons	Polychlorinated biphenyls (PCBs), polybrominated biphenyls (PBBs), dioxin (TCDD), dibenzofurans, hexachlorobenzene
Plasticizers and plastic monomers	Diisocyanates, organotin compounds, vinyl chloride, styrene, anhydrides, formaldehyde
Aromatic hydrocarbons	Benzene and other solvents
Aromatic amines	Benzidine
Airborne pollutants	Ozone, nitrogen dioxide, sulfur dioxide, asbestos, silica, volcanic ash, diesel engine emissions, cigarette smoke
Physical agents	Radiation

[a]Data from references 17, 26, 41, 44, 46, 68, 184, and 187.

ogy (169). Immunotoxicology deals with the adverse effects of xenobiotic exposure on the immune system and on the mechanisms involved in immunotoxicity. Research in immunotoxicology has been enhanced by use of both traditional toxicological methods and modern immunologic techniques.

One of the goals of immunotoxicology is to develop methods that assess the potential immunotoxicity of chemicals. In light of the widespread distribution of agents that are potentially immunotoxic, screening of such agents before their use or release into the environment is of importance. Because of the complexity and diverse functions of the immune system and of the varied immunotoxic reactions that may follow chemical exposure, a wide spectrum of tests are required to assess immunotoxicity (39,41,102). Table 23-2 presents examples of various tests used to detect immunotoxicity (41,163).

Assessing chemicals for their immunotoxic effects includes procedures for evaluating immunopathology, humoral immunity, cell-mediated immunity, macrophage function, and host resistance. A multitiered approach using a battery of sensitive in vivo and in vitro assays in rodents has been developed for this purpose (42,58,122,184). The initial screening or tier I testing generally includes an assessment of the major components of the immune system. This includes examining the histopathology of the spleen, thymus, bone marrow, and lymph nodes and detecting changes in cell-mediated and humoral immunity (41,102). Agents found to cause immunologic damage, at dose levels that are not overtly toxic, are further evaluated using a more comprehensive battery of tests (tier II). (See Table 23-2.)

Tier II testing examines the mechanism(s) underlying immunotoxicity. Cell-mediated immunity, humoral immunity, and nonspecific immunity are examined in depth. Since immune function is best evidenced by environmental challenge, tier II testing includes a series of assays that measure changes in host resistance to pathogens and tumor cells after chemical exposure (24,60,164). In this way information is gained about the functional reserve of the immune system. Dean and his co-workers devised a means of assessing the functional reserve of the immune system. Rodents are exposed to multiple doses of immunosuppressive chemicals. The degree of depression of certain immune functions is correlated with changes in susceptibility to challenge with infectious agents or transplantable tumors (44). Host resistance models in rodents provide the only means of assessing the functional integrity of the immune system.

Although a large number of tests are available to monitor immunotoxicity in animals, most are directed toward detecting immunosuppression. Immunopotentiation, which may result in hypersensitivity or autoimmunity, is not well addressed by animal models. At present, a reliable method for testing the hypersensitivity potential of chemicals uses the guinea pig to assess delayed hypersensitivity skin reactions (4,127). An experimental model has been developed to study sensitization to toluene diisocyanate (TDI). Guinea pigs exposed to TDI develop essentially all of the features seen in humans with TDI-induced respiratory allergy (93). Although animal models for the study of autoimmune disease have been difficult to develop, a rodent

TABLE 23-2. Tests Used for Detecting Immunotoxic Effects in Laboratory Animals[a]

Modality evaluated	Procedure
Tier I (mouse or rat)	
Immunopathology	Routine hematology, lymphoid organ weights (spleen and thymus), histology (spleen, thymus, lymph nodes), cellularity (spleen and bone marrow)
Cell-mediated immunity	
Proliferation	Mixed leukocyte response
Tumoricidal	NK[b]-cell activity
Humoral immunity	Antibody plaque-forming cell response to sheep erythrocytes (IgM) or specific immunoglobin level
Tier II (mouse only)	
Immunopathology	Quantification of lymphocyte subpopulation using surface markers (monoclonal antibody reagents)
Host-resistance challenge models	Susceptibility to transplantable syngeneic tumor (PYB6 sarcoma, B16F10 melanoma) *Listeria monocytogenes*, *Streptococcus*, or influenza virus challenge
Cell-mediated immunity	
Proliferation	Mitogen response
Tumoricidal	Cytotoxic T-cell cytolysis
Macrophage function	Phagocytosis, macrophage ectoenzyme levels

[a]From Dean et al. (41) as modified and presented by Dean et al. (44).
[b]Natural killer.

model involving exposure to mercury evidenced features of autoimmune disease with glomerulonephritis (51). Additional experimental models are needed to aid our understanding of chemically induced allergic and autoimmune disease and to permit the testing of industrial and environmental chemicals for their potential in this direction.

In summary, highly sensitive, quantitative, and reproducible immunoassays have been developed in animals to detect immunotoxicity induced by industrial and environmental chemicals. As with other forms of toxicity testing, estimating human risk from the effects observed in animals is complicated by such problems as differences in species susceptibility, differences in the route of exposure, intensity of exposure, and differences in age and nutritional status of the host. Concomitant exposure to additional agents in the workplace and general environment and variations in certain host factors further complicate extrapolations from animal experimental data. However, in light of the data now at hand, there is a general consensus that immunotoxic testing has a role in the safety assessment of xenobiotics.

EPIDEMIOLOGY

A number of clinical studies have pointed out the relationship between exposure to industrial chemicals and the development of hypersensitivity diseases. However, relatively few epidemiologic studies have assessed the immunotoxic effects of environmental and occupational chemicals. Immune function has been investigated in a few groups exposed to outdoor air pollution or pesticides or accidentally exposed to such agents as polychlorinated biphenyls, dibenzofurans, and other contaminants present in mixtures of polychlorinated biphenyls, polybrominated biphenyls, 2,3,7,8-tetrachlorodibenzo-p-dioxin (TCDD or dioxin), methyl isocyanate, and adulterated rapeseed oil (10–14,30–32,57,62,77,81,117). The immunotoxic effects of benzene are discussed in Chapter 21. Studies of immune function have also been done in groups exposed to asbestos (14,108–110,131,132). Few prospective epidemologic studies have been performed. Thus, the predictive value of immunoxic events in terms of disease development such as cancer is uncertain (11,57).

Occupational Exposures Associated with Allergic and Autoimmune Reactions

Allergic Asthma and Contact Skin Allergy

It is well recognized that immunologic illness occurring in an occupational setting notably afflicts the respiratory tract and the skin. Allergic reactions affecting the lung are reflected in the onset of asthma and hypersensitivity pneumonitis. In the skin, they are manifest as urticaria and contact sensitivity. Studies of various occupational exposures have linked a wide variety of industrial agents in the development of immune-mediated asthma and hypersensitivity lung disease (18,27,33,74,139,140, 145,156,157,193). Early reports cited plant and animal proteins as causal agents. As new materials are introduced into the workplace and general environment, the list of agents capable of inducing respiratory disorders based on immunologic mechanisms continues to grow (Table 23-3). The incidence of asthma induced by low-molecular-weight organic or inorganic chemicals is rapidly increasing (18,19, 27,74,145,156). In addition, a wide variety of industrial and environmental chemicals such as metals and solvents may cause cutaneous contact hypersensitivity reactions (1,125). A further discussion of cutaneous hypersensitivity is found in Chapter 15.

Glomerulonephritis

There is evidence that mercury exposure in humans may result in glomerulonephritis mediated through an autoimmune response. Membranous glomerulonephritis, which implies immunologically mediated disease, has been reported in mercury-exposed workers (50,96,180). Membranous glomerulonephritis has also been observed in cases of mercury poisoning or exposure to mercury-containing drugs or cosmetics (61).

There is also some evidence to suggest that solvent-induced glomerulonephritis may occur in humans and that it may be immunologically mediated. Case reports have linked Goodpasture's syndrome, characterized in part by proliferative and extracapillary glomerulonephritis, to solvent exposure in an occupational setting (98). The glomerulonephritis found in this syndrome is associated with circulating and tissue-bound antibodies to glomerular basement membrane (79). Other clinical reports have noted the importance of solvent exposure in patients with chronic glomerulonephritis (9,53,107,198).

Scleroderma-like Syndrome

Although nonmalignant liver function abnormalities and hemangiosarcoma of the liver have been reported in vinyl chloride polymerization workers, a scleroderma-like syndrome has been described. This illness was found to occur in genetically susceptible exposed individuals (23).

TABLE 23-3. Chemical Agents Causing Occupational Asthma[a]

Agent	Irritant	Pharmacological	Immunologic
		Mechanism	
Organic chemicals			
Amines (ethylene diamine and paraphenylenediamine)	?		?
Formaldehyde	+		?
Diisocyanates	?	+	+
Phthalic anhydride	?		
Plexiglas dust	?		
Sulfone chloramines	?	+	+
Sulfone chloramide	?	+	+
Trimellitic anhydride	+		+
Polyvinyl chloride (phthalic anhydride)	?		+
Carmine (coccus cactus extract)	?		
Furan binders (furfurol alcohol resin containing paraformaldehyde)	?		
Plicatic acid (wood dusts)		+	+
Colophony (vegetable gums and resins)		+	+
Plant enzymes (papain)			+
Microbial enzymes (*Bacillus subtilis*)			+
Bromelin			+
Pancreatin			+
Antibodies and pharmaceuticals			
Cimetidine		?	
Penicillins (ampicillin, benzyl penicillin, 6-aminopenicillic acid)			?
Phenyl glycine acid hydrochloride			+
Spiramycin			?
Sulfathiazole powder			?
Sulfathiazine			?
Tetracycline			?
Inorganic chemicals			
Chromium salts?	?		?
Nickel salts			+
Platinum salts		?	+
Amprolium hydrochloride	?		
Stainless steel fumes (chromium, nickel)	?		?
Ethylene oxide gas			+
Chloramine			+
Metabisulfites	?	?	?
Aluminum soldering flux (amino ethylethanolamine)	?		

[a]From Salvaggio et al. (157).

Environmental Exposures Associated with Allergic Reactions

Inhalation Allergies

The extent and potential risk to the general population of allergic reactions induced by environmental pollutants is unknown and difficult to determine. It is noteworthy that observers are beginning to note an increase in inhalation allergies in industrialized countries (5,92,134,136,174).

Before 1950, allergic rhinitis caused by cedar pollens was extremely rare in Japan. Epidemiologic studies in the past three decades reveal that the incidence of this disorder has increased dramatically. Allergic rhinitis caused by pollens is much higher among school children in urban districts with high levels of automobile exhaust than in less-polluted districts. In 1980 the prevalence of allergic rhinitis in children living in highly polluted areas reached 33% (92).

The striking increase that occurred in urban areas with high levels of air pollutants coincided with a rapid growth in the number of diesel cars used in Japan. The increase in allergic rhinitis appeared even though the pollen count of Japanese cedar is much lower in urban than in rural areas (134). The link between the development of IgE-mediated allergic response and exposure to air pollutants is also raised by the findings of other epidemiologic studies. In these studies IgE concentration in the serum of healthy children from polluted areas was higher than that found in less-polluted areas (16,76).

Cigarette Smoking and Hypersensitivity Reactions

A number of surveys have reported increased IgE levels in smokers. In addition, smokers in a number of different occupational settings are much more likely than nonsmokers to have increased IgE antibody production in conjunction with the development of asthmatic symptoms. Occupational allergens include such agents as coffee bean dust, phthalic anhydride present in plastics-manufacturing plants, and bacterial enzymes used in the production of detergents (75,82,83,128,133,142,183,197).

Environmental and Occupational Exposure Accidents Associated with Changes in Immune Function

During the past 15 years episodes of environmental contamination resulted in human exposure to a number of halogenated aromatic hydrocarbons that are reported to be immunotoxic in animals. These exposure accidents permitted the immunologic evaluation of exposed individuals.

Polybrominated Biphenyls

In 1973, in the state of Michigan, a mixture of polybrominated biphenyls (PBBs) was mistakenly added to a special feed supplement for lactating cows. This accident, in which 500 to 1000 lb of PBBs were accidently substituted for a magnesium oxide feed supplement, resulted in widespread contamination and disease of livestock and the death of large numbers of farm animals. Widespread pollution of the food chain occurred, with dairy farmers and their families being most heavily exposed. Contaminated meat and dairy products continued to be distributed throughout the state of Michigan for a number of months before the extent of the problem was fully appreciated (95,195).

In 1976, Bekesi et al. investigated the effects of PBB exposure on the immune system of Michigan dairy farmers. When compared with Wisconsin farm families, the Michigan dairy farmers exhibited abnormalities in a number of immune parameters (10–14). A decrease in the number of circulating T lymphocytes, a concomitant increase of T lymphocytes without detectable membrane surface markers (null cells), and a reduced response to antigen stimulation were observed.

When the Michigan farm residents were reexamined in 1981, the immunologic abnormalities were found to persist (14). Low numbers of T lymphocytes with impaired function were observed in Michigan dairy farmers some 8 years after their initial exposure to PBB. Immunologic abnormalities clustered in families. There were significant correlations between the prevalence of neurological, musculoskeletal, dermatologic, and gastrointestinal symptoms and immunologic findings. Although no correlation was found between immune dysfunction and PBB serum concentration, which ranged between 0.6 and 70 ppb, the PBB content of white blood cells, particularly in the apolipoprotein-B fraction, appeared to correlate with the most severe immune dysfunction (150). It is noteworthy that the toxic chemicals were detected in the target cells. This finding explained why the serum concentration of PBBs did not correlate with pathophysiological events.

Polychlorinated Biphenyls and Related Substances

The ingestion of contaminated rice oil resulted in two outbreaks of accidental human exposure to polychlorinated biphenyls (PCBs), polychlorinated dibenzofurans (PCDFs), and polychlorinated quaterphenyls (PCQs). Over 1000 people were poisoned in Japan in 1968, and over 2000 people were poisoned in Taiwan in 1979. According to estimates, the total amount of PCBs, PCDFs, and PCQs consumed in Japan was, on the average, 633 mg, 3.4 mg, and 596 mg, respectively (105). In Taiwan, the average total intake of PCBs was estimated to range from 0.77 to 1.8 mg. In both episodes the clinical manifestations included chloracne, pigmentation of the skin, nails, and mucous membranes, swelling of the eyelids, jaundice, fever, and numbness of the limbs. Based on the evidence provided by many investigators, PCDFs are now considered the primary cause of Japanese "Yusho" (oil disease) and Taiwanese "Yu-Cheng" (oil disease) (104). Based on these findings, "PCB poisoning" may not be the correct term for the conditions.

Immunologic studies were also performed on exposed individuals in both the Japanese and Taiwanese incidents. In Japan, Shigematsu et al. studied patients with "PCB poisoning." In 1970, 2 years after exposure, the patients were noted to have a decreased level of serum IgA and IgM and an increased level of IgG. The levels had returned to normal on retesting in 1972. The incidence of respiratory symptoms, which included cough, expectoration, and wheezing, correlated well with the concentration of PCBs in the blood (106,165).

In a study of similarly exposed individuals in Taiwan, Chang noted that suppression of cellular immunity, as assessed by response to recall antigens, was significantly correlated with the severity of the dermal lesions induced by PCB exposure (32). Additional studies revealed the PCB-poisoned individuals had a decreased percentage of active T cells, and a reduction in serum IgA and IgM levels, but normal serum IgG levels (30). Four years after exposure, Yu-Cheng patients were found to have a lower T-helper/T-suppressor ratio than did the controls (106,117). In both episodes, exposure appears to have been to multiple compounds, and the precise association between agent(s) and immune dysfunction is difficult to establish.

2,3,7,8-Tetrachlorodibenzo-*p*-dioxin

In 1976, an industrial accident in Seveso, in northern Italy, released a cloud containing 2,3,7,8-tetrachlorodibenzodioxin (TCDD or dioxin) over a wide area. This resulted in contamination of the surrounding farmland and exposure of the residents and farm animals. The total amount of TCDD in the contaminated areas was estimated to be about 300 g. A few days after this disaster, domestic animals began to die, and cases of dermatitis appeared, particularly in children. A portion of the population received sufficient exposure to TCDD to produce chloracne, a skin condition characteristic of exposure to certain halogenated aromatic compounds.

Immunologic studies were performed on 45 children who were present in the area maximally exposed to dioxin. Twenty of these children, ranging in age from 3 to 7 years, had chloracne. Immunologic testing began in 1976 and was repeated several times over a 5-year period. Serum immunoglobulins were found to be normal. Increased complement hemolytic activity was consistently present and higher in cases of chloracne, whereas in vitro lymphoproliferative responses were not consistently increased (148).

In 1971, sludge wastes contaminated with TCDD were mixed with waste oils and sprayed for dust control in various locations in the state of Missouri. No action was taken to reduce dioxin exposure at any of the locations until 1982. The residents at the Quail Run Mobile Home were selected for study because high levels of dioxins (up to 2200 ppb) were found at this site. A comprehensive medical evaluation, which included studies of cellular immune function, was performed on 154 individuals who lived in the dioxin-contaminated mobile park for at least 6 months between 1971 and 1983. A similar number of unexposed persons were also studied. The exposed group was reported to have an increased frequency of anergy and altered T-lymphocyte subsets but no excess of clinical illness such as prolonged or repeated infections (81). When a nonrepresentative sample of the persons with depressed cellular immunity were reexamined in 1986, no evidence of anergy was found. Other immunologic parameters generally remained the same (57).

In another study Webb et al. measured adipose tissue levels of TCDD in 51 individuals with a history of TCDD exposure in residential, recreational, or occupational settings (192). No anergy was found, even in those subjects with adipose tissue levels of TCDD greater than 60 ppt. Altered T-lymphocyte subsets were found in 7 of 12 individuals with TCDD greater than 60 ppt. No evidence of clinical immunosupression (e.g., increase in the frequency of infectious disease, antibiotic use, weight loss, or lymphadenopathy) was found.

Methyl Isocyanate

In 1984, a runaway chemical reaction at a chemical factory in Bhopal, India released a gas cloud composed of methyl isocyanate. The eyes and respiratory tract of exposed individuals were most severely affected (45). Deo et al. performed immunologic studies on 67 individuals who received sufficient methyl isocyanate exposure to cause conjunctivitis, breathlessness, temporary unconsciousness, and, in some instances, pulmonary edema and skin rashes. An increase in the number of T-helper lymphocytes and total T cells but a decrease in lymphocyte mitogenesis were noted when compared with controls (45).

Spanish Toxic Oil Syndrome

In 1981 in Spain, large numbers of individuals living in the northwest region of Madrid became ill after consuming adulterated rapeseed oil (29,97). The rapeseed oil, denatured with anilines and intended only for industrial use, was imported into Spain. Because of its low price, some companies (illegally) attempted to remove the anilines and sold the oil for human use. Although there is no definite proof, many of the clinical, pathological, and laboratory features of the toxic oil syndrome have allergic and autoimmune characteristics. In spite of intensive efforts, a search for the specific agent(s) causing the problem has been unsuccessful (72).

The acute phase of the syndrome, which appeared some 2 to 3 weeks after the ingestion of the toxic oil, affected about 20,000 people. Those afflicted developed a wide spectrum of symptoms and signs. These included rashes, fever, itching, gastrointestinal symptoms, interstitial pneumonitis, and pleuropericarditis; facial edema, arthralgias, myalgias, intrahepatic cholestasis, eosinophilia, and thrombocytopenia were also found. Although a few patients died of thromboembolic episodes, most recovered from the acute phase, which appeared to be self-limited. Three to 4 months after the onset of the toxic oil syndrome, about 15% of those affected developed a new set of serious problems. This chronic phase was characterized by a neuromuscular syndrome with peripheral neuropathy and inflammatory myopathy, a scleroderma-like syndrome, Sjögren's syndrome, Raynaud phenomenon, acroosteolysis, and pulmonary hypertension. Women were more frequently afflicted with the chronic phase of the toxic oil syndrome (72,89,97,176).

Although the clinical picture of the toxic oil syndrome varied widely, the pathology, in both the early and late phases of the illness, was characterized by a nonnecrotizing vasculitis. The vasculitis involved all types of vessels and was associated with perivascular, medial, and intimal infiltration with mononuclear cells and eosinophils (126).

Immunologic studies during the acute phase of the toxic oil syndrome showed the presence of elevated nonspecific IgE antibody levels. Subsequent studies failed to demonstrate specific IgE antibodies against agents suspected of having contaminated the ingested rapeseed oil (25). Marked eosinophilia was present in 50% to 98% of the patients during the early months of the illness. The total number of lymphocytes and T-helper cells were normal, but a decrease in T-suppressor cells was noted. During the course of the disease many different types of autoantibodies were detected. During the early phase of the illness higher levels of antinuclear, antilymphocyte, and anticollagen antibodies were detected than during the chronic phase (72). In the chronic phase of the toxic oil syndrome, the presence of antibodies was not related to the severity of the disease (72).

Pesticides

In 1986, the immune responses of 27 women with chronic exposure to aldicarb from contaminated ground water were compared with those of 27 women whose drinking water had come from an uncontaminated source. The estimated aldicarb ingestion was 0.3 to 48.2 µg/day. The exposed group was found to have increased numbers of T-suppressor lymphocytes and a decreased ratio of T-helper to T-suppressor lymphocytes. Thus, with aldicarb exposure, the T-helper to T-suppressor ratio was low because of an absolute increase in the number of T-suppressor cells. There was no other clinical evidence of immunodeficiency in the aldicarb-exposed subjects (62).

Evidence of immune-associated hemolytic anemia in an individual exposed to the pesticide dieldrin has been reported. Blood analysis revealed antidieldrin antibodies bound to red blood cells. This phenomenon was presumed to be related to the autoimmune destruction of the red blood cells (77).

Asbestos

Asbestos-induced disease has emerged as a major occupational and public health problem in many countries during the 20th century. It is overwhelmingly apparent that asbestos exposure is implicated in the development of malignant diseases such as lung cancer and malignant pleural and peritoneal mesothelioma(s) in addition to other nonmalignant conditions, i.e., interstitial pulmonary fibrosis (asbestosis) and pleural thickening and calcification (159). A series of clinical studies has revealed a variety of alterations in humoral and cellular immune responses in patients with asbestos-related diseases and in asymptomatic individuals exposed to airborne asbestos (28,49,87,88,131,155,190).

The most consistent responses have been decreased cell-mediated immunity and increased humoral immunity. Impaired expressions of cellular immunity include anergy to recall antigens, depressed total circulating T lymphocytes, inverted T-helper/T-suppressor ratio, and reduced lymphocyte responsiveness to phytohemagglutinin (PHA), concanavalin A (Con A), and pokeweed mitogen (PWM) (47,78,87,132). Hyperactive humoral immune responses are reflected in increased immunoglobulins, nonspecific autoantibodies, and the presence of rheumatoid factor(s) (85,108–110,147,181,196).

Investigations of the primary host immune response [i.e., natural killer (NK)-cell activity] in patients with asbestos exposure have shown that over half of 20 patients with malignant mesothelioma had profound deficiency in NK-cell activity that correlated with their clinical course. It is unclear whether the impairment of NK-cell activity is a contributing factor in the pathogenesis of asbestos-associated diseases (112). Impairment in the activity of NK cells in asbestos-exposed workers has also been reported by others. These abnormalities were not correlated with age, smoking history, or duration of exposure but were associated with chest x-ray evidence of asbestos-associated effects (179).

Summary

In summary, epidemiologic studies increasingly point to a link between exposure to occupational and environmental chemicals and changes in the immune response. Thus far, except for hypersensitivity reactions, there are little data to support or refute the clinical relevance of immunologic changes induced by exposure to chemicals. The potential for immunosuppression is suggested from the study of populations exposed to halogenated hydrocarbons, asbestos, and benzene, whereas the potential for immunopotentiation is reflected in the toxic-oil syndrome induced by adulterated rapeseed oil.

Assessing the immunologic effects of exposure and determining the associated health effects are complex problems that warrant intensified efforts. With low levels of exposure in particular, changes in immune function are likely to be subtle and therefore difficult to measure. The long-term effects of immune dysfunction must also be addressed, especially the question of whether environmentally induced immunosuppression is associated with increased susceptibility to infection and cancer. Populations with past exposure to PCBs, PCDFs, PBB, and TCDD thus require continued epidemiologic surveillance. Epidemiologic investigations of immunotoxic effects of chemical exposure on populations with a particularly vulnerable immune system (i.e., fetus, infant, aged, and malnourished) are also of great importance.

PATHOLOGICAL PHYSIOLOGY

In a relatively short period of time enormous progress has been made in understanding the basic components of the immune system and its structure, function, and secretory products. A brief review of this complex system is presented with a view to helping the reader understand the mechanisms potentially involved in the development of immunotoxic phenomena.

The Immune System

The immune system (15,20,84,141,143,153,154) comprises a network of cellular components widely dispersed throughout the body. To protect the host against microorganisms and the development and spread of cancer, the immune system undergoes continued renewal, activation, and differentiation. The overall responsiveness of the immune system is governed by the genetic capabilities of the host; amplified and regulated by the action of lymphocytes, macrophages (and related cells), and their secretory products; and moderated by signals from the endocrine and nervous systems.

Immune function is carried out by lymphocytes and by accessory cell populations, including macrophages and a series of related cells. The cells involved in the immune response are found in organized organs and tissues termed the lymphoid system. The lymphoid system can be divided into primary or central and secondary or peripheral lymphoid organs.

In the primary lymphoid organs, the bone marrow and thymus, lymphocytes are generated and differentiated into functional T and B lymphocytes. The thymus produces T lymphocytes, and the bone marrow and fetal liver produce B lymphocytes, both of which migrate to the secondary lymphoid organs. The secondary lymphoid organs include the lymph nodes, spleen, and mucosal-associated lymphoid tissue. Here, lymphocytes react with each other, with antigens, with antigen-presenting cells,

and with secretory products to produce an immune response. Figure 23-2 shows the cellular components of the immune system and their functions.

Apart from the lymphocytes, the cellular populations involved in the immune response form the mononuclear phagocyte system. Cells of the mononuclear phagocyte lineage, formerly assigned to the reticuloendothelial system, are related by origin, morphology, and function. They consist of monocytes and macrophages, fixed tissue histiocytes, dendritic cells, Langerhans cells, and Kupffer cells. Though highest in concentration in lymph nodes and spleen, these cells are present in the blood and in all tissues including the portals of entry, i.e., the respiratory, gastrointestinal, and genitourinary tracts as well as the skin. Cells of the mononuclear phagocytic system play a vital role in the immune response by acting as antigen-presenting cells that capture and process microorganisms for presentation to antigen-sensitive lymphocytes. Phagocytic macrophages also play a role in inflammation and in the removal of foreign materials.

Immune defenses are formed by two interrelated tiers. The first tier is a nonspecific innate immune response. The second tier is a specific adaptive immune response. The innate immune response is characterized by phagocytosis and the inflammatory reaction. These responses involve phagocytes, natural killer cells, and such chemical mediators as complement components, vasoactive amines, lysosomal enzymes, and lymphocyte products. If the nonspecific part of the immune defense proves inadequate, the adaptive immune defense is initiated. The adaptive immune response leads to the recognition of and specific reaction against each infectious agent. It depends on an encounter between antigens from the invading microbe and cells of the immune system, i.e., lymphocytes and macrophages.

Two interrelated immune reactions, mediated through different populations of lymphocytes, pinpoint the immunologic assault. Humoral immunity, characterized by the production and secretion of antigen-specific antibodies, is carried out by plasma cells of the B-lymphocyte series. Cell-mediated immunity depends on thymus-derived or T lymphocytes (T cells). These cells secrete a variety of factors known collectively as lymphokines, which are of importance in mediating the immune response. T cells are effectors of cellular defense and fundamental regulators of immune function.

The T lymphocytes contain various specialized subpopulations, which include one subset known as the CD8 or T8 suppressor/cytotoxic T lymphocytes and another subset known as CD4 or T4-positive helper/inducer T lymphocytes. The regulatory function of T lymphocytes, though modified by the genetic capabilities of the host, includes their

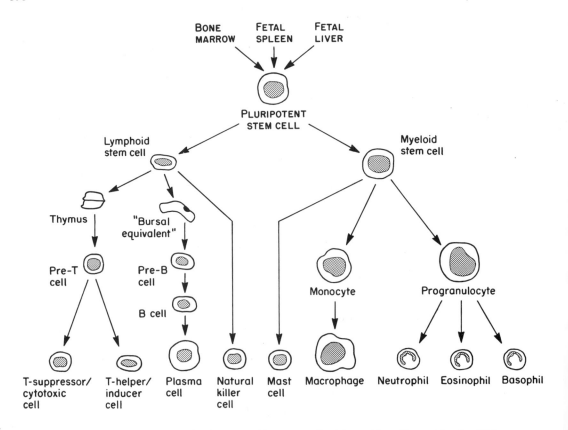

FIGURE 23-2. Origin and development of immune cells. Adapted from Vos and Luster (187).

ability to stimulate cell-mediated cytotoxicity by other T cells and immunoglobulin production by plasma cells, which are the mature cells of the B-cell series. In addition to stimulating immune responses, T cells also have the ability to suppress immune responses.

The immune response involves a series of carefully orchestrated and controlled events built on specificity, memory, and the recognition of self and nonself. A detailed account of immune function is beyond the scope of this chapter. The reader is referred to several books and articles for a more extensive discussion of this topic (15,20,84,141, 143,153,154).

Immune System as a Target for Toxicity

The immune system, with its varied cellular make-up, its wide dispersion throughout the body, and its complex function, provides immunotoxic agents with a vast number of potential targets. Foreign chemicals may adversely affect the organs in which the constituents of the immune system originate or reside, i.e., the bone marrow, thymus, spleen, lymph nodes, and mucosal-associated lymphoid tissue, or the actual cells, the macrophages, monocytes, natural killer cells, lymphocytes of various types, and their subsets. Xenobiotics may also affect the intercellular interactions and molecular events that underlie the immune response (17, 26,41,44,56,68).

Xenobiotics differ widely in their immunotoxic effects. Some agents affect one immunocyte population more than others, whereas other agents selectively injure discrete lymphoid organs (i.e., thymus or bone marrow). Some chemicals may have competitive effects on immune cells and processes. Other agents, particularly drugs, may modify immunotoxic events by modulating the various steps in immune expression. In addition, a single chemical can exert diverse immunomodulatory effects by selectively compromising a particular component or several components of the immune response. The type of immunologic injury induced by a xenobiotic can also vary markedly with the dose. It has been observed, for example, that some agents cause immunosuppression or immunostimulation depending on the dose or duration of exposure (102,121,

162,163,170,171,194). Immunotoxicity is also markedly affected by such host factors as gender, nutrition, age, stress, neuroendocrine status, concomitant disease, and genetic make up (2,135,166). The immune system and the role of nutrition on immune function are discussed in Chapter 10.

The remarkable functional reserve of the immune system allows immunotoxic chemicals to alter one or more components of the immune response without compromising immune function enough to affect host defenses against infections or malignant disease (44). The extent of this functional reserve determines the point at which chemically induced immune modulation leads to increased host susceptibility (43). In contrast to such organs as the heart and kidney, the widespread dispersion, cellular complexity, and rapid regenerative capacity of the immune system make assessment of its functional reserve unusually difficult. However, determination of functional reserve and degree of reversibility is essential in assessing immunotoxicity.

Adverse Immune Reactions Induced by Chemicals

In some instances, agents affect the immune system directly and preferentially, thereby modulating the immune response. In other instances, a foreign chemical may evoke a specific immune response or induce a reaction against the body's own constituents (autoimmunity). As previously noted, the consequences of immune modulation may be immunosuppression or immunoenhancement (70) (Fig. 23-1). Immunosuppression may be followed by

increased susceptibility to infectious and to neoplastic disease (41,144). Immunoenhancement, although not necessarily followed by an adverse outcome, may increase the likelihood of allergic or autoimmune reactions (21,22,41,70,91,102,163,184).

Chemically induced autoimmune and allergic diseases have features in common. The border between them may at times be unclear. In both cases, genetically controlled mechanisms allow the immune system to react to chemical exposure with responses that cause tissue injury. However, chemically induced allergic and autoimmune reactions can be distinguished from each other. In cases of allergy, the injurious immune response is confined to the offending exogenous agent encountered in the tissue, whereas in chemically induced autoimmunity, the injurious immune response is not confined to the chemical instigating the response but also involves responses to self-antigens (70).

Mechanisms of Immunotoxicity

Immunotoxic agents may adversely affect immune function by the following general mechanisms: (1) destruction of immune cells or disruption of their renewal and maturation, (2) interference with cellular immunocompetence, (3) interference with immunoregulatory processes dependent on intercellular interaction and the elaboration of soluble factors, and (4) indirect alteration of immune function by effecting changes in neuroendocrine status (40,163,170,171,184). Potential mechanisms by which xenobiotics may modulate the immune response are shown in Table 23-4.

TABLE 23-4. Immunotoxic Mechanisms Potentially Involved
in the Modulation of the Immune Response

Destruction of immune cells or disruption of their renewal and maturation affects:
  The production and/or differentiation of precursor immunocytes
  Cells needed in the development of lymphoid cells (e.g., thymic epithelial cells and their products)
  The absolute or relative number of helper, suppressor, and/or effector immune cells (T, B lymphocytes; monocytes–
    macrophages; NK (natural killer) cells, and others) in lymphoid organs and/or in other peripheral sites
  Platelets and neutrophils
Interference with cellular immunocompetence affects:
  Antigen distribution and/or persistence in the body
  Antigen processing by accessory cells (i.e., macrophages)
  Antigen presentation to lymphocytes
  Activation-thresholds of immunocytes to antigen
  Growth-differentiating factors (e.g., expression of receptors for lymphokines)
  Routing and recirculation of immunocytes
Interference with immunoregulatory processes affects:
  The production, release, and/or metabolism of immune mediators (e.g., lymphokines and cytokines)
  Other substances modulating immune cell function
  The quantity, quality, persistence, and distribution of effector–regulatory immune products (e.g., antibody, comple-
    ment)
Indirect effects on immune function affect:
  Neuroendocrine status

---

[a]From Dean et al. (44) and Spreafico (170).

Immunosuppression, for example, may be achieved not only through the depletion or inhibition of immunocompetent cells but also by stimulating the effect of immunocytes engaged in down-regulating the immune response (170). In light of the subtle immune events that may accompany xenobiotic exposure, viewing immunotoxic responses in terms of immunosuppression or immunopotentiation is an arbitrary division that is frequently quite blurred (170). Thus, immunotoxic events, by influencing regulatory mechanisms, may transform an immunosuppressive response to one of immunopotentiation or reverse this process.

As previously noted, chemically induced toxicity of the immune system may be reflected in allergic and autoimmune diseases. Under these conditions, inflammatory immune responses, which ordinarily play a central role in protecting the body from foreign antigens, give rise to tissue injury. These immune responses are involved in the immunopathogenesis of many human diseases (64). Although the mechanisms by which immunotoxic chemicals induce allergic and autoimmune reactions are poorly understood, the following general events may take place: (1) a low-molecular-weight chemical normally incapable of inducing an immune response becomes capable of inducing an immune response by acting as a hapten that combines with serum or tissue proteins; (2) a hapten bound to a structural antigen leads to the creation of a new antigenic determinant, which is then recognized as nonself by the immune system; and (3) a foreign chemical may act by dysregulating the immune system (21,50,91).

It should be noted that apparently healthy persons commonly exhibit autoimmune reactions. The appearance of serum autoantibodies therefore does not necessarily imply the existence of autoimmune disease. The production of autoantibodies may have little clinical impact and indeed may even be viewed as an inherent condition of the normal immune system (158).

In some instances, the application of modern immunologic techniques has uncovered mechanisms involved in the development of chemically induced allergic and autoimmune reactions. The discovery that low-molecular-weight chemicals, acting as haptens, acquire a sensitizing potential after combining with carrier molecules has aided our understanding of allergic asthma induced by certain occupational chemicals (18,71,145). Such haptens include phthalic anhydride, trimellitic anhydride, toluene diisocyanate (TDI), and methylene diphenyl diisocyanate (MDI), as well as nickel, platinum, and chromium salts (18,71,74,157). Animal models developed for the study of the respiratory effects of isocyanate sensitivity have been useful (93,94).

Chemically induced autoimmune reactions,

particularly those linked to drugs, have drawn the attention of a number of investigators (21,70,90,91). A growing list of drugs and chemicals has been implicated in the formation of autoantibodies and autoimmune disease in humans, yet little is known about the autoimmunizing potential of occupational and environmental chemicals (21,91). A recently developed model of mercury-induced autoimmune glomerulonephritis in genetically susceptible rodents has been useful in studying autoimmune reactions induced by metals (51). Although research into chemically induced autoimmune reactions is being actively pursued, and many possible mechanisms are being proposed, the means by which chemical compounds induce autoimmune disease remain largely obscure (3,21,69).

Classification of Adverse Immune Reactions on the Basis of Their Pathogenesis

In contrast to our relatively limited grasp of the mechanisms that underlie chemically induced immunotoxic tissue injury, considerable progress has been made in elucidating the pathogenesis of allergic and autoimmune disease (86,158,168,172). In 1963, Gell and Coombs classified immunologically mediated adverse tissue reactions into four major types (67). The simplified classification provides a useful framework for organizing concepts about the immunopathogenesis of tissue injury. It does not imply that only one such response will be operating in an individual.

Type I, allergic, reaginic, or immediate hypersensitivity is observed when certain antigens or haptens bound to protein stimulate the production of IgE antibodies. The binding of antigen to IgE antibodies at the surface of mast cells and basophils results in the liberation of histamine, leukotrienes, and other mediators that are responsible for such allergic phenomena as urticaria, seasonal rhinitis, asthma, and anaphylactic reactions. There is evidence that foreign chemicals similarly induce the formation of IgE antibodies in humans and in experimental animals. Some industrial chemicals that are known or presumed to cause immunologic lung disease are acid anhydrides, isocyanates, and pyrolysis products of polyvinyl chloride (15,64,153).

Type II, cytotoxic antibody reaction, is characterized by the destruction of cells after binding with specific antibodies. The accumulation of inflammatory cells (neutrophils), together with complement activation, leads to the destruction of target cells. The destruction of tissues in Goodpasture's syndrome in autoimmune hemolytic anemia and immune-mediated thrombocytopenia of systemic lupus erythematosus are examples of cytotoxic hypersensitivity (15,64,153).

Type III, immune complex reaction, is characterized by the deposition of circulating immune complexes in tissues. This is a common feature of rheumatic disorders. The introduction of large amounts of antigen, as occurs after the administration of heterologous serum, may be followed by a serum sickness reaction. This condition entails the deposition of circulating immune complexes in the walls of small blood vessels. There are several descriptions of glomerular lesions (membranous glomerulonephritis) in humans and animals following exposure to mercury and gold (15,50,64,69,153).

Type IV, cell-mediated delayed hypersensitivity, may follow the interaction of antigen with T lymphocytes. This designation is related to the kinetics of the inflammatory process following the deposition of antigen in the skin. Allergic reactions occur within seconds to minutes of exposure, whereas delayed-type hypersensitivity reactions peak at 48 to 72 h after the intradermal deposition of antigen. This response is encountered in cases of allergic contact dermatitis. Delayed hypersensitivity reactions may occur following sensitization to a variety of chemicals including nickel, chromium, organomercurials, perfumes, hair dyes, resin, dyes in clothing, pesticides, photographic chemicals, and a wide variety of industrial chemicals (15,64,153).

Experimental Studies of Immunotoxicity

Most research in immunotoxicology has focused on the immunosuppressive action of environmental chemicals in animal models. In some cases the underlying mechanisms have been well defined; in most cases, however, the site(s) of action and the biochemical processes that form the basis of immunotoxic injury are poorly understood. In contrast to the large number of experiments dealing with immunosuppression, relatively few laboratory studies have investigated the allergic and autoimmunizing potential of foreign chemicals. The gap stems from the difficulty experienced in developing animal models for this purpose. The guinea pig model of skin sensitization has been a prime example of an animal model used to study delayed hypersensitivity. Only recently have animal models been developed to study chemically induced respiratory allergy and autoimmune disease (50,51, 93,178).

Of interest are the studies of Miyamoto et al. (134). These workers showed that the IgE antibody response is enhanced in mice after immunization, either intraperitoneally or intranasally, with antigens together with diesel exhaust particles. These findings suggest that, after being inhaled, atmospheric particles may exert an adjuvant effect for IgE antibody production. These results may also help to explain the increased incidence of allergic rhinitis

to cedar pollen that has taken place in Japan in relation to increased air pollution from diesel car exhausts (134).

The following discussion focuses on the classes of environmental chemicals that show evidence of immunotoxicity. These classes include polycyclic aromatic hydrocarbons, polyhalogenated aromatic hydrocarbons, heavy metals, pesticides, and inhaled pollutants. The list of chemicals reported to influence the integrity of the immune system is continually growing. The immunotoxic effects of industrial chemicals, pesticides, air pollutants, and drugs have been reviewed by a number of authors (41,46,55,60,65,66,99,100–103,111,114,124,163,184, 186,187,191).

Polycyclic Aromatic Hydrocarbons

Polycyclic aromatic hydrocarbons (PAHs), which arise from fossil fuels, motor vehicle exhaust, and refuse burning, are widely dispersed in the environment. Human exposure to these agents occurs through breathing polluted air and ingesting contaminated food and water (see Chapters 2–4).

The PAHs have been shown to be immunosuppressive in animal studies. Their immunosuppressive effects were observed especially in relation to the production of specific antibodies. The age of the animal at the time of exposure appears related to the degree of immunosuppression. Of interest is that many carcinogenic PAHs are noted to be immunosuppressive, whereas their noncarcinogenic analogues are not. Studies of host resistance following exposure to benzo[a]pyrene, a potent tumor initiator, showed no evidence of increased susceptibility to tumor challenge or infection (121,191). However, most PAHs seem to affect humoral immunity.

Polyhalogenated Aromatic Hydrocarbons

Polyhalogenated aromatic hydrocarbons (PHAs) are a family of compounds widely dispersed throughout the occupational and general environment. they are industrial chemicals that arise in the manufacture of pesticides and phenols. Some halogenated biphenyls are no longer manufactured in the United States but may still be encountered in the environment. These agents have been used in plasticizers, as flame retardants, and as heat transfer agents. The PHAs have evidenced considerable toxicity in experimental animals, and there is concern about their carcinogenic potential in human populations. The PHAs include such compounds as polychlorinated biphenyls (PCBs), polybrominated biphenyls (PBBs), and 2,3,7,8-tetrachlorodibenzo-*p*-dioxin (TCDD or dioxin).

Some investigators have shown that certain congeners of PCBs suppress immune responses in animals. Experimental exposure to some PCBs commonly leads to atrophy of the primary and secondary lymphoid organs. There is also evidence of depressed humoral immunity, decreased specific antibody responses, and decreased host resistance to a number of infectious agents. The PCBs have been reported both to augment and to suppress cell-mediated immunity (40,115,167,185,189).

Animals experimentally exposed to PBBs have shown immunosuppression. There is suppression of antibody responses as well as a reduction of delayed-type hypersensitivity. It should be noted that the effects on cell-mediated immunity occur at or near exposure levels that produce signs of more generalized toxicity. However, PBB-exposed mice failed to evidence decreased resistance to infectious challenge (63,119).

The immunotoxic effects of 2,3,7,8-tetrachlorodibenzo-p-dioxin (TCDD) have been extensively investigated. In common with other polyhalogenated hydrocarbons, TCDD suppresses the immune system of animals. In most species studied thus far, the dominant features of TCDD toxicity are lymphoid atrophy, immunosuppression, and impaired host resistance when challenged by infectious agents or transplantable tumor cells.

The specific immunotoxic effects of TCDD exposure depend, in large part, on the age of the animal at the time of exposure. The administration of TCDD in utero results in a persistent suppression of cellular immunity. Similar exposure in adult animals, although it causes some suppression of cellular immunity, does not result in the marked and persistent suppression of T-cell function noted in neonates. In adult animals, TCDD exposure transiently reduces rapidly proliferating cell populations, which include hematopoietic stem cells and B lymphocytes (59,60,120,187,188). The mechanisms involved in TCDD toxicity have been reviewed by numerous authors (41,44,121). Species differences are very prominent with regard to TCDD-related toxic effects (120).

Metals

A number of investigators have shown that heavy metals such as lead, cadmium, and mercury affect the immune system in animals (99,101,103, 111,175,177). Immunosuppression or immunopotentiation may occur depending on the species studied, the dose administered, the route of exposure, the particular metal salt tested, and the assay system employed (44,111,121). One of the most consistent effects of heavy metal exposure in animals is a decreased resistance to infectious organisms (80, 99,111,175).

There is evidence that certain heavy metals, particularly mercury, induce autoimmunity. As previously noted, studies have been done using Brown–Norway rats as a model for mercury-induced autoimmunity. In this genetically susceptible model, a highly reproducible autoimmune glomerulonephritis develops after the subcutaneous injection of mercuric chloride (51). Antinuclear antibodies and glomerular deposits of immunoglobulins have been observed in Brown–Norway and other strains of rats receiving gold salts (149). Newly developed animal models hold promise of providing considerable insight into the mechanisms underlying autoimmune reactions.

Pesticides

A number of pesticides have been examined for their immunotoxic potential in animals. In general, the organophosphates appear to suppress the immune response. Their immunotoxicity, however, appears to be relatively low because of their rapid detoxification. Of interest is the presence of certain contaminants formed, during the manufacture of some organophosphates, that appear to have greater immunotoxic potential than the pesticide itself (151,152). Studies done to date suggest that organochlorine pesticides such as DDT, captan, and chlordane also can alter immune function in animals. As noted, the effects of pesticide exposure on the immune system have been reviewed in detail by a number of authors (41,44,163,173).

Inhaled Pollutants

Experimental data show that animals exposed to such noxious gases as NO_2 and O_3, at concentrations routinely found in polluted ambient air, have increased respiratory infections when challenged by pathogenic organisms. Moreover, mice forced to exercise during O_3 exposure exhibit increased mortality when similarly challenged (65,130). This increased susceptibility has been linked to altered immune function (7). A number of animal studies reveal that acute exposure to O_3 markedly impairs the function of alveolar macrophages (66,73). Exposure to NO_2 produces effects similar to those encountered with O_3 exposure except that the concentration required to affect host resistance to pathogenic organisms is much greater (66,137). There is also evidence that animals exposed to airborne metals, which include cadmium, nickel, manganese, zinc, and lead, have significantly increased susceptibility to laboratory-induced bacterial pneumonia (54). This increased susceptibility has been correlated with impaired alveolar macrophage function (6). The reader is referred to Chapters 7 and 16, respectively, for discussions of pulmonary defenses against pollutant exposure and of disorders of the lungs related to pollutant exposure.

CLINICAL ASPECTS OF EXPOSURE TO ENVIRONMENTAL AND INDUSTRIAL CHEMICALS ON THE IMMUNE SYSTEM

Clinicians are well aware that exposure to environmental and industrial chemicals can transiently or permanently impair immune function. In susceptible individuals, these agents are known to cause allergic and hypersensitivity reactions especially affecting the lungs and skin. Given the recent developments in immunotoxicology, however, clinicians must become aware of other immune dysfunctions that may potentially arise from exposure to occupational and environmental chemicals. Even though there is currently little supporting epidemiologic or clinical evidence, physicians should be aware that animal studies point to the immunosuppressive and autoimmunizing potential of industrial chemicals. Developing a broad understanding of immunotoxic events encourages physicians to examine for impaired immune function in patients with known toxic exposures and to search for toxic exposure in patients suffering from a wide range of immune disorders. At present many chemically induced immune disorders either go unrecognized or are considered idiopathic.

The Medical History

The clinical assessment of chemically induced immunologic dysfunction usually begins when the physician suspects that the patient has an immunologically mediated disorder. Once the diagnosis is established, the next step is to consider exposure to occupational and environmental chemicals in the etiology. This consideration is justified because the manifestations of many immune disorders induced by industrial chemicals are indistinguishable from those that arise spontaneously from drugs or for unknown reasons.

Since the skin and respiratory tract take the brunt of the body's exposure to environmental chemicals, the response of these organs to such assault is frequently readily apparent to physicians and patients alike. On this basis, skin and respiratory disorders arising from exposure to industrial chemicals have received considerably more attention from investigators and clinicians than similar problems arising in other organs (see Chapters 15 and 16). In line with these efforts, particular attention is directed to the clinical assessment of immunologically mediated lung and skin diseases induced by industrial agents (34,52,125).

In the discussion that follows, asthma, which develops on an allergic basis, is used as an example of a common ailment that can arise from chemically induced immune dysfunction. Although the topic is briefly presented, the clinical approach used to investigate the problem is also applicable to other disorders that may arise from environmentally induced immune dysfunction. The potential role of industrial chemicals in immunosuppression and autoimmune disease is also considered.

Allergic Asthma

The medical history is fundamental to the assessment of immune dysfunction stemming from exposure to industrial chemicals. It can be especially helpful in uncovering exposure conditions that lead to symptoms suggestive of immunologic lung disease. A prime example of such a disorder is asthma. It should be appreciated, however, that asthmatic reactions occurring in the workplace and general environment are induced by both immunologic and nonimmunologic mechanisms. It is likely that asthma induced by work and environmental exposures is induced by a combination of a number of different mechanisms (e.g., immunologic, irritant, toxic, and/or pharmacological). Immunologic methods alone are therefore often incapable or insufficient to establish a diagnosis of occupational and environmental asthma (18; see also Chapter 16).

The diagnostic value of a careful medical, occupational, and environmental history in patients with asthma is increased enormously when the physician is aware of the broad spectrum of agents that have been associated with this disorder (Table 23-3). This knowledge allows the physician to inquire about the patient's exposure to specific agents and to suggest that the patient make inquiry into the exact nature of his or her occupation and environmental exposures.

The medical history should include information on the presence of plant and animal antigens, gases, vapors, respiratory irritants, organic and inorganic dusts, and chemical agents in the patient's work, home, and community environment. Since inhalant allergens are well recognized in an occupational setting and are generally more easily identified than environmental exposures, a description of current and past jobs with information about specific exposures, their duration, and the type of respiratory protection used is essential.

Important clues are provided by information on the onset of respiratory symptoms in relation to a new job or a new industrial agent or process, the improvement of symptoms during weekends or time off from work, the occurrence of symptoms only during working hours, and the fact that other workers are experiencing similar problems. In some cases, respiratory symptoms develop several hours after exposure; this type of response may cloud the impact of exposure. The tendency for patients to seek medical help only after respiratory symptoms become severe also tends to obscure the link between exposure and symptoms. It is therefore important to sort out the conditions that existed when the illness began.

Since asthma is well known to be induced and exacerbated by outdoor and indoor air pollutants, the effect of such agents as pollens and molds and the degree and type of outdoor air pollution come under investigation. The particular effects of local industrial sources of air pollution should be considered. Indoor air pollution, with its complement of respirable particles, pollutant and organic gases, and biological contaminants (e.g., bacteria, viruses, mites, animal proteins, fungal spores, mold, mildew, pollen), must also be taken into account (182; see also Chapters 2, 16, and 28).

The personal and family history provides information about atopy or allergic disease. Such a history is important because it may indicate that an individual is more likely to develop allergic asthma. Other contributing factors such as smoking should also be noted. The physical examination may provide important supporting data. However, a normal physical examination does not exclude the possibility that the patient has occupational or environmental asthma.

In the clinical setting, certain historical features help to identify asthma that develops on an immunologic basis. Allergic asthma may be more prone to occur in individuals with a personal or family history of allergy. A period of symptomless exposure exists during which the sensitization takes place. Following sensitization, reactions are provoked by minimal, often minute, exposures that are far lower than the amounts required for sensitization. This feature helps to distinguish allergic reactions from the effects of nonspecific respiratory irritants. When reexposure to the sensitizing agent takes place after an exposure-free interval, symptoms immediately recur, often with increased intensity (18,145).

Once the history suggests that an occupational or environmental agent is responsible for the asthma and the diagnosis is substantiated, its etiology and pathogenesis are addressed through a series of tests. These include serum immunologic tests, skin testing, and bronchoprovocation tests. Although immunologic studies may be an easier means of defining specific reactivity than bronchoprovocation tests, the lack of an immunologic marker for many sensitizing substances limits their usefulness. Skin test reagents for such known occupational allergens as diisocyanates and acid anhydrides (chemically conjugated to carrier human serum albumins) are available at research centers. Bronchoprovocation tests should be approached with caution. Such testing is best performed in specialized centers experienced in their use.

Investigating the environmental etiology of asthma is often a complex problem requiring the expertise of experienced clinicians. For a detailed discussion of occupational and environmental immunologic lung disease, the reader is directed to a number of excellent reviews of this subject (18,71, 74,145,146,156,157). The diagnostic approaches used in the evaluation of occupational lung disease can be found in several references (34,116). There are also reviews of the diagnostic testing and immunotherapy for allergic diseases (35–37,113,129).

Immunosuppression

As previously noted, the immunosuppressive effects of occupational and environmental chemicals observed in animals find limited correlates in the few epidemiologic studies that have addressed this problem (123,124). The dearth of epidemiologic and clinical data surrounding this issue relates to the recent development of the discipline along with a number of other difficulties. Apart from the problem of documenting exposure, which faces most occupational and environmental studies, the unusual reserve capacity of the immune system makes it difficult to assess the immunosuppressive effects of exposure to industrial chemicals, particularly at low doses. Moreover, there is no battery of tests that is diagnostic or pathognomonic of chemically induced injury to the immune system. In addition, for many of the determinations used to assess immune function, there are uncertainties about the establishment of ranges of normal values in humans.

These problems notwithstanding, physicians should be attentive to the possibility of exposure to occupational and environmental chemicals in all patients with evidence of secondary or acquired immunosuppression. In many cases, the etiology of the immunodeficiency disorder will be apparent. It may be secondary to underlying disease or infections or be related to such exogenous factors as the administration of steroids or chemotherapeutic or immunosuppressive agents. Malnutrition or the extremes of age (e.g., the newborn or the aged) may also play a role (see Chapter 10). In some cases, however, immunosuppression may appear without apparent cause.

When immunosuppression occurs in patients for unknown reasons, it is essential that the physician search for a history of exposure to occupational and environmental agents. However, even cases of immunodeficiency that occur for known reasons merit inquiry regarding chemical exposures that could further compromise immune function. Clearly, the importance of identifying such exposure(s) resides in the likelihood of reversing the immunosuppressive process once the exposure is stopped. Physicians should be alert to the fact that the immune systems of the young, the old, and the malnourished are especially susceptible to the effects of immunosuppressive chemicals (see Chapter 10).

Autoimmune Disease

As previously noted, there is a sharp contrast between the advances that have been made in our understanding of the pathogenesis of autoimmune diseases and the little that is known regarding their etiology. In those cases in which an etiological agent has been defined, it is most often a drug. Little is known about the autoimmune potential of occupational and environmental chemicals. Identifying the possibility of such a relationship is of major clinical importance. Its importance stems from the observation that drug-induced autoimmune symptoms usually disappear after withdrawal of the drug

(70,91). A similar response might be hoped for after stopping exposure to an inciting industrial chemical. This favorable response is quite different from the natural history of idiopathic autoimmune disease, which often progresses or has periods of exacerbations and remissions (70,91).

Laboratory Testing

Although laboratory tests cannot define immune suppression or autoimmune disease induced by chemical exposure, a number of laboratory procedures are available for evaluating immune com-

TABLE 23-5. Tests of Immunologic Function[a]

Nonspecific immune response	Specific immune response	Tissue-damaging immune response
Tests of inflammatory response and phagocytic cell function	Enumeration of B lymphocytes	Tests of Reagin (IgE) hypersensitivity
WBC count and differential	(EA and EAC rosettes, SMIg, monoclonal antibodies)	Direct measurement of total IgE globulins (PRIST)
Sedimentation rate		IgE specific antibody (RAST)
C-reactive protein	Enumeration of T lymphocytes and subsets	Immediate hypersensitivity skin tests
Complement activity	(E rosettes, monoclonal antibodies)	Histamine release
Rebuck skin window technique		
Quantitative or histochemical NBT test	Tests of humoral (antibody) function	Tests of cytotoxic injury
Chemiluminescence	Quantitation of immunoglobulins and IgG subclasses	Red cell agglutinins
Chemotactic assay	Specific antibody responses: prior sensitization, isohemagglutinins (IgM), DPT, poliovirus, or measles (IgG)	Antiglobulin test (Coombs')
Phagocytic index		
Bactericidal activity		Tests of Ag–Ab complex injury
Phagocytic cell adherence	Schick and Dick tests (IgG)	Rheumatoid factor (RF)
Measurement of specific WBC enzymes	Specific antibody responses: de novo sensitization, *Salmonella* O (IgM); H (IgG)	Antinuclear factor (ANF)
		Serum complement (Clq, C3, C5)
		Tissue biopsy (localization of IgG and C components by immunofluorescence)
	Tests of cell-mediated (delayed hypersensitivity) function	
	In vivo	Tests of injury caused by delayed hypersensitivity
	Skin tests (prior sensitization), *Candida*, *Trichophyton*	Tissue biopsy, infiltration of lymphocytes in areas of injury
	Skin tests (de novo sensitization), DNCB	Skin tests (patch) in contact hypersensitivity
	Skin grafts	
	In vitro	
	Lymphocyte stimulation: nonspecific (PHA); specific (antigen)	
	Measurement of effector molecules (MIF)	
	Mixed lymphocyte culture (MLC)	
	Natural killer (NK) cell activity	
	Antibody-dependent cellular cytotoxicity (ADCC) or killer (K) cell activity	
	Lymph node biopsy	

[a]From Bellanti and Peters (15).

petence in individuals with suspected immuno-deficiencies and for investigating the presence of autoimmune disease (Table 23-5). For a detailed discussion of the use and interpretation of diagnostic immunologic laboratory tests, several references are recommended (15,48).

In some cases, uncovering the cause of immune dysfunction is aided through the use of laboratory tests that provide evidence of immunotoxic exposure. The biological monitoring of exposure to heavy metals, for example, may be helpful (8; see also Chapter 27).

SUMMARY

The immune system is geared to defend the body against infectious agents and spontaneously arising neoplasms. Animal studies have shown that a variety of chemicals commonly found in the workplace and widely distributed in the environment have induced changes in immune function. Disruption of immune function may result in immunosuppression or immunopotentiation. Immunosuppression may be associated with severe infection and cancer, whereas immunopotentiation may be associated with allergic or autoimmune disease. The immunotoxic effects noted in animals have been increasingly supported by epidemiologic studies that point to a link between exposure to certain occupational and environmental chemicals and alterations in the immune response. As individuals are increasingly exposed to chemicals with immunotoxic potential, clinicians must pay attention to the possibility of chemically induced damage to the immune system. Indeed, a major challenge for the future will be the search for environmental exposures that trigger the development of immune disorders.

REFERENCES

1. Adams RM (ed.): Occupational Skin Disease, 2nd ed., WB Saunders, Philadelphia, 1989.
2. Ahmed SA, Penhale WJ, Talal N: Sex hormones, immune responses, and autoimmune disease. Am J Pathol 121:531, 1983.
3. Allison AC: Theories of self tolerance and autoimmunity. In: Autoimmunity and Toxicology, p 67, Kammuller ME, Bloksma N, Seinen W (eds.), Elsevier, Amsterdam, 1989.
4. Andersen KE, Maibach HI (eds.): Current Problems in Dermatology. Vol 14, Contact Allergy. Predictive Tests in Guinea Pigs, S Karger, Basel, 1985.
5. Andrae S, Axelson O, Björksten BD, et al: Symptoms of bronchial hyperactivity and asthma in relation to environmental factors. Arch Dis Child 63:473, 1988.
6. Aranyi C, Miller FJ, Andres S, et al: Cytotoxicity on

7. Aranyi C, Vana SC, Thomas PT, et al: Effects of subchronic exposure to a mixture of O_3, SO_2, $(NH_4)_2$ SO_4 on host defenses in mice. Environ Res 12:55, 1983.
8. Baselt RC, Cravey RH: Disposition of Toxic Drugs and Chemicals in Man, 3rd ed., Year Book Medical Publishers, Chicago, 1989.
9. Beirne G: Glomerulonephritis associated with hydrocarbon solvents. Environ Res 23:422, 1980.
10. Bekesi JG, Roboz JP, Solomon S, et al: Altered immune function in Michigan residents exposed to polybrominated biphenyls. In: Immunotoxicology, p 181, Gibson GG, Hubbard R, Parke D (eds.), Academic Press, Orlando, 1983.
11. Bekesi JG, Roboz JP, Solomon S, et al: Persistent immune dysfunction in Michigan dairy farm residents exposed to polybrominated biphenyls. In: Advances in Immunopharmacology, p 55, Hadden JW, Chedid L, Dukor P, et al. (eds.), Pergamon Press, New York, 1983.
12. Bekesi JG, Holland JF, Anderson HA, et al: Lymphocyte function of Michigan dairy farmers exposed to polybrominated biphenyls. Science 199:1207, 1978.
13. Bekesi JG, Roboz JP, Fischbein A, et al: Immunotoxicology: Environmental contamination by polybrominated biphenyls and immune dysfunction among residents of the state of Michigan. Cancer Detect Prev 1 (Suppl):29, 1987.
14. Bekesi JG, Roboz JP, Fischbein A, et al: Clinical immunology studies in individuals exposed to environmental chemicals. In: Immunotoxicology, p 347, Berlin A, Dean J, Draper MH, et al. (eds.), Martinus Nijhoff, The Hague, 1987.
15. Bellanti JA, Peters SM: Diagnostic applications of immunology. In: Immunology III, p 558, Bellanti JA (ed.), WB Saunders, Philadelphia, 1985.
16. Berciano FA, Crespo M, Bao CG, et al: Serum levels of total IgE in nonallergic children. Allergy 24:276, 1987.
17. Berlin A, Dean J, Draper MH, et al. (eds.): Immunotoxicology, Martinus Nijhoff, The Hague, 1987.
18. Bernstein IL: Occupational asthma. Clin Chest Med 2:255, 1981.
19. Biagini RE, Bernstein IL, Gallagher JS, et al: The diversity of reaginic immune response to platinum and platinum metallic salts. J Allergy Clin Immunol 76:794, 1985.
20. Bick PH: The immune system: Organization and function. In: Immunotoxicology and Immunopharmacology, p 1, Dean JH, Luster MI, Munson AE, et al. (eds.), Raven Press, New York, 1985.
21. Bigazzi PE: Mechanisms of chemical-induced autoimmunity. In: Immunotoxicology and Immunopharmacology, p 277, Dean JH, Luster MI, Munson AE, et al. (eds.), Raven Press, New York, 1985.
22. Bigazzi PE: Autoimmunity induced by chemicals. Clin Toxicol 26:125, 1988.
23. Black CM, Welsh KI, Walker AE, et al: Genetic susceptibility to scleroderma-like syndrome induced by vinyl chloride. Lancet 1:53, 1983.
24. Bradley SG, Morahan PS: Approaches to assessing host resistance. Environ Health Perspect 43:61, 1982.
25. Brostoff J, Blanca M, Boulton P, et al: Absence of

specific IgE antibodies in toxic oil syndrome. Lancet 1:277, 1982.

26. Burger EJ, Tardiff RG, Bellanti JA (eds.): Environmental Chemical Exposures and Immune System Integrity. Princeton Scientific Publishing, Princeton, 1987.

27. Butcher B, Salvaggio J: Occupational asthma. J Allergy Clin Immunol 78:547, 1986.

28. Campbell MJ, Wagner MMF, Scott MP, et al: Sequential immunological studies in an asbestos exposed population II. Factors affecting lymphocyte function. Clin Exp Immunol 39:176, 1980.

29. Catala FJ, Mata de la Torre JN: Epidemiologia de sindrome toxico. In: Simposium Nacional Sindrome Toxico, p 143, Ministerio de Sanidad y Consumo, Madrid, 1982.

30. Chang KJ, Hsieh KH, Lee TP, et al: Immunologic evaluation of patients with polychlorinated biphenyl poisoning: Determination of lymphocyte subpopulations. Toxicol Appl Pharmacol 61:58, 1981.

31. Chang KJ, Hsieh KH, Lee TP, et al: Immunologic evaluation of patients with polychlorinated biphenyl poisoning: Determination of phagocyte Fc and complement receptors. Environ Res 28:329, 1982.

32. Chang KJ, Hsieh KH, Tang SY: Immunologic evaluation of patients with polychlorinated biphenyl poisoning: Evaluation of delayed-type skin hypersensitivity response and its relation to clinical studies. J Toxicol Environ Health 9:217, 1982.

33. Chan-Yeung M, Malo JL: Occupational asthma. Chest 91(Suppl):130S, 1987.

34. Committee on Occupational Lung Disease of the American Academy of Allergy and Immunology: Guidelines for the diagnosis and evaluation of occupational immunologic lung disease. J Allergy Clin Immunology 84:791–839, 1989.

35. Council on Scientific Affairs: In vivo diagnostic testing and immunotherapy for allergy, report I, part I, of the allergy panel. JAMA 258:1363, 1987.

36. Council on Scientific Affairs: In vivo diagnostic testing and immunotherapy for allergy, report I, part II, of the allergy panel. JAMA 258:1505, 1987.

37. Council on Scientific Affairs: In vitro testing for allergy, report II of the allergy panel. JAMA 258:1639, 1987.

38. Cullen MR (ed.): Workers with multiple chemical sensitivities. Occup Med 2:655, 1987.

39. Dean JH, Padarathsingh M (eds.): Biological Relevance of Immune Suppression as Induced by Genetic, Therapeutic and Environmental Factors. Van Nostrand Reinhold, New York, 1981.

40. Dean JH, Luster MI, Boorman GA: Immunotoxicology. In: Immunopharmacology, p 349, Sirois P, Rola-Pieszgyski M (eds.), Elsevier, Amsterdam, 1982.

41. Dean JH, Murray MJ, Ward EC: Toxic responses of the immune system. In: Casarett and Doull's Toxicology, 3rd ed., p 245, Klaassen CD, Amdur MO, Doull J (eds.), Macmillan, New York, 1986.

42. Dean JH, Lauer LD, House RV, et al: Experience with validation of methodology for immunotoxicity assessment in rodents. In: Immunotoxicology, p 135, Berlin A, Dean J, Draper MH, et al. (eds.), Martinus Nijhoff, The Hague, 1987.

43. Dean JH, Thurmond LM, Lauer LD, et al: Comparative toxicology and correlative immunotoxicology. In:

Environmental Chemical Exposures and Immune System Integrity, p 85, Burger EJ, Tardiff RG, Bellanti JA (eds.), Princeton Scientific Publishing, Princeton, 1987.

44. Dean JH, Cornacoff JB, Luster MI: Toxicity of the immune system: A review. In: Immunopharmacology reviews, Vol 1, p 377, Hadden JW, Szentivanyi A (eds.), Plenum Press, New York, 1990.

45. Deo M, Gangal S, Bhisey AN, et al: Immunological mutagenic and genotoxic investigations in gas exposed population of Bhopal. Indian J Med Res 86:63, 1987.

46. Descotes J: Immunotoxicology of Drugs and Chemicals, 2nd ed., Elsevier, Amsterdam, 1988.

47. deShazo RD, Norberg J, Baser Y, et al: Analysis of depressed cell-mediated immunity in asbestos workers. J Allergy Clin Immunol 71:418, 1983.

48. deShazo RD, Lopez M, Salvaggio JE: Use and interpretation of diagnostic immunologic laboratory tests. JAMA 258:3011, 1987.

49. Doll NJ, Diem JE, Jones RN, et al: Humoral immunologic abnormalities in workers exposed to asbestos cement dust. J Allergy Clin Immunol 72:509, 1983.

50. Druet P, Hirsch F, Pelletier L, et al: Mechanisms of chemical-induced glomerulonephritis. In: Mechanisms of Cell Injury: Implications for Human Health, p 153, Fowler BA (ed.), John Wiley & Son, New York, 1987.

51. Druet P, Pelletier L, Rossert J, et al: Autoimmune reactions induced by metals. In: Autoimmunity and Toxicology, p 337, Kammuller ME, Bloksma N, Seinen W (eds.), Elsevier, Amsterdam, 1989.

52. Dupis G, Benezra C: Allergic Contact Dermatitis to Simple Chemicals, Marcel Dekker, New York, 1982.

53. Ehrenreich T, Yunis SL, Churg J: Membranous nephropathy following exposure to volatile hydrocarbons. Environ Res 14:35, 1977.

54. Ehrlich R: Interaction between environmental pollutants and respiratory infections. Environ Health Perspect 35:89, 1980.

55. Ercegovich CD: Relationship of pesticides to immune responses. Fed Proc 32:2010, 1973.

56. Estabrook RW, Lindenlaub E, Oesch F, et al. (eds.): Toxicological and Immunological Aspects of Drug Metabolism and Environmental Chemicals, Symposia Medical Hoechst 22, FK Schattauer Verlag, Stuttgart, 1988.

57. Evans RG, Webb KB, Knutsen AP, et al: A medical follow-up of the health effects of long-term exposure to 2,3,7,8-tetrachlorodibenzo-p-dioxin. Arch Environ Health 43:273, 1988.

58. Exon JH, Koller LD, Talcott PA, et al: Immunotoxicity testing: An economical multiple assay approach. Fund Appl Toxicol 7:387, 1986.

59. Faith RE, Luster MI: Investigation on the effects of 2,3,7,8-tetrachlorodibenzo-p-dioxin on parameters of various immune function. Ann NY Acad Sci 320:564, 1979.

60. Faith RE, Luster MI, Vos JG: Effects on immunocompetence by chemicals of environmental concern. In: Review in Biochemical Toxicology 2, p 173, Hodgson E, Bend JR, Philpot RM (eds.), Elsevier/North Holland, Amsterdam, 1980.

61. Fillastre JP, Mery JP, Morel-Maroger L, et al: Drug-

induced glomerulonephritis. In: Acute Renal Failure, p 389, Solez K, Whelton A (eds.), Marcel Dekker, New York, 1985.

62. Fiore MC, Anderson HA, Hong R, et al: Chronic exposure to aldicarb-contaminated groundwater and human immune function. Environ Res 41:653, 1986.

63. Fries GF: The PBB-episode in Michigan: An overall appraisal. CRC Crit Rev Toxicol 16:105, 1986.

64. Gallin JI, Goldstein IA, Syderman R (eds.): Inflammation: Basic Principles and Clinical Correlates, Raven Press, New York, 1988.

65. Gardner DE: Effects of environmental chemicals on host defense responses of the lung. In: Biological Relevance of Immune Suppression as Induced by Genetic, Therapeutic and Environmental Factors, p 275, Dean JH, Padarathsingh ML (eds.), Van Nostrand Reinhold, New York, 1981.

66. Gardner DE, Graham JA: Altered immune function and host resistance following exposure to common airborne pollutants. In: Immunotoxicology, p 234, Berlin A, Dean J, Draper MH, et al. (eds.), Martinus Nijhoff, The Hague, 1987.

67. Gell PGH, Coombs RRA: Clinical Aspects of Immunology, Blackwell, London, 1963.

68. Gibson GG, Hubbard R, Parke DV (eds.): Immunotoxicology, Academic Press, Orlando, 1983.

69. Gleichmann E, Vogeler S, Mirtschewa J, et al: Possible pathogenic pathways of chemically induced autoimmunity: Experimental studies in animals. In: Toxicology and Immunological Aspects of Drug Metabolism and Environmental Chemicals, Symposia Medica Hoechst 22, p 419, Estabrook RW, Lindenlaub E, Oesch F, et al. (eds.), FK Schattauer Verlag, Stuttgart, 1988.

70. Gleichmann E, Kimber I, Purchase IFH: Immunotoxicology: Suppressive and stimulatory effects of drugs and environmental chemicals on the immune system. Arch Toxicol 63:257, 1989.

71. Goldstein RA, Sogn DD, Ayres J: Occupational and environmental immunologic lung disease. In: Immunotoxicology and Immunopharmacology, p 489, Dean J, Luster MI, Munson AE, et al. (eds.), Raven Press, New York, 1985.

72. Gomez-Reino JJ: Immune system disorders associated with adulterated cooking oil. In: Immunotoxicology, p 376, Berlin A, Dean J, Draper MH, et al. (eds.), Martinus Nijhoff, The Hague, 1987.

73. Graham JA, Gardner DE: Immunotoxicity of air pollutants. In: Immunotoxicology and immunopharmacology, p 367, Dean J, Luster MI, Munson AE, et al. (eds.), Raven Press, New York, 1985.

74. Grammer LC, Patterson R: Occupational immunologic lung disease. Ann Allergy 58:151, 1987.

75. Greenburg M, Milne MF, Watt A: A survey of workers exposed to dusts containing derivatives of Bacillus subtilis. Br Med J 11:629, 1970.

76. Hallauer JF, Krämer U, Stiller-Winkler R, et al: Concentration of IgE in sera of children from residential areas with different air pollution. Zentralbl Bakteriol Hyg 184:432, 1987.

77. Hamilton HE, Morgan DP, Simmons A: A pesticide (Dieldrin)-induced hemolytic anemia. Environ Res 17:155, 1978.

78. Hasllam PL, Lukoszek A, Merchant JA, et al: Lymphocyte responses to phytohaemagglutinin in patients with asbestosis and pleural mesothelioma. Clin Exp Immunol 31:178, 1978.

79. Heale WF, Matthiesson AM, Naill JF: Lung hemorrhage and nephritis (Goodpasture's syndrome). Med J Aust 2:355, 1969.

80. Hemphill FE, Kaeberle ML, Buck WB: Lead suppression of mouse resistance to Salmonella typhimurium. Science 172:1031, 1971.

81. Hoffman RE, Stehr-Green PA, Webb KB, et al: Health effects of long-term exposure to 2,3,7,8-tetrachlorodibenzo-p-dioxin. JAMA 255:2031, 1986.

82. Holt PG: Immune and inflammatory function in cigarette smokers. Thorax 42:241, 1987.

83. Holt PG: Environmental pollutants as co-factors in IgE production. Curr Opin Immunol 1:653, 1989.

84. Hubbard R: Fundamentals of immunology. In: Immunotoxicology, p 5, Gibson GG, Hubbard R, Parke DV (eds.), Academic Press, Orlando, 1983.

85. Huuskonen MS, Rasanen YA, Harkonen A, et al: Asbestos exposure as a cause of immunological stimulation. Scand J Respir Dis 59:326, 1978.

86. Ishizaka K, Ishizaka T: Allergy. In: Fundamental Immunology, 2nd ed, p 867, Paul WE (ed.), Raven Press, New York, 1989.

87. Kagan E, Solomon A, Cochrane JC, et al: Immunologic studies of patients with asbestosis I: Studies of cell-mediated immunity. Clin Exp Immunol 28:261, 1977.

88. Kagan E, Solomon A, Cochrane JC, et al: Immunological studies of patients with asbestosis. II: Studies of circulating lymphoid cell numbers and humoral immunity. Clin Exp Immunol 28:268, 1977.

89. Kammuller ME, Bloksma N, Seinen W: Chemical-induced autoimmune reactions and Spanish toxic oil syndrome. Focus on hydantoins and related compounds. Clin Toxicol 26:157, 1988.

90. Kammuller ME, Bloksma N, Seinen W (eds.): Autoimmunity and Toxicology, Elsevier, Amsterdam, 1989.

91. Kammuller ME, Bloksma N, Seinen W: Autoimmunity and toxicology, immune disregulation induced by drugs and chemicals. In: Autoimmunity and Toxicology, p 3, Kammuller ME, Bloksma N, Seinen W (eds.), Elsevier, Amsterdam, 1989.

92. Kaneko S, Shimada K, Horiuchi H, et al: Nasal allergy and air pollution. Oto-Rhino-Laryngology (Tokyo) 23(Suppl 4):270, 1980.

93. Karol MH: Hypersensitivity to isocyanates. In: Immunotoxicology and Immunopharmacology, p 475, Dean JH, Luster MI, Munson AE, et al. (eds.), Raven Press, New York, 1985.

94. Karol MH: Respiratory effects of inhaled isocyanate. CRC Crit Rev Toxicol 16:349, 1986.

95. Kay K: Polybrominated biphenyls (PBBs) environmental contamination in Michigan, 1973–1976. Environ Res 13:74, 1977.

96. Kazantzis G: Industrial hazards to the kidney and urinary tract. In: Sixth Symposium on Advanced Medicine, p 263, States JDH (ed.), Pittman Medical, London, 1970.

97. Kilbourne EM, Rigau-Perez J, Heath CM, et al: Clinical epidemiology of toxic-oil syndrome. Manifestations of a new illness. N Engl J Med 309:1408, 1983.

98. Klavis G, Drommer W: Goodpasture's syndrome and effects of benzene. Arch Toxikol 26:40, 1970.

99. Koller LD: Immunosuppression produced by lead, cadmium and mercury. Am J Vet Res 34:1457, 1973.

100. Koller LD: Effects of environmental contaminants on the immune system. Adv Vet Sci Comp Med 23:267, 1979.

101. Koller LD: Immunotoxicology of heavy metals. Int J Immunopharmacol 2:269, 1980.

102. Koller LD: Immunotoxicology today. Toxicol Pathol 15:346, 1987.

103. Koller LD, Vos JG: Immunologic effects of metals. In: Immunologic Consideration in Toxicology, Vol 1, p 67, Sharma RP (ed.), CRC Press, Boca Raton, 1981.

104. Kunita N, Kashimoto T, Miyata H, et al: Causal agents of Yusho. In: PCB Poisoning in Japan, p 45, Kuratsume M, Shapiro RE (eds.), Alan R Liss, New York, 1984.

105. Kuratsume M: Yusho. In: Halogenated Biphenyls, Terphenyls, Napthalenes, Dibenzodioxins and Related Products, p 287, Kimbrough RD (ed.), Elsevier, Amsterdam, 1980.

106. Kuratsume M: Yusho, with Reference to Yu-Cheng. In: Halogenated Biphenyls, Terphenyls, Naphthalenes, Dibenzodioxins and Related Products, 2nd ed., p 381, Kimbrough RD, Jensen AA (eds.), Elsevier, Amsterdam, 1989.

107. Lagrue G, Kamalodine T, Hirbec G, et al: Role de l'inhalation de substances toxiques dans la genese des glomerulonephrites. Nouv Presse Med 6:3609, 1977.

108. Lange A: An epidemiological survey of immunological abnormalities in asbestos workers. I. Non-organ and organ specific autoantibodies. Environ Res 22:162, 1980.

109. Lange A: An epidemiological survey of immunological abnormalities in asbestos workers. II. Serum immunoglobins levels. Environ Res 22:170, 1980.

110. Lange A, Smolik R, Zatonski W, et al: Autoantibodies and serum immunoglobulin levels in asbestos workers. Arch Arbeitsmed 32:313, 1974.

111. Lawrence DA: Immunotoxicity of heavy metals. In: Immunotoxiology and immunopharmacology, p 341, Dean JH, Luster MI, Munson AE, et al. (eds.), Raven Press, New York, 1985.

112. Lew F, Tsang P, Holland JF, et al: High frequency of immune dysfunction in asbestos workers and in patients with malignant mesothelioma. J Clin Immunol 6:225, 1986.

113. Lockey RF (ed.), Bukhantz SC (assoc. ed.): Primer on allergic and immunologic diseases—second edition. JAMA 258:2829–3034, 1987.

114. Loose LD, Pittman KA, Benitz JB, et al: Environmental chemical-induced immune dysfunction. Ecotoxicol Environ Safety 2:173, 1978.

115. Loose LC, Silkworth JB, Pittman KA, et al: Impaired host resistance to endotoxin and malaria in polychlorinated biphenyl- and hexachlorobenzene-treated mice. Infect Immun 20:30, 1978.

116. Lopez M, Salvaggio JE: Diagnostic method of occupational allergic lung disease. Clin Rev Allergy 4:289, 1986.

117. Lu YC, Wu YC: Clinical findings and immunological abnormalities in Yu-Cheng patients. Environ Health Perspect 59:17, 1985.

118. Luster MI, Dean JH: Immunological hypersensitivity resulting from environmental or occupational exposure to chemicals: A state-of-the-art workshop summary. Fund Appl Toxicol 2:327, 1982.

119. Luster MI, Faith RE, Moore JA: Effects of polybrominated biphenyls (PBB) on immune response in rodents. Environ Health Perspect 23:227, 1978.

120. Luster MI, Boorman GA, Dean JH, et al: Examination of bone marrow immunologic parameters and host susceptibility following pre- and post-natal exposure to 2,3,7,8-tetrachlorodibenzo-p-dioxin. Int J Immunopharmacol 2:301, 1980.

121. Luster MI, Blank JA, Dean JH: Molecular and cellular basis of chemically induced immunotoxicity. Annu Rev Pharmacol Toxicol 27:23, 1987.

122. Luster MI, Munson AE, Thomas PT, et al: Methods evaluation development of a testing battery to assess chemical-induced immunity: National Toxicology Program's guidelines for immunotoxicity evaluation in mice. Fund Appl Toxicol 10:2, 1988.

123. Luster MI, Germolec DR, Rosenthal GL: Immunotoxicology: Review of current status. Ann Allergy 64:427, 1990.

124. Luster MI, Wierda D, Rosenthal GJ: Environmentally related disorders of hematologic and immune systems. Med Clin North Am 72:2, 1990.

125. Maibach HI, Epstein E: Contact skin allergy. In: Allergy Principles and Practice, 3rd ed., Vol 2, p 1429, Middleton E Jr, Reed CE, Ellis EF, et al. (eds.), CV Mosby, St Louis, 1988.

126. Martinez-Tello P, Navas-Palacios J, Ricoy JR, et al: Pathology of a new toxic syndrome caused by adulterated oil in Spain. Virchows Arch Pathol Anat 397:261, 1982.

127. Marzulli FN, Maibach HI: Human predictive tests for allergic contact dermatitis. In: Occupational and Industrial Dermatology, p 227, Maibach HI (ed.), Year Book Medical Publishers, Chicago, 1987.

128. McSharry C, Wilkinson PC: Serum IgG and IgE antibody against aerosolised antigens from Nephrops norvegius among seafood process workers. Adv Exp Med Biol 216:865, 1987.

129. Middleton E Jr, Reed CE, Ellis EF, et al. (eds.): Allergy Principles and Practice, 3rd ed., Vols 1 and 2, CV Mosby, St Louis, 1988.

130. Miller FJ, Gardner DE, Graham JA: Effects of urban ozone levels on laboratory induced respiratory infections. Toxicol Lett 2:163, 1978.

131. Miller K, Brown RC: The immune system and asbestos-associated diseases. In: Immunotoxicology and Immunopharmacology, p 429, Dean JH, Luster MI, Munson AE, et al. (eds.), Raven Press, New York, 1985.

132. Miller LG, Sparrow D, Ginn LC: Asbestos exposure correlates with alterations in circulating T-cell subsets. Clin Exp Immunol 51:110, 1983.

133. Mitchell CA, Gandevia B: Respiratory symptoms and skin reactivity in workers exposed to proteolytic enzymes in the detergent enzymes. Am Rev Respir Dis 104:1, 1971.

134. Miyamoto T, Takafuji S, Suzuki S, et al: Environmental factors in the development of allergic reactions. In: Toxicological and Immunological Aspects of Drug Metabolism and Environmental Chemicals, p 553, Estabrook RW, Lindenlaub E, Oesch F, et al. (eds.), FK Schattauer Verlag, Stuttgart, 1988.

135. Monjan AA, Collector MI: Stress-induced modulation of the immune response. Science 196:307, 1977.

136. Morrison Smith J, Harding LK, Cumming G: The changing prevalence of asthma in school children. Clin Allergy 1:57, 1971.

137. Morrow PE: Toxicological data on NO_2: An overview. J Toxicol Environ Health 13:205, 1984.

138. Mullen PW (ed.): Immunotoxicology: A Current Perspective of Principles and Practice, Springer-Verlag, Berlin, 1984.

139. Murdoch RD, Pepys J, Hughes EG: IgE antibody responses to platinum group metals: A large scale refinery survey. Br J Ind Med 43:37, 1986.

140. Newman Taylor AJ, Venable KM, Durham SR, et al: Acid anhydrides and asthma. Int Arch Allergy Appl Immunol 82:435, 1987.

141. Nossal GJV: Current concepts: Immunology. The basic components of the immune system. N Engl J Med 316:1320, 1987.

142. Osterman K, Johansson SGO, Zetterstrom O: Allergy to coffee bean dust. Allergy 33:350, 1976.

143. Paul WE (ed.): Fundamental Immunology, Raven Press, New York, 1989.

144. Penn I: The neoplastic consequences of immunodepression. In: Immunotoxicology, p 69, Berlin A, Dean J, Draper MH, et al. (eds.), Martinus Nijhoff, The Hague, 1987.

145. Pepys J: Allergic reactions of the respiratory tract to low molecular weight chemicals. In: Immunotoxicology, p 107, Gibson GG, Hubbard R, Parke DV (eds.), Academic Press, Orlando, 1983.

146. Pepys J: Occupational allergic lung disease caused by organic agents. J Allergy Clin Immunol 78:1058, 1986.

147. Pernis B, Vigliane EC, Selikoff IJ: Rheumatoid factor in serum of individuals exposed to asbestos. Ann NY Acad Sci 132:117, 1965.

148. Reggiani G: Medical survey techniques in the Seveso TCDD exposure. J Appl Toxicol 1:323, 1981.

149. Robinson CJG, Balazs T, Egorov IK: Mercuric chloride, gold sodium thiomalate and d-penicillamine-induced antinuclear antibodies in mice. Toxicol Appl Pharmacol 86:159, 1986.

150. Roboz J, Suzuki RK, Bekesi JG, et al: Mass spectral identification and quantification of polybrominated biphenyls in blood compartments of exposed Michigan chemical workers. J Environ Pathol Toxicol Oncol 3:362, 1980.

151. Rodgers KE, Imamura T, Devans BH: Effects of subchronic treatment with O,O,S-trimethyl phosphorothioate on cellular and humoral immune response systems. Toxicol Appl Pharmacol 81:310, 1985.

152. Rodgers KE, Imamura T, Devans BH: Investigations into the mechanisms of immunosuppression caused by acute treatment with O,O,S-trimethyl phosphorothioate. I, Characterization of the immune cell population affects. Immunopharmacology 10:171, 1985.

153. Roitt IM (ed.): Essential Immunology, 7th ed., Blackwell Scientific Publishers, London, 1991.

154. Roitt I, Brostoff J, Male D: Immunology, 2nd ed., Gower Medical Publishing, London, 1989.

155. Rola-Peszczynski M, Masse S, Sirois P, et al: Early effects of low doses exposure to asbestos on local cellular immune responses in the lung. J Immunol 127:2535, 1981.

156. Salvaggio JE: Overview of occupational immunologic lung disease. J Allergy Clin Immunol 70:5, 1982.

157. Salvaggio JE, Butcher BT, O'Neil CE: Occupational asthma due to chemical agents. J Allergy Clin Immunol 78:1053, 1986.

158. Schwartz RS, Datta SK: Autoimmunity and autoimmune diseases. In: Fundamental Immunology, 2nd ed., p 819, Paul WE (ed.), Raven Press, New York, 1989.

159. Selikoff IJ: Occupational respiratory disease. In: Public Health and Preventive Medicine, 11th ed., p 568, Last JM (ed.), Appleton-Century-Crofts, New York, 1980.

160. Sharma RP: Immunity and the immune system. In: Immunologic Considerations in Toxicology, p 9, Sharma RP (ed.), CRC Press, Boca Raton, 1981.

161. Sharma RP (ed.): Immunologic Considerations in Toxicology, Vols I and II, CRC Press, Boca Raton, 1981.

162. Sharma RP: Chemical interactions and compromised immune system. Fund Appl Toxicol 4:345, 1984.

163. Sharma RP, Reddy RV: Toxic effects of chemicals on the immune system. In: Handbook of Toxicology, p 555, Haley TJ, Berndt WO (eds.), Hemisphere, Washington, 1987.

164. Sharma RP, Zeeman MG: Immunologic alterations by environmental chemicals: Relevance of studying mechanisms versus effects. J Immunopharmacol 2: 285, 1980.

165. Shigematsu N, Ishimaru S, Saito R, et al: Respiratory involvement in PCB poisoning. Environ Res 16:92, 1978.

166. Shoham J: Vulnerability to toxic or therapeutic immunomodulation—as two complementary aspects of age and nutrition dependent immunodeficiency. In: Immunotoxicology, p 389, Berlin A, Dean J, Draper MH, et al. (eds.), Martinus Nijhoff, The Hague, 1987.

167. Silkworth JB, Loose LC: Cell-mediated immunity in mice fed either Aroclor 1016 or hexachlorobenzene. Toxicol Appl Pharmacol 45:326, 1978.

168. Sinha AA, Lopez T, McDevitt HO: Autoimmune diseases: The failure of self tolerance. Science 248: 1380, 1990.

169. Spreafico F: Immunomodulation by xenobiotics. The open field of immunotoxicity. In: Immunomodulation New Frontiers and Advances, p 311, Fudenberg HH, Whitten MD, Ambrogi F (eds.), Plenum Press, New York, 1984.

170. Spreafico F: Immunotoxicology in 1987: Problems and challenges. Fund Clin Pharmacol 2:353, 1988.

171. Spreafico F, Merendino A, Braceschi L, et al: Immunodepressive drugs as prototype immunotoxicants. In: Immunotoxicology, p 192, Berlin A, Dean J, Draper MH, et al. (eds.), Martinus Nijhoff, The Hague, 1987.

172. Stanworth DR: Current concepts of hypersensitivity. In: Immunotoxicology and Immunopharmacology, p 91, Dean JH, Luster MI, Munson AE, et al. (eds.), Raven Press, New York, 1985.

173. Street JC: Pesticides and the immune system. Immunologic Consideration in Toxicology, Vol 1, p 45, Sharma RP (ed.), CRC Press, Boca Raton, 1981.

174. Taylor B, Wadsworth J, Wadsworth M, et al: Changes in the reported prevalence of childhood eczema since the 1939–45 war. Lancet 1:1255, 1984.

175. Thomas PT, Tatajczak HV, Aranyi C, et al: Evaluation of host resistance and immune function in cadmium-exposed mice. Toxicol Appl Pharmacol 80:446, 1986.

176. Toxic Epidemic Syndrome Study Group: Toxic epidemic syndrome, Spain, 1981. Lancet 2:697, 1982.

177. Treagan L: Metals and immunity. In: Metal Ions in Biological Systems, p 27, Sigel H (ed.), Marcel Dekker, New York, 1983.

178. Trizio D, Basketter DA, Botham PH, et al: Identification of immunotoxic effects of chemicals and assessment of their relevance to man. Fund Chem Toxicol 26:527, 1988.

179. Tsang PH, Chu FN, Fischbein A, et al: Impairments in functional subsets of T-suppressor (CD8) lymphocytes, monocytes, and natural killer cells among asbestos-exposed workers. Clin Immunol Immunopathol 47:323, 1988.

180. Tubbs RR, Gephardt GN, McMahon JT, et al: Membranous glomerulonephritis associated with industrial mercury exposure. Study of pathogenic mechanisms. Am J Clin Pathol 77:409, 1982.

181. Turner-Warwick M, Parkes WL: Circulating rheumatoid and antinuclear factors in asbestos workers. Br Med J 3:492, 1970.

182. US Environmental Protection Agency: The Inside Story: A guide to Indoor Air Quality, EPA 400/1-88/004, USEPA, Washington, 1988.

183. Venables KM, Topping MD, Howe W, et al: Interaction of smoking and atopy in producing specific IgE antibody against a hapten protein conjugate. Br Med J 290:201, 1985.

184. Vos JG: Immune suppression as related to toxicology. CRC Crit Rev Toxicol 5:67, 1977.

185. Vos JG: Immunotoxicology assessment: Screening and function studies. Arch Toxicol 4(Suppl):95, 1980.

186. Vos JG, Krajnc EI: Immunotoxicology of pesticides. In: Developments in the Science and Practice of Toxicology, p 229, Hayers AW, Schnell RC, Miya TS (eds.), Elsevier, Amsterdam, 1983.

187. Vos JG, Luster MI: Immune alterations. In: Halogenated Biphenyls, Terphenyls, Naphthalenes, Dibenzodioxins and Related Products, 2nd ed., p 295, Kimbrough RD, Jensen AA (eds.), Elsevier, Amsterdam, 1989.

188. Vos JG, Moore JA: Suppression of cellular immunity in rats and mice by maternal treatment with 2,3,7,8-tetrachlorodibenzo-p-dioxin. Int Arch Allergy Appl Immunol 47:777, 1974.

189. Vos JG, Van Driel-Grootenhuis L: PCB-induced suppression of humoral and cell-mediated immunity in guinea pigs. Sci Total Environ 1:289, 1972.

190. Wagner MMF, Campbell MJ, Edwards RF: Sequential immunologic studies of an asbestos exposed population I. Factors affecting peripheral blood leucocytes and T lymphocytes. Clin Exp Immunol 38:323, 1979.

191. Ward EC, Murray MJ, Dean JH: Immunotoxicity of nonhalogenated polycyclic aromatic hydrocarbons. In: Immunotoxicology and Immunopharmacology, p 291, Dean JH, Luster MI, Munson AE, et al (eds.), Raven Press, New York, 1985.

192. Webb KB, Evans D, Knutsen AP, et al: Medical evaluation of subjects with known body levels of 2,3,7,8-tetrachlorodibenzo-p-dioxin. J Toxicol Environ Health 28:183, 1989.

193. Wenfors M, Nielson J, Schutz A, et al: Phthalic anhydride-induced occupational asthma. Int Arch Allergy Appl Immunol 79:77, 1986.

194. Winkelstein A: Immune suppression resulting from various cytotoxic agents. Clin Immunol Allergy 4:295, 1984.

195. Wolff MS, Anderson HA, Selikoff I: Human tissue burdens of halogenated aromatic chemicals in Michigan. JAMA 247:2112, 1982.

196. Zerva CV, Constantopoulos SH, Moutsopoulos HM: Humoral immunity alterations after environmental asbestos exposure. Respiration 55:237, 1989.

197. Zetterström O, Osterman K, Machado L, et al: Another smoking hazard: Raised serum IgE concentration and increased risk of occupational allergy. Br Med J 283:1215, 1981.

198. Zimmerman SW, Groehler K, Beirne GJ: Hydrocarbon exposure and chronic glomerulonephritis. Lancet 2:199, 1975.

RECOMMENDED READINGS

Abbas AK, Lichtman AR, Pober JS: Cellular and Molecular Immunology, W.B. Saunders, Philadelphia, 1991.

Berlin A, Dean J, Draper MH, et al. (eds.): Immunotoxicology, Martinus Nijhoff, The Hague, 1987.

Committee on Biologic Markers, National Research Council: Biological Markers in Immunotoxicology, National Academy Press, Washington, 1991.

Dean JH, Luster MI, Munson AE, et al. (eds.): Immunotoxicology and Immunopharmacology, Raven Press, New York, 1985.

Dean JH, Cornacoff JB, Luster MI: Toxicity to the immune system: A review. In: Immunopharmacology Reviews, Vol 1, p 377, Hadden JW, Szentivanyi A (eds.), Plenum Press, New York, 1990.

Descotes J: Immunotoxicology of Drugs and Chemicals, 2nd ed., Elsevier, Amsterdam, 1988.

Gibson GG, Hubbard R, Parke DV (eds.): Immunotoxicology, Academic Press, Orlando, 1983.

Paul WE (ed.): Fundamental Immunology, 2nd ed., Raven Press, New York, 1989.

24. DISORDERS OF THE FEMALE REPRODUCTIVE SYSTEM AND DEVELOPMENTAL DISORDERS

Richard B. Kurzel

INTRODUCTION

Contrary to popular belief, the adverse effects of environmental chemicals on human reproduction are not a new problem but rather an old one rediscovered. Chemicals and toxins have been used since antiquity as abortifacients. The adverse reproductive effects of workplace exposure have been well documented since the industrial revolution. Careful recording of such events and their sequelae, as well as the results of accidental poisonings, constitutes the clinical core of reproductive toxicology and teratology. Over the years, clinicians have alerted the medical community to the reproductive hazards of toxic exposure. Although this surveillance is now supplemented by epidemiologic and animal studies, there is little doubt that the alert clinician will continue to be among the first to detect the reproductive hazards of toxic exposure. Clearly the aim of such observations is to reduce fetal loss, infant malformation, and infant debility.

Exposure to chemicals found in the workplace and general environment can be associated with a broad spectrum of reproductive hazards (6,26,68, 119,134,142,164). Toxic agents may adversely affect the reproductive system and/or the developing fetus.

Reproductive toxicology has been defined as the study of dysfunctions induced by chemical (as well as physical and biological) agents that affect

Principles and Practice of Environmental Medicine, edited by Alyce Bezman Tarcher. Plenum Medical Book Company, New York, 1992.

gametogenesis from its earliest stage to implantation of the conceptus in the mother (34). A reproductive toxicant may interfere with reproductive and/or sexual function. Toxic assault on the reproductive system can damage the germ cells and lead to infertility or aberrant fetal development. Toxic assault may also result in impotence and irregular menstrual cycles (34).

Developmental toxicology is concerned with adverse effects on development that occur from conception to puberty (164). Developmental toxicants have four principal effects on the offspring: (1) death of the conceptus, (2) structural malformations, (3) altered growth, and (4) functional deficiency (181).

Toxic assault on the fetus can lead to such problems as intrauterine death, spontaneous abortion, and congenital malformations. At times toxic assault can lead to a significant alteration in fetal or neonatal organ or body weight. This is termed "altered growth." It can be induced at any stage of development and be reversible or result in permanent damage. At times untoward effects on the embryo/fetus are not recognized at birth but become apparent later in life. Exposures during the embryo/fetal period, for example, can be linked to such problems as the induction of childhood and adult-onset tumors, reproductive dysfunction, and alterations in physical and mental development (10,102).

Embryotoxicity and fetotoxicity refer to toxic effects on the conceptus that occur during prenatal exposure. The critical difference between the terms is the period during which the insult occurs. These terms include such adverse effects as malformation, altered growth, and in utero death.

Study of the adverse effects of the environment on development is termed teratology. Developmental defects, malformations, congenital abnormalities, or anomalies all fall within the purview of this discipline. Under some conditions environmental exposure produces embryotoxicity without teratogenesis. Because abnormal development is increasingly being explained in toxicological terms, it has been suggested that teratogenesis reflects a special form of embryotoxicity (111).

Traditionally the identification of a teratogenic agent was based primarily on its ability to produce structural defects in the embryo/fetus. More recently the concept of teratogenesis has been expanded to include those agents acting during embryonic or fetal development that produce abnormal function (functional teratogenesis). Thus, the teratogenic effects of occupational and environmental exposures can include growth retardation, developmental abnormalities, and behavioral disorders as well as structural defects.

ENVIRONMENTAL CHEMICALS ASSOCIATED WITH DEVELOPMENTAL DISORDERS AND ADVERSE EFFECTS ON THE FEMALE REPRODUCTIVE SYSTEM

Adverse reproductive effects in animals can be induced by over 800 chemicals. In man such effects are known to occur after exposure to about 25 agents, most of them pharmaceuticals. Environmental and occupational chemicals adversely affecting human reproduction are listed in Table 24-1. Table 24-2 contains agents reported to be toxic to the female reproductive system.

Distribution

Although there is a general awareness that workplace exposures to such agents as solvents, heavy metals, and pharmaceuticals can be dangerous to the pregnant woman, less attention has been directed to the effects of chemical exposure in the general environment (6,26,68,119). The pregnant woman, however, is exposed to a vast array of pollutants in air, water, and food. The pollutants vary from the products of combustion found in indoor and outdoor air to complex organic chemicals and toxic metals present in hazardous waste sites (see Chapters 2–5).

The area in and around the home, in particular, may be an important source of chemical exposure for the pregnant woman, the fetus, and the newborn. Toxic chemicals may be found in such consumer products as paints, cleansers, solvents, propellants, and plastics and in such building materials as resins and insulation (20). Volatile organic compounds used in hobbies or heavy metals that vaporize from kilns may also contaminate the home. A study by the National Academy of Sciences found that homeowners in the United States use 5.3 to 10.6 lb of pesticide per acre per year. This figure is often many times the amount applied by farmers to corn and soybean crops (37). Chemicals from the workplace may also be brought home inadvertently on soiled clothing. Excessive lead and asbestos exposures have resulted from this practice (2,4). Proximity to industry and to hazardous waste sites may also be a potential source of contamination in and around the home. The home can also be subject to contamination with insecticides and aerial sprayings with herbicides.

TABLE 24-1. Environmental and Occupational Chemicals Associated
with Adverse Effects on Human Reproduction[a]

Agent	Effects
Anesthetic gases	Abortions, decreased birth weight, stillbirths, and congenital malformations
Carbon disulfide	Abortions, premature births, menstrual disorders
Carbon monoxide	Fetal death, severe neurological impairment
Formaldehyde	Low birth weight
Hexachlorobenzene	Stillbirths, increased death rate in infants
Laboratory chemicals (including organic solvents)	Abortions, congenital malformations
Lead and other smelter emissions	Abortions, decreased birth weights, stillbirths, neonatal deaths, and neurological impairment
Methyl mercury	Gross impairment in mental and motor development, cerebral palsy
Pesticides	?Miscarriages, low birth weights, toxemia, postpartum hemorrhage
Polychlorinated biphenyls (PCBs)	Stillbirths, low birth weight, developmental defects, cola-colored skin
Vinyl chloride	?Fetal death

[a]Data in table derived from Barlow and Sullivan (6) and Nisbet and Karch (119).

TABLE 24-2. Environmental and Occupational Chemicals Associated with Adverse Effects on the Female Reproductive System[a]

Agent	Effects
Metals	
Chromium	Altered menses, amenorrhea
Lead	Abnormal menses
Mercury	Menstrual disorders
Pesticides	
Organochlorines:	Abnormal menses, menorrhagia, hypermenorrhea, toxemia of pregnancy
DDT, toxaphene, lindane	
Organophosphates	Hypermenorrhea, oligomenorrhea
Organic compounds	
Gasoline	Altered menses, impaired fertility
Benzene, toluene, xylene	Prolonged menstrual bleeding
Miscellaneous compounds	
Carbon disulfide	Menstrual disorders
Formaldehyde	Abnormal menses, toxemia and anemia in pregnancy
Phthalate esters	Abnormal menses, ?anovulation
Vinyl chloride	Irregular menses
Rubber industry	Irregular menses

[a]Data in table derived from Mattison (98) and Nisbet and Karch (119).

Toxicology

Developmental Toxicology

The fetal response to toxic agents depends on such factors as the agent, the dose, the duration of exposure, the species involved, and the timing of the insult relative to fetal development (77). It has been repeatedly observed that high embryotoxicity may be associated with minimal maternal toxicity (181). Thus, the embryo is generally more sensitive to chemical exposure than the mother (Fig. 24-1).

In general, acute exposures are thought to have greater teratogenic potential than chronic exposures. As with other toxic responses, teratogenic effects are expected to follow a dose-response curve that is generally quite steep. Thus far every carefully tested teratogen has demonstrated a threshold below which no adverse morphological effects were observed (180). For most agents, however, the dose thresholds for teratogenicity are generally unknown. Exposure to multiple agents may alter developmental toxicity. Animal studies have demonstrated that exposure to multiple agents, each of which is nonteratogenic, can cause a high incidence of malformations. For example, a high incidence of birth defects follows exposure to a mixture of cyclophosphamide, actinomycin, and 5-fluorouracil. Individually these agents are nonteratogenic (178). In some animal models, susceptibility to teratogens may be seasonal or exhibit a circadian rhythm.

The timing of toxic exposure relative to fetal development is most important. During the early

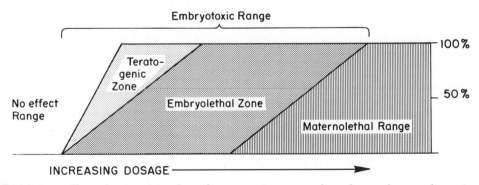

FIGURE 24-1. Toxic effects of an increasing dose of a teratogenic agent on the embryo and maternal organism. From Wilson (181).

preimplantation period, when the blastocyst is free within the uterus, toxic exposures are most likely to be lethal. Toxic exposure occurring during organogenesis, the interval between implantation and the 55th day in humans, is most likely to produce malformations (181) (Fig. 24-2). Species differences are associated with divergent reactions to teratogenic agents. A most notable example of this phenomenon is the response to thalidomide. The human embryo is extremely vulnerable to the deforming effects of this agent, whereas the rat is resistant (147).

Maternal Factors There are many metabolic events that intervene between the maternal exposure to toxic agents and the fetal exposure to toxic agents. The maternal distribution, detoxication, and excretion of foreign chemicals coupled with the protective action of the placenta all serve to reduce fetal exposure.

Once the developmental toxicant is absorbed by the mother, it is distributed within the maternal circulation and tissues. When the agent is sequestered in maternal tissues, circulating levels may be reduced. Lipophilic pollutants such as 2,2-bis(p-chlorophenyl)-1,1,1-trichloroethane (DDT), polychlorinated biphenyls (PCBs), and polybrominated biphenyls (PBBs) are stored in adipose tissue, and lead may accumulate in bone. Maternal detoxication of foreign compounds further reduces fetal exposure.

On occasion, however, such reactions within the mother may produce metabolites that are more toxic than the original compound. Under these circumstances, the biotransformations taking place in the mother can increase the toxic assault on the fetus (75). The reproductive toxicity attributed to polycyclic hydrocarbons, i.e., benzo[a]pyrene, carbon monoxide, cyanide, and nicotine depends on this process (102,132,148). It has also been shown that xenobiotics such as polycyclic hydrocarbons induce microsomal enzyme activity. This in turn can lead to increased toxicity through the production of bioactive metabolites. The extent to which maternal metabolism increases fetal exposure to developmental toxicants is not known. Clearly, much work remains to be done in this important area.

The maternal excretion of foreign chemicals (xenobiotics) also reduces fetal exposure to such agents. The excretory capacity of the maternal lung, kidney, and biliary and gastrointestinal tracts is therefore of vital importance to the developing embryo.

It is evident that fetal exposure to toxic agents is closely linked to the mother's ability to detoxify and excrete foreign chemicals. Any condition that alters this process would tend to affect the environmental assault received by the fetus. Thus, the age of the mother and her nutritional status, general health, and well-being all affect her capacity to protect the developing embryo.

Placental Factors Although the placenta has long been known to guard the fetus from environmental assault, there is ample evidence that many chemicals traverse the placenta (36). The critical question relative to fetal toxicity is the rate at which foreign chemicals traverse the placenta. Transfer may occur by simple diffusion, by facilitated diffusion, by filtration, by active transport, or by pinocytosis.

A number of factors affect the rate of transfer. The maternal plasma concentration is most impor-

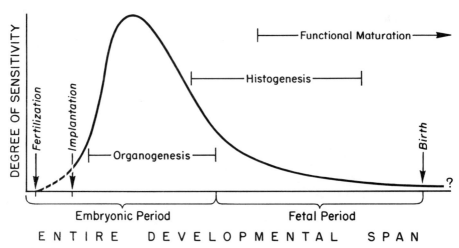

FIGURE 24-2. Sensitivity to toxicity across entire developmental span. From Wilson (179).

tant. So too are lipid solubility, molecular weight, and electrical charge. Compounds with high lipid solubility, low molecular weight, and low charge generally move across the placenta with ease. Water-soluble agents and those bound to serum albumin move less easily. Circulatory flow on either side of the placenta also influences the transplacental flux of molecules (73). In some instances agents may be preferentially concentrated in the fetus. Under such circumstances the fetus is exposed to a higher dose than is the mother. Methyl mercury is an example of an agent that is preferentially concentrated in the fetus.

Since the placenta is known to have all of the common detoxication mechanisms, it is possible that the transplacental movement of foreign chemicals could be affected by such reactions. It appears, however, that the placental metabolism of xenobiotics is not sufficient to significantly affect their transfer across this organ (71,75). There is some concern, however, that placental metabolism may generate bioactive metabolites that may be toxic to the embryo/fetus. Although our knowledge of the placental metabolism is fragmentary, it has been reported that maternal exposure to polychlorinated biphenyls can induce microsomal enzymes in the human placenta (184).

Embryonic Factors The presence of xenobiotic metabolism in the fetus is established. Very little data exist on the ability of early mammalian embryos to metabolize foreign compounds. It has been shown, however, that the preimplantation mouse embryo can metabolize benzo[a]pyrene (49). At midgestation, the livers of human fetuses are capable of oxidizing a wide variety of foreign compounds. Hydrolytic and conjugative reactions are also present in the human liver at this time (133). It appears, however, that the fetal capacity to detoxify foreign chemicals that have crossed the placenta is limited (75,76,131). Subsequent studies, however, indicate that this capacity may be greater than was formerly appreciated (74). The evidence that the fetus itself produces reactive metabolites from the metabolism of xenobiotics points out yet another potential source of harm to the fetus.

Xenobiotic-metabolizing enzymes found in the fetal liver and other tissues can be induced by perinatal exposure to foreign chemicals (132). Although the increase in fetal enzyme activity, relative to the basal state, may be marked, it is much lower than that found in the adult liver. The implications of induced fetal enzyme activity, particularly in relationship to fetotoxicity produced by the generation of reactive metabolites, is a matter of speculation.

In summary, fetal exposure to a foreign chemical is the net result of a complex and delicate interplay among many forces, i.e., maternal absorption, distribution (sequestration), metabolism, excretion, placental transport and metabolism, and fetal distribution, metabolism, and excretion. The implications of xenobiotic metabolism in the mother, placenta, and embryo/fetus are a topic of current investigation.

Reproductive Toxicology

The ability to reproduce depends on the structural and functional integration of a number of systems. Consequently, there are a number of ways in which reproductive function can be impaired either directly or indirectly. Environmental assault may affect the genetic determinants of sex, gametogenesis, sexual development and reproductive tract differentiation, and the postnatal integration of endocrine function necessary for procreation (34). The effects of exposure to environmental agents on sexual differentiation and reproductive capacity are largely unknown. A number of agents, however, have been shown to affect hormone synthesis and function (33).

Increasingly, biological markers that define cellular, biochemical, or molecular alterations that are measurable in tissues are being used to determine the extent of exposure and its effects. Developments in this field, particularly as related to the current status and potential markers in female reproductive toxicology, have been reviewed (156).

Animal Testing to Determine Reproductive Hazards

Since agents suspected of having reproductive toxicity can seldom if ever be tested in people, most data must come from animal and laboratory experimentation. Animal testing is the single most important method used to predict human reproductive risk associated with toxic exposure. Animal testing also provides fundamental access to the basic biology of abnormal development.

Animal studies for identifying reproductive hazards are divided into four segments, which are applied to two or more animal species at several chemical concentrations. The first segment looks at fertility and general reproductive performance in both sexes. The second segment studies embryotoxicity and teratogenicity in pregnant females during the period of organogenesis. The third segment assesses late injuries during the fetal and postnatal periods and during lactation. The fourth segment involves multigeneration testing. These studies are intended to assess such areas as gonadal function, conception, abortion, maternal behavior, fetal development, and postpartum growth over more than one generation (172).

Clearly, the major purpose of animal testing is

to assess human risk. Although there are caveats that must be applied before the results of animal teratogenicity testing can be applied to humans, it is notable that almost all chemicals considered to cause human malformations have induced embryotoxicity in some animal species. The teratogenic effects may differ among animal species and frequently differ from those observed in humans.

When assessing human risk, animal testing attempts to answer three questions. (1) Does the agent induce developmental defects (teratogenic potential)? (2) Over what dose ranges are birth defects produced (teratogenic potency)? (3) What is the relationship between developmental toxicity and adult toxicity? The details of these important concepts and their relationship to human risk estimation have recently been addressed (44).

The current animal-testing procedures for teratogens—all of which are expensive, time consuming, and wasteful of animals—have spurred interest in screening tests for teratogenesis. The in vitro systems currently under investigation for teratogenicity testing include whole-organ culture (embryonic limb bud) and whole (postimplantation) embryo culture (118,154). If successful, such tests may allow the rapid and inexpensive mass screening of chemicals. The in vitro approach to teratogenicity testing has been reviewed by Brown and Fabro (14).

EPIDEMIOLOGY

Epidemiologic methods are used to define and document a potential relationship between exposure and reproductive failure or developmental defects. Observational studies of human populations are the core of this discipline. Although epidemiologic studies have elucidated many etiologic factors in human disease, they generally demonstrate a statistical association between pollutant exposure and an adverse health effect, rather than proving causation.

Epidemiologic investigation of the adverse reproductive effects of human exposure to environmental agents can be divided into two general categories. The first is concerned with the distribution of disease. The second focuses on its determinants. The latter, often called analytical epidemiology, includes cohort and case-control studies. In the cohort study (prospective and retrospective), the frequency of adverse outcome is compared between exposed and unexposed individuals. In the case-control study, the frequency of exposure among individuals with the disease is compared with those who are free of the disease. Some epidemiologic studies concerned with reproductive outcome have searched for evidence of toxic exposure in mothers of malformed children or looked for defects in the off-

spring of exposed mothers. Other studies have examined the reproductive function of populations involved in episodes of contamination and those living near factories or hazardous waste sites.

Before the epidemiologic methods can be applied to the study of reproductive dysfunction, reproductive performance and exposure must be assessed (12). Table 24-3 lists the markers that can be used to monitor reproductive failure associated with environmental exposures. In some cases the adverse effects occur early and are quite easily measured; in others they are subtle and/or delayed. It is relatively easy, for example, to monitor such endpoints as decreased birth weight or infant death but much more difficult to monitor sexual dysfunction, behavioral disorders, learning disabilities, or transplacental malignancies, which appear in the offspring long after their in utero exposure to the causal agent. A study of behavioral disorders in the offspring is referred to as behavioral teratology. In recent years greater attention has been given to subtle postnatal changes induced by fetal exposure to hazardous substances (10; see also Chapter 14).

All epidemiologic studies have inherent limitations. Some relate to the method itself, whereas others are specific to the study of reproductive effects. One of the major limitations of case-control studies is recall bias. A mother who has a poor reproductive outcome or a defective child will be more likely to remember exposures than one who has had a normal child. If the exposure history is obtained from an interview, there is the additional problem of faulty recall because of the time that has elapsed. Cohort studies also have limitations. These include the time required for completion of the study and attrition of the exposed group that is being followed.

Epidemiologic studies of reproductive effects

TABLE 24-3. Markers of Reproductive Dysfunction[a]

Sexual dysfunction: libido, potency
Sperm abnormalities: number, motility, shape
Decreased fertility
Illness during pregnancy
Abortions
Stillbirths
Infant deaths
Birth defects: major, minor, mutations
Chromosomal abnormalities
Decreased birth weight
Premature or postmature births
Altered sex ratio
Childhood morbidity and developmental disabilities
Childhood malignancies
Age at menopause

[a]Table derived from Bloom (12).

must take into account certain special considerations. First, reproductive outcome is related to exposure of the father as well as the mother. Second, some reproductive impairments and losses are difficult to measure and record. Reproductive failure resulting from impotence or infertility, for example, is difficult to assess and not usually recorded. Early spontaneous abortions may go unnoticed, and those occurring during the first trimester are not routinely recorded. Third, the control of confounding variables—factors that are independently associated with the toxic exposure and adverse reproductive effects—are nearly all related to maternal exposures and characteristics (Table 24-4). When attributes of the sperm and/or semen are being studied for their effect on reproduction, male characteristics and exposures are pertinent. It is noteworthy that male characteristics, exposures, attributes of the sperm and semen are also pertinent with regard to their effects on reproduction (see Chapter 25).

The epidemiologist investigating the effects of environmental exposure on reproduction clearly confronts major problems in controlling for confounding variables. For example, loss of libido or potency may be psychogenic. Attention must be directed to this possibility before attributing reproductive effects to chemical exposure. Hyperthermia in the male may give rise to oligospermia. Hyperthermia, physical stress, and anxiety in the female may cause anovulation, menstrual irregularities, and decreased fertility (34,164).

Exposure to drugs is one of the most important variables to be considered in the study of reproductive dysfunction. This includes the use of cigarettes, alcohol, and prescription and nonprescription drugs. The reproductive difficulties that follow the use of these agents have been well documented (58,86).

Maternal age is another variable that must be considered when studying adverse reproductive effects. Women at both extremes of their reproductive years have decreased fertility because of anovulation. The very young are reported to give birth to

TABLE 24-4. Confounding Factors in the Study of Toxic Exposure and Adverse Reproductive Effects

Concurrent drug exposure (cigarettes, alcohol, pharmaceuticals)
Contraceptive use
Surgical procedures (vasectomy, tubal ligation)
Maternal age and parity; paternal age
Geographic and social factors
Genetic factors
Infectious disease and concurrent illness
Metabolic diseases
Nutritional deficiencies

offspring with a higher incidence of birth defects. Increasing maternal age is also correlated with a greater risk of having children with chromosomal abnormalities. Higher abortion rates might also be expected with advancing maternal age. Advancing paternal age has been shown to increase spontaneous abortions. For example, when the association between paternal occupational exposure to vinyl chloride was studied in relation to fetal loss, Clemmensen demonstrated that the increase in fetal loss could be explained by the confounding effect of paternal age (18).

Other exposures, in themselves teratogenic, must also be considered for their confounding effect. These include viral illnesses with such agents as Herpes simplex, rubella, and cytomegalic virus. Syphilitic infections and toxoplasmosis may also cause birth defects.

Various metabolic derangements may predispose to teratogenesis. The best known of these are nutritional deficiencies and diabetes mellitus. Deficiencies of protein and vitamins A, B_2, and E have been shown to give rise to birth defects in animals. Diabetes mellitus is associated not only with lowered fertility and increased fetal loss but also with an increased incidence of birth defects.

Variations in the effects of exposure on reproduction may sometimes be accounted for by variations in the duration and intensity of exposure or by the complex interactions between multiple exposures. As previously mentioned, exposure to multiple toxic agents may enhance their teratogenic effect. It is possible, for example, that the teratogenic effects of some chemicals may be enhanced by exposure to agents commonly present in cigarette smoke.

Apart from the problems mentioned above, the epidemiologist generally encounters difficulties in assessing exposure. Frequently, little if any information is available on exposure. Exposures are often multiple. In addition, the populations under investigation are often so small that the study has limited ability to detect an effect, if in fact an adverse reproductive effect exists. For these reasons, and the problems cited previously, the lack of epidemiologic evidence affirming an untoward reproductive effect of certain environmental exposures should not be taken as proof that no such effect exists.

Most foreign compounds have not been critically evaluated for their effect on reproduction. Studies thus far have generally focused on the reproductive hazards of drugs and chemicals found in the workplace. Exposures are generally higher and more easily monitored under these conditions. A few studies have explored the reproductive effects of environmental exposure to heavy metals, polyhalogenated biphenyls, pesticides, Agent Orange, herbicides, dioxin, solvents, carbon monoxide, and hazardous waste sites. In some instances, particularly with episodes of environmental contamination, there is evidence of adverse reproductive effects. In other instances adverse effects have not been established.

This discussion is limited to the untoward reproductive effects of maternal exposure and exposure of both parents. The adverse reproductive effects of paternal exposure are discussed in Chapter 25.

Developmental Effects

Heavy Metals

Lead   Lead is widely distributed in the environment. Metallic lead produced from ore is used in a wide variety of industries, where it is cast or molded into shape or used as solder. It is a major component of many alloys. Metallic lead and its compounds have a wide variety of uses as paint pigments, in storage batteries, and in ceramics. Tetraethyl lead is used as an antiknock agent in gasoline.

The adverse effect of lead on reproduction has been known since the mid-1800s. Exposure to lead may result in decreased fertility in both sexes; it may increase the frequency of abnormal pregnancies, spontaneous abortions, and stillbirths (21,26,56). During the industrial revolution, women employed in lead factories had a high incidence of spontaneous abortions and stillbirths (128). It is of interest that the abortifacient effect of lead was so well known around the turn of the century that in England and Denmark it was administered for this purpose (55).

Maternal exposure to lead during the course of gestation results in a broad spectrum of adverse fetal effects. There may be neurological damage, often with mental retardation, or there may be intrauterine or postnatal growth retardation. A higher proportion of retarded infants were born to women who drank water containing excessive amounts of lead during their pregnancy (177). Increased concentrations of lead have been found in the placentae of stillbirths and infants with congenital malformations (175). The concentration of umbilical cord blood lead was discovered to be associated, in a dose-related fashion, with an increased risk for minor anomalies (114).

Bellinger et al. performed a prospective cohort study of children from birth to 2 years of age that assessed the relationship between prenatal and postnatal lead exposure and early cognitive development (10). The results of this study indicate that lead levels in the umbilical cord blood between 10 and 25 μg/dL (0.5–1.2 μmol/L) were associated with slower mental growth than expected by the age of 2. These findings, along with the results of other studies, indicate that adverse effects occur at blood lead concentrations that were formerly thought to be safe (31,92,149) (see Chapters 13 and 14). It has been suggested that the teratogenic effects of lead represent a paradigm for transplacental toxicants (113).

Occupational studies and case reports of poisonings from drinking lead-contaminated water or tainted moonshine whiskey or from inhaling lead fumes from the burning of battery cases have also confirmed the reproductive hazards of lead exposure (15,129).

Evidence is accumulating that lead may be toxic to the placenta and thus affect the course of the pregnancy. Catz and Jaffee noted a relationship between placental hemorrhage and lead-induced abortion (16). An epidemiologic study of pregnant women living near a lead mine in Missouri correlated the levels of lead in the placenta, in the amniotic membranes, and in the fetus with premature rupture of the membranes and premature delivery (45).

Methyl Mercury   Mercury is widely used in industry and agriculture. It is used in the electrolytic preparation of chlorine and caustic soda. It is also used in electrical apparatus and in such control instruments as thermometers and barometers. Mercury is used in agriculture as a fungicide for grain. The extensive use of mercury has resulted in substantial environmental contamination. Of particular concern is the environmental pollution that occurs in proximity to industrial plants that discharge mercury.

Methyl mercury is firmly established as a toxin to the developing fetus (120). The adverse reproductive effects of this compound were demonstrated by an epidemic of mercury poisoning that occurred in the 1950s in Minimata Japan. The epidemic developed when fish, contaminated with methyl mercury from the effluent of a nearby factory, were eaten by the local inhabitants. Cerebral palsy and mental retardation occurred in the offspring of women who ate the contaminated fish. The enhanced vulnerability of the fetal brain was clearly evidenced by the severe neurological symptoms found in the offspring of mothers who exhibited few symptoms (173). The neurological impairment affecting the newborn and the inhabitants of the area came to be known as "Minimata disease" (103).

Other episodes have been reported of mercury poisoning caused by the accidental ingestion of contaminated food. In 1964 an epidemic of poisoning linked to eating mercury-contaminated fish was reported in Niigata, Japan. There have also been reports of accidental poisoning by the ingestion of seeds tainted with fungicides containing alkyl or phenyl mercury compounds. Such events have been reported in Sweden, Guatemala, Pakistan, Iraq, and in the United States in New Mexico. The fetal neurological sequelae of these episodes were similar to those found in Minimata, Japan.

Studies suggest that exposure to mercury compounds in the workplace can be associated with menstrual disorders and with such reproductive disorders as growth retardation (53,105).

Multiple Exposures

Swedish studies have described such reproductive problems as reduction in birth weight, spontaneous abortion, and congenital malformations in female employees of a metal smelter in northern Sweden (9,123–126). The major products of the smelter were arsenic, copper, lead, sulfuric acid and sulfur dioxide. One study drew attention to the increased reproductive risk that might occur when the father as well as the mother was employed at the smelter (125).

Hemminki et al. were the first to study the contributions of both parents to an adverse reproductive outcome (62). These investigators, using national hospital discharge and census tract data, examined the incidence of spontaneous abortion in a single Finnish community with over 30,000 inhabitants. Spontaneous abortions were analyzed according to the occupations and workplaces of both the women and their husbands. A significant increase in the rate of spontaneous abortions was noted in women who worked in a textile plant. This increased risk varied with the husband's workplace. Thus, a further increase in the rate of spontaneous abortions among women textile workers was noted when their husbands worked at a large metallurgical factory. Little change was observed in those women whose husbands worked elsewhere. These data suggest that events taking place in both parents can act in a synergistic manner to increase the risk of an adverse reproductive outcome.

Polyhalogenated Hydrocarbons

Polychlorinated Biphenyls The polychlorinated biphenyls (PCBs), produced commercially since 1929, are a mixture of a number of chlorobiphenyl isomers. These compounds have great chemical and thermal stability. The PCBs have been used extensively in capacitors and high-voltage transformers, as plasticizers in paints, inks, and paper, as hydraulic fluids, and as heat-transfer agents. Animal studies show that the PCBs affect fetal and postnatal growth and development (6,101). The PCBs persist in the environment and are found in ambient air, water, and many foods. It has been estimated that about 90% of the general population have detectable levels of PCBs in their adipose tissue. PCBs are no longer produced in the United States.

In 1968, an industrial accident in southern Japan resulted in large-scale human poisoning with PCB (85). "Yusho" (rice oil disease) was linked to the ingestion of cooking rice oil that was accidentally contaminated with PCBs during its refining process (84). There were over 1,200 cases of "Yusho" disease. The major manifestations included chloracne—a cystic, relatively noninflammatory acne-like rash—headache, anorexia, nausea, and diarrhea. Thirteen of the infants exposed in utero were examined. Two were stillborn, and the others showed growth retardation, conjunctivitis, neonatal jaundice, and dark cola-colored pigmentation of the skin, gingiva, and nails. Another episode of human poisoning from PCB-contaminated food has been recorded in Taiwan (84).

The PCB-contaminated rice oil also contained polychlorodibenzofurans (PCDFs) and polychlorinated quaterphenyls (PCQs). Because PCDFs are more toxic in animals models, these agents are now considered the major cause of Yusho. The polychlorodibenzofurans are also thought to play an important role in the episode of PCB poisoning that occurred in Taiwan (17,93).

Fein et al. were the first to study the effects of maternal exposure to ordinary dietary levels of PCB on the human infant (46). In this study, 242 newborn infants whose mothers consumed moderate quantities of Lake Michigan fish and 71 infants whose mothers did not eat such fish were examined during the immediate postpartum period. The ingestion of Lake Michigan fish was taken as an indicator of PCB exposure and as a source of transplacental exposure. Evidence of fetal PCB exposure was based on a maternal history of eating contaminated fish and the detection of PCB in umbilical cord blood. Increased fetal PCB exposure was associated with lower birth weight and smaller head circumference. None of the effects were attributable to such potential confounding variables as socioeconomic status, maternal age, and smoking during pregnancy. These findings are in keeping with the research on rhesus monkeys (7,96).

In 1985, evidence of congenital poisoning by polychlorinated biphenyls (PCBs) and their contaminants surfaced in Taiwan. These events were related to an episode of mass poisoning from contaminated cooking oil that occurred in 1979. Because PCBs and their contaminants persist in human tissue, children born to women after the outbreak were exposed in utero. The exposed offspring were shorter and lighter than controls and had abnormalities of the gingiva, skin, nails, teeth, and lungs (138).

In addition to being exposed to PCBs that cross the placenta, the infant may also receive exposure through breast milk. Surveys of nonoccupationally exposed mothers in the United States and other parts of the world have revealed contamination of their milk with PCBs, DDT, and other similar agents (136,137). A 1975 survey of pesticides found in 1,038 samples of mother's milk showed 1% with no PCB contamination, 69% with levels below 0.05 ppm, and 30% with levels above 0.05 ppm. Of the latter group about 20% have levels of PCBs above 0.1 ppm (141). The PCBs, being lipophilic and difficult to excrete, are normally stored in fat. During lactation, they are excreted in breast milk, which is about 3% fat.

Polybrominated Biphenyls Polybrominated biphenyls (PBBs), like PCBs, are polyhalogenated aromatic hydrocarbons that are lipophilic, poorly metabolized, and slowly excreted. These highly brominated compounds have been used as flame retardants, mainly in plastics requiring high heat resistance. The PBBs are reported to be fetotoxic and teratogenic in animal studies (6). They are no longer manufactured in the United States.

In 1973, the food supply of the state of Michigan was inadvertently contaminated with PBB. A fire retardant, Firemaster, containing PBBs was accidently mixed with cattle feed. By the time the PBB contamination was detected a year later, large numbers of Michigan residents had eaten contaminated farm and dairy products. Numerous studies, including those of reproductive dysfunction, have been done to evaluate the health impact of this episode of environmental contamination.

The neuropsychological development of young children conceived, born, and/or breast fed during the period of maximal PBB exposure has been studied (144,145). Seagull studied children between the ages of 2½ and 4 years, whereas Schwartz and Rae studied them between the ages of 4 and 6 years. From the initial report it appeared that PBB exposure, based on PBB levels in a fat biopsy, had a significant adverse effect on neuropsychological development. This finding, however, was not confirmed by the follow-up study done 2 years later. The disparity between the findings could be related to the different conditions of testing and the small numbers involved. It could also reflect diminishing of the PBB effect with time (112). These studies emphasize that attention must be directed to the subtle and latent reproductive effects of pollutant exposure, which may be difficult to evaluate by epidemiologic methods.

Studies of fetal mortality in relation to PBB contamination reveal little or no effect (67). The misclassification of exposure status and the absence of information on early spontaneous abortions represent serious methodological problems in this study.

Pesticides

Although many pesticides have been shown to be teratogenic in animals, few studies have explored the reproductive hazards of pesticide exposure in humans (142). Increased fetal loss and malformations of the extremities have been reported in Japan following the high-level spraying of organophosphorus pesticides on field workers (127). Nora et al. reported two offspring with malformations in a group of 50 mothers exposed to insecticides during their first trimester (121). Additional epidemiologic studies are clearly needed to evaluate the reproductive risks of pesticide exposure in the home and agricultural setting.

Agent Orange, Dioxin, and Phenoxy Herbicides

Agent Orange Agent Orange, the most widely used herbicide in Vietnam, was composed of a mixture of equal parts 2,4-dichlorophenoxyacetic acid (2,4-D) and 2,4,5-trichlorophenoxyacetic acid (2,4,5-T). It was reported that the 2,4,5-T in Agent Orange contained about 2 ppm of 2,3,7,8-tetrachlorodibenzo-*p*-dioxin (TCDD) or "dioxin" (189). Although there are 75 chlorodioxins, TCDD or "dioxin" is considered to be the most toxic of this group. It is estimated that about 25 million kilograms of 2,4-D, 20 million kilograms of 2,4,5-T, and 166 kg of TCDD were released in Vietnam (189).

The phenoxy herbicides, which include 2,4-D and 2,4,5-T, gained wide acceptance as weed control agents in the early 1940s. TCDD is a contaminant produced in the manufacture of the herbicide 2,4,5-T. For this reason 2,4,5-T and all of its products may be contaminated with TCDD. Between 1948 and 1970 vast amounts of 2,4,5-T (contaminated with TCDD) was used in forestry, farming, and along roadsides to control weeds. In 1979 the Environmental Protection Agency suspended the use of 2,4,5-T in forestry, rights of way, and pastures (166).

Experimental studies reveal that TCDD and 2,4,5-T (with or without TCDD) adversely affect reproduction in animals. TCDD is an extremely potent teratogen and fetotoxic agent. It produces cleft palate in mice in doses lower than those found with any other agent (27). TCDD is fetotoxic to a number of animals including rats, sheep, monkeys, rabbits, and hamsters (52,100,116,151). TCDD also causes diminished fertility, decreased litter size, survival, growth after birth, and immunologic defects (107,171). Animal studies also show that 2,4,5-T, with or without TCDD contamination, is embryopathic and teratogenic in rodents, producing cleft palates, renal anomalies, and perhaps skeletal malformations (28,29,65,116). Exposure to 2,4-D has been teratogenic and fetotoxic in some studies but not in others (187). It is of interest that the administration of 2,4,5-T to incubating chicken eggs, in environmentally relevant doses, altered behavior in chickens after hatching (140). Several comprehensive reviews of the toxicology and teratogenic effects of Agent Orange, TCDD, and the phenoxy herbicides have been published (24,25,50,167).

A great deal of concern exists about the potential adverse reproductive effects of exposure to Agent Orange and the phenoxy herbicides. Vast numbers of people have been exposed to these agents, which animal studies have identified as teratogens. Epidemiologic studies of the Vietnamese population show no clear teratogenic hazard related to Agent Orange exposure. It has been suggested, however, that the offspring of Vietnamese women who were exposed to herbicides have an increased incidence of congenital malformations (30). A review of Vietnamese hospital records between 1962 and 1973 revealed no increased frequency of birth defects in the children of women who may have been exposed to herbicides (83). These studies are, unfortunately, seriously flawed on methodological grounds.

The traditional concern for adverse effects in the offspring from maternal exposure now includes an awareness that untoward reproductive events may also be mediated through the father (30,39, 41,60,62,88,150,157,162). The issue of birth defects mediated through exposure of the father is discussed in Chapter 25.

Dioxin and Phenoxy Herbicides Widespread environmental exposure to dioxin occurred in 1976 in Seveso, Italy as a result of a runaway chemical reaction at a factory synthesizing trichlorophenol. Over 37,000 individuals were potentially exposed to varying amounts of this agent. The seriousness of this accident was not appreciated until birds, plants, and animals began to show signs of severe toxicity a few days after the accident. Nine days after the accident dioxin was found in the area. Investigating the incidence of congenital abnormalities among children whose mothers were exposed to dioxin was difficult for a number of reasons. There was a lack of reliable indicators of exposure, an absence of good base-line data for the period prior to the accident, a sparsity of reproductive events in the area of highest exposure, a firm recommendation on contraception, a high rate of elective abortions, and a delay in implementing the studies. Follow-up studies, however, reported no evidence of a significant teratologic effect related to TCDD exposure (23,92).

A number of epidemiologic studies have looked at the reproductive effects of environmental exposure of both sexes to phenoxy herbicides and dioxin (35,50,57,115,160,161). Thomas, conducting a study in Hungary, reported that although 2,4,5-T use has increased over 26-fold between 1969 and 1975 there was no associated increase in the incidence of cleft palate and lip or of cystic kidney disease (160). A more recent Hungarian study by Thomas and Czeizel revealed no relationship between rates of miscarriage and birth defects and herbicide consumption (161).

Another study in the United States by Nelson et al. revealed no relationship between agricultural use of 2,4,5-T and the incidence of cleft palate in the state of Arkansas (115). An investigation of the rate of birth defects in New Zealand offered no evidence that aerial spraying with 2,4,5-T was associated with any malformation of the central nervous system, including spina bifida. A significant association between spraying of 2,4,5-T and the occurrence of talipes was noted however (57). An Australian study performed by Field and Kerr demonstrated a significant association between the amount of 2,4,5-T used and the rates of neural tube defects (48). An EPA study examining the frequency of spontaneous abortions in an area of Oregon subjected to aerial spraying with 2,4,5-T containing dioxin reported a positive relationship between spontaneous abortions and 2,4,5-T use (165).

Unfortunately, all epidemiologic studies concerned with the reproductive effects of herbicides and dioxin exposure are faulted by such serious methodological problems as inadequate assessment of exposure, mixed exposures, inadequate information on the background incidence of spontaneous abortions and other abnormal reproductive outcomes, and inadequate assessment of confounding variables.

Organic Solvents

Although adverse reproductive effects in humans have not been clearly linked to solvent exposure, preliminary studies suggest that they may pose a hazard to reproduction. Apart from occupational exposures to such agents as benzene, toluene, and glycol ethers, excessive exposure to organic solvents occurs with substance abuse. Substances that are sniffed to achieve an altered state of mind and intoxication include plastic, model, and household cements, fingernail polish remover, lacquer thinner, lighter fluid, and gasoline. The principal solvents in these substances are *n*-hexane, toluene, ethyl acetate, acetone, and benzene.

The adverse reproductive effects of glue sniffing were observed by Suzuki et al. (158). These workers observed that four women who sniffed glue containing toluene gave birth to premature infants. Three of the infants had birth defects, which included cardiac defects and facial and nail abnormalities. Hunter et al. also suggested a link between solvent exposure and birth defects (69). This suggestion was based on the dysmorphic features and mental retardation seen in the offspring of two pregnant women who inhaled gasoline. The gasoline contained tetraethyl lead as well as hydrocarbons.

During an 8-year period in Czechoslovakia,

Kucera noted that the mothers of five of the nine infants born with sacral agenesis had close contact with organic solvents during their pregnancy (82). The solvents in question were acetone, xylene, trichlorethylene, methyl chloride, and gasoline. Hemminki et al. noted that the rate of spontaneous abortion among women chemical workers in Finland was significantly higher than among other women. Women working with pharmaceuticals, plastics, especially styrene, and viscose rayon had the greatest risk (59). In another study, no differences in neurobehavioral development were noted in the children of mothers who worked with organic solvents during their pregnancy (40). Additional epidemiologic studies are needed to confirm these findings and to determine the effect of organic solvent exposure on the pregnancy and the fetus.

In animal studies, organic solvents such as chloroform, carbon tetrachloride, methyl ethyl ketone, and perchloroethylene cause intrauterine death or growth retardation (182).

Carbon Monoxide

Carbon monoxide, formed by the incomplete combustion of organic fuels, has been shown to have adverse effects on the fetus. There is clear evidence that carbon monoxide poisoning in humans can result in fetal death or severe neurological damage (22,89). Fetal effects appear to be related to the intensity of maternal exposure. Carbon monoxide poisoning in the mother severe enough to cause unconsciousness is associated with great risk to the fetus. Under these conditions fetal death or severe neurological damage may occur. Because the fetus is more sensitive to anoxia than is the mother, levels of carbon monoxide that are tolerated by the mother may produce fetal toxicity. It is well known that maternal smoking results in low birth weights. Maternal smoking is also reported to be associated with increased perinatal death and congenital heart disease (6,89,139). Whether these adverse effects are related to the increased maternal levels of carbon monoxide that occur with smoking is unknown.

Hazardous Waste Sites

Thus far there is little evidence of a definite reproductive hazard among individuals living near a hazardous waste site. Investigators exploring this problem generally find that the contents of the chemical site have not been adequately identified, that it is difficult if not impossible to document individual exposure, and that the population at risk is small (155,168).

The Love Canal site with the presence of over 82 organic chemicals and metals has been the subject of numerous epidemiologic studies. One study demonstrated a statistically significant excess of low birth weight among live-born infants in the houses located on the natural drainage pathways in the area. This occurred during the period of active dumping from 1940 to 1953. Another study raised the question of an association between an increase in spontaneous abortion and chemical exposure from the Love Canal site (169,170).

Irradiation

Human exposure to ionizing radiation is derived primarily from natural background radiation, from irradiation used in the treatment of malignant tumors, and from the medical use of x rays. Other sources include atmospheric weapons testing and nuclear power plant operation.

Much of our understanding of the teratogenic effects of ionizing radiation on fetal and postnatal development is derived from the epidemiologic studies performed on the offspring of women who were exposed to the atomic bomb in Hiroshima and Nagasaki (19,106,185,188). Microcephaly occurred in the offspring of women exposed to levels between 5 and 10 rads (104). Severe mental retardation also followed prenatal exposure to the atomic bomb (106). Evidence exists of increase risk of leukemia and other cancers following prenatal exposure to irradiation; at present, however, there is no agreement that this finding is related to irradiation (90,91,106).

Reproductive Effects

Traditionally, studies of reproductive hazards have focused on the embryo, fetus, and placenta. It is increasingly apparent that attention must be directed to the toxic effects of environmental chemicals on the male and female reproductive system.

Although our knowledge of the toxic effects of xenobiotics on the female reproductive system is fragmentary, there are reports that suggest that certain occupational exposures are associated with menstrual disturbances, ovarian toxicity, abnormal hormonal production, uterine toxicity, and impaired fertility (98). Very little information is available on the effects of toxic exposure on the cervix and the vagina.

Exposure to pesticides that contain halogenated hydrocarbons and organophosphorus compounds are reported to be linked to abnormal menses, temporary infertility, and a change in ovarian function (Table 24-2). Many of the heavy metals also appear to alter the menstrual cycle in women (97,99). Exposures to various hydrocarbons have also been reported to affect female reproductive function (98) (Table 24-2).

Irradiation may affect the female reproductive

potential. Exposure of the oocytes to ionizing radiation during gestation or following birth may result in reproductive disorders (5).

PATHOLOGY AND PATHOLOGICAL PHYSIOLOGY

Birth defects may arise in 2–3% of all births. Of these, 25% have underlying genetic causes, and 5–10% are caused by teratogenic agents. The remaining 60% to 65% are of unknown cause (180).

Environmental teratogens may be classified as follows: biological agents (viruses, bacteria, and protozoa), physical agents (radiation, hyperthermia), habitual practices (smoking and drinking), nutritional factors, and chemicals (drugs and toxic exposures in the workplace and general environment). Of the birth defects caused by exposure to environmental agents, it is estimated that 4–6% may result from exposure to chemicals.

As previously mentioned, chemicals may adversely affect reproduction in a number of ways. Toxic exposure during adult life can adversely affect fertility directly, by acting on the gonads, or indirectly, by altering the body's metabolism. Toxic exposure during pregnancy can cause intrauterine death, congenital malformation, cancer in the offspring, or abnormal postnatal development (Table 24-5).

TABLE 24-5. Adverse Effects of Chemical Exposure on Reproduction

Reproductive effects
  Abnormal menses
  Impaired fertility
  ?Early menopause
Developmental effects
  Fetotoxicity
    Abortion
    Stillbirths
    Neonatal deaths
  Teratogenic effects
    Birth defects
    Prenatal and postnatal retardation in morphological
      development
    Developmental disabilities compromising the function of such systems as immune, reproductive, endocrine, and including behavior disorders
    Transplacental carcinogenesis
Effects on pregnancy
  Bleeding disorders
  Toxemia
  Premature rupture of membranes
  Premature labor

Female Reproductive System

The female reproductive system—composed of the hypothalamus, pituitary, ovary, fallopian tubes, uterus, and cervix—functions through a number of complex interactions. A normal hormonal balance must exist along the hypothalamic-pituitary-ovarian-uterine axis if reproduction is to take place. Most xenobiotics have not been carefully studied for their effect on the female reproductive system. It is becoming apparent, however, that exposure to environmental chemicals may interrupt the reproductive process at a number of points (Table 24-5).

Certain xenobiotics, for example, may disrupt the normal balance of the hypothalamic-pituitary-ovarian-uterine axis. Other xenobiotics may adversely affect the oocyte (96,98). Reproductive toxins may act directly because of their similarity to such endogenous compounds as hormones or because of their chemical reactivity, as with alkylating agents. Reproductive toxins may act indirectly by interrupting the physiological control mechanisms of reproduction (96).

The prenatal exposure to environmental chemicals can have adverse effects on the reproductive function of the offspring (34). During intrauterine development, chemicals may act directly, by affecting the gonads and reproductive tract, and/or indirectly, by inhibiting growth-promoting factors. In mammals, the female is particularly vulnerable to agents that damage germ cells in utero because all oocytes appear before birth. The future reproductive capacity of the female may thereby be compromised by toxic exposure that occurs during the prenatal period. The effects of prenatal exposure to environmental chemicals on the reproductive capacity of the offspring is an important topic for future investigation.

Kimbrough and Jensen have postulated that the reproductive toxicity of halogenated polycyclic hydrocarbons is related, in part, to their hormone agonist activity (79). The estrogen agonist activity of polychlorinated biphenyls is supported by the observation that exposed animals have early opening of the vagina and persistent estrus (51). DDT, given to neonatal rats, also produces a premature vaginal opening and a persistent estrus, which are dose dependent (15,174). Although the reproductive effects of human exposure to organic compounds have not been well studied, it is of interest that abnormal menses have been reported in women with occupational exposure to organochlorine compounds (Table 24-2).

Polycyclic aromatic hydrocarbons (PAHs), which are widely dispersed pollutants produced from the combustion of fossil fuels, can also interrupt the sequence of events necessary for the menstrual cycle. Exposure to PAHs destroys oocytes in rats and mice (94), and PAH exposure of a pregnant rat will destroy oocytes in a female fetus (47). Since the ovary possesses the microsomal enzymes necessary for xenobiotic metabolism, the ovarian toxicity and oocyte destruction that follow PAH exposure may be related to the bioactive products of their metabolism (95).

Although no information is available on the reproductive effects of PAH exposure in humans, there is evidence that women who smoke have an earlier menopause and find it much more difficult to become pregnant than do nonsmokers (3,66,70). It is not known if these adverse reproductive effects are linked to the PAHs, carbon monoxide, heavy metals, or other pollutants present in cigarette smoke.

Little is known about the effect of xenobiotics on ovum transport, fertilization, implantation, and parturition.

Concepts in Teratology

About 4% to 6% of known or suspected causes of human malformations are attributable to chemicals and drugs. The mechanisms by which chemicals induce teratogenic actions are in general unknown. The effects, however, are likely to be varied, depending on the chemistry, the dose, and the time of administration. In many instances, depending on intensity of exposure, an agent may be abortifacient, a teratogen, or a carcinogen. Chemicals may act directly on the fetus or indirectly, by interfering with maternal, placental, or fetal functions. The specific mechanisms thought to be involved in teratogenesis have been discussed by a number of authors (8,72, 176,180,181).

Three factors affect the action of a teratogenic agent on the embryo: (1) the developmental stage of the embryo, (2) the genetic susceptibility of the embryo, and (3) the physiological or pathological status of the mother (163). A teratogenic effect in an embryo will not be transmitted to the next generation; only mutations in germ cells can be passed on to the offspring.

Developmental Factors

Three well-defined stages of fetal development are susceptible to xenobiotic exposure—the preimplantation, the embryonic, and the fetal stages (Fig. 24-2). During the preimplantation stage, from conception to 17 days, fertilization, blastulation, gastrulation, and erosion of the uterine wall take place. During the embryonic stage, from 18 to 55 days after conception, the process of organogenesis occurs. During the fetal phase, from the end of the embryonic stage to birth, histogenesis, function maturation, and growth take place (Fig. 24-2).

During the preimplantation phase, when the cells are still totipotential, the embryo may be killed or may recover from an environmental insult. The preimplantation period has been described as the "all-or-none period" in that the embryo will continue to grow normally if it is not destroyed by an insult (178). When the embryo perishes during the preimplantation stage, it is obviously difficult to perceive this loss. Such events may be couched in terms of impaired fertility associated with irregular or late periods.

During the embryonic phase, the greatest amount of cellular differentiation takes place. With organogenesis the embryo becomes susceptible to most teratogenic agents. Each organ system has its own critical period of vulnerability to injury. The appearance of birth defects will depend on the agent, the dose, and the timing of the insult. Embryos also may be killed during the period of organogenesis. When lethal effects occur during the embryonic period, the loss is recognized as an abortion or miscarriage.

Toxic assault during the fetal period, when histogenesis, functional maturation, and growth are taking place, can lead to growth retardation, functional deficits, and transplacental carcinogenesis. As the central nervous system continues to develop throughout the pregnancy, injury during the fetal period may give rise to functional or psychomotor deficits. Specifically, interference with development at this time may give rise to sensory or motor deficits as well as to learning, memory, and problem-solving disabilities (10). The urogenital, immune, and endocrine systems also continue to develop during the fetal period. Toxic exposure during this interval may therefore result in functional deficits in these systems (102). Increased attention is now directed to the more subtle functional changes produced by prenatal exposures. Fetal loss occurring during the fetal period is termed a stillbirth.

Death may also occur in the neonatal or postpartum period as a result of birth defects or of cumulative toxicity to vital organs. After birth the newborn must depend on its own defenses to withstand environmental assault. With relatively immature defense mechanisms, the neonate is more susceptible to exposure. Increased susceptibility to drugs and other xenobiotics is therefore present at this time (102). During the neonatal period the infant may be exposed to numerous xenobiotics through the ingestion of breast milk (136,137).

The embryo/fetus is clearly more susceptible to environmental assault than is the mother. High embryotoxicity associated with minimal maternal toxicity has been repeatedly observed in experimental studies and in humans (178). Pregnant women have been little affected by such potent teratogens as thalidomide, steroid hormones, and folic acid antagonists (11,159).

Transplacental Carcinogenesis

Transplacental carcinogenesis is defined as the appearance of cancer in the offspring of females exposed to chemical agents during their pregnancy. It is increasingly evident that fetal exposure to environmental agents may induce childhood or adult-onset tumors. The transplacental induction of cancer was demonstrated in animals long before it was discovered in man. The dose that results in the malignant transformation of fetal tissues is frequently much less than that required for adult tissues. High cellular replication rates and low immunocompetence may contribute to this susceptibility. Although all sites of the developing fetus may be affected, the tissues most likely to exhibit a neoplastic response to carcinogens administered during pregnancy are the nervous system, lung, and kidney. The type of tumor induced in the offspring by a particular carcinogen differs among species.

To date, approximately 60 compounds have been shown to induce transplacental carcinogenesis in animals (80,135). These compounds are found in the following major classes of chemical carcinogens: nitroso compounds, polycyclic aromatic hydrocarbons, and aminoazo compounds. This is in marked contrast to the findings in humans. Thus far there is convincing epidemiologic evidence of transplacental cancer induction in humans for only one compound: only maternal treatment with diethylstilbestrol has been shown to induce vaginal adenocarcinoma in young women (54,64). The topic of perinatal and multigeneration carcinogenesis has been reviewed (109).

A number of compounds have exhibited both carcinogenic and teratogenic properties. The connection between transplacental carcinogenesis and teratogenesis has been reviewed (80,81). The findings thus far reveal that teratogenic activity has not been observed for every carcinogen. This does not, however, indicate that teratogenesis and carcinogenesis are mutually exclusive processes. Clinicians have observed that children with cancer appear to have a higher incidence of congenital malformations. Certain types of cancer are reported to be associated with specific teratogenic syndromes. For example, adrenal carcinoma and neuroblastoma have been linked to the fetal alcohol syndrome (1).

Genetic Susceptibility

The embryo's susceptibility to teratogenesis depends on its genetic constitution. This principle has been demonstrated repeatedly in animals. This sus-

ceptibility varies not only between different species but also within a species and among animals of the same litter (181). Information on the mechanism underlying the genetic variation in teratogenic susceptibility is fragmentary.

Physiological and Pathological Status of the Mother

Since the maternal organism plays a vital role in nurturing and defending the embryo during its development, any condition that compromises these functions would tend to enhance the action of a teratogenic agent. Thus, as mentioned previously, the age of the mother and her nutritional and hormonal status, as well as the presence of disease and metabolic abnormalities, will affect the action of teratogenic agents.

CLINICAL ASPECTS OF EXPOSURE TO ENVIRONMENTAL CHEMICALS AND PHYSICAL AGENTS ON REPRODUCTIVE AND DEVELOPMENTAL DISORDERS

Clinical recognition of the adverse effects of environmental exposure on reproduction assumes major importance when it is appreciated that (1) a number of environmental agents such as lead, mercury, PCBs, ionizing radiation, cigarette smoking, alcohol, infection, and drugs (alkylating agents, estrogenic and androgenic hormones, anesthetic gases, anticonvulsants, and coumarin) are known to be teratogenic, (2) others including insecticides, herbicides, fungicides, and solvents are suspected of having teratogenic effects, (3) between 5% and 7% of all newborns in the United States have birth defects, (4) over 500,000 spontaneous abortions, stillbirths, and infant deaths are recorded each year (110), (5) between 10% and 20% of pregnancies end in spontaneous abortion, (6) 10–15% of couples who wish to become parents are infertile, and (7) 60% to 65% of birth defects occur for unknown causes (183).

There is increasing concern that environmental factors may play a causal role in the large percentage of birth defects that occur without known cause. The multiplicity of chemical and drug exposures received by both parents add to this concern. Experimental evidence indicates that simultaneous exposure to multiple agents may be teratogenic, whereas exposure to a single agent is not (181). Epidemiologic evidence also raises the issue that when both parents receive chemical exposure, each may contribute to the increased risk of an adverse reproductive outcome (62).

Clinical evaluation of the reproductive effects of environmental exposure begins with a good medical history. Documenting past and present medications and occupational and environmental exposures for both parents is an integral part of a thorough evaluation. As the type and degree of susceptibility to teratogenic agents are related to the developmental stage of the conceptus, the specific date of the last period and the exact timing of exposure are critical. As previously stated, with exposure to teratogenic agents the embryo is most apt to sustain morphological defects during organogenesis (18 to 55 days after fertilization). After this time the fetus is less apt to incur morphological defects but more apt to suffer such functional changes as alterations in psychological development.

Information must be obtained on the type and degree of exposure. Was the exposure acute or chronic? Was it associated with evidence of maternal toxicity? Exposure of the male must also be evaluated in relation to female reproductive dysfunction. Obstetricians, gynecologists, and urologists must pay particular attention to the adverse reproductive effects of environmental exposure on reproduction. Family practitioners, internists, and pediatricians, however, may be the first to uncover the untoward reproductive effects of chemical exposure, particularly if they routinely take an occupational and environmental history and remain alert to the problems of infertility, abnormal menstrual patterns, and untoward reproductive events.

The clinical evaluation of reproductive dysfunction caused by toxic exposure may be approached in three ways: (1) disorders of the female reproductive system, (2) developmental disorders occurring in the embryo/fetus, and (3) disorders of the male reproductive system resulting in an adverse reproductive outcome.

Disorders of the Female Reproductive System

This discussion is directed to problems of infertility. It must be emphasized, however, that toxic exposure may be linked to troubling disorders apart from infertility. These include menstrual disorders with frequent and heavy bleeding and early menopause.

Female infertility may result from reproductive and/or fetal problems. Female infertility may be secondary to disruption of the normal hormonal balance of the hypothalamic-pituitary-gonadal-uterine axis, to untoward events in the oocyte (resulting in pre- or postimplantation fetal loss), or to toxic effects on the embryo. As previously mentioned, early fetal loss may be difficult to differentiate from a "late period." Only an early positive serum pregnancy test can clarify this point.

Our knowledge of the toxic effects of environmental agents on the female reproductive system is fragmentary. It appears, however, that infertility

may be linked to such menstrual disturbances as hypermenorrhea, polymenorrhea, oligomenorrhea, or amenorrhea, all of which have been observed in occupationally exposed women (Table 24-2). These disturbances may, in part, be explained by a decrease in ovarian hormone output, luteal-phase defects, and anovulation.

A medical history with a careful exposure history is the best method of investigating a link between toxic exposure and menstrual dysfunction, infertility, and fetal loss. The patient should be encouraged to keep a diary of her menstrual pattern in relation to occupational/environmental exposures. The return of normal function and fertility following a cessation of exposure helps to substantiate a causal relationship.

An infertility work-up must be performed in the standard fashion, keeping in mind possible toxic influences. The traditional and common causes of infertility and anovulation must be considered (153). Evidence of anovulation in an exposed female is obtained by recording basal body temperatures, by measuring serum progesterone level, and by obtaining an endometrial biopsy during the luteal phase. When ovulation occurs, a luteal-phase defect may be determined by observing the absence of a sustained rise of basal body temperatures, by measuring the serum progesterone, or by obtaining an endometrial biopsy.

Toxic effects on the ovaries may be evidenced by hypogonadal function. Patients who suffer such toxic effects are anovulatory and oligomenorrheic or amenorrheic. They have decreased concentration of total serum or urinary estrogens and an elevation of serum follicle-stimulating hormone (FSH) and luteinizing hormone (LH) to menopausal ranges. Hypogonadal function secondary to adverse effects on the hypothalamus or pituitary will be reflected in low levels of FSH and LH. To determine the specific defect, it may be necessary to measure the luteinizing hormone-releasing hormone (LHRH). At times, the presence of toxic agent(s) in the patient's blood, urine, expired air, hair, etc. may be helpful in determining if her reproductive dysfunction is related to such exposure (see Chapter 27).

When adverse reproductive effects are linked to toxic exposure, removing the patient from the toxic source is the cornerstone of management. Although little data are available, it appears that, depending on the agent and severity of injury, the effects of toxic exposure are in general reversible, and the prognosis for a return of normal function is good. The medical treatment for anovulation and for luteal-phase defects secondary to toxic exposure is no different from that for other etiologies. For anovulation, ovulatory drugs may be given (clomiphene citrate, pergonal). For luteal-phase defects treatment may include administration of progesterone, injections of human chorionic gonadotropin (hCG), or treatments with clomiphene or human menopausal gonadotropins (153).

Developmental Disorders

A prenatal history, like the history that searches for the cause(s) of infertility, must include questions about present and past exposures of both parents. Exposures present in the workplace, home, and community must be noted. Specific data on working conditions, tasks, and exposures are particularly important. Information on medication, life style, and hobbies must be recorded. Information on the exposures of both parents to toxic agents should also be assessed. Simultaneous exposure to multiple agents is often important (186).

If a woman has a history of having had a child with a birth defect, it is vital to obtain a detailed exposure history. When obtaining the exposure history, the physician must try to sort out the various factors that may be linked to the development of birth defects. These include maternal age, disease, infection, medication, nutritional problems, smoking, alcohol consumption, the use of recreational drugs, and a family history of birth defects. The physician must also keep in mind a tendency for recall bias in mothers who have had infants with birth defects.

At times the clinician may see a pregnant woman with a clear history of chemical exposure or one with evidence of acute toxicity. In both instances the mother may be at increased risk of having an infant with a birth defect. Confirmation of the presence of birth defects in the developing embryo is fraught with uncertainty.

Visualization of the fetus can be performed noninvasively through the use of ultrasonography. This procedure, without apparent risk to fetus or mother, is one of the most important diagnostic advances available to the physician. Ultrasonography can detect such gross malformations as hydrocephalus, anencephaly, spina bifida, abdominal wall defects, phocomelia, and renal agenesis. Finer morphological defects may be ascertained by fetoscopy. Fetoscopy involves viewing the fetus by means of a fetoscope that has been introduced into the uterus. This procedure, in the best hands, may result in a fetal loss of at least 5%. The prenatal diagnosis of inherited chromosomal abnormalities, fetal disease, and metabolic deficiencies requires invasive intervention. Amniocentesis, the removal of amniotic fluid from the uterus, can usually be performed with reasonable safety during the midtrimester of pregnancy. This procedure allows the assessment of chromosomal abnormalities and cytogenetic studies. In addition to direct chromosomal analysis, recombinant DNA technology now allows the diagnosis of a number of genetic disorders. Amniocentesis has been used to evaluate the risk for neural tube defects (42).

If a fetal malformation is discovered, the mother may be given the option of terminating the pregnancy, depending on the defect, the teratogen, and the nature and degree of exposure. Maternal exposure to methyl mercury, lead, or carbon monoxide, especially with evidence of maternal toxicity, is cause for concern. In such cases the embryo would be at substantial risk. There are, however, no absolutes in making predictions. An exposed mother without toxic symptoms may have an affected child, as with methyl mercury exposure, whereas an exposed mother with severe toxic symptoms may have a normal infant, as has been reported in an exceptional case of carbon monoxide poisoning (22). The decisions made by the physician and mother clearly depend on the particular conditions present.

Once a toxic exposure has taken place, there is no medical treatment that prevents or minimizes the teratogenic risk. Chelating agents, used in the management of heavy metal poisoning, have not prevented the teratogenic effects of these metals. The cornerstone in the management of teratogenesis is preventing exposure. A patient who is contemplating pregnancy should speak with her physician. Environmental and occupational exposures that may be hazardous to a developing embryo should be discussed at this time.

For infertile couples and women who habitually abort, sperm analysis and chromosomal studies should be offered. It has been suggested that evaluating the abortuses for evidence of toxic exposure may provide diagnostic clues. This, however, is rarely done. The value of analyzing preserved specimens was dramatically demonstrated in the case of methyl mercury poisoning that occurred in Minimata Bay, Japan. The dried umbilical stump, kept by the Japanese family for decades, was analyzed from those children born in the 1950s during an epidemic of mercury poisoning. These analyses revealed that the concentration of mercury in the umbilical stump paralleled the industrial discharge of mercury into Minimata Bay (118).

Disorders of the Male Reproductive System Resulting in an Adverse Reproductive Outcome

In the past, investigations of reproductive problems linked to toxic exposure have focused on the female. It is now clear that attention must also be directed to the male. Information on male-mediated reproductive effects is limited. A few reports indicate that reproductive dysfunction in the female, including infertility, spontaneous abortion, and the development of cancer in the offspring, may be mediated through the male (60–62).

Data from the United States and Great Britain reveal an increase in birth defects among the children of male anesthetists (152). Beckman and Nordström observed an increased fetal death rate in women whose husbands worked in a Swedish copper smelter (9). A study from Israel reported an increase in spontaneous abortions among the wives of men exposed to dibromochloropropane (DBCP) (78). Abnormalities in sperm count, morphology, and motility have been reported in lead-exposed workers (87). Increased chromosomal abnormalities in somatic cells have been reported in men with occupational exposure to lead (32,122,143). Finnish investigators report that the children of men working as motor vehicle drivers, farmers, machine repairers, and painters appear to have an increased risk of cancer (61). The adverse reproductive effects of paternal exposure have been reviewed by Fabro (41).

Clinicians must also be aware that male-mediated reproductive problems may ensue when a women is inadvertently exposed to pollutants brought home on her mate's soiled clothing.

Sources of Information

There are a few reference books that will be of help to the clinician and patient. Shepard's *Catalog of Teratogenic Agents* (147) contains a bibliography of potential human and animal teratogenic agents including chemicals, drugs, physical agents, and viruses. This catalogue is updated regularly. Schardein's *Chemically Induced Birth Defects* (142) is an exhaustive review of the teratogenic effects of chemicals. It correlates the laboratory and clinical teratogenic properties of environmental chemicals. Heinonen, Slone, and Shapiro have published information on birth defects and drugs in pregnancy (58). Reproductive hazards have also been reviewed by other authors (63,130). Information on reproductive toxicology is available to clinicians from the Reproductive Toxicology Center, Columbia Hospital for Women, Washington, D.C. 20037.

The methods used and theories of teratology are well covered in the *Handbook of Teratology* edited by Wilson and Fraser (183). The fundamentals of reproductive and developmental toxicology along with information on drugs and chemicals suspected of adversely affecting the embryo/fetus, and their alternatives are presented in *Drug and Chemical Action in Pregnancy* edited by Fabro and Scialli (43). Information can also be obtained from the Environment Teratology Information Center (ETIC) (38) maintained by the National Institute of Environmental Health Sciences. Brent has reviewed the effects of embryonic and fetal exposure to x rays, microwaves, and ultrasound (13). In general, the relative teratogenic risks of the various exposures are not available. The interested reader is directed to an article by Shepard that deals with the counseling of pregnant women exposed to potentially harmful agents during pregnancy (146).

SUMMARY

Exposure to chemicals present in the workplace and the general environment can be associated with a variety of reproductive hazards. Toxic agents may adversely affect the reproductive system and/or produce developmental abnormalities in the offspring. Agents adversely affecting reproduction interfere with reproductive and/or sexual function, whereas those adversely affecting development give rise to teratogenic effects. These include growth retardation, developmental abnormalities, and behavioral disorders, as well as structural defects. Transplacental carcinogenesis also occurs as the result of fetal exposure to environmental agents. It is increasingly evident that attention must be directed to the father as well as to the mother in relationship to adverse reproductive outcome. In light of the foregoing information, it is essential that physicians counsel both parents about exposures to potentially harmful agents prior to and during pregnancy.

REFERENCES

1. Allen RW Jr, Ogden B, Bently FL, et al: Fetal hydantoin syndrome, neuroblastoma, and hemorrhagic disease in a neonate. JAMA 244:1464, 1980.
2. Anderson HA, Lilis R, Daum SM, et al: Household contact asbestos neoplastic risk. Ann NY Acad Sci 271:311, 1976.
3. Baird DD, Wilcox AJ: Cigarette smoking associated with delayed conception. JAMA 253:2979, 1985.
4. Baker EL, Follard DS, Taylor TA, et al: Lead poisoning in children of lead workers: Home contamination with industrial dust. N Engl J Med 296:260, 1977.
5. Baker TG, Neal P: Action of ionizing radiation on the mammalian ovary. In: The Ovary, Vol 3, p 1, Zuckerman S, Weir BJ (eds.), Academic Press, New York, 1977.
6. Barlow SM, Sullivan FM: Reproductive Hazards of Industrial Chemicals, Academic Press, Orlando, 1982.
7. Barsotti DA, Marier RJ, Allen J Jr: Reproductive dysfunction in rhesus monkeys exposed to low levels of polychlorinated biphenyls (Aroclor 1248). Food Cosmet Toxicol 14:99, 1976.
8. Beckman DA, Brent RL: Mechanisms of teratogenesis. Annu Rev Pharmacol Toxicol 24:483, 1984.
9. Beckman L, Nordström S: Occupational and environmental risks in and around a smelter in northern Sweden. IX. Fetal mortality among wives of smelter workers. Hereditas 97:1, 1982.

10. Bellinger D, Leviton A, Waternaux C, et al: Longitudinal analyses of prenatal and postnatal lead exposure and early cognitive development. N Engl J Med 316:1037, 1987.

11. Biggs R, Rose E: The familial incidence of adrenal hypertrophy and female pseudohermaphroditism. J Obstet Gynaecol Br Emp 54:369, 1947.

12. Bloom AD (ed.): Guidelines for Studies of Human Populations Exposed to Mutagenic and Reproductive Hazards. March of Dimes Birth Defects Foundations, New York, 1981.

13. Brent RL: The effect of embryonic and fetal exposure to X-ray, microwaves, and ultrasound: Counseling the pregnant and nonpregnant patient about these risks. Semin Oncol 16:347, 1989.

14. Brown NA, Fabro S: The in vitro approach to teratogenicity testing. In: Developmental Toxicology, p 165, Snell K (ed.), Praeger, London, 1982.

15. Bulger WH, Kupfer D: Estrogenic action of DDT analogs. Am J Ind Med 4:163, 1983.

16. Catz CS, Jaffee SJ: Environmental factors: Pharmacology. In: Prevention of Embryonic, Fetal and Perinatal Disease, Vol 3, p 119, Brent RL, Harris MI (eds.), John E Fogarty International Center for Advanced Study in the Health Sciences, NIH, Bethesda, 1976.

17. Chen PHS, Luo MI, Wong CK, et al: Polychlorinated biphenyls, dibenzofurans and quaterphenyls in the toxic rice-bran oil and PCBs in the blood of patients with PCB poisoning in Taiwan. Am J Ind Med 5:133, 1984.

18. Clemmensen J: Mutagenicity and teratogenicity of vinyl chloride monomers: Epidemiological evidence. Mutat Res 98:97, 1982.

19. Committee on the Biologic Effects of Ionizing Radiation, National Research Council: Health Effects of Exposure to Low Levels of Ionizing Radiation, BIER V, National Academy Press, Washington, 1990.

20. Committee on Indoor Air Pollutants, National Research Council: Indoor Pollutants, National Academy Press, Washington, 1981.

21. Committee on Lead in the Environment, National Research Council: Lead in the Human Environment, National Academy Press, Washington, 1980.

22. Copel J, Bowen F, Bolognese R: Carbon monoxide intoxication in early pregnancy. Obstet Gynecol 59(Suppl 6):265, 1982.

23. Coulston F, Pocchiari F (eds.): Accidental Exposure to Dioxins, Academic Press, Orlando, 1983.

24. Council on Scientific Affairs: The Health Effects of "Agent Orange" and Polychlorinated Dioxin Contaminants, American Medical Association, Chicago, 1981.

25. Council on Scientific Affairs: The Health Effects of "Agent Orange" and Polychlorinated Dioxins Contaminants: An Update, 1984, American Medical Association, Chicago, 1984.

26. Council on Scientific Affairs: Effects of toxic chemicals on the reproductive system. JAMA 253:3431, 1985.

27. Courtney KD: Mouse teratology studies with chlorodibenzo-p-dioxins. Bull Environ Contam Toxicol 16:674, 1976.

28. Courtney KD: Prenatal effects of herbicides: Evaluation by the prenatal development index. Arch Environ Contam Toxicol 6:33, 1977.

29. Courtney KD, Moore JA: Tetratology studies with 2,4,5-trichlorophenoxyacetic acid and 2,3,7,8-tetrachlorodibenzo-p-dioxin. Toxicol Appl Pharmacol 20:396, 1971.

30. Cutting RT, Phuoc TH, Ballo JM, et al: Congenital malformations, hydatidiform moles in the Republic of Vietnam 1960–1969, US Government Printing Office, Washington, 1970.

31. Davis JM, Svendsgaard DJ: Lead and child development. Nature 329:297, 1987.

32. Deknudt GH, Leonard A, Ivanov B: Chromosome aberrations observed in male workers occupationally exposed to lead. Environ Physiol Biochem 3:132, 1973.

33. Dixon RL: Potential of environmental factors to affect the development of reproductive systems. Fund Appl Toxicol 2:5, 1982.

34. Dixon RL: Toxic responses of the reproductive system. In: Casarett and Doull's Toxicology, The Basic Science of Poisons, 3rd ed., p 432, Klaassen CD, Amdur MO, Doull J (eds.), Macmillan, New York, 1986.

35. Donovan JW: Case-Control Study of Congenital Anomalies and Vietnam Service, Commonwealth Institute of Health, University of Sydney, Sydney, Australia, 1983.

36. Dowty BJ, Laseter J, Storer J: The transplacental migration and accumulation in blood of volatile organic constituents. Pediatr Res 10:696, 1976.

37. Environmental Studies Board, Commission on Natural Resources: Urban Pest Management, National Academy Press, Washington, 1980.

38. Environmental Teratogen Information Center (ETIC): National Institute of Environmental Health Sciences, Research Triangle Park, NC.

39. Erickson JD, Mulinare J, McClain PW, et al: Vietnam veteran's risk for fathering babies with birth defects. JAMA 252:903, 1984.

40. Eskenazi B, Gaylord L, Bracken MB, et al: In utero exposure to organic solvents and human neurodevelopment. Dev Med Child Neurol 30:492, 1988.

41. Fabro S (ed.): Paternally induced adverse pregnancy effects. Reprod Toxicol 3:13, 1984.

42. Fabro S, Scialli AR: The role of the obstetrician in the prevention and treatment of birth defects. In: Issues and Reviews in Teratology, Vol 3, p 1, Kalter H (ed.), Plenum Press, New York, 1985.

43. Fabro S, Scialli AR (eds.): Drug and Chemical Action in Pregnancy, Marcel Dekker, New York, 1986.

44. Fabro S, Shull G, Brown NA: The relative teratogenic index and teratogenic potency: Proposed components of developmental toxicity risk assessment. Teratogen Carcinogen Mutagen 2:61, 1982.

45. Fahim MS, Fahim Z, Hall DG: Effects of subtoxic lead levels on pregnant women in the state of Missouri. Res Commun Chem Pharmacol 13:309, 1976.

46. Fein GG, Jacobson JL, Jacobson SW, et al: Prenatal exposure to polychlorinated biphenyls: Effects on birth size and gestational age. J Pediatr 105:315, 1984.

47. Felton JS, Kwan TC, Wuebbles BJ, et al: Genetic differences in polycyclic aromatic hydrocarbon metabolism and their effects on oocyte killing in developing mice. In: DOE Symposium Series, Vol 47: Developmental Toxicology of Energy Related Pollutants, p 1526, Mahlum DD, Sikov MR, Hackett PL, et

al. (eds.), U.S. Department of Energy, Washington, 1978.

48. Field B, Kerr C: Herbicide use and the incidence of neural-tube defects. Lancet 1:1341, 1979.

49. Filler R, Lew KJ: Developmental onset of mixed-function oxidase activity in preimplantation mouse embryos. Proc Natl Acad Sci USA 78:6991, 1981.

50. Friedman JM: Does agent orange cause birth defects? Tetratology 29:193, 1984.

51. Gellert RJ: Uterotrophic activity of polychlorinated biphenyls (PCB) and induction of precocious reproductive aging in neonatally treated female rats. Environ Res 16:123, 1978.

52. Giavini R, Prati M, Vismara C: Rabbit teratology study with 2,3,7,8-tetrachlorodibenzo-p-dioxin. Environ Res 27:74, 1982.

53. Goncharuk GA: Hygiene of women working in the mercury industry. Gig Truda Prof Zabol 21:17, 1977.

54. Greenwald P, Barlow JJ, Nasca P, et al: Vaginal cancer after maternal treatment with synthetic estrogens. N Engl J Med 287:1259, 1971.

55. Hall A: The increasing use of lead as an abortifacient. Br Med J 1:584, 1905.

56. Hamilton A: Women in Lead Industries, US Bureau of Labor Statistics, Washington, 1919.

57. Hanify JA, Metcalf P, Nobbs CL, et al: Aerial spraying of 2,4,5-T and human birth malformation: An epidemiologic investigation. Science 212:349, 1981.

58. Heinonen OP, Slone D, Shapiro S: Birth Defects and Drugs in Pregnancy, Publishing Sciences Group, Littleton, MA, 1977.

59. Hemminki K, Frassila E, Vaino H: Spontaneous abortions among female chemical workers in Finland. Int Arch Occup Environ Health 45(2):123, 1980.

60. Hemminki K, Saloneimi I, Luoma T, et al: Transplacental carcinogens and mutagens: Childhood cancer, malformations and abortions as risk factors. J Toxicol Environ Health 6:1115, 1980.

61. Hemminki K, Saloniemi I, Salonen T, et al: Childhood cancer and parental occupation in Finland. J Epidemiol Commun Health 35:11, 1981.

62. Hemminki K, Kyyronen P, Niemi ML, et al: Spontaneous abortions in an industrial community in Finland. Am J Public Health 73:32, 1983.

63. Hemminki K, Sorsa M, Vainio H (eds.): Occupational Hazards and Reproduction, Hemisphere Publishing, Washington, 1985.

64. Herbst AL, Ulfelder H, Poskanzer DC: Adenocarcinoma of the vagina: Association of maternal stilbestrol therapy with tumor appearance in young women. N Engl J Med 284:878, 1971.

65. Highman B, Gaines TB, Schumacher HJ: Retarded development of fetal renal alkaline phosphatase in mice given 2,4,5-trichlorophenoxyacetic acid. J Toxicol Environ Health 2:1007, 1977.

66. Howe G, Westhoff C, Vessey M, et al: Effects of age, cigarette smoking, and other factors on fertility: Findings in a large prospective study. Br Med J 290:1697, 1985.

67. Humble CG, Speizer FE: Polybrominated biphenyls and fetal mortality in Michigan. Am J Public Health 74:1130, 1984.

68. Hunt VR: Work and the Health of Women, CRC Press, Boca Raton, 1978.

69. Hunter A, Thompson D, Evans J: Is there a fetal gasoline syndrome? Teratology 20:75, 1979.

70. Jick H, Porter J, Morrison AS: Relationship between smoking and age of natural menopause. Lancet 1:1354, 1977.

71. Juchau MR: Drug biotransformation in the placenta. Pharmacol Ther 8:501, 1980.

72. Juchau MR: The Biochemical Basis of Chemical Teratogenesis, Elsevier-North-Holland, New York, 1981.

73. Juchau MR: The role of the placenta in developmental toxicology. In: Developmental Toxicology, p 189, Snell K (ed.), Praeger, London, 1982.

74. Juchau MR: Bioactivation in chemical teratogenesis. Annu Rev Pharmacol Toxicol 29:165, 1989.

75. Juchau MR, Faustman-Watts E: Pharmacokinetic considerations in the maternal-placental-fetal unit. Clin Obstet Gynecol 26:379, 1983.

76. Juchau MR, Chao ST, Omiecinski CJ: Drug metabolism by the human fetus. Clin Pharmacokinet 5:320, 1980.

77. Karnaofsky DA: Drugs as teratogens in animals and man. Annu Rev Pharmacol 5:447, 1965.

78. Kharrazi M, Potashnik G, Goldsmith JR: Reproductive effects of dibromochloropropane. Israel J Med Sci 10:403, 1980.

79. Kimbrough RD, Jensen AA (eds.): Halogenated Biphenyls, Terphenyl, Naphthalene, Dibenzodioxins and Related Products, 2nd ed., Elsevier, Amsterdam, 1989.

80. Kleihues P: Developmental carcinogenicity. In: Developmental Toxicology, p 211, Snell K (ed.), Praeger, London, 1982.

81. Kleihues P, Lantos PL, Magee PN: Chemical carcinogenesis in the nervous system. Int Rev Exp Pathol 15:153, 1976.

82. Kucera J: Exposure to fat solvents: A possible cause of sacral agenesis in man. J Pediatr 72:857, 1968.

83. Kunstadter P: A Study of Herbicides and Birth Defects in the Republic of Vietnam: An Analysis of Hospital Records, National Academy Press, Washington, 1982.

84. Kuratsune M, Shapiro RE (eds.): PCB Poisoning in Japan and Taiwan, Alan R Liss, New York, 1984.

85. Kuratsune M, Yoshimura T, Matsuzaka J, et al: Epidemiologic study of Yusho, a poisoning caused by ingestion of rice bran oil contaminated with a commercial brand of polychlorinated biphenyls. Environ Health Perspect 1:119, 1972.

86. Kurzel RB: Substance abuse in pregnancy. In: The Problem Oriented Medical Record for High Risk Obstetrics, p 76, Cetrulo CL, Sbara A (eds.), Plenum Press, New York, 1984.

87. Lancranjan I, Popescu H, Gavanescu O, et al: Reproductive ability of workmen occupationally exposed to lead. Arch Environ Health 30:396, 1975.

88. Lathrop GD, Wolfe WH, Albanese RA, et al: Project Ranch Hand II: An Epidemiologic Investigation of Health Effects in Air Force Personnel Following Exposure to Herbicides: Baseline Morbidity Study Results, US Air Force School of Aerospace Medicine, Aerospace Medical Division, Brooks Air Force Base, San Antonio, 1983.

89. Longo LD: The biological effects of carbon monoxide on the pregnant woman, fetus and newborn infant. Am J Obstet Gynecol 129:69, 1977.

90. MacMahon B: Prenatal X-ray exposure and twins. N Engl J Med 312:576, 1985.

91. MacMahon B: Some recent issues in low-exposure radiation epidemiology. Environ Health Perspect 81: 131, 1989.

92. Mastrolacovo P, Spagnolo A, Marni E, et al: Birth defects in the Seveso area after TCDD contamination. JAMA 259:1668, 1988.

93. Masuda Y, Yoshimura H: Polychlorinated biphenyls and dibenzofurans in patients with Yusho and their toxicological significance: A review. Am J Ind Med 5: 32, 1984.

94. Mattison DR: Difference in sensitivity of rat and mouse primordial oocyte to destruction by polycyclic aromatic hydrocarbons. Chem Biol Interact 28:133, 1979.

95. Mattison DR: Effects of biologically foreign compounds on reproduction. In: Drugs During Pregnancy: Clinical Perspective, p 101, Abdul-Karim RW (ed.), George F Stickely, Philadelphia, 1981.

96. Mattison DR: The mechanisms of action of reproductive toxins. Am J Ind Med 4:65, 1983.

97. Mattison DR: Ovarian toxicity: Effects on sexual maturation. In: Reproductive and Developmental Toxicity of Metals, p 317, Clarkson T, Nordberg G, and Sager P, Plenum Press, New York, 1983.

98. Mattison DR: Clinical manifestations of ovarian toxicity. In: Reproductive Toxicology, p 109, Dixon RL (ed.), Raven Press, New York, 1985.

99. Mattison DR, Gates AH, Leonard A, et al: Reproductive and developmental toxicity of metals: Female reproductive system. In: Reproductive and Developmental Toxicity of Metals, p 41, Clarkson T, Nordberg G, Sager P (eds.), Plenum Press, New York, 1983.

100. McNulty WP: Chronic toxicity of TCDD for rhesus macques. Food Cosmet Toxicol 19(1):57, 1981.

101. Merson MH, Kirkpatrick RL: Reproductive performance of captive white-footed mice fed a PCB. Bull Environ Contam Toxicol 16:392, 1976.

102. Miller RK: Perinatal toxicology: Its recognition and fundamentals. Am J Ind Med 4:205, 1983.

103. Miller RW: Areawide chemical contamination: Lessons from case histories. JAMA 245:1548, 1981.

104. Miller RW, Mulvihill JJ: Small head size after atomic radiation. Teratology 14:355, 1976.

105. Mishonova VN, Stepanova PA, Zarudin VV: Characteristics of the course of pregnancy and parturition in women occupationally exposed to low concentrations of metallic mercury vapors. Gig Truda Prof Zabol 24: 21, 1980.

106. Mole RH: Irradiation of the embryo and fetus. Br J Radiol 60:17, 1987.

107. Murray FJ, Smith FA, Nitschke KD, et al: Three-generation reproduction study of rats given 2,3,7,8-tetrachlorodibenzo-p-dioxin (TCDD) in the diet. Toxicol Appl Pharmacol 50:241, 1979.

108. Mushak P, Davis JM, Crocetti AF, et al: Prenatal and postnatal effects of low-level lead exposure: integrated summary of a report to the US congress on childhood lead poisoning. Environ Res 50:11, 1989.

109. Napalkov NP, Rice JM, Tomatis L, et al. (eds.): Perinatal and Multigeneration Carcinogenesis. IARC Scientific Publication No 96, International Agency for Research on Cancer, Lyon, 1989.

110. National Foundation/March of Dimes: Facts, National Foundation, New York, 1975.

111. Nebert DW, Merker HJ, Kohler E, et al: Biochemical aspects of teratology. In: Advances in the Biosciences, Vol 6, p 575, Raspe G (ed.), Peragamon Press, London, 1970.

112. Nebert DW, Eiashoff JD, Wilcox KR: Possible effect of neonatal polybrominated biphenyl exposure on the developmental abilities of children. Am J Public Health 73:286, 1983.

113. Needelman HL: The neurotoxic, teratogenic and behavioral teratogen effects of lead at low dose: A paradigm for transplacental toxicants. In: Transplacental Effects on Fetal Health, p 279, Scarpelli DG, Migaki G (eds.), Alan R Liss, New York, 1989.

114. Needleman HL, Rabinowitz M, Leviton A, et al: The relationship between prenatal exposure to lead and congenital anomalies. JAMA 251:2956, 1984.

115. Nelson CJ, Holson JF, Green HG, et al: Retrospective study of the relationship between agricultural use of 2,4,5-T and cleft palate occurrence in Arkansas. Teratology 19:377, 1979.

116. Neubert D, Dillmann I: Embryotoxic effects of mice treated with 2,4,5-trichlorophenoxyacetic acid and 2,3,7,8-tetrachlorodibenzo-p-dioxin. Arch Pharmacol 272:243, 1972.

117. Neubert DW, Zens P, Rothenwaller A, et al: A survey of the embryotoxic effects of TCDD in mammalian species. Environ Health Perspect 5:67, 1973.

118. New DAT: Techniques for assessment of teratologic effects: Embryo culture. Environ Health Perspect 18: 105, 1976.

119. Nisbet ICT, Karch NJ: Chemical Hazards to Human Reproduction, Noyes Data Corporation, Park Ridge, New Jersey, 1983.

120. Nishigaka S, Harada M: Methylmercury and selenium in umbilical cords of inhabitants of the Minamata area. Nature 258:324, 1975.

121. Nora JJ, Nora AH, Sommerville RJ, et al: Maternal exposure potential teratogens. JAMA 202:1065, 1967.

122. Nordenson I, Beckman G, Beckman L, et al: Occupational and environmental risks in and around a smelter in northern Sweden: IV. Chromosomal aberrations in workers exposed to lead. Hereditas 88:263, 1978.

123. Nordström S, Beckman L, Nordenson I: Occupational and environmental risks in and around a smelter in northern Sweden: I. Variations in birth weight. Hereditas 88:43, 1978.

124. Nordström S, Beckman L, Nordenson I: Occupational and environmental risks in and around a smelter in northern Sweden: III. Frequencies of spontaneous abortion. Hereditas 88:51, 1978.

125. Nordström S, Beckman L, Nordenson I: Occupational and environmental risks in and around a smelter in northern Sweden: V. Spontaneous abortion among female employees and decreased birth weight in their offspring. Hereditas 90:291, 1979.

126. Nordström S, Beckman L, Nordenson I: Occupational and environmental risks in and around a smelter in northern Sweden: VI. Congenital malformations. Hereditas 90:297, 1979.

127. Ogi D, Hamada A: Case reports on fetal deaths and malformation of extremities probably related to in

secticide poisoning. J Jpn Obstet Gynecol Soc 17:569, 1965.

128. Oliver T: A lecture on lead poisoning and race. Br Med J 1:1096, 1911.

129. Palmisano P, Sneed R, Cassady G: Untaxed whiskey and fetal lead exposure. J Pediatr 75:869, 1969.

130. Paul M, Himmelstein J: Reproductive hazards in the workplace: What the practitioner needs to know about chemical exposure. Obstet Gynecol 71:921, 1988.

131. Pelkonen O: Biotransformation of xenobiotics in the fetus. Pharmacol Ther 10:261, 1980.

132. Pelkonen O: Environmental influences on human fetal and placental xenobiotic metabolism. Eur J Clin Pharmacol 18:17, 1980.

133. Pelkonen O: The differentiation of drug metabolism in relation to developmental toxicology. In: Developmental Toxicology, p 167, Snell K (ed.), Praeger, London, 1982.

134. Pruett JG, Winslow SG: Health Effects of Environmental Chemicals on the Adult Human Reproductive System. A Selected Bibliography with Abstracts, 1963–1981. FASEB Special Publication NLM/TIRC-82/1 FASEB, 9000 Rockville Pike, Bethesda, MD, 1982.

135. Rice J: Effects of prenatal exposure to chemical carcinogens and methods for their detection. In: Developmental Toxicology, p 191, Kimmel CA, Buelke-Sam J (eds.), Raven Press, New York, 1981.

136. Rogan WJ, Bagniewska A, Damstra T: Pollutants in breast milk. N Engl J Med 302:1450, 1980.

137. Rogan WJ, Gladen BC, McKinney JD, et al: Polychlorinated biphenyls (PCBs) and dichlorodiphenyl dichloroethene (DDE) in human milk: Effects of maternal factors and previous lactation. Am J Public Health 76:172, 1986.

138. Rogan WJ, Gladen BC, Hung KL, et al: Congenital poisoning by polychlorinated biphenyls and their contaminants in Taiwan. Science 241:334, 1988.

139. Rylander R, Vesterlund J: Carbon monoxide criteria effects on the fetus. Scand J Work Environ Health 7: 25, 1981.

140. Sanderson CA, Rogers LJ: 2,4,5-Trichlorophenoxyacetic acid causes behavioral effects in chickens at environmentally relevant doses. Science 211:593, 1981.

141. Savage EP: National study to determine levels of chlorinated hydrocarbon insecticides in human milk, 1975–1976, and supplementary report to the national milk study: 1975–1976, National Technical Information Service, Springfield, VA, 1977.

142. Schardein JL: Chemically Induced Birth Defects, Marcel Dekker, New York, 1985.

143. Schwanitz G, Lehnert G, Gebhart E: Chromosomal injury due to occupational lead poisoning. Ger Med Month 15:738, 1970.

144. Schwartz EM, Rae WA: Effect of polybrominated biphenyls (PBB) on developmental abilities in young children. Am J Public Health 73:277, 1983.

145. Seagull EAW: Developmental abilities of children exposed to polybrominated biphenyls (PBB). Am J Public Health 73:281, 1983.

146. Shepard TH: Counseling pregnant women exposed to potentially harmful agents during pregnancy. Clin Obstet Gynecol 26(2):478, 1983.

147. Shepard TH: Catalog of teratogenic agents, 7th ed., The Johns Hopkins University Press, Baltimore, 1992.

148. Shum S, Jensen NM, Nebert DM: The murine Ah locus: in uterotoxicity and teratogenesis associated with genetic differences in benzo[a]pyrene metabolism. Teratology 20:365, 1979.

149. Smith MA, Grant LD, Sors AI (eds.): Lead Exposure and Child Development, Kluwer Academic Publishers, Dordrecht, 1989.

150. Soyka LF, Joffe JM: Male mediated drug effects on offspring. In: Drug and Chemical Risks to the Fetus and Newborn, p 49, Schwarz RH, Yaffe SJ (eds.), Alan R Liss, New York, 1980.

151. Sparschu GL, Dunn FL, Rowe VK: Study of the teratogenicity of 2,3,7,8-tetrachlorodibenzo-p-dioxin in the rat. Food Cosmet Toxicol 9:405, 1971.

152. Spence AA, Cohen EN, Brown BW, et al: Occupational hazards for operating room-based physicians: Analysis of data from the United States and United Kingdom. JAMA 238:955, 1977.

153. Speroff L, Glass RH, Kase NG (eds): Clinical Gynecologic Endocrinology and Infertility, 4th ed., Williams & Wilkins, Baltimore, 1989.

154. Spielmann H, Eibe HG, Jacob-Muller U: In-vitro method for the study of the effects of teratogens on pre-implantation embryos. Acta Morphol Acad Sci Hung 28:105, 1980.

155. Stein Z, Hatch M, Kline J, et al: Epidemiological considerations in assessing health effects. In: Assessment of Health Effects at Chemical Disposal Sites, p 125, Lowrance WW (ed.), The Rockefeller University, New York, 1981.

156. Subcommittee on Reproductive and Neurodevelopmental Toxicology, National Research Council: Biologic Markers in Reproductive Toxicology. National Academy Press, Washington, 1989.

157. Suskind RR, Hertzberg VS: Human health effects of 2,4,5-T and its toxic contaminants. JAMA 251:2372, 1984.

158. Suzuki K, Gipe B, Hammil H: Glue-sniffing gravida at risk for premie with severe acidosis. Obstet Gynecol New 17:8, 1982.

159. Thiersch JB: Therapeutic abortion with a folic acid antagonist 4-aminoteroylglutamic acid (4-amino PGA) administered by the oral route. Am J Obstet Gynecol 63:1298, 1952.

160. Thomas HF: 2,4,5-T use and congenital malformation rates in Hungary. Lancet 2:214, 1980.

161. Thomas HF, Czeizel A: Safe as 2,4,5-T? Nature 295: 276, 1982.

162. Townsend JC, Bodner KM, Van Peene PFD, et al: Survey of reproductive events in wives of employees exposed to chlorinated dioxins. Am J Epidemiol 115: 695, 1982.

163. Tuchmann-Duplessis H: The teratogenic risk. Am J Ind Med 4:245, 1983.

164. US Congress, Office of Technology Assessment: Reproductive Health Hazards in the Workplace. US Government Printing Office, OTA-BA-266, Washington, 1985.

165. United States Environmental Protection Agency: Six years spontaneous abortion rates in Oregon areas in relationship to forest 2,4,5-T spray practices, USEPA, Washington, 1979.

166. United States Environmental Protection Agency: Suspended, Cancelled and Restricted Pesticides, 3rd rev, USEPA, Washington, 1985.

167. United States Government Printing Office: Review of literature on herbicides including phenoxy herbicides and associated dioxins, Vols 4 and 6 (stock numbers 051-000-00165-6, 051-000-00174-5), US Government Printing Office, Washington, 1984–1985.

168. Universities Associated for Research and Education in Pathology: Health Aspects of the Disposal of Waste Chemicals, Peragamon Press, London, 1986.

169. Vianna NJ: Adverse pregnancy outcomes — potential endpoints of human toxicity in the Love Canal: Preliminary results, In: Human Embryonic and Fetal Death, p 165, Porter IH, Hook EB (eds.), Academic Press, Orlando, 1980.

170. Vianna NJ, Polan AK: Incidence of low birth weight among Love Canal residents. Science 226:1217, 1984.

171. Vos JG, Moore JA: Suppression of cellular immunity in rats and mice by maternal treatment with 2,3,7,8-tetrachlorodibenzo-*p*-dioxin. Int Arch Allergy Appl Immunol 47:777, 1974.

172. Vouk VB, Sheehan PJ (eds.): Methods for Assessing the Effects of Chemicals on Reproductive Functions. Scientific Group on Methodologies for the Safety Evaluation of Chemicals. John Wiley & Sons, New York, 1983.

173. Weiss B, Clarkson TW: Mercury toxicity in children. In: Chemical and Radiation Hazards to Children. Ross Conferences on Pediatric Research, Ross Laboratory, Columbus, OH, 1982.

174. Welch RM, Levin W, Connery AH: Estrogenic action of DDT and its analogs. Toxicol Appl Pharmacol 14: 358, 1969.

175. Wibberly DG, Khere AK, Edwards JH, et al: Lead levels in human placentae from normal and malformed births. J Med Genet 14:339, 1977.

176. Williams KE: Biochemical mechanisms of teratogenesis. In: Developmental Toxicology, p 95, Snell K (ed.), Praeger, London, 1982.

177. Wilson AT: Effects of abnormal lead content of water supplies on maternity patients. Scott Med J 11:73, 1966.

178. Wilson JG: Teratogenic interaction of chemical agents in the rat. J Pharmacol Exp Ther 144:429, 1964.

179. Wilson JG: Environmental effects on development—teratology. In: Patho-physiology of Gestation, p 269, Vol 2, Assali NS (ed.), Academic Press, New York, 1972.

180. Wilson JG: Mechanisms of teratogenesis. Am J Anat 136:129, 1973.

181. Wilson JG: Environment and Birth Defects, Academic Press, New York, 1973.

182. Wilson JG: Teratogenic effects of environmental chemicals. Fed Proc 36:1698, 1977.

183. Wilson JG, Fraser FE (eds.): Handbook of Teratology, Vol 1, Plenum Press, New York, 1977.

184. Wong TK, Everson RB, Hsu ST: Potent induction of human placental mono-oxygenase activity by previous dietary exposure to polychlorinated biphenyls and their thermal degradation products. Lancet 1: 721, 1985.

185. Wood JW, Johnson Y, Omori S: In-utero exposure to Hiroshima atomic bomb: An evaluation of head size and mental retardation 27 years later. Pediatrics 39: 385, 1967.

186. World Health Organization: Health Effects of Combined Exposure in the Work Environment. WHO Technical Reports Series, no. 662, World Health Organization, Geneva, 1981.

187. World Health Organization: 2,4-Dichlorophenoxyacetic acid. Environmental health criteria 29, World Health Organization, Geneva, 1984.

188. Yamasaki JN, Wright SW, Wright PM: Outcome of pregnancy in women exposed to the atomic bomb in Nagasaki. Am J Dis Child 87:448, 1954.

189. Young AL, Calcagani JA, Thalken CE, et al: The Toxicology, Environmental Fate and Human Risk of Herbicide Orange and Its Associated Dioxin. US Air Force Occupational and Environmental Health Laboratory (OEHL) Technical Report TR-78-92, Aerospace Medical Division, Brooks, TX, 1978.

RECOMMENDED READINGS

Barlow SM, Sullivan FM: Reproductive Hazards of Industrial Chemicals, Academic Press, Orlando, 1982.

Clarkson TW, Nordberg GF, Sager PR (eds.): Reproductive and Developmental Toxicology of Metals, Plenum Press, New York, 1983.

Hemminki K, Sorsa M, Vainio H (eds.): Occupational Hazards and Reproduction, Hemisphere Publications, Washington, 1985.

Napalkov NP, Rice JM, Tomatis T, et al: Perinatal and Multigeneration Carcinogenesis, IARC Scientific Publication No. 96, International Agency for Research on Cancer, Lyon, 1989.

Schardein JL: Chemically Induced Birth Defects, Marcel Dekker, New York, 1985.

Shepard TH: Catalog of Teratogenic Agents, 7th ed., The Johns Hopkins University Press, Baltimore, 1992.

Subcommittee on Reproductive and Neurodevelopmental Toxicology, National Research Council: Biologic Markers in Reproductive Toxicology, National Academy Press, Washington, 1989.

25. DISORDERS OF THE MALE REPRODUCTIVE SYSTEM

Emil Steinberger

INTRODUCTION

The last decade has witnessed an increased awareness of the reproductive hazards associated with exposure to chemicals commonly found in the environment. In the past, concern for the harmful reproductive effects of toxic exposure focused mainly on the pregnant woman and her fetus. A number of recent events have drawn attention to the adverse effects of occupational and environmental exposures on the male reproductive system. In 1976 an explosion at a chemical plant in Seveso, Italy released a cloud of dioxin, a known reproductive toxin in test animals. This industrial accident aroused concern for the reproductive health of the exposed workers and the general population (14). In 1977 Whorton et al. reported that occupational exposure to dibromochloropropane (DBCP) was linked to profound testicular toxicity without evidence of other adverse effects (147). Later in the same decade large numbers of Vietnam veterans were alarmed by the disclosure that exposure to Agent Orange might increase their risk for fathering offspring with birth defects.

Unfortunately, relatively few of the chemicals found in the workplace and general environment have been tested for their effect on the reproductive

system in experimental animals or humans. Most of our knowledge about the toxic effects of chemicals on the testes is a byproduct of studies investigating their actions as carcinogens, mutagens, or anticancer, alkylating, or contraceptive agents. Additional information comes from studies that examined the possible spermatotoxic side effects of therapeutic agents.

A wide variety of pharmacological agents are known to affect the male reproductive system. A number of clinical and laboratory studies indicate that substances that alter hormone balance adversely affect male reproductive capacity. Among these substances are testosterone, progesterone, estrogen, prednisone, and antiestrogen, antiandrogen agents (121,128,141); alkylating agents, i.e., triethylenephosphoramide (TEPA) (20,113,117), busulfan (Myeleran®) (42), cyclophosphamide (Cytoxan), chlorambucil, methotrexate, and nitroamino compounds, i.e., nitrofurans and nitropyrroles (80).

There are a number of problems inherent in studying the toxic effects of chemicals on the male reproductive system. These include (1) difficulties in assessing the affected population because of moral, legal, and ethical considerations (These considerations are magnified by emotionally charged attitudes toward the target tissue.); (2) the lack of precise and acceptable procedures for measuring male reproductive potential (This dilemma is reflected in a disagreement among investigators as to which semen characteristics, i.e., ejaculate volume, sperm density, motility, morphology, etc., con-

Principles and Practice of Environmental Medicine, edited by Alyce Bezman Tarcher. Plenum Medical Book Company, New York, 1992.

stitute the best indicators of infertility potential.); (3) marked differences among laboratories and among investigators in their ability to assess adequately the male reproductive function. (The test results of semen characteristics and the interpretation of testicular biopsies, for example, frequently vary from laboratory to laboratory.); and (4) the fact that the basic physiological parameters of normality have still not been established for the human male. In spite of a number of attempts to define semen characteristics in populations of "normal" individuals, there are still no acceptable norms (110,136). In addition, the influence of ethnic background, geographic location, and socioeconomic factors on the sperm output is not known.

There is general agreement that the hazards of toxic exposure on the male reproductive system must be vigorously investigated through laboratory and epidemiologic studies. Such studies require more investigators trained in male reproductive physiology and toxicology and more laboratories with expertise in these areas. The perceptive observations of an individual physician must continue to alert the medical and scientific communities to the dangers of toxic exposure. To discover a link between exposure and reproductive dysfunction, the clinician must maintain a high level of awareness and have some understanding of the hazards of toxic exposure for reproduction.

The study of toxic assault on reproductive and sexual functioning can be divided into reproductive and developmental toxicology. Reproductive toxicology assesses the effects of toxic exposure on the reproductive or sexual functioning of the adult from puberty through adulthood. Developmental toxicology assesses the effects of toxic exposure on the offspring from conception to puberty (136).

This chapter focuses on the toxicology of the male reproductive system. It explores the effect of exposure to environmental chemicals on reproduction in the male. Since the contribution of the father may play a role in fetal development, this aspect of developmental toxicology is also considered. The chapter begins with a discussion of those chemicals found in the workplace and in the general environment that adversely affect the male reproductive system. It continues with a discussion of epidemiology and pathological physiology and concludes with a discussion of the clinical implications of exposure to environmental and industrial chemicals on the male reproductive system.

ENVIRONMENTAL CHEMICALS ASSOCIATED WITH ADVERSE EFFECTS ON THE MALE REPRODUCTIVE SYSTEM

Reproductive toxicology is a relatively new discipline. Our current knowledge of occupational and environmental hazards to reproduction is incomplete for a number of reasons. Most foreign chemicals found in the workplace and in the general environment have not been systematically assayed for their mutagenicity, for their effects on the endocrine and reproductive systems, and for their effects on fertility. In most cases, only animal data are available, and only one sex has been studied under conditions of acute exposure. Many epidemiologic studies of the reproductive hazards in human populations are inadequate because of methodological problems.

Human data, in most cases, are inconclusive or nonexistent. Only a few occupational and environmental chemicals have been shown, with any assurance, to cause adverse reproductive effects in humans (4,27,49,99,146). In contrast, a relatively large number of chemicals and drugs have been reported to affect the reproductive system of male laboratory animals (4,23,81,124,136). Table 25-1 lists occupational and environmental agents shown to affect the male reproductive system adversely in humans and in animals. Table 25-2 lists the adverse reproductive effects reported from the occupational exposure of male workers.

The results of animal studies are presented in Table 25-1 to alert the reader that agents found to have adverse reproductive effects in laboratory animals must be considered a potential hazard to human reproduction. The agents cited, although not exhaustive, represent substances commonly found in the workplace and general environment. Some agents, e.g., dibromochloropropane (DBCP) and chlordecone (Kepone®), are no longer used in the United States. Nonetheless, these agents are considered because an awareness of their adverse reproductive effects increases our understanding of reproductive toxicology.

Distribution

Animal studies clearly indicate that many metals, agricultural chemicals, polyhalogenated biphenyls, organic solvents, and industrial chemicals pose a reproductive hazard to the male reproductive system (4,81,136). In humans, the adverse reproductive effects of exposure to environmental chemicals have generally been noted in the workplace, where exposures are usually more defined and higher. It should be recognized, however, that exposure to toxic agents in air, food, and water may adversely affect the male reproductive system.

Toxic metals such as lead, cadmium, and mercury are widely dispersed in the environment. Lead is used in automobile batteries, gasoline additives, pigments, and paints. Environmental exposure occurs primarily through food and air. Cadmium is used in paint pigments, batteries, catalysts, antiseptics, and fungicides, and as an additive to rubber and plastic. Cadmium accumulates in soil through

TABLE 25-1. Occupational and Environmental Chemicals Associated with Reproductive Dysfunction in the Male[a]

Man		Animals
Carbon disulfide	Metals and trace elements	Herbicides
Chlordecone (Kepone)	Aluminum	Chlorinated phenoxyacetic acids (2,4-D, 2,4,5-T)
Dibromochlorochloropropane	Arsenic	Diquat
(DBCP)	Boron	Paraquat
Lead	Cadmium	Fungicides
	Lead	Captan
	Manganese	Carbon disulfide
	Mercury, methyl mercury	Dibromochloropropane (DBCP)
	Molybdenum	Ethylene dibromide (EDB)
	Nickel	Ethylene oxide
	Silver	Thiocarbamates (cineb, maneb)
	Uranium	Triphenyltin
	Solvents	Industrial chemicals
	Benzene	Benzo[a]pyrene
	Carbon disulfide	Chloroform
	Carbon tetrachloride	Chloroprene
	Glycol ethers	Dioxin (TCDD)
	Hexane	Dimethylbenzanthracene (DMBA)
	Thiophene	Epichlorohydrin
	Trichloroethylene	Polybrominated biphenyls (PBBs)
	Toluene	Polychlorinated biphenyls (PCBs)
	Xylene	Phthalate esters
	Insecticides	Vinyl chloride
	Benzene hexachloride	
	Carbaryl	
	Chlordecone (Kepone)	
	Chlordane	
	Dieldrin	
	Dichlorvos (DDVP)	
	DDT	
	Methoxychlor	

[a]Adapted from references 4, 23, 81, 100, 124, 136.

the use of phosphate fertilizers, sludge application, and air deposition. Food represents the major source of cadmium exposure (91). Human exposure to mercury occurs via methyl mercury. Exposure to this compound comes almost entirely by way of consuming fish and seafood. There is growing concern that acid rain may increase the concentration of such toxic metals as lead, cadmium, and mercury in food and water (83).

Exposure to agricultural chemicals occurs not only during their manufacture and distribution but in the home as well. It has been estimated, for example, that homeowners in the United States use many times the amounts of pesticides applied to crops of corn and soybeans (31). Solvents are also widely used in the home in such agents as paints, paint thinners, furniture polish, cleansers, glues, and inks. Proximity to hazardous waste sites and industry may also provide a potential environmental source of pollutant exposure.

TABLE 25-2. Adverse Reproductive Effects Associated with Exposure of the Father to Occupational and Environmental Chemicals[a]

Agent	Effects
Anesthetic gases	Spontaneous abortion, congenital abnormalities
Carbon disulfide	Decreased libido, impotence, increased sperm abnormalities
Dibromochloropropane (DBCP)	Infertility, azoospermia, oligospermia
Lead and/or other smelter exposures	Infertility, spontaneous abortions, premature births

[a]Adapted from references 4 and 81.

Toxicology

There is evidence that a number of xenobiotics (foreign compounds) gain entrance into the male reproductive tract in humans. Tris, a mutagenic flame retardant formerly used on children's clothing, has been found in human seminal plasma (51). Other xenobiotics such as alcohol, cadmium, DBCP, pesticides, and lithium have also been found in human seminal fluid (30).

The toxicity of a chemical on the testes and on accessory sex organs is determined by its passage into these tissues and by the ability of the tissues to detoxify and excrete the xenobiotic and to repair any somatic or genetic damage that has been done (21,25,52). Animal studies reveal the presence of a blood-testis barrier that limits the transfer of drugs and environmental agents from the blood into the lumen of the seminiferous tubules (85,104). This distinctive feature of testicular anatomy allows germ cells in the seminiferous tubules to proliferate in a relatively protected environment. The transfer of compounds across the barrier depends on their molecular size and lipid solubility. The permeability characteristics of the blood-testis barrier is similar to the characteristic of membranes present in the central nervous system and in the gastrointestinal tract (25). It has been reported that the blood-testis barrier system is less effective in immature and newborn animals and in later life (22).

The biotransformation of xenobiotics from insoluble lipophilic compounds to soluble metabolites that can be easily excreted is, in large part, the body's defense against chemical assault. A number of studies have shown that the testes contain the microsomal enzyme system required to detoxify exogenous chemicals (25,26,78). This membrane-bound enzyme system possesses mixed-function oxidases, which are capable of metabolizing a broad range of substrates. These include both endogenous compounds such as hormones and exogenous compounds such as drugs and environmental chemicals. In some instances, the process of biotransformation potentiates the toxicity of certain chemicals. The highly reactive metabolites so formed can lead to tissue injury (see Chapter 9).

Animal studies demonstrate that exposure to such xenobiotics as 2,3,7,8-tetrachlorobenzo-p-dioxin (TCDD) and benzo[a]pyrene induces the microsomal enzymes in the testes and prostate (23). The toxicological significance of these findings is not fully understood. It is speculated, however, that the toxic assault on the germ cells and accessory sex organs is influenced by exposure to environmental chemicals that affect the production of reactive metabolites.

There is evidence that physical and chemical agents can induce damage to DNA molecules. Such damage, unless repaired, can lead to lethal mutations (cell death), mutations that result in transformed cells, or mutations that are inheritable. Lethal and dominant mutations in germ cells result in nonviable offspring. Adverse mutations in somatic cells may alter gene expression and thus initiate cancer. Adverse mutation in germ cells may affect subsequent generations (125).

Fortunately, biochemical studies reveal that cells are able to repair the DNA damage induced by environmental chemicals and radiation. DNA repair mechanisms have been reviewed in detail (43). A number of workers have studied the capacity of spermatogenic cells to repair the nucleic acid damage brought on by environmental assault (61,63, 101,153). The normal nucleic acid structure is restored by a number of local excision–repair mechanisms. The DNA repair system appears to be both dose and time dependent. Thus, exposure that overtaxes the repair mechanisms could result in a larger number of germinal cell mutations that escape DNA repair mechanisms.

Animal Testing for the Determination of Reproductive Hazards

The single most important method of assessing potential reproductive hazards to humans is through animal testing. Such studies evaluate the effects of exposure at varying doses under controlled conditions. A major disadvantage of animal studies is the necessity of extrapolating the results to humans. The laboratory assessment of male reproductive hazards must therefore be viewed in light of the species differences in anatomy, morphology, and functional activity of the male reproductive tract. Adequate methods for extrapolating the results of reproductive studies done in animals to humans are not available. Efforts are now being made to remedy this situation.

As with all toxicological studies, assessing the effects of toxic assault on the male reproductive system must include a consideration of the species selected, the dosage, the route, and the timing of exposure. The timing of exposure is particularly important when assessing the effects of chronic exposure on the male reproductive tract.

Regardless of the system used for testing, the agent under investigation must be administered during the entire process of spermatogenesis. Spermatogenesis, the time from spermatogonial division to mature spermatozoa, has been well worked out in a number of species. Mature spermatozoa are provided by divisions of the seminiferous epithelium, which occur cyclically and synchronously. The length of the cycle of the seminiferous epithelium varies among species. In order to detect the effects of toxic exposure on spermatogenesis, an agent must be given for six complete cycles of the seminiferous epithelium, i.e., 77 days in the rat and 65 days in the rabbit (23). This principle is related to the observation that a decreased sperm count caused by a toxic effect on A-type spermatogonia may not be detectable for a time equal to approximately six cycles of the seminiferous epithelium. When reversibility is monitored, the animals should be exposed to the toxic agent for six cycles and examined 12 cycles after termination of exposure. Although recovery periods in man are longer, animal data may indicate whether the testicular damage induced by each agent is potentially reversible in man (23,74).

Reproductive Capacity and Outcome

The laboratory assessment of male reproductive hazards focuses on reproductive capacity and reproductive outcome. Substances that pose a male reproductive hazard can decrease the fertilizing capacity of the spermatozoa. They may also induce chromosomal alterations in the sperm. Such alterations may be associated with fetal death or abnormal development (81).

The ultimate index of male reproductive capacity is the ability to induce pregnancy and normal offspring. Animal studies assessing reproductive function are practical only with rodent species. Reproductive capacity is tested by mating a male that has been treated with a selected chemical to an untreated female. The assay, which includes recording the number of dead and live births and the percentage litter loss, has been described in detail (50,81). If mutations in the male germ cells are suspected, a dominant lethal assay can be made. This assay is performed in a female that has been mated with a male treated with the test agent.

Early embryonic death is one endpoint in animal tests for mutagens. It is generally considered to be the expression of a dominant lethal genetic trait in the paternal genome caused by a chemical-induced chromosomal aberration. Dominant lethal mutations are evidenced by an increased number of dead or resorbed embryos or by a reduction in the total number of fetuses (81). Tests for reproductive and developmental toxicity may be single- or multigeneration studies. Multigeneration studies, now considered the cornerstone of reproductive toxicity testing of chemicals, are designed to assess the cumulative effects of chronic exposure to chemical agents (159).

Mating studies that evaluate the effect of toxic exposure on male reproductive function are of value in assessing human risk. Animal studies, however, are time consuming, costly, and an insensitive measure of the adverse effects of toxic exposure on the male reproductive system. It has been shown, for example, that simple mating procedures show no evidence of reduced fertility in the rat even after the sperm available for ejaculation are reduced by 70% (50). In addition, the dominant lethal assay is considered a crude measure of mutagenic damage to male germ cells.

Morphologic Changes

Other means of identifying the adverse effects of chemicals on the male reproductive system include evidence of gross and microscopic changes in the gonads and accessory organs of reproduction and interference with spermatogenesis. Semen analysis, although performed in the rabbit, is not usually done in rodent studies of reproductive toxicity. Advances are being made in this area, however (154). Morphological changes, though frequently used to assess reproductive toxicity, are frequently an inadequate marker of reproductive function. New analytic tests applying computer-vision methods to analyze sperm morphology and motion are currently under development. In general, laboratory methods now available are unable to identify subtle reproductive hazards.

Other Techniques

New laboratory methods are being developed to assess the impact of chemicals on male reproductive function. These include in vitro fertilization assays and techniques for evaluating mutagenicity using sperm cells (24,39,125,137,156). Investigation of genetic damage in humans is directed to developing biological markers of germinal mutation in sperm and heritable mutations (125,137,156). Thus far the link between induced sperm anomalies and reduced fertility and heritable genetic defects is unclear (125,154). New techniques of assessing reproductive toxicity in the male are needed. These include a need for cell separation techniques and organ culture systems that permit the in vitro study of toxic effects on germ cells and reproductive tract tissues. New methods designed to identify heritable genetic damage are also needed. The interested reader is urged to consult the National Research Council's review of biological markers in reproductive toxicology (125) (see Chapter 1 for a discussion of biological markers).

EPIDEMIOLOGY

Epidemiologic methods provide the most useful means of studying the relationship between exposure and reproductive dysfunction in human populations. In order to assess reproductive hazards, epidemiologic studies must monitor exposure in relation to reproductive capacity and reproductive outcome.

The epidemiologist frequently encounters major problems in assessing exposure. Adequate information on exposure is frequently unavailable. Individuals are continuously exposed to a wide variety of agents, mostly at low concentrations. The inability to assess exposure adequately makes it difficult to identify reproductive toxins. Often when exposure is well established, the population is so small that there is little likelihood of detecting a significant difference in effect between experimental and control groups. At times, defining the control population poses a greater dilemma than selecting the exposed population.

Endpoints Used to Monitor Male Reproductive Function

Epidemiologists also have difficulty in determining if potential reproductive hazards have actually affected the reproductive capacity of the exposed individuals. A number of endpoints have been used by epidemiologists to monitor reproductive function in males exposed to occupational and environmental chemicals (Table 25-3). These include the assessment of fertility, reproductive outcome, sexual function, and semen analysis. The effects of a reproductive toxin may also be assessed by biopsying the testis. This invasive procedure is rarely performed in epidemiologic studies of reproductive hazards. Unfortunately, reproductive endpoints currently measured, particularly in the male, are often unreliable and unsure clues to reproductive performance. In addition, a reproductive history may be inaccurate, particularly if based only on information obtained from the husband.

Assessment of Fertility

A reproductive history is one of the most direct means of assessing fertility. It has been suggested that information on live births gained from a short questionnaire or from existing medical, employment, or insurance records can be used as a noninvasive, inexpensive means of assessing the repro-

TABLE 25-3. Endpoints Used to Monitor Male Reproductive Function

Assessment of fertility
Reproductive outcome
Sexual function
Semen analyses
Testicular histopathology
Hormone analyses

ductive effects of chemical exposure (65,66,151,152). Data on the number of live births that occurred in the exposed group are compared, after proper statistical adjustments, with national fertility rates in the United States. Using this method, investigators detected a significant decrease in fertility in exposed workers (152). The method is capable of examining, either retrospectively or prospectively, the fertility of exposed women or of the wives of exposed men. It can also take into account the effects of exposure of both mates (152). Apart from being noninvasive and relatively inexpensive, the method has the additional advantage of depending on a clear reproductive endpoint, i.e., the number of live births.

One of the method's major limitations stems from the means used to determine the fertility of the exposed population. This is usually done by comparing the fertility rates of the exposed population with those of the general United States population (79). Such comparisons may not be valid, as national fertility rates provide no information on the fertility of a number of ethnic groups, many of which have higher fertility than the national average. In addition, regional differences, religious preferences, contraceptive practices, educational levels, socioeconomic classes, and life styles are other neglected variables in the national fertility rates. Further discussion of the methodology and the advantages and limitations of the reproductive surveillance program described above has been published (152).

Reproductive Outcome

There is increasing concern that paternal exposure may play a role in such adverse reproductive effects as spontaneous abortions and congenital abnormalities. These adverse effects may be linked to chemically induced damage to the father's germ cells (45,124). At present, germ cell genotoxicity tests, which are time consuming and costly, have had little use in human epidemiology studies (39). Some investigators have assessed chromosomal aberrations in the lymphocytes of exposed workers (19,84). The relationship between chromosomal aberration in somatic cells, and germ cells and their ultimate effect on fertility and embryo/fetal development, is unclear. Exposure to a known mutagen (such as ionizing radiation) at high doses (as in Hiroshima and Nagasaki), which causes considerable residual chromosomal damage, has not been linked to an increase in spontaneous abortions or to birth defects. It must be assumed that such effects do occur, but their incidence is very low. To date there are no epidemiologic data that support the occurrence of heritable chromosomal abnormalities (7,131).

Some investigators have monitored for the adverse effects of paternal exposure on reproduction. These include the potential for spontaneous abortion, abnormal fetal development, and cancer in the offspring (32,36,40,47,48,55,77,98,112,150). Monitoring reproductive outcome, however, is difficult, as many adverse reproductive effects are subtle and difficult to measure. Assessing the incidence of spontaneous abortions, for example, is extremely difficult. Many women who have spontaneous abortions are not hospitalized, and others are unaware that they were pregnant. Assessing the delayed effects of reproductive toxins, which may appear as developmental disorders in the offspring, is also difficult.

Semen Analysis

Semen analysis, which includes an examination of sperm density, motility, and morphology, has long been used as a marker of male reproductive function (10). Semen analysis is obviously important in the identification of male reproductive hazards. It has the advantage of being a noninvasive means of examining germ cells and evaluating toxic injury to the testes.

Any study that depends on semen analysis, however, faces many problems. It is often difficult to get the cooperation of the group under study unless there is an obvious hazard. Semen analysis is expensive and often difficult to perform properly. Obtaining a suitable control population frequently poses a problem. Finally, semen analysis offers the epidemiologist no sure clue to male fertility because marked differences in semen characteristics are compatible with reproduction.

The most important measure of fertility potential currently available in the human male is the concentration of motile sperm in the ejaculate. Evaluating sperm output and motility in relation to male fertility is fraught with potential pitfalls. There is no valid standard for "normal semen" that can be used for comparative purposes. The influence of ethnic background, geographic location, and socioeconomic factors on sperm production has not been determined (117). Without population frequencies for semen quality, it is difficult for the epidemiologist to place an individual sperm count within the context of normality for the population being investigated.

Wide variations exist in semen characteristics. Laboratory error and physiological fluctuations in semen quality contribute to these variations in the following manner. (1) Under "normal" conditions, in all men, the quality and quantity of semen vary significantly. In addition, a sperm count may change appreciably in samples taken from the same person at different times. (2) Illness, personal habits, seasonal change, and abstinence also affect semen characteristics. For example, sperm output may

drop sporadically because of stress, allergic reactions, or systemic or localized viral or bacterial infections (70,71). Heat exposure associated with an elevation in scrotal temperature and personal habits such as heavy alcohol consumption may also affect sperm production. Seasonal changes in sperm output have been reported (132). The sperm count may also be affected by the frequency of ejaculation in the days and weeks before the sample was obtained (34). (4) Differences between laboratories in their assessment of sperm characteristics may add to the wide fluctuations in semen characteristics and make it impossible to compare data between laboratories. (5) Improper collection and handling of the semen sample and failure to analyze the specimen promptly also introduce large variations in the results of semen analysis.

It is apparent that alterations in sperm counts frequently offer little help in assessing fertility or in detecting a mild degree of testicular toxicity. In contrast, severely suppressed sperm counts or the absence of sperm over a period of months strongly suggest that normal spermatogenesis has been affected. Such findings in a group of exposed individuals clearly support the presence of a reproductive toxin. Although low sperm counts are compatible with fertility, a reduced sperm count does increase the risk of infertility. Individuals with sperm counts below 10 million per milliliter carry a risk of infertility that is ten times greater than that of men having sperm counts between 60 and 160 million per milliliter. Men with sperm counts from 10 to 20 million and from 20 to 40 million per milliliter carry a risk of infertility that is five and three times greater, respectively, than for men with counts of 60 to 160 million per milliliter (18,110,160).

Evaluation of morphological characteristics of spermatozoa is another parameter of semen analysis. Sperm malformations are easily discernible under the microscope. The visual assessment of sperm morphology, however, is a subjective qualitative judgment, which makes the comparison of data among laboratories difficult. Although a number of factors may affect sperm morphology, the occurrence of gross morphological abnormalities of the spermatozoa may signal the presence of a noxious agent that is inducing significant damage to the spermatogenic process. The relationship between chemically induced sperm anomalies and reduced fertility and heritable, genetic defects is unclear (155). Human studies focusing on the relationships among chemical exposure, sperm morphology, and reproductive function are needed.

Reproductive Effects of Paternal Exposure

Relatively few epidemiologic studies have looked at male reproductive function in relation to chemical exposure in the workplace and the environment. Most studies have focused on the effects of toxic exposure on the developing embryo/fetus without consideration of the male component. Apart from the essential complexity of performing valid epidemiologic studies, the lack of simple reliable tests of male reproductive function undoubtedly contributes to the limited data available on male reproductive hazards. Most epidemiologic studies concerned with the male reproductive effects of exposure to environmental chemicals were performed in the workplace where exposures are higher and more easily assessed. The agents studied include heavy metals, polyhalogenated biphenyls, pesticides, Agent Orange, herbicides, dioxin, solvents, hydrocarbons, petroleum, paints, industrial chemicals, and ionizing radiation. In some cases adverse reproductive effects have been confirmed. In most cases the adverse effects have not been established (4,52,94,99,100,136). Increased attention is being given to the developmental and carcinogenic risks faced by the offspring of fathers exposed to toxic chemicals (8,33,36,40,46,48,77,98,112,124, 150). Savitz and Chen have reviewed the epidemiologic studies of parental occupation and childhood cancer (98).

Metals

Exposure to a number of metals such as arsenic, boron, cadmium, lead, and mercury can cause male reproductive dysfunction in animals (4,5,136). With the exception of lead, the human data are so limited that no assessment can be made regarding the effect of metals on male reproductive function. In view of the many reproductive ills elicited by metal exposure in experimental animals, it is critical to perform reproductive studies of exposed human populations.

As previously noted, both inorganic and organic lead are widespread contaminants in the workplace and general environment. Inorganic lead has long been recognized as a reproductive hazard. It has been used as a spermicide as well as an abortifacient (129). A number of reports support the conclusion that lead is a male reproductive toxin (5,136,140). In 1975, Lancranjan et al., studying 150 lead workers, reported dose-related sperm abnormalities. Workers with blood lead concentrations between 23 and 75 μg/100 mL exhibited asthenospermia, oligospermia, and teratospermia. Workers having blood lead levels around 75 μg/100 mL suffered from impaired fertility (59). Semen analysis in workers exposed to lead in a storage battery factory revealed sperm with lowered chromatic stability. Decreased secretory function of the accessory genital glands was also reported (149).

A number of early reports indicate that paternal lead exposure adversely affects pregnancy outcome. Past studies based on occupational exposure to high levels of lead noted increased numbers of spontaneous abortions and stillbirths in the wives of lead workers. Decreased survival time of the offspring was also seen (86,145).

Polyhalogenated Hydrocarbons

The polychlorinated biphenyls (PCBs) and polybrominated biphenyls (PBBs) are polyhalogenated aromatic hydrocarbons. The chemical stability, low volatility, and low flammability of these compounds were highly prized in the manufacture of flame retardants and heat transfer agents. Since 1979, all manufacture, processing, and distribution of PCBs and PBBs have been banned in the United States. This decision, in part, was based on their persistence in the environment and a concern for their reproductive toxicity.

To date there are no reports on the effects of PCB exposure on reproduction in the human male. One study has examined semen quality in men exposed to PBBs (95). This study by Rosenman et al. was performed in the wake of an episode of PBB contamination that occurred in Michigan. In 1973 PBB inadvertently added to cattle feed led to widespread contamination of the food chain. Semen quality was analyzed in 52 men who were exposed to PBB in the workplace or who ingested contaminated food. The study showed no differences in sperm counts, motility, or morphology between the exposed group and a group of male university students. Since this study was done 4 years after the episode of contamination, an earlier reversible effect on semen quality could have been missed.

Pesticides

Few agricultural chemicals have been well studied for their effects on reproduction. Epidemiologic studies are difficult to perform, particularly when exposure occurs in the field. Under such circumstances exposure is poorly characterized, and long-term follow-up often presents an insurmountable problem. The wide use of pesticides, their ubiquitous presence, and their selected persistence in the environment emphasize the importance of obtaining information on their reproductive effects. The heightened awareness of the reproductive hazards of agricultural chemicals stemmed from the profound testicular toxicity induced by the nematocide dibromochloropropane (DBCP) (146).

Dibromochloropropane

Dibromochloropropane, a soil fumigant and nematocide, was widely used in the United States and abroad from the mid-1950s until 1979, when its use was banned except in Hawaiian pineapple fields. Although DBCP was noted to be a testicular toxin in experimental animals in 1961, its effects in humans were not discovered until 16 years later. In 1977, Whorton et al. described the adverse reproductive effects of DBCP in humans (147). Prior to this report no agent, in concentrations found in the workplace, was shown to produce infertility and sterility in otherwise healthy men. This report stemmed from observations on workers employed in a California pesticide formulation plant. The men noted that they fathered fewer children after their employment in the agricultural chemical division of the pesticide factory. DBCP had been formulated in this division since 1962. All of the workers in this division were examined for semen quality. Of the 25 workers examined, 14 were azoospermic or oligospermic. There were no other abnormal physical or laboratory findings apart from elevated levels of follicle-stimulating hormone and luteinizing hormone in men with low or absent sperm count. Testosterone levels were normal. There was a direct relationship between the length of DBCP exposure and abnormally low sperm counts (147).

A number of studies subsequently performed on DBCP-exposed men, i.e., formulators, applicators, and farmers, confirmed these initial observations (29,67,92,97,148). Men exposed to DBCP, whether as workers in factories or as field workers, suffered a reduction in sperm counts and testicular damage. The extent of testicular damage was directly related to both the duration and the degree of exposure. All segments of the spermatogenic process, including the spermatogonia, were affected. Sertoli cells and Leydig cells appeared morphologically intact. In the most severely affected cases there was destruction of spermatogonial stem cells with no sign of recovery even after 5 years. In cases where effects were less severe and associated with oligospermia, some recovery took place after 3 years. In men with testicular damage no other signs of toxicity were present. There was no loss of libido or potency. Plasma levels of FSH were elevated in men with oligo- or azoospermia. There were inconsistent increases in levels of LH. Blood levels of testosterone were not affected (29,67,148). The interested reader is referred to a comprehensive review of the subject (146).

Few studies have examined the reproductive outcome in wives of men exposed to DBCP. An Israeli study compared the rate of spontaneous abortions in the wives of DBCP-exposed banana farmers before and after exposure. Examination of the medical records revealed a threefold increase in spontaneous abortions when the pregnancy began after the father's exposure to DBCP (55). A more recent study of the reproductive outcome of DBCP-exposed men

has been published by Israeli investigators. The families of 30 workers employed in a plant that until 1977 produced DBCP were monitored for 5 years. Of 13 men who were azoospermic in 1977, four recovered spermatogenesis, and two fathered children. Of eight men who were oligospermic in 1977, all fathered children. No increase in spontaneous abortion was observed in the wives of the exposed men. No infant or fetal deaths and no congenital abnormalities occurred among 12 children born to the wives of DBCP-exposed men (38).

Chlordecone (Kepone®)

Kepone® is a chlorinated hydrocarbon insecticide that was used against leaf-eating insects, ants, cockroaches, and the larvae of flies until its use was banned in 1977. In the late 1970s an epidemic of Kepone® poisoning occurred in the Life Sciences Products Company in Hopewell, Virginia. The symptoms of intoxication were mainly neurological, characterized by nervousness, tremor, and visual disturbances. However, reduced sperm count and motility and abnormal sperm morphology were also reported. As blood chlordecone levels decreased after exposure stopped, sperm counts increased. These findings indicated that the oligospermia induced by chlordecone poisoning was reversible (11).

Agent Orange, Dioxin, and Phenoxy Herbicides

Agent Orange, composed of equal parts 2,4-dichlorophenoxyacetic acid (2,4,-D) and 2,4,5-trichlorophenoxyacetic acid (2,4,5-T), was used as a defoliant in Vietnam from the mid-1960s until 1971. The 2,4,5-T in Agent Orange contained about 2 ppm of dioxin or TCDD (2,3,7,8-tetrachlorodibenzo-p-dioxin). TCDD is an extremely toxic chemical for certain animal species (75). About 166 kg of TCDD was released in Vietnam (157). The phenoxy herbicide 2,4,5-T was widely used between 1948 and 1970 for weed control in forestry, farming, family gardens, and along roadsides.

Animal studies show that TCDD and 2,3,4-T (with or without TCDD) are teratogenic and fetotoxic (35,37). It is unclear whether TCDD affects spermatogenesis in lower animals (143). The evidence that 2,4,5-T exposure leads to birth defects in animals, and the concern for its effects on human reproduction, led the Environmental Protection Agency, in 1979, to suspend its use in forestry, rights of way, and pastures (138). A number of comprehensive reviews dealing with the toxicology and the reproductive effects of Agent Orange, TCDD, and the phenoxy herbicides have been published (15, 16,35,139).

The widespread use of Agent Orange during the Vietnam war caused concern about its possible adverse reproductive effects among Vietnam veterans. Large-scale epidemiologic studies to investigate this issue were designed and performed by the United States Air Force and by the Centers for Disease Control (32,60). Attention was directed to the possibility of paternally induced birth defects.

A series of reports have come from the long-range epidemiologic study being done by the United States Air Force. Code-named Ranch Hand, this study, still in progress, searched for evidence of reproductive dysfunction in Ranch Hand participants, i.e., pilots, crew members, and support personnel, who had received substantial exposure, on almost a daily basis, to herbicides and dioxin. The findings in 1,174 Ranch Hand participants were compared with a matched group of nonexposed personnel who served in Southeast Asia during the same period. Thus far no significant differences were reported in fertility, infertility, miscarriages, stillbirths, or live births between the exposed and unexposed groups. Neonatal and infant deaths (age 1–28 days) were higher among children born to Ranch Hand personnel. An increase in minor birth defects, primarily birthmarks, and a slightly higher number of physical handicaps were also reported in the offspring of Ranch Hand personnel. These associations are based on self-reported findings and therefore must be ruled tentative until the data can be confirmed by an examination of the medical records (60). Semen specimens obtained from those willing to provide one showed no group difference with respect to total sperm count or percentage abnormal sperm.

In a study from the Centers for Disease Control, Erickson et al. looked at the relative risk for Vietnam veterans of fathering children with serious congenital malformations. The study was based on the experiences of parents of babies born in metropolitan Atlanta from 1968 to 1980 (32). Information regarding military service in Vietnam was obtained from review of the military records and from interviews with the mothers and the fathers of babies in the case and control groups. There were 7133 babies in the case group and 4246 babies in the control group. The results of this study indicate that, in general, Vietnam veterans do not have a greater risk than other men for fathering babies with serious structural birth defects. But Vietnam veterans with greater estimated exposure to Agent Orange do seem to be at increased risk for fathering children with a few specific types of defects, i.e., spinal bifida, certain types of tumors, and cleft lip with or without cleft palate. An Australian study of the offspring of Australian Vietnam veterans showed no evidence of an increased incidence of morphological birth defects (28).

Other investigators have looked at the reproductive effects of occupational exposure to herbicides and dioxin. Townsend et al. reported that the wives of men exposed to TCDD in the workplace faced no significant increased risk of spontaneous abortion, perinatal death, or congenital malformations (134). Suskind and Hertzberg reported on the long-term effects of occupational exposure to 2,4,5-T and its contaminants, including dioxin (126). Information on reproductive factors and on birth defects was obtained from the male participants. No significant differences were reported in the number of pregnancies, live births, infant deaths, miscarriages, birth defects, or stillbirths between the exposed and control populations.

A number of epidemiologic studies have focused on the reproductive effects of environmental exposure to phenoxy herbicides and dioxin on both sexes. The results of these studies are presented in Chapter 24, which deals with reproductive hazards in the female.

Organic Solvents

A wide variety of organic solvents such as benzene, carbon disulfide, carbon tetrachloride, styrene, xylene, and toluene have been used for many years in manufacturing and in the chemical industry. The electronic industry provides an important, relatively new, source of solvent exposure (58). Organic solvents form a major portion of the chemicals used by the microelectronics industry. Solvents are also widely used in schools, in chemistry laboratories, and in the home. They are used in reagents, in cleaning and thinning agents, in household cements, in wood stains, varnishes, paints, and inks. It is estimated that 10 million individuals are exposed to solvents in the workplace alone (136).

Few epidemiologic studies have examined the reproductive effects of solvent exposure in the male. Cook et al. studied men exposed to a group of chemical solvents known as glycol ethers. Although this study failed to document reproductive toxicity in the exposed group, the results are difficult to interpret because of the small number of participants (13). Since a number of organic solvents such as carbon disulfide, carbon tetrachloride, and glycol ethers are known to be harmful to the reproductive systems of male and female test animals, attention must be focused on the potentially adverse reproductive effects of solvent exposure in humans (4,44,99,100,136).

Hydrocarbons, Petroleum, Paints, and Industrial Chemicals

Fetal loss was assessed in the wives of men employed in a waste treatment plant of a major oil company. In the course of processing the contaminated water, these workers were exposed to a wide range of substances at low concentrations. Information on fetal loss, i.e., miscarriage or stillbirth, was obtained from the wives of 89 exposed workers and verified by hospital records. The relative risk of fetal loss was found to be increased when paternal exposure in the waste-water treatment plant occurred at about the time of conception (77).

In 1974, Fabia and Thuy attempted to determine whether there was a link between the cancer deaths of 386 children before the age of 5 and the occupations of their fathers at the time of the children's birth. The cases were traced from death certificates, hospital records, and data on fathers' occupations and residences. In the children who had died of malignant disease there was a significant increase in the number of fathers employed in jobs having exposure to hydrocarbons, i.e., motor-vehicle mechanics, machinists, miners, and painters (33). Some studies using different populations, techniques, and age groups support these findings, although others did not (41,46,54,90,112,158).

Ionizing Radiation

Data on the effects of ionizing radiation on the human male reproductive system come from four sources: (1) individuals involved in radiation accidents, (2) patients whose testes were irradiated during radiotherapy for malignant tumors, (3) volunteers who received graded doses of irradiation to the gonads during controlled experiments, and (4) workers exposed to radiation in an occupational setting.

Radiation Accidents

Information obtained from studies of those involved in radiation accidents is of limited value because exposure levels are not precise, and the status of the reproductive systems of the victims prior to the accident is unknown.

Radiotherapy

Radiotherapy is a commonly used mode of treatment for patients with Hodgkin disease, lymphosarcoma, and testicular tumors. In a study of 11 patients aged 18 to 49 who received total doses to the testes of 118 to 228 rad, azoospermia was observed in all subjects approximately 3 months after irradiation. In three patients, sperm production rose to fertile levels 11 to 18 months after irradiation. In two patients, sperm count reached "subfertile" levels 25 to 41 months after irradiation. Five were not followed long enough to assess spermatogenic recovery, and one patient had a bilateral orchidectomy (3). In another study of ten patients who had received irradiation therapy for Hodgkin disease, the testes had received doses of 5 to 15 rad in 14 to 26 daily fractions. All of these patients developed azoospermia, and no spermatogenic recovery was noted after

a follow-up of 40 months (3). In a group of 44 patients ranging in age from 21 to 56 years who had received radiation therapy, all developed azoospermia. Recovery of spermatogenic function was related to the duration and level of exposure. In this group, the induction of azoospermia occurred at a total dose as low as 35 rad. At doses from 35 to 97 rad, spermatogenic function recovered within 18 months after irradiation in most patients and after 2 to 3 years in all patients. Among those receiving 105 to 160 rad, spermatogenic recovery began 13 to 38 months after irradiation. Recovery of spermatogenesis was observed 12 to 14 years post-irradiation among a group receiving 210 to 312 rad. Out of all the 44 cases, 15 eventually produced a total of 22 children. An important observation in all of the clinical studies is the finding that fractionated irradiation may be more harmful that acute exposure (3). The effects of gonadal irradiation in clinical radiation therapy have been reviewed (69).

Graded Doses of Ionizing Radiation

Investigation of the effect of ionizing radiation on normal men involved a group of volunteers who received single doses of testicular irradiation varying between 8 and 600 rad. At all dose levels except 8 rad, type B spermatogonia were the most radiosensitive cells. At the dose level of 200 to 300 rad, spermatocytes were unable to complete maturation division. This resulted in a decrease in spermatids. At dose levels of 400 to 600 rads, spermatocytes showed visible damage. Although spermatids showed no overt damage, the numbers of spermatozoa were significantly reduced after exposure to 400 to 600 rad. At all dose levels above 78 rad, azoospermia occurred after 67 days. At doses of 50 to 78 rad, there was marked oligospermia (2 million per milliliter) (96).

Complete recovery of sperm concentrations to preirradiated concentrations varied with the degree of radiation exposure. With doses of 100 rad or less, recovery was complete within 9 to 18 months; with doses of 200 to 400 rad, recovery occurred 30 months after exposure; with doses of 400 to 600 rad, recovery occurred 5 years or more after exposure (96).

The success of radiotherapy and the survival of cancer patients, along with the realization that even after exposure to relatively high doses of irradiation spermatogenic recovery can occur, has raised concern regarding genetic defects in progeny of exposed individuals. This issue has been discussed (12).

Occupational Exposure to Ionizing Radiation

A British study by Gardner et al. showed that men receiving external radiation in the workplace had a higher than expected number of children with leukemia. The children were seven to eight times more likely to develop leukemia if their father had been exposed to external radiation before the child's conception. This study was performed in response to a documented increased incidence of childhood leukemia that appeared near the Sellafield nuclear plant in West Cumbria, England. This is the first time that childhood leukemia has been associated with the father's occupational exposure to radiation (36).

PATHOLOGY AND PATHOLOGICAL PHYSIOLOGY

The function of the male reproductive system depends on a vast number of critical molecular and cellular processes that are highly vulnerable to toxic injury. Toxic assault on these processes during adult life may lead to decreased fertility and abnormal fetal development. Toxic assault during embryonic and fetal life may adversely affect reproductive capacity and sexual behavior (4,118,136).

A reproductive toxin may have a direct effect because of its structural similarity to an endogenous compound (hormone or nutrient) or because of its chemical reactivity. Toxins possessing structural similarity to physiologically active molecules may operate by misleading the cell or organism. Compounds of this type are usually agonists or antagonists of endogenous hormones (9). Direct-acting toxins that are chemically reactive are usually nonspecific at their site of action. They are frequently toxic, mutagenic, or carcinogenic in a number of organ systems; their reproductive toxicity may be overlooked.

Toxins may act indirectly by altering physiological control mechanisms or by exerting their effect only after being metabolized. Indirect-acting toxins may be metabolized to form toxic metabolites that are chemically reactive. They may also mimic endogenous molecules. Compounds such as dibromochloropropane and the polycyclic aromatic hydrocarbons become reproductive toxins when they are transformed to chemically reactive metabolites (62, 73). Toxins may also indirectly affect the reproductive system by inducing or inhibiting enzymes that alter physiological control systems (74). The action of many halogenated hydrocarbon pesticides, such as DDT, polychlorinated biphenyls (PBCs), and polybrominated biphenyls, is based in part on this mechanism.

To date no serious attempt has been made to elucidate the biochemical mechanisms responsible for the adverse effects of chemically induced injury to the male reproductive tract. Our understanding of reproductive toxicology depends primarily on identifying the site of injury. In most cases this is accomplished by relatively crude means. Even when progress has been made in understanding the normal biochemical mechanisms of reproduction, as with testicular function, little attention has been directed to the biochemical mechanisms underlying testicular injury. In most instances, the assessment of chemically induced testicular injury in animals is still limited to measuring testicular weight, evaluating the histology of the testes, determining sperm output and fertility, and measuring hormonal levels in the blood (114,117,122).

The reproductive process involves a complex series of steps that may be interrupted at any point by toxic exposure. In the male, for example, reproduction depends on hypothalamo-pituitary-gonadal interactions, hormonal synthesis and action, spermatogenesis, gene integrity, and normal accessory sex organs and sexual function. Interference with any of these processes may lead to a disturbance in reproductive function. The complexity of the reproductive and developmental process often makes it difficult to determine the exact site(s) of action of a reproductive toxin. In some instances the target site susceptible to chemical injury has received a good deal of attention, as with the testes. In others (i.e., accessory sex glands and secretion) little information is available (142). In the male, by far the greatest attention has been given to toxic injury to the testes, and this discussion focuses on chemically induced injury to the testes. The effects of a few selected agents found in the workplace and general environment are examined. The interested reader is referred to several reviews of this subject (105,142).

Chemically Induced Testicular Injury

The testes are a critical site of toxic injury. They serve two main purposes in the adult male: the production of spermatozoa and the production of male hormones, primarily testosterone. Spermatogenesis occurs in the seminiferous tubules (Fig. 25-1). Between the seminiferous tubules are interstitial compartments that include the Leydig (interstitial) cells. Androgen biosynthesis takes place in the Leydig cells. Sertoli cells, the only nongerm cells of the seminiferous tubule, appear to play a role in the initiation, maintenance, and control of spermatogenesis. Spermatogenesis and androgen production are interrelated, as testosterone is necessary for sperm production, for the integrity of secondary sexual characteristics (male accessory glands and external genitalia), and for sexual behavior. The anterior pituitary, through the production of follicle-stimulating hormone (FSH) and luteinizing hormone (LH), exerts control on spermatogenesis and androgen production, respectively (87).

Adult reproductive capacity may be compromised by any testicular toxin that disrupts the pro-

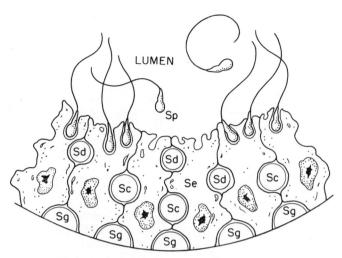

FIGURE 25-1. Seminiferous tubule. Sc, spermatocyte; Sd, spermatid; Se, Sertoli cell; Sg, spermatogonium; Sp, spermatozoon. From Waller et al. (142).

cess of germ cell replication or gametogenesis. It is important to appreciate the differences between the male and female in this process, as these differences may affect the action of a reproductive toxin. In the female, the germ cells or oocytes appear prenatally; no new germ cells are formed after birth. Thus, during the prenatal period, the female is especially vulnerable to any chemically induced changes that would be toxic to meiosis and mitosis. The male germ cells, on the other hand, go into mitotic arrest in the perinatal period and fail to enter meiosis until puberty. It is estimated that from puberty through the human male's reproductive life span a quadrillion spermatozoa are produced. Prenatal exposure of the male may result in interference with gamete production along with possible mutagenic effects (118). Spermatogenesis, a continuous process in the adult male, is vulnerable throughout the reproductive life span.

The inhibition of spermatogenesis appears to be one of the major effects of the nematocide DBCP. After DBCP exposure, evidence of testicular toxicity was found in rabbits, guinea pigs, and rats (133). As mentioned previously, workers exposed to DBCP have decreased sperm counts and degeneration of the seminiferous epithelium. The mechanism of DBCP toxicity on the testes is unknown. It has been suggested that metabolism of DBCP produces a reactive metabolite that acts directly on germ cells (6). Ethylene dibromide (EDB), formerly used as a grain and soil fumigant, is another agent that alters spermatogenesis in experimental animals (2,107). To date, limited data have not clearly linked human exposure to EDB with testicular toxicity.

The industrial agent di-(2-ethylhexyl)phthalate (DEHP), a phthalate ester widely used to plasticize (i.e., improve the flexibility of) polyvinyl chloride, produces testicular atrophy and degeneration in experimental animals (130). Finished plastics such as auto and household upholstery, garden hose, shower curtains, and dialysis and blood transfusion tubing may be composed of as much as 50% phthalate esters. To date, no information is available on the reproductive effects of phthalate ester exposure in humans.

Glycol ethers, widely used as industrial solvents and present in wood stains, varnishes, paints, and ink, produce testicular atrophy and sperm head abnormalities in rodents. These adverse effects were noted after male rodents were treated with such glycol ethers as ethylene glycol monomethyl ether (Methyl Cellosolve®), ethylene glycol monoethyl ether (Cellosolve®), or diethylene glycol monoethyl ether (76). It is not known if these effects occur in humans.

A number of metals such as boron, lead, and cadmium are known to cause testicular injury. Animal studies show dose-related effects of boron exposure on the testes. Male rats fed borax developed testicular atrophy that was associated with a decrease in seminiferous tubular diameter and a marked reduction of spermatocytes and spermatogenic cells (27,144). Recently scientists in Russia have expressed concern regarding the toxic effects of high boron concentrations on male reproductive function. Russian studies report oligospermia and decreased libido in men working in factories producing boric acid and in men living in communities where boron concentrations are high in drinking water (57,127).

Studies in a variety of animals show that parenteral administration of cadmium produces severe damage to both the seminiferous tubules and the interstitial portion of the testes (88,89). The effects of cadmium exposure on male reproductive function in humans are unclear. There is limited evidence that cadmium may induce testicular damage in humans (108). Lead produces seminiferous tubular damage with the inhibition of spermatogenesis, an increased number of abnormal sperm, and oligospermia in a number of animal species including man (64,129). Decreased fertility and increased frequency of asthenospermia, hypospermia, and teratospermia are reported in men exposed to lead in the workplace (59).

Adverse Reproductive Outcome

Chemical exposure of the male, apart from interrupting reproductive function, may adversely affect reproductive outcome (40,47,124). This can occur in two ways: (1) chemicals present in the seminal fluid or bound to spermatozoa can be transported to the maternal environment and thereby affect the reproductive process, and/or (2) chemical exposure of the male can induce genetic damage in germ cells, thereby increasing the risk of infertility, abnormal development in the embryo/fetus or offspring, or the development of childhood cancer.

It is well established that toxic chemicals find their way into the male reproductive tract. Compounds such as heavy metals, pesticides, and flame retardants have been identified in semen (17,72). What effect toxic chemicals in the male reproductive tract have on fertility and the development of the embryo/fetus and offspring is unknown.

Since half of the genetic information is derived from the father, injury to the male gamete may adversely affect the development of the embryo/fetus and offspring. Recent studies show that exposing male laboratory animals to agents that induce genetic damage produces congenital malformations in their offspring. Thus, irradiation or treatment of male mice with urethane is linked to an increased incidence of malformations in their offspring (56,82,102,103). Trasler et al., treating male rats with cyclophosphamide, a mutagenic drug used in the treatment of cancer, produced birth defects in their offspring (135).

Not all embryos produced by genetically damaged germ cells have congenital malformations. Early embryonic death, occurring shortly after implantation, may take place. Such deaths, it is assumed, are the expression of a "dominant lethal" genetic trait. Chemical injury to the DNA of spermatocytes or precursor cells may cause a lethal and dominant mutation and a nonviable offspring (8, 39,52).

Cancer in the offspring may theoretically be produced by paternal exposure to an agent that alters the germ cells. Experimental evidence suggests that, in mice, paternal exposure to mutagenic agents leads to an increased incidence of cancer in their offspring (81). As noted, a number of epidemiologic studies have looked at the relationship between childhood cancer and the occupation of the father (36,40,46,47,112,150). Cancer in the offspring, linked to parental exposure, will undoubtedly be the focus of many future investigative efforts.

CLINICAL ASPECTS OF EXPOSURE TO ENVIRONMENTAL CHEMICALS AND PHYSICAL AGENTS ON THE MALE REPRODUCTIVE SYSTEM

The medical history provides a means of obtaining information on past, current, and future exposures. The physician must inquire about present and past occupational exposures, focusing on specific agents and on the duration and intensity of the exposure. The pattern of exposure in the home and neighborhood should be considered. The nature of an individual's hobby, for example, is particularly pertinent if it entails the heavy use of solvents in a poorly ventilated setting. Information on medication and life style is important. The timing of exposures is sometimes critical to reproductive events. Since spermatogenesis is a continuous process, paternal exposures occurring shortly before conception deserve particular attention. The exposure patterns of both mates must also be considered.

Assessing the reproductive hazards of toxic exposure in men is unfortunately frustrated by a limited understanding of male reproductive physiology and by a lack of easily measured indicators of male reproductive function. As previously mentioned, the range of normality for the male reproductive system can be very broad, and the primary indicator of reproductive function, namely, sperm production, can be seriously diminished for unknown reasons. In other words, the incidence of idiopathic oligospermia is very high in the general population. Exposure to toxic substances may also cause sexual dysfunction (e.g., impotence or decreased libido), which is difficult to assess. These factors clearly make it difficult for the clinician to identify the adverse effects of toxic exposure on the male reproductive system. The problem is compounded by the fact that most medical school curricula and residency programs do not include even rudimentary instruction concerning the effect of toxic substances on the male reproductive system. Even more remarkable, most medical school curricula contain minimal or no information concerning the physiology and the pathophysiology of the male reproductive system (1,68).

Reproductive dysfunction caused by toxic exposure of the male may be viewed in two ways: (1) disorders of the male reproductive system affecting fertility and (2) adverse reproductive outcome mediated through the father.

Disorders of the Male Reproductive System

The most commonly available methods used to assess reproductive function in the human male are (1) a medical history that includes a reproductive and sexual history, (2) a physical examination, (3) semen analysis, (4) hormone assay with determinations of the plasma levels of testosterone, luteinizing hormone (LH), and follicle-stimulating hormone (FSH), and (5) a testicular biopsy.

Reproductive and Sexual History

A reproductive and sexual history need not be an extensive exercise. It requires gathering information regarding the development of the reproductive system. It includes a pubertal history, information on possible congenital or developmental disorders of the reproductive system, a history of sexual performance, data on sexually transmitted diseases previously contracted by the patient, a marital history, the number of offspring, the outcome of pregnancies, and some information concerning the reproductive normality of the sexual partner. Information on exposure to toxins, pharmacological agents, recreational drugs (including alcohol), irradiation, and excessive heat (hot tubs) should also be included.

Physical Examination

A complete physical examination includes an assessment of masculine development (i.e., the male habitus, hair distribution, musculature, development of the penis, scrotum, and testes). Examination of the scrotal contents includes palpation for the presence of the vas deferens, of varicocele, spermatocele, or other pathological structures in the scrotum, the presence and normality of the epididymis, and the size and consistency of the testicles. The rectal examination includes a determination of the size, consistency, and degree of tenderness of the prostate.

Semen Analysis

Semen analysis is of major importance in evaluating male fertility. Of the various semen characteristics measured, the concentration of motile sperm (sperm count times percentage motility) in the ejaculate appears to be more closely related to pregnancy rates than either the sperm count or the "percentage motility" alone (111). As mentioned previously, evaluation of the sperm count is fraught with problems, which range from collecting the specimen properly to placing an individual sperm count within the context of normality for the population being investigated (106,110,116,160). Apart from the wide variations in sperm concentration and characteristics compatible with fertility, a sperm count may vary appreciably in samples taken from the same person at different times. Sperm output may also drop sporadically as a result of systemic or localized viral or bacterial infections or allergic reactions (70,71). The sperm count at a given time may also be affected by the frequency of ejaculation in the days and weeks before the sample was obtained (34).

In an initial assessment of sperm output, at least three specimens, collected at monthly intervals, should be examined. The preferred method of obtaining the ejaculate is by masturbation. It is important to collect the entire ejaculate because sperm cells are not equally distributed throughout the ejaculate. Samples should be collected after 2 or 3 days of sexual abstinence, since recent ejaculation may lower the sperm count. The semen should be delivered to a laboratory within 1–2 h after collection and should be analyzed promptly. For commonly used techniques for performance of semen analysis, see Smith and Rodriguez-Rigau (109).

Hormone Assay

The measurement of circulating hormone levels has some relevance to studies of spermatogenic function. For the following reasons, however, its usefulness is generally limited to the detection of serious disturbances in spermatogenesis. Although elevated plasma FSH levels are reported in men with damage to the germinal epithelium, "normal" FSH levels are seen in men with serious disturbances of spermatogenesis (93,116). Testosterone levels within the normal range are often considered to reflect normal Leydig cell function. However, Leydig cells with intrinsic cell damage may compensate and produce levels of circulating testosterone that fall within "normal" ranges. The importance of this phenomenon is apparent for assessment of the effects of chemicals that may cause injury to the Leydig cells.

Testicular Biopsy

The spermatogenic function of the testes can often be evaluated by means of a testicular biopsy. This invasive procedure requires the proper procurement and preparation of tissues for microscopic evaluation, as damaged tissue specimens are of little diagnostic value (117). The interpretation of biopsy material must be done by individuals trained in the pathomorphology of the testes. A number of investigators have demonstrated the effectiveness of carefully performed testicular biopsies, particularly in the quantitative evaluation of human spermatogenesis (53,120).

Evaluation of Fertility

Reduced fertility is one of the major concerns of toxic insult to the male reproductive system. It is therefore important to have some idea of the fertility expectation before drawing conclusions concerning effects of a toxicant. There are several factors to consider when assessing the likelihood of pregnancy in fertile couples. The prevalence of infertility among couples at reproductive age in the general population is estimated to be from 0.3% to about 15% (115). It is necessary to examine the probability of conception for each month of unprotected intercourse in fertile couples at various ages. With this information the probability of a couple's achieving a pregnancy within a specified period of time can be calculated.

Among women in their early 20s with average fertility potential, there is a monthly probability of conception between 20% and 25%. This means that within a year between 93% and 97% of these women will get pregnant. Among women in their late 20s and early 30s, the monthly probability of pregnancy is between 10% and 15%. Therefore, between 70% and 85% of these women could be expected to be pregnant within a year. There is one study showing that in a large population of fertile couples of all ages, 80% had achieved a pregnancy within 1 year and 90% had done so within 1½ years (119,123).

As mentioned previously, male fertility cannot be assessed independently of the fertility of the partner. Fertility reflects the potential of a couple. If the reproductive potential of the male is assessed in isolation, the possibility exists of erroneously attributing a couple's lowered fertility potential solely to the adverse effects of exposure on the male. Thus, a group of males having a history of low fertility or childlessness and "low" sperm counts may be considered the cause of impaired reproductive capacity until it is discovered that their partners have a high level of ovulatory dysfunction or other disturbance of their reproductive potential.

Diagnosis and Treatment

In most instances, there are no specific clinical or pathological findings that reflect the adverse effects of a particular agent on the male reproductive system. This lack of specificity clearly poses a problem for the clinician seeking to uncover the effects of toxic exposure on the male reproductive system. When entertaining the possibility that male reproductive dysfunction may be related to toxic exposure, the clinician must consider other factors that can adversely affect reproductive function. These include local or generalized infections, medications, and the use of recreational drugs and/or alcohol.

When investigating the presence of a reproductive hazard, clinicians should attempt to answer the following questions. (1) Has reproductive dysfunction been clearly established? (2) Has exposure been established to a reasonable extent by a careful occupational and environmental history? (3) Do environmental or occupational monitoring data and/or clinical laboratory determinations provide evidence of exposure? (4) Has similar exposure been shown to cause a comparable disease in animal or human studies? (5) Does stopping the exposure improve the condition?

In many instances it will be impossible to answer each of these questions satisfactorily, and the role of toxic exposure may be unclear. However, a physician who is mindful that his or her patient is subjected to toxic assault can increase the patient's awareness of such assault. Informing the patient of his increased risk is clearly the first step in reducing that risk. Since no specific method exists for treating toxic injuries of the male reproductive system, treatment must depend on avoiding, decreasing, or stopping the toxic exposure. Under these circumstances, the importance of prevention is evident. Thus, from the viewpoint of prevention, diagnosis, and treatment, clinicians must routinely obtain an adequate reproductive and sexual history in conjunction with a history of toxic exposure.

Adverse Reproductive Outcome Mediated through the Father

In the past, the potential for abnormal development of the fetus and offspring focused primarily on the risks posed by toxic exposure of the pregnant woman. As noted, it is now appreciated that the offspring of fathers exposed to toxic agents may be at increased risk for abnormal development and cancer. The clinician must have an awareness of this potential. When there is a history of spontaneous abortion, abnormal development of the embryo/fetus and offspring, or cancer in the offspring, paternal as well as maternal exposure requires careful attention. Because spermatogenesis is a continuous process, paternal exposures occurring shortly before conception are of particular importance in relation to reproductive outcome.

It is often recommended that a woman contemplating pregnancy speak with her physician in order to assess her health and her exposure to hazardous agents. The susceptibility of the male reproductive system to toxic substances and the potential for adverse reproductive outcome linked to paternal exposure means that a similar recommendation is now in order for a man who is contemplating fatherhood.

REFERENCES

1. Amador A, Bartke A: Teaching of andrology in medical schools of the USA and Canada. J Androl 3:42, 1982.
2. Amir D, Volcani R: The effects of dietary ethylene dibromide on bull semen. Nature 206:99, 1965.
3. Ash P: The influence of radiation infertility in man. Br J Radiol 53:271, 1980.
4. Barlow SM, Sullivan FM: Reproductive Hazards of Industrial Chemicals, Academic Press, Orlando, 1982.
5. Berlin M, Insu PL, Russell LD: Effects of metals on male reproduction. In: Reproductive and Developmental Toxicity of Metals, p 41, Clarkson TW, Nordberg GF, Sager PR (eds.), Plenum Press, New York, 1983.
6. Biava CG, Smuckler EA, Whorton D: The testicular morphology of individuals exposed to dibromochloropropane. Exp Mol Pathol 29:448, 1978.
7. Bloom AD (ed.): Guidelines for Studies of Human Populations Exposed to Mutagenic and Reproductive Hazards, March of Dimes Birth Defects Foundation, New York, 1981.
8. Brown NA: Are offspring at risk from their father's exposure to toxins? Nature 316:110, 1985.
9. Bulger WH, Kupfer D: Estrogenic activity of pesticides and other xenobiotics on the uterus and male reproductive tract. In: Endocrine Toxicology, p 1, Thomas JA, Korach KS, McLachlan JA (eds.), Raven Press, New York, 1985.
10. Burger EJ Jr, Tardiff RG, Scialli AR, et al: Sperm Measures and Reproductive Success, Alan R Liss, New York, 1989.
11. Cohn WJ, Boylan JJ, Blanke RV, et al: Treatment of chlordecone (Kepone) toxicity with cholestyramine: Results of a controlled clinical trial. N Engl J Med 298:243, 1978.
12. Committee on the Biological Effects of Ionizing Radiations, National Research Council: Health Effects of Exposure to Low Levels of Ionizing Radiation, BIER V, National Academy Press, Washington, 1990.
13. Cook RR, Bodner KM, Kolesar R, et al: A cross-sectional study of ethylene glycol monomethyl ether process employees. Arch Environ Health 37:346, 1982.
14. Coulston F, Pocchiari F (eds.): Accidental Exposure to Dioxins, Academic Press, Orlando, 1983.
15. Council on Scientific Affairs: The Health Effects of "Agent Orange" and Polychlorinated Dioxin Contaminants. Technical Report, American Medical Association, Chicago, 1981.
16. Council on Scientific Affairs: The Health Effects of "Agent Orange" and Polychlorinated Dioxin Contaminants: An Update, 1984. Technical Report, American Medical Association, Chicago, 1984.
17. Danielsson BRG, Dencker A, Lindgren J, et al: Accumulation of toxic metals in male reproductive organs. Arch Toxicol Suppl 7:177, 1984.
18. David G, Jouannet P, Martin-Boyce A, et al: Sperm counts in fertile and infertile men. Fertil Steril 31:453, 1979.
19. DeKnudt G, Leonard A, Ivanov B: Chromosome aberrations observed in male workers occupationally exposed to lead. Environ Physiol Biochem 3:132, 1973.
20. de Rooij DG, Kramer M: The effects of three alkylating agents on the seminiferous epithelium of rodents. 1. Depletory effect. Virchows Arch B 4:267, 1970.
21. Dixon RL: Pharmacological principles of reproductive toxicity. In: Reproductive Toxicology, p 287, Dixon RL (ed.), Raven Press, New York, 1985.
22. Dixon RL: Aspects of male reproductive toxicology. In: Occupational Hazards and Reproduction, p 57, Hemminki K, Sorse M, Vainio H (eds.), Hemisphere Publishing, Washington, 1985.
23. Dixon RL: Toxic response of the reproductive system. In: Casarett and Doull's Toxicology: The Basic Science of Poisons, 3rd ed., p 432, Klaassen CE, Amdur MO, Doull J (eds.), Macmillan, New York, 1986.
24. Dixon RL, Hall JL: Reproductive toxicology. In: Principles and Methods of Toxicology, p 107, Hayes AW (ed.), Raven Press, New York, 1982.
25. Dixon RL, Lee IP: Pharmacokinetic and adaptation factors involved in testicular toxicity. Fed Proc 39:66, 1980.
26. Dixon RL, Lee IP: Metabolism of benzo(a)pyrene by isolated perfused testis and testicular homogenate. Life Sci 27:2439, 1980.
27. Dixon RL, Sherins, RJ, Lee IP: Assessment of environmental factors affecting male fertility. Environ Health Perspect 30:53, 1979.
28. Donovan JW: Case-control study of congenital anomalies and Vietnam service, Commonwealth Institute of Health, University of Sydney, Sydney, Australia, 1983.
29. Egnatz DG, Ott MG, Townsend RD, et al: DBCP and testicular function in chemical workers: An epidemiological survey in Midland, Michigan. J Occup Med 22:727, 1980.
30. Eliasson R: Clinical effects of chemicals on male reproduction. In: Reproductive Toxicology, p 161, Dixon RL (ed.), Raven Press, New York, 1985.
31. Environmental Studies Board, Commission on Natural Resources, National Research Council: Urban Pest Management, National Academy Press, Washington, 1980.
32. Erickson JD, Mulinare J, McClain PW, et al: Vietnam veteran's risk for fathering babies with birth defects. JAMA 252:903, 1984.
33. Fabia J, Thuy TD: Occupation of father at time of birth of children dying of malignant diseases. Br J Prev Soc Med 28:98, 1974.
34. Freund M: Effect of frequency of emission on semen output and an estimate of daily sperm production in man. J Reprod Fertil 6:269, 1963.

35. Friedman JM: Does Agent Orange cause birth defects? Teratology 29:193, 1984.

36. Gardner MJ, Snee MP, Hall AJ, et al: Results of case-control study of leukaemia and lymphoma among young people near Sella field nuclear plant in West Cumbria. Br Med J 300:423, 1990.

37. Giavini R, Prati M, Vismara C: Rabbit teratology with 2,3,6,7-tetrachlorodibenzo-*p*-dioxin. Environ Res 27:74, 1982.

38. Goldsmith JR, Potashnik G, Israeli R: Reproductive outcomes in families of DBCP-exposed men. Arch Environ Health 39:85, 1984.

39. Goodman DR, James RC, Harbison RD: Assessment of mutagenicity using germ cells and the application of test results. In: Reproductive Toxicology, p 267, Dixon RL (ed.), Raven Press, New York, 1985.

40. Haas JF, Schottenfeld D: Risks to the offspring from parental occupational exposures. J Occup Med 21:607, 1979.

41. Hakulinen T, Salonen T, Teppo L: Cancer in the offspring of fathers in hydro-carbon-related occupations. Br J Prev Soc Med 30:138, 1976.

42. Hall RW, Gomes WR: Testosterone levels in the serum and testes of growing rats following prenatal exposure to busulfan. J Reprod Fertil 35:131, 1973.

43. Hanawalt PC, Cooper PK, Ganesan AK, et al: Repair responses to DNA damage: Enzymatic pathways in *E. coli* and human cells. In: Mechanisms of Chemical Carcinogenesis, p. 275, Harris CC, Cerutti PA (eds.), Alan R Liss, New York, 1982.

44. Hardin BD: Reproductive toxicity of the glycol ethers. Toxicology 27:91, 1983.

45. Hemminki K, Sorsa M, Vainio H: Genetic risks caused by occupational chemicals. Scand J Work Environ Health 5:307, 1979.

46. Hemminki K, Saloniemi I, Luoma K, et al: Transplacental carcinogens and mutagens: Childhood cancer, malformations and abortions as risk indicators. J Toxicol Environ Health 6:1115, 1980.

47. Hemminki K, Saloniemi I, Salonen T, et al: Childhood cancer and parental occupation in Finland. J Epidemiol Commun Health 35:11, 1981.

48. Hemminki K, Kyyronen P, Nieme ML, et al: Spontaneous abortions in an industrialized community in Finland. Am J Public Health 73:32, 1983.

49. Henderson J, Baker HWG, Hanna PJ: Occupation-related male infertility: A review. Clin Reprod Fertil 4:87, 1986.

50. Heywood R, James RW: Current laboratory approaches for assessing male reproductive toxicity: Testicular toxicity in laboratory animals. In: Reproductive Toxicology, p 147, Dixon RL (ed.), Raven Press, New York, 1985.

51. Hudec T, Thean J, Kuehl G, et al: Tris(dichloropropyl)phosphate, a mutagenic flame retardant: Frequent occurrence in human seminal plasma. Science 211:951, 1981.

52. Jackson H, Schnieden H: Aspects of male reproductive pharmacology and toxicology. Rev Pure Appl Pharmacol Sci 3:1, 1982.

53. Johnson SG: Testicular biopsy score count or method for registration of spermatogenesis in human testes: Normal values and results in 335 hypogonadal males. Hormone 1:2, 1970.

54. Kantor AF, McCrea-Curnen MG, Meigs JW: Occupations of fathers of patients with Wilms's tumour. J Epidemiol Commun Health 33:253, 1979.

55. Kharrazi M, Potashnik G, Goldsmith JR: Reproductive effects of dibromochloropropane. Israel J Med Sci 10:403, 1980.

56. Kirk KM, Lyon MF: Induction of congenital malformation in the offspring of male mice treated with X-rays at pre-meiotic and post-meiotic stages. Mutat Res 125:74, 1984.

57. Krasovskil GN, Varshavskaya SP, Borisov AI: Toxic and gonadotropic effects of cadmium and boron relative to standards for these substances in drinking water. Environ Health Perspect 13:69, 1976.

58. LaDou J (ed.): The microelectronic industry. Occup Med 1:1, 1986.

59. Lancranjan I, Popescu HI, Gavanescu O, et al: Reproductive ability of workmen occupationally exposed to lead. Arch Environ Health 30:396, 1975.

60. Lathrop GD, Wolfe WH, Albanese MD, et al: Project Ranch Hand II. An Epidemiologic Investigation of Health Effects in Air Force Personnel Following Exposure to Herbicides: Baseline Morbidity Study Results, US Air Force School of Aerospace Medicine, Brooks Air Force Base, Texas, 1984.

61. Lee IP: Adaptive biochemical repair response toward germ cell DNA damage. Am J Ind Med 4:135, 1983.

62. Lee IP, Dixon RL: Factors influencing reproductive and genetic toxic effects on male gonads. Environ Health Perspect 24:117, 1978.

63. Lee IP, Suzuki K: Differential DNA repair in prespermiogenic cells of various mouse strains. Mutat Res 80:201, 1981.

64. Leonard A, Gerber GB, Jacquet P: Effects of lead on reproductive capacity and development of mammals. In: Reproductive and Developmental Toxicity of Metals, p 357, Clarkson TW, Nordberg GF, Sager PR (eds.), Plenum Press, New York, 1983.

65. Levine RJ, Symons MJ, Balogh SA, et al: A method for monitoring the fertility of workers 2. Validation of the method among workers exposed to dibromochloropropane. J Occup Med 23:183, 1981.

66. Levine RJ, Blunden PB, Calcorso RD, et al: Superiority of reproductive history to sperm counts in detecting infertility in a dibromochloropropane manufacturing plant. J Occup Med 25:591, 1983.

67. Lipshultz LI, Ross CE, Whorton D, et al: Dibromochloropropane and its effect on testicular function in man. J Urol 124:464, 1980.

68. Lloyd JA, Steinberger E: Survey and analysis of education efforts in reproductive biology and human sexuality in American medical schools. J Reprod Med 24:17, 1980.

69. Lushbaugh CC, Casarett GW: The effects of gonadal irradiation in clinical radiation therapy: A review. Cancer 37:111, 1976.

70. Macleod J: Effect of chickenpox and pneumonia on semen quality. Fertil Steril 2:523, 1951.

71. Macleod J: A testicular response during and following a severe allergic reaction. Fertil Steril 2:531, 1962.

72. Mann T, Lutwak-Mann C: Passage of chemicals into human and animal semen: Mechanism and significance. CRC Crit Rev Toxicol 11:1, 1982.

73. Mattson DR: Effects of biologically foreign com-

pounds on reproduction. In: Drugs During Pregnancy, p 101, Abdul-Karim RW (ed.), G. F. Stickley Co., Philadelphia, 1981.

74. Mattson DR (ed.): Reproductive Toxicology, Alan R. Liss, New York, 1983.

75. McConnell EE, Moore JA, Jaseman J, et al: The comparative toxicity of chlorinated dibenzo-*p*-dioxins in mice and guinea pigs. Toxicol Appl Pharmacol 44: 335, 1978.

76. Millar JD: Glycol ethers 2-methoxyethanol and 2-ethoxyethanol, NIOSH Current Intelligence Bulletin 39, US Dept Health and Human Services, Pub No. 83–112, DHHS, Washington, 1983.

77. Morgan RW, Kheifets MA, Obrinsky DL, et al: Fetal loss and work in a waste water treatment plant. Am J Public Health 74:499, 1984.

78. Mukhtar H, Lee IP, Foureman GL, et al: Epoxide metabolizing enzyme activities in rat testis: Postnatal development and relative activity in interstitial and spermatogenic cell compartments. Chem Biol Interact 22:153, 1978.

79. National Center for Health Statistics: Fertility Tables for Birth Cohorts of Color: United States, 1917–1973, US Government Printing Office, Washington, 1976.

80. Nelson WO, Steinberger E, Boccabella A: Effects of nitrofurans on reproduction. In: Proceedings XIX International Physiological Congress, p 105, Acta, Montreal, 1953.

81. Nisbet ICT, Karch NJ: Chemical Hazards to Human Reproduction, Noyes Data Corp, Park Ridge, New Jersey, 1983.

82. Nomura T: Paternal exposure to x-rays and chemicals induces heritable tumours and anomalies in mice. Nature 296:575, 1982.

83. Nordberg GF, Goyer RA, Clarkson TW: Impact of effects of acid precipitation on toxicity of metals. Environ Health Perspect 63:169, 1985.

84. Nordenson I, Beckman G, Beckman L, et al: Occupational and environmental risks in and around a smelter in northern Sweden II. Chromosomal aberrations in workers exposed to arsenic. Hereditas 88:47, 1978.

85. Okumura K, Lee IP, Dixon RL: Permeability of selected drugs and chemicals across the blood-testis barrier of the rat. J Pharmacol Exp Ther 194:89, 1975.

86. Oliver T: Lead poisoning and the race. Br Med J 1:1096, 1911.

87. Overstreet JW, Blazak WF: The biology of human male reproduction: An overview. Am J Ind Med 4:5, 1983.

88. Parizek J: Sterilization of the male by cadmium salts. J Reprod Fertil 1:294, 1960.

89. Parizek J, Zahor Z: Effect of cadmium salts on testicular tissue. Nature 177:1036, 1956.

90. Peters JM, Preston-Martin S, Yu MC: Brain tumors in children and occupational exposure of parents. Science 213:235, 1981.

91. Piscator M: Dietary exposure to cadmium and health effects: Impact of environmental changes. Environ Health Perspect 63:127, 1985.

92. Potashnik G, Yanai-Inbar I, Sacks MI, et al: Effect of dibromochloropropane on human testicular function. Israel J Med Sci 15:438, 1979.

93. Rodriguez-Rigau IJ, Smith KD, Steinberger E: Possible relation between elevated FSH levels and Leydig cell dysfunction in azoospermic and oligospermic men. J Androl 1:127, 1980.

94. Rosenberg MJ, Feldblum PJ, Marshall EG: Occupational influences on reproduction: A review of recent literature. J Occup Med 29:584, 1987.

95. Rosenman KD, Anderson HA, Selikoff IJ, et al: Spermatogenesis in men exposed to polybrominated biphenyl. Fertil Steril 32:209, 1979.

96. Rowley MJ, Leach DR, Warner GA, et al: Effects of graded doses of ionizing radiation on the human testes. Radiat Res 59:665, 1974.

97. Sandifer SH, Wilkins RI, Loadholt CB, et al: Spermatogenesis in agricultural workers exposed to dibromochloropropane (DBCP). Bull Environ Contam Toxicol 23:703, 1979.

98. Savitz DA, Chen J: Parental occupation and childhood cancer: Review of epidemiological studies. Environ Health Perspect 88:325, 1990.

99. Schrag SD, Dixon RL: Occupational exposure associated with male reproductive dysfunction. Annu Rev Pharmacol Toxicol 25:567, 1985.

100. Schrag SD, Dixon RL: Reproductive effects of chemical agents. In: Reproductive Toxicology, p 301, Dixon RL (ed.), Raven Press, New York, 1985.

101. Sega GA: DNA repair in spermatocytes and spermatids of the mouse. In: Indicators of Genotoxic Exposure, Banbury Report 13, p 503, Bridges BA, Butterworth BE, Weinstein IB (eds.), Cold Spring Harbor Laboratory, New York, 1982.

102. Selby PB, Selby PR: Gamma-ray-induced dominant mutations that cause skeletal abnormalities in mice. I. Plan, summary of results and discussion. Mutat Res 43(3):357, 1977.

103. Selby PB, Selby PR: Gamma-ray-induced dominant mutations that cause skeletal abnormalities in mice. II. Description of proved mutations. Mutat Res 51(2):199, 1978.

104. Setchell BP, Voglmayr JK, Waites GMH: A blood-testis barrier restricting passage from blood lymph into the rete testis fluid but not into the lymph. J Physiol (Lond) 200:73, 1969.

105. Sever LE, Hessol NA: Toxic effects of occupational and environmental chemicals on the testes. In: Endocrine Toxicology, p 211, Thomas JA, Korach, KS, McLachlan JA (eds.), Raven Press, New York, 1985.

106. Sherins RJ, Brightwell D, Sternthal P: Longitudinal analysis of semen of fertile and infertile men. In: The Testis in Normal and Infertile Men, p 473, Troen P, Nankin HR (eds.), Raven Press, New York, 1977.

107. Short RD, Winston JM, Wong CB, et al: Effects of ethylene dibromide on reproduction in male and female rats. Toxicol Appl Pharmacol 49:97, 1979.

108. Smith JP, Smith JC, McCall AJ: Chronic poisoning from cadmium fumes. J Pathol Bacteriol 80:287, 1960.

109. Smith KD, Rodriguez-Rigau LJ: Laboratory evaluation of testicular function. In: Endocrinology, Vol 3, p 1539, DeGroot LJ, Cahill GF Jr, Martini L, et al. (eds.), Grune & Stratton, New York, 1979.

110. Smith KD, Steinberger E: What is oligospermia? In: The Testis in Normal and Infertile Men, p 489, Troen P, Nankin HR (eds.), Raven Press, New York, 1977.

111. Smith KD, Rodriguez-Rigau LJ, Steinberger E: Relation between indices of semen analysis and preg

nancy rate in infertile couples. Fertil Steril 28:1314, 1977.

112. Spitz MR, Johnson CC: Neuroblastoma and paternal occupation: A case-control analysis. Am J Epidemiol 121:924, 1985.

113. Steinberger E: A quantitative study of the effect of an alkylating agent (triethylenemelamine) on the seminiferous epithelium of rats. J Reprod Fertil 3:250, 1962.

114. Steinberger E: Hormonal control of spermatogenesis. In: Endocrinology, Vol 3, p 1535, DeGroot LJ, Cahill GF Jr, Martini L, et al. (eds.), Grune & Stratton, New York, 1979.

115. Steinberger E: Male Infertility. In: Endocrinology, Vol 3, p 1567, DeGroot LJ, Cahill GF Jr, Martini L, et al (eds.), Grune & Stratton, New York, 1979.

116. Steinberger E: Management of male reproductive dysfunction. Clin Obstet Gynecol 22:187, 1979.

117. Steinberger E: Current status of studies concerned with evaluation of toxic effects of chemicals on the testes. Environ Health Perspect 38:29, 1981.

118. Steinberger E, Lloyd JA: Chemicals affecting the development of reproductive capacity. In: Reproductive Toxicology, p 1, Dixon RL (ed.), Raven Press, New York, 1985.

119. Steinberger E, Rodriguez-Rigau LJ: The infertile couple. J Androl 4:111, 1983.

120. Steinberger E, Tjioe DY: A method for quantitative analysis of human seminiferous epithelium. Fertil Steril 19:960, 1968.

121. Steinberger E, Smith KD, Rodriguez-Rigau LJ: Suppression and recovery of sperm production in men treated with testosterone enanthate for one year. A study of a possible reversible male contraceptive. Int J Androl 2 (Suppl):748, 1978.

122. Steinberger E, Steinberger A, Sanborn BM: Molecular mechanisms concerned with hormonal control of the seminiferous epithelium. In: Recent Progress in Andrology, p 143, Fabrini A, Steinberger E (eds.), Academic Press, New York, 1978.

123. Steinberger E, Rodriguez-Rigau LJ, Smith KD: The infertile couple: A quantitative approach to the evaluation of each partner. In: Advances in Diagnosis and Treatment of Infertility, p 179, Insler V, Bettendorf C (eds.), Elsevier-North-Holland, Amsterdam, 1981.

124. Strobino BR, Kline J, Stein Z: Chemical and physical exposures of parents: Effects on human reproduction and offspring. Early Hum Dev 1:371, 1978.

125. Subcommittee on Reproductive and Neurodevelopmental Toxicology, National Research Council: Biologic Markers in Reproductive Toxicology, National Academy Press, Washington, 1989.

126. Suskind RR, Hertzberg VS: Human health effects of 2,4,5-T and its toxic contaminants. JAMA 251:2372, 1984.

127. Tarasenko NY, Kasparov AA, Strongina OM: The effect of boric acid on the generative function in males. Gig Tr Prof Sabol 16:13, 1972.

128. Tcholakian RK, Chowdhury M, Steinberger E: Time of action of oestradiol-17 on luteinizing hormone and testosterone. J Endocrinol 63:122, 1974.

129. Thomas JA, Brogan WC III: Some actions of lead on the sperm and on the male reproductive system. Am J Ind Med 4:127, 1983.

130. Thomas JA, Northus SJ: Toxicity and metabolism of monoethylhexyl phthalate and diethylhexyl phthalate: A survey of the recent literature. J Toxicol Environ Health 9:141, 1982.

131. Tice RR: An overview of occupational studies directed at assessing genetic damage. In: Reproduction: The New Frontier in Occupational and Environmental Health Research, p 429, Lockey JE, Lemasters GK, Keye WR (eds.), Alan R Liss, New York, 1984.

132. Tjoa WS, Smolensky MH, Hsi BP, et al: Circannual rhythm in human sperm count revealed by serially independent sampling. Fertil Steril 38:454, 1982.

133. Torkelson TR, Sadek SE, Rowe VK, et al: Toxicologic investigations of 1,2-dibromo-3-chloropropane. Toxicol Appl Pharmacol 3:545, 1961.

134. Townsend JC, Bodner KM, Van Peene PFD, et al: Survey of reproductive events in wives of employees exposed to chlorinated dioxins. Am J Epidemiol 115:695, 1982.

135. Trasler JM, Hales BF, Robaire B: Paternal cyclophosphamide treatment of rats causes fetal loss and malformation without affecting male fertility. Nature 316:144, 1985.

136. US Congress, Office of Technology Assessment: Reproductive Health Hazards in the Workplace, OTA-BA-266, US Government Printing Office, Washington, 1985.

137. US Congress, Office of Technology Assessment: Technologies for Detecting Heritable Mutations in Human Beings, NTIS #Pb 87–140158/AS, US Government Printing Office, Washington, 1986.

138. US Environmental Protection Agency: Suspended, Cancelled and Restricted Pesticides, 3rd ed., USEPA, Washington, 1985.

139. US Government Printing Office: Review of Literature on Herbicides Including Phenoxy Herbicides and Associated Dioxins, Vols 4 and 6 (stock nos. 051–000–00165–6, 051–000–00174–5), USGPO, Washington, 1984 and 1985.

140. Uzych L: Teratogenesis and mutagenesis associated with exposure of human males to lead: A review. Yale J Biol Med 58:9, 1985.

141. Verjans HJ, Eik-Nes KB, AaFjes JH, et al: Effect of oestradiol benzoate on pituitary and testis function in the normal adult male rat. Acta Endocrinol (Kbh) 77:636, 1974.

142. Waller DP, Killinger JM, Zaneveld LJD: Physiology and toxicology of the male reproductive tract. In: Endocrine Toxicology, p 269, Thomas JA, Korach KS, McLachlan JA (eds.), Raven Press, New York, 1985.

143. Wassom JS, Huff JE, Loprieno N: A review of the genetic toxicology of chlorinated dibenzo-p-dioxins. Mutat Res 47:141, 1977/78.

144. Weir RJ, Fisher RS: Toxicologic studies on borax and boric acid. Toxicol Appl Pharmacol 23:351, 1972.

145. Weller CV: The blastophthoric effect of chronic lead poisoning. J Med Res 33:271, 1915.

146. Whorton MD, Foliart DE: Mutagenicity, carcinogenicity and reproductive effects of dibromochloropropane (DBCP). Mutat Res 123:13, 1983.

147. Whorton MD, Krauss RM, Marshall R, et al: Infertility in male pesticide workers. Lancet 2:1259, 1977.

148. Whorton MD, Milby TH, Krauss RM, et al: Testicular function in DBCP-exposed pesticide workers. J Occup Med 21:161, 1979.

149. Wildt K, Eliasson R, Berlin M: Effects of occupational exposure to lead on sperm and semen. In: Reproductive and Developmental Toxicity of Metals, p 279, Clarkson TW, Nordberg GF, Sager PR (eds.), Plenum Press, New York, 1983.
150. Wilkins JR III, Koutras RA: Paternal occupation and brain cancer in offspring: A mortality-based case control study. Am J Ind Med 14:299, 1988.
151. Wong O, Utidjian HMD, Karten VS: Retrospective evaluation of reproductive performance of workers exposed to ethylene dibromide (EDB). J Occup Med 21:98, 1979.
152. Wong O, Morgan RW, Whorton MD: An epidemiologic surveillance program for evaluating occupational reproductive hazards. Am J Ind Med 7:295, 1985.
153. Working PK, Butterworth BE: An assay to detect chemically induced DNA repair in rat spermatocytes. Environ Mutagen 6:273, 1984.
154. Wyrobek AJ, Gordon LA, Burkhart JG, et al: An evaluation of the mouse sperm morphology and other sperm tests in nonhuman mammals. A report of the US Environmental Protection Agency Gene-Tox Program. Mutat Res 115:1, 1983.
155. Wyrobek AJ, Watchmaker G, Gordon L: Evaluation of sperm tests as indicators of germ-cell damage in men exposed to chemical or physical agents. In: Reproduction: The New Frontier in Occupational and Environmental Health Research, p 385, Lockey JE, Lemasters GK, Keye WR (eds.), Alan R Liss, New York, 1984.
156. Wyrobek AJ, Currie M, Stilwell JL, et al: Detecting specific locus mutations in human sperm. In: Biology of Mammalian Germ Cell Mutagenesis, Banbury Report 34, p 93, Allen JW, Bridges BA, Lyon MF, et al (eds.), Cold Spring Harbor Laboratory Press, New York, 1990.

157. Young AI, Calcagani JA, Thalken CE, et al: The Toxicology, Environmental Fate and Human Risk of Herbicide Orange and Its Associated Dioxin. US Air Force Occupational and Environmental Health Laboratory (OEHL) Technical Report TR-78–92, Aerospace Medical Division, Brooks, TX, 1978.
158. Zack M, Cannon S, Lloyd D, et al: Cancer in children of parents exposed to hydrocarbons-related industries and occupations. Am J Epidemiol 111:329, 1980.
159. Zenick H, Cleeg ED: Assessment of male reproductive toxicity: A risk assessment approach. In: Principles and Methods in Toxicology, 2nd ed., p 275, Hayes AW (ed.), Raven Press, New York, 1989.
160. Zuckerman Z, Rodriguez-Rigau LJ, Weiss DB, et al: Quantitative analysis of the seminiferous epithelium in human testicular biopsies and the relation of spermatogenesis to sperm density. Fertil Steril 30:448, 1978.

RECOMMENDED READINGS

Barlow SM, Sullivan FM: Reproductive Hazards of Industrial Chemicals, Academic Press, Orlando, 1982.
Lamb JC IV, Foster PMD (eds.): Physiology and Toxicology of Male Reproduction, Academic Press, Orlando, 1988.
Nisbet ICT, Karch NJ: Chemical hazards to human reproduction, Noyes Data Corp, Park Ridge, New Jersey, 1983.
Schrag SD, Dixon RL: Occupational exposure associated with male reproductive dysfunction. Annu Rev Pharmacol Toxicol 25:567, 1985.
Subcommittee on Reproductive and Neurobehavioral Toxicology, National Research Council: Biologic Markers in Reproductive Toxicology, National Academy Press, Washington, 1989.

26. THE ROLE OF ENVIRONMENTAL CHEMICALS IN HUMAN CANCER CAUSATION

Howard M. Kipen and I. Bernard Weinstein

INTRODUCTION

In 1775 Sir Percival Pott first defined the role of environmental chemicals as etiological agents in human cancer. Pott, a London surgeon, drew attention to the unique susceptibility of chimney sweeps to scrotal skin cancer (205). He attributed their increased cancer risk to chronic soot exposure. It is now appreciated, many years later, that soot contains chemical substances known as polycyclic aromatic hydrocarbons (PAHs), which are potent carcinogens. Among these PAHs is benzo[a]pyrene (BaP), a ubiquitous environmental pollutant found in cigarette smoke, automobile exhaust, and urban air. This substance has been demonstrated to be a potent skin carcinogen in experimental animals.

In contrast to the large amount of information available on chemical carcinogens from animal experiments, there is remarkably little data in man. This is undoubtedly because of the difficulties inherent in the epidemiologic investigation of the health effects of exposure to environmental chemicals. One of the major problems encountered is the

complex nature of chemical exposure. Epidemiologic studies may implicate an exposure situation or occupation in the genesis of human cancer, but it is rarely possible to incriminate a specific compound by such investigation (107).

In a sense cancer epidemiology today is analogous to the field of infectious diseases in the 1870s. Bacteria were discovered about 1800, and tuberculosis had been observed for centuries, but it was not until 1882 that Robert Koch first demonstrated that a particular bacterium could reliably cause tuberculosis. There followed the attack on infectious disease through advances in sanitation, hygiene, immunization, and antibiotic therapy. Infectious disease, which was formerly a leading cause of death in the developed world, has been replaced by cancer. We are now presented with the challenge of identifying the causes of cancer and implementing new approaches to cancer prevention.

This chapter focuses on environmental factors in human cancer causation. Methods of identifying environmental carcinogens are discussed. Particular attention is given to chemical carcinogenesis, the agents involved, and their sources and distribution in the environment. Cancer epidemiology in relation to environmental pollution is considered. The biological and biochemical principles of carcinogenesis are reviewed. New techniques that may provide a basis for evaluating the biological effect of carcinogen

Principles and Practice of Environmental Medicine, edited by Alyce Bezman Tarcher. Plenum Medical Book Company, New York, 1992.

exposure in humans are presented. The chapter concludes with some guidelines for cancer prevention.

EVIDENCE FOR THE ROLE OF ENVIRONMENTAL FACTORS IN THE GENESIS OF CANCER

Cancer accounts for about 20% of all deaths in the developed world. About 30% of individuals living in these countries will develop cancer at some time in their lives (3,172). Although there have been important advances in our understanding of the molecular biology of cancer, the specific causes of most forms of human cancer are unknown. It is estimated, however, that 60% to 90% of human cancer is attributable to environmental rather than inborn or genetic factors, even though the carcinogenesis process undoubtedly involves disturbances in genetic mechanisms (90,232). Environmental factors include foreign and naturally occurring chemicals in air, water, and food, radiation, workplace exposure, and such personal factors as smoking, alcohol ingestion, and dietary patterns.

The grounds for attributing a high proportion of human cancer to environmental factors rest on the following lines of evidence: (1) differences in the incidence of specific types of cancer between different communities, (2) changes in the incidence of cancer in community members who migrate, (3) changes in the incidence of specific cancers over time, and (4) specific exposures that result in a higher incidence of malignancy in well-defined groups of exposed persons (49,92).

There are many examples of differences in the incidence of particular cancers among communities. The Japanese, for example, have a high incidence of stomach cancer and a low incidence of breast cancer. The population of West Africa demonstrates a high incidence of liver cancer coupled with a low incidence of lung, colon, and rectal cancer. The population of the United States has a high incidence of lung, breast, colon, and rectal cancer and a low incidence of liver cancer.

Changes in the incidence of cancer with migration are reflected in the Japanese who moved to Hawaii. After migration, incidence of cancer in this group approaches that of the host population, deviating markedly from that of those who did not leave Japan. A similar example of the migration phenomenon is reflected in the observation that blacks in the United States have an incidence of cancer closer to that of American whites than to black West Africans. Table 26-1 illustrates that the age-standardized rate of liver cancer is fourfold lower in American blacks than in Nigerians. Colon cancer shows the opposite trend, with American blacks having ten times the incidence of blacks living in Nigeria.

TABLE 26-1. Cancer Incidence Rates for Ibadan, Nigeria and for Blacks and Whites of the San Francisco Bay Area[a]

| | Annual incidence per million people | | |
| | Ibadan, Nigeria | San Francisco 1969–1973 | |
Primary site of cancer	1960–1969	Blacks	Whites
Male colon	34	349	294
Male liver	272	67	39
Male pancreas	55	200	126
Male lung	27	1546	983
Prostate	134	724	318
Female breast	337	1268	1828
Uterine cervix	559	507	249
Uterine body	42	235	695
Male lymphosarcoma (less than 15 years)	133	10	4

[a]Modified from Doll and Peto (49).

This comparison may be discredited because black Americans could come from parts of Africa having a cancer incidence different from that noted in Nigeria. The dramatic difference in the incidence of cancer, however, is clearly best explained by new factors introduced with migration.

Changes in the incidence of stomach and lung cancer during the past few decades in the United States also reflect the role of environmental factors (Fig. 26-1). Clearly, genetic changes would not act on a broad population within such a short period of time. The identification of specific causes of cancer lends additional support to the influence of external factors. There is, for example, convincing evidence that the current dramatic increase in lung cancer is related to cigarette smoking (77). Occupational exposure to certain chemicals has also been linked to an increased incidence of cancer (107). A report on age-specific trends in cancer mortality in France, West Germany, Italy, Japan, England, Wales, and the United States notes that, except for lung and stomach, which together comprise between 20% and 43% of all cancer in males in these countries, all forms of cancer are increasing in persons over the age of 54 (45). Efforts must be made to explain these findings.

Epidemiologic studies demonstrate that a number of environmental factors contribute to the genesis of cancer. These include smoking, occupation, sunlight, ionizing radiation, drugs, diet, alcohol, and reproductive and social behavior (49,191). The relative contributions made by various environmental factors to the incidence of cancer in the United States have been estimated by a number of workers (49,92,231).

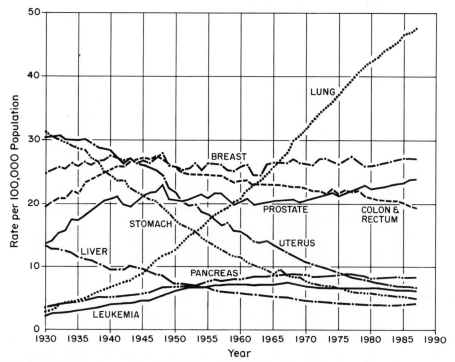

FIGURE 26-1. Cancer death rates by site, United States, 1930–1987. Rate for the population standardized for age on the 1970 U.S. population. Rates are for both sexes combined except breast and uterus (female population only) and prostate (male only). From American Cancer Society (3).

Diet and smoking are estimated to be the major environmental factors involved in cancer causation in the United States. Although the data on the role of tobacco in the genesis of cancer are very sound, the percentages attributed to other environmental factors are only estimates. It is generally accepted that about 30% of cancer deaths are caused by tobacco. Doll and Peto estimate that occupation, pollution, and industrial products have 4%, 2%, and less than 1% effects, respectively, on current cancer mortality (49). Given the fact that there are approximately 400,000 cancer deaths per year in the United States, an attributable fraction of 4% means that occupational exposures may account for over 16,000 cancer deaths per year. Other experts estimate that as many as 20% of cancers in the near term and future may be linked to carcinogens found in the workplace (44, 140). The variation in carcinogenic risks noted likely stems from the fact that various studies used different criteria to define exposure, and a variable proportion of the population studied were exposed to carcinogenic agents.

It bears emphasis that current cancer patterns reflect past exposures to carcinogens. This is because of the long latent period that exists between the initial exposure to a carcinogen and the clinical appearance of cancer. The relatively recent introduction of many carcinogens into the environment coupled with a latency period that is rarely less than 10 to 20 years makes it impossible, by epidemiologic methods, to estimate the future carcinogenic effects of such exposures (49).

METHODS FOR IDENTIFYING ENVIRONMENTAL CARCINOGENS

Four methods are used for identifying carcinogens: clinical observations, epidemiologic studies, animal bioassays, and short-term in vitro tests (Table 26-2). Each of these methods, with its particular strengths and weaknesses, is discussed.

Clinical Observations

Almost invariably, the perceptive observations of an alert clinician are the first to define a new syndrome or a relationship between disease and the environment. Clinical observations, lacking statistical significance, must be confirmed by experimental

TABLE 26-2. Methods for
Detecting Carcinogens[a]

Methods in vivo
  Clinical observations by astute physicians and patients
  Epidemiologic studies
  Experimental animal bioassays
Short-term tests
  Mutagenesis assays
    Bacteria: Ames test
    Mammalian cell cultures
    Other eukaryotes: yeast, *Drosophila*, mice
  Assays for cell transformation
  Assays for DNA binding, damage, and repair and binding to other macromolecules
  Assays for chromosomal abnormalities and sister chromatid exchange

[a]From Weinstein (217).

and epidemiologic studies. The sequence of detecting environmental effects frequently begins with the clinical observation, followed by epidemiologic confirmation and then animal experimentation (133).

One of the first associations between an occupational exposure and cancer was that by the English surgeon Sir Percival Pott, whose classic description of cancer of the scrotum in chimney sweeps was written over 200 years ago (205). Since then astute clinical observations have provided the first clue to a number of other human carcinogens including the association between cigarette smoking and lung cancer, asbestos exposure and mesothelioma, and transplacental exposure to diethylstilbestrol (DES) and vaginal carcinoma (89,203).

Epidemiologic Methods

Epidemiology is the scientific discipline that studies the determinants of the frequency and distribution of disease in population groups. Cancer epidemiology is directed to the discovery and interpretation of the frequency of cancer in humans. Epidemiologic studies are unique in that they are concerned with health problems that arise under real-life situations.

The major strength of epidemiologic studies is that they investigate, in humans, the effects of exposures as they occur. Such studies can investigate a wide range of acute and chronic health effects, many of which cannot be studied in the laboratory. Epidemiologic studies also provide fundamental information on current rates and trends in cancer incidence and mortality. Such studies avoid the pitfalls of animal experimentation, which must be extrapolated to humans. Epidemiologic studies have drawn attention to carcinogenic hazards associated with smoking, x rays, asbestos, and many chemical agents. Under special circumstances, epidemiologists may successfully identify specific human carcinogens, particularly when the investigation is directed to groups showing an unusual frequency of cancer or having an unusually high exposure to a suspected carcinogen. The data on chemical carcinogens encountered in the workplace reflect such studies. In some instances epidemiologic studies have provided sufficient quantitative exposure data to permit the carcinogenic risk assessment of various exposures (37).

The major criteria for identifying an environmental agent as a human carcinogen come from epidemiologic studies of an exposed population. Such studies attempt to define a cause-effect relationship by associating particular exposures with the development of cancer. On this basis cancer epidemiology and other epidemiologic studies are highly dependent on the measurement and documentation of exposure and the occurrence of cancer.

Cancer epidemiology is generally impeded by difficulties in measuring the degree of individual exposure. Environmental exposures are myriad and difficult to quantify. For most studies, the dose is estimated from rather crude exposure data such as proximity of a residence to the exposure site. More precise exposure information can be obtained from direct measurement of the compound in question or its metabolites in body tissues. Determining the dose of a carcinogen from the tissue concentration of the parent compound can be misleading, however. Many known chemical carcinogens must be metabolized within the cell before they can exert their carcinogenic effects. In addition, many known chemical carcinogens are readily metabolized or excreted, thus mitigating the effects of their exposure (155). New approaches that may overcome these limitations are discussed later in this chapter.

Epidemiologic studies have some important limitations. Being essentially observational rather than experimental, they provide evidence for an association rather than for an identification of specific causative factors. In addition, they are open to a variety of interpretations. The epidemiologist is constantly confronted with the problem of separating out the influence of biased information, the confounding of two or more factors, and discriminating between cause and effect. For these reasons, most epidemiologic studies have limited sensitivity (11). It has been observed that epidemiologic methods can usually monitor twofold or greater relative risk if the exposed and unexposed groups are clearly identified and of sufficient size. Epidemiologic methods can rarely detect a 10% increase in risk unless a very large-scale investigation is undertaken (157).

Epidemiology is likely to miss the carcinogenic effects of specific chemical agents found in the environment. The multiple exposures at relatively low concentrations and the likely low carcinogenic risk expected for each agent at low concentrations make it almost impossible for epidemiologists to evaluate the specific carcinogenic potential of an individual environmental chemical (91). Epidemiologic studies, however, may be useful in evaluating the additional impact of the overall burden of chemicals in a particular environment by relating cancer trends in different environments. In this way the sum total of the increased risks can be assessed (91).

Another limitation inherent in epidemiologic studies is that they are largely retrospective rather than predictive. They cannot detect the effects of a carcinogen until there is clinical evidence of cancer. The long latent period between the initial exposure to a carcinogen and the clinical appearance of cancer hinders the epidemiologist in establishing a cause-and-effect relationship between exposure and cancer. It also means that carcinogens may be in the environment for a number of years before they are detected by epidemiologic methods. By that time large populations may have experienced irreversible damage.

The importance placed on epidemiologic studies in defining human carcinogens merits some discussion of the guidelines that can be used to assess such studies (54). An excellent summary of the guidelines used for evaluation of clinical and epidemiologic studies is provided by the International Agency for Research on Cancer (IARC). This report provides guidelines for evaluating positive as well as negative findings (104).

Particular attention should be directed to studies that are reported to show negative results. It cannot be concluded from studies that show no relationship between exposure and an adverse health effect that no damage has occurred in the exposed population. When the validity of a negative study is assessed, attention is directed to the study design, the size of the population studied, and the latency period involved (122,204).

The study design should be searched for such flaws as the inclusion of an unexposed population with the exposed group or the exclusion of exposed populations, i.e., workers who left for reasons other than retirement. The documentation of exposure must be carefully assessed. The latency period between exposure and the appearance of disease must always be considered. Clearly, the effects of exposure will not be evident if the subjects are examined when the health effects of exposure are still in a period of latency. Premature examination of the subjects is of particular importance in epidemiologic studies concerned with the genesis of cancer. Frequently the exposed population studied will be small. Under such conditions the study will have difficulty in detecting cause-effect relationships, even if adverse health effects exist. Such studies

have low statistical power, which is defined as the probability that a study will be able to demonstrate an effect if an effect is present in a population. The statistical power of a negative study must therefore be assessed. Indeed, it has been recommended that all epidemiologic studies include a statement regarding the statistical power of the study to observe an increased frequency of a given disease (54).

A study that shows a positive association between an agent and an effect must also be scrutinized carefully. The study design, for example, must be reviewed for such flaws as a positive bias, which would lead to a more strongly positive association between an agent and disease than actually exists. The possibility of positive confounding must also be considered. Under such circumstances, the relationship between an agent and a disease is rendered more strongly positive than it is in fact. This can stem from an association between the agent and another agent that either causes or prevents the disease (54).

In summary, it bears emphasis that it cannot be concluded that exposure to a particular substance is free of adverse health effects in humans unless epidemiologic studies have shown that heavy exposure of a large, well-defined group to that substance for two or three decades is without apparent effect (49).

Experimental Animal Bioassays

Much of our knowledge about cancer has come from laboratory studies, especially studies using mice and rats. At present the long-term administration of a substance to laboratory animals is the most reliable method for determining whether that substance is carcinogenic. The details necessary for the proper conduct and interpretation of animal bioassays are discussed elsewhere (141,188).

There is now extensive experience with animal studies that assess the carcinogenic potential of various chemical agents. The validity of such studies has been demonstrated in several ways (188). Almost all of the known human carcinogens have been shown to cause cancer in the rodent bioassay. In addition, rodent bioassays predicted the carcinogenicity of certain compounds that subsequently proved to be carcinogenic in humans [e.g., diethylstilbestrol, vinyl chloride aflatoxin, bis(chloromethyl)-ether, and 4-aminobiphenyl] (188,189).

Animal bioassays, however, have certain major limitations. There can be marked variations between strains and species in their responses to specific carcinogens. Thus, if 2-naphthylamine, a known human bladder carcinogen, had first been tested in mice, it would be considered a liver carcinogen; if first tested in rats, it would be thought to be noncarcinogenic. It is only from studies with hamsters that this agent would be suspected to be a bladder carcinogen in humans (217).

Another drawback of animal bioassays is the high doses to which the animals must be exposed. The usual approach to increasing the sensitivity of rodent bioassays without using thousands of animals is to use doses many times that to which humans might be exposed. A major difficulty with this approach is our current limited knowledge on how to extrapolate accurately the results obtained in the laboratory at high doses to those that would be expected to occur at low doses in an environmental setting. These uncertainties are illustrated schematically in Fig. 26-2. Whether or not carcinogens display a threshold (or no-effect dose level) and the precise shape of the dose-response curve are unresolved issues. Until information is available to the contrary, it seems prudent to assume that a threshold does not exist. Even if a threshold exists in theory, this has little practical importance unless we have accurate knowledge of what the threshold dose is in humans. The reader is referred to several references for detailed discussions of risk extrapolation (8,37,98,121,131,190,202).

Another problem cited by some critics is that the high doses used in animal carcinogen testing lead to misleading results (6). Ames et al. state that the methodology exaggerates cancer risk. They contend that conducting animal tests for long periods of time at maximum tolerated doses can cause chronic mitogenesis, which in turn leads to far too large a fraction of chemicals so assayed to show up as carcinogens (6). Although there is little dispute that increased cell proliferation plays some role in carcinogenesis, the process is complex, takes place in multiple stages, and generally involves genetic changes (32,218,222) (see Biological and Biochemical Principles of Carcinogenesis, discussed in this chapter).

Another area of difficulty in extrapolating from laboratory carcinogenesis experiments to humans is that animals are generally exposed to one agent, whereas humans are typically exposed each day to thousands of compounds, which include carcinogens, as well as to agents that either promote or inhibit carcinogenesis (5).

Despite its limitations, positive results for carcinogenicity in a rodent bioassay must be taken as strong evidence that the substance in question is likely to pose a carcinogenic hazard to humans.

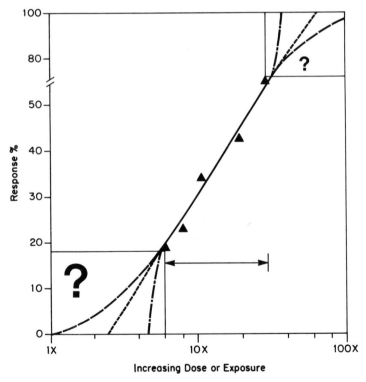

FIGURE 26-2. Possible dose–response curves, with the interrupted lines at the low and high ends of the curve indicating the usual types of uncertainty in dose extrapolation. From Gehring and Blau (61).

Negative results, as with most negative data, are more difficult to interpret because of the problem of species specificity and the limited sensitivity of studies that may employ 100 animals per group. The absence of tumors in a study in which 100 animals were given the test substance does not exclude the possibility that the compound is carcinogenic. Under these conditions carcinogenic response occurring in fewer than 1% of the animals tested would not be evident. Yet an agent that induces cancer in even 0.1% of a human population of several million would be considered a major health hazard.

Short-Term Tests

The rodent lifetime bioassay is clearly too expensive and lengthy to be used in evaluating all of the thousands of chemicals in our environment. Great effort has therefore been directed to developing simple tests that may be used as predictors of carcinogenicity. Within the past decade there has been a major advance, indeed a revolution, in our methodology for detecting potential carcinogens through the use of short-term in vitro tests. Such tests utilize biological or biochemical endpoints other than the induction of tumors in the whole animal.

Most short-term tests do not measure carcinogenicity directly. They usually determine if the agent in question can cause gene mutations, chromosome loss or damage, or primary structural damage to DNA. Short-term tests, therefore, generally demonstrate mutagenesis or other forms of chemical interaction with DNA. Existing data indicate that there is a good but not an absolute correlation between mutagenesis and carcinogenesis. The current types of short-term tests are listed in Table 26-2. A number of references provide a comprehensive review of the subject (4,5,50,57,99).

Mutagenesis Assay

The ability of many carcinogens to generate electrophilic compounds that bind to cellular DNA has provided the rationale for utilizing metagenesis as a screening tool in bacterial or mammalian cell cultures. The most extensively studied and validated assay of this type is the *Salmonella typhimurium* system developed by Ames and colleagues (4). The Ames test has been widely used since it was introduced in the mid-1970s.

This system utilizes *Salmonella* strains that contain mutants in a gene involved in the biosynthesis of the amino acid, histidine. Such mutant bacteria can not grow on a substrate that lacks histidine unless the mutant gene reverts and regains the ability to synthesize histidine. If a large number of such histidine-mutant bacteria are plated on a sub-

strate that lacks histidine, a few colonies will be formed, representing spontaneous revertant mutations. The addition of a mutagenic agent, however, increases the number of revertant colonies. The endpoint of the Ames test consists of counting the number of colonies on histidine-deficient media to which the test substance has been added. Results are obtained in 3 to 4 days.

A crucial element in the Ames system is that it metabolizes potential carcinogens as occurs in mammals. This link is necessary, as most carcinogens are not active until they are metabolized into carcinogenic forms by the microsomal enzymes that are present in a number of tissues (132,155). This requirement was successfully incorporated into the *Salmonella* reversion test by adding a liver homogenate and cofactors to the bacterial growth medium. The liver homogenate provides a microsomal enzyme source that activates the test compound to intermediates that react with the DNA of the bacteria. The use of "activating" enzymes is both a strength and a weakness of the bacterial test system. Because of the known species and tissue variations in metabolism, there is concern that activating enzymes taken from a single source (usually rat liver) and assayed under specific conditions may not duplicate the conditions found in the intact animal. This situation could be a source of false-negative or false-positive results. It also means that the relative potency of a compound in the assay in vitro may not always reflect its potency as a carcinogen in the intact animal (57).

Cell Transformation

A different type of short-term test uses, as its endpoint, the morphological transformation of mammalian cells in culture (57,99). Such tests can be performed within a few weeks. The transformed cells, when injected into appropriate hosts, often generate tumors, thus indicating that the in vitro endpoint correlates with the neoplastic process. It would be desirable to utilize epithelial cells from specific organs and also human cells for in vitro cell transformation studies. Promising advances are being made in these areas (57).

Assays for DNA Binding

Recently developed assays can detect carcinogenic molecules chemically linked to DNA. With antibody techniques, DNA adducts can now be detected with a high degree of sensitivity (160,161). An antibody to a benzo[a]pyrene-DNA adduct, for example, can detect as little as one of these adducts in 10^7 normal nucleotides in cellular DNA. Such antibodies may be useful in the monitoring of high-risk individuals for the occurrence of carcinogen-DNA adducts in their tissues (151,152,155,156).

Assays for Chromosomal Abnormalities

Another short-term test, the sister chromatid exchange (SCE), measures changes induced in the morphology of chromosomes. This test, using special staining techniques that differentiate the sister chromatids, permits the exchange of genetic material between them to be visualized. This process often increases with exposure to agents that damage DNA. Sister chromatid exchanges are subtle and do not affect gross chromosomal structure. The SCE test can be performed with a number of human cell types. The test is able to monitor the exposure of human cells and tissues by in vivo as well as in vitro means. For example, tests for SCE and chromosomal aberrations may be performed on cells in culture after exposure to toxins in vitro. They may also be performed on phlebotomized human peripheral blood lymphocytes to assess the effects of in vivo exposure to genotoxicants. Assays for chromosomal abnormalities and SCE have been reviewed (17,226).

Validity of Short-Term Tests

How reliable are these short-term tests for monitoring carcinogenic agents? The predictive value of short-term tests that have been assessed in comparison to rodent carcinogenicity studies ranges from 60% to 90%, depending on the type of chemical assayed (4,57,99,187). The disparity between the carcinogenicity in rodent bioassays and the results of short-term tests most likely resides in the proportion of chemicals being tested that act through other than mutagenic mechanisms (165,187).

Short-term assay for potential carcinogens may be useful for classifying carcinogenic agents according to their mechanism of action. Certain agents known to induce cancer in animals and/or humans, such as asbestos, dioxin, PCBs, and diethylstilbesterol (DES), are negative in the Ames assay (4). Such agents may be examples of carcinogens that act through nonmutagenic mechanisms. It is possible that carcinogens that are negative in short-term assays for mutagenesis enhance tumor formation by acting as promoting rather than initiating agents. Animal studies, in part, lend support to this conclusion (50,155). A detailed discussion of cancer initiators and promoters is presented in the section on Biological and Biochemical Principles of Carcinogenesis.

There are few studies available on the validation of cell transformation systems as a screen for chemical carcinogens. However, on the basis of a study using more than 100 compounds, the hamster em-bryo transformation system looks quite promising (158). It is difficult to perform this test on a routine basis. Short-term tests based on sister chromatid exchanges and other chromosomal abnormalities require further validation. At present, there is no evidence linking such mutagenic changes to an increased risk of developing cancer in the human population.

There is general agreement that a battery of short-term tests must be used to screen for potential carcinogens. Such tests can provide a quick and inexpensive means of providing clues to new and potentially carcinogenic compounds before they enter the environment. Such testing may also serve to highlight agents that deserve a high priority for testing in rodent carcinogen assays.

CHEMICALS, INDUSTRIAL PROCESSES, AND INDUSTRIES ASSOCIATED WITH CANCER IN HUMANS

A carcinogen is broadly defined as a substance that results in an increased age-specific incidence of cancer in the exposed experimental animal or in humans. Although several carcinogen classification schemes have been developed over the past three decades, the World Health Organization, International Agency for Research on Cancer (IARC) classification is used in this chapter because of its rigorous scientific base, its extensive documentation, and its international viewpoint (107).

In this system chemicals and complex exposure situations (including manufacturing processes) are ranked into three groups according to their documented and inferred carcinogenic risk to humans. The IARC schema does not consider the potency of the carcinogenic effect or the mechanism involved.

According to the IARC classification, chemicals, groups of chemicals, industrial processes or occupational exposures are assigned to the following groups. Group 1 includes exposure situations or specific chemicals for which there is sufficient epidemiologic evidence to support a causal association between the exposure and the occurrence of cancer in humans. Group 2 includes exposure situations or specific chemicals for which there is evidence for carcinogenicity in animals, but the evidence in humans is not certain. This grouping is further divided into 2A and 2B depending on the degree of evidence for human carcinogenicity. In group 2A the evidence for human carcinogenicity is almost sufficient. In group 2B epidemiologic data in humans are poor or nonexistent. The data from studies in experimental animals play a large part in the criteria used for group 2, particularly group 2B. Sufficient evidence of carcinogenicity in animals combined with inadequate data in humans usually results in a classification of 2B. Group 3 is used when the chemical, group of chemicals, industrial process, or occupational exposure cannot be classified as to carcinogenicity to humans. In the IARC classification scheme the results of tests for genetic and related effects may be used in the overall evaluation of carcinogenicity to humans, but they carry much less weight than epidemiologic or rodent bioassay data (107).

Tables 26-3 through 26-5 depict the IARC evaluation of the carcinogenic risk of chemicals to humans. The data are derived from *IARC Monographs* 1–42 (107–109,191,199). Table 26-3 shows group 1, chemicals and industrial processes that have been causally associated with human cancer. Table 26-4 shows group 2A, chemicals or groups of chemicals and industrial processes that are probably carcinogenic to humans. Table 26-5 shows group 2B, chemicals or groups of chemicals and industrial processes or occupations that are possibly carcinogenic to humans. The *IARC Monographs* program for evaluating the carcinogenic risk of chemicals and industrial processes to humans is constantly being updated. The interested reader is urged to consult recent publications.

The list of known carcinogens is remarkable for its structural and chemical heterogeneity as well as for the diverse conditions of exposure. Carcinogens are found in many chemical classes of compounds. These include polycyclic aromatic hydrocarbons, aromatic amines, nitrosamines, nitrosoureas, alkylating agents, alkyl and aryl halides, steroid hormones, mycotoxins, heavy metals, and mineral fibers. Known carcinogens include such chemicals as benzene, DES, and vinyl chloride and such naturally occurring substances as aflatoxin, asbestos, and elemental arsenic.

SOURCES AND DISTRIBUTION OF CARCINOGENS IN THE ENVIRONMENT

Known and suspected human chemical carcinogens are distributed widely in the environment (156). They are present in air, water, food, soil, and consumer products. This discussion, which focuses on the sources and the distribution of chemical carcinogens found in the environment, is not meant to assign actual risks to humans of such exposure. Risk assessment is a particularly difficult task requiring vast amounts of complex information. For example, assessing the carcinogenic risk of a particular exposure entails consideration of such factors as the dose, duration, and extent of exposure, the enhancing or inhibiting effects of other agents, and the sensitivity of the exposed population. Risk assessment also entails a knowledge of dose-response relationships. In addition, for environmental (non-

TABLE 26-3. Agents That Are Carcinogenic in Humans (Group 1)[a]

Aflatoxins
Aluminum production
4-Aminobiphenyl
Analgesic mixtures containing phenacetin
Arsenic and arsenic compounds[b]
Asbestos
Auramine, manufacture of
Azathioprine
Benzene
Benzidine
Betel quid with tobacco
N,N-Bis(2-chloroethyl)-2-naphthylamine (Chlornaphazine)
Bis(chloromethyl)-ether and chloromethyl methyl ether (technical grade)
Boot and shoe manufacture and repair
1,4-Butanediol dimethanesulphonate (Myleran)
Chlorambucil
1-(2-Chloroethyl)-3-(4-methylcyclohexyl)-1-nitrosourea (Methyl-CCNU)
Chromium compounds, hexavalent[b]
Coal gasification
Coal-tar pitches
Coal tars
Coke production
Cyclophosphamide
Diethylstilbestrol
Erionite
Estrogen replacement therapy
Estrogens, nonsteroidal[b]
Estrogens, steroidal[b]
Furniture and cabinet making
Hematite mining, underground, with exposure to radon
Iron and steel founding
Isopropyl alcohol manufacture, strong-acid process
Magenta, manufacture of
Melphalan
8-Methoxypsoralen (Methoxsalen) plus ultraviolet radiation
Mineral oils, untreated and mildly treated
MOPP (combined therapy with nitrogen mustard, vincristine, procarbazine, and prednisone) and other combined chemotherapy including alkylating agents
Mustard gas (sulfur mustard)
2-Naphthylamine
Nickel and nickel compounds[b]
Oral contraceptives, combined[c]
Oral contraceptives, sequential
The rubber industry
Shale-oils
Soots
Talc containing asbestiform fibers
Tobacco products, smokeless
Tobacco smoke
Treosulfan
Vinyl chloride

[a]From IARC (109).
[b]This evaluation applies to the group of chemicals as a whole and not necessarily to all individual chemicals within the group.
[c]There is also conclusive evidence that these agents have a protective effect against cancers of the ovary and endometrium.

TABLE 26-4. Agents That Are Probably Carcinogenic in Humans (Group 2A)[a]

Acrylonitrile
Adriamycin
Androgenic (anabolic) steroids
Benz[a]anthracene
Benzidine-based dyes
Benzo[a]pyrene
Beryllium and beryllium compounds
Bischloroethyl nitrosourea (BCNU)
Cadmium and cadmium compounds
1-(2-Chloroethyl)-3-cyclohexyl-1-nitrosourea (CCNU)
Cisplatin
Creosotes
Dibenz[a,h]anthracene
Diethyl sulfate
Dimethylcarbamoyl chloride
Dimethyl sulfate
Epichlorohydrin
Ethylene dibromide
Ethylene oxide
N-Ethyl-N-nitrosourea
Formaldehyde
5-Methoxypsoralen
4,4'-Methylene bis(2-chloroaniline) (MOCA)
N-Methyl-N'-nitro-N-nitrosoguanidine (MNNG)
N-Methyl-N-nitrosourea
Nitrogen mustard
N-Nitrosodiethylamine
N-Nitrosodimethylamine
Phenacetin
Polychlorinated biphenyls
Procarbazine hydrochloride
Propylene oxide
Silica, crystalline
Styrene oxide
Tris(1-aziridinyl)phosphine sulfide (Thiotepa)
Tris(2,3-dibromopropyl) phosphate
Vinyl bromide

[a]From IARC (109).

occupational) exposures, assumptions about the magnitude of effects at low doses introduce significant problems into risk assessment. For these reasons, no simple or generally recognized method exists for quantitatively evaluating the risk of environmental exposures to specific agents with respect to cancer or, indeed, to other environmentally related diseases. Often each specific exposure situation must be evaluated on its own, and even then, only broad estimates can be made of individual risk. With these caveats in mind, the probable major environmental sources and the distribution of known and suspected human carcinogens are discussed.

The environmental and occupational distribution and sources of known human chemical carcinogens are noted in Tables 26-6 through 26-12. The list of agents is based on the IARC classification of human chemical carcinogens. Data on the sources

and distribution of these agents were derived primarily from the *IARC Monographs on the Evaluation of Carcinogenic Risk of Chemicals to Humans.* Although the assignments noted in Tables 26-6 through 26-12 are at times somewhat discretionary, they do serve to emphasize the wide distribution, the differing sources, and the broad range of chemicals that can be involved in human cancer causation.

Outdoor Air

A number of known chemical carcinogens are present in outdoor air (Table 26-6). Arsenic (as arsenic trioxide), often formed as a byproduct of the smelting process (18), is found near lead and other smelters. It has also been detected in the outdoor air of communities adjacent to a smelter. For example, near a smelter in Tacoma Washington, the levels of arsenic were as high as 1.46 $\mu g/m^3$ (143). Benzene is present in outdoor air. The concentrations of this known human carcinogen is dependent on local industry, automobile traffic, geography, and weather (100).

Low levels of asbestos are widely distributed in many urban and rural areas throughout the world. Asbestos has been detected at concentrations of nanograms per cubic meter of air in virtually all of the major cities in the United States (37). Asbestos consists of the commercially marketed varieties of several silicate minerals. The chrysotile variety accounts for approximately 95% of the asbestos most recently sold in the United States. Asbestos in the outdoor urban air results from the wearing down of brake shoes and, clutches and from other industrial products containing asbestos. Asbestos is also liberated into the air during the application or removal of asbestos insulation, especially the spray varieties (126). Some rural roads have also been surfaced with tailings from asbestos mines (123). Chrysotile asbestos fibers have been found in human lungs in a random series of autopsies performed on New York City residents (173).

Indoor Air

Known human chemical carcinogens that may be found in indoor air in a nonoccupational setting are listed in Table 26-7. An EPA-sponsored study revealed that exposure to 11 common toxic air pollutants is greater in the home than outdoors (206,207). Included in this list of pollutants is benzene, a known human carcinogen. Possible sources of this agent in indoor air include such consumer products as paints, varnishes, glues, lacquers, and cleaners.

Vinyl chloride, a potent inducer of hepatic angiosarcomas in the occupational setting, has been used as an aerosol propellant in numerous products including hair sprays and deodorants. Vinyl chlo-

TABLE 26-5. Agents That Are Possibly Carcinogenic in Humans (Group 2B)[a]

A-α-C (2-Amino-9H-pyrido[2,3-b]indole)
Acetaldehyde
Acetamide
Acrylamide
AF-2[2-(2-Furyl)-3-(5-nitro-2-furyl)acrylamide]
para-Aminoazobenzene
ortho-Aminoazotoluene
2-Amino-5-(5-nitro-2-furyl)-1,3,4-thiadiazole
Amitrole
ortho-Anisidine
Aramite®
Auramine, technical grade
Azaserine
Benzo[b]fluoranthene
Benzo[j]fluoranthene
Benzo[k]fluoranthene
Benzyl violet 4B
Bitumens, extracts of steam-refined and air-refined
Bleomycins
Bracken fern
1,3-Butadiene
Butylated hydroxyanisole (BHA)
β-Butyrolactone
Carbon-black extracts
Carbon tetrachloride
Carpentry and joinery
Carrageenan, degraded
Chloramphenicol
Chlordecone (Kepone)
α-Chlorinated toluenes
Chloroform
Chlorophenols
Chlorophenoxy herbicides
4-Chloro-ortho-phenylenediamine
para-Chloro-ortho-toluidine
Citrus Red No. 2
para-Cresidine
Cycasin
Dacarbazine
Daunomycin
DDT
N,N'-Diacetylbenzidine
2,4-Diaminoanisole
4,4'-Diaminodiphenyl ether
2,4-Diaminotoluene
Dibenz[a,h]acridine
Dibenz[a,j]acridine
7H-Dibenzo[c,g]carbazole
Dibenzo[a,e]pyrene
Dibenzo[a,h]pyrene
Dibenzo[a,i]pyrene
Dibenzo[a,l]pyrene
1,2-Dibromo-3-chloropropane
para-Dichlorobenzene
3,3'-Dichlorobenzidine
3,3'-Dichloro-4,4'-diaminodiphenyl ether
1,2-Dichloroethane
Dichloromethane

1,3-Dichloropropene (technical-grade)
Diepoxybutane
Di(2-ethylhexyl)phthalate
1,2-Diethylhydrazine
Diglycidyl resorcinol ether
Dihydrosafrole
3,3'-Dimethoxybenzidine (ortho-Dianisidine)
para-Dimethylaminoazobenzene
trans-2-[(Dimethylamino)methyl-imino]-5-[2-(5-nitro-2-furyl)-vinyl]-1,3,4-oxadiazole
3,3'-Dimethylbenzidine (ortho-Tolidine)
1,1-Dimethylhydrazine
1,2-Dimethylhydrazine
1,4-Dioxane
Ethyl acrylate
Ethylene thiourea
Ethyl methanesulphonate
2-(2-Formylhydrazino)-4-(5-nitro-2-furyl)thiazole
Glu-P-1 (2-Amino-6-methyldipyrido-[1,2-a:3',2'-d]imidazole)
Glu-P-2(2-Aminodipyrido[1,2-a:3',2'-d]-imidazole)
Glycidaldehyde
Griseofulvin
Hexachlorobenzene
Hexachlorocyclohexanes
Hexamethylphosphoramide
Hydrazine
Indeno[1,2,3-cd]pyrene
IQ (2-Amino-3-methylimidazo[4,5-f]quinoline)
Iron–dextran complex
Lasiocarpine
Lead and lead compounds, inorganic
MeA-α-C (2-Amino-3-methyl-9H-pyrido[2,3-b]indole)
Medroxyprogesterone acetate
Merphalan
2-Methylaziridine
Methylazoxymethanol and its acetate
5-Methylchrysene
4,4'-Methylene bis(2-methylaniline)
4,4'-Methylenedianiline
Methyl methanesulphonate
2-Methyl-1 nitroanthraquinone (uncertain purity)
N-Methyl-N-nitrosourethane
Methylthiouracil
Metronidazole
Mirex
Mitomycin C
Monocrotaline
5-(Morpholinomethyl)-3-[(5-nitrofur-furylidene)amino]-2-oxazolidinone
Nafenopin

Niridazole
5-Nitroacenaphthene
Nitrofen (technical-grade)
1-[(5-Nitrofurfurylidene)amino]-2-imidazolidinone
N[4-(5-Nitro-2-furyl)-2-thiazolyl]-acetamide
Nitrogen mustard N-oxide
2-Nitropropane
N-Nitrosodi-n-butylamine
N-Nitrosodiethanolamine
N-Nitrosodi-n-propylamine
3-(N-Nitrosomethylamino)propio-nitrile
4-(N-Nitrosomethylamino)-1-(3-pyridyl)-1-butanone (NNK)
N-Nitrosomethylethylamine
N-Nitrosomethylvinylamine
N-Nitrosomorpholine
N'-Nitrosonornicotine
N-Nitrosopiperidine
N-Nitrosopyrrolidine
N-Nitrososarcosine
Oil Orange SS
Panfuran S (containing dihydroxy-methylfuratrizine)
Phenazopyridine hydrochloride
Phenobarbital
Phenoxybenzamine hydrochloride
Phenytoin
Polybrominated biphenyls
Ponceau MX
Ponceau 3R
Potassium bromate
Progestins
1,3-Propane sultone
β-Propiolactone
Propylthiouracil
Saccharin
Safrole
Sodium ortho-phenylphenate
Sterigmatocystin
Streptozotocin
Styrene
Sulfallate
2,3,7,8-Tetrachlorodibenzo-para-dioxin (TCDD)
Tetrachloroethylene
Thioacetamide
4,4'-Thiodianiline
Thiourea
Toluene diisocyanates
ortho-Toluidine
Toxaphene (Polychlorinated cam-phenes)
Trp-P-1 (3-Amino-1,4-dimethyl-5H-pyrido[4,3-b]indole)
Trp-P-2 (3-Amino-1-methyl-5H-pyrido[4,3-b]indole)
Trypan blue
Uracil mustard
Urethane

[a]From IARC (109).

TABLE 26-6. Agents Found in Outdoor Air That Are Carcinogenic in Humans[a]

Agent	Sources of exposure
Arsenic and arsenic compounds	Copper and lead smelter emissions, pesticides
Asbestos	Building and friction materials
Benzene	Gasoline combustion, industrial emissions
Chromium and certain chromium compounds	Plating and alloy industry
Nickel and certain nickel compounds	Emissions from coal- and oil-fired boilers, coke ovens, diesel fuel burning, and gray-iron foundries
Soots, shale oils	Power plants, fossil fuel processing
Vinyl chloride	Emissions from plastic industry

[a]From IARC (109) and USDHHS (197).

ride was banned from consumer products in the United States in 1974 because it was found to be a human carcinogen (60).

Other agents classified as probably carcinogenic to humans and found in indoor air (apart from the workplace) include formaldehyde, which may arise from urea-formaldehyde insulation and certain consumer products, and PCBs, which during fires can be released into indoor air from enclosed systems such as electrical capacitors, transformers, and hydraulic equipment (154,181) (Table 26-4). Chloroform, which is classified as possibly carcinogenic in humans, can be found in indoor air from its volatilization from drinking water (27).

Office buildings and schools constructed with asbestos-containing materials may contain from 9 to 1990 ng/m³ of chrysotile, depending on the conditions of the building material (37). The deterioration of asbestos-containing ceilings and walls installed in the 1940s, 1950s, and 1960s accounts for the problem. Exposures in asbestos-insulated school buildings, in particular, have caused considerable concern. Even though the asbestos levels found in indoor air in a nonoccupational setting are on the whole very low when compared with those found in the workplace, it has been shown that asbestos is a carcinogen even at low concentrations (7,144). The nonoccupational health risks of asbestos exposure have been comprehensively reviewed (37).

Tobacco smoke is a carcinogen found in indoor air. It is the major air pollutant linked to cancer in cigarette smokers. Recent studies that demonstrate an increased lung cancer risk in certain populations exposed to environmental tobacco smoke support the conclusion that passive or involuntary smoking is also a cause of cancer (38,41,59,94,193,196). Chapter 2 contains a detailed discussion of the pollutants found in indoor and outdoor air.

Water

Known human chemical carcinogens that may be found in drinking water are listed in Table 26-8. Within the IARC classification of chemical carcinogens, there are three major groups of carcinogenic contaminants of water: (1) solid fibers or particulates, such as asbestos; (2) inorganic solutes, such as arsenic, and chromium; and (3) organic chemicals, such as benzene.

Drinking water may be contaminated with asbestos from the leachate from rocks or asbestos pipes, from deposition of airborne asbestos, or by runoff from dumps or ore deposits. The character of the rocks and soils present in the water supply basin markedly affects the asbestos content of the drinking water. For example, natural asbestos leachate is present in much of the San Francisco Bay Area drinking water. In San Francisco, concentrations as high as 3 million fibers/L have been reported. It has been difficult to document a carcinogenic hazard from ingested asbestos (37,85,115).

Cadmium, a probable human carcinogen, in

TABLE 26-7. Agents Found in Indoor Air That Are Carcinogenic in Humans[a]

Agent	Sources of exposure
Asbestos	Deteriorating building materials
Benzene	Paints, varnishes, glues, lacquers, cleaners
2-Naphthylamine	Cigarette smoke
Soots	Fireplace smoke
Tobacco smoke	Cigarettes, pipes, cigars
Vinyl chloride	Aerosol sprays (banned in U.S.), cigarette smoke, volatilization of vinyl chloride from vinyl polymers within car interiors (greater in new cars)

[a]From IARC (109) and USDHHS (197).

TABLE 26-8. Agents Found in Water That Are Carcinogenic in Humans[a]

Agent	Sources of exposure
Arsenic and arsenic compounds	Pesticide runoff
Asbestos	Asbestos–cement pipe, geologic formations
Chromium and chromium compounds	Plating and alloy industry
Benzene	Industrial discharges
Bis(chloromethyl)ether	Industrial discharges
Nickel and certain nickel compounds	Industrial discharges
Vinyl chloride	Industrial discharges

[a]From IARC (109) and USDHHS (197).

drinking water usually stems from the corrosion of galvanized pipes and fittings. Increased levels of arsenic in water can be related to pollution from smelters and from natural sources. High levels of arsenic have been found in the drinking water in certain areas of Taiwan and Chile. This finding may be linked to an increase in the incidence of skin cancer (194,236). The occurrence of excess chromium in drinking water is usually the result of pollution by industrial wastes.

Organic chemicals enter the water supply from such sources as industrial and municipal discharges, agricultural runoff, hazardous waste sites, and the decomposition of organic matter (humus). Synthetic organic chemicals are widely found in both raw and finished drinking water. They are found in water systems using ground as well as surface water. Many treatment facilities in the United States are not designed to remove soluble organic agents from water (227). In addition, the use of chlorine in the water treatment process creates halogenated organic compounds that were not originally present in the untreated water. In 1974, Rook et al. reported the formation of chloroform from a reaction between chlorine and organic materials present in water (167). Chloroform was later shown to be an animal carcinogen. An EPA survey found chloroform in almost every chlorinated water supply in the United States (27). Chloroform and chlorophenols formed during the chlorination of drinking water are listed in the IARC classification as possible human carcinogens (Table 26-5). For a detailed discussion of drinking water disinfection and disinfectant byproducts the interested reader is referred to a recent report (185).

Chapter 4 contains a detailed discussion of the chemical contaminants in water.

Food

Food contaminants known to be human chemical carcinogens are shown in Table 26-9 (39). Vinyl chloride has been reported to leach from polyvinyl chloride food-wrapping material (106). Agents that are classified as probably carcinogenic to humans include PCBs, cadmium, ethylene dibromide, and benzo[a]pyrene (BaP). The PCBs are often found in fish (105) (Table 26-4). Cadmium may be present in seafood, grains, vegetables, and organ meats (103). The pesticide ethylene dibromide (EDB) has been reported at levels in excess of 1 ppb in many grain products and in citrus fruits. Extremely high BaP levels on the surface of meat and fish can be a consequence of broiling or charring. These methods of cooking can also lead to the formation of highly mutagenic and carcinogenic amino acid pyrolysis products (5). Chapter 3 contains a detailed discussion of the pollutants found in food.

Consumer Products

Humans are increasingly exposed to chemical agents via such consumer products as construction materials, appliances, containers and packaging materials, clothing, pesticides, and preservatives. It is important to consider consumer products as well as air, water, and food as sources of potentially hazardous exposures. Table 26-10 provides examples of consumer products that may contain known human

TABLE 26-9. Agents Found as Food Contaminants That Are Carcinogenic in Humans[a]

Agent	Sources of exposure
Aflatoxin	Products of fungi that grow on peanuts, grains, and other foods
Arsenic, some arsenic compounds	Arsenic-containing pesticides
Nickel and certain nickel-containing compounds	Food processing may cause leaching from nickel-containing alloys

[a]From IARC (109) and USDHHS (197).

TABLE 26-10. Agents Found in Consumer Products That Are Carcinogenic in Humans[a]

Agent	Sources of exposure
Asbestos	Asbestos-containing talc, formerly used as insulation in home appliances such as hair dryers
Benzene	Contaminant of gasoline and such consumer products as paints, varnishes, glues, enamels, lacquers, and cleaners
Benzidine	Benzidine-based dyes (production being reduced)
Smokeless tobacco products	Oral use of tobacco
Tobacco smoke	Cigarettes, pipes, cigars
Vinyl chloride	Upholstery in new cars (see Table 26-7)

[a]From IARC (109) and USDHHS (197).

chemical carcinogens. The list, though not exhaustive, serves to emphasize the magnitude of the problem and the need to evaluate carefully the potential health hazards of consumer products.

Pharmaceutical Agents

Therapeutic drugs known to be human carcinogens are shown in Table 26-11. It is essential that physicians be aware of the potential carcinogenic hazards of drugs, that they carefully evaluate the benefits versus the risks of using drugs known to be carcinogenic, and that they seek alternative medications when available. This subject has been thoroughly reviewed (183).

Occupational Exposure

A vast majority of the known or suspected human carcinogens were first identified in the workplace. Indeed, occupational exposures linked to the causation of specific cancers are the cornerstone of the field of environmental carcinogenesis. Chemicals and groups of chemicals causally associated with human cancer in which exposure has occurred primarily in the workplace are shown in Table 26-12.

Radiation

An extensive discussion of radiation sources and their potential carcinogenicity is beyond the scope of this chapter. Certain salient features, however, are discussed because radiation is a well-recognized human carcinogen. Exposure to ionizing radiation may occur in the therapeutic or diagnostic medical setting (x rays). The potential for occupational radiation exposure is present for certain health-care workers and for workers in certain high-technology and service industries. Exposure to radiation in the general environment is also of concern. The health effects of exposure to ionizing radiation have been reviewed in detail (34).

Radon, a gaseous radioactive decay product of uranium, can be found in indoor air. The indoor air levels of radon depend on the concentration of radon in the underlying soil, the type of construction material used, and the type of ventilation. There is evidence that much of the radon in indoor air is derived from the soil beneath the building. Radon may also enter the home through the water supply. Radon production in soil is influenced by the distribution of uranium, which varies widely throughout the earth's crust. It is found in large amounts in soils and rocks containing uranium, shale, granite, pitchblende, and phosphate.

Concern for the presence of radon indoors is related to the measurable excesses of lung cancer related to inhalation of radon that occurs in workers who mine uranium, hematite, and certain other ores

TABLE 26-11. Drugs Causally Associated with Human Cancer[a]

Analgesic mixtures containing phenacetin
Azathioprine
N,N-Bis(2-chloroethyl)-2-naphthylamine (Chlornaphazine)
1,4-Butanediol dimethanesulfonate (Myleran)
Chlorambucil
1-(2-Chloroethyl)-3(4-methylcyclohexyl)-1-nitrosourea (Methyl-CCNU)
Cyclophosphamide
Diethylstilbestrol
Estrogen replacement therapy
Estrogens, nonsteroidal
Estrogens, steroidal
Melphalan
8-Methoxypsoralen (Methoxsalen) plus UV radiation
MOPP and other combined chemotherapy including alkylating agents
Oral contraceptives, combined
Oral contraceptives, sequential
Treosulfan

[a]The evaluation of carcinogenicity in humans applies to the group of chemicals as a whole and not necessarily to all individual chemicals within the group. From IARC (109), Tomatis et al. (191), and USDHHS (197).

TABLE 26-12. Chemicals, Groups of Chemicals, and Industrial Processes Causally Associated with Cancer in Which Exposure Has Been Mostly Occupational[a]

Agent	Sources of exposure
4-Aminobiphenyl	Manufacture of dyes, antioxidant in rubber (no longer used in U.S. commerce)
Arsenic and arsenic compounds[b]	Pesticides, metal smelters, manufacture of glass and ceramics
Asbestos	Building, friction, and insulating materials
Benzene	Oil refining, gasoline production, manufacture of chemicals, paints, plastics, widely used as a solvent
Benzidine	Laboratory reagent, manufacture of dyes
Bis(chloromethyl)ether	Manufacture of chemicals and plastics
Chromium compounds, hexavalent[b]	Manufacture of metal alloys, pigments for paints, electroplating, welding
Coal tars	Coke production, coal gasification, aluminum production, foundries
Coal-tar pitches	Pavement tar, roofing tar, coal-tar paints
Mineral oils, untreated and mildly treated	Manufacture of cars, airplanes, steel products, engine repair, newspapers, commercial printing
Mustard gas	Weapons production
2-Naphthylamine	Manufacture of dyes and rubber
Nickel and nickel compounds[b]	Battery manufacture, ceramic makers, electroplating, refineries, smelters
Shale oils	Manufacture of coal tar, creosote, crude mineral oils, cutting oils
Soots	Used in the recovery of trace metals in the metallurgical industry
Talc containing asbestiform fibers	Mining of talc containing asbestiform tremolite
Vinyl chloride	Manufacture of plastics

Industrial processes
   Aluminum production
   Auramine manufacture (manufacture of dyes)
   Boot and shoe manufacture and repair
   Coal gasification
   Coke production
   Furniture and cabinet making
   Hematite mining, underground, and exposure to radon
   Iron and steel founding
   Isopropyl alcohol manufacture (strong-acid process)
   Magenta, manufacture of
   Painters (occupational exposure)
   Rubber industry

[a]From IARC (109), Tomatis et al. (191), and USDHHS (197).
[b]The evaluation of carcinogenicity in humans applies to the group of chemicals as a whole and not necessarily to individual chemicals within the group.

(169,170). The α-emitting radon daughters must be inhaled to be carcinogenic (179). Excessive levels of radon, approaching those found in some mining situations, have been recorded in some homes, particularly those with poorly ventilated basement areas, in certain areas of the United States and Scandinavia (169). Although indoor radon may represent a problem in virtually every state, public health concerns in the United States have been focused on the homes built on a natural rock formation in New Jersey, Pennsylvania, and New York.

At times the improper disposal of radiotherapy equipment can result in widespread exposure to radiation. Such an episode occurred in 1983 in Juarez, Mexico, when junkyard workers unwittingly opened a cancer therapy device. This error released over 6000 tiny cylinders, each containing about 70 μCi of cobalt-60, which were then widely dispersed. This event was discovered only by chance and long after the contaminated scrap metal had found its way into reinforcing rods used for home construction (130).

Solar radiation, from exposure to ultraviolet light, poses a cancer threat. Sun exposure is associated with squamous and basal cell carcinomas of the skin. Most of these nonmelanoma skin cancers occur on sun-exposed body areas of individuals, particularly Caucasians, who spend a great deal of time outdoors. The incidence of ultraviolet-induced skin cancer is inversely correlated with geographic latitude, i.e., the closer to the equator the more frequent the incidence of skin cancers (52) (see Chapter 15).

EPIDEMIOLOGY OF ENVIRONMENTAL CANCER

It is often relatively easy for epidemiologists to investigate the effects of high-level or point-source occupational exposures. Assessing the effects of low-dose environmental exposures, however, is very difficult. Environmental exposure to carcinogens may be divided into three categories: exposure in the general outdoor and indoor environment, exposure near known sources of carcinogens within the community, and exposure through the use of consumer products. Attempts have been made to assess the carcinogenic effects of air and water pollution in the general environment by correlating cancer patterns with industrialization and population density. Similar assessments have been made in communities where there are significant sources of carcinogens either from industry or from hazardous waste sites.

General Environment

Air Pollution: Urban-Rural Differences

As previously noted, a number of pollutants in indoor and outdoor air are human carcinogens (Tables 26-6 and 26-7). The concentrations of these pollutants vary from one locale to another depending on a large number of geographic, geological, meteorological, and industrial factors. The question arises, is there evidence that these compounds, acting either singly, additively, or synergistically at concentrations found in ambient air, increase the incidence of cancer in exposed populations?

A number of studies demonstrate a variable (up to ninefold) increase in lung cancer mortality for men and women living in urban centers when compared to those living in rural areas, even after the effects of cigarette smoking have been controlled (22,47,182). Although most studies that have controlled for the effects of smoking find that lung cancer is still more common in urban than in rural areas, not all studies show this relationship (95). All epidemiologic studies concerned with the possible carcinogenic risk of air pollution, however, are flawed by a lack of data on personal exposure to pollutants and, in particular, by an absence of direct measurements of ambient levels of known carcinogens. The results of the studies noted above and others have been well summarized by Shy and Struba (175).

Studies of migrant populations support the importance of a delayed, or latent, effect that may be linked to environmental pollution. Eastcott first noted that, despite comparable smoking habits, migrants from the United Kingdom to New Zealand showed lung cancer patterns that were higher than those of the indigenous population. The incidence of lung cancer was higher in migrants who left Britain after the age of 30 than in those who left before that age (51). Similar observations have been made on other migrant populations (46).

In aggregate, most studies suggest the presence of an "urban factor" apart from smoking that increases the incidence of lung cancer. They also suggest that exposure to this factor at a younger age has a greater adverse effect than exposure at an older age. The exact nature of the "urban factor" is unclear. It may be related to one or a combination of factors. These include occupational exposures, indoor and outdoor air pollution, and exposure to specific consumer products and, to a lesser extent, water pollution. Other components of an urban environment may also be important. Thus far, however, the role of the "urban factor" in lung cancer causation appears to be notably weaker than the effects of cigarette smoke. Certain authorities seriously question whether urban air pollution plays a role in lung cancer causation (49). The interested reader is referred to a detailed monograph on the factors that may contribute to urban-rural differences in cancer mortality (68).

Efforts have been made to quantify the risk of lung cancer from air pollution using benzo[a]pyrene (BaP) as the indicator of air pollution (29,33). Benzo[a]pyrene has been used as a convenient index of air pollution because it is a well-characterized experimental carcinogen and is easily measured in ambient air (171). Such estimates are associated with many uncertainties. These include the absence of quantitative data on individual exposures, a lack of evidence that links exposure to the occurrence of lung cancer, and a lack of evidence that BaP is itself an appropriate index of air pollution.

Water Pollution

There is concern that various chemical agents found in drinking water may increase the risk of cancer. This concern is based on the finding that drinking water contains many chemicals that are known or suspected human carcinogens.

The majority of the epidemiologic studies concerned with the relationship between chemical contaminants of drinking water and cancer are based on mortality rates in specific geographic areas, i.e., counties, cities, or states. Such studies generally seek associations between cancer mortality and water quality for the geographic areas under analysis. Since 1974 over 20 epidemiologic studies have examined the relationship between various aspects of water quality (surface versus ground water, chlorinated versus nonchlorinated, estimates of trihalomethanes, etc.) and cancer mortality and morbidity (175,227). Geographic correlation studies and case-control studies suggest a relationship between exposure to organic chemicals in water and the occurrence of cancers of the urinary bladder and gastrointestinal tract, especially the colon and rectum (1,114).

The above studies rely on very uncertain estimates of exposure. This uncertainty is coupled with such complex and interrelated factors as age, race, mobility, socioeconomic class, and the synergistic effects of occupational and/or recreational exposures, all of which are operative in complex urban settings where contaminated surface waters often occur. On the basis of the current epidemiologic studies, it has been concluded that there is preliminary evidence for an association between chemical contaminants in drinking water and certain cancers; the magnitude of this association, however, is not expected to be large (175).

Community Exposure Near Known Sources of Carcinogens

Asbestos

An increased risk of mesothelioma in nonasbestos workers was first reported in 1960 in a region surrounding the asbestos mines of the northwest Cape Province of South Africa (203). In the more urban setting of London, England, a case-control study of pleural and peritoneal mesothelioma by Newhouse and Thompson demonstrated an increased risk of mesothelioma for asbestos workers as well as their family members and for individuals living near asbestos factories (144). Clusters of pleural mesothelioma have also been reported in rural areas of Turkey in association with x-ray changes characteristic of asbestos exposure. Mineralogical data in these areas have not consistently shown asbestos in the environment, although other fibers of similar shape and size (zeolite) have been found (9). It is likely that these occurrences of mesothelioma provide another example of fiber-induced environmental cancer unrelated to occupational exposure.

The increased carcinogenic risk associated with community exposure to asbestos from nearby industrial sources is in keeping with the high cancer risk noted from occupational exposure to asbestos. Insulation workers in the construction industry have an approximately fivefold increase in lung cancer mortality. In a large ongoing cohort study of over 17,000 asbestos workers, approximately 20% eventually develop lung cancer, and another 10% die of mesothelioma (174). The risk of developing mesothelioma is exceedingly low in the absence of asbestos exposure. Cigarette smokers who were also asbestos workers were found to have over a 50-fold excess of lung cancer deaths (78,79). A quantitative

assessment of the risks for mesothelioma and lung cancer from environmental (nonoccupational) exposure to asbestiform fibers has been published (37). This publication provides an excellent example of the method used in risk assessment.

Dioxin and Phenoxy Herbicides

There is a concern about the possible long-term health effects of exposure to 2,3,7,8-tetrachlorodibenzo-p-dioxin (TCDD) or "dioxin" and phenoxy herbicides (21,200). Dioxin is generated as a contaminant during the chemical manufacture of such agents as hexachlorophene and trichlorophenol, and the herbicide 2,4,5-trichlorophenoxyacetic acid (2,4,5-T). Chlorinated dioxins can also be formed during the combustion of organic material. They have been identified in fly ash from municipal incinerators, in industrial heating facilities, and in the effluent from paper mills (24). TCDD is one of 75 chlorinated dioxins. Animal studies show that TCDD is both a carcinogen and a tetratogen (43, 121,144). Although this agent is considered to be the most toxic synthetic poison known, there are large species differences in its toxicity.

Widespread exposure to dioxin occurred during the Vietnam War with the use of Agent Orange as an aerial defoliant. Agent Orange (or Herbicide Orange) was made up of a 1:1 mixture of 2,4,5-T and 2,4-dichlorophenoxyacetic acid (2,4-D). As a result of contamination of 2,4,5-T with TCDD, the concentration of TCDD in Agent Orange ranged between 0.02 and 15 ppm, with a weighted mean of 1.98 ppm. It is estimated that about 25 million kilograms of 2,4-D, 20 million kilograms of 2,4,5-T, and 166 kg of TCDD were released in Vietnam between January 1962 and February 1971 (233). Most of the spraying was done between 1967 and 1969 as part of "Operation Ranch Hand."

Major ongoing epidemiologic investigations of populations exposed to TCDD-contaminated phenoxy herbicides involve Vietnam veterans. Particular attention is being directed to long-term health effects on Air Force members who were herbicide loaders or herbicide specialists in connection with aerial spraying missions in Southeast Asia (Operation Ranch Hand). The Air Force Health Study compares the mortality and morbidity of 1174 Air Force "Ranch Hand" personnel to a matched control group. The study is designed to evaluate mortality and morbidity over a 20-year period beginning in 1982. Mortality reports published in 1983, 1984, 1985, and 1986 failed to reveal any statistically significant differences in the number of deaths between the Ranch Hand group and their matched controls (124,228–230). The death rate at the time of these reports, however, is low, 4–5%.

A second phase of the study designed to determine the incidence of such problems as cancer, reproductive dysfunction, and hepatic, dermatologic, cardiovascular, immunologic, hematological, pulmonary, renal, and endocrine abnormalities was reported in 1984 (125). On the basis of data collected thus far through questionnaires and physical examinations, no significant differences were found between the Ranch Hand personnel and controls with regard to the incidence of systemic cancers, clinically significant blood abnormalities, or cardiovascular, renal, pulmonary, hepatic, and neurological effects. Using the same participants, periodic follow-up examinations will be done.

Thus far no association between soft tissue sarcoma and military service in Vietnam has been noted (109). It should be appreciated that although the Air Force study is in its early phase, insufficient time has elapsed to reveal such long-term health effects of exposure to heavily TCDD-contaminated chlorophenoxy herbicide as the development of cancer. Comprehensive reviews of this subject have been published (21,42,233).

In 1976, the residents of Seveso, Italy received excessive exposure to TCDD as the result of an industrial accident. In 1986, 15 cases of soft-tissue sarcoma were reported in the exposed population. This figure is not excessive when compared with the rates encountered in the unexposed population. The incidence of this tumor was high in the Seveso area before the episode of environmental TCDD contamination, possibly related to earlier emissions (164). In 1989, a 10-year mortality experience of the population in the contaminated Seveso area was reported. Although the relative risks for malignancies as a whole were not increased, mortality from specific cancers was increased. The increases, often based on small numbers, were noted in liver and hepatobiliary cancers in women and lymphatic and hematopoietic cancers (particularly leukemia) in men. Suggestive increases in melanoma and soft-tissue tumors were also observed (13).

The health effects of exposure to chlorophenoxy herbicides and TCDD-contaminated products have been reported chiefly in workers (40,136,137, 148,231,232). The effect most often observed as the clinical marker of exposure to TCDD-contaminated materials is chloracne, which is an acneform eruption characterized by dense large blackheads and skin-colored cystic lesions. Abnormal liver function, peripheral neuropathy, nervousness, irritability, personality changes, porphyria cutanea tarda, hypertrichosis, and hyperpigmentation have also been observed. Laboratory abnormalities include elevated blood cholesterol, triglycerides, and liver enzymes and prolonged prothrombin time (136,186).

Thus far several small mortality analyses of U.S. industrial workers exposed to TCDD-contaminated phenoxy herbicides reveal no increased mortality or pattern of death from cancer (40,148,234, 235). A large Danish study of workers involved in the manufacture of phenoxy herbicides demonstrated some excess of soft-tissue sarcomas (129). A study in Germany described increased cancer mortality in men employed in a herbicide plant that was heavily contaminated with TCDD (129A). Other investigators have reported some excesses of nasal cancer and non-Hodgkin lymphoma in workers exposed to phenoxy herbicides (31,166). Noteworthy in the foregoing studies and the Danish study is the fact that some excess cancers developed among phenoxy-herbicide-exposed workers when little if any exposure to TCDD was likely.

Swedish studies were the first to suggest that workers in forestry, farming, and wood and paper mills who received exposure to phenoxyacetic acid herbicides and chlorophenols are at increased risk of developing soft-tissue sarcoma, Hodgkin disease, and non-Hodgkin lymphoma (55,81–84). These findings caused concern because the phenoxy herbicides had been widely used. Vast amounts of 2,4,5-T, contaminated with varying amounts of TCDD, were used from 1948 to 1970 in farming, family gardens, forest management, and for weed control along roadsides. It is estimated that in 1964 in the United States, 9.8 million pounds of 2,4,5-T was produced for domestic use alone. In 1979 the Environmental Protection Agency suspended the use of 2,4,5-T in forestry, rights of way, and pastures (198). Vast amounts of 2,4-D continue to be used. This herbicide has been used widely for the past 35 years. Nearly 40 million pounds of 2,4-D is used annually in the United States by agriculture (39). There is no evidence that 2,4-D is contaminated with TCDD.

In 1977 seven cases of soft-tissue sarcoma were described among Swedish lumberjacks who previously had heavy exposure to phenoxy herbicides (81). This clinical observation led Swedish researchers to conduct case-control studies of workers in occupations (i.e., forestry, farming, wood, and paper mills) that utilize phenoxyacetic acids and chlorophenols (83). These workers found that persons with occupational exposure to phenoxyacetic acids or chlorophenols had a sixfold increased risk of developing soft-tissue sarcoma. This increased tumor risk was attributed to such impurities as TCDD, which was present in phenoxy acids and chlorophenols. Subsequent case-control studies, however, revealed about a five- to sixfold increased risk of soft-tissue sarcoma and lymphoma with exposure to phenoxy acids and chlorophenols irrespective of contamination with dioxin (55,84). A case-control study on soft-tissue sarcoma, performed to see if the above findings could be reproduced, revealed that exposure to phenoxy acids gave roughly a threefold increase for soft-tissue sarcoma. Soft-tissue sarcoma was not associated with exposure to chlorophenols in this study (82).

A case-control study from New Zealand failed to demonstrate any increased risk of soft-tissue sarcoma in people exposed to phenoxy herbicides (176). The degree to which the phenoxy herbicides were contaminated with TCDD is unknown.

A large population-based case-control study was performed in Kansas, a major U.S. wheat-producing state where large quantities of phenoxy herbicides have been in use for many years. Herbicide exposure was examined in relation to newly diagnosed cases of soft-tissue sarcoma, Hodgkin disease, and non-Hodgkin lymphoma. A sixfold increase in non-Hodgkin lymphoma was found in farmers exposed to herbicides more than 20 days per year. The increased risk was associated specifically with the use of 2,4-D (96). These findings are consistent with the Swedish studies and other reports that suggest an increased risk for lymphoma among agricultural workers exposed to phenoxyacetic acid herbicides (23,25,28,150,184).

The work of Wigle et al. provides additional data supporting the tenet that exposure to herbicides increases the risk of non-Hodgkin lymphoma among farmers (15,225). This study of Canadian farmers analyzed mortality records pertaining to nearly 70,000 male farmers in Saskatchewan. As has been noted previously, the mortality among farmers is considerably lower than that of the general population (16,225). Nonetheless, mortality from non-Hodgkin lymphoma rose significantly with increasing number of acres sprayed with herbicides, particularly on smaller farms where the farmer was more likely to have personally engaged in herbicide application. Although the study provided no information on the specific herbicide used, the authors indicate that the phenoxy herbicide 2,4-D accounted for 75% of the weight of all herbicide active ingredients used in agriculture in Saskatchewan in 1970, and a larger percentage in 1960 (225).

The inappropriate disposal of phenoxyacetic herbicides and TCDD-contaminated material can be an important source of community exposure. The events occurring in the United States at Times Beach, Missouri typify this problem. In the early 1970s about 29 kg of TCDD-contaminated waste, mixed with waste oils, was applied to the soil for dust control at numerous sites in Missouri. One site, an urban residential area called Times Beach, contained soil samples with levels of dioxin as high as 98 ppm (117). Because there were no adequate human dose-response data that could be used to estimate the TCDD exposure level associated with reasonable risk, extrapolations from chronic animal toxicity data were used. On the basis of these calculation, 1 ppb of TCDD in residential soil was chosen

as a level of concern (117,120,142). The high level of TCDD soil contamination led to a near-total evacuation of the town. The exposed population is currently under study.

On the basis of the epidemiologic studies done thus far, the International Agency for Research on Cancer (IARC) has concluded that there is limited evidence that persons exposed to phenoxy herbicides and chlorophenols may be at increased risk of soft-tissue sarcoma and lymphoma. There are inadequate data to conclude that TCDD is carcinogenic to humans, although the evidence of its carcinogenicity in animals is sufficient (109). A comprehensive overview of 2,4-D, 2,4,5-T, and TCDD has been published (128).

Organochlorine Insecticides and Fumigants

A population-based case-referent study in Kansas examined the relationship between exposure to insecticides and the development of soft-tissue sarcoma and Hodgkin disease (97). Soft-tissue sarcoma was associated with the use of insecticides on animals but not on crops. Hodgkin disease was not significantly associated with either use. Soft-tissue sarcoma risk was noted to be higher among the farmers who themselves mixed or applied insecticides to animals than among those who did not. In addition, farmers who failed to use any protective equipment to reduce insecticide exposure were at significantly increased risk of soft-tissue sarcoma. Chlorinated hydrocarbon insecticides known to have been used in the early 1940s include DDT, benzene hexachloride, heptachlor, lindane, methoxychlor, and toxaphene.

Alavanja et al. studied the morality experience during the period 1955–1985 among over 22,000 white males who were enrolled in the life insurance program of the American Federation of Grain Millers. Excess risks for developing non-Hodgkin lymphoma, leukemia, and pancreatic cancer were noted in workers employed in flour mills where pesticides were used more frequently than in other segments of the industry. Within the flour mills, the workers who had ever worked in the maintenance department or in the elevator department were at increased risk of developing non-Hodgkin lymphoma. Workers who more frequently used grain fumigants, including carbon tetrachloride, carbon disulfide, and phosphine, appeared to be at greater risk for non-Hodgkin lymphoma (2).

Other Exposures

Attempts to demonstrate a relationship between an industrial process and an increased cancer incidence in the surrounding community have been unsuccessful except for the case of industrial sources of asbestos. However, one study of communities near vinyl chloride polymerization plants suggests an increase in central nervous system and lymphatic cancers (102). This finding requires further study and confirmation. Future epidemiologic studies must be directed to the investigation of a possible link between the location of major industrial plants and the incidence of cancer in the surrounding area. Such studies should monitor actual exposure levels.

Hazardous Waste Sites

Considerable concern exists about the potential carcinogenic hazards of chemical dump sites (71). The Love Canal site near Niagara Falls, New York has caused particular alarm. This site, which typifies many dump sites, contained more than 80 chemicals, many of which are human carcinogens. In 1981 Janerich et al. using the data in the New York Cancer Registry, concluded that the incidence of liver cancer, lymphoma, or leukemia in the census tracts adjacent to the Love Canal site was similar to that found in the upstate New York area (111). Lung cancer appeared to be more frequent among the Love Canal area residents. However, this finding did not appear to be related to chemical exposure at the site, because Niagara Falls residents, in upstate New York, have a high baseline rate of respiratory cancer when compared with the rest of New York State. The authors emphasized that the uncertain latency period for cancer and the small size of the study population are major deficiencies in their study.

Heath et al. in 1984 studied the frequency of chromosomal aberrations or sister chromatid exchange between residents living close to Love Canal and controls living in other parts of the Niagara Falls region (86). The analyses were performed on peripheral blood from 46 present or past residents of the Love Canal area. No significant differences were found in the frequency of chromosomal aberration or sister chromatid exchange when compared with controls. Cigarette smoking in both groups was associated with an increase in the frequency of sister chromatid exchange, a finding noted in other studies (177).

Thus far relatively few studies have evaluated the possible health effects of exposure to hazardous wastes, and few have yielded meaningful results (195). The epidemiologist investigating this question generally encounters major problems. Little if any information is available on exposure. Multiple exposures are present. The group under investigation is frequently so small that it is almost impossible to detect an adverse health effect. When the incidence of cancer is studied, the problem is further complicated by the long latent period between the initial exposure to a carcinogen and the clinical appearance of cancer.

BIOLOGICAL AND BIOCHEMICAL PRINCIPLES OF CARCINOGENESIS

Interaction between Environmental and Host Factors

Considerable emphasis has been placed on the importance of environmental factors in the causation of cancer. Environmental factors linked to cancer include chemical, physical, microbial, and viral agents. Such agents are found in the workplace, in the general environment, in the home, and in consumer products. Most cancers result from a complex interaction among environmental and host factors (90). An understanding of carcinogenesis must therefore include a knowledge of host as well as environmental factors. Host factors are defined as those elements present in the individual that influence his or her risk of developing cancer.

Some of the major host factors known to play a role in cancer causation in experimental animals and/or in humans are listed in Table 26-13 (218). Host factors can be inherited or acquired. They include such conditions as age, sex, genetic constitution, nutritional, hormonal, and immunologic status, prior exposure to environmental carcinogens, and the presence of disease. Although studies of carcinogen-metabolizing enzymes, DNA repair enzymes, and cell growth control processes are providing new insights into the mechanisms that underlie host factors in carcinogenesis, the mechanisms underlying the influence of most host factors (genetics, aging, nutritional status, immunologic status, etc.) are not well understood.

Particular attention has been directed to the interaction between genetic and environmental factors (138,147). The term ecogenetics was coined to describe the study of genetically determined variation in susceptibility to environmental agents (147). There are numerous well-documented examples of genetically determined differences in response to a variety of chemical exposures (113). These include genetic factors that influence an individual's susceptibility to environmentally induced cancer (146,178).

A rare but striking example of inherited susceptibility to cancer is the autosomal recessive genetic disease, xeroderma pigmentosum. This condition reflects an unusual sensitivity to solar radiation. It is characterized by the early onset of multiple skin cancers at sites exposed to sunlight. Xeroderma pigmentosum is linked to a genetic defect that diminishes the individual's ability to repair DNA that has been damaged by ultraviolet light. Another example of an inherited susceptibility to cancer is found in patients with ataxia telangiectasia. Such patients have increased susceptibility to γ-irradiation-induced malignancy. These are rare hereditary disorders, but they suggest that, within the general

TABLE 26-13.   Host Factors in Carcinogenesis[a]

Host factor	Genetic	Acquired	Genetic/acquired
Age	+		
Sex	+		
Hormones, growth factors, and receptors			+
Immunologic factors			+
Nutritional status		+	
Acquired diseases		+	
Prior exposure to environmental carcinogens (initiators, etc.)		+	
Carcinogen metabolism			+
DNA repair	+		
Chromosomal defects	+		
Cellular proliferation		+	
State of differentiation and gene expression		+	
Oncogenes and tumor suppressor genes	+		

[a]Modified from Weinstein (218).

population, less striking hereditary variations in DNA repair may influence susceptibility to specific types of environmental carcinogens.

Oncogenes

Early in the 1970s, molecular biologists studying retroviruses that cause cancer in animals discovered a set of genes that could induce cancer. These "oncogenes" were first found in viruses. Subsequently, however, investigation demonstrated that these genes were closely related to a similar set of genes, termed proto-oncogenes, that are normally found in the cells of higher animals and humans (14). A proto-oncogene is a gene that normally plays a major role in the control of growth and/or differentiation. It is a gene that has the capacity when mutated or "activated" to become an "oncogene," i.e., a gene that contributes to the abnormal behavior of tumor cells. New oncogenes continue to be identified each year. The current number of known oncogenes is about 50 (14). When normal cells are infected by viruses that carry activated forms of these oncogenes, perhaps originally derived from normal cells, they can be transformed into cancer cells. There is increasing evidence that cellular oncogenes are involved in the transformation of cells by chemical carcinogens. Under these conditions, the DNA damage induced by exposure to the carcinogen triggers rearrangements, mutations, and/or switching-on of the inactive proto-oncogene to form an active oncogene. These changes can occur in the absence of a virus vector. Should this hypothesis be correct, it might be possible to identify rapidly the cellular genes involved in environmental carcinogenesis. Indeed, recent studies implicate specific cellular oncogenes in the causation of a number of human cancers including bladder and lung cancer (48,64,149,201). It is noteworthy that oncogenes play

a role in only part of the multistep process of carcinogenesis. Negative gene regulators or tumor suppressor genes have also been identified (213).

Clearly, a major challenge to future research in carcinogenesis is to identify the specific cellular genes involved in the transformation of cells by chemical and physical agents. Because of the multistep nature of the carcinogenic process and the complex interactions between environmental and host factors, it seems likely that multiple genes are involved in this process (224). Indeed, studies indicate that the multistage carcinogenic process is often associated with the progressive accumulation of activating mutations in cellular oncogenes and inactivating mutations or deletions in tumor suppressor genes (14,27A,176A,213,220).

Diet and Cancer

There is evidence that host factors, acting at a systemic level or directly on the cells undergoing malignant change, may enhance or inhibit the carcinogenic process. Of particular importance is the influence of the host's nutrition (35,36). Epidemiologic studies reveal that variations in the incidence of specific types of cancer in different populations can often be correlated with differences in diet (35,36,49). These findings are further buttressed by animal studies showing marked dietary influences on the incidence of specific cancers. An understanding of the relationship between diet and cancer could be of great practical importance because dietary changes may provide a powerful means of preventing specific types of cancer. The interested reader is referred to a comprehensive review of this subject (36).

During the past decade it has been shown that the induction of cancer in experimental animals by specific chemicals can be inhibited by a number of compounds contained in food (208,210,212). These compounds, which include indoles, flavones, phenols, and aromatic isothiocyanates, are natural constituents of a number of vegetables. Cruciferous vegetables, which include Brussels sprouts, cabbage, broccoli, and cauliflower, are particularly rich in these agents (36,209). Animals fed such plants (or given the specific chemicals mentioned above) and then treated with such known carcinogens as benzo[a]pyrene (BaP) or dimethylbenz[a]anthracene (DMBA) develop fewer cancers than the control group. Other inhibitors include coumarins and simple lactones present in a wide variety of vegetables and fruits. The synthetic antioxidant butylated hydroxyanisole (BHA), widely used as a food additive, also inhibits chemical carcinogenesis (210,211).

There is evidence that such diverse compounds as indoles, phenols, flavones, and aromatic isothiocyanates inhibit chemical carcinogenesis by interfering with the metabolism of carcinogens. Some inhibitors may block the enzymatic activation of the carcinogen to its reactive carcinogenic form, whereas others may interact directly with the reactive carcinogen and thus act as scavengers (211).

Epidemiologic studies suggest that inhibitors present in the diet also play a role in preventing human cancer. A number of epidemiologic studies reveal an inverse relationship between the consumption of vegetables containing naturally occurring inhibitors and the risk of gastrointestinal cancer (36). Graham et al. reported that consumption of such raw vegetables as cole slaw and red cabbage was associated with a lower incidence of stomach cancer (66). An inverse relationship between the consumption of vegetables and the risk of stomach cancer has been reported (75,76).

Attention has also been directed to the role of vitamins in cancer prevention. The strongest evidence relates to the role of vitamin A and other retinoids in the prevention of malignancy. Retinoids have been shown to be effective in inhibiting chemical carcinogenesis in experimental animals. These agents are particularly effective in preventing breast, bladder, and skin cancer (20,134,135,180). Epidemiologic evidence also indicates that there is an inverse relationship between the consumption of vitamin A and its precursors and the risk of cancer (36). Limited epidemiologic studies on the effect of vitamin C in relation to the incidence of cancer suggest that consumption of foods high in this vitamin reduces the risk for gastric and esophageal cancer (36).

Metabolism of Chemical Carcinogens

Metabolic Activation

A basic principle in the biochemistry of carcinogenesis is that a number of chemical carcinogens must be metabolized in order to exert their carcinogenic effect. The carcinogenic potential of many compounds is achieved when they undergo metabolic activation to electrophilic and highly reactive intermediates that are capable of reacting with cellular macromolecules to form covalent adducts (87, 132,216). The critical event in this process is most likely covalent binding to DNA. The term "reactive" is used to describe a chemically unstable molecule that, in order to reach a more stable state, rapidly interacts with suitable nearby molecules. This process generally involves the sharing of electrons and the formation of a covalent bond.

The metabolism of the polycyclic aromatic hydrocarbon benzo[a]pyrene, a known carcinogen, provides an excellent example of the process of activation. This agent is not highly reactive chemically: when mixed with nucleic acid or protein, it will not form covalent bonds. The metabolic action of the enzymes present in the endoplasmic reticulum dramatically changes this condition. These microsomal enzymes, which also function to detoxify many environmental pollutants by converting them to water-soluble excretable compounds, activate benzo[a]pyrene by converting it to a mixture of epoxides. These highly reactive intermediates, unless further metabolized, will interact with cellular DNA and other macromolecules to form covalent adducts. It has been shown, using a group of polycyclic aromatic hydrocarbons, that the ability of a chemical substance to bind covalently to DNA of mouse skin correlates with its carcinogenic potency (65). In the case of benzo[a]pyrene, the major reactive intermediate is a specific diol epoxide that interacts with guanine residues in cellular DNA (Fig. 26-3). The

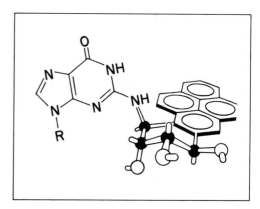

FIGURE 26-3. Structure of an adduct formed by a guanine base in DNA shown on the left linked to an epoxide derivative of benzo[a]pyrene shown on the right. From Weinstein (214).

pathway described above for BaP can be generalized to a number of other carcinogens that are activated by the microsomal enzyme system (62,112,132,216).

It is becoming clear that the metabolism of carcinogens within the organism often represents a balance between metabolic detoxication and activation. The choice between detoxication and activation—the latter process resulting in carcinogenic molecules linked to DNA—depends on the nature of the chemical, its concentration, and the animal species involved. The host's genetic background, previous exposure history, nutritional status, parallel exposure to other agents, and tissue-specific factors also determine whether a chemical carcinogen will be activated and attach to cellular macromolecules or be detoxified and excreted. The process of detoxication and activation is discussed in detail in Chapter 9.

DNA Adducts

Although the above discussion has focused on BaP, the chemistry, metabolism, and nucleic acid interactions of several other types of carcinogens are now understood in considerable detail (72,74,132). Different carcinogens can attack different sites on the DNA, and a single carcinogen can form multiple adducts. These conditions complicate attempts to formulate a unified theory relating specific types of DNA damage to the mechanism of carcinogenesis. There is evidence, however, that the major carcinogen-DNA adducts, in diverse species and tissues, are generally the same. This finding provides some unity to the comparative chemistry of carcinogen-DNA adducts (216). In vitro studies provide direct evidence that modification of DNA and RNA by carcinogens impairs their template activities during replication, transcription, and translation (73).

Free Radicals

The mechanism of chemical carcinogenesis may, in addition to being linked to the formation of carcinogen-DNA adducts, also be dependent on the generation of free radicals (5,192). Free radicals are atomic or molecular species that, by virtue of possessing unpaired electrons, are extremely reactive. Free radicals may produce carcinogenic effects by inducing strand breaks in DNA. There is evidence that free radicals are produced with membrane lipid and radiation damage, with exposure to a variety of toxic chemicals, and during the metabolism of chemical carcinogens (5,139). The possibility that the reactive species in the induction of cancer may be oxidants or free radicals is supported by the inhibition of chemical carcinogenesis by antioxidants and free-radical scavengers (5,210).

DNA Repair

Fortunately, cells are capable of repairing the cellular DNA damage induced by environmental chemicals and radiation. Biochemical studies reveal that a number of local excision-repair mechanisms restore the normal nucleic acid structure of DNA. The multiplicity of excision mechanisms and enzymes that have evolved to protect the DNA from the onslaught of environmental chemicals is somewhat reassuring. But there remains the danger that the environment may become sufficiently polluted to overtax these defenses. A detailed review of DNA repair mechanisms can be found in a publication by Hanawalt et al. (80).

Perhaps the strongest evidence to support the concept that DNA repair mechanisms are important in the prevention of cancer is the high incidence of skin cancer in patients with xeroderma pigmentosum. Individuals affected by this condition have an autosomal recessive disease that results in a marked inability to repair DNA damage caused by ultraviolet light (80). Other types of deficiencies in DNA repair mechanisms may, in part, explain individual differences in carcinogen susceptibility.

Presumably, the carcinogenic process is initiated when unrepaired DNA damage, including DNA-chemical adducts, produces heritable gene mutations and alterations in gene expression. The level and persistence of some DNA adducts are appreciable (30). It seems likely that complex cellular responses to altered DNA exist in higher organisms and play a key role in carcinogenesis (110,216). Studies are in progress to determine whether the net results include such heritable changes in oncogenes as point mutations, sequence deletions, gene amplications, or gross chromosomal rearrangements.

Stages of Carcinogenesis

It is now apparent that carcinogenesis is a multistage process that can proceed during a large portion of an individual's life span. Chemically induced carcinogenesis is characterized, in certain model systems, as a two-stage process. The first stage is identified as initiation; the second stage as promotion. A third stage of tumor progression is also recognized in the vast majority of malignant neoplasms (12,58). The multistage development of cancer underlines the importance of understanding the agents involved in tumor initiation, promotion, and progression and of monitoring the environment for chemicals that exert these effects. An overview of the molecular and cellular mechanisms by which various chemical agents influence the multistage carcinogenic process is given by Weinstein (219,220).

The most powerful paradigm for understanding the complex two-stage phenomenon has been the model of cancer produced in mouse skin. Studies of epidermal carcinogenesis in the mouse clearly demonstrate the two stages of cancer development. The first stage, initiation, takes place when a single application of a known carcinogen, such as benzo[a]pyrene, is directly applied to the skin at a low dose. If the animal receives no further treatment, no neoplasms are formed. The second stage, promotion, takes place when a second noncarcinogenic agent such as the potent tumor promoter 12-O-tetradecanoylphorbol-13-acetate (TPA) is repeatedly applied to the skin following the initial treatment with the carcinogen. In specific strains of mice, this combination of initiation and promotion results in the occurrence of multiple skin tumors, both papillomas and carcinomas. Tumors are produced even if the interval between the initial application of the initiator and that of the promoter is as long as a year. Repeated applications of the promoter alone or before treatment with the carcinogen produce transient hyperplasia but no tumors. There is evidence that liver cancer, bladder cancer, colon cancer, and breast cancer also proceed via processes analogous to the two-stage mechanism of carcinogenesis. A graphic representation of the experiments performed on mouse skin, demonstrating the properties of cancer initiation and promotion, is shown in Fig. 26-4.

The existence of a latent period between the initial application of a carcinogen and the appearance of a neoplasm has been known for many years. This latency period can occupy over 50% of the animal's life span and has been found with all of the known carcinogens. Support for the view that the latency period consists of the initiation and promotion phases in cancer development is based on a variety of experimental studies.

There is no direct evidence that the stages of initiation and promotion apply to human cancer, but there are indications that similar processes may be operable in man. There is ample evidence that a latent period exists between the initial exposure to a carcinogen and the clinical appearance of cancer. A latent period is clearly demonstrated in the development of bronchogenic carcinoma associated with smoking and of cancers resulting from exposure to radiation or to occupational carcinogens. Epidemiologic studies also support the concept that certain agents have a cancer-promoting action. It has been shown, for example, that smokers who consume large amounts of alcohol have a significantly increased risk of developing cancer of the larynx, esophagus, and oral cavity (231). Cigarette smoking, when combined with asbestos exposure, dramatically increases the incidence of lung cancer (78). Experimental evidence indicates that alcohol per se is not carcinogenic; cigarette smoke possesses both initiating and promoting properties.

Features of Cancer Initiation, Promotion, and Progression

Studies on skin cancer in the mouse indicate that tumor initiation involves biological and bio-

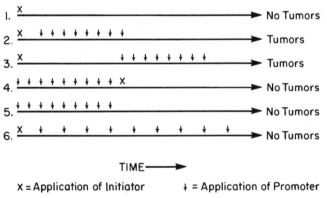

FIGURE 26-4. Outline of experiments demonstrating initiation and promotion as developed from studies of carcinogenesis of mouse skin. Each line represents an experimental condition in which there is either no application or a single application (x) of the initiating agent, usually a carcinogenic polycyclic hydrocarbon. The multiple vertical arrows represent multiple applications of the promoting agent (croton oil, phorbol ester, or other known promoters for mouse skin). The time span may extend from 15 to more than 70 weeks, depending on the dosages of the initiator and promoter used, the mouse strain employed, or the format of the experiment. In line 3, the delay between initiation and promotion may be more than a year. In line 6, the time intervals between application of the promoting agent may be 4 weeks or more, whereas in the other experiments the promoting agent is applied twice weekly. From Pitot (163).

chemical processes that are quite distinct from those of tumor promotion (Table 26-14) (217). The major difference is that initiation appears to involve DNA damage, whereas promotion does not. It appears that covalent binding of the initiating agent to DNA is the critical event in the action of the initiating agent. Irreversibility and the absence of a measurable threshold below which no tumors are produced are also important features of the initiation process. The major portion of this chapter has been concerned with chemical agents that initiate the carcinogenic process.

In contrast, tumor promoters do not bind covalently to cellular macromolecules and are not mutagenic. Tumor promotion can be reversed in its early stage, and promoting agents require repeated applications at frequent intervals to exert their effects (Fig. 26-4). A number of initiating agents, when administered in large or repeated doses, act as complete carcinogens, suggesting that they can also act as promoters. Promoting agents when given alone may induce a small number of tumors, perhaps because of the spontaneous occurrence of initiation.

Until recently there were very few specific cellular or biochemical markers for the action of tumor promoters. Much of our understanding has come from studies with the phorbol ester promoting agents in cell culture systems and on mouse skin. Studies indicate that the phorbol ester tumor promoters act by binding to a specific enzyme, protein kinase C, an enzyme that plays a key role in signal transduction (27A,220). This induces alterations in cellular growth, gene expression, and differentiation (19). These effects are mediated through the phosphorylation of serine and threonine residues on specific cellular proteins (27A,145). Much less is known about the mechanism of action of other classes of tumor promoters and about the specific biochemical events associated with tumor promotion in tissues other than the skin, e.g., the liver, breast, colon, bladder (67). The discovery that these processes also involve the activation of protein kinases would provide a general approach to detecting tumor promoters in the environment.

A number of agents, in addition to the phorbol esters, have been identified as promoters of carcinogenesis. These include such substances as dietary fat, alcohol, cigarette smoke, halogenated hydrocarbons (dioxin, PCBs), and synthetic estrogens (Table 26-15) (163). Epidemiologic studies indicate that some of these agents are important factors in the development of cancer in humans. There is considerable evidence, for example, that high dietary lipids increase the risk for breast and colon cancer and that alcohol increases the risk for esophageal, gastric, and hepatic cancer (127). There is also evidence that suggests that hormones play a role in the genesis of human breast cancer. Thus, women have a much greater risk of breast cancer than men. The disease is absent before puberty; premenopausal castration reduces its incidence; and an early age of first pregnancy is protective (116,118).

A third stage of cancer development, termed progression, has been defined (12,58). During this stage tumors acquire increasing degrees of malignancy and invasiveness. Their growth rate and metastatic frequency also increase. Tumor progression and the evolution of tumors into more heterogeneous cell populations is often associated with chromosomal abnormalities visible by light microscopy and gene amplification. The list of chromosomal abnormalities associated with specific types of human cancer is growing rapidly (119,168). Gross chromosomal changes may play an important role in the multistep development of cancer, particularly during the later stages of the process. The basic biological and biochemical facts related to chemical carcinogenesis are summarized in Table 26-16 (215, 222).

Chemical-Viral Interactions

There are several examples in which initiating carcinogens, tumor promoters, or other chemical and physical agents interact synergistically with viruses in the carcinogenic process. This interaction, which occurs in vivo and in cell culture, has recently been reviewed (56,67,221). It seems likely that cer-

TABLE 26-14. Biological Properties of Initiating and Promoting Agents[a]

Initiating agents	Promoting agents
1. Carcinogenic by themselves, "solitary carcinogens"	1. Not carcinogenic alone
2. Must be given before promoting agent	2. Must be given after the initiating agent
3. Single exposure sufficient	3. Require prolonged exposure
4. Action "irreversible" and additive	4. Action reversible (at early stage) and not additive
5. No apparent threshold	5. Possible threshold
6. Yield electrophiles that bind covalently to cell macromolecules	6. No evidence of covalent binding
7. Mutagenic	7. Not mutagenic

[a]Modified from Weinstein (217).

TABLE 26-15. Promoting Agents in the Human Environment and the Neoplasms Associated with Prolonged Contact with Those Agents[a]

Agent	Resultant neoplasm
Dietary fat (calories)	Increased cancer incidence in general with excess caloric intake
	Mammary adenocarcinoma
Cigarette smoke	Bronchogenic carcinoma
	Esophageal and bladder cancer
Asbestos	Bronchogenic carcinoma and mesothelioma
Halogenated hydrocarbons (TCDD, PCBs)	Liver
Saccharin	Bladder
Phenobarbital	Liver
Prolactin	Mammary adenocarcinoma
Synthetic estrogens	Liver adenomas
Alcoholic beverages	Liver and esophageal cancer, oral cancer

[a]From Pitot (163).

tain human cancers may be caused by interactions between environmental chemicals and certain types of viruses that alone would have little or no oncogenic potential. This appears to be the case for liver cancer in Africa, nasopharyngeal cancer in Asia, and Burkitt lymphoma. Hepatitis B virus infection (probably in combination with exposure to aflatoxin) appears to be a causative factor in the high incidence of liver cancer in Africa. Epstein-Barr virus (in combination with unknown environmental factors) has been implicated in nasopharyngeal cancer in Asia and in Burkitt lymphoma in Africa. Recent studies suggest that papilloma viruses, in combination with certain environmental agents, may be involved in the causation of human cervical cancer (63). Greater progress might be made in designing studies concerned with cancer causation and prevention if there were an awareness that certain human cancers may result from complex interactions between viruses and chemicals and that the final pathways by which both classes of agents produce cell transformation may be quite similar.

NEW METHODS OF ASSESSING CARCINOGEN EXPOSURE AND DETECTING INCREASED CANCER RISK

Although conventional approaches in cancer epidemiology have provided a wealth of information, they are seriously limited in their ability to detect and evaluate carcinogenic hazards. Animal bioassays and the newly developed short-term tests, although extremely sensitive and useful for detecting potential human carcinogens, are flawed by the paucity of information on how such data can be extrapolated to humans (155,216).

Clearly, the solution to these problems will not come from performing more of the same types of studies. Rather, it must come from applying new

methods to the study of human carcinogenesis. Epidemiologic methods combined with newly developed laboratory procedures that provide biological markers of molecular or biochemical events linked to carcinogen exposure supply a new approach to the study of human cancer causation. This approach has been termed "molecular cancer epidemiology" (151,152,155). The goal of molecular cancer

TABLE 26-16. Chemical Carcinogens: Basic Biologic and Biochemical Facts[a]

1. Carcinogenesis is dose dependent: the larger the dose, the greater the incidence of tumors, and the shorter the lag. There is no evidence of a threshold dose below which a carcinogen is safe.
2. There is a long lag between exposure and the appearance of tumors. In humans this is about 5–30 years. In various species the lag is generally proportional to the life span of the species. Carcinogens can act transplacentally, with tumors appearing only later in the adult progeny.
3. Conversion of a normal tissue to a malignant neoplasm is a multistep process.
4. The action of certain types of carcinogens, so-called initiating agents, is markedly enhanced by promoting agents, hormonal agents, and various cofactors.
5. Cellular proliferation enhances carcinogenesis.
6. Neoplasms induced by the same chemical carcinogen often display antigenic diversity as well as a general diversity of phenotypes in terms of growth rate, degree of differentiation, cell surface properties, enzyme profiles, etc.
7. Carcinogens are subject to both metabolic activation and detoxication in vivo.
8. The metabolically activated forms of carcinogens are highly reactive electrophiles that bind covalently to nucleophilic residues in cellular proteins and nucleic acids.

[a]Modified from Weinstein (215).

epidemiology is to identify specific carcinogenic hazards in the environment, to assess their biologically effective dose and biological effect, and to provide a means of appraising host factors that modify susceptibility. With such data in hand the risks associated with carcinogen exposure can be estimated with greater accuracy and precision.

From an epidemiologic perspective, the term "biochemical" or "molecular" epidemiology indicates that biological markers have been used in analytic epidemiologic research (101). Biological markers that provide evidence of cellular biochemical, or molecular changes in tissues, cells, or fluids have long been used in epidemiologic research. For example, serum cholesterol, lipids, and lipoprotein fractions have aided epidemiologists in the study of cardiovascular disease. The recent development of a variety of highly sensitive and specific laboratory procedures now promises to aid the cancer epidemiologist by providing markers of (1) genetic and acquired host susceptibility (139,148), (2) metabolism and tissue levels of carcinogens (160), (3) levels of carcinogen molecules chemically linked to DNA (30,151,152,155), and (4) early cellular responses to carcinogen exposure, e.g., sister chromatid exchange, DNA repair, altered gene expression, gene mutations, oncogene activation. Thus far all of the current markers of carcinogenic dose reflect genetic damage to the DNA or the chromosome. No methods are currently available for routinely screening individuals for genetic traits that predispose to cancer.

A particularly promising tool of molecular cancer epidemiology is the highly sensitive immunoassay for carcinogen-DNA adducts (153,155,160,161). These assays may provide a tissue dosimeter of carcinogen exposure. Such assays, because they take into account such complex pharmacodynamic parameters as the metabolic activation of the carcinogen in question, would be more valid measures of exposure than the simple measurement of ambient levels. Research studies are in progress to assess the levels of carcinogen-DNA adducts in individuals exposed to various carcinogens. Utilizing the DNA collected from white blood cells, placenta, or tissue specimens obtained from surgical biopsy or autopsy material, investigators are examining the data to see if they correlate with the risk of developing cancer.

It is hoped that as methodological problems are solved and protocols are standardized, assays of carcinogen molecules chemically linked to DNA will be widely applied to clinical and epidemiologic studies (10). Such studies are currently being performed (88). At the present time there are no simple tests to detect, in human samples, the action of tumor promoters or cofactors. Basic research in this area is proceeding rapidly.

Several carcinogens form covalent adducts with proteins. Ehrenberg and co-workers have shown that the covalent modification of hemoglobin can be used as a monitor of carcinogen exposure. Hemoglobin serves as a convenient "trapping" agent for assessing the levels of activated carcinogens in vivo. It can be obtained in large amounts from red blood cells, has a long half-life, and is readily purified and analyzed. The covalent modification of hemoglobin has been used to estimate the extent of exposure and disease risk in workers exposed to ethylene oxide (26,53) (see Chapter 27 for further discussion of biological monitoring of genotoxic agents).

PREVENTION OF CANCER

The obvious goal of understanding the complex subject of environmental carcinogenesis is to develop a sound rationale for cancer prevention (69,223). At present, our understanding of the genesis of cancer is incomplete, and we are often thwarted in our attempts to demonstrate cancer causation at the level of individual compounds. It is well to remember, however, that preventive measures can and should be initiated before the pathogenesis of cancer is completely understood. Such measures are based on what is known at present (36,69,70,212). Smoking cessation, reduction of exposure to hazardous chemicals in the workplace, reduction of environmental pollution, and alterations in our diet are examples of such preventive measures.

Although efforts for cancer prevention related to the workplace or the general environment must, in large part, fall within the realm of government and industry, there are several personal measures that are useful in reducing the risk of cancer. These are listed in Table 26-17. Specific dietary recommendations from the American Cancer Society are listed

TABLE 26-17. Ten Personal Measures for Cancer Prevention

1. Avoid cigarette smoking (could prevent 30% of cancer deaths)
2. Avoid excessive exposure to sunlight
3. Avoid dietary excesses—alcohol, high-fat diet, unnecessary food additives and preservatives
4. Avoid unnecessary drug exposure
5. Avoid exposure to pesticides, chemical fumes, dusts
6. Avoid unnecessary diagnostic x rays
7. Avoid exposure to toxic materials in the workplace
8. Protect the fetus from drugs, various chemicals, radiation
9. Be well informed on the benefits and risks of consumer products
10. Read the labels of consumer products and maintain a high index of suspicion of the safety of new products

TABLE 26-18.   Nutrition and Cancer: American Cancer Society Recommendations[a]

1. Avoid obesity
2. Cut down on total fat intake
3. Eat more high-fiber foods, such as whole-grain cereals, fruits, and vegetables
4. Include foods rich in vitamins A and C in the daily diet
5. Include cruciferous vegetables, such as cabbage, broccoli, Brussels sprouts, kohlrabi, and cauliflower, in the diet
6. Be moderate in consumption of alcoholic beverages
7. Be moderate in consumption of salt-cured, smoked, and nitrite-cured foods

[a]From American Cancer Society (3).

in Table 26-18 (3). Similar dietary recommendations have been made by the National Research Council in their report, *Diet Nutrition and Cancer* (36).

REFERENCES

1. Alavanja M, Goldstein I, Susser M: A case-control study of gastrointestinal and urinary tract cancer mortality and drinking water chlorination. In: Water Chlorination. Environmental Impact and Health Effects, Vol 2, p 395, Jolley RL, Goirchev H, Hamilton DH Jr (eds.), Ann Arbor Science Publishers, Ann Arbor, 1978.
2. Alavanja MCR, Blair A, Master MN: Cancer mortality in U.S. flour industry. J Natl Cancer Inst 82:840, 1990.
3. American Cancer Society: Cancer Facts and Figures, ACS, Washington, 1991.
4. Ames BN: Identification of environmental chemicals causing mutations and cancer. Science 204:587, 1979.
5. Ames BN: Dietary carcinogens and anticarcinogens: Oxygen radicals and degenerative diseases. Science 221:1256, 1983.
6. Ames BN, Gold LS: Too many rodent carcinogens: Mitogenesis increases mutagenesis. Science 249:970, 1990.
7. Anderson HA, Lilis R, Daum SM, et al: Household-contact asbestos neoplastic risk. Ann NY Acad Sci 271:311, 1976.
8. Bailar JC III, Crouch AC, Shaikh D, et al: One-hit models of carcinogenesis: Conservative or not? Risk Anal 8:485, 1988.
9. Baris YI, Artvinli M, Sahin AA: Environmental mesothelioma in Turkey. Ann NY Acad Sci 330:423, 1979.
10. Bartsch H, Hemminki K, O'Neill LK (eds.): Methods for Detecting DNA Damaging Agents in Humans: Application in Cancer Epidemiology and Prevention, IARC Scientific Publication No. 89, International Agency for Research on Cancer, Lyon, 1988.
11. Beaumont JJ, Breslow NE: Power considerations in epidemiologic studies of vinyl chloride workers. Am J Epidemiol 114:725, 1981.
12. Berenblum I: Sequential aspects of chemical carcinogenesis: Skin. In: Cancer: A Comprehensive Treatise, 2nd ed., Vol 1, p 451, Becker FF (ed.), Plenum Press, New York, 1982.
13. Bertazzi PA, Zocchetti C, Pesatori AC, et al: Ten-year mortality study of the population involved in the Seveso incident in 1976. Am J Epidemiol 129:1187, 1989.
14. Bishop JM: Molecular themes in oncogenesis. Cell 64:235, 1991.
15. Blair A: Herbicides and non-Hodgkin's lymphoma: New evidence from a study of Saskatchewan farmers. J Natl Cancer Inst 82:544, 1990.
16. Blair A, Malker H, Cantor KP, et al: Cancer among farmers: A review. Scand J Work Environ Health 11:397, 1985.
17. Bloom AD (ed.): Guidelines for Studies of Human Populations Exposed to Mutagenic and Reproductive Hazards. March of Dimes Birth Defects Foundation, New York, 1981.
18. Blot WJ, Fraumeni JF Jr: Arsenical air pollution and lung cancer. Lancet 2:142, 1975.
19. Blumberg PM, Delclos KB, Dunn JA, et al: Phorbol ester receptors and the in vitro effects of tumor promoters. Ann NY Acad Sci 407:303, 1983.
20. Bollag W: Prophylaxis of chemically induced benign and malignant epithelial tumors by vitamin A acid (retinoic acid). Eur J Cancer 8:689, 1972.
21. Boyle CA, Decoufle P, O'Brien TR: Long-term health consequences of military service in Vietnam. Epidemiol Rev 11:3, 1989.
22. Buell P: Relative impact of smoking and air pollution on lung cancer. Arch Environ Health 15:291, 1967.
23. Buesching DP, Wollstadt L: Cancer mortality among farmers. J Natl Cancer Inst 72:503, 1984.
24. Bumb RR, Crummett WB, Cutie SS, et al: Trace chemistries of fire: Source of chlorinated dioxins. Science 210:385, 1980.
25. Burmeister LF, Everett GD, Van Lier SF, et al: Selected cancer mortality and farm practices in Iowa. Am J Epidemiol 118:72, 1983.
26. Calleman CJ, Ehrenberg L, Jansson B, et al: Monitoring and risk assessment by means of alkyl groups in hemoglobin in persons occupationally exposed to ethylene oxide. J Environ Pathol Toxicol 2:427, 1978.
27. Cantor KP: Epidemiological evidence of carcinogenicity of chlorinated organics in drinking water. Environ Health Perspect 46:187, 1982.
27A. Cantley LC, Auger KR, Carpenter C, et al: Oncogenes and signal transduction. Cell 64:281, 1991.
28. Cantor KP: Farming and mortality from non-Hodgkin's lymphoma: A case-control study. Int J Cancer 29:239, 1982.
29. Carnow BW, Meier P: Air pollution and pulmonary cancer. Arch Environ Health 27:207, 1973.
30. Cerutti P: Persistence of carcinogen-DNA adducts in cultured mammalian cells. In: Mechanisms of Chemical Carcinogenesis, p 419, Harris CC, Cerutti PA (eds.), Alan R Liss, New York, 1982.
31. Coggon D, Pannett B, Winter PD, et al: Mortality of workers exposed to 2-methyl-4-chlorophenoxy acetic acid. Scand J Work Environ Health 12:448, 1986.
32. Cohen SM, Ellwein LB: Cell proliferation and carcinogenesis. Science 249:1007, 1990.

33. Committee on Biological Effects of Atmospheric Pollutants, National Research Council: Particulate Polycyclic Organic Matter, National Academy Press, Washington, 1972.

34. Committee on the Biological Effects of Ionizing Radiations: Health Effects of Exposure to Low Levels of Ionizing Radiation, BIER V, National Academy Press, Washington, 1990.

35. Committee on Diet and Health, National Research Council: Diet and Health, National Academy Press, Washington, 1989.

36. Committee on Diet, Nutrition and Cancer, National Research Council: Diet, Nutrition, and Cancer, National Academy Press, Washington, 1982.

37. Committee on Nonoccupational Health Risks of Asbestiform Fibers, National Research Council: Asbestiform Fibers: Nonoccupational Health Risks, National Academy Press, Washington, 1984.

38. Committee on Passive Smoking, National Research Council: Environmental Tobacco Smoke: Measuring Exposure and Assessing Health Effects, National Academy Press, Washington, 1986.

39. Committee on Scientific and Regulatory Issues Underlying Pesticide Use Patterns and Agricultural Innovation, National Research Council: Regulating Pesticides in Food, National Academy Press, Washington, 1987.

40. Cook RR, Townsend JC, Ott MG, et al: Mortality experience of employees exposed to 2,3,7,8-tetrachlorodibenzo-p-dioxin (TCDD). J Occup Med 22:530, 1980.

41. Correa P, Fontham E, Pickle LW, et al: Passive smoking and lung cancer. Lancet 2:595, 1983.

42. Council of Scientific Affairs: The Health Effects of "Agent Orange" and Polychlorinated Dioxin Contaminants: An Update, 1984, Technical Report, American Medical Association, Chicago, 1984.

43. Courtney KD, Moore JA: Teratology studies with 2,4,5-trichlorophenoxyacetic acid and 2,3,7,8-tetrachlorodibenzo-p-dioxin. Toxicol Appl Pharmacol 20:396, 1971.

44. Davis DL, Bridbord K, Schneiderman M: Cancer prevention: Assessing causes, exposures, and recent trends in mortality for U.S. males 1968–1978. Teratogen Carcinogen Mutagen 2:105, 1982.

45. Davis DL, Hoel D, Fox J, et al: International trends in cancer mortality in France, West Germany, Italy, Japan, England and Wales, and the USA. Lancet 2:474, 1990.

46. Dean G: Lung cancer in South Africans and British immigrants. Proc R Soc Med 57:984, 1964.

47. Dean G: Lung cancer and bronchitis in Northern Ireland, 1960–1962. Br Med J 1:1506, 1966.

48. Der CJ, Krontiris TG, Cooper GM: Transforming genes of human bladder and lung carcinoma cell lines are homologous to the ras gene of Harvey and Kirsten sarcoma viruses. Proc Natl Acad Sci USA 79:3637, 1982.

49. Doll R, Peto R: The Causes of Cancer: Quantitative Estimates of Avoidable Risks of Cancer in the United States Today, Oxford University Press, New York, 1981.

50. Douglas JF (ed.): Carcinogenesis and Mutagenesis Testing, Humana Press, Clifton, New Jersey, 1984.

51. Eastcott DF: The epidemiology of lung cancer in New Zealand. Lancet 1:37, 1956.

52. Editorial: The aetiology of melanoma. Lancet 1:253, 1981.

53. Ehrenberg L: Risk assessment of ethylene oxide and other compounds. In: Assessing Chemical Mutagens: The Risk to Humans, Banbury Report 1, p 157, McElheny VK, Abrahamson S (eds.), Cold Spring Harbor Laboratory, New York, 1979.

54. Epidemiology Work Group of the Interagency Regulatory Liaison Group: Guidelines for documentation of epidemiologic studies. Am J Epidemiol 114:609, 1981.

55. Eriksson M, Hardell L, Berg NO, et al: Soft-tissue sarcomas and exposure to chemical substances: A case-referent study. Br J Ind Med 38:27, 1981.

56. Fisher PB, Weinstein IB: Chemical viral interactions and multistep aspects of cell transformation. In: Molecular and Cellular Aspects of Carcinogen Screening Tests, p 76, Montesano R, Bartsch H, Tomatis L (eds.), IARC Scientific Publications, Lyon, 1980.

57. Fisher PB, Weinstein IB: In vitro screening tests for potential carcinogens. In: Carcinogens in the Environment and Industry, p 113, Sontag JM (ed.), Marcell Dekker, New York, 1981.

58. Foulds L: Neoplastic Development, Vol 1, Academic Press, New York, 1969.

59. Garfinkel L: Time trends in lung cancer mortality among nonsmokers and a note on passive smoking. J Natl Cancer Inst 66:1061, 1981.

60. Gay BW Jr, Lonneman WA, Bridbord K, et al: Measurements of vinyl chloride from aerosol sprays. Ann NY Acad Sci 246:286, 1975.

61. Gehring PJ, Blau GE: Mechanisms of carcinogenesis: Dose response. Cancer Bull 29:152, 1977.

62. Gelboin HV, Ts'o POP (eds.): Polycyclic Hydrocarbons and Cancer, Vols 1 and 2, Academic Press, New York, 1978.

63. Gissmann L, Boshart M, Durst M, et al: Presence of human papillomavirus in genital tumors. J Invest Dermatol 83(1 Suppl):26s, 1984.

64. Goldfarb M, Shimizu K, Perucho M, et al: Isolation and preliminary characterization of a human transforming gene from T24 bladder carcinoma cells. Nature 296:404, 1982.

65. Goshman LM, Heidelberger C: Binding of tritium-labeled polycyclic hydrocarbons to DNA of mouse skin. Cancer Res 72:1678, 1961.

66. Graham S, Schotz W, Martino P: Alimentary factors in the epidemiology of gastric cancer. Cancer 30:927, 1972.

67. Greenbaum E, Weinstein IB: Relevance of the concept of tumor promotion to the causation of human cancer. Progress in Surgical Pathology 2:27, 1981.

68. Greenberg MR: Urbanization and Cancer Mortality: The United States Experience, 1950–1975, Oxford University Press, New York, 1983.

69. Greenwald P: Principles of Cancer Prevention: Diet and Nutrition. In: Cancer Principles and Practice of Oncology, 3rd ed., p 167, DeVita VT, Hellman S, Rosenberg SA (eds.), Lippincott, Philadelphia, 1989.

70. Greenwald P, Sondik E, Lynch BS: Diet and chemoprevention in NCI's research strategy to achieve na-

tional cancer control objectives. Annu Rev Public Health 7:267, 1986.

71. Grisham JW (ed.): Health Aspects of the Disposal of Waste Chemicals, Pergamon Press, New York, 1986.

72. Grover P (ed.): Chemical Carcinogens and DNA, CRC Press, Boca Raton, 1979.

73. Grunberger D, Weinstein IB: Biochemical effects of the modification of nucleic acids by certain polycyclic aromatic carcinogens. In: Progress in Nucleic Acid Research and Molecular Biology, p 105, Cohn WE (ed.), Academic Press, Orlando, 1979.

74. Grunberger D, Weinstein IB: Conformational changes in nucleic acids modified by chemical carcinogens. In: Chemical Carcinogens and DNA, Vol 1, p 59, Grover P (ed.), CRC Press, Boca Raton, 1979.

75. Haenszel W, Kurihara M, Segi M, et al: Stomach cancer among Japanese in Hawaii. J Natl Cancer Inst 49:969, 1972.

76. Haenszel W, Kurihara M, Lock FB, et al: Stomach cancer in Japan. J Natl Cancer Inst 56:265, 1976.

77. Hammond EC, Horn D: Smoking and death rates: Report on forty-four months of follow-up of 187,783 men. JAMA 166:1294, 1958; reprinted JAMA 251:2840, 1984.

78. Hammond EC, Selikoff IJ: Asbestos exposure, smoking and neoplasia. JAMA 204:104, 1968.

79. Hammond EC, Selikoff IJ, Seidman H: Asbestos exposure, cigarette smoking and death rates. Ann NY Acad Sci 330:473, 1979.

80. Hanawalt PC, Cooper PK, Ganesan AK, et al: Repair responses to DNA damage; Enzymatic pathways in E. coli and human cells. In: Mechanisms of Chemical Carcinogenesis, p 275, Harris CC, Cerutti PA (eds.), Alan R Liss, New York, 1982.

81. Hardell L: Malignant mesenchymal tumours and exposure to phenoxy acids—a clinical observation [Swed]. Lakartidningen 74:2753, 1977.

82. Hardell L, Eriksson M: The association between soft tissue sarcomas and exposure to phenoxyacetic acids. Cancer 62:652, 1988.

83. Hardell L, Sandstrom A: A case-control study: Soft-tissue sarcomas and exposure to phenoxyacetic acids or chlorophenols. Br J Cancer 39:711, 1979.

84. Hardell L, Eriksson M, Lenner P, et al: Malignant lymphoma and exposure to chemicals, especially organic solvents, chlorophenols and phenoxy acids: A case-control study. Br J Cancer 43:169, 1981.

85. Harrington JM, Craun GF, Meigs JW, et al: An investigation of the use of asbestos cement pipe for public water supply and the incidence of gastrointestinal cancer in Connecticut, 1935–1973. Am J Epidemiol 107:96, 1978.

86. Heath CW, Nadel MR, Zack MM, et al: Cytogenetic findings in persons living near the Love Canal. JAMA 251:1437, 1984.

87. Heidelberger C: Chemical carcinogenesis. Annu Rev Biochem 44:79, 1975.

88. Hemminki K, Grzybowska E, Chorazy M, et al: DNA adducts in humans environmentally exposed to aromatic compounds in an industrial city in Poland. Carcinogenesis 11:1229, 1990.

89. Herbst AL, Ulfelder H, Poskanzer DC: Adenocarcinoma of the vagina: Association of maternal stilbestrol therapy with tumor appearance in young women. N Engl J Med 284:878, 1971.

90. Hiatt HH, Watson JD, Winsten JA (eds.): Origins of Human Cancer, Book A: Incidence of Cancer in Humans, Cold Spring Harbor Laboratory, New York, 1977.

91. Higginson J: Rethinking the environmental causation of human cancer. Food Cosmet Toxicol 19:539, 1981.

92. Higginson J, Muir CS: Environmental carcinogenesis: Misconceptions and limitations to cancer control [Editorial]. J Natl Cancer Inst 63:1291, 1979.

93. Higginson J, Jensen OM, Muir CS: Environmental Carcinogenesis—A Global Problem, Year Book Medical Publishers, Chicago, 1981.

94. Hirayama T: Non-smoking wives of heavy smokers have a higher risk of lung cancer: A study from Japan. Br Med J 282:183, 1981.

95. Hitosugi M: Epidemiological study of lung cancer with special reference to the effect of air pollution and smoking habits. Bull Inst Public Health 17:237, 1968.

96. Hoar SK, Blair A, Holmes FF, et al: Agricultural herbicide use and risk of lymphoma and soft-tissue sarcoma. JAMA 256:1141, 1986.

97. Hoar SK, Blair A, Holmes FF, et al: A case-referent study of soft-tissue sarcoma and Hodgkin's disease. Scand J Work Environ Health 14:224, 1988.

98. Hoel DG, Gaylor DW, Kirschstein RL, et al: Estimation of risk of irreversible delayed toxicity. J Toxicol Environ Health 1:133, 1975.

99. Hollstein M, McCann J, Angelosanto FA, et al: Short term tests for carcinogens and mutagens. Mutat Res 65:133, 1979.

100. Holmberg B, Ahlborg U (eds.): Consensus report: Mutagenicity and carcinogenicity of car exhausts and coal combustion emission. Environ Health Perspect 47:1, 1983.

101. Hulka BS, Wilcosky TC, Griffith JD: Biological Markers in Epidemiology, Oxford University Press, Oxford, 1990.

102. Infante PF, Wagoner JK, Waxweile RJ: Carcinogenic, mutagenic and teratogenic risks associated with vinyl chloride. Mutat Res 41:131, 1976.

103. International Agency for Research on Cancer: IARC Monographs on the Evaluation of the Carcinogenic Risk of Chemicals to Man: Vol 11 Cadmium, Nickel, Some Epoxides, Miscellaneous Industrial Chemicals and General Considerations on Volatile Anesthetics, IARC, Lyon, 1976.

104. International Agency for Research on Cancer: IARC Monographs on the Evaluation of Carcinogenic Risks of Chemicals to Humans, Preface, IARC, Lyon, 1978.

105. International Agency for Research on Cancer: IARC Monographs on the Evaluation of the Carcinogenic Risk of Chemicals to Humans, Vol 18, Polychlorinated Biphenyls and Polybrominated Biphenyls, IARC, Lyon, 1978.

106. International Agency for Research on Cancer: IARC Monographs on the Evaluation of the Carcinogenic Risk of Chemicals to Humans, Vol 19, Some Monomers, Plastics, and Synthetic Elastomers, and Acrolein, IARC, Lyon, 1979.

107. International Agency for Research on Cancer: IARC Monographs on the Evaluation of the Carcinogenic

Risk of Chemicals to Humans, Vols 1–29, Chemicals, Industrial Processes and Industries Associated with Cancer in Humans, Suppl 4, IARC, Lyon, 1982.

108. International Agency for Research on Cancer: IARC Monographs on the Evaluation of the Carcinogenic Risks of Chemicals to Humans, Vol 41, Some Halogenated Hydrocarbons and Pesticide Exposure, IARC, Lyon, 1986.

109. International Agency for Research on Cancer: IARC Monographs on the Evaluation of Carcinogenic Risks of Chemicals to Humans, Vols 1–42, Suppl 7, IARC, Lyon, 1987.

110. Ivanovic V, Weinstein IB: Genetic factors in *Escherichia coli* that affect cell killing and mutagenesis induced by benzo[a]pyrene-7,8-dihydrodiol 9,10-oxide. Cancer Res 40:3508, 1980.

111. Janerich D: Cancer incidence in the Love Canal area. Science 212:1404, 1981.

112. Jeffey AM, Kinoshita T, Santella RM, et al: The chemistry of polycyclic aromatic hydrocarbon-DNA adducts. In: Carcinogenesis: Fundamental Mechanisms and Environmental Effects, p 565, Pullman B, Ts'o POP, Gelboin H (eds.), D Reidel, Amsterdam, 1980.

113. Kalow W, Goedde HW, Agarwal DP (eds.): Ethnic Differences in Reactions to Drugs and Xenobiotics, Alan R Liss, New York, 1986.

114. Kanarek MS, Young TB: Drinking water treatment and risk of cancer death in Wisconsin. Environ Health Perspect 46:179, 1982.

115. Kanarek MS, Conforti PM, Jackson LA, et al: Asbestos in drinking water and cancer incidence in the San Francisco Bay area. Am J Epidemiol 112:54, 1980.

116. Kelsey JL: A review of the epidemiology of human breast cancer. Epidemiol Rev 1:74, 1979.

117. Kimbrough RD, Falk H, Stehr P, et al: Health implications of 2,3,7,8-tetrachlorodibenzodioxin (TCDD) contamination of residential soil. J Toxicol Environ Health 14:47, 1984.

118. Kirschner MA: The role of hormones in the etiology of human breast cancer. Cancer 39:2716, 1977.

119. Klein G: The role of gene dosage and genetic transpositions in carcinogenesis. Nature 294:313, 1981.

120. Kociba RJ, Keyes DG, Beyer JE, et al: Results of a two-year chronic toxicity and oncogenicity study of 2,3,7,8-tetrachlorodibenzo-p-dioxin in rats. Toxicol Appl Pharmacol 46:279, 1978.

121. Land CE: Estimating cancer risks from low doses of ionizing radiation. Science 209:1197, 1980.

122. Landrigan PJ: Epidemiologic approaches to persons with exposure to waste chemicals. Environ Health Perspect 48:93, 1983.

123. Langer AM: Environmental asbestos pollution related to use of quarried serpentine rock. Science 196:1322, 1977.

124. Lathrop GD, Wolfe WH, Albanese RA, et al: Project Ranch Hand II. An Epidemiologic Investigation of Health Effects in Air Force Personnel Following Exposure to Herbicides; Baseline Mortality Study Results, USAF School of Aerospace Medicine, Brooks Air Force Base, TX, 1983.

125. Lathrop GD, Wolfe WH, Albanese RA, et al: Air Force Health Study, Project Ranch Hand II. An Epidemiologic Investigation of Health Effects in Air

Force Personnel Following Exposure to Herbicides; Baseline Morbidity Study Results, USAF School of Aerospace Medicine, Brooks Air Force Base, TX, 1984.

126. Levine RJ (ed.): Asbestos: An Information Resource, DHEW No. (NIH) 78–1681, US Government Printing Office, Washington, 1981.

127. Lieber CS, Seitz HK, Garro AJ, et al: Alcohol-related diseases and carcinogenesis. Cancer Res 39:2863, 1979.

128. Lilienfeld DE, Gallo MA: 2,4-D, 2,4,5-T, and 2,3,7,8-TCDD: An overview. Epidemiol Rev 11:28, 1989.

129. Lynge E: A follow-up study of cancer incidence among workers in manufacture of phenoxy herbicides in Denmark. Br J Cancer 52:259, 1985.

129A. Manz A, Berger J, Dwyer JH, et al: Cancer mortality among workers in a chemical plant contaminated with dioxin. Lancet 338:959, 1991.

130. Marshall E: Juarez: An unprecedented radiation accident. Science 223:1152, 1984.

131. Maugh TH: Chemical carcinogens: How dangerous are low doses? Science 202:37, 1978.

132. Miller EC: Some current perspectives on chemical carcinogenesis in humans and experimental animals. Cancer Res 38:1479, 1978.

133. Miller RW: Pollutants and children: Lessons from case histories. In: Guidelines for Studies of Human Populations Exposed to Mutagenic and Reproductive Hazards, p 155, Bloom AD (ed.), March of Dimes Birth Defects Foundation, New York, 1981.

134. Moon RC, Grubbs CJ, Sporn MB: Inhibition of 7,12-dimethylbenz(a)anthracene-induced mammary carcinogenesis by retinyl acetate. Cancer Res 36:2626, 1976.

135. Moon RC, McCormick DL, Mehta G: Inhibition of carcinogenesis by retinoids. Cancer Res 43 (Suppl): 2469s, 1983.

136. Moses M, Selikoff IJ: Soft tissue sarcomas, phenoxy herbicides, and chlorinated phenols. Lancet 1:1370, 1981.

137. Moses M, Lilis R, Crow KD, et al: Health status of workers with past exposure to 2,3,7,8-tetrachlorodibenzo-p-dioxin in the manufacture of 2,4,5-trichlorophenoxy-acetic acid; comparison of findings in and without chloracne. Am J Ind Med 5:161, 1984.

138. Mulvihill JJ: Clinical observations of ecogenetics in human cancer. Ann Intern Med 92:809, 1980.

139. Nagata C, Kodama M, Ioki Y, et al: Free radicals produced from chemical carcinogens and their significance in carcinogenesis. In: Free Radicals and Cancer, p 1, Floyd RA (ed.), Marcel Dekker, New York, 1982.

140. National Cancer Institute: Estimates of the fraction of cancer in the U.S. related to occupational factors. Prepared by National Cancer Institute, National Institute of Environmental Health Sciences, National Institute for Occupational Safety and Health, US Government Printing Office, Washington, 1978.

141. National Toxicology Program: General Statement of Work for the Conduct of Toxicity and Carcinogenicity Studies in Laboratory Animals. Available from National Institute of Environmental Health Sciences, Central Data Management A001, PO Box 12233, Research Triangle Park, NC 27709.

142. National Toxicology Program: Carcinogenesis Bio-assay of 2,3,7,8-Tetrachlorodibenzo-*p*-dioxin (CAS 1746–01–6) in Osborne-Mendel Rats and B6C3f1 mice (gavage study). DHEW Publication No. (NIH) 82–1765, p 195, Washington, 1982.

143. Nelson KW: Industrial contributions of arsenic to the environment. Environ Health Perspect 19:31, 1977.

144. Newhouse ML, Thompson H: Mesothelioma of pleura and peritoneum following exposure to asbestos in the London area. Br J Ind Med 22:261, 1965.

145. Nishizuka Y: The role of protein kinase C in cell surface signal transduction and tumour promotion. Nature 308:693, 1984.

146. Omenn GS, Gelboin HV (eds.): Genetic Variability in Responses to Chemical Exposure. Banbury Report 16, Cold Spring Harbor Laboratory, New York, 1984.

147. Omenn GS, Motulsky AG: Eco-genetics: Genetic variations in susceptibility to environmental agents. In: Genetic Issues in Public health and Medicine, p 83, Cohen BH, Lilienfeld AM, Huang PC (eds.), Charles C Thomas, Springfield, IL, 1979.

148. Ott MG, Holder BB, Olson RD: A mortality analysis of employees engaged in the manufacture of 2,4,5-trichlorophenoxyacetic acid. J Occup Med 22:47, 1980.

149. Parada LF, Tabin CJ, Shih C, et al: Human *EJ* bladder carcinoma oncogene is homologue of Harvey sarcoma virus *ras* gene. Nature 297:474, 1982.

150. Pearce NE, Smith AH, Fisher DO: Malignant lymphoma and multiple myeloma linked with agricultural occupations in a New Zealand cancer registry-based study. Am J Epidemiol 121:225, 1985.

151. Perera FP: Molecular epidemiology: A novel approach to the investigation of pollutant-related chronic disease. In: Environmental Impact on Human Health: An Agenda for Long Term Research and Development, p. 61, Draggan S, Cohrssen JJ, Morrison RE (eds.), Praeger, London, 1986.

152. Perera FP: Molecular cancer epidemiology: A new tool in cancer prevention. J Natl Cancer Inst 78:887, 1987.

153. Perera FP: The significance of DNA and protein adducts in human biomonitoring studies. Mutat Res 205:255, 1988.

154. Perera FP, Petito C: Formaldehyde: A question of cancer policy? Science 216:1285, 1982.

155. Perera FP, Weinstein IB: Molecular epidemiology and carcinogen-DNA adduct detection: New approaches to studies of human cancer causation. J Chron Dis 35:581, 1982.

156. Perera FP, Boffetto P, Nisbet ICT: What are the major carcinogens in the etiology of human cancer? Imp Adv Oncol 249:65, 1989.

157. Peto R: Detection of risk of cancer to man. Proc R Soc Lond [Biol] 205:111, 1979.

158. Pienta RJ: Transformation of Syrian hamster embryo cells by diverse chemicals and correlation with their reported carcinogenic and mutagenic activities. In: Chemical Mutagens: Principles and Methods for Their Detection, Vol VI, p 175, deSerres FF, Hollaender A (eds.), Plenum Press, New York, 1980.

159. Piotrowski JK: Individual exposure and biological monitoring. In: Methods for Estimating Risk of Chemical Injury: Human and Nonhuman Biota and Ecosystems, p 123, Vouk V, Butler GC, Hoel DG, et al. (eds.), John Wiley & Sons, New York, 1985.

160. Poirier MC, Yuspa SH, Weinstein IB, et al: Detection of carcinogen DNA adducts by radioimmunoassay. Nature 270:186, 1977.

161. Poirier MC, Santella R, Weinstein IB, et al: Quantitation of benzo(a)pyrene-deoxyguanosine adducts by radioimmunoassay. Cancer Res 40:412, 1980.

162. Pitot HC: Fundamentals of Oncology, 3rd ed., Marcel Dekker, New York, 1986.

163. Pitot HC, Goldsworthy T, Moran S: Natural history of carcinogenesis. J Supramol Struct Cell Biochem 17:133, 1981.

164. Puntoni R, Merlo F, Fini A, et al: Soft tissue sarcoma in Seveso. Lancet 2:525, 1986.

165. Purchase IF: Range of experimental evidence in assessing potential human carcinogenicity. Arch Toxicol 3 Suppl:283, 1980.

166. Riihimaki V, Asp S, Pukkala E, et al: Mortality and cancer morbidity among chlorinated phenoxyacid applicators in Finland. Chemosphere 12:779, 1983.

167. Rook JJ: Formation of haloforms during chlorination of natural waters. Water Treat Exam 23(2):234, 1974.

168. Rowley JD, Testa JR: Chromosome abnormalities in malignant hemotologic diseases. Adv Cancer Res 36:103, 1982.

169. Samet JM, Hornung RW: Review of radon and lung cancer risk. Risk Anal 10:65, 1990.

170. Samet JM, Kutvirt DM, Waxweiler RJ: Uranium mining and lung cancer in Navajo men. N Engl J Med 310:1481, 1984.

171. Sawicki E, Elbert WC, Hauser TR, et al: Benzo[a]pyrene content of American communities. Am Ind Hyg Assoc J 21:443, 1960.

172. Schottenfeld D, Fraumeni JF Jr (eds.): Cancer Epidemiology and Prevention, WB Saunders, Philadelphia, 1982.

173. Selikoff IJ, Nicholson WJ, Langer AM: Asbestos air pollution. Arch Environ Health 25:1, 1972.

174. Selikoff IJ, Hammond EC, Seidman H: Mortality experience of insulation workers in the United States and Canada, 1943–1876. Ann NY Acad Sci 330:91, 1979.

175. Shy CM, Struba RJ: Air and water pollution. In: Cancer Epidemiology and Prevention, p 336, Schottenfeld D, Fraumeni JF (eds.), WB Saunders, Philadelphia, 1982.

176. Smith AH, Pearce NE, Fisher D, et al: Soft tissue sarcoma and exposure to phenoxy-herbicides and chlorophenols in New Zealand. J Natl Cancer Inst 73:1111, 1984.

176A. Solomon E, Borrow J, Goddard AD: Chromosome aberrations and cancer. Science 254:1153, 1991.

177. Soper KA, Stolley PD, Galloway SM, et al: Sister chromatid exchange (SCE) report on control subjects in a study of occupationally exposed workers. Mutat Res 129:77, 1984.

178. Spatz L, Bloom AD, Paul HW: Detection of Cancer Predisposition: Laboratory Approaches, March of Dimes Birth Defects Foundation, New York, 1990.

179. Spengler JD, Sexton K: Indoor air pollution: A public health perspective. Science 221:9, 1983.

180. Sporn MB, Squire RA, Brown CC, et al: 13-*cis*-Retinoic acid: Inhibition of bladder carcinogenesis in the rat. Science 195:487, 1977.

181. Sterling DA: Volatile organic compounds in indoor air: An overview of sources, concentration, and health effects. In: Indoor Air and Human Health, p 387, Gammage RB, Kaye SV (eds.), Lewis Publishers, Chelsea, Michigan, 1985.

182. Stocks P, Campbell MJ: Lung cancer death rates among nonsmokers and pipe and cigarette smokers. An evaluation in relation to air pollution by benzpyrene and other substances. Br Med J 2:923, 1955.

183. Stolley PD, Hibberd PL: Drugs. In: Cancer Epidemiology and Prevention, p 44, Schottenfeld DF, Fraumeni JF Jr. (eds.), WB Saunders, Philadelphia, 1982.

184. Stubbs HA, Harris J, Spear RC: A proportionate mortality analysis of California agricultural workers, 1978–1979. Am J Ind Med 6:305, 1984.

185. Subcommittee on Disinfectants and Disinfectant By-Products, Safe Drinking Water Committee, National Research Council: Drinking Water and Health, Vol 7: Disinfectants and Disinfectant By-Products, National Academy Press, Washington, 1987.

186. Suskind RR, Hertzberg VS: Human health effects of 2,4,5-T and its toxic contaminants. JAMA 257:2372, 1984.

187. Tennant RW, Margolin BH, Shelby MD, et al: Prediction of chemical carcinogenicity in rodents from in vitro genetic toxicity assays. Science 236:933, 1989.

188. Tomatis L: The predictive value of rodent carcinogenicity tests in the evaluation of human risks. Annu Rev Pharmacol Toxicol 19:511, 1979.

189. Tomatis L: Environmental cancer risk factors. A review. Acta Oncol 27:5, 1988.

190. Tomatis L, Breslow NE, Bartsch H: Experimental studies in the assessment of human risk. In: Cancer Epidemiology and Prevention, p 304, Schottenfeld D, Fraumeni JF Jr. (eds.), WB Saunders, Philadelphia, 1982.

191. Tomatis L, Aitio A, Wilbourn J, et al: Human carcinogens so far identified. Jpn J Cancer Res 80:795, 1989.

192. Totter JR: Spontaneous cancer and its possible relationship to oxygen metabolism. Proc Natl Acad Sci USA 77:1763, 1980.

193. Trichopoulos D, Kalandidi A, Sparros L, et al: Lung cancer and passive smoking. Int J Cancer 27:1, 1981.

194. Tseng WP, Chu HM, How SW, et al: Prevalence of skin cancer in an endemic area of chronic arsenicism in Taiwan. J Natl Cancer Inst 40:453, 1968.

195. Upton AC, Kneip T, Toniolo P: Public health aspects of toxic chemical disposal sites. Annu Rev Public Health 10:1, 1989.

196. US Department of Health and Human Services: The Health Consequences of Involuntary Smoking: A Report to the Surgeon General, DHHS, Washington, 1986.

197. US Department of Health and Human Services: Sixth Annual Report on Carcinogens, Summary 1991, National Toxicology Program, NTP, DHHS, Washington, 1991.

198. US Environmental Protection Agency: Suspended, Cancelled and Restricted Pesticides, 3rd rev, USEPA, Washington, 1985.

199. Vainio H, Hemminki K, Wilborn J: Data on the carcinogenicity of chemicals in the IARC Monographs Programme. Carcinogenesis 6:1653, 1985.

200. Vainio H, Hesso A, Jappinen P: Chlorinated dioxins and dibenzofurans in the environment—a hazard to public health? Scand J Work Environ Health 15:377, 1989.

201. Vande Woude GF, Levine AJ, Topp WC, et al: Cancer Cells, Vol II, Oncogenes and Viral Genes, Cold Spring Harbor Laboratory, New York, 1984.

202. Van Ryzin J: Quantitative risk assessment. J Occup Med 22:321, 1980.

203. Wagner JC, Sleggs CA, Marchand P: Diffuse pleural mesothelioma and asbestos exposure in the North Western Cape Province. Br J Ind Med 17:260, 1960.

204. Wald NJ, Doll R (eds.): Interpretation of Negative Epidemiological Evidence for Carcinogenicity, IARC Scientific Publication No. 65, International Agency for Research on Cancer, Lyon, 1985.

205. Waldron HA: A brief history of scrotal cancer. Br J Ind Med 40:390, 1983.

206. Wallace LA, Pellizzari E, Hartwell T, et al: Personal exposure to volatile organic compounds: I. Direct measurement in breathing zone air, drinking water, food, exhaled breath. Environ Res 35:293, 1984.

207. Wallace L, Pellizzari E, Leaderer BP, et al: Personal exposures, indoor-outdoor relationships and breath levels of toxic air pollutants measured for 355 persons in New Jersey. Atmos Environ 19:1651, 1985.

208. Wattenberg LW: Naturally occurring inhibitors of chemical carcinogenesis. In: Naturally Occurring Carcinogens—Mutagens and Modulators of Carcinogenesis, p 315, Miller EC, Miller JA, Hirono I, et al. (eds.), Japan Science Social Press, Tokyo University Park Press, Baltimore, 1979.

209. Wattenberg LW: Increasing evidence of anti-carcinogens. J Environ Pathol Toxicol 3:35, 1980.

210. Wattenberg LW: Inhibition of chemical carcinogenesis by antioxidants. In: Carcinogenesis, Vol 5: Modifiers of Chemical Carcinogenesis, p 85, Slaga TJ (ed.), Raven Press, New York, 1980.

211. Wattenberg LW: Inhibitors of chemical carcinogens. In: Cancer: Achievements, Challenges, and Prospects for the 1980s, Vol 1, p 517, Burchenal JH, Oettgen HF (eds.), Grune & Stratton, Orlando, 1981.

212. Wattenberg LW: Chemoprevention of cancer. Cancer Res 45:1, 1985.

213. Weinberg RA: Positive and negative controls on cell growth. Biochemistry 26:8263, 1989.

214. Weinstein IB: Benzo(2)pyrene diol epoxides as intermediates in nucleic acid binding in vitro and vivo. Science 193:592, 1976.

215. Weinstein IB: Molecular and cellular mechanisms of chemical carcinogenesis. In: Cancer and Chemotherapy, Vol 1, p 169, Academic Press, Orlando, 1980.

216. Weinstein IB: Current concepts and controversies in chemical carcinogenesis. J Supramol Struct Cell Biochem 17:99, 1981.

217. Weinstein IB: The scientific basis for carcinogen detection and primary cancer prevention. Cancer 47:1133, 1981.

218. Weinstein IB: Carcinogenesis as a multistage process—experimental evidence. In: Host Factors in

Human Carcinogenesis, p 9, Bartsch H, Armstrong B (eds.), IARC Scientific Publication no. 39, IARC, Lyon, 1982.

219. Weinstein IB: Growth factors, oncogenes, and multi-stage carcinogens. J Cell Biochem 33:213, 1987.

220. Weinstein IB: The origins of human cancer: Molecular mechanisms of carcinogenesis and their implication for cancer prevention and treatment. Twenty-seventh G.H.A. Clowes Memorial Award Lecture. Cancer Res 48:4135, 1988.

221. Weinstein IB: Synergistic interactions between chemical carcinogens, tumor promoters and viruses and their relevance to human liver cancer. In: Pathogenesis and Prevention of Hepatocellular Carcinoma Cancer Detection and Prevention 14:253, 1989.

222. Weinstein IB: Mitogenesis is only one factor in carcinogenesis. Science 251:387, 1991.

223. Weinstein IB: Cancer Prevention: Recent Progress and Future Opportunities. Cancer Res. 51(Suppl): 5080S, 1991.

224. Weinstein IB, Gattoni-Celli S, Kirschmeier P, et al: Multistage carcinogenesis involves genes and multiple mechanisms. In: Cancer Cells 1: The Transformed Phenotype, p 229, Levine AJ, Vande Woude GF, Topp WC, et al. (eds.), Cold Spring Harbor Laboratory, New York, 1984.

225. Wigle DT, Semenciw RM, Wildkins K, et al: Mortality study of Canadian male farm operators: Non-Hodgkin's lymphoma mortality and agricultural practices in Saskatchewan. J Natl Cancer Inst 82:575, 1990.

226. Wilcosky TC, Rynard SM: Sister chromatid exchanges. In: Biological Markers in Epidemiology, p 105, Hulka BS, Wilcosky TC, Griffith JD (eds.), Oxford University Press, Oxford, 1990.

227. Wilkins JR, Reiches NA, Kruse CW: Organic chemical contaminants in drinking water and cancer. Am J Epidemiol 110:420, 1979.

228. Wolfe WH, Michalek JE: Project Ranch Hand II. An Epidemiologic Investigation of the Health Effects in Air Force Personnel Following Exposure to Herbicides. Mortality Update, USAF School of Aerospace Medicine, Brooks Air Force Base, TX, 1985.

229. Wolfe WH, Michalek JE, Albanese RA, et al: Project Ranch Hand II. An Epidemiologic Investigation of the Health Effects in Air Force Personnel Following Exposure to Herbicides. Mortality Update, USAF School of Aerospace Medicine, Brooks Air Force Base, TX, 1984.

230. Wolfe WH, Michalek JE, Miner JC, et al: Air Force Health Study, Project Ranch Hand II. An Epidemiologic Investigation of Health Effects in Air Force Personnel Following Exposure to Herbicides. Mortality Update, USAF School of Aerospace Medicine, Brooks Air Force Base, TX, 1986.

231. Wynder EL: The environment and cancer prevention. J Environ Pathol Toxicol 3:171, 1980.

232. Wynder EL, Gori GB: Contribution of the environment to cancer incidence: An epidemiologic exercise. J Natl Cancer Inst 58:825, 1977.

233. Young AL, Calcagni JA, Thalken CE, et al: The Toxicology, Environmental Fate and Human Risk of Herbicide Orange and Its Associated Dioxin, Technical Report TR-78–92, Final Report, USAF Occupational and Environmental Health Laboratory, Aerospace Medical Division (AFSC), Brooks Air Force Base, TX, 1978.

234. Zack JA, Gaffey WR: A mortality study of workers employed at the Monsanto plant in Nitro, West Virginia. Environ Sci Res 26:575, 1983.

235. Zack JA, Suskind RR: The mortality experience of workers exposed to tetrachlorodibenzo-p-dioxin in a trichlorophenol process accident. J Occup Med 22:11, 1980.

236. Zaldivar R: Arsenic contamination of drinking water and food-stuffs causing endemic chronic poisoning. Beitr Pathol 151:384, 1974.

RECOMMENDED READINGS

Bartsch H, Hemminki K, O'Neill LK (eds.): Methods for Detecting DNA Damaging Agents in Humans: Application in Cancer Epidemiology and Prevention, IARC Scientific Publication No. 89, International Agency for Research in Cancer, Lyon, 1988.

Bishop JM: Molecular themes in oncogenesis. Cell 64:235, 1991.

International Agency for Research in Cancer: IARC Monographs on the Evaluation of Carcinogenic Risks of Chemicals to Humans. IARC Monograph, Vols 1–42, Suppl 7, IARC, Lyon, 1987.

Pitot HC: Fundamentals of Oncology, 3rd ed., Marcel Dekker, New York, 1986.

Montesano R, Bartsch H, Vainio H, et al: Long-Term and Short-Term Assays for Carcinogens: A Critical Appraisal, IARC Scientific Publication No. 83, International Agency for Research on Cancer, Lyon, 1986.

Schottenfeld D, Fraumeni JF Jr (eds.): Cancer Epidemiology and Prevention, WB Saunders, Philadelphia, 1982.

US Department of Health and Human Services: Sixth Annual Report on Carcinogens, Summary 1991, National Toxicology Program NTP, DHHS, Washington, 1991.

Weinstein IB: Cancer prevention: Recent Progress and Future Opportunities. Cancer Res 51(Suppl):5080S, 1991.

Weinstein IB: The origins of human cancer: Molecular mechanisms of carcinogenesis and their implication for cancer prevention and treatment. Twenty-seventh G.H.A. Clowes Memorial Award Lecture. Cancer Res 48:4135, 1988.

Part VI

ASSESSING EXPOSURE TO ENVIRONMENTAL CHEMICALS

27. ENVIRONMENTAL AND BIOLOGICAL MONITORING

John D. Osterloh and Alyce Bezman Tarcher

INTRODUCTION

Human populations are increasingly exposed to large numbers of chemicals that pose potential health risks. To understand and prevent the hazards of exposure to a chemical, precise information is required concerning its concentration in the environment and its concentration within the body in relation to its adverse health effects. It is widely acknowledged that assessment of the health risks of pollutant exposure is greatly impeded by imprecise exposure data (97,191,204,206).

This chapter is written to give the reader an understanding of the methods used to monitor chemical exposure. It focuses primarily on biological monitoring, which assesses exposure within the body. The first portion of the chapter deals with the biological monitoring of specific hazardous chemicals. An overview of each chemical is presented along with the monitoring data. The second portion of the chapter focuses on the assessment of exposure to carcinogens by measuring their genotoxic actions.

Chemical exposure can be assessed in two ways: environmental (ambient) and biological mon-

itoring. Environmental monitoring assesses exposure to a chemical agent by measuring its concentration in the environment (i.e., air, food, water). Biological monitoring assesses internal exposure to a chemical agent by measuring the chemical, its metabolites, and/or a nonadverse biological response in body tissues, fluids, expired air, and/or excreta. Biological monitoring offers a more accurate measure of individual exposure than does environmental monitoring. Each method, however, has its advantages and disadvantages. Since biological monitoring is in many ways complementary to environmental monitoring, more meaningful information is gained when both methods are used together.

Environmental Monitoring

Monitoring levels of pollutants in air, water, and food and identifying their emission sources is and continues to be the most important means of evaluating, reducing, preventing, and regulating such exposure.

Environmental monitoring has certain advantages. It often can be quickly applied to potentially hazardous conditions. If hazardous conditions are found, preventive measures can be instituted before severe toxicity occurs. In addition, a single environmental monitoring operation may protect many individuals. The analytic methodology needed for

Principles and Practice of Environmental Medicine, edited by Alyce Bezman Tarcher. Plenum Medical Book Company, New York, 1992.

environmental monitoring is often less complex than that needed for biological monitoring. Because the chemicals to be tested are present in such simple media as air and water, little preparation of the sample is needed prior to analysis. Measuring chlorinated hydrocarbons in the air using infrared spectroscopy, for example, requires no isolation of the analyte, whereas extraction, trapping, and chromatographic separation are required to measure chlorinated hydrocarbons or their metabolites in the blood or urine. Because environmental monitoring has a long history, a body of information on the relationship between environmental exposure and adverse health effects is available for many chemicals. With the development of new analytic devices for measuring personal exposure to pollutants, environmental monitoring is becoming increasingly sophisticated.

The major disadvantage of measuring the ambient concentration of a chemical is that such measurements may not closely reflect the amount that is actually absorbed. Apart from differences in absorption among individuals, their varied exposure patterns, use of protective devices, activities, and life style make it impossible for environmental monitoring techniques to provide exact information on internal exposure.

Biological Monitoring

The aim of biological monitoring is to provide a biological marker of exposure. This may be the identification of an exogenous substance within the body, an interactive product between a xenobiotic agent and endogenous components, or other events in the body that are related to exposure. Biological monitoring provides a better measure of internal dose than does ambient monitoring. Its major advantage lies in the fact that the measurement of internal exposure is more likely to be directly related to adverse health effects than is the measurement of external exposure. In addition, the data obtained through biological monitoring are independent of such factors as the route of absorption, biovariability in absorption, variation in exposure patterns, and life styles (145,147,212,302).

Biological monitoring is used to assure that current or past exposures do not represent unacceptable health risks and/or to detect potentially excessive exposure before adverse health effects become apparent (2,145,147,255,302). Biological monitoring may also provide some guidance in the use and effectiveness of therapy for exposure to toxic chemicals (e.g., chelation therapy for heavy metal exposure and pharmacological therapy for organophosphate exposure). It can also be used to document exposure; such documentation may be necessary for legal and/or regulatory purposes.

The major limitations of biological monitoring of chemical exposure are (1) limited availability of valid and practical methods, (2) insufficient knowledge of the disposition and time course (toxicokinetics) and the quantitative relationships among external exposure, internal exposure, and adverse effects (toxicodynamics), (3) greater difficulty in obtaining biological samples and possible increased risk to the individual when invasive techniques are used (i.e., adipose tissue biopsy), and (4) high costs, particularly when individual test results may not be applicable to others experiencing similar exposure.

Biological monitoring should be distinguished from diagnostic testing and health surveillance. Diagnostic testing is used to confirm the presence of adverse health effects that are clinically apparent. Health surveillance entails the periodic medical–physiological examination of exposed individuals, primarily workers, with the purpose of protecting health and preventing disease (Fig. 27-1). It should be appreciated, however, that there is a continuum between markers of exposure and markers of health status. Biological markers that define cellular, biochemical, or molecular events that are measurable in human tissues are tools that are increasingly being used to clarify the relationship between exposure to foreign compounds and adverse health effects (83,113).

REQUIREMENTS FOR THE EFFECTIVE USE OF BIOLOGICAL MONITORING

After absorption, a chemical is distributed within the body, metabolized, and excreted (Fig. 27-2). Depending on the tests performed and the conditions of investigation, internal dose may have different meanings: the amount of a chemical that has been recently absorbed (recent exposure), the amount stored in the body (body burden or integrated exposure), or the amount interacting with such critical cellular targets such as DNA, RNA, and protein (target dose or biological effective dose). Although the biological effective dose may be the best indicator of health risk, it is difficult to measure because the critical cellular targets are generally in tissues that are not readily accessible to sampling (145,203,204,206).

External Exposure, Internal Exposure, and Adverse Health Effects: Their Relationships

A number of conditions must be met before biological monitoring can be used to assess exposure and before the results can be used to assess potential health risk. Obvious requisites include (1) an understanding of the relationship between external and internal exposure and (2) an understanding

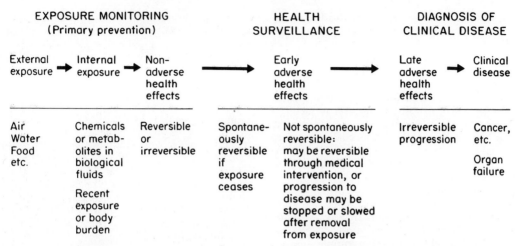

FIGURE 27-1. Monitoring, surveillance, and diagnosis. Adapted from Lohman (154).

of the relationship between the biological markers of internal exposure and adverse health effects (dose–response relationship). The effective prevention of adverse health effects linked to chemical exposure depends in part on sufficient dose–response information. Unfortunately, for most chemicals, such information is not available.

Under ideal conditions, the biological markers of exposure should (1) vary consistently and quantitatively with the intensity of exposure, (2) accurately distinguish between exposed and unexposed individuals, particularly at low doses, (3) be specific for the exposure under investigation, (4) be present in tissues or fluids suitable for sampling, (5) provide evidence of past and cumulative exposure, and (6) be sufficiently stable to be stored for a period of time (53).

Toxicokinetic and Toxicodynamic Information

Effective biological monitoring also depends on a body of toxicological information about the fate (absorption, metabolism, distribution, excretion) and mechanism of action of the chemical being monitored. Such information is essential in determining the biological media to sample, the best conditions for sampling (time and frequency), and the form of the chemical to be analyzed. Kinetic data are also vital in establishing whether the biological parameter being measured reflects recent exposure or integrated exposure (body burden).

Knowledge of the metabolism and excretion of the chemical being monitored, particularly the form that produces the toxic effects, is of help in determining what compound to analyze. The parent chemical often is analyzed when it undergoes little or no change within the body. This is the case for

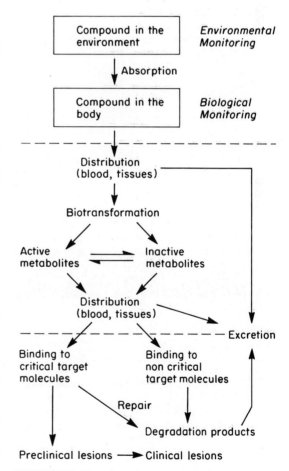

FIGURE 27-2. Fate of xenobiotics in the body. From Lauwerys (147).

many inorganic chemicals such as lead, cyanide, and fluoride. If a compound is extensively metabolized and excreted, then specific metabolites may be analyzed in the blood and/or urine. For example, trichloroethylene is extensively metabolized to trichloroethanol and trichloroacetic acid, which are excreted in the urine. However, exposures to trichloroethylene, trichloroethane, and tetrachloroethylene all result in the excretion of trichloroacetic acid in the urine. Of these chlorinated hydrocarbons, only trichloroethylene is extensively metabolized to trichloroacetic acid. This information is important in interpreting the levels of trichloroacetic acid present in the urine after exposure to these agents (116).

Toxicokinetic information that reveals how quickly the chemical being monitored enters and leaves the body helps in determining the time and frequency of sampling. For example, the rapid absorption and short biological half-life of low-molecular-weight volatile solvents require that sampling be performed within hours after exposure. Because these agents are rapidly metabolized, only recent exposure would be determined by biological monitoring. With chemicals having a long biological half-life, such as lead or polychlorinated hydrocarbons (PCBs), a sample taken shortly after exposure may reflect recent exposure, whereas later samples may reflect cumulative or integrated exposure (body burden). For example, the relationship between the concentration of polychlorinated biphenyls (PCBs) in the blood to body burden depends on how quickly a particular PCB leaves the blood (34). The lower chlorine-containing PCBs are more easily metabolized and excreted, whereas the more highly chlorinated and more lipid-soluble PCBs are slowly metabolized. Lipid solubility and resistance to metabolic transformation are reflected in a long biological half-life (120,247). Once the slowly metabolized PCBs have equilibrated between adipose tissue and blood, blood levels correlate with adipose tissue concentrations (31). The measurement of PCBs in blood and adipose tissue after their equilibration reflects the accumulated exposure to the more chlorinated isomers of PCB. Unfortunately, with many chemicals so little is known about their toxicokinetics, it is difficult to know to what degree the biological marker of exposure reflects recent exposure and/or body burden.

Understanding the mechanism of action of the chemical being monitored is always of value in monitoring internal exposure. This is well illustrated in the case of lead exposure. Erythrocyte protoporphyrin levels are often measured in blood as a screening test for lead exposure. A critical concentration of lead causes the inhibition of the enzyme ferro-chelatase, which results in the accumulation of protoporphyrin within red blood cells. Because it takes time for lead to accumulate within the developing red blood cells and time for the protoporphyrin-laden red blood cells to accumulate in the circulation, red cell protophorphyrin determinations done immediately after acute lead exposure do not reflect this exposure (46,47).

Analytic Factors

Effective biological monitoring depends on the availability of sensitive, precise, accurate, and practical techniques for analyzing the biological marker(s) of exposure. The analytic requirements are often quite rigorous. At this time, proficiency-testing programs for the biological monitoring of industrial or environmental chemicals are rare.

Analytic problems hampering the use of biological monitoring include lack of testing availability, poor interlaboratory agreement, and slow turnaround times. Strict standardization of the specimen collection (i.e., time, nutritional state, etc.) is needed to minimize sampling variation. Other problems include the misapplication of testing procedures. The matrix to which the assay is being applied will affect the accuracy of the assay. Some laboratories, by applying methods developed for water or soil to such biological media as blood or urine, have obtained erroneous results. Contamination is another formative problem encountered in biological monitoring, particularly the monitoring of lead. Glass and various plastic containers, for example, may contain varying amounts of lead and other heavy metals.

Interindividual variation is also an important consideration in establishing abnormal biological responses. When the variability among individuals is large, as in the case of cholinesterase activity, which is used to assess organophosphate exposure, marked changes may occur within an individual and yet be within the range observed for all normal individuals. For such situations, base-line determinations are required to detect changes within an individual over time.

Interpreting the Results

Reference values are usually required to interpret the results. Reference ranges should be specific for the population under study. Levels of urine arsenic, for example, are higher in people drinking certain well waters than for urban populations (136). Occupationally exposed populations differ from nonoccupationally exposed populations. Attention is being directed to the reference values obtained from biological monitoring of environmental pollutants in nonoccupationally exposed individuals in the general population (182,229,263).

For further practical and theoretical discussions of biological monitoring and analytic procedures the reader is referred to several works (2,3,18,19,23, 144,145,147,244,302).

BIOLOGICAL MONITORING OF ENVIRONMENTAL CHEMICALS

Based on knowledge currently available, biological monitoring can be carried out for a limited number of environmental pollutants (3,18) (Table 27-1). The limited availability of appropriate reference data puts significant constraints on the usefulness of biological monitoring in evaluating exposure and health risk. The World Health Organization (WHO) has proposed a few health-based reference values. These values are defined as levels in blood, urine, or other biological media not linked to any detectable adverse toxic effects. Such values have been defined for lead, mercury, cadmium, a few solvents, and some pesticides. As new data are forthcoming, these values are subject to change. The American Conference of Governmental Industrial Hygienists (ACGIH) has established biological exposure indices (BEIs) for about 20 compounds. These indices are based on occupational exposure in a healthy adult workforce (6). To interpret the results of biological monitoring, the medical investigator often must depend on data in the current literature. Such data must be interpreted with an understanding of the statistical, methodological, and pharmacological pitfalls.

Certain of the chemicals chosen for discussion have been studied sufficiently to permit some meaningful interpretation of the findings. These agents (lead, trichloroethylene, carbon monoxide, etc.) afford good examples of biological monitoring. Other chemicals chosen for discussion are currently being studied for the feasibility of assessing their exposure by biological monitoring techniques. More detailed background information on each chemical is found in other chapters of this book and in general toxicology textbooks. Further information on methodology and the interpretation of test findings has been published (13,19,145,244).

Arsenic

Occurrence

Exposure to arsenic may occur in the manufacture of pesticides, in the smelting of metals, in the use of antifouling paints, and in drinking from contaminated water supplies. Absorption may occur through ingestion, dermal exposure, or by the inhalation of dust or fumes in the workplace. Most arsenic in nature exists in the pentavalent state (arsenate). Industrially produced arsenic, usually in the trivalent form (arsenite), is more toxic than pentavalent arsenic (234). Organic arsenic, although present in many foods and highest in seafoods, is much less toxic.

Disposition

Once absorbed, arsenic is distributed predominantly into muscle, liver, skin, and hair. Arsenic has a biological half-life of 30–60 h (60,161). About 60–70% of an oral dose of inorganic arsenic is excreted in the urine in 4 days (32). Inorganic arsenic is methylated rapidly and excreted as mono- and di-

TABLE 27-1. Pollutants Amenable to Biological Monitoring in Various Tissues[a]

Tissues/media	As	Cd	Cr	Pb	Hg	RHg	CO	OCP	OP	PCB	TCE	Bz	CPH	TCDD
Adipose tissue								x		x				x
Blood	x	x		x	x	x	x	x	x	x	x	x	x	x
Bone				x										
Brain					x	x								
Expired air							x				x	x		
Feces		x												
Hair	x					x								
Kidney		x		x	x									
Liver		x		x	x									
Milk								x		x				x
Placenta		x		x										
Teeth				x										
Urine	x	x	x	x	x				x		x	x	x	

[a]Modified from Berlin et al. (18).
As, Arsenic; Cd, Cadmium; Cr, Chromium; Pb, Lead; Hg, Inorganic mercury; RHg, Methyl mercury; CO, Carbon monoxide; OCP, Organochlorine pesticides; OP, Organophosphorus pesticides; PCB, Polychlorinated biphenyls; TCE, Trichloroethylene; Bz, Benzene; CPH, Chlorophenoxy herbicides; TCDD (dioxin).

methylated products (32,60). About half is excreted as dimethylarsinic acid, up to one-quarter as methylarsonic acid, and less than 10% as arsenite and arsenate forms (32,33). Organoarsenic compounds, as found in seafood, are excreted in the urine unchanged (60).

Health Effects

Arsenic inhibits the activity of many enzymes by reacting with sulfhydryl groups and interfering with phosphate metabolism. Such reactions are considered responsible for much of the toxic action of arsenicals. Arsenic toxicity may produce gastrointestinal pain, diarrhea, anemia, peripheral neuropathy, hepatic cirrhosis, and dermal keratosis. Exposure to inorganic arsenic compounds in drugs, drinking water, and occupational environments is causally associated with the development of skin cancer and possibly lung cancer (115).

Kreiss et al., studying a population exposed to arsenic-contaminated well water, reported that total urine arsenic concentrations increased in proportion to the amount of arsenic ingested (136). Some of those exposed had abnormal nerve conduction, but this abnormality was not clearly related to the amount of arsenic ingested or excreted. In another study, electromyographic changes were seen in persons drinking well water with greater than 0.05 ppm arsenic (111). In smelter workers with documented exposure to arsenic, about 40% had evidence of clinical neuropathy (84).

Biological Monitoring

Arsenic concentration in blood and urine primarily reflects recent exposure to arsenic. In populations without industrial exposure, urinary arsenic is related to the arsenic present in drinking water and food. On the basis of limited data, the reference value 0.3–0.5 μmol (20–40 μg) As/L has been proposed for urinary arsenic (32). Exposure to air concentrations of 0.03 μmol (2 μg)/m^3 will not increase base-line urine levels. Urine arsenic will exceed 2.7 μmol (200 μg)/L when air concentrations exceed 0.7 μmol (50 μg)/m^3 (145).

Analysis

Ideally, the biological monitoring of arsenic in urine would measure arsenite (As^{3+}), arsenate (As^{5+}), methylarsonic acid (MAA), and dimethylarsinic acid (DMAA). Separation of various arsenic metabolites by selective extraction or chromatography has been performed but has not been put to widespread use. In most clinical laboratories, all arsenic species are commonly measured by atomic absorption spectrometry and included as total arsenic (i.e., organic and inorganic arsenic). Seafood ingestion results in a marked increase in total urinary arsenic (13,21).

Arsenic in the hair provides a reasonably good index of internal exposure to inorganic arsenic when external contamination is unlikely. Arsenic determination in hair has been used for forensic purposes and may be useful for evaluating past exposure to arsenic. In an industrial setting, determining the concentration of arsenic in hair is of little value because of the external contamination of the hair shaft by arsenic in the air, in bath water, and in sweat. Hair concentrations less than 0.3 mmol (2 mg)/kg suggest lack of internal and external exposure (279).

Cadmium

Occurrence

Cadmium exposure occurs in alloy production, in plating processes, in the manufacture of ammunition and batteries, and wherever lead and zinc are mined or processed. Industrial exposure is mainly by inhalation of vapors or dusts. Environmental pollution occurs from motor vehicle exhaust and cigarette smoking. Cadmium is a contaminant of superphosphate fertilizers and sewer sludge used for agricultural purposes. The major source of cadmium for the general population is its presence in food (90).

Disposition

Cadmium is absorbed from the digestive tract and by inhalation. Seventy percent of cadmium in whole blood is bound to red blood cells. The main tissue binding protein is metallothionein. The major organs of cadmium storage are the kidney and the liver. The renal cortex may contain one-third of the total cadmium body burden. The renal cortex appears to be the target organ for cadmium accumulation from low-level dietary exposure (68,226).

Health Effects

Studies suggest that human exposure to cadmium may be associated with increased risks of respiratory and genitourinary cancers (115). Cadmium exposure may also be a risk factor in the development of hypertension (209).

As the body burden of cadmium increases, urinary cadmium tends to increase slightly but is not a good predictor of exposure or of renal function status (227). Neutron activation analysis of kidney cortices indicates that renal dysfunction occurs when cortical levels of cadmium exceed 215 to 385 ppm. These levels correspond to a urinary excretion of 0.09–0.16 μmol (10 to 18 μg) Cd/g creatinine (145).

It has been suggested that the no-effect level of long-term cadmium exposure is a blood cadmium level of 0.09 μmol (10 μg)/L or less (145). Subjects without occupational exposure demonstrate an average of 0.04 umoles (4 μg) Cd/L in whole blood (10).

Biological Monitoring

After exposure begins, the cadmium blood levels of occupationally exposed workers increases linearly up to 120 days and then levels off. This suggests that after equilibrium occurs, cadmium blood levels may be a good indicator of recent exposure (148,227).

When the cadmium-binding capacity of the kidney is reached, proteinuria ensues, cadmium and metallothionein excretion increase, and cortical or total kidney cadmium concentrations begin to decrease (68,226,227). Although cadmium excretion increases slightly after the onset of renal dysfunction, its urinary concentration may still be very low. Because of the wide variation in urinary cadmium levels among exposed individuals, some with and some without renal failure, this determination cannot be used to predict renal injury in a particular individual (81,82,227,263). However, urinary cadmium below 0.09 μmol (10 μg) per gram of creatinine is thought to be associated with a low risk of cadmium-induced renal disease.

Urinary β_2-microglobulin determinations have generally been recommended for assessing the early adverse renal effects of cadmium in exposed workers (81,82). β_2-microglobulin, however, is unstable in an acid urine (14). The determination of retinol-binding globulin in the urine has been used as an indicator of renal damage secondary to cadmium exposure (22,145). Retinol-binding protein has the advantage of being stable in the urine. The determination of urinary metallothionein has been used to monitor cadmium exposure, since urinary cadmium is bound primarily to this protein. Metallothionein excretion appears roughly proportional to kidney and liver burdens of cadmium (242). Although urinary metallothionein excretion may reflect cadmium-induced renal injury, it should not be taken as evidence of the intensity of recent exposure (81).

Analysis

The amount of cadmium in body fluids is determined by two atomic absorption methods. One method, involving flame atomic absorption spectrometry, is adequate for determining toxic levels of cadmium. The other, dependent on the flameless detection of cadmium, is sufficiently sensitive to determine blood and urinary cadmium in unexposed populations (13,21). The presence of cadmium contamination in laboratory reagents and in glassware presents a common analytic problem. Many commercial laboratories do not perform blood cadmium analyses to the required sensitivity. A lab measuring blood cadmium concentrations should be able to discriminate between 0 and 0.04 μmol/L (0 and 5 μg/L) of blood.

Lead

Occurrence

Of all toxic metals, lead is the most widely dispersed by human activity. Chemical forms causing toxicity include metallic lead, lead salts, lead oxides, and alkyl lead. Occupational sources of lead exposure include mining, smelting, radiator repair, lead paint removal, and the manufacture of batteries. Environmental lead is found in the air, in dust and soil, in food, and in water. Nearly all lead in the environment is inorganic. Airborne lead is derived from mining and smelting activities and from leaded gasoline. Flaking lead-based indoor paint and lead-containing dust in old homes are an important source or exposure. Lead occurs in food, particularly in crops grown near heavily traveled roads or near stationary sources of lead pollution. For children, soil and dust contaminated with lead from automotive and industrial activities are often important sources of lead exposure. This is true particularly for children who live near major sources of airborne lead pollution. Lead pipes and soldered joints are an important source of lead in drinking water, particularly soft water having an acidic pH. Lead in certain imported dinnerware may also be a source of lead exposure (41,47).

Disposition

Adults absorb 5–10% of ingested lead, whereas young children absorb about 50% of ingested lead. The total intake of lead is variable from less than 0.5 μmol/day (0.1 mg/day) to more than 9.7 μmol/day (2 mg/day). Absorption of lead dusts and oxides may also occur through the respiratory system. Up to 75% of the absorbed dose can be excreted in the urine, with another 10% being excreted in the sweat and gastrointestinal tract. Total body lead in man is distributed in essentially three compartments: blood, soft tissue, and bone (218). The biological half-life of lead in the blood and soft tissue is 35–40 days. The biological half-life of lead in bone is about 20 years. Ninety percent of the body burden of lead is found in bone. Blood lead levels represent, to a variable extent, recent exposure and some degree of previous exposure to the metal (1). In whole blood, 90% of the lead is bound to red blood cells (21,47).

Health Effects

Lead adversely affects the red blood cells and their precursors, the central and peripheral nervous system, the kidney, the gastrointestinal tract, and reproduction in both sexes (46,47,50,54,140,185,187) (Table 27-2). Lead may also play a limited role in the pathogenesis of hypertension. Animal studies and a number of recent human studies have noted a positive association between blood lead and blood pressure (265).

Lead exposure interferes with the heme biosynthetic pathway at several stages (Fig. 27-3). This biological disturbance results in a pattern of events that is characteristic of excessive lead exposure. This includes inhibition of porphobilinogen synthase (formerly δ-aminolevulinic acid dehydrase) in erythrocytes, increased erythrocyte protoporphyrin, and an increased excretion of δ-aminolevulinic acid and coproporphyrin in the urine (46). Inhibition of ferrochelatase, which catalyzes the incorporation of iron into protoporphyrin IX to form heme, results in the accumulation of protophorphyrin in red blood cells. It has been shown that the non-iron-bound protoporphyrin that accumulates in red blood cells during excessive lead exposure is chelated with zinc at the site usually occupied by iron.

By using electrophysiological measurement of nerve conduction velocities, a number of workers have demonstrated subclinical evidence of nerve dysfunction related to lead exposure (27,238–240, 246,256). Changes in nerve conduction velocities were well correlated with blood lead levels greater than 80 μg/dL (3.8 μmol/L) (27,246).

A number of investigators have demonstrated that low-level lead exposure affects behavior and learning in children (167,185,187,250,300,301). The blood lead level at which subclinical behavioral and learning deficits are described is as low as 15 μg/dL (7 μmol/L) (1,300). There is also a growing body of evidence that indicates that low birth weight and deficits in postnatal behavioral development are more likely to occur with maternal or cord blood levels exceeding 10–20 μg/dL (0.5–1.0 μmol/L) (Table 27-2) (16,17,62). The level of fetal lead exposure needed to produce these adverse effects is lower than that needed to produce impaired behavioral development in the infant or young child.

TABLE 27-2.   Adverse Effects of Lead[a]

Lowest-observed-effect level(PbB)[b]		Heme synthesis hematological effect	Neurological effects	Reproductive effects	Other effects
(μmol/L)	(μg/dL)				
3.8–4.8	80–100		Encephalopathy		Chronic nephropathy, colic, and other GI effects
3.4	70	Frank anemia	Peripheral neuropathy	Female reproductive effect	
2.4	50			Altered testicular function	
1.9	40	Reduced hemoglobin, elevated CP[d] an ALA-U[e]			
1.4	30		Slowed nerve conduction velocity		
1.2	25		Lower IQ, slower reaction time		
0.7–1	15–20	EP[c] elevation			
0.5–0.7	10–15	ALA-D[f] inhibition	Deficits in neurobehavioral development	Reduced gestational age and weight at birth; reduced size to age 7–8 years	

[a]Adapted from references 1, 175, and 273.
[b]PbB, blood lead concentration.
[c]EP, erythrocyte protoporphyrin.
[d]CP, coproporphyrin.
[e]ALA-U, aminolevulinic acid in urine.
[f]ALA-D, aminolevulinic acid dehydrase, now porphobiliogen synthase.

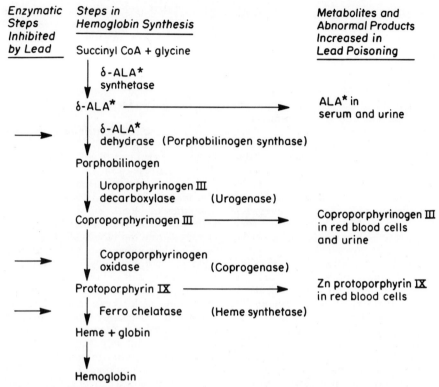

| Enzymatic Steps Inhibited by Lead | Steps in Hemoglobin Synthesis | Metabolites and Abnormal Products Increased in Lead Poisoning |

FIGURE 27-3. Effects of lead on heme biosynthesis. ALA, aminolevulinic acid.

Biological Monitoring

Biological monitoring of lead exposure relies on both the measurement of lead and its biological effects. As noted, blood lead concentrations represent to a variable extent recent exposure along with some degree of equilibration with the lead present in soft tissues and active bone. Blood lead correlates with surface or trabecular bone lead but may not represent accumulated lead stored deep within the cortical bone compartment (47,48,100,218). Although x-ray fluorescence has been used to measure the lead content of bones, there is, at present, no routine test that directly reflects the total body burden of lead (146). Shed deciduous teeth have been used as markers of past lead exposure (186).

The calcium disodium edetate (EDTA) lead-mobilization test may provide evidence of an excessive body burden of lead. Though the results of this test generally correlate quite well with equilibrated blood lead determinations, this test may be of value in assessing past lead exposure in persons who are no longer exposed (5). In subjects without excessive lead exposure, the urinary excretion of lead during the 24 h following the injection of EDTA is less than 3 μmol (600 μg) (70,283,284).

The dose–response relationships observed between blood lead and changes in various heme precursors make it possible to identify persons in the general population with increased lead exposure before the advent of serious toxicity (Table 27-2). It is well established that lead is most harmful to children under 6 years of age. Screening asymptomatic children in this age group for evidence of excessive lead exposure therefore offers a means of preventing serious toxicity (41,46).

The most useful screening tests for excessive lead exposure in adults are blood lead and erthyrocyte protoporphyrin (EP). The blood lead provides evidence of lead absorption, whereas EP provides evidence of impaired heme synthesis from lead toxicity. The EP will begin to rise when equilibrated blood lead concentrations reach about 20 μg/dL (1.0 μmol/L). Elevations of EP do not occur immediately after an acute single exposure, since time is required for lead to accumulate within the red blood cells. Inhibition of porphobilinogen synthase (formerly δ-aminolevulinic acid dehydrase) occurs more quickly and is evident at blood lead concentrations of 10–20 μg/dL (.05–1.0 μmol/L). Since the EP level is also elevated in cases of iron deficiency anemia, an elevation in EP alone cannot be considered to be diagnostic of lead toxicity; iron deficiency anemia must be ruled out.

EP concentrations are not useful in screening for low-level exposure to lead, e.g., blood lead levels less than 25 µg/dL (1.20 µmol/L). Thus blood lead determinations should be used as the primary screening method for children and newborns (41). Blood lead determinations also provide definite evidence of absorption and are the determinations used for chelation therapy (41).

The adverse effects of lead are noted across a broad range of blood lead concentrations (Table 27-2) (1,40,110,160,175,198,211,291,300). It should be appreciated that the adverse effects of lead, particularly long-term neurobehavioral, cognitive, and developmental effects, are increasingly being seen in children with lead levels much lower than were previously believed to be harmful (see Chapter 14) (41).

In 1991, the Centers for Disease Control replaced the single definition of childhood lead poisoning with the following multitier approach (41). It was recommended that community prevention activities be initiated by blood lead levels of ≥ 10 µg/dL (0.5 µmol/L). All children with blood lead levels ≥ 15 µg/dL (0.7 µmol/L) should receive individual case management, including nutritional and educational interventions and more frequent screening. Medical evaluation and environmental investigation and remediation should be done for all children with blood lead levels ≥ 20 µg/dL (1.0 µmol/L). A child with > 45 µg/dL (2.2 µmol/L) requires both medical and environmental interventions including chelation therapy. A blood lead level ≥ 70 µg/dL (3.4 µmol/L) is considered a medical emergency requiring immediate medical and environmental management (41). The interested reader is urged to consult the Statement by the Centers for Disease Control (41; see Chapters 13 and 14).

A national survey of blood lead levels in the United States conducted between 1976 and 1980 revealed the average blood lead level of the US population to be about 10 µg/dL (0.5 µmol/L) (159). Among preschool children, 9.1% had blood lead levels of 25 µg/dL (1.2 µmol/L) or more. Almost 25% of black children had blood lead levels of 25 µg/dL (1.2 µmol/L) or more (159). In adults, a blood lead concentration of 40 µg/dL (1.9 µmol/L) is considered harmful to hematopoietic, renal, and most likely reproductive function and thereby necessitates removal of a worker from exposure (140,184).

Analysis

Blood lead can be analyzed by atomic absorption spectrometry or anodic stripping voltammetry to a sensitivity of 0.1 µmol/L (2 µg/dL). Contamination is a major problem when performing a lead analysis in blood and urine. Dust particles may contain from 1000 to 30,000 ppm (0.1–3%) lead. Often the reagent solutions used in analytic laboratories contain 30–200 ppb. The leaching of lead may occur when samples are stored in certain glass containers, and lead may be absorbed into certain types of plastic. Specially designed sample containers are available for lead analysis in urine or whole blood (13,21).

Red blood cells containing zinc-protoporphyrin are intensely fluorescent. The concentration of zinc protoporphyrin can therefore be measured by the direct fluorescence of intact red blood cells or by fluorometry after its extraction from red blood cells. The analysis is very easy to perform on finger-stick quantities of blood. Zinc protoporphyrin is converted to erythrocyte protoporphyrin after being extracted from red blood cells (21).

The determination of urinary coproporphyrinogen and porphobilinogen, the presence of basophilic stippling of red blood cells, and the appearance of anemia cannot be used in the biological monitoring of lead exposure. These findings are nonspecific and usually appear when lead toxicity is clinically apparent. Measurement of lead in hair has not been a useful indicator of lead absorption. The ubiquitousness of environmental lead dust results in its adsorption on the surface of the hair. Current analytic capabilities cannot readily discriminate between lead incorporated into the hair and lead adsorbed on its surface.

Mercury

Occurrence

Humans may be exposed to mercury in its metallic, inorganic, and organic forms. The vapor of metallic mercury is found predominantly in the workplace, whereas organic mercury is present in the food chain, primarily in fish and fish products (290).

Exposure to metallic mercury by routes other than inhalation is rare. Metallic mercury is used industrially, particularly in manometric and electric switching devices and in amalgams used in dentistry. Inorganic mercury is used in industrial chemical processing, particularly for synthetic reactions. The waste water of industrial plants using mercury compounds may be polluted with significant amounts of mercury compounds. Elemental mercury or inorganic mercury dumped into bodies of water can be alkylated by microorganisms and concentrated in the food chain. Organic forms of mercury have been widely used in the production of pesticides to prevent fungal growth. Episodes of mercury intoxication have been recorded as a result of the consumption of mercury-contaminated fish and seed grain treated with mercury-containing fungicides. Exposure to environmental mercury results primarily from ingestion of food in which there has been the bioaccumulation of organic mercury. Mercury-contaminated fish is a notable example of this phenomenon (11,151,290).

Metallic mercury has a high vapor pressure and is only slightly soluble in water but over 1000 times more soluble in organic solvents such as pentane. Inorganic mercury salts may be monovalent (mercurous) or divalent (mercuric). Monovalent mercury salts are much less soluble than divalent mercury salts and are therefore less well absorbed and less toxic. Divalent mercury is more toxic, more water soluble, and has greater reactivity with sulfhydryl groups. Organic mercury compounds are lipid soluble and also react with sulfhydryl groups (290).

Disposition

Elemental mercury is absorbed from the vapor phase in a monoatomic form by the pulmonary route. Less than 0.01% of elemental mercury is absorbed from the gastrointestinal tract in liquid form. After absorption, elemental mercury enters red blood cells, and a portion is transported to the brain. It has a biological half-life that ranges from 35 to 90 days. Elemental mercury is oxidized to divalent mercury both in red blood cells and in the brain. Aerosolization and pulmonary absorption of inorganic mercury and organic mercury are possible but rarely encountered. Less than 10% of inorganic mercury salts are absorbed from the gastrointestinal tract, whereas organic mercury is readily absorbed. Absorbed inorganic mercury is deposited principally in the kidney. It is excreted by exfoliation of kidney tubular cells and in the feces and has a biological half-life of about 40 days. Organic mercury is lipid soluble and deposits in the brain. Methyl mercury is excreted primarily in the bile and by exfoliation of gastrointestinal cells. About 90% of absorbed methyl mercury is found in the feces. The biological half-life of methyl mercury is about 70 days (49,145,290).

Health Effects

Elemental mercury and methyl mercury adversely affect the central nervous system. Elemental mercury may produce such neuropsychiatric symptoms as depression and emotional instability. Central nervous effects of methyl mercury include alteration of visual fields, decreased coordination, and decreased senses of taste, smell, and hearing. Mercuric (divalent) mercury primarily affects the kidney. The clinical picture is that of acute tubular necrosis. Gastrointestinal toxicity from inorganic mercury includes stomatitis, gingivitis, corrosive ulceration, and necrosis. Mercurous (monvalent) mercury, as mentioned, is less toxic than the mercuric salts. However, mercurous mercury, through its past use in teething powders, has been incriminated in acrodynia or "pink disease" of children.

Biological Monitoring

Mercury levels in blood and urine can be used to assess exposure to inhaled and inorganic mercury. In unexposed persons the concentration of mercury in blood is rarely greater than 0.10 μmol/L (2 μg/dL) (145). Unexposed individuals generally excrete less than 0.02 μmol (5 μg) Hg per gram of creatinine (15,145). Abnormal psychomotor tests have been described at levels ranging between 0.25 and 2.50 μmol (50–500 μg) Hg per gram of creatinine (141,228). To prevent the development of central nervous system effects, it has been suggested that the level of urinary mercury not exceed 0.25 μmol (50 μg) Hg per gram creatinine (228). Variations in the urinary excretion of mercury in a given subject and among individuals require that urinary concentrations be corrected for dilution and urine flow (281).

Since methyl mercury is excreted primarily in the feces, urine samples are of little value in determining exposure or body burden (11,49). Blood determinations provide an indication of recent or long-term exposure to methyl mercury compounds (49). Early signs of methyl mercury intoxication may appear when blood levels of Hg exceed 1.0 μmol/L (20 μg/dL) (293). To prevent toxicity in persons exposed to alkyl mercury, the concentration of blood mercury should not exceed 0.5 μmol/L (10 μg/dL). Mercury blood levels may vary considerably among populations, higher levels being present in fish-eating peoples.

Mercury in hair is an important indicator of methyl mercury exposure but is not satisfactory for evaluating exposure to mercury vapor (49). During exposure to methyl mercury, the concentration of mercury in hair correlates well with blood concentration (49). At the time of its emergence from the scalp, mercury concentration in hair is approximately 250 to 300 times that in the blood (49,158). It has been estimated that symptoms of mercury intoxication appear when mercury in hair exceeds 0.25 μmol (50 μg) Hg/g (290).

Analysis

All forms of mercury are measured in toto by atomic absorption methodologies. Inorganic and organic mercury in biological media are reduced to elemental mercury. The released mercury vapor is then analyzed by an atomic absorption spectrometer. In commercial laboratories, the sensitivity is rarely better than 0.05 μmol (10 μg) Hg per gram of creatinine or liter of urine. Methyl mercury can be extracted from blood and also be determined by electron-capture gas chromatography (11,21).

Benzene

Occurrence

Benzene is a byproduct of the petroleum industry and the coking process. It is extensively used in industry in the manufacture of solvents, paints, paint removers, pesticides, and detergents. Benzene is the starting material for the synthesis of many organic chemicals. Because of its antiknock properties, benzene is a constituent of high-octane gasoline. With the elimination of alkyl lead compounds from gasoline, a mixture of benzene-rich aromatics had been added to gasoline. Consumers can be exposed to benzene through products containing petroleum distillates (i.e., paint removers, contact adhesives). The general population is exposed to benzene in urban air from such sources as automobile gasoline, coke ovens, and chemical plants. Benzene has been detected in cigarette smoke (142,212,251).

Disposition

Benzene exposure occurs primarily through inhalation. Dermal exposure may also take place by direct contact with petroleum products. A portion of the inhaled benzene is exhaled unchanged. Benzene is metabolized in the liver and bone marrow to more water-soluble products including phenol, catechol, muconic acid, and hydroquinone (199). The toxicity of benzene depends on one or more of its metabolites rather than on benzene itself (142, 145,251).

Health Effects

Benzene toxicity can be classified as acute or chronic. Acute exposures to high concentrations of benzene produce depression of the central nervous system. Chronic benzene exposure (10 to 1000 ppm) affects the hematopoietic system. Its toxicity is characterized by bone marrow depression resulting in pancytopenia and eventual aplastic anemia. Chronic benzene exposure is also associated with leukemia, particularly acute myelogenous leukemia (114,225) (see Chapter 21).

Biological Monitoring

Benzene exposure can be assessed by determining the urinary excretion of phenol. Over 50% of the absorbed benzene is excreted within 48 h as phenol. Elevated urinary phenol levels confirm re-cent benzene exposure but are not predictive of future hematological disease. Unexposed individuals excrete variable quantities of phenol and phenol-like substances in their urine, usually less than 0.11 μmol (10 mg)/L. The ingestion of phenol-producing medications (Pepto-Bismol®, Chloraseptic®, and others) can dramatically increase urinary phenol excretion (86,233). New methods for measuring muconic acid are likely to be more specific indicators of benzene exposure.

Benzene levels in expired air can be used for monitoring exposure (20,200). In nonoccupationally exposed persons, the concentration of benzene in exhaled air ranges between 0.001 and 0.002 ppm. Because benzene is present in cigarette smoke, smokers have a slightly higher level (20). The measurement of benzene in blood provides a sensitive means of detecting low-level benzene exposure. Few studies have used this approach, however.

Analysis

Urinary phenol and muconic acid levels are determined by gas chromatography. Simple colorimetric techniques for phenol determinations are also used, but these are insensitive and cross-react with phenol-like substances. Determinations of benzene in blood and expired air are performed by gas chromatography (13,17,202).

Trichloroethylene

Occurrence

Trichloroethylene is used for degreasing metal parts and as a solvent for dyes, spot removers, and rug cleaners. Trichloroethylene was formerly widely used as a dry-cleaning agent. It has been supplanted by tetrachloroethylene (perchloroethylene). Trichloroethylene has reportedly been found to be one of the most frequent contaminants of ground water in the United States (55).

Disposition

Trichloroethylene is a volatile liquid of low flammability. Exposure is primarily inhalational. Up to 75% of inhaled trichloroethylene is retained, and less than 12% is excreted in the breath (85,176). Most trichloroethylene is metabolized to trichloroethanol and trichloroacetic acid, which are then excreted in the urine. Tetrachloroethylene and trichloroethane are also metabolized to trichloroacetic acid, but to a much lesser extent. Both trichloroethanol and trichloroacetic acid have longer half-lives than the parent compound, i.e., 10–15 h and 70–100 h, respectively (74).

Health Effects

In cases of acute exposure to high concentrations, trichloroethylene produces cardiac arrhythmias, anesthetic-like effects on the central nervous system, and hepatotoxicity. Trichloroethylene may produce alcohol intolerance, and alcohol potentiates the hepatotoxicity of trichloroethylene. Long-term effects include hepatocellular and lung cancer in mice (234,260).

Biological Monitoring

Urine levels of trichloroethanol and trichloroacetic acid correlate well with ambient air concentrations of trichloroethylene. Most individuals exposed to 50 ppm of trichloroethylene during a 5-workday period can be expected to have urine levels of trichloroethanol and trichloroacetic acid exceeding 0.84 and 0.31 μmol (125 and 50 mg)/L (74,180,181). Because trichloroacetic acid and trichloroethanol accumulate during the work week, urinary measurements of these agents provide a means of monitoring exposure that occurred during the previous week. Blood levels of trichloroethanol and trichloroacetic acid, though less frequently monitored than urine levels, also reflect current or accumulated exposure to trichloroethylene. For example, during an exposure of 100 ppm, the blood trichloroethylene concentration will average 9.2 μmol/L (1.2 μg/mL) (85,145,260).

Analysis

The colorimetric method used for analysis of trichloroethanol and trichloroacetic acid is not sufficiently sensitive to be used for modern-day occupational exposure. Gas chromatographic methods are commonly preferred (13,181).

Carbon Monoxide

Occurrence

Carbon monoxide is formed when fossil fuels, including gasoline, are incompletely burned. Automotive exhausts, boilers, furnaces, and fires are sources of carbon monoxide. When all sources are considered (automotive, industrial, and energy production), carbon monoxide is one of the major pollutants in ambient air and one of the five common air pollutants for which the U.S. Environmental Protection Agency has established national ambient air quality standards. Levels above these standards are considered threats to public health. Primary ambient standards for carbon monoxide specify both an 8-h average (9 ppm) and a 1-h level (35 ppm) not to be exceeded. An EPA-sponsored study in Washington revealed that over one-third of those individuals who spent the most time on the road were exposed to CO levels greater than the 8-h primary ambient standard (105).

High concentrations of carbon monoxide are encountered in heavy downtown traffic in urban areas and in underground garages. Urban air concentrations of carbon monoxide may exceed 50 ppm during some smog alerts. Carbon monoxide is a common pollutant of indoor air. Unvented combustion appliances such as space heaters, ranges, and stoves, defective furnaces, garages connected to living quarters, and cigarette smoke are all sources of carbon monoxide in the home environment. Hazardous concentrations are most likely to develop in confined spaces. Paint removers containing methylene chloride provide a source of carbon monoxide exposure. Once inhaled, methylene chloride is metabolized to carbon monoxide (261).

Disposition

Carbon monoxide is a transparent, tasteless, and odorless gas. It combines reversibly with hemoglobin (Hb) to form carboxyhemoglobin (COHb). Human hemoglobin has an affinity for carbon monoxide approximately 220 times greater than its affinity for oxygen. The carboxyhemoglobin so formed is not available to carry oxygen. Carboxyhemoglobin concentrations are proportional to the concentration of carbon monoxide in inspired air, the length of exposure, and the breathing rate (259). Because carbon monoxide has a high affinity for hemoglobin, increased levels of COHb can result from continued exposure to relatively low carbon monoxide levels. For example, breathing 0.05% (500 ppm) carbon monoxide for 200 min in a sedentary state at atmospheric pressure and normal oxygen concentrations (21%) produces 50% carboxyhemoglobin. Once carboxyhemoglobin is formed, it has a biological half-life of 4–5 h. The inhalation of 100% oxygen reduces its biological half-life to 1.5 h.

Health Effects

The toxic action of carbon monoxide stems from hypoxemia (292). The organs most susceptible to hypoxia are the central nervous system and heart. Certain population groups are particularly vulnerable to low-level carbon monoxide exposure. These include the developing fetus, young infants, and individuals with angina, peripheral vascular disease, chronic lung disease, and anemia (271).

Typical early symptoms and signs of exposure to high concentrations of carbon monoxide are headache, dizziness, drowsiness, nausea, and vomiting. As exposure levels rise, increasing weakness, obtundation, and coma occur. Acute carbon monoxide poisoning may be followed by the delayed onset of neurological deterioration related to posthypoxic damage to the white matter (leukoencephalopathy). Carbon monoxide exposure may adversely affect individuals with angina pectoris (8). Debate exists regarding the effects of chronic exposure to low levels of carbon monoxide. Although the results of numerous studies are conflicting, it appears that low-level CO exposure leads to some impairment in human performance, particularly the execution of complex, visually demanding tasks (122). Laties and Merigan have reviewed the neurobehavioral effects of CO exposure (143).

Biological Monitoring

Blood levels of carboxyhemoglobin reflect the degree of exposure and the direct pathological effect (hypoxemia). Central nervous symptoms have been reported to occur at COHb levels of 5% to 17%. These symptoms include the impairment of vigilance, visual perception, manual dexterity, learning ability, and the performance of complex tasks (271). There is evidence that aggravation of angina may occur at COHb levels in the range of 3.0% to 4.5% (8). Carboxyhemoglobin levels of 15% to 25% produce symptoms of headache, dizziness, and nausea. Levels greater than 50% COHb are life threatening (292).

The biological monitoring of CO exposure is done by determining COHb in blood and CO in blood or expired air. Carboxyhemoglobin levels in unexposed nonsmokers should be less than 2%. Endogenous production of carbon monoxide produces carboxyhemoglobin levels usually less than 0.7%. The median value of COHb for smokers is approximately 5%. However, COHb values of 10% are not uncommon in smokers.

Analysis

Carboxyhemoglobin levels are determined by differential spectrophotometry after the hemoglobin and carboxyhemoglobin are converted to cyanomethemoglobin and reduced hemoglobin. Automated techniques are sufficiently reproducible and sensitive to levels of 1% to 2% carboxyhemoglobin. After the carbon monoxide has been liberated, blood carbon monoxide content can be determined by gas chromatography. Blood carbon monoxide content correlates with carboxyhemoglobin levels, but this analysis is a less sensitive determination (63). Carbon monoxide levels in exhaled air correlate with blood carboxyhemoglobin levels and can be easily measured with infrared spectrometry (117). Other volatile chemicals exhaled in the breath must be excluded in this technique.

Formaldehyde

Formaldehyde is a byproduct of many chemical reactions in industry. It is used as an embalming fluid and as a viral disinfectant in dialysis machines (193). Formaldehyde is used in the manufacture of adhesive resins widely used in the production of plywood and particle board. The textile industry uses formaldehyde for producing crease-resistant and shrinkproof fabrics. Formaldehyde has also been used in the production of urea–formaldehyde foam insulation. Formaldehyde is found throughout the environment (223). In outdoor air, it comes from incinerators and engine exhaust; it is also a component of industrial and automotive smog. In indoor air, formaldehyde is released from such sources as urea–formaldehyde foam insulation, plywood, particleboard, permapress fabrics, and foam-backed carpets. Particularly high levels of formaldehyde have been recorded in new buildings and mobile homes. Formaldehyde levels in residential indoor air have, at times, exceeded occupational standards (169) (see Chapter 2).

Disposition

Formaldehyde is a volatile, highly reactive, water-soluble chemical. It is metabolized to an unknown extent to formic acid, particularly in the liver and red blood cells (223). A portion is excreted in the urine. Formaldehyde is also formed endogenously from the oxidation of glycine and from demethylation reactions.

Health Effects

Formaldehyde has an odor detection threshold of 0.5–1 ppm. Its irritant effects are intolerable above 5 ppm. Increased pulmonary resistance occurs at concentrations greater than 0.3 ppm for 1 h. Its respiratory effects are similar to those noted with sulfur dioxide. Chronic exposure to formaldehyde vapor induces nasal cancer in rats and mice in concentrations of 3.5 to 15 ppm (125). Occupational exposure to formaldehyde may pose some increased risk of cancer of various organs. When coupled with particulate exposure, formaldehyde may pose a specific risk of cancer of the nasopharynx and oropharnyx (24,25).

Biological Monitoring

Preliminary efforts have been made to monitor worker exposure to formaldehyde by measuring formaldehyde in the blood and formic acid in the urine. Determination of blood formaldehyde levels offers little help in monitoring exposure. Formaldehyde is poorly recovered from the blood, and studies thus far show no correlation between blood concentrations and exposure (145,212). Formic acid concentrations in the blood or urine are insensitive indicators of ambient exposure (98). Therefore, at present, formaldehyde exposure is poorly assessed by biological monitoring.

Organophosphorus Pesticides

Occurrence

Because of their shorter-lived residues and lower environmental persistence, organophosphorus pesticides (OPs) continue to replace the organochlorine pesticides. The OPs are used as agricultural and domestic insecticides. Some common OPs include malathion, parathion, diazinon, and chlorpyrifos. Occupational and environmental exposure occurs during the synthesis and formulation processes, during the application, and early reentry into pesticide-treated fields, gardens, and buildings.

Disposition

Exposure to OPs occurs via dermal, pulmonary, and gastrointestinal routes. The OPs easily pass across biological membranes and rapidly undergo oxidation or hydrolysis. Although a diverse number of organophosphorus pesticides have been synthetized, their major biological effect is mediated through the inhibition of cholinesterases. The inhibition of acetylcholinesterase results in an accumulation of acetylcholine in nerve tissue and effector organs. The various OPs have different pharmacokinetic properties and varying capacity to produce toxicity. For example, the oral LD50 in male rats is 13 mg/kg for parathion and 108 mg/kg and 1375 mg/kg for diazinon and malathion, respectively (106).

Health Effects

The acute toxicity that follows exposure to OPs reflects the muscarinic, nicotinic, and central nervous system actions of acetylcholine. Muscarinic effects include bradycardia (which can progress to heart block), miosis, wheezing, increased bronchial secretions, sweating, nausea, gastrointestinal cramping, diarrhea, and increased urination. Nicotinic effects include skeletal muscle fasciculation, tremor, and muscular cramps. Central nervous system effects include restlessness, headache, insomnia, impaired consciousness, convulsions, and coma (106). Some OPs can induce a delayed peripheral neuropathy that develops several weeks after acute exposure. This condition is not dependent on the inhibition of cholinesterase activity (4,91,123,243). The chronic effects of acute or long-term organophosphate exposure are less well established than their acute effects. Neurobehavioral abnormalities

such as impairment of memory, difficulty in thinking, and visual disturbances have been described in individuals exposed to OPs (28,168,266). Investigators have also described symptoms of anxiety, depression, irritability, headache, and memory difficulties in connection with chronic OP exposure (96,296) (see Chapter 14).

Biological Monitoring

Biological monitoring of exposure to OPs can be done by measuring their biological effects or their metabolites in urine (58,59,106). The biological effect of exposure to OPs is assessed by determining cholinesterase activity in blood. As mentioned, many esterases are inhibited by OPs. These esterases include two types of cholinesterase in blood: erythrocyte acetylcholinesterase (true cholinesterase) and plasma cholinesterase, which is also known as pseudocholinesterase or butyrylcholinesterase. Inhibition of erythrocyte cholinesterase more adequately reflects the biological effects of OP exposure since this enzyme is identical to that found in nervous tissues.

Depression of plasma and erythrocyte cholinesterase activity has traditionally been used to estimate OPs and their effects on exposed workers. After OP exposure, the red blood cell cholinesterase is depressed less rapidly than is the plasma cholinesterase, and the plasma cholinesterase levels return to normal more rapidly than the red blood cell cholinesterase levels (150). Recovery rates vary considerably in exposed agricultural workers and may take several months to return to normal after OP exposure has stopped (58).

The development of symptoms depends on the rate and the degree of cholinesterase inhibition. For example, workers may have 70% to 80% inhibition after a few weeks of moderate OP exposure without symptoms, whereas acute exposure resulting in a sudden decrease of 30% in cholinesterase activity is often accompanied by symptoms (58,106).

The interpretation of cholinesterase activity levels is complicated by wide interindividual variation and imprecision in laboratory analyses (224, 297). Since the intraindividual variation in cholinesterase activity is small in comparison to the variation encountered in the laboratory analysis, changes of less than 20% in cholinesterase activity in the same person may not represent a true change in enzyme activity (287). Because of the wide range of normal interindividual variation, it is possible for an individual's cholinesterase activity to decrease 50% but still be within the normal range. The best evidence of OP effect is provided by a comparison of postexposure cholinesterase activity with preexposure levels. A reduction of 25% or more is strong evidence of excessive OP absorption (178).

A more sensitive approach to detecting OP exposure is offered by determining the presence of the intact pesticide and/or its metabolites in the urine (59,89,155,164,222). Under conditions of a single exposure to certain OPs, a high correlation has been shown between exposure and excretion products (89,179). Thus far, however, the usefulness of measuring pesticide excretion products is limited, as few relationships have been established between pesticide exposure and the excretion of pesticide metabolites in the urine. In addition, interpreting the significance of urinary pesticide metabolite levels often presents a dilemma because the relationship between these levels and adverse health effects is usually unknown. For many pesticides currently in use, no methods are available for monitoring exposure.

Exposure to certain dimethyl or diethyl OPs can be detected by measuring alkyl phosphate metabolites in the urine (59,89,155,164,222). Urinary metabolites of OPs are excreted soon after exposure and can be detected for several days after exposure. Increased urinary levels of alkyl phosphates are detectable before there is evidence of inhibition of cholinesterase in erythrocytes or plasma (89). Other compounds found in the urine after OP exposure include p-nitrophenol, a metabolite or parathion, and p-nitro-m-cresol, a metabolite of fenitrothion (13,289).

It is of interest that the California Department of Food and Agriculture now requires a pesticide manufacturer to specify a urinary metabolite that can be used to monitor exposure before registering a new pesticide. Those readers interested in biological monitoring of pesticide exposure are referred to several references (270,295).

Analysis

Methods for determining cholinesterase activity in red cells and plasma fall into two general categories: those based on the electrometric method developed by Michel and those based on the colorimetric method developed by Ellman (69,170). The same analytic procedure should always be used to determine any change in the levels of cholinesterase activity in the same person.

The gas chromatographic method developed by Shafik et al. is a method for determining a number of alkyl phosphates in the urine (241). This method can detect such alkyl phosphates as dimethyl or diethyl phosphates and phosphorothionates.

Organochlorine Pesticides

Occurrence

The best-known example of an organochlorine pesticide is dichlorodiphenyltrichloroethane (DDT). Other examples include such compounds as aldrin,

dieldrin, chlordane, hepatochlor, and toxaphene. The organochlorine pesticides were in wide use for three decades until the early 1970s. DDT production in the United States, for example, rose to a peak of 179 million pounds in 1963 (257). Although occupational exposure provides the greatest risk of pesticide exposure, the general population is exposed to pesticides from many sources. Pesticide residues on foods are ingested, pesticide laden dusts are inhaled, and dermal absorption occurs from the use of pesticides in the home and garden.

Disposition

After absorption, the long biological half-life of certain of the lipophilic organochlorine pesticides has resulted in their storage in adipose tissue (138). Residues of these compounds also can be detected in urine, blood, and milk (43,182,230).

The organochlorine pesticides, as a group, are generally considered less acutely toxic than the organophosphorus and carbamate pesticides. They have come into disfavor because of their persistence in the environment, their accumulation in the food chain, their harmful ecological effects, and their persistence in humans. The potential long-term effects of organochlorine pesticides are of particular concern because a great number of these agents are documented animal carcinogens (115). Beginning in 1972, the EPA canceled or severely restricted the use of such organochlorine pesticides as DDT, aldrin, dieldrin, chlordane, hepatochlor, and toxaphene (272). The export of canceled and restricted pesticides to developing countries, along with their subsequent reentry into the United States as pesticide residues on imported fruits and vegetables has caused concern (72).

DDT is the most widely known example of the organochlorine pesticides. DDT is dechlorinated to form dichlorodiphenyldichloroethylene (DDE), a major metabolic product that also accumulates in adipose tissue. DDT is also dechlorinated to form dichlorodiphenyldichloroethane (DDD), which is transformed to dichlorodiphenylacetic acid (DDA), the major urinary metabolite of DDT (183).

Health Effects

Information on the long-term health effects of environmental exposure to organochlorine pesticides has not been adequately investigated (243). One study of a rural population excessively exposed to DDT residues through the ingestion of contaminated fish was performed by Kriess et al. (135). These workers noted a steady increase of serum DDT levels with advancing age. High DDT serum levels were positively associated with increases in serum cholesterol, triglycerides, and γ-glutamyl transpeptidase. The geometric mean level of total DDT in serum samples was 0.22 μmol/mL (76.2 ng/ml). This figure is more than five times than that noted in a national survey sponsored by the EPA. DDE accounts for an average of 86.7% of the total DDT. The study by Kriess et al. was not designed to address the long-term health effects of DDT exposure.

The International Agency for Research on Cancer (IARC), after assessing the available human and animal studies, concluded that DDT is possibly carcinogenic for humans. DDT's carcinogenic potential has been inadequately assessed in humans. Animals studies, however, have adequately shown that DDT is carcinogenic (115).

Biological Monitoring

In 1969 the EPA developed, and has since continued, a human monitoring program. This program is designed to determine, on a national scale, the incidence, level, and trends of pesticide exposure experienced by the general population (182, 229,269). A broadly based EPA survey conducted between 1976 and 1980 revealed that nearly all blood samples tested had detectable levels of DDT and its analogues (limits of detection 0.003–0.006 μmol (1–2 μg)L. Between 4% and 14% of the blood samples had detectable levels of residues from such organochlorine pesticides as aldrin, dieldrin, benzene hexachloride, and chlordane (limits of detection 0.003–0.006 μmol (1–2 μg)/L. A National Human Adipose Tissue Monitoring Survey in 1978 revealed that all samples contained DDT and its analogues, and over 90% of the specimens contained evidence of chlordane, hepatochlor, aldrin, dieldrin, and benzene hexachloride (limits of detection 0.03–0.06 μmol (10–20 μg)/L. Between 1972 and 1977, analyses of adipose tissue showed declining levels of DDT residues. However, the levels of aldrin, dieldrin, chlordane, and hepatochlor remained constant (126,182).

DDT blood levels—which include DDT, DDE, and DDD—in nonoccupationally exposed normal individuals are usually less than 0.04 μmol (15 μg)/L, whereas occupationally exposed pesticide workers average about 0.16 μmol/L (57 ppb) (262). Once DDT in the blood has equilibrated with the lipid-soluble compartment, some estimate of the extent and magnitude of exposure to this agent may be made by monitoring blood levels (229). Recent exposures to DDT can be estimated by measuring dichlorodiphenylacetic acid (DDA) in the urine shortly after exposure (13,212). Workers whose average daily intake of DDT was estimated to be 18 mg excreted 3.59 μmol (1.27 mg)/L of DDA in their urine (149).

Analysis

All analyses of organochlorine pesticides require the careful extraction of organochlorine pesticides and their metabolites from biological material. The analyses are performed by gas chromatography with electron capture, photometic, or mass-selective detector systems. To avoid contamination with organochlorines that interfere with the analysis, sampling must be carefully done. The quality of performance among laboratories varies considerably. A compilation of methods used in pesticide-monitoring programs is given by the U.S. EPA (270).

Polychlorinated Biphenyls

Occurrence

Polychlorinated biphenyls (PCBs) are a group of compounds belonging to the class of chlorinated aromatic hydrocarbons. Commercial PCBs are complex mixtures of chlorinated biphenyls, which may also contain polychlorinated dibenzofurans (PCDFs) and chlorinated quaterphenyls (PCQs) as impurities. Commercial mixtures of PCBs manufactured by Monsanto in the United States were numerically identified according to their chlorine content. Thus, Aroclor 1254 contained about 54% chlorine, and Aroclor 1260 about 60% chlorine. The PCBs do not occur naturally. Introduced in the 1930s, the flame-retardant and insulating properties of PCBs led to their extensive use by the electrical industry in capacitors and transformers; PCBs were also used in carbonless duplicating paper and in plastics, oils, and paints (129).

Although the EPA banned the production and commercial use of PCBs in the late 1970s, human exposure continues. Resistance to degradation and their wide use have resulted in worldwide PCBs contamination involving rivers, lakes, the atmosphere, fish, and wildlife. Like DDT residues, PCBs accumulate and are concentrated in the food chain. In the United States, environmental exposure to PCBs occurs primarily from eating fish from contaminated waters (234,237). Human exposure has also been the consequence of fires involving PCBs (87,195). Concern about the environmental persistence and human accumulation of PCBs is based on their ability to cause liver cancer in rodents, reproductive problems in humans and other species, and alterations in immune function in certain species (129,130).

Disposition

The primary routes of exposure to PCBs are oral and pulmonary. The PCBs are highly lipid-soluable compounds. Those PCBs that accumulate in adipose tissue are more highly chlorinated and less readily metabolized. The more readily metabolized chlorinated biphenyls have adjacent unsubstituted carbon atoms in the 3–4 position (163,247). The readily metabolized PCBs are tranformed to more polar compounds and excreted. The PCBs can also be eliminated from the body, unmetabolized, in association with agents having a high lipid content (i.e., milk, eggs). Because PCBs readily cross the placenta, these agents are present in the fetus (163).

Health Effects

Polychlorinated biphenyls are not considered acutely toxic. In rodents the acute oral LD50 is 9 g/kg of body weight. Animal studies have demonstrated that commercial PCBs produce a wide range of chronic toxic effects, which include decreased immunocompetence, reproductive problems, liver damage, and alteration in lipid metabolism (128). The PCBs have produced hepatocellular carcinomas in rodents (128,192). Isomers of PCBs vary greatly in toxicity. The more toxic isomers are generally the more persistent, highly chlorinated compounds (130,192). The toxicity of PCB mixtures also depends on the extent of contamination. In early animal studies conducted with PCBs, these agents were contaminated with polychlorinated dibenzofuans (PBDFs) and polychlorinated dibenzodioxins (PCDDs). Since these compounds are many times more toxic than PCBs, many toxic effects attributed to PCBs are now considered to have been caused by PCDFs and PCDDs (130,165).

Much of our knowledge about the adverse health effects of exposure to PCBs and their impurities in humans stems from two large-scale poisoning episodes that occurred in Japan in 1968 and in Taiwan in 1979. In Japan the mass poisoning was called "Yusho"; in Taiwan it was called "Yu Cheng." These epidemics were related to the accidental ingestion of rice cooking oil that had been contaminated with PCBs. Further analysis revealed that the rice oil had also been contaminated with polychlorinated dibenzofurans (PCDFs) and polychlorinated quaterphenyls. Recent studies indicate that the clinical manifestations seen in the Yusho and Yu Cheng patients were most likely caused by the ingestion of PCDFs (162).

Ingesting PCB-contaminated rice oil produced chloracne, characterized by pustules, comedos, and straw-colored cysts. Hyperpigmentation of the skin and nails, hypersecretion of the Meibomian glands, abnormalities in serum lipid concentrations, and increased porphyrin excretion also occurred (52, 137). Nonspecific symptoms included anorexia, fatigue, and weight loss. Severely afflicted individuals were noted to have abnormal liver function tests (137). Abnormalities in the immune response were found in the Yu Cheng patients (44,45). A fetal PCB syndrome was also described (299).

A follow-up study of the offspring of women exposed to PCBs and dibenzofurans during the Taiwan epidemic revealed that offspring from pregnancies that occurred after maternal exposure had ceased showed evidence of delayed development and abnormalities of the gingiva, skin, nails, teeth, and lung. The long persistence of PCBs and dibenzofurans in maternal tissue results in the in utero exposure of the fetus, which gives rise to afflicted offspring (231).

Epidemiologic studies of workers with occupational exposure to PCBs do not demonstrate the severe clinical manifestations found in the Yusho and Yu Cheng patients. The PCB exposure of the Yusho and Yu Cheng patients is not directly comparable to occupational PCB exposure. Much lower levels of exposure were generally encountered in an occupational setting. In addition, PCB mixtures manufactured in the United States were, for the most part, not contaminated with PCDFs (133).

Several studies of PCB-exposed workers reveal the presence of chloracne and increased urinary uroporphyrin excretion (52,130). Several chlorinated hydrocarbons, including PCBs inhibit uroporphyrinogen decarboxylase and thereby cause an increase in uroporphyrin excretion (52). A number of investigators observed a correlation between serum PCB levels and changes in the blood levels of certain hepatic enzymes (133). A positive association between serum PCB levels and elevated levels of triglycerides, serum cholesterol, and blood pressure was noted by some workers (130,134). The association between serum PCBs and serum lipid levels disappears when PCB levels are expressed as a function of fat in serum rather than of whole serum.

Based on a review of epidemiologic studies of occupational populations and of populations accidently exposed to PCB mixtures, the IARC has listed PCBs as probably carcinogenic to humans. The available studies point to a relationship between PCBs and cancer, particularly hepatobiliary cancer (115). The evidence is limited, since the number of individuals studied was small, dose–response relationships could not be evaluated, and the role of compounds other than PCBs could not be excluded (115).

Biological Monitoring

Many reports have shown that PCBs are widely present in human tissues (133,229,230). These reports include EPA-sponsored national surveys (270). Monitoring studies in the United States show that populations without occupational exposure to PCBs have mean serum levels between 0.01 and 0.02 μmol/L (4 and 8 ng/mL), with 95% of individuals having mean serum levels below 0.06 μmol/L (20 ng/mL). Populations with increased environmental exposure to PCBs (i.e., those consuming fish from contaminated waters) have mean serum PCB levels several times greater than those of the general population, often reaching levels found in exposed workers (133). The concentration of PCBs in adipose tissue and milk is 100–300 times that found in serum (119).

Although no firm relationship between PCB dose and tissue levels has been established, monitoring blood levels of PCBs permits some qualitative estimate of the extent and magnitude of exposure to these agents. Studies of PCB-exposed workers reveal that the blood concentration of PCBs correlated with the degree and duration of exposure (71). After the absorbed PCBs equilibrate with adipose tissue, serum PCB concentrations correlate reasonably with adipose tissue levels (31). Because of this equilibration, blood sampling, rather than adipose tissue biopsy, can be used to roughly assess the body burden of PCBs. At present it is impossible to assign a health risk to a particular PCB tissue concentration.

Analysis

Serum and adipose tissue PCB levels may be analyzed by gas chromatography with electron capture and mass-selective detection (13,36). Containers for collecting serum to be analyzed for PCBs should be pure silica glass (acid and hexane washed). No plastic products (plastic syringes, rubber stoppers, plungers) should come in contact with the sample.

Chlorophenoxyacetic Acid Herbicides and Dioxin

Occurrence

Chlorophenoxyacetic acids, which include 2,4-dichlorophenoxyacetic acid (2,4-D) and 2,4,5-trichlorophenoxyacetic acid (2,4,5-T), have been widely used as herbicides since the 1940s. These agents are economically important chemicals used for weed control in forestry, agriculture, home lawns, and gardens. Other major uses include weed control along highways, railroad rights-of-way, waterways, and public recreation areas.

Concern about exposure to the phenoxy herbicides has focused particularly on 2,4,5-T, which contains traces of an unwanted contaminant, 2,3,7,8-tetrachlorodibenzo-p-dioxin (TCDD) or "dioxin." TCDD is considered to be one of the most powerful poisons for lower animals. There is considerable species variation in response to this agent (129). In the 1960s, during the Vietnam War, "Agent Orange" was widely used as a defoliant. This herbicidal mixture was composed of equal parts 2,4-D and 2,4,5-T, the latter being contaminated with varying amounts of TCDD. In 1979, the use of 2,4,5-T was severely restricted by the EPA. It has also been banned in other parts of the world. Now 2,4-D continues to be the most widely used phenoxy herbicide in agriculture and forestry. There is no evidence that 2,4-D contains TCDD (56).

The phenoxy herbicides are generally applied as esters in organic solvents or as basic salts dissolved in water. Though regarded as nonpersistent compounds, they have been detected in some soil samples as long as 1 year after their application. The phenoxy herbicides undergo photochemical decomposition as well as degradation by soil bacteria. Under conditions favoring bacterial growth, such as warmth, moisture, and nutrient availability, the phenoxy herbicides are more rapidly degraded (56).

Studies reveal that TCDD is extremely photosensitive, breaking down quickly in the presence of ultraviolet radiation. There is a progressive dechlorination of the aromatic ring. As the chlorine is removed, the product becomes more biodegradable. Since only the dioxin at the surface of the soil or aquatic system is exposed to ultraviolet radiation, it may persist several years in the soil and aquatic ecosystems (56). TCDD may also be found at sites formerly producing 2,4,5-T, and in fly ash from municipal incinerators and industrial heating facilities.

Disposition

Exposure to the phenoxyacetic acids is predominantly dermal. Pulmonary and oral absorption are also possible. In a matter of a few days after absorption, most phenoxy herbicides are eliminated in the urine, largely unchanged. For example, in human volunteers given 0.02 mmol/kg (5 mg/kg) of 2,4-D, 82% was excreted as free 2,4-D, and 13% was excreted as a 2,4-D conjugate. The average biological half-life was about 18 h (236). Human volunteers given 0.02 mmol/kg (5 mg/kg) of 2,4,5-T absorbed essentially all of the orally administered dose and excreted it unchanged in the urine. Nearly 90% of the administered dose of 2,4,5-T was excreted in the urine by the end of 96 h (95). In each case no detectable short-term effects were observed.

Rodent studies using ^{14}C-labeled TCDD determined that after absorption over 50% was excreted in the feces, with small amounts being eliminated in the urine and expired air. TCDD has a half-life of 1 month in rodents and accumulates in the adipose tissue and liver (219,232).

The advent of new technology permitting the measurement of TCDD in adipose tissue and serum provides a means of assessing exposure and biological half-life of this agent in humans. This technology has been applied to U.S. Army Vietnam-era veterans, Agent-Orange-exposed Vietnam veterans, and participants in the U.S. Air Force "Ranch

Hand" study of Vietnam veterans who were herbicide loaders or herbicide specialists (42,43,124). From these studies the biological half-life of TCDD in humans has been calculated to be approximately 7 years (213).

Health Effects

The acute toxicity of 2,4-D and 2,4,5-T, in their uncontaminated forms, is relatively low. The LD50s range from 300 to over 1000 mg/kg in many species. In humans, accidental skin exposure to high concentrations of 2,4-D has produced acute toxicity with symptoms of nausea, vomiting, diarrhea, headache, vertigo, and weakness. Under conditions of heavy dermal exposure, peripheral neuropathy has been documented. There is little information on the acute toxicity and/or chronic toxicity in humans associated with 2,4,5-T itself. In the past, essentially all 2,4,5-T contained varying quantities of TCDD. AT present the TCDD content in 2,4,5-T is regulated at 0.1 ppm or less.

It was thought that the fetotoxic effects of 2,4,5-T were probably related to its contamination with TCDD, but subsequent studies have revealed that purified 2,4,5-T is teratogenic and fetotoxic (188). Some studies have shown exposure to 2,4-D to be teratogenic, but other studies have not (294). Thus far, animal studies provide no conclusive evidence that 2,4-D and 2,4,5-T are carcinogenic (115).

Animal studies indicate that TCDD is one of the most potent chemical toxins, having LD50s of 0.07 mmol/kg (0.022 mg/kg) for rats and 0.002 μmol/kg (0.0006 mg/kg) for guinea pigs. Toxic effects in animals include wasting, debilitation, hepatotoxicity, skin lesions, and thymic atrophy (129). It is noteworthy that there are large species variations in the toxicity of TCDD.

The acute health effects of human exposure to TCDD-contaminated material in the workplace or through episodes of environmental contamination, as occurred in Seveso, Italy and in the state of Missouri, include chloracne, some abnormal liver tests, disordered lipid metabolism, and complaints of sensory neuropathy (121,131,214,264). Chloracne was noted to be the most persistent health effect. However, when exposure ceased, most health effects appeared to improve or subside completely.

Concern has centered on the potential reproductive and carcinogenic hazards of phenoxy herbicide exposure, particularly exposure to TCDD-contaminated 2,4,5-T. In animals, TCDD is an extremely potent teratogen and fetotoxic agent (57). There is also evidence that TCDD produces cancer in animals (115).

Numerous epidemiologic studies have investigated the relationship between exposure to the phenoxy herbicides and the development of cancer

(73,101–103,112,115,156,243). Based on a review of these studies, the International Agency for Research on Cancer (IARC) has concluded that there is limited evidence that persons exposed to phenoxy herbicides and chlorophenols may be at increased risk of soft-tissue sarcoma and lymphoma (115). Of note is the finding that some excesses of these cancers occurred under conditions of exposure to phenoxy herbicides in which no substantial TCDD exposure was likely to have occurred (51,112,127,157).

After a review of the studies investigating the relationship between TCDD exposure and cancer, the IARC classified this agent as a possible human carcinogen. As noted, there is sufficient evidence for carcinogenicity in animals but inadequate evidence for carcinogenicity in humans (115). Three cases of soft-tissue sarcoma have been reported thus far in Vietnam veterans exposed to TCDD-containing "Agent Orange" during the 1960s (235). Limited observations suggest a possible increased number of soft-tissue sarcomas in Seveso, Italy as a result of the accidental exposure of the residents to TCDD. This exposure occurred in 1976 with a runaway chemical reaction at a plant producing trichlorophenol (217). Populations exposed to TCDD must continue to be followed carefully because of the well-established latent period that exists between the initial exposure to a carcinogen and the clinical appearance of cancer.

A number of epidemiologic studies have investigated the reproductive effects of exposure to phenoxy herbicides and dioxin. The results of these studies are discussed in Chapter 24.

Biological Monitoring

Relatively little biological monitoring data are available for groups with occupational exposure to phenoxy herbicides (2). No definite guidelines thus exist for what constitutes excessive exposure to phenoxy herbicides. At the end of the day, workers spraying these compounds have urinary levels ranging between 0.2 and 70 μmol (44–15,470 μg)/L (132).

The development of methods to measure TCDD levels in blood and tissue provides a means of monitoring exposure to this agent (200). Blood and adipose tissue levels of TCDD were measured in Agent-Orange-exposed Vietnam veterans and in matched controls. The results of these studies indicate that 15 to 20 years after their exposure the levels of TCDD in Vietnam veterans heavily exposed to Agent Orange exceeded the levels found in matched controls (124). In all heavily exposed subjects, the TCDD levels in adipose tissue exceeded 0.05 pmol (15pg)/g. None of the control subjects exceeded that level (124). Further study of serum TCDD levels in "Ranch Hand" subjects who sustained heavy herbicide exposure during the Vietnam war revealed that their mean serum TCDD level was 49 parts per trillion (ppt). Nearly two-thirds of this group had TCDD serum levels above 20 ppt, the figure considered the upper limit for U.S. residents without known TCDD exposure (35). Another study found that serum TCDD levels of U.S. Army Vietnam-era veterans who did not handle herbicides were nearly identical to those found in non-Vietnam-veterans (43).

These results indicate that heavily exposed individuals have higher TCDD blood and adipose levels than do other individuals. Of note is the finding that adipose tissue and blood levels of TCDD are highly correlated (124,201). This correlation makes it likely that blood sampling will supplant the adipose tissue biopsy in assessing the body burden of TCDD. As yet, no threshold level has been determined for the health effects of TCDD in humans. In view of the biological monitoring data that are rapidly accumulating, it seems likely that blood measurements of TCDD will be an aid in establishing cohorts of exposed and unexposed individuals for epidemiologic study of the health effects of such exposure.

Analysis

Phenoxy herbicides in serum and urine can be measured by gas chromatographic and high-pressure liquid chromatographic methods (13,194). These methods are not widely available commercially. High-resolution gas chromatography/mass spectrometry is used in the determination of TCDD (200,249).

BIOLOGICAL MONITORING OF EXPOSURE TO CARCINOGENIC AND MUTAGENIC AGENTS

Introduction

Humans are exposed to carcinogenic and mutagenic substances, both natural and man-made, that are found in air, water, and food (7,114). The detection and assessment of human risk from exposure to environmental carcinogens are currently based on animal bioassay and epidemiologic studies. Short-term in vitro assays as predictors of carcinogenicity have been under intensive investigation for a number of years. Because of methodological limitations, these tools have limited usefulness in accurately predicting human carcinogenic risk (177,206).

Animal experiments are commonly conducted on relatively few animals with exposure levels many times those normally encountered by humans. The results must be extrapolated to low doses that correspond to human exposure. Extrapolations to low-dose exposure and between species are steps ac

companied by large uncertainties. Epidemiologic studies furnish important human data but give limited assessment of carcinogenic risk. Though such studies avoid the pitfalls of species extrapolation, they are frequently limited by a lack of critical exposure information, by many confounding factors, and by the long interval between the initial exposure to a carcinogen and the clinical appearance of cancer. Because of this latent period, epidemiologic studies cannot provide an early warning of carcinogenic risk. Short-term in vitro screening tests may provide some information on the potential carcinogenicity of chemicals. Such testing, however, is not applicable to all carcinogens. In addition, it is difficult to extrapolate the results of short-term in vitro testing to humans and to gain information on carcinogenic potency. When these limitations are considered, it is apparent that new methods are needed to detect carcinogenic hazards in a timely manner.

This need has spurred investigators to develop biological monitoring techniques that provide an early warning of mutagenic and/or carcinogenic risk to human populations. Their goal is twofold: the detection of exposure to carcinogens and mutagens before irreversible effects have occurred and the more precise estimation of risk from such exposure. The benefits of biological monitoring methods are realized when they are combined with epidemiologic methods (113). Under these conditions, conventional epidemiologic studies should have increased power to detect carcinogenic or other health risks earlier, more precisely, and at lower exposures (203,204,206,271). The term "molecular cancer epidemiology" was used by Perera and Weinstein to describe the integration of advanced laboratory methods with analytic epidemiology to identify at the biochemical or molecular level specific exogenous or endogenous factors that play a role in human cancer causation (204,206). From an epidemiologic view "biochemical or molecular epidemiology" incorporates biological markers into analytic epidemiologic investigation. This methodology can be used in the epidemiologic study of diseases other than cancer. There are several reviews of this subject (92,113,174,203,204,206,282,286) (see Chapter 1).

Indicators of Genotoxic Exposure

The best indicator of risk is the amount of the chemical or its active metabolites that has reacted with critical cellular targets (biologically effective dose or target dose). With carcinogenic chemicals, the biological effective dose refers to the amount of carcinogen or its active metabolite that has interacted with critical cellular macromolecules (DNA, RNA, and protein). In an attempt to assess mutagenic and carcinogenic risks, methods of quantifying the biological effective dose have been developed and applied, almost exclusively, to genotoxic agents (12,92,203,204,206,245).

Investigators have developed a number of methods to assay human cells and tissues for genetic changes linked to chemical and radiation exposure. Current monitoring methods are based on biochemical and cytogenetic markers of genotoxic exposure. Biochemical markers of exposure are reflected in the level of genotoxic chemicals, their metabolites, and derivatives present in body tissues and fluids. Cytogenetic markers of exposure represent the visible changes found in chromosomes. Specific monitoring techniques include relatively new methods of measuring DNA and protein modifications as well as the more established methods of cytogenetic monitoring (i.e., chromosomal aberrations and sister chromatid exchanges (Table 27-3) (12,92,154,204,206,253–255,274–277,286).

Thus far, the application of biological monitoring methods that assess genotoxic changes associated with exposure to mutagens and carcinogens has been relatively limited. The effective application of such methods to large-scale epidemiologic studies requires that extensive efforts be made to develop simple assay techniques and to validate their use. Work is proceeding rapidly in this area, and the interested reader is urged to consult the most recent publications in this field.

Advantages of Genotoxic Monitoring

Determining the biologically effective dose of a mutagen or carcinogen has a number of potential advantages. It could (1) provide direct evidence of the extent of exposure to carcinogenic and mutagenic agents in occupational and environmental settings, (2) identify, in a timely manner, potentially

carcinogenic hazards, (3) increase the power of epidemiologic studies to assess the risk of exposure to carcinogenic agents, (4) monitor the effectiveness of control measures for reducing exposure to carcinogens, and (5) provide clues to the mechanisms involved in carcinogenesis (204,206,253).

Rapid technical advancements in assessing the interaction of carcinogens with critical cellular macromolecules hold the promise of monitoring low-dose exposure to carcinogens and mutagens in humans. Assessing genotoxic changes may also provide a means of estimating relative carcinogenic potency of different chemicals. It is evident that all carcinogenic and mutagenic agents are not equally harmful. With potencies ranging over a factor as high as 10^7, any meaningful interpretation of human exposure to carcinogens must consider this factor (278).

Limitations of Genotoxic Monitoring

Nearly all present techniques developed for monitoring mutagens and carcinogens deal with the effects of exposure on genetic material. They thereby provide a gauge of early or initiating events in the carcinogenic process. Events that occur later, i.e., promotion and progression, are not evaluated (see Chapter 26 for a detailed discussion of the stages of carcinogenesis).

One of the major problems encountered when monitoring cells and tissues for genotoxic changes is the lack of background data or knowledge of normal variability in unexposed populations. Obtaining such data is complicated by the fact that normal populations are exposed to a variety of chemicals, viruses, and pharmaceuticals, which may confound genotoxic changes associated with exposure to chemical carcinogens present in the workplace and general environment (177,205,286).

Monitoring genotoxic exposure is most commonly performed in such somatic cells as peripheral blood lymphocytes and in maturing erythrocytes of the bone marrow. Though the findings noted in these somatic cells may provide a window to the damage taking place in other somatic cells, information obtained thus far suggests that there may be organ and tissue specificity with regard to the induction of DNA damage (12). It is not known if the genotoxic effects noted in somatic cells reflect the types of damage taking place in germ cells. Little if any information is available on the response of the germ cell line chromosomes to damage by environmental chemicals (76).

The following discussion focuses on biochemical and cytogenetic markers used to detect exposure to carcinogens and mutagens based on their genotoxic action. Table 27-4 presents an evaluation of some of these markers. As noted, each has its ad-

TABLE 27-3. Biological Monitoring of Exposure to Carcinogens and Mutagens Based on Their Genotoxic Effects

Types of markers	Examples
Adduct formation with nucleic acids	Acetylaminofluorene–DNA Benzo[a]pyrene–DNA
Adduct formation with protein	Alkylation of hemoglobin (e.g., by ethylene oxide)
Urinary excretion of excised DNA adducts	Excretion of chemical–nucleoside adducts
Cytogenetic damage	Chromosomal aberrations Sister chromatid exchanges Numerical alterations Micronuclei

TABLE 27-4. Evaluation of Markers Used to Assess Human Exposure to Carcinogenic and Mutagenic Agents[a]

Method of biological monitoring	Exposure assessment			Health effect assessment	
	Recent internal dose	Long-term body burden	Dose at target site	Nonadverse (reversible)	Adverse
Determination of chemical/ metabolite in body	+[b]	±	−	±	±
Determination of mutagenic activity in excreta	(+)	−	−	−	?
Detection of blood protein adducts	+	(+)	−	(−)	(−)
Detection of DNA adducts in somatic cells	+	(+)	+	(−)	(−)
Analysis of chromosomal aberrations in somatic cells	(+)	+	−	+	(+)
Analysis of sister chromatid exchanges in somatic cells	(+)	+	−	+	(+)
Analysis of micronucleated cells	?	?	−	?	?

[a]From references 12 and 154.
[b]+, applicable/true; (+), probably applicable/probably true; −, not applicable/not true; (−) not presently applicable/not presently true; ±, cannot be generalized; ?, unknown.

vantages and limitations, depending on the monitoring goal.

Biochemical Markers

Exposure to chemical carcinogens and mutagens can be monitored by measuring their interaction with critical cellular macromolecules (DNA and protein). This interaction results in the formation of DNA and/or protein adducts, which can be detected in human tissues and fluids (12,65,109,205,277,285).

DNA Adducts

There is much support for measuring DNA adducts as a relevant indicator or marker of the biological effective dose of exposure to carcinogenic chemicals. Carcinogenic chemicals yield electrophiles capable of forming covalent adducts with cellular DNA. The formation of DNA adducts represents a critical event leading to mutations and/or malignant transformation (30,171–173). The degree of adduct formation appears to correlate with carcinogenic potency and tumor-initiating activity (30, 156,205,248).

The potential usefulness of measuring DNA adducts or protein adducts ultimately depends on their reliability as an index of target cell exposure and carcinogenic risk. The most important unanswered question is how carcinogenic risk in humans is quantitatively related to the extent of DNA binding. The answer to this question depends on a large body of knowledge, which includes an understanding of the kinetics of DNA adduct formation and repair in human tissues. Information is needed on adduct stability and on the rate of adduct formation in relation to dose and the number of doses received. The rate of DNA repair is important, for if human cells are adept in DNA repair, adducts, though formed, will not be detected. These critical issues are currently under investigation (12,109, 205,286).

From laboratory investigations and preliminary studies in humans done thus far, it generally appears that the degree of binding of carcinogen to DNA targets reflects the administered dose. Because of rapid DNA repair processes, it is unclear to what extent the presence of carcinogen–DNA adducts reflects recent exposure (286). There is no threshold or level of exposure below which adducts are not formed (205).

In recent years highly sensitive techniques have been developed for measuring DNA adducts. These methods include the use of immunoassays and postlabeling techniques. Immunoassays are based on antibodies induced in rabbits or monoclonal antibodies that specifically recognize a number of carcinogen-modified nucleic acid residues (205,285, 286). Postlabeling techniques entail the enzymatic incorporation of radiolabeled ^{32}P into the DNA to be tested for the presence of covalent adducts. The radiolabeled nucleosides are separated into normal and adducted nucleotides by chromatographic migration and then subjected to scintillation assay. Radioactive ^{32}P postlabeling techniques are done without giving radioactive compounds to the subjects under study (109). Immunoassays are quantitative and highly specific, whereas ^{32}P can be used to search for genotoxic components in crude environmental mixtures and to monitor human exposure to DNA-damaging agents.

Though the sensitivities of these procedures vary, immunologic techniques are sensitive enough to detect about one in 10^7 nucleotides of DNA. Each human cell is known to contain about 3×10^9 nucleotides of DNA. This figure is equivalent to about 300 carcinogen residues per cell. If the sensitivity of the immunoassay for specific carcinogen–DNA adducts can be increased 300-fold, which seems likely, then a negative test would indicate that there is less than one carcinogen residue per cell (286). Postlabeling techniques can detect one adduct in about 10^{10} normal nucleotides (109). In some instances, ultrasensitive physicochemical methods based on fluorescence properties have been used to detect carcinogen–DNA adducts in humans. For a detailed discussion of the methods used for the detection and estimation of DNA adducts in biological material, the reader is referred to relevant references (104,109,118,156,215,216,220).

Measurements of DNA and protein adducts can be performed in humans in peripheral blood cells and in the cells of other tissues obtained through biopsy or autopsy. DNA and protein adducts from peripheral blood cells have been used to reflect the biological effective dose of chemical carcinogens. However, for most carcinogens, comparisons between the genotoxic effects observed in peripheral blood cells and in target sites have not been studied.

DNA adducts can also be monitored in the urine. Their presence results from the fact that adducts removed from cellular nucleic acids are excreted in the urine. The detection of DNA adducts in urine could provide qualitative information on recent exposure to specific carcinogens (288).

Thus far, a limited number of pilot studies have attempted to validate the use of DNA adducts in the biological monitoring of chemical carcinogens. DNA adducts have been measured in such groups as treated cancer patients, smokers, and coke oven workers (104,207,221). Studies thus far reveal variability in adduct formation among persons with similar exposures (205).

Protein Adducts

The covalent binding of a large group of genotoxic chemicals results in the alkylation of proteins. Direct information on exposure to mutagens and carcinogens is therefore provided by measuring alkylated proteins (276,277). In 1974, Ehrenberg and his co-workers first proposed that the reaction products of alkylating agents with circulating proteins might provide a marker of genotoxic exposure. This approach has been validated in animal experiments and is now being applied to human populations exposed to genotoxic compounds (64–66,268).

Hemoglobin adducts were proposed as a surrogate for DNA–carcinogen adducts because modified amino acids are more easily measured than are corresponding changes in DNA. Moreover, hemoglobin and other blood proteins are more readily available in much larger quantities than is DNA (197). The long life span of hemoglobin offers the special advantage of providing an index of total genotoxic exposure over its 4-month life span (99). The validity of using the hemoglobin molecule as dose monitor for genotoxic exposure is supported by (1) a proportionality between the rate of formation of hemoglobin adducts and the rate of formation of DNA adducts over a wide dose range, (2) the stability of hemoglobin adducts throughout the life span of the erythrocyte, and (3) the large numbers of mutagens and cancer initiators that have been shown to bind covalently to hemoglobin (37,67,183, 189,190,208).

Hemoglobin alkylation has been measured in the blood of workers exposed to ethylene oxide (38). It was possible to measure and isolate alkylated residues of the amino acid histidine in the hemoglobin of workers whose exposure to ethylene oxide was as low as 5 to 10 ppm. The concentration of alkylated hemoglobin was shown to reflect accurately exposure to ethylene oxide and adequately reflect DNA adduct formation. A subsequent study of workers who had low-level ethylene oxide exposure (less than 0.05 ppm) failed to show a correlation between exposure and hemoglobin adduct formation (280).

Analysis of human hemoglobin adducts can be performed by nonradioactive methods using gas chromatography/mass spectrometry (267). The present detection limit of hemoglobin adduct determination in human samples (0.1 nmol $^{-1}$) is approximately the same as has been given for the determination of DNA adducts by radioimmunoassay techniques (196).

Mutagens

The introduction of relatively simple bacterial mutagenicity assays allows human body fluids to be assayed for mutagenic agents (299). Mutagenicity assays have been most widely performed on urine. The monitoring or urinary mutagenic activity is a nonspecific technique for assessing exposure to carcinogens and mutagens. It is therefore most useful when exposure to these agents is suspected but the specific chemical is unknown. Advantages of the urinary mutagenicity assay include its noninvasive nature and the relative ease of obtaining, storing, and analyzing the sample. The disadvantages include its unknown biological significance, its application to only certain classes of mutagens, and the interference in the analysis by substances normally present in the urine (92,278).

The observation by Yamasaki and Ames in 1977 that the urine of smokers is mutagenic prompted a number of studies in this area (298). Human studies have reported urinary mutagens among various occupational groups, patients receiving cancer chemotherapy, and passive smokers (80,166,298). Thus far, no correlation between the excretion of mutagens and presumed exposure has been found (92,93). When mutagenicity in the urine is used to monitor occupational exposures to genotoxic chemicals, smoking, diet, alcohol, drugs, and other life-style factors must be considered as possible confounding conditions.

Cytogenetic Markers

Biological monitoring of exposure to mutagens and carcinogens can be done by assessing visible chromosome damage. This is based on the observation that most chemicals that cause chromosome damage (i.e., that are clastogenic) are known or suspected carcinogens. Chromosome damage in humans exposed to mutagens can be detected by structural chromosomal alterations, chromosome numerical changes, sister chromatid exchanges (SCE), or as micronucleated cells. These alterations represent early responses to DNA damage. Although early cytogenetic responses are considered indicators of potential cancer risk, they cannot presently be used for the quantitative assessment of such risk (154,276).

Chromosomal Aberrations

Monitoring structural changes in chromosomes in peripheral blood lymphocytes was one of the earliest methods of identifying genetic injury. Cytogenetic monitoring was initially and effectively applied to monitor populations exposed to ionizing radiation. Chromosomal aberrations in humans appear after relatively low levels of radiation exposure. Aberration frequency is strictly dependent on absorbed dose. Damaged cells survive for many years after exposure. Scoring chromosomal aberrations has proved to be specific and sensitive enough to monitor populations exposed to ionizing radiation (i.e., survivors of the atomic bombings of Hiroshima and Nagasaki, uranium miners, and nuclear dockworkers) (9,29,78,153).

In contrast, it is presently impossible to monitor the degree of exposure to carcinogenic and mutagenic chemicals by assaying structural chromosome aberrations. The cytogenetic effects of exposure to chemical mutagens appear more complex than those seen with radiation exposure. In distinction to radiation, mutagenic chemicals induce a wide variety of lesions associated with large differences in responses among individuals (76). Chromosomal aberrations are not a specific response to a particular agent. They are considered a means of detecting the total chromosome-damaging effect of exposure to a mixture of chemicals, which in turn may be related to carcinogenic risk (153). Thus far the application of cytogenetic monitoring of populations exposed to occupational and environmental mutagens and carcinogens is still limited and qualitative (61,79, 92,277).

The technique most commonly used for monitoring exposure to agents producing chromosomal damage involves short-term cultures of blood samples. This entails the metaphase chromosome analysis of mitogen-stimulated lymphocytes (77). The disadvantages of this method relate to the fact that the scoring of chromosomal aberrations is laborious, subjective, time consuming, and expensive (88).

Sister Chromatid Exchanges

Sister chromatid exchanges (SCEs) represent an interchange between DNA molecules at homologous loci within a replicating chromosome. This rearrangement does not result in alteration of the chromosomal morphology or the genetic information. The rationale for using SCEs as markers of exposure to mutagens and carcinogens lies in the observation that a large number of mutagens and chromosome-damaging agents have been shown to induce SCEs. For a number of agents, increases in the number of SCEs are associated with increases in gene mutation (94,258). To date, however, there is no evidence that SCEs are predictive of adverse health effects (26,153).

Since the first visualization of SCEs in 1958, numerous technical advances have been made in their detection. With the introduction of harlequin staining methods, it is now possible to visualize a SCE in the replicating chromosome (210). The test is much easier, quicker, and cheaper to perform than that used to detect chromosome aberrations. In vitro tests indicate that the increases in SCEs are detectable at levels of exposure far below those required to increase chromosome aberrations (252, 255,277). Thus far the monitoring of SCEs has had limited use as a cytogenetic monitoring tool in humans. Its widest application has been in cancer patients undergoing chemotherapy (139).

Micronuclei

Micronuclei are fragments of the cell nucleus consisting of acentric chromosome fragments or lagging whole chromosomes. They are usually located in the cytoplasm and, though smaller than the main nucleus, have similar staining properties. They may be microscopically observed in a number of tissues. These include maturing erythrocytes of the bone marrow and lymphocytes from peripheral blood (252). Micronucleus formation appears to be related to chromosome breakage or loss (108). Formation of micronuclei appears to provide evidence of clastogenic effects (107). The scoring of micronuclei is less difficult and less time consuming than that of other cytogenetic markers.

The method has had limited application thus far. Studies have been performed on the cells of the buccal mucosa in betel chewers, on cultured lymphocytes of certain occupationally exposed groups, and on bone marrow of patients undergoing chemotherapy. The method has not been validated for purposes of biological monitoring (153,252).

SUMMARY

Exposure to occupational and environmental chemicals is assessed by environmental and biological monitoring. Each method has its advantages and disadvantages.

Environmental monitoring, which examines exposure to a particular chemical by measuring its concentration in the environment, has traditionally been used to assess exposure to chemicals in the workplace and general environment. Monitoring the concentration of pollutants in air, water, and food and identifying their emission sources continue to be the most important means of evaluating, reducing, preventing, and regulating such exposure.

Biological monitoring, by assessing the internal dose, provides more direct and precise evidence of chemical exposure than does environmental monitoring. Its primary goal is to assure that current or past exposures do not entail unacceptable health risks and/or to detect potentially excessive exposure before adverse health effects become apparent. When biological monitoring methods are incorporated into conventional epidemiologic studies, such studies can have increased power to detect and quantitate health risk.

Based on current knowledge, it is possible to conduct biological monitoring programs for a relatively small number of chemical pollutants. For the most part, the findings are not yet applicable to the individual.

Many methods are now available to detect the genotoxic effects of exposure to mutagens and carcinogens. At present, no method provides a means of quantifying carcinogenic or mutagenic risk in exposed populations. Present methods are not applicable to large-scale epidemiologic studies. As the methods for assessing carcinogenic exposure are validated and become simpler, more reliable, and less expensive, there is promise that they will provide a means of estimating carcinogenic risk in exposed populations and, perhaps ultimately, in the individual.

REFERENCES

1. Agency for Toxic Substances and Disease Registry: The Nature and Extent of Lead Poisoning in Children in the United States: A Report to Congress, US Department of Health and Human Services, Public Health Services, Washington, 1988.
2. Aitio A, Riihimäki V, Vainio H (eds.): Biological Monitoring and Surveillance of Workers Exposed to Chemicals, Hemisphere Publishing, Washington, 1984.
3. Aitio A, Järvisalo J, Riihimäki V, et al: Biological monitoring. In: Occupational Medicine: Principles and Practical Applications, 2nd ed, p 178, Zenz C (ed.), Year Book Medical Publishers, Chicago, 1988.
4. Aldridge WN, Barnes JM, Johnson MK: Studies on delayed neurotoxicity produced by some organophosphate compounds. Ann NY Acad Sci 160:314, 1969.
5. Alessio L, Castoldi MR, Monelli O, et al: Indicators of internal dose in current and past exposure to lead. Int Arch Occup Environ Health 44:127, 1979.
6. American Conference of Governmental Industrial Hygienists: Threshold Limit Values and Biological Exposure Indices for 1987–1988, American Conference of Governmental Industrial Hygienists, Cincinnati, Ohio, 1987.
7. Ames BN: Dietary carcinogens and anticarcinogens. Science 221:1256, 1983.
8. Anderson EW, Andelman JM, Strauch NJ, et al: Effect of low-level carbon monoxide exposure on onset and duration of angina pectoris: A study on 10 patients with ischemic heart disease. Ann Intern Med 79:46, 1973.
9. Awa AA, Sofuni T, Honda T, et al: Relationship between the radiation dose and chromosome aberrations in atomic bomb survivors of Hiroshima and Nagasaki. J Radiat Res (Toyko) 19:126, 1978.
10. Baker EL Jr, Peterson WA, Holtz JL, et al: Subacute cadmium intoxication in jewelry workers: An evaluation of diagnostic procedures. Arch Environ Health 34:73, 1979.
11. Bakir F, Damluji SF, Amin-Zaki L, et al: Methylmercury poisoning in Iraq. Science 181:230, 1973.
12. Bartsch H, Hemminki K, O'Neill IK (eds.): Methods for Detecting DNA Damaging Agents in Humans: Applications in Cancer Epidemiology and Prevention, IARC Scientific Publication 89, International Agency for Research on Cancer, Lyon, 1988.
13. Baselt RC, Cravey RH: Disposition of Toxic Drugs and Chemicals in Man, 3rd ed., Year Book Medical Publishers, Chicago, 1989.
14. Bastable MD: β 2-Microglobulin in urine: Not suitable for assessing renal tubular function. Clin Chem 29:996, 1983.

15. Bell ZG, Lovejoy HB, Vizena TR: Mercury exposure evaluations and their correlations with mercury excretions. J Occup Med 15:501, 1973.
16. Bellinger D, Leviton A, Needleman HL, et al: Low-level lead exposure and infant development in the first year. Neurobehav Toxicol Teratol 8:151, 1986.
17. Bellinger D, Leviton A, Waternaux C, et al: Longitudinal analyses of prenatal and postnatal lead exposure and early cognitive development. N Engl J Med 316:1037, 1987.
18. Berlin A, Wolff AH, Hasegawa Y (eds.): The Use of Biological Specimens for the Assessment of Human Exposure to Environmental Pollutants, Martinus Nijhoff, The Hague, 1979.
19. Berlin A, Draper M, Kemminki K, et al. (eds.): Monitoring Human Exposure to Carcinogenic and Mutagenic Agents. International Agency for Research on Cancer, Lyon, 1984.
20. Berlin M, Gage JC, Gullberg B, et al: Breath concentration as an index of the health risk from benzene. Scand J Work Environ Health 6:104, 1980.
21. Berman E: Toxic Metals and their Analysis, Heyden and Son, London, 1980.
22. Bernard AM, Lauwerys RR: Retinol binding protein in urine: A more practical index than urinary β_2-microglobulin for the routine screening of renal tubular function. Clin Chem 27:1781, 1981.
23. Bernard AM, Lauwerys MD: Present status and trends in biological monitoring of exposure to industrial chemicals. J Occup Med 28:558, 1986.
24. Blair A, Stewart P, O'Berg M, et al: Mortality among industrial workers exposed to formaldehyde. J Natl Cancer Inst 76:1071, 1986.
25. Blair A, Stewart P, Hoover RN, et al: Letter to the editor: Cancer of the nasopharynx and oropharynx and exposure to formaldehyde. J Natl Cancer Inst 78:191, 1987.
26. Bloom DA (ed.): Guidelines for Studies of Human Populations Exposed to Mutagenic and Reproductive Hazards, March of Dimes Birth Defects Foundation, New York, 1981.
27. Bordo B, Mossetto N, Musicco M, et al: Electrophysiologic changes in workers with "low" blood lead levels. Am J Ind Med 3:23, 1982.
28. Bowers MB, Goodman E, Sim VM: Some behavioral changes in man following anticholinesterase administration. J Nerv Ment Dis 138:383–389, 1964.
29. Brandom WF, Saccomanno G, Archer PG, et al: Chromosome aberrations as a biological dose response indicator of radiation exposure in uranium miners. Radiat Res 76:159, 1978.
30. Brookes P, Lawley PD: Evidence for the binding of polynuclear aromatic hydrocarbons to the nucleic acids of mouse skin: Relation between carcinogenic power of hydrocarbons and their binding of deoxyribonucleic acid. Nature 202:781, 1964.
31. Brown JF Jr, Lawton RV: Polychlorinated biphenyl (PCB) partitioning between adipose tissue and serum. Bull Environ Contam Toxicol 33:277, 1984.
32. Buchet JP, Lauwerys R, Roels H: Comparison of the urinary excretion of arsenic metabolites after a single dose of sodium arsenite, monomethylarsonate, or dimethylarsinite in man. Int Arch Occup Environ Health 48:71, 1981.
33. Buchet JP, Lauwerys R, Roels H: Urinary excretion of inorganic arsenic and its metabolites after repeated ingestion of sodium metaarsenite by volunteers. Int Arch Occup Environ Health 48:111, 1981.
34. Burse VW, Kimbrough RD, Villanueva EC, et al: Polychlorinated biphenyls. Storage, distribution, excretion, and recovery: Liver morphology after prolonged dietary ingestion. Arch Environ Health 29:301, 1974.
35. Byard JL: The toxicological significance of 2,3,7,8-tetrachlorodibenzo-p-dioxin and related compounds in human adipose tissue. J Toxicol Environ Health 22:381, 1987.
36. Cairns T, Siegmund EG: PCBs: Regulatory history and analytical problems. Anal Chem 53:1183A, 1981.
37. Calleman CJ: Monitoring of background levels of hydroxyethyl adducts in human hemoglobin. In: Genetic Toxicology of Environmental Chemicals, Part B: Genetic Effects and Applied Mutagenesis, p 261, Ramel C, Lambert B, Magnusson J (eds.), Alan R Liss, New York, 1986.
38. Calleman CJ, Ehrenberg L, Jansson B, et al: Monitoring and risk assessment by means of alkygroups in hemoglobin in persons occupationally exposed to ethylene oxide. J Environ Pathol Toxicol 2:427, 1978.
39. Catton MJ, Harrison MJ, Fullerton PM, et al: Subclinical neuropathy in lead workers. Br Med J 2:80, 1970.
40. Cavalleri A, Baruffini A, Minola C, et al: Biological response of children to low levels of inorganic lead. Environ Res 25:415, 1981.
41. Centers for Disease Control: Preventing Lead Poisoning in Young Children: A Statement by the Centers for Disease Control, Centers for Disease Control, Atlanta, 1991.
42. Centers for Disease Control: Leads from the MMWR. Serum 2,3,7,8-tetrachloride benzo-p-dioxin levels in Air Force health study participants, preliminary report. JAMA 259:3533, 1988.
43. Centers for Disease Control: Serum 2,3,7,8-tetrachlorodibenzo-p-dioxin levels in US Army Vietnam-era veterans. JAMA 260:1249, 1988.
44. Chang KJ, Hsieh KH, Lee TP, et al: Immunologic evaluation of patients with polychlorinated biphenyl poisoning: Determination of lymphocyte subpopulations. Toxicol Appl Pharmacol 61:58, 1981.
45. Chang KJ, Hsieh KH, Tang S, et al: Immunologic evaluation of patient with polychlorinated biphenyl poisoning: Evaluation of delayed-type skin hypersensitivity and its relation to clinical studies: J Toxicol Environ Health 9:217, 1982.
46. Chisolm JJ Jr: Lead poisoning. In: Pediatrics, 18th ed., p 732, Rudolph AM (ed.), Hoffman JIE (co-ed.), Axelrod S (asst. ed.), Appleton & Lange, Norwalk, Connecticut, 1987.
47. Chisolm JJ, O'Hara DM: Lead absorption in children—management, clinical and environmental aspects, Urban & Schwarzenberg, Baltimore, 1982.
48. Christofferson JO, Schütz A, Ahlgren L, et al: Lead in finger-bone analyzed in vivo in active and retired workers. Am J Ind Med 6:447, 1984.
49. Clarkson TW, Greenwood MR: Mercury, biological specimen collections. In: The Use of Biological Specimens for the Assessment of Human Exposure to Environmental Pollutants, p 109, Berlin A, Wolff AH,

Hasegawa Y (eds.), Martinus Nijhoff, The Hague, 1979.

50. Clarkson TW, Nordberg GF, Sager PR: Reproductive and Developmental Toxicity of Metals, Plenum Press, New York, 1983.

51. Coggon D, Pannett B, Winter PC, et al: Mortality of workers exposed to 2-methyl-4-chlorophenoxyacetic acid. Scand J Work Environ Health 12:448, 1986.

52. Colombi A, Maroni M, Ferioli A, et al: Increases in urinary porphyrin excretion in workers exposed to polychlorinated biphenyls. J Appl Toxicol 2:117, 1982.

53. Committee on Biological Markers of the National Research Council: Biological Markers in Environmental Health Research. Environ Health Perspect 74:3, 1987.

54. Committee on Lead in the Human Environment, National Research Council: Lead in the Human Environment. National Academy of Sciences, Washington, 1980.

55. Council on Environmental Quality: Contamination of Ground Water by Toxic Organic Chemicals, US Government Printing Office, Washington, 1981.

56. Council on Scientific Affairs: The Health Effects of "Agent Orange" and Polychlorinated Dioxin Contaminants: An Update, 1984, American Medical Association, Chicago, 1984.

57. Courtney KD: Mouse teratology studies with chlorodibenzo-p-dioxins. Bull Environ Contam Toxicol 16:674, 1976.

58. Coye MJ, Lowe JA, Maddy KT: Biological monitoring of agricultural workers exposed to pesticides I. Cholinesterase activity determinations. J Occup Med 28:619, 1986.

59. Coye MJ, Lowe JA, Maddy KT: Biological monitoring of agricultural workers exposed to pesticides. II. Monitoring of intact pesticides and their metabolites. J Occup Med 28:629, 1986

60. Crecelius EA: Changes in the chemical speciation of arsenic following ingestion by man. Environ Health Perspect 19:147, 1977.

61. Dabney BJ: The role of human genetic monitoring in the workplace. J Occup Med 23:626, 1981.

62. Dietrich KN, Krafft KM, Bornschein RL, et al: Low-level fetal lead exposure effect on neurobehavioral development in early infancy. Pediatrics 80:721, 1987.

63. Dubowski KM, Luke JL: Measurement of carboxyhemoglobin and carbon monoxide in blood. Ann Clin Lab Sci 3:53, 1973.

64. Ehrenberg L: Risk assessment of ethylene oxide and other compounds. In: Assessing Chemical Mutagens: The Risk to Humans, Banbury Report 1, p 157, McElhen VK, Abrahamson S (eds.), Cold Spring Harbor Laboratory, New York, 1979.

65. Ehrenberg L: Covalent binding of genotoxic agents to proteins and nucleic acids. In: Monitoring Human Exposure to Carcinogenic and Mutagenic Agents, p 107, Berlin A, Draper M, Hemminki K, et al. (eds.), International Agency for Research on Cancer, Lyon, 1984.

66. Ehrenberg L, Hiesche KD, Osterman-Golkar S, et al: Evaluation of genetic risks of alkylating agents: Tissue doses in the mouse from air contaminated with ethylene oxide. Mutat Res 24:83, 1974.

67. Ehrenberg L, Moustacchi E, Osterman-Golkar S, et al: Dosimetry of genotoxic agents and dose response relationship of their effects. Mutat Res 123:121, 1983.

68. Ellis KJ, Morgan WD, Zauzi I, et al: Critical concentrations of cadmium in human renal cortex: Dose–effect studies in cadmium smelter workers. J Toxicol Environ Health 7:691, 1981.

69. Ellman GL, Courtney KD, Andres V, et al: A new and rapid colorimetric determination of acetylcholinesterase activity. Biochem Pharmacol 7:88, 1961.

70. Emmerson BT: Chronic lead nephropathy. Kidney Int 4:1, 1973.

71. Emmett EA, Maroni M, Jeffery J, et al: Studies of transformer repair workers exposed to PCBs: II. Results of clinical laboratory investigations. Am J Ind Med 14:47, 1988.

72. Environmental Quality: 16th Report, p 227, Council on Environmental Quality, Washington, DC, 1985.

73. Eriksson M, Hardell L, Berg NO, et al: Soft tissue sarcomas and exposure to chemical substances. A case referent study. Br J Ind Med 38:27, 1981.

74. Ertie T, Henschler D, Muller G: Metabolism of trichloroethylene in man. I. The significance of trichloroethanol in long-term exposure conditions. Arch Toxikol 29:171, 1972.

75. Evans HJ: The role of human cytogenetics in study of mutagenesis and carcinogenesis. In: Genetic Toxicology of Environmental Chemicals. Part A: Basic Principles and Mechanisms of Action, p 41, Ramel C, Lambert B, Magnusson J (eds.), Alan R Liss, New York, 1986.

76. Evans HJ: What has been achieved with cytogenetic monitoring? In: Monitoring of Occupational Genotoxicants, p 3, Sorsa M, Norppa H (eds.), Alan R Liss, New York, 1986.

77. Evans HJ, O'Riordan ML: Human peripheral blood lymphocytes for the analysis of chromosome aberrations in mutagen tests. Mutat Res 31:135, 1975.

78. Evans HJ, Buckton KE, Hamilton GE, et al: Radiation-induced chromosome aberrations in nuclear dockyard workers. Nature 277:531, 1979.

79. Fabricant JC, Legator MS: Etiology, role and detection of chromosome aberrations in man. J Occup Med 23:617, 1981.

80. Falck K, Grohn P, Sorsa H, et al: Mutagenicity in urine of nurses handling cytostatic drugs. Lancet 1:1250, 1979.

81. Falck FY, Fine LJ, Smith RG, et al: Metallothionein and occupational exposure to cadmium. Br J Ind Med 40:305, 1983.

82. Falck FY, Fine LJ, Smith RB, et al: Occupational cadmium exposure and renal status. Am J Ind Med 4:541, 1983.

83. Faó V, Emmett EA, Maroni M, et al. (eds.): Occupational and Environmental Chemical Hazards: Cellular and Biochemical Indices for Monitoring Toxicity, John Wiley & Sons, New York, 1987.

84. Feldman RG, Niles CA, Kelly-Hayes M, et al: Peripheral neuropathy in arsenic smelter workers. Neurology 29:939, 1979.

85. Fernandez JG, Humbert BE, Droz PO, et al: Exposition au trichloroethylene. Bilan de l'absorption, de l'excretion et du metabolisme sur des sujets hu-

mains. Arch Mal Prof Med Trav Securite Soc (Paris) 36:397, 1975.

86. Fishbeck WA, Langner RR, Kociba RJ: Elevated urinary phenol levels not related to benzene exposure. Am Ind Hyg Assoc J 36:820, 1975.

87. Fitzgerald EF, Standfast SJ, Youngblood LG, et al: Assessing the health effects of potential exposure to PCBs, dioxins, and furans from electrical transformer fires: The Binghamton State Office Building Medical Surveillance Program. Arch Environ Health 41:368, 1986.

88. Forni A: Chromosomal aberrations in monitoring exposure to mutagens–carcinogens. In: Monitoring Human Exposure to Carcinogenic and Mutagenic Agents, p 325, Berlin A, Draper M, Hemminki K, et al. (eds.), International Agency for Research on Cancer, Lyon, 1984.

89. Franklin CA, Fenske RA, Greenhalgh R, et al: Correlation of urinary pesticide metabolite excretion with estimated dermal contact in the course of occupational exposure to guthion. J Toxicol Environ Health 7:715, 1981.

90. Friberg L: Cadmium. Annu Rev Public Health 4:367, 1983.

91. Gadoth N, Fisher A: Late onset of neuromuscular block in organophosphate poisoning. Ann Intern Med 88:654, 1978.

92. Garner RC: Assessment of carcinogen exposure in man. Carcinogenesis 6:1071, 1985.

93. Garner RC, Mould AJ, Lindsay-Smith V, et al: Mutagenic urine from bladder cancer patients. Lancet 2: 398, 1982.

94. Gebhart E: Sister chromatid exchange (SCE) and structural chromosome aberration in mutagenicity testing. Hum Genet 58:235, 1981.

95. Gehring PJ, Dramer CG, Schwetz BA, et al: The fate of 2,4,5-trichlorophenoxyacetic acid following oral administration to man. Toxicol Appl Pharmacol 26: 352, 1973.

96. Gershon S, Shaw FB: Psychiatric sequelae of chronic exposure to organophosphorus insecticides. Lancet 1:1371, 1961.

97. Goldstein IF: The use of biological markers in studies of health effects of pollutants. Environ Res 25:236, 1981.

98. Gottschling LM, Beaulieu HJ, Melvin WW: Monitoring of formic acid in urine of humans exposed to low levels of formaldehyde. Am Ind Hyg Assoc 45:19, 1984.

99. Green LC, Skipper PI, Turesky RJ, et al: In vivo dosimetry of 4-aminobiphenyl in rats via a cysteine adduct in hemoglobin. Cancer Res 44:4254, 1984.

100. Hammond PB, Lerner SI, Gartside PS, et al: The relationship of biological indices of lead exposure to the health status of workers in a secondary lead smelter. J Occup Med 22:475, 1980.

101. Hardell L, Eriksson M: The association between soft-tissue sarcomas and exposure to phenoxyacetic acids. Cancer 62:652, 1988.

102. Hardell L, Sandstrom A: Case-control study: Soft-tissue sarcomas and exposure to phenoxyacetic acids or chlorophenols. Br J Cancer 39:711, 1979.

103. Hardell L, Eriksson M, Lenner P: Malignant lymphoma and exposure to chemicals, especially organic

solvent, chlorophenols and phenoxyacids: A case control study. Br J Cancer 43:169, 1981.

104. Harris CC, Vahakangas K, Newman MJ, et al: Detection of benzo(a)pyrene diol epoxide–DNA adducts in peripheral blood lymphocytes and antibodies to the adducts in serum from coke oven workers. Proc Natl Acad Sci USA 82:6672, 1985.

105. Hartwell TC, et al: Study of Carbon Monoxide Exposure of Residents of Washington, DC and Denver, CO Prepared for US Environmental Protection Agency, Environmental Monitoring Systems Laboratory, Research Triangle Park, NC, 1984.

106. Hayes WJ Jr: Pesticide Studies in Man, Williams & Wilkins, Baltimore, 1982.

107. Heddle JA, Blakey DH, Duncan AMV, et al: Micronuclei and related nuclear anomalies as a short-term assay for colon carcinogens. In: Indicators of Genotoxic Exposure, Banbury Report 13, p 367, Bridges BA, Butterworth BE, Weinstein IB (eds.), Cold Spring Harbor Laboratory, New York, 1982.

108. Heddle JA, Hite M, Kirkhart B, et al: The induction of micronuclei as a measure of genotoxicity. Mutat Res 123:61, 1983.

109. Hemminki K, Randerath K: Detection of genetic interaction of chemicals by biochemical methods: Determination of DNA and protein adducts. In: Mechanisms of Cell Injury: Implications for Human Health, p 209, Fowler BA (ed.), John Wiley & Sons, New York, 1987.

110. Hernberg S, Nakkanen J, Mellin G, et al: γ-Aminolevulinic acid dehydrase as a measure of lead exposure. Arch Environ Health 21:140, 1970.

111. Hindmarsh JT, McLetchie OR, Leroy MD, et al. Electromyographic abnormalities in chronic environmental arsenicalism. J Anal Toxicol 1:270, 1977.

112. Hoar SK, Blair A, Holmes FF, et al: Agricultural herbicide use and risk of lymphoma and soft-tissue sarcoma JAMA 256:1141, 1986.

113. Hulka BS, Wilcosky TC, Griffith JD: Biological Markers in Epidemiology, Oxford University Press, 1990.

114. International Agency for Research on Cancer: Benzene. In: Monographs on the Evaluation of the Carcinogenic Risk of Chemicals to Humans, Vol 29, Some Chemicals and Dyestuffs, p 93, IARC, Lyon, 1982.

115. International Agency for Research on Cancer: Monographs on the Evaluation of Carcinogenic Risk to Humans, Suppl 7, Overall Evaluation of Carcinogenicity: An Updating of IARC Monographs Vol 1–42, IARC, Lyon, 1987.

116. Ikeda M, Otsumi H, Imamura T, et al: Urinary excretion of total trichloro compounds, trichloroethanol, and trichloroacetic acid as a measure of exposure to trichloroethylene and tetrachloroethylene. Br J Ind Med 29:328, 1972.

117. Jabara JW, Baaulieu HJ, Buchan RM, et al: Carbon monoxide: Dosimetry in occupational exposures in Denver, Colorado. Arch Environ Health 35:198, 1980.

118. Jeffery AM, Weinstein IB, Jennette KW, et al: Structures of benzo(a)pyrene–nucleic acid adducts formed in human and bovine bronchial explants. Nature 269: 348, 1977.

119. Jensen AA: Chemical contaminants in human milk. Residue Rev 89:1, 1983.

120. Jensen S, Sundstrom G: Structure and levels of most chlorobiphenyls in two technical PCB products and in human adipose tissue. Ambio 3:70, 1974.

121. Jirasek L, Kalensky J, Kubec K, et al: Chloracne, porphyria cutanea tarda and other manifestations of general poisonings during the manufacture of herbicides. Cesk Dermatol 49:145, 1974.

122. Johnson BL (ed.): Prevention of Neurotoxic Illness in Working Populations, John Wiley & Sons, New York, 1987.

123. Johnson MK: Mechanism of protection against delayed neurotoxic effects of organo-phosphorous ester. Fed Proc 31:73, 1976.

124. Kahn PC, Gochfeld M, Nygren M, et al: Dioxins and dibenzofurans in blood and adipose tissue of Agent Orange-exposed Vietnam veterans and matched controls. JAMA 259:1661, 1988.

125. Kerns WD, Pavkov KL, Donofrio DJ, et al: Carcinogenicity of formaldehyde in rats and mice after long-term inhalation exposure. Cancer Res 43:4582, 1983.

126. Khan MAQ, Stanton RH (eds.): Toxicology of Halogenated Hydrocarbons: Health and Ecological Effects, p 38, Pergamon Press, New York, 1981.

127. Kiihimäki V, Asp S, Pukkala E, et al: Mortality and cancer morbidity among chlorinated phenoxyacid applicators in Finland. Chemosphere 12:779, 1983.

128. Kimbrough RD: The toxicity of polychlorinated polycyclic compounds and related compounds. CRC Crit Rev Toxicol 2:445, 1974.

129. Kimbrough RD, Jensen AA (eds.): Halogenated Biphenyls, Terphenyls, Naphthalene, Dibenzodioxins and Related Products, 2nd Ed., Elsevier/North Holland, Amsterdam, 1989.

130. Kimbrough RD; Human health effects of polychlorinated biphenyls (PCBs) and polybrominated biphenyls (PBBs). Annu Rev Pharmacol Toxicol 27:87, 1987.

131. Kimbrough RD, Carter CD, Liddle JA, et al: Epidemiology and pathology of a tetrachlorodibenzodioxin poisoning episode. Arch Environ Health 32:77, 1977.

132. Kolmodin-Hedman G, Höglund S, Åkerblom M: Studies on phenoxyacid herbicides. 1. Field study: Occupational exposure to phenoxyacid herbicides (MCPA, dichlorprop, mecroprop, and 2,4-D) in agriculture. Arch Toxicol 54:257, 1983.

133. Kreiss K: Studies on populations exposed to polychlorinated biphenyls. Environ Health Perspect 60: 193, 1985.

134. Kreiss K, Zack MM, Kimbrough RD, et al: Association of blood pressure and polychlorinated biphenyl levels. JAMA 245:2505, 1981.

135. Kreiss K, Zack MM, Kimbrough RD, et al: Cross-sectional study of a community with exceptional exposure to DDT. JAMA 245:926, 1981.

136. Kreiss K, Zach MM, Landrigan PJ, et al: Neurologic evaluation of a population exposed to arsenic in Alaskan well water. Arch Environ Health 38:116, 1983.

137. Kuratsume M, Shapiro RE (eds.): PCB Poisoning in Japan and Taiwan, Alan R Liss, New York, 1984.

138. Kutz FW, Yobs AR, Strassman SC, et al: Effects of reducing DDT usage on total DDT storage in humans. Pesticide Monit J 11:61, 1977.

139. Lambert B, Lindblad A, Homberg E, et al: The use of sister chromatid exchange to monitor human populations for exposure to toxicologically harmful agents. In: Sister Chromatid Exchange, p 149, Wolff S (ed.), John Wiley & Sons, New York, 1982.

140. Lancranjan I, Popescu HI, Gavanescu O, et al: Reproductive ability of workman occupationally exposed to lead. Arch Environ Health 30:396, 1975.

141. Langolf GD, Chaffin R, Henderson R, et al: Evaluation of workers exposed to elemental mercury using quantitative tests of tremor and neuromuscular functions. Am Ind Hyg Assoc J 39:976, 1978.

142. Laskin S, Goldstein BD (eds.): Benzene toxicity: A critical evaluation. Toxicol Environ Health 2(Suppl): 1977.

143. Laties VG, Merigan WH: Behavioral effects of carbon monoxide on animals and man. Annu Rev Pharmacol Toxicol 19:357, 1979.

144. Lauwerys R: Biological criteria for selected industrial toxic chemicals: A review. Scand J Work Environ Health 1:139, 1975.

145. Lauwerys RR: Industrial Chemical Exposure—Guidelines for Biological Monitoring, Biomedical Publications, Davis, CA, 1983.

146. Lauwerys RR: In vivo tests to monitor body burdens of toxic metals in man. In: Chemical Toxicology and Clinical Chemistry of Metals, p 113, Brown SS, Savory J (eds.), Academic Press, Orlando, 1983.

147. Lauwerys R: Basic concepts of monitoring human exposure. In: Monitoring Human Exposure to Carcinogenic and Mutagenic Agents, p 31, Berlin A, Draper M, Kemminki K, et al. (eds.), International Agency for Research on Cancer, Lyon, 1984.

148. Lauwerys R, Roels H, Regniers M, et al: Significance of cadmium concentration in blood and in urine in workers exposed to cadmium. Environ Res 20:375, 1979.

149. Laws ER, Curley A, Biros FJ: Men with intensive occupational exposure to DDT. Arch Environ Health 15:766, 1967.

150. Lewalter J, Koralius U: Erythrocyte protein conjugates as a principle of biological monitoring for pesticides. Toxicol Lett 33:153, 1986.

151. Lindstedt G: Individual mercury exposure of chlor-alkali workers and its relation to blood and urinary mercury levels. Scand J Work Environ Health 5:59, 1979.

152. Lloyd DC: An overview of radiation dosimetry by conventional cytogenetic methods. In: Biological Dosimetry, p 3, Eisert WG, Mendelsohn ML (eds.), Springer-Verlag, Berlin, 1984.

153. Lohman PHM, Jansen JD, Baan RA: Comparison of various methodologies with respect to specificity and sensitivity in biomonitoring occupational exposure to mutagens and carcinogens. In: Monitoring Human Exposure to Carcinogenic and Mutagenic Agents, p 259, Berlin A, Draper M, Hemminki K, et al. (eds.), International Agency for Research on Cancer, Lyon, 1984.

154. Lohman PHM, Lauwerys R, Sorsa M: Overview: Methods of monitoring human exposure to carcinogenic and mutagenic agents. In: Monitoring Human Exposure to Carcinogenic and Mutagenic Agents, p 423, Berlin A, Draper M, Hemminki K, et al. (eds.),

International Agency for Research on Cancer, Lyon, 1984.

155. Lores EM, Bradway DE, Moseman RF: Organophosphorus pesticide poisonings in humans: Determination of residues and metabolites in tissues and urine. Arch Environ Health 33:270, 1978.

156. Lutz WK: In vivo covalent binding of organic chemicals to DNA as a quantitative indicator in the process of chemical carcinogenesis. Mutat Res 65:289, 1979.

157. Lynge E: A follow-up study of cancer incidence among workers in manufacture of phenoxy herbicides in Denmark. Br J Cancer 52:259, 1985.

158. Magos L: Biological methods of defining human exposures. In: Health Effects from Hazardous Waste Sites, p 122, Andelman JB, Underhill DW (eds.), Lewis Publishers, Boca Raton, 1987.

159. Mahaffey KR, Annest JL, Roberts MS, et al: National estimates of blood lead levels. United States 1976–1980. N Engl J Med 307:573, 1982.

160. Mahaffey KR, Annest JL, Roberts MS, et al: Association between age, blood lead concentration and serum 1,25-dihydroxycholecaliferol levels in children. Am J Clin Nutr 35:1327, 1982.

161. Mahieu P, Buchet JP, Roels HA, et al: The metabolism of arsenic in humans acutely intoxicated by AsO_3. Its significance for the duration of BAL therapy. Clin Toxicol 18:1067, 1981.

162. Masuda Y, Kuroki H, Karaguchi K, et al: PCB and PCDF congeners in the blood and tissues of yusho and yu-cheng patients. Environ Health Perspect 59:53, 1985.

163. Matthews HB, Dedrick RL: Pharmacokinetics of PCBs. Annu Rev Pharmacol Toxicol 24:85, 1984.

164. Mattson AM, Sedlak VA: Ether-extractable urinary phosphates in man and rats derived from malathion and similar compounds. J Agr Food Chem 8:107, 1960.

165. McConnell EE: Comparative toxicity of PCBs and related compounds in various species of animals. Environ Health Perspect 60:29, 1985.

166. McCoy EC, Hankel R, Robins R, et al: Presence of mutagenic substances in the urines of anesthesiologists. Mutat Res 53:71, 1978.

167. McMichael AJ, Baghurst PA, Wigg NR, et al: Port Pirie cohort study: Environmental exposure to lead and children's abilities at the age of four years. N Engl J Med 319:468, 1988.

168. Metcalf DR, Holmes JH: EEG, psychological and neurological alterations in humans with organophosphate exposure. Ann NY Acad Sci 160:357, 1969.

169. Meyer B: Indoor Air Quality, Addison-Wesley, Reading, MA, 1983.

170. Michel HO: An electrometric method for the determination of red blood cell and plasma cholinesterase activity. J Lab Clin Med 34:1564, 1949.

171. Miller EC, Miller JA: Mechanisms of chemical carcinogenesis: Nature of proximate carcinogens and interactions with macromolecules. Pharmacol Rev 18:805, 1966.

172. Miller EC, Miller JA: Mechanisms of chemical carcinogenesis. Cancer 47:1055, 1981.

173. Miller JA, Miller EC: Ultimate chemical carcinogens as reactive mutagenic electrophiles. In: Origins of Human Cancer, p 605, Hiatt HH, Watson JD, Winsten

AA (eds.), Cold Spring Harbor Laboratory, New York, 1977.

174. Milman HA, Sell S (eds.): Application of Biological Markers to Carcinogen Testing, Plenum Press, New York, 1982.

175. Morbidity and Mortality Weekly Report: Childhood lead poisoning—United States: Report to the Congress by the Agency for Toxic Substances and Disease Registry. Morbid Mortal Week Rep 37(32):461, 1988.

176. Monster AC, Boersma G, Duba WC: Kinetics of trichloroethylene in repeated exposure of volunteers. Int Arch Occup Environ Health 42:283, 1979.

177. Montesano R, Bartsch H, Vainio H, et al: Long-Term and Short-Term Assays for Carcinogens: A Critical Appraisal, IARC Scientific Publication no. 83, International Agency for Research on Cancer, Lyon, 1986.

178. Morgan DP: Recognition and Management of Pesticide Poisonings, 4th Ed., EPA-540/9-88-001 US EPA, Washington, 1989.

179. Morgan DP, Hetzler HL, Sclach EE, et al: Urinary excretion of paranitrophenol and alkylphosphates following ingestion of methyl or ethyl parathion by human subjects. Arch Environ Contam Toxicol 6:153, 1977.

180. Muller G, Spassovski M, Henschler D: Trichloroethylene exposure and trichloroethylene metabolites in urine and blood. Arch Toxikol 29:335, 1972.

181. Muller G, Spassovski M, Henschler D: Metabolism of trichloroethylene in man. II. Pharmacokinetics of metabolites. Arch Toxicol 32:283, 1974.

182. Murphy RS, Kutz FW, Strassman SC: Selected pesticide residues or metabolites in blood and urine. Specimens from a general population survey. Environ Health Perspect 48:81, 1983.

183. Murthy MSS, Calleman CJ, Osterman-Golkar S, et al: Relationships between ethylation of hemoglobin, ethylation of DNA and administered amount of ethyl methanesulfonate in the mouse. Mutat Res 127:1, 1984.

184. National Institute of Occupational Safety and Health: Criteria for Recommended Standard Occupational Exposure to Inorganic Lead. Revised Criteria, US DHEW (NIOSH), Pub #78-158, Washington, 1978.

185. Needleman HL: Low level lead exposure in the fetus and young child. Neurotoxicology 8:389, 1987.

186. Needleman HL, Tuncay O, Shapiro IM: Lead levels in deciduous teeth of urban and suburban children. Nature 235:111, 1972.

187. Needleman HL, Gunnoe C, Leviton A, et al: Deficits in psychologic and classroom performance of children with elevated dentine lead levels. N Engl J Med 300:689, 1979.

188. Neubert D, Dillmann I: Embryotoxic effects on mice treated with 2,4,5-trichlorophenoxyacetic acid and 2,3,7,8-tetrachlorodibenzo-p-dioxin. Arch Pharmacol 272:243, 1972.

189. Neumann HG: Dose–response relationship in the primary lesion of strong electrophilic carcinogens. Arch Toxicol 3 (Suppl):69, 1980.

190. Neumann HG: Analysis of hemoglobin as a dose monitor for alkylating and arylating agents. Arch Toxicol 56:1, 1984.

191. Newmann HG: Concepts for assessing the internal dose of chemicals in vivo. In: Mechanisms of Cell

Injury: Implications for Human Health, p 241, Fowler BA (ed.), John Wiley & Sons, New York, 1987.

192. Norbach DH, Weltman RH: Polychlorinated biphenyl induction of hepatocellular carcinoma in the Sprague–Dawley rat. Environ Health Perspect 60:97, 1985.

193. Osterloh J, Kaysen G, Becker C: Handling of formalin in dialysis units. Transplant Dialysis 12:353, 1983.

194. Osterloh J, Lotti M, Pond SM: Toxicological studies in a fatal overdose of 2,4-D, MCPP, and chlorpyrifos. J Anal Toxicol 7:125, 1983.

195. Osterloh J, Cone J, Harrison R, et al: Pilot survey of urinary porphyrin from persons transiently exposed to a PCB transformer fire. J Toxicol Clin Toxicol 24:533, 1987.

196. Osterman-Golkar S, Ehrenberg L: Dosimetry of electrophilic compounds by means of hemoglobin alkylation. Annu Rev Public Health 4:397, 1983.

197. Osterman-Golkar S, Ehrenberg L, Segerbäch D, et al: Evaluation of genetic risks of alkylating agents II. Haemoglobin as a dose monitor. Mutat Res 34:1, 1976.

198. Otto D, Robinson G, Baumann S, et al: 5-year follow-up study of children with low-to-moderate lead absorption: Electrophysiological evaluation. Environ Res 38:168, 1985.

199. Park DV, Williams RT: Studies in detoxication. The metabolism of benzene containing $_{14}$C. Biochem J 54:231, 1953.

200. Patterson DG Jr, Hampton L, Lapeza CR Jr, et al: High-resolution mass spectrometric analysis of human serum on a whole-weight and lipid basis for 2,3,7,8-tetrachlorodibenzo-p-dioxin. Anal Chem 59:2000, 1987.

201. Patterson DG Jr, Needham LL, Pirkle JL, et al: Correlation between serum and adipose tissue levels of 2,3,7,8-tetrachlorodibenzo-p-dioxin in 50 persons from Missouri. Arch Environ Contam Toxicol 17:139, 1988.

202. Perbellini L, Faccini GB, Pasini F, et al: Environmental and occupational exposure to benzene by analysis of breath and blood. Br J Ind Med 45:345, 1988.

203. Perera F: Molecular epidemiology: A novel approach to the investigation of pollutant-related chronic disease. In: Environmental Impacts on Human Health: Agenda for Long-Term Research and Development, p 61, Draggan S, Cohrssen JJ, Morrison RE (eds.), Praeger, London, 1987.

204. Perera FP: Molecular cancer epidemiology: A new tool in cancer prevention. J Natl Cancer Inst 78:887, 1987.

205. Perera FP: The significance of DNA and protein adducts in human biomonitoring studies. Mutat Res 205:255, 1988.

206. Perera F, Weinstein IB: Molecular epidemiology and carcinogen–DNA adduct detection: New approaches to studies of human cancer causation. J Chron Dis 35:581, 1982.

207. Perera F, Santella RM, Brenner D, et al: DNA adducts, protein adducts, and sister chromatic exchange in cigarette smokers and nonsmokers. J Natl Cancer Inst 79:449, 1987.

208. Periera MA, Chang LW: Binding of chemical carcinogens and mutagens to rat hemoglobin. Chem Biol Interact 33:301, 1981.

209. Perry HM, Gurdarsham S, Thind MD, et al: The biology of cadmium. Symposium on Trace Elements. Med Clin North Am 60:759, 1976.

210. Perry P, Wolff S: New Giemsa method for differential staining of sister chromatids. Nature 261:156 1974.

211. Piomelli S, Seamen C, Zullow D, et al: Threshold for lead damage to heme synthesis in urban children. Proc Natl Acad Sci USA 79:3335, 1982.

212. Piotrowski JK: Exposure Tests for Organic Compounds in Industrial Toxicology, US Government Printing Office, Washington, 1977.

213. Pirkle JL, Wolfe WH, Patterson DG Jr, et al: Estimates of the half-life of 2,3,7,8-tetrachlorodibenzo-p-dioxin in Ranch Hand veterans. Presented at the Seventh International Symposium on Clorinated Dioxins and Related Compounds, Las Vegas, Nevada, October 7, 1987.

214. Pocchiari F, Silano V, Zamplieri A: Human health effects from accidental release of tetrachlorodibenzo-p-dioxin (TCDD) at Seveso, Italy. Ann NY Acad Sci 275:311, 1979.

215. Poirier MC: Antibodies to carcinogen–DNA adducts. J Natl Cancer Inst 67:515, 1981.

216. Poirier MC, Stanley JR, Beckwith JB, et al: Indirect immunofluorescent localization of benzo(a)pyrene adducts to nucleic acids in cultured mouse keratinocyte nuclei. Carcinogenesis 3:345, 1982.

217. Putoni R, Merio F, Fini A, et al: Soft-tissue sarcomas in Seveso. Lancet 2:525, 1986.

218. Rabinowitz MB, Wetherill GW, Kopple JM: Kinetic analysis of lead metabolism in healthy humans. J Clin Invest 58:260, 1976.

219. Ramsey JC, Hefner JG, Karbowski RJ, et al: The in-vivo biotransformation of 2,3,7,8-tetrachlorordibenzo-p-dioxin in the rat. Toxicol Appl Pharmacol 48(1)(part2):A162, 1979.

220. Reddy MV, Gupta RC, Randerath EV, et al: ^{32}P-Postlabelling test for covalent DNA binding of aromatic carcinogens and methylating agents. Carcinogenesis 5:231, 1984.

221. Reed E, Yuspa SH, Swelling LA, et al: Quantitation of cis-diaminedichloroplatinum II (cisplatin)–DNA-intrastrand adducts in testicular and ovarian cancer patients receiving cis-platin chemotherapy. J Clin Invest 77:545, 1986.

222. Reid SJ, Watts RR: A method for the determination of dialkylphosphate residues in urine. J Anal Toxicol 5:1264, 1981.

223. Report of the Federal Panel on Formaldehyde: Environ Health Perspect 43:139, 1982.

224. Rider JA, Hodges JL, Swader J, et al: Plasma and red cell cholinesterase in 800 "healthy" blood donors. J Lab Clin Med 50:376, 1957.

225. Rinsky RA, Young RJ, Smith AB: Leukemia in benzene workers. Am J Ind Med 2:217, 1981.

226. Roels H, Bernard A, Buchet JP, et al: Critical concentration of cadmium in renal cortex and urine. Lancet 1:221, 1979.

227. Roels HA, Lauwerys RR, Buchet JP, et al: In vivo measurement of liver and kidney cadmium in workers exposed to this metal: Its significance with respect to cadmium in blood and urine. Environ Res 26:217, 1981.

228. Roels H, Lauwery R, Buchet JP, et al: Comparison of renal function and psychomotor performance in workers exposed to elemental mercury. Int Arch Occup Environ Health 50:77, 1982.

229. Rogan WJ: Persistent pesticides and polychlorinated biphenyls. Annu Rev Public Health 4:381, 1983.

230. Rogan WJ, Bagniewski A, Damstra T: Pollutants in breast milk. N Engl J Med 302:1450, 1980.

231. Rogan WJ, Gladen BC, Hung KL, et al: Congenital poisoning by polychlorinated biphenyls and their contaminants in Taiwan. Science 241:334, 1988.

232. Rose JQ, Ramsey JC, Wentzler TH, et al: The fate of TCDD following single and repeated oral doses to the rat. Toxicol Appl Pharmacol 36:209, 1976.

233. Roush GJ, Ott MG: A study of benzene exposure versus urinary phenol levels. Am Ind Hyg Assoc J 38:67, 1977.

234. Safe Drinking Water Committee, National Research Council: Drinking Water and Health, National Academy of Sciences, Washington, 1977.

235. Sarma PR, Jacobs J: Thoracic soft-tissue sarcoma in Vietnam veterans exposed to Agent Orange. N Engl J Med 306:1109, 1982.

236. Sauerhoff MW, Braun WH, Blau GE, et al: The fate of 2,4-dichlorophenoxyacetic acid (2,4-D) following oral administration to man. Toxicology 8:3, 1977.

237. Schwartz PM, Jacobson SW, Fein GG, et al: Lake Michigan fish consumption as a source of polychlorinated biphenyls in human cord serum, maternal serum and milk. Am J Public Health 73:293, 1983.

238. Seppäläinen Am, Hernberg SA: A follow-up study of nerve conduction velocities in lead exposed workers. Neurobehav Toxicol Teratol 4:721, 1982.

239. Seppäläinen AM, Tola S, Hernberg S, et al: Subclinical neuropathy at "safe" levels of lead exposure. Arch Environ Health 30:180, 1975.

240. Seppäläinen AM, Hernberg S, Vesanto R, et al: Early neurotoxic effects of occupational lead exposure: A prospective study. Neurotoxicology 4:181, 1983.

241. Shafik T, Bradway DE, Enos HF, et al: Human exposure to organophosphate pesticides. A modified procedure for gas liquid chromatographic analysis of alkyl phosphate metabolites in urine. J Agr Food Chem 21:625, 1973.

242. Shaikh ZA, Tohyama C: Urinary metallothionein as an indicator of cadmium body burden and of cadmium-induced nephrotoxicity. Environ Health Perspect 54:171, 1984.

243. Sharp DS, Eskenazi B, Harrison R, et al: Delayed health hazards of pesticide exposure. Annu Rev Public Health 7:441, 1986.

244. Sheldon L, Umana M, Bursey J, et al: Biological Monitoring Techniques for Human Exposure to Industrial Chemicals: Analysis of Human Fat, Skin, Nails, Hair, Blood, Urine, and Breath, Noyes Publications, Park Ridge, New Jersey, 1986.

245. Silbergeld EK: Exposures: Uptake, tissue and target dose. In: Mechanisms of Cell Injury: Implications for Human Health, p 405, Fowler BA (ed.), John Wiley & Sons, New York, 1987.

246. Singer R, Valciukas JA, Lilis R: Lead exposure and nerve conduction velocity: The differential time course of sensory and motor nerve effects. Neurotoxicology 4:193, 1983.

247. Sipes IG, Slocum ML, Perry DF, et al: 2,4,5,2',4',5'-Hexachlorobiphenyl: Distribution, metabolism and excretion in the dog and the monkey. Toxicol Appl Pharmacol 65:264, 1982.

248. Slaga TJ, Fischer SM, Weeks CE, et al: Studies on the mechanism involved in multistage carcinogenesis in mouse skin. In: Mechanisms of Chemical Carcinogenesis, p 207, Harris CC, Cerutti PA (eds.), Alan R Liss, New York, 1983.

249. Smith LM, Stalling DL, Johnson JL: Determination of part-per-trillion levels of polychlorinated dibenzo-furans and dioxins in environmental samples. Anal Chem 56:1830, 1984.

250. Smith M: Recent work on low level lead exposure and its impact on behavior, intelligence and learning: A review. J Am Acad Child Psychiatry 24:24, 1985.

251. Snyder R, Longacre SL, Witmer CM, et al: Biochemical toxicology of benzene. (Revised) Biochem Toxicol 3:132, 1981.

252. Sorsa M: Sister chromatid exchange and micronuclei as monitoring methods. In: Monitoring of Human Exposure to Carcinogenic and Mutagenic Agents, p 339, Berlin A, Draper M, Hemminki K, et al. (eds.), International Agency for Research in Cancer, Lyon, 1984.

253. Sorsa M: Occupational genotoxicology. In: Occupational Medicine Principles and Practical Applications, p 806, Zenz C (ed.), Year Book Medical Publishers, Chicago, 1988.

254. Sorsa M, Norppa H (eds.): Monitoring of Occupational Genotoxicants, Alan R Liss, New York, 1986.

255. Sorsa M, Kemminki K, Vainio H: Biological monitoring of exposure to chemical mutagens in the occupational environment. Teratogen Carcinogen Mutagen 2:137, 1982.

256. Spivey GH: Subclinical effects of chronic increased lead absorption: A prospective study. J Occup Med 22:607, 1980.

257. State of the Environment: A View Toward the Nineties, p 135, The Conservation Foundation, Washington, DC, 1987.

258. Stetka DG, Wolff S: Sister chromatid exchange as an assay for genetic damage induced by mutagen–carcinogens. I. In vivo test for compounds requiring metabolic activation. Mutat Res 41:333, 1976.

259. Stewart RD: The effect of carbon monoxide on humans. Annu Rev Pharmacol 15:409, 1975.

260. Stewart RD, Dodd HC, Gay HH, et al: Experimental human exposure to trichloroethylene. Arch Environ Health 20:64, 1970.

261. Stewart RD, Fisher TN, Hosko MJ, et al: Experimental human exposure to methylene chloride. Arch Environ Health 25:342, 1972.

262. Strassman SC, Kutz FW: Trends of organochlorine pesticide residues in human tissues. In: Toxicology of Halogenated Hydrocarbons, p 38, Khan MAQ, Stanton RH (eds.), Pergamon Press, New York, 1981.

263. Subramanian KS, Meranger JE: Diurnal variations in the concentration of cadmium in urine. Clin Chem 30:1110, 1984.

264. Suskind RR, Hertzberg VS: Human health effects of 2,4,5-T and its toxic contaminants. JAMA 251:2372, 1984.

265. Symposium on lead–blood pressure relationship. Environ Health Perspect 78:3–139, 1988.

266. Tabershaw IR, Cooper WC: Sequela of acute organic phosphate poisoning. J Occup Med 8:5, 1966.

267. Tornqvist M, Mowrer J, Jensen S, et al: Monitoring of environmental cancer initiators through hemoglobin adducts by a modified Edman degradation method. Anal Biochem 154:255, 1986.

268. Tornqvist M, Osterman-Golkar A, Kautiainen S, et al: Tissue doses of ethylene oxide in cigarette smokers determined from adduct levels in hemoglobin. Carcinogenesis 7:1519, 1986.

269. US EPA: Levels of Chemical Contaminants in Nonoccupational Exposed US Residents, EPA 000/1-80-002, EPA, Washington, 1980. Available from the National Technical Information Service, Springfield, VA 22161.

270. US EPA: Manual of Analytical Methods for the Analysis of Pesticides in Humans and Environmental Samples, Health Effects Research Laboratory, EPA-600/8-80-038, US EPA, Washington, 1980.

271. US EPA: Review of the NAAQS for Carbon Monoxide: Reassessment of Scientific and Technical Information. EPA-450/5-84-004, Office of Air Quality Planning Standards, US EPA, Washington, 1984.

272. US EPA: Suspended, Cancelled and Restricted Pesticides, 3rd rev, US EPA, Washington, 1985.

273. US EPA: Air Quality Criteria for Lead 6/86 and Addendum 9/86, EPA-600/8-83-018F, Office of Health and Environmental Assessment, US EPA, Washington, 1986.

274. Vainio H: Current trends in the biological monitoring of exposure to carcinogens. Scand J Work Environ Health 11:1, 1985.

275. Vainio H, Sorsa M: Application of cytogenetic methods for biological monitoring. Annu Rev Public Health 4:403, 1983.

276. Vainio H, Sorsa M, Rantanen J, et al: Biological monitoring in the identification of the cancer risk of individuals exposed to chemical carcinogens. Scand J Work Environ Health 7:241, 1981.

277. Vainio H, Sorsa M, Kemminki K: Biological monitoring in surveillance of exposure to genotoxicants. Am J Ind Med 4:87, 1983.

278. Vainio H, Sorsa M, Falck K: Bacterial urinary assay in monitoring exposure to mutagens and carcinogens. In: Monitoring of Human Exposure to Carcinogenic and Mutagenic Agents, p 247, Berlin A, Draper M, Hemminki K, et al. (eds.), International Agency for Research on Cancer, Lyon, 1984.

279. Valentine JL, Kang HK, Spivey G: Arsenic levels in human blood, urine and hair in response to exposure via drinking water. Environ Res 20:24, 1979.

280. Van Sittert NJ, de Jong G, Clare MG, et al: Cytogenetic, immunological and hematological effects in workers in an ethylene oxide manufacturing plant. Br J Ind Med 42:19, 1985.

281. Wallis G, Barber T: Variability in urinary mercury excretion. J Occup Med 24:590, 1982.

282. Warren AJ, Beck BD: Screening and monitoring for exposure and susceptibility to carcinogen. In: Variations in Susceptibility to Inhaled Pollutants, p 376, Brain JD, Beck BD, Warren AJ, et al. (eds.), The Johns Hopkins University Press, Baltimore, 1988.

283. Wedeen RP, Maesaka JK, Weiner B, et al: Occupational lead nephropathy. Am J Med 59:630, 1975.

284. Wedeen RP, Malik DK, Batuman V: Detection and treatment of occupational lead nephropathy. Arch Intern Med 139:53, 1979.

285. Weinstein IB: The monitoring of DNA adducts as an approach to carcinogen detection. Annu Rev Public Health 4:409, 1983.

286. Weinstein IB: Molecular cancer epidemiology: The use of new laboratory methods in studies on human cancer causation. In: Epidemiology and Health Risk Assessment, p 159, Gordis L (ed.), Oxford University Press, Oxford, 1988.

287. Wetstone HJ, LaMotta RV: The clinical stability of serum cholinesterase activity. Clin Chem 11:653, 1965.

288. Wogan GN, Gorelick NJ: Chemical and biochemical dosimetry of exposure to genotoxic chemicals. Environ Health Perspect 62:5, 1985.

289. Wolfe HR, Durham WF, Armstrong JF: Urinary excretion of insecticide metabolites—excretion of para-nitrophenol and DDA as indicators of exposure to parathion. Arch Environ Health 21:711, 1970.

290. World Health Organization: Environmental Health Criteria 1, Mercury, World Health Organization, Geneva, 1976.

291. World Health Organization: Environmental Health Criteria 3, Lead, WHO, Geneva, 1977.

292. World Health Organization: Environmental Health Criteria 13, Carbon Monoxide, World Health Organization, Geneva, 1979.

293. World Health Organization: Report of a Study Group: Recommended Health-Based Limits in Occupational Exposure to Heavy Metals. Technical Report Series 647, World Health Organization, Geneva, 1980.

294. World Health Organization: Environmental Health Criteria 29, 2,4-Dichlorophenoxyacetic Acid, World Health Organization, Geneva, 1981.

295. World Health Organization: Field Surveys of Exposure to Pesticides: Standard Protocol, Division of Vector Biology and Control, World Health Organization, Geneva, 1982.

296. Xintaras C, Johnson BL, deGroot I (eds.): Behavioral Toxicology: Early Detection of Occupational Hazards, NIOSH Publication 74-126, US DHEW, Washington, 1974.

297. Yager J, McLean H, Hudes M, et al: Components of variability in blood cholinesterase assay results. J Occup Med 18:242, 1976.

298. Yamasaki E, Ames BN: Concentration of mutagens from urine by absorption with nonpolar resin XAD-2: Cigarette smokers have mutagenic urine. Proc Natl Acad Sci USA, 74:3555, 1977.

299. Yamashita F, Hayaski M: Fetal PCB syndrome: Clinical features, intrauterine growth retardation and possible alteration in calcium metabolism. Environ Health Perspect 59:41, 1985.

300. Yule W, Rutter MI: Effect of lead on children's behavior and cognitive performance: A critical review. In: Dietary and Environmental Lead: Human Health Effects, p 2, Mahaffey KR (ed.), Elsevier Press, Amsterdam, 1985.

301. Yule W, Lansdown R, Millar IB, et al: The relationship between blood lead concentrations, intelligence

and attainment in a school population: A pilot study. Dev Med Child Neurol 23:567, 1981.

302. Zielhuis RL: Biological monitoring. Scand J Work Environ Health 4:1, 1978.

RECOMMENDED READINGS

Aitio A, Järvisalo J, Riihlmäki V, et al: Biological monitoring. In: Occupational Medicine Principles and Practical Applications, 2nd ed., p 178, Zenz C (ed.), Year Bood Medical Publishers, Chicago, 1988.

Bartsch H, Hemminki K, O'Neill IK (eds.): Methods for Detecting DNA Damaging Agents in Humans: Applications in Cancer Epidemiology and Prevention, IARC Scientific Publication 89, International Agency For Research on Cancer, Lyon, 1988.

Berlin A, Wolff AH, Hasegawa Y (eds.): The Use of Biological Specimens for the Assessment of Human Exposure to Environmental Pollutants, Martinus Nijhoff, The Hague, 1979.

Committee on National Monitoring of Human Tissues, National Research Council: Monitoring Human Tissues for Toxic Substances, National Academy Press, 1991.

Garner RC, Farmer PB, Steel GT, et al. (eds.): Human Carcinogen Exposure. Biomonitoring and Risk Asessment. Oxford University Press, Oxford, 1991.

Hulka BS, Wilcosky TC, Griffith JD: Biological Markers in Epidemiology, Oxford University Press, Oxford, 1990.

Lauwerys RR: Industrial Chemical Exposure—Guidelines for Biological Monitoring, Biomedical Publications, Davis, California, 1983.

Sorsa M, Norppa H (eds.): Monitoring of Occupational Genotoxicants, Alan R Liss, New York, 1986.

Part VII

CONTROLLING EXPOSURE TO ENVIRONMENTAL CHEMICALS AND PHYSICAL AGENTS

28. PERSONAL METHODS OF CONTROLLING EXPOSURE TO INDOOR AIR POLLUTION

Anthony V. Nero, Jr.

INTRODUCTION

Indoor air pollution has been a part of the human condition since humans first began to live indoors. The pollutants found indoors are similar to those found outdoors and in some instances actually come from outdoor sources. In the absence of indoor sources, the concentrations of combustion products are typically somewhat less than those in outdoor air. Yet the pollutants measured in highest concentrations are measured indoors and originate from within buildings. Only in recent years have we become aware of the dimensions of the problem and the relevance of indoor air quality for health. A number of factors combined to produce this awareness: complaints of eye, nose, and throat irritation and other symptoms by occupants of new or recently remodeled office buildings; the presence of deteriorating asbestos in public schools; the problem of radon in homes; and the symptoms evidenced by the occupants of houses insulated with urea–formaldehyde foam. The past decade has therefore witnessed the growth of an immense body of literature dealing with the source, concentrations, control, health effects, and engineering and policy aspects of indoor air pollution (1,9,23,24). For many

airborne pollutants, such as combustion-generated contaminants, volatile organic compounds, pesticides, asbestos, lead, radon, and biological agents, the greatest potential for human exposures takes place not outdoors but inside homes, offices, and other nonindustrial buildings. Indoor concentrations of these pollutants often exceed those found outdoors. Moreover, most people in developed countries spend more of their time indoors than outdoors.

There are many gaps in our understanding of the health effects of indoor air pollution as well as great uncertainty about what concentrations and periods of exposure are needed to produce specific health effects. The wide range of pollutant types and concentrations entails a correspondingly wide range of potential health risks. Health risks fall into two categories: those that take place immediately after exposure, e.g., acute eye, nose, and throat irritation and hypersensitivity reactions; and those that may appear many years after exposure or only after repeated periods of exposure, e.g., impaired cardiopulmonary function and cancer (1,23,24).

The indoor air quality problems currently of greatest health concern relate to passive exposure to tobacco smoke, NO_2 exposure from gas-fueled cooking stoves, formaldehyde exposure, radon decay products, and the health problems encountered by workers in newly sealed and renovated office buildings (23). In only a relatively few instances, such as hypersensitivity pneumonitis and carbon

Principles and Practice of Environmental Medicine, edited by Alyce Bezman Tarcher. Plenum Medical Book Company, New York, 1992.

monoxide poisoning, is there a clear-cut relationship between a given exposure to an indoor air pollutant and an associated health effect. As with other exposures, the health risks of indoor air pollution are determined by the nature and level of exposure as well as by individual susceptibility. Thus, the likelihood of an individual developing an adverse reaction to indoor air pollutants depends, in part, on such factors as age, health status, and other conditions that effect susceptibility (see Chapter 12). Noteworthy is the fact that the very young, the elderly, and the chronically ill, especially those suffering from respiratory or cardiovascular disease, are those who usually spend the greatest amount of time indoors.

There is agreement that it is prudent to attempt to improve the quality of indoor air, particularly in those situations where the concentrations of one or more pollutants are substantially higher than average. Because it is generally much easier to improve the quality of indoor air than that of outdoor air, the fact that the levels of many pollutants are greater indoors than outdoors gives the individual greater personal control of airborne pollutant exposures. Depending on the situation and the amount of exposure, the reduction required may be large, modest, or undetermined. As discussed below, the potential for reduction in concentration or exposure can depend substantially on the pollutant class, on the particular circumstances, and on the methods available.

Even so, there are limitations. An individual has a different degree of control at home than in a place of work. This is true even if we exclude industrial environments with a potential for exposures specifically associated with manufacturing or other industrial processes. A typical nonindustrial work environment is that of an office. Although an individual has some degree of control over an office environment, a substantial amount of control resides with the architect and builder, the operator of the building, and the company for which the individual works. Similarly, even at home, where greater control can be exercised, there are limitations in what individuals are able to do, either because they are not the owner of the building or because some of the possible options are too costly or uncertain in effect. It is noteworthy that, to some degree, individuals can influence what happens to their air, regardless of who actually carries out a particular control measure. The discussion below addresses the range of options, whether implemented by an individual occupant, a building owner, or a company.

It is useful, before discussing methods of control specific for each class of pollutants, to roughly frame each class, note the factors that affect their concentration indoors, describe the general methods of control, and provide a simple guide for judging whether a home has, or could develop, indoor air problems.

CLASSES OF INDOOR AIR POLLUTANTS

The pollutants measured in highest concentrations indoors may be classified as combustion emissions, environmental tobacco smoke, organic chemicals, asbestos, lead, radon, and biogenic agents. A brief discussion of these sources of indoor air pollution is presented below. For a more complete discussion the reader is referred to Chapter 2.

Combustion Emissions

The most easily appreciated class of pollutants, partly because they are so widespread and partly because of their similarity to pollutants of principal concern in outdoor air, is combustion emissions. These include oxides of nitrogen (NO_2, NO), carbon (CO_2, CO), and sometimes sulfur (SO_2) as well as more complex particles and gases arising from incomplete combustion. Among the sources of these substances are combustion appliances, outdoor air, and especially smoking. Commonly used combustion appliances are gas cooking or wood-burning stoves, unvented kerosene heaters, and fireplaces. Smoking is in a class by itself in terms of the amount of complex chemicals produced (1,31,35). Not surprisingly, the presence of smokers or of unvented combustion appliances can raise the levels of indoor air pollutants significantly. In developing countries, major sources of indoor combustion emissions are the use of peat and dung as fuels.

Organic Compounds

Organic chemicals, gaseous or on airborne particles, constitute another class of concern and include most of the more complex substances emitted from combustion. But organic compounds can also arise from several other sources, including building materials, furnishings, household and personal care products, tobacco smoking, hobbies, and pesticide use. The types and amounts of organics present indoors vary widely in number, sources, and concentration. In recent years, hundreds of volatile organic compounds (VOCs), including formaldehyde, have been identified in homes and commercial buildings (12,36). The concentrations of many organic compounds indoors generally range from two to 20 times outdoor levels. The use of such products as room deodorizers may increase the levels considerably (12,36). Because it is time consuming and expensive to identify and quantify VOCs, identifying their source, in many cases, poses a difficult problem. It is noteworthy that a wide range of health risks may be linked to VOCs. Some are known human carcinogens, and others have respiratory and neurotoxic effects (see Chapters 13, 14, 16, and 26).

Asbestos

Certain special substances arise from materials present in many homes and buildings and have significant health effects but do not fall into the classes already mentioned. Important examples are asbestos and lead. Both arise from materials that were, until recently, used in building interiors and are therefore present in a large number of homes, schools, and offices. In the past, asbestos was most often used in homes as thermal insulation on furnaces and pipes. It was also used in vinyl floor tiles or linoleum, textured paints, and other coating materials. Asbestos fibers used in building materials, under conditions of normal use and maintenance, generally pose no problem. However, respirable fibers of asbestos can be released indoors, particularly from asbestos-containing materials that are damaged or undergoing deterioration. Thus, asbestos presents a hazard when asbestos-containing materials are disturbed during repair or remodeling activities (1,27,31). Most homes built before 1975 are likely to contain asbestos in some building materials. It has long been recognized that asbestos fibers produce such diseases as asbestosis, lung cancer, and malignant mesothelioma (see Chapter 16).

Lead

The inhalation of lead dust can be an important means of exposure to this element. High concentrations develop when lead-based paint is removed by sanding or open-flame burning. Lead can also be brought into the home from the workplace. Outdoor sources such as the incursion of contaminated soil and indoor activities such as soldering, stained-glass artwork, and electronics repair can also result in high indoor concentrations of airborne lead. In the United States prior to 1940, lead paint was widely used in homes. This use was greatly reduced between 1940 and 1960 and essentially abandoned thereafter. Moreover, since 1975, when the EPA mandated a 95% reduction in the use of lead in gasoline, the influx of lead-contaminated outdoor air into indoor air has dropped dramatically. Airborne lead is well recognized as a pollutant of indoor air, especially harmful for the fetus and young children (see Chapters 13, 14, and 24).

Radon

Radon and its daughters constitute an important class of pollutants that do not produce immediate symptoms. Because it comes directly from the ground on which the house is built, indoor air pollution with radon is perhaps the most disconcerting problem for the occupants of many homes. This radioactive gas is generated naturally as a product of the nuclear decay of radium, a member of the decay series of uranium. Radon in turn decays into a series of short-lived solid isotopes referred to as radon decay products or sometimes as radon "daughters." The health effect potentially resulting from excessive radiation exposures from radon daughters is lung cancer. Reducing such exposure must therefore be looked on as a preventive measure (16).

Biogenic Particles

A distinctly different class of indoor air pollutant includes living organisms such as bacteria, fungi, dust mites, and pollens. It also includes such products of living organisms as animal saliva, urine, and dander, human dander, and insect parts and wastes. The sources of biogenic particles include wet or moist walls, ceilings, carpets and furnishings; poorly maintained dehumidifiers and air conditioners; bedding; and household pets (1). To some degree, biogenic particles may be considered outside the class of what we consider to be pollutants; i.e., they include infectious agents and allergenic substances whose mode of action is quite distinct from chemical and physical agents. On the other hand, biological contaminants are important sources of indoor air pollution, and some of the measures used for their control are similar to those employed for chemical agents. Infectious disease does not fall within the scope of indoor air quality or building-related health concerns except perhaps for Legionnaires' disease, which has been linked to contaminated air-conditioning systems.

FACTORS THAT DETERMINE INDOOR AIR POLLUTANT CONCENTRATIONS

The above classes of pollutants are almost always present in indoor air. However, their concentrations vary widely depending on (1) the rate at which each pollutant is emitted into the indoor atmosphere, (2) the ventilation rate, (3) the rate at which a particular pollutant reacts with other airborne species, and (4) the behavior of the occupants. Other conditions influencing the concentration of indoor contaminants include the type, condition, and use of the source(s) of contamination, indoor temperature and relative humidity, air mixing, and the season of the year (1,9).

Large differences in the concentration of indoor pollutants are often noted from one building to another and among various types of buildings such as offices, homes, and schools. Large differences also exist from one time to another in a given building. The variability depends primarily on the rate at which each pollutant is emitted into the indoor atmosphere. This is true even for pollutants arising from sources that do not depend on occupant behavior. Substances that arise from the use of particular appliances or consumer products are particularly subject to variability in time.

The variability in exposure patterns that exists from one building to another often arises from factors that are not obvious to the occupants. Such sources as the building structure, the furnishings, or even materials underlying the building give rise to a range of pollutants whose emission rates may vary tremendously depending on specific materials or building design (9). Even a knowledgeable environmental scientist cannot estimate emission rates without actual measurements of pollutant concentrations or information on the specific materials and designs used. Surprisingly, the concentration of a specific pollutant can easily vary by a factor of 100 from one building to another, often because of differences in source characteristics that cannot be determined from superficial examination (9).

As might be expected, ventilation also plays a role in indoor air quality. Thus, as energy-conscious homeowners in the United States and elsewhere began to reduce ventilation rates by roughly 10% to 30% through weather stripping, plugging openings in the building's shell, and caulking around the windows and doors, a modest increase in the concentrations of indoor air pollutants occurred. As ventilation rates were reduced in newer structures containing materials having high emission rates of formaldehyde and other organic compounds, the increased concentrations of indoor air pollutants became a matter of concern. In new "tight" homes, the air-exchange rate, especially during the winter months, can be reduced by 50% (9).

Another but much less obvious factor that determines indoor air pollutant concentration is the rate at which a particular pollutant reacts with other airborne species or interior surfaces. Nitrogen dioxide, for example, is found to be removed from indoor air as much by such reactions as by ventilation. The chemical forms and concentrations of radon daughters (isotopes of polonium, lead, and bismuth) also depend on the amount of airborne particles as well as on the pattern of air movement. Many other potentially important aspects of indoor-air chemistry remain virtually unexplored (16).

Finally, the behavior of the building occupants can affect indoor air quality. It is often this factor, more than any other, that ultimately determines the success or failure of any program instituted to control indoor air quality. Yet the occupants of a building are often unaware of potential health problems that stem from the way they use certain appliances or substances. Even building managers may be unaware of activities for which the building was originally designed or how the ventilation equipment was meant to be used. The original design of the equipment may have been altered, or poorly trained operators may be in charge. Frequently environmental tobacco smoke significantly compromises indoor air quality. Changing behavior is therefore often one of the simplest, least expensive, and most effective means of improving indoor air quality. Prohibiting smoking indoors or completely isolating a smoking area is undoubtedly one of the most effective means of immediately and dramatically improving indoor air quality. The maintenance of gas appliances and the proper storage of cleaning materials, paints, and solvents also improve indoor air quality (1).

GENERAL METHODS OF CONTROLLING INDOOR AIR POLLUTION

Indoor air pollution may, in principle, be controlled by three types of measures: (1) reducing the rate of emission from sources (including removal of the sources); (2) supplying additional ventilation; and (3) cleaning the indoor air by filtration or other means (Table 28-1). Depending on the circumstances, these approaches are applicable to varying degrees to all pollutant classes. In general, the methods of control are stated in the order of effectiveness, with the control of pollutants at the source being the most effective strategy for maintaining the quality of indoor air.

TABLE 28-1. Methods of Controlling Indoor Air Pollution

Source control
Eliminating, reducing, or isolating sources that emit pollutants
Ventilation
Increasing ventilation to the entire structure and/or to a local area
Air cleaning
Using various devices to remove particles and/or gases

Source Control

The importance of controlling the sources of indoor air contamination is supported by the observation that the wide variability in pollutant concentrations from one building to another is related primarily to differences in the presence of pollutant sources. It has been noted that the marked divergence, with factors ranging from 100 to 1000, in the pollutant concentrations measured in U.S. buildings is reflected in the emission rates of pollution sources. Moreover, for most buildings, especially homes with excessive pollutant concentrations, the origin of the problem is most often associated with high emissions from the pollution source. The clearest quantitative example of this overall behavior is that of radon (18,19). It is also seen with environmental tobacco smoke, VOCs such as pesticides, and other pollutants, such as lead, whose indoor concentrations depend on whether the source is present or not.

Unusually low ventilation rates can have an adverse effect, but the disparity in ventilation rates is typically not as large as the range of indoor pollutant levels noted among residential and office buildings. A reduction in indoor air pollutant concentration by a factor of ten or more can often be achieved by attention to the pollution sources, whereas a comparable reduction by ventilation measures would require a tenfold increase in ventilation rate. The required increase in ventilation rate is typically more difficult and much more expensive to achieve than eliminating or reducing the source of pollution. Similarly, air cleaners, which provide an alternative means of control, suffer from the same limitations as ventilation in that the marked reduction in pollutant concentrations often needed would require high rates of air processing. Such an approach is not practical because of cost, size, and maintenance requirements.

As shown in Table 28-2, the methods available for controlling the sources of indoor air pollution cover a broad range of options. The methods used depend on the nature of the particular pollutant and the type of problem. Often it is helpful to use a combination of methods. The application of these methods is described below in the context of problems that arise from specific classes of pollutants.

Ventilation

Although ventilation is often thought of as either air movement within a building or the introduction of outdoor air, it is, in fact, a combination of processes involved in the supply and removal of air from inside a building. These processes typically include the entry of outdoor air, its mixture with

TABLE 28-2. Methods of Controlling the Sources of Indoor Air Pollution

Using building materials, funishings, and consumer products with low emissions rates
Physical removal of offending materials
Isolating, encapsulating, or controlling emission sources
Local venting of pollutants at the point of emission (e.g., range hood, substructure radon control system)
Behavioral changes that reduce the number and strength of pollutant sources and/or modify their use (e.g., no smoking, maintenance of cooking and heating systems, using agents with lower emissions)
Controlling indoor environment (e.g., temperature, relative humidity)

some portion of indoor air, its distribution within the building, and finally the release of some portion of the indoor air to the outside. The quality of indoor air may deteriorate when one or more of these processes are inadequate.

Outdoor air enters and leaves a structure in three ways: infiltration occurs through cracks around windows and doors and openings for pipes and wiring; natural ventilation occurs when windows or doors are opened; and mechanical ventilation occurs through the use of fans and other devices. The rate at which outdoor air replaces indoor air is defined as the air-exchange rate. The ventilation rate is the rate at which outside air enters and leaves a building. It is expressed in two ways: the number of changes of outside air per unit of time or the rate at which a volume of outside air enters per unit of time.

Ventilation improves the quality of indoor air by diluting the level of most pollutants. Ventilation is therefore most effective when the source of the pollutant(s) is indoors and when outdoor concentrations are relatively low in comparison to those present indoors. The ventilation rate, though generally not the major factor in determining the concentration of indoor pollutants, may be an important contributing factor. Many are surprised to learn that the air inside most homes and other buildings exchanges with outside air about once an hour, and even more often with the windows open or with mechanical ventilation systems. In relatively "tight" homes, the average exchange rate can be as low as 0.3 air changes per hour. In contrast, in "leaky" homes, it may be as high as two air changes per hour. It should be understood that an air exchange rate of 1 per hour does not imply that all indoor contaminants will be removed in this time. Pollutants typically continue to be emitted, and, as noted, ventilation allows the dilution and gradual removal of airborne pollutants (9).

The general ventilation of small structures such as houses stems primarily from the infiltration of outside air into the interior. Opening windows and doors increases the natural influx of outdoor air and is thereby the fastest and simplest means of increasing ventilation. Mechanical ventilation can also be used in the home, but usually to a limited extent. Thus, natural ventilation may be augmented by use of outdoor-vented fans, including those that are simply placed in windows. Since increasing ventilation provides a general, albeit usually modest, improvement in indoor air quality, opening windows and doors and loosening the building shell are sometimes the most appropriate control measures, particularly in the case of tight homes with low air-exchange rates. The concentration of indoor air pollutants can also be decreased by providing mechanical ventilation in local areas with the greatest concentration of indoor pollutants. Bathroom and kitchen exhaust fans are important in this regard.

Opening windows or using fans, although often helpful, has the disadvantage that energy is lost or drafts created. To avoid these difficulties, a more sophisticated form of ventilation transfers heat between air leaving the building and that entering. This is done by a mechanical ventilation system that employs an air-to-air heat exchanger (also known as heat recovery ventilators). Such a system may be incorporated into a central air system or installed as a small window air conditioner. A variety of measurements have demonstrated the effectiveness of these systems in terms of both providing effective ventilation of the interior space and recovering most of the energy that would otherwise be lost through ordinary ventilation (6). Such systems are particularly attractive in colder climates, where energy saving is relatively important.

In contrast to the ventilation methods found in homes, large structures such as office buildings generally rely on mechanical ventilation to maintain the quality of indoor air. For the newly constructed sealed office buildings, mechanical ventilation systems that exchange indoor air with outdoor air provide the only means of maintaining indoor air quality. As new buildings become less and less permeable in order to conserve energy, the importance of supplying outside air to mechanical ventilating systems is increased. Mechanical heating, ventilation, and air-conditioning (HVAC) systems are designed to provide air at comfortable temperature and humidity levels, free of harmful concentrations of air pollutants. In many cases, the systems are complex, requiring the attention of well-trained operators (1).

As might be expected, if the the HVAC system is inadequately designed, installed, operated, or maintained, the concentration of internally generated pollutants increases. Some common problems include installation of air supply vents too close to building exhaust vents and/or the placement of outdoor air supply vents near sources of pollution (e.g., loading docks, parking and heavy traffic areas); failure to maintain proper temperature, humidity, and air movement; failure to supply a sufficient quantity of outside air (e.g., reducing or eliminating the amount of outdoor air during hot and cold spells reduces the cost of cooling and heating the air); and failure to operate the HVAC system before the occupants arrive and/or shutting it off before the end of the work day. In some cases, the ventilation system itself becomes the source of contaminants. For example, continuously moist mechanical components generate airborne microorganisms, and dirty filters may emit volatile components of environmental tobacco smoke (1,33).

Air Cleaners

Air cleaning is another means of controlling indoor pollutants, especially particles from combustion (including environmental tobacco smoke) and other sources (e.g., dust, fabric lint). Particulate matter or dust is enough of a problem in many large buildings and in spaces occupied by individuals with special sensitivities to merit some degree of air cleaning. Because no air-cleaning system effectively removes all pollutants from indoor air, this measure should be considered an adjunct to source control and ventilation. Air cleaners, usually classified by the method employed to remove particles of various sizes from the air, operate on a range of different principles. Types of air cleaners include mechanical filters, electronic air cleaners, and hybrid devices using two or more particle removal devices. Air-cleaning devices come in many types and sizes ranging from movable inexpensive tabletop models to sophisticated expensive systems incorporated into heating, air-conditioning, or ventilation systems (9).

Mechanical filters contain materials that retain particles by physical collection. Mechanical filters used for air cleaning are of two major types: flat or panel filters and pleated or extended-surface filters. Flat or panel filters usually consist of a low packing density of coarse glass fibers, animal hair, vegetable fibers, or synthetic fibers, often coated with a viscous substance to act as an adhesive for particulate material. The flat filter is the typical furnace filter installed in the central heat and/or air-conditioning system used in many homes. Flat filters efficiently collect large particles, but only a small portion of the respirable-sized particles are removed. Pleated or extended-surface filters have greater surface areas, which allows the use of smaller fibers and increased packing density of the filter without a large drop in air flow rate. Extended-surface filters such as high-efficiency particulate filters (HEPA) are effective in removing particles having a wide range of sizes (34).

Electronic air cleaners trap charged particles using an electrical field. In electrostatic precipitators, particles are charged and then collected on a surface with the opposite charge. These devices are effective in removing large particles, which include pollens and large mold spores. They are less effective in removing smaller particles, which include residues from house dust mites, animal allergens, and particles found in tobacco smoke (1,34). Ion generators also use static charges to remove particles from indoor air. Charges are generated that adhere to the particles. Once charged, the particles in a room are attracted to walls, floors, tabletops, draperies, and occupants. These devices are available only in portable units. In some cases, ion generators contain a collector to attract the charged particles back to the unit. Of note is the fact that ion generators and electrostatic precipitators may produce ozone (1,34).

For the removal of gaseous pollutants, air cleaners may contain absorbent materials and/or reactive materials (14). As might be expected, the efficiency of devices that function through absorption and adsorption depends on such factors as air flow through the sorbent and the sorption capacity and affinity. The most commonly used sorbents are activated carbon, activated alumina, and silica gel. Organic gases of moderate molecular weight are generally effectively adsorbed. Activated carbon, however, does not efficiently adsorb volatile, low-molecular-weight gases (5,35). Moreover, the ability of carbon to remit trapped pollutants is of concern (34). Special sorbents, often impregnated with chemically active materials, have been developed to remove specific gaseous pollutants. These sorbents include such materials as potassium permanganate or copper oxide. Formaldehyde, for example, can be removed by alumina activated with potassium permanganate. In general, air cleaners containing specialized sorbents are more effective in removing gaseous pollutants than are those containing activated carbon alone. As sorbents become saturated, they must be replaced on a regular basis. Air cleaners that do not contain sorbent materials will not remove gaseous materials from indoor air (34).

How well an air cleaner works in removing pollutants from the air depends on both the percentage of the pollutant removed (expressed as a percentage efficiency rate) and how much air is handled through the cleaning and filtering mechanism (expressed as cubic feet per minute). Thus, a highly effective cleaner has both a high circulation rate and an efficient collector. Although there is no generally defined method for comparing air-cleaning devices, the results of some studies of portable air-cleaning units have been expressed as an "effective cleaning rate" (ECR). The ECR is the product of the unit efficiency and the air flow rate and is a measure of the number of cubic feet per minute of air it effectively cleans for a specific material. Knowledge of both the ECR and the unit efficiency is helpful in choosing a device for use in removing pollutants from a specific source. It should be appreciated that, in general, the effectiveness of any portable device is increased by its location near the source of pollution (34).

Direct measurements performed on portable air cleaners have demonstrated that such systems have a wide range of effectiveness, as assessed by the removal of particulates in environmental tobacco smoke from indoor air (Table 28-3) (1,4,21). It is not surprising that the relatively popular, small, and inexpensive cleaners have been found to be almost completely ineffective in removing particulates (21, 34). The reasons for poor removal rates of these small devices is fairly clear: (1) they tend to have relatively low flow rates, so that even if they were 100% efficient, their cleaning rate would be relatively low; (2) they often contain a flat-panel particulate filter, which tends to be inefficient for the removal of respirable particles; and (3) they may be constructed such that much of the air drawn through the system bypasses the filter, especially if substantial care is not employed in their design and production.

In contrast, larger and more expensive systems usually have increased flow rates, a better collection medium, and more careful design and construction. Some systems have been found to provide air-cleaning rates, at least for respirable particles, that are comparable to or greater than the removal from ordinary ventilation rates (34). Thus, in many instances, air-cleaning systems can be expected to provide a substantial reduction in indoor particle concentrations, though still not as substantial as elimination of the pollution source. The most effective devices for particle cleaning are those employing extended-surface filters, such as HEPA (high-efficiency particulate) filters, or electrostatic precipitation. Both types of air cleaners require some degree of maintenance in terms of filter replacement or cleaning, but not to a degree that is overly burdensome.

Apart from considering the ability of an air cleaner to reduce the concentrations of indoor air pollutants under the condition of use, the following factors should also be kept in mind: installation requirements; use and need for maintenance; cost; noise; possible production or redispersal of such pollutants as ozone and trapped gaseous agents; the inability of air cleaners designed for particle removal to control gaseous pollutants; and the possible soiling of surfaces by charged particles produced by ion generators (34).

TABLE 28-3. Comparison of Modular Environmental Tobacco Smoke-Cleaning Devices[a]

	Units tested (n)	Costs of device[b]	Replacement filter costs[b]	Flow rate (cfm)[c]	Particulate ECR (cfm)	Gas cleaning
Flat filter	LBL 3	$30–$40	$4–$6	10–29	0–3	Not effective
	CR 12	$15–$100	$4–$6 ($15–$41)	20–100	2–8 (14)	
With ion generator	LBL 1	$150	$12	17	7	Not effective
	CR 1	$299	$16	40–60	47	
Pleated filter	LBL 1	$395	$77	157	180	Not effective
	CR 4	$45–140	$5–$20	10–90	6–33	
With ion generator	LBL 1	$295	$16	66	57	Not effective
	CR 2	$100	$7–$15	20–100	13–47	
Electrostatic precipitators	LBL 2	$370–$395	$15	200–215	116–122	Not effective
	CR 1	$158	$7	40–90	19	
Ion generators	LBL 2	$80–$120	—	—	1–30	Not effective
	CR 3	$44–$79	—	—	13–58	
Fan	LBL 1	$52	—	1800	1	
	CR				2	

[a]From American Thoracic Society (1). ETS, environmental tobacco smoke; ECR, effective cleaning rate; LBL, Lawrence Berkeley Laboratory (21); CR, Consumer Reports (4).
[b]These costs are presented to give the reader information on relative costs.
[c]cfm = cubic feet per minute.

ASSESSING THE GENERAL STATUS OF INDOOR AIR QUALITY IN THE HOME

It is widely agreed that even in the absence of symptoms, it is prudent to attempt to improve the indoor air quality of one's home. This is especially true if there are indications that the concentrations of any pollutants are significantly higher than average. It is also clear that sensitive individuals, e.g., those suffering from allergies associated with indoor pollutants, should make a special effort to improve the quality of indoor air to which they are exposed. As a guide to assessing the general status of indoor air quality in the home, it is useful to evaluate the following: (1) potential sources of indoor air pollution; (2) problems with ventilation; and (3) behavior that increases indoor air pollution (Table 28-4). It is noteworthy that certain building conditions are especially likely to be associated with problems of indoor air quality. These include remodeling or renovation, acquisition of new furnishings, pesticide application, the presence of environmental tobacco smoke, and strict energy-conserving measures. In some instances, particularly when clinical problems arise or major indoor air quality problems are evidenced by poor air flow or specific pollutant sources, it may be helpful to assess actual concentrations and sources. This can be done either by direct measurement or by detailed characterization of potential sources. Since testing for many indoor air pollutants requires special knowledge and apparatus and can be expensive, monitoring should be done in consultation with state or local health departments or with a professional trained in dealing with indoor air quality problems. However, for such pollutants as radon, NO_2, and formaldehyde, inexpensive and easily used detectors are available along with public information on their use.

METHODS OF CONTROLLING SPECIFIC INDOOR AIR POLLUTANTS

Combustion Emissions

Some combustion products come from appliances, primarily heaters and stoves. Others come from smokers, and a narrower range of substances come from outdoors. Controlling emissions at their source is generally the best solution to the problem, although, to some degree, general ventilation and air cleaning also apply. Table 28-5 shows a checklist that may help one discover a combustion-related indoor air quality problem.

If they are not vented to the outdoors, indoor combustion appliances can be substantial sources of combustion products. Although central furnaces are invariably vented, usually via a chimney or by a flue to the outside air, it is well to have them inspected at regular intervals. If significant amounts of combustion products are entering the indoor atmosphere from the central heating system, a failure of the heat exchanger or flue is implied, and these should be repaired. Other combustion sources include improperly vented gas water heaters and driers.

TABLE 28-4. A Guide for Assessing the General Status of Indoor Air Quality in the Home

Sources of indoor air pollutants
 New, well-insulated home containing new furnishings including furniture, carpets, and draperies that emit formaldehyde and other volatile organic compounds
 Polyurethane or urea–formaldehyde insulation
 Deteriorated asbestos insulation or other asbestos-containing materials
 Chipped or peeling lead-based paint (e.g., in a home built before 1960)
 Recent ongoing or planned renovation or remodeling
 Unvented or malfunctioning stoves, furnaces, or space heaters
 Gas heating or cooking appliances with flames that appear yellow instead of blue
Problems with ventilation
 Unusual and noticeable odors
 Stale air
 Lack of air movement
 Dirty central heating and air-cooling equipment
 Damaged flues and chimneys
 Moisture condensation on cold surfaces
 Mold and mildew growth
Behavioral factors
 Tobacco smoke present indoors
 Pesticides used indoors
 Hobbies involving ceramics, jewelry making, painting, photography, stained-glass making, and woodworking
 Cleaning agents and solvents used and stored improperly
 Gas oven used for heating purposes

TABLE 28-5. Combustion-related Indoor Air Pollution Checklist[a]

1. Are the flames in the appliance yellow, and/or are they lifting off the burner assembly?
2. Are there any unvented space-heating appliances in the home?
3. Are the flues of "vented" appliances properly connected and free of obstruction? Do they meet code specifications for size and vertical and horizontal slope?
4. Is the heat exchanger in the forced-air furnace system cracked? Can oil or combustion odors be detected inside the house? Does the house have excess moisture?
5. Is the inside wall above the fireplace or areas around exhaust ducts covered with soot?
6. Is the cooking range used for heat?
7. Are cars, lawn mowers, snow blowers, or combustion generators used in or near indoor environments?
8. Is the smell of wood smoke noticeable indoors when the wood stove is operating?
9. Is the wood stove airtight?
10. Is there a range hood in the kitchen? Is it used?

[a]From American Thoracic Society (1).

An increase in the levels of combustion products can occur when appliances are used for purposes far beyond their design parameters, as when an oven is used for heating the kitchen or larger spaces. A more common cause of an increase in indoor combustion emissions is the use of an unvented heating or cooking appliance. Small kerosene heaters of the type that have become very popular in the last 15 years are a major example (13,26). Pollution of the indoor atmosphere from this source can be prevented by avoiding the use of such devices. If their use is essential, adequate ventilation, e.g., by opening the door(s) and window(s), must be provided. Moreover, care should be taken to use manufacturer-specified fuels and a unit properly sized for the space in which it is to operate. An oversized unit will have higher total emissions, as a greater amount of fuel is used. The same general principles apply to the use of unvented gas-fired heaters (9).

Gas ranges or ovens are a somewhat different case, since a means of venting the products of combustion or cooking is usually present. It has been shown that the concentration of combustion emissions is substantially reduced by use of a range hood (9). Pilot lights on cooking ranges and ovens should be turned off or eliminated, and appliances should be properly adjusted. Emission rates are reduced by using gas ranges and ovens with electronic ignition. The proper adjustment of a gas heating or cooking appliance, as evidenced by a blue rather than a yellow flame, also reduces emissions. An obvious alternative to venting, in cases where occupants have a very low tolerance for combustion products, is replacement of gas ranges or ovens by electric appliances. Other combustion sources include wood and coal stoves that are not airtight. Care must be taken, therefore, to ascertain that only properly vented and airtight stoves be used. Unvented gas fireplaces are another pollution source. When one is in use, the flues must be open. Emissions from vehicles in attached garages can permeate indoors. Care must be taken not to idle cars inside the garage.

The final source of indoor combustion emissions to be mentioned is outdoor air. Outdoor emissions include nitrogen oxides, carbon monoxide, and respirable particles, all of which have widely varying indoor/outdoor ratios, depending primarily on the presence of indoor pollution sources. In certain situations, where outdoor concentrations are high, the building shell can actually provide a shield against exposure. This applies to sulfur dioxide (SO_2) and ozone (O_3), whose indoor concentrations are only a fraction of those found outdoors. When SO_2 comes from an indoor source, it is commonly derived from a kerosene heater using fuel with a high sulfur content. When O_3 comes from an indoor source, that source is generally an electronic air cleaner or a photocopy machine.

Environmental Tobacco Smoke

Smoking is the other source of combustion emissions of major, often dominant, importance. Since it arises directly from a personal habit, it is in a different class than most other pollutants considered here. In recent years exposure to environmental tobacco smoke (ETS) has been linked to a myriad of adverse health effects, which have been summarized in reports by the U.S. Surgeon General and the National Research Council (3,28) (see Chapter 16). The public health impact of passive smoking makes it abundantly clear that such exposure should be avoided. Moreover, in certain individuals, the acute effects of ETS makes it necessary for them to reduce or eliminate such exposure.

In a space over which an individual has control, smoking may simply be prohibited. In other circumstances, some reduction may be achieved by ventilation or air cleaning. A comparison of the relative effectiveness of portable air-cleaning devices for environmental tobacco smoke is shown in Table 28-3 (4,5,34). The comparison presented deals only with particulate components of environmental tobacco smoke. Air-cleaning devices for residential use, which remove both the particulate and gaseous constituents, are currently being sold. These units typically consist of filters to remove both large and small particulates and sorbents to remove gas-phase components. The effectiveness of such units has not yet been fully evaluated.

Restricting smoking to a certain area may reduce the concentration of environmental tobacco smoke, but indoor air contamination will continue unless the area is physically isolated from the rest of the home or building. Smoking in a restricted area connected to a heating, ventilation, or air-conditioning system that recirculates air, results in the smoke contamination of other areas. Although air contaminated with tobacco smoke can theoretically be cleaned and then recirculated, the complexity of the mixture requires a multistage process. Its implementation either as a part of a HVAC or as a standalone unit is both difficult and costly. Beyond doubt, the control strategy having the greatest public health benefits is that of totally eliminating tobacco smoking (1).

Formaldehyde and Other Volatile Organic Compounds

Semivolatile and volatile organic compounds (VOCs), including formaldehyde, derived from building materials, furnishings, cleaning materials, and personal care products, are ubiquitous indoors.

It is noteworthy that most of the materials that emit formaldehyde significantly (e.g., a variety of pressed wood products) can also emit a wide range of organic compounds. Controlling the indoor concentrations of VOCs may be a difficult matter because these agents are often emitted from the structure of the building, and methods of sealing in or removing their emissions in situ are not well developed. Similarly, removing the structural materials themselves is usually difficult.

Since, in theory, source control offers the best means of eliminating or greatly reducing exposure, it should be considered first. With regard to formaldehyde, a primary means of source control is to avoid the use of products with high formaldehyde emission rates. Products having the strongest emissions of formaldehyde include those bonded with urea–formaldehyde resins, e.g., hardwood plywood paneling, particleboard, medium-density fiberboard, and urea–formaldehyde foam insulation (UFFI). Substitutes for these products are available and should be considered (9). Because high formaldehyde levels are associated with the use of particleboard as subflooring, it is advisable to avoid this use. It should be noted, however, that since the late 1970s in North America and Europe, there has been a significant reduction in formaldehyde emissions from urea–formaldehyde-based wood products.

Interior furnishings such as tables, sofas, and cabinets often incorporate pressed-wood products as major components, leading to the same potential for emission of formaldehyde and other organics as associated with the building structure. In general, the same principles for control apply, except that removal of the source material, perhaps only during the period with large emission rates, is typically a more practical option. Since the home furnishings likely to be the most significant sources of formaldehyde are cabinets and furniture made of pressed-wood products, another means of control rests on the restricted use of high-formaldehyde-emitting furnishings. A single piece of furniture made of hardwood plywood, medium-density fiberboard, or particleboard may have a negligible effect on indoor air quality in a large, well-ventilated room. In contrast, the effect of using many pieces of formaldehyde-emitting furniture in a small, poorly ventilated bedroom is significant.

Because it is often impractical or impossible to remove the source of formaldehyde emissions, another approach would depend on isolating the source through chemical or physical measures. This entails the application of a coating material or using a physical barrier to encapsulate the emitting surface. A variety of surface coatings have been used. A single application of Valspar formaldehyde sealant reduced formaldehyde levels 78–87%; two applications of nitrocellulase-based varnish reduced formaldehyde levels by 70%. Valspar is no longer commercially available, and the use of nitrocellulase-based varnishes is limited by their high emissions of volatile vehicle materials (9). A variety of potential formaldehyde permeation barriers have been used. Vinyl linoleum and polyethylene have proved effective, reducing formaldehyde emissions by 90% and 80%, respectively. This subject has been reviewed in detail by Godish (9).

Ammonia fumigation has been used to reduce formaldehyde levels. Thus far this measure appears to be the most effective and inexpensive retrofit control measure available for mobile homes (11). The odious nature of such treatment, however, restricts its use. Another method developed to hasten formaldehyde emission rates and thereby more quickly improve the air quality of new commercial buildings involves elevating indoor temperatures prior to occupancy. This "baking-out" process has had limited use, apparently with some success (8).

Climate control, by reducing indoor temperature and relative humidity, can effectively reduce indoor formaldehyde levels (9). Reducing temperature from 30° to 20°C reduced formaldehyde levels by 70%. A 40% reduction was noted when the relative humidity levels were reduced from 70% to 30%. Temperature reductions may provide a means of reducing both formaldehyde levels and energy costs (10). Aging of the furnishing and the materials is another factor that significantly reduces formaldehyde and other organic emissions from building materials and furnishings. Typically, formaldehyde emissions decrease significantly during the first 6 to 12 months after their manufacture (9). This decay can result in major decreases in formaldehyde levels. A control strategy may thereby focus on the period during which emission rates are high.

As with formaldehyde, the best means of controlling exposure to total VOCs is to avoid or reduce emission sources. Sources having high emission rates include adhesive and filler products such as ethylene vinyl acetate and polyvinyl acetate, vinyl, plastic, and rubber-type floor coverings, varnishes, and oil-based paints (9). Certain substances may liberate specific VOCs that are of particular concern. For example, vinyl floor and wall covering may emit residual monomers of vinyl chloride and plasticizers such as diisobutyl phthalate and butyl benzyl phthalate (22). It is of interest that measurements reveal that it may be erroneous to assume that water-based products are lower in VOC emissions than are solvent-based products (7). The decay rates for VOCs are typically more rapid than that noted with formaldehyde. The indoor concentration of VOCs generally decreases markedly or completely within 6 months or less (9).

In the case of formaldehyde, and perhaps other organic compounds, ventilating or cleaning the air to obtain lower concentrations alters the equilibrium between the source material and the air and effects a higher emission rate. As a result, the airborne concentration is not lowered as much as might otherwise be expected. Thus, although the use of mechanical ventilation with an air-to-air heat exchanger lowers the concentration of VOCs to some degree, this measure may not be as effective as for other types of pollutants. Nonetheless, short of avoiding or removing source materials, ventilation or air cleaning offers the main opportunity for lowering indoor concentrations of semivolatile and volatile compounds. It is noteworthy that formaldehyde is the only VOC for which an easy measurement method is available, at least at levels that are often encountered in ordinary nonindustrial environments. An inexpensive method is needed to measure total VOCs.

Apart from combustion emissions and environmental tobacco smoke, already discussed, home and consumer products can contribute significantly to indoor concentrations of semivolatile and volatile organic compounds. Diverse household chemicals, frequently liquid, are used for cleaning, painting or stripping, pest control, hobbies, and other purposes. Many of these products contain substances that are known to be potential health hazards. These agents often carry warning labels indicating that they must be used only under well-ventilated conditions. Nonetheless, even with good ventilation, the concentrations encountered can be very high. The presence of these substances is often quite obvious, from smell alone, to a person who walks into a room in which the substance is being used.

A pitfall to be avoided when using household chemicals is to assume that there is no hazard if there is no smell. A substance of concern may not have a significant odor, and, even if it does, the olfactory system very rapidly accommodates. This accounts for the fact that after only a short period of exposure, one may no longer be aware of an odor that would be quite apparent to someone entering the room afresh.

Methods for reducing exposure to VOCs in household chemicals are straightforward: careful selection of such products; avoiding them where possible; limiting the frequency and period of exposure; and providing substantial ventilation, via open windows, fans, or other means, during and often after the period of use. Specifically, the following measures are encouraged: pesticide use indoors should be avoided as much as possible; moth repellants and room air fresheners such as paradichlorobenzene should be avoided; vessels containing such agents as paints, solvents, and other gasoline-related aromatics should be carefully stored, preferably in an external shed; clothing should be aired out after its return from the dry cleaners; and cleaning agents, especially those containing VOCs, should be used only as necessary and with sufficient ventilation.

Equipment used at work, or increasingly in the home, is another pollution source. Devices such as photocopiers, typewriters, or computer output terminals may have a range of specific emissions, including VOCs, associated with their presence. Control can be accomplished by changing their use or location or, as usual, by appropriate ventilation and possible air-cleaning measures. Practical methods of controlling VOCs emphasize ventilation or special air-cleaning systems. In the latter case, air-cleaning devices that use sorbents are most effective in removing volatile organic compounds. Small, inexpensive devices, generally without sorbents, are likely to be inefficient and to have so low an air flow rate as to be ineffective for practical purposes (34).

Asbestos

Asbestos is unique in that the only satisfactory method of controlling exposure to this agent is at its source. However, because asbestos fibers are not released through ordinary use and maintenance, it is unlikely that asbestos-containing materials in the home pose significant exposure problems. There is therefore no need to remove asbestos-containing floor tiles, decorative ceilings, or insulation on furnace ducts or pipes if these are in good condition. Undamaged materials should not be disturbed, damaged, or touched. Periodic inspection is advised. In cases where difficulties are thought to exist, it is important for the occupants to be aware of the various control options (27,31). If a question exists about the inhalation of asbestos dust, if asbestos-containing materials are badly deteriorated, or if remodeling is planned, it is exceedingly important that a professional be consulted. A list of professionals trained in handling asbestos-containing materials can be obtained from state or county health departments or from the local American Industrial Hygiene Association.

Table 28-6 presents the advantages and disadvantages of asbestos control measures available to the homeowner (1). It is important for homeowners to be aware that the improper removal of asbestos can result in a badly contaminated dwelling. Thus, whenever possible, it is best to seal, rewrap, paint, or otherwise encapsulate asbestos-containing materials. When it becomes necessary to remove asbestos or take other actions, it is exceedingly important that the contractors chosen to do the work present both a license to do this type of work and evidence of having taken an EPA-approved course in asbestos abatement (1,27).

Lead

Lead paint represents a primary source of indoor lead. As noted previously, many houses built prior to 1940 and some built between 1940 and 1960 used lead paint. It is therefore wise for occupants living in such structures to determine if lead paint is present. Health departments may offer some help in locating laboratories that test for lead in paint.

Lead-based paint in good condition and unlikely to be eaten by children should not be disturbed. If the paint is cracked or peeling, it should be considered an immediate lead hazard for children. It should be abated whenever possible. This includes encapsulating, replacing, or removing the lead-based paint (2). At times, it may also be possible to replace painted surfaces. Under no circumstances should lead paint be removed by scraping, sanding, or burning. Such techniques result in very high indoor lead levels. Because these steps are often necessary prior to painting, repainting areas covered with lead-based paint is not advised. Consideration should be given to having lead-painted woodwork, such as doors and molding, taken out for off-site lead removal. If the removal of lead-based paint in situ is the only option, then only well-trained protected workers involved in the removal process should remain in the house. A thorough and proper clean-up is essential, as ordinary household measures are ineffective in removing the lead dust produced by sanding and scraping. Moreover, in ordinary vacuum cleaners, lead dust particles pass through the filtering system. The topic of lead abatement has been reviewed (2).

Radon and Its Decay Products

It is now understood that small differences in air pressure between indoors and outdoors permit radon-bearing air from the underlying soil to enter structures. The most effective means of reducing the entry of radon is therefore to lower the air pressure under the building. This will reverse the pressure gradient that draws the gas from the soil into the house. It can be done by driving one or more pipes through the basement floor and then using small fans to exhaust air from the underlying soil to the outdoors. As this measure lowers the air pressure in the soil near the basement, radon is no longer sucked into the house (15–17,20,32). Radon entering through a sump system can be removed by a similar approach: cover the sump, connect a pipe to it, and pull air outdoors with a small fan. If radon enters through a crawl space, a homeowner can remove it by actively ventilating the space (16,17). Measures have also been proposed for radon reduction in new construction (30).

TABLE 28-6.   Advantages and Disadvantages of Control Options for Asbestos[a]

Control	Advantages	Disadvantages
Leave in place, but control activities that might release fibers	No immediate cost No risk of contamination by improper removal or repair	Material remains in place with some risk of future damage or deterioration Cost of removal will be faced later by current or future owner
Encapsulate, enclose, or otherwise seal asbestos	Higher degree of safety from inadvertent release Can usually be done for pipe covering at reasonable cost with low risk of contamination (if current damage is not great)	Moderate cost Some risk of contamination during encapsulation work Cost of future removal still remains Encapsulated material may become difficult to remove later
Removal	Building is free of asbestos	Most costly Greatest risk of contamination from improper work Need to replace material removed

[a]From American Thoracic Society (2).

An alternative control measure involves reducing the openings in the understructure by which radon enters the house. Unfortunately, sealing the understructure of a house does not protect adequately against a pressure-driven flow of radon. Even if 90% of the entry points are sealed, the amount of radon drawn into the house remains almost unchanged. Moreover, as the house settles, seals can deteriorate, and new entry points can appear (16,17).

Increased ventilation also proves to be a relatively impractical remedy for most radon problems. By illustration, assume a house with five times (740 Bq/m^3 or 20 pCi/L) the EPA-recommended guideline of radon and an ordinary infiltration rate of one air change per hour and a half. Any attempt to lower the concentration of radon fivefold simply by increasing the ventilation rate would cause great discomfort. Five times as much air flowing through the house not only would make the house drafty but would double or triple the heating bills (16). The only way to avoid this would be to use a heat exchanger that recovers heat from the outgoing air. Indoor radon, its causes, and control strategies are discussed in several references (15,20).

Several measuring devices are available to determine the level of indoor radon. The two most commonly used are the charcoal canister and the α-track detector. Both of these devices are exposed to the air within the house for a specified period. A short-term measurement, for less than 1 week, has been recommended by the EPA for screening for high radon concentrations. These devices are sent to a laboratory for analysis, and measured concentrations of radon gas are reported as becquerels per cubic meter (Bq/m^3) or picocuries per liter (pCi/L)— 1 Bq equals 27 pCi. By this means an occupant can determine, without excessive cost, whether or not

a potential radon problem exists (29). Most scientists, however, recommend long-term measurements because short-term measurements are unreliable indicators of radon exposure over a long period of time.

There are no clear guidelines for testing. Nonetheless, average radon concentrations above 148–370 Bq/m^3 (4–10 pCi/L) in homes in the vicinity indicate that testing should be performed. Such information can often be obtained from local health agencies. At present, no one knows which homes are likely to have highly elevated radon levels, and no program has been instituted to systematically identify high-radon areas. In 1988, the EPA issued an advisory urging that most houses in the United States be tested for radon (25). There is significant dissent among some members of the scientific community on this point (25).

Although it is clear that very high levels of radon must be quickly reduced, interpreting the health risks associated with lower levels of indoor radon is difficult, and no consensus exists (25). The EPA and other groups have provided guidelines (17,29): the EPA has recommended 148 Bq/m^3 (4 pCi/L) as a guideline for the annual average concentrations in homes. The following actions are recommended by the EPA: with a screening measurement greater than about 7400 Bq/m^3 (200 pCi/L), a follow-up measurement of no more than 1 week should be performed as soon as possible, and steps taken immediately to reduce radon levels; with a screening measurement of about 740–7400 Bq/m^3 (20–200 pCi/L), a follow-up measurement for no more than 3 months should be performed; with a screening measurement of about 148–740 Bq/m^3 (4 pCi/L to about 20 pCi/L), a follow-up measurement for 1 year or no more than 1 week during each of the four seasons should be performed; with a screening measurement of less than about 148 Bq/m^3 (4 pCi/L), follow-up measurements are not suggested (29).

Biogenic Particles

Biological contaminants are so diverse that generalization is difficult. Moreover, as with combustion products, certain of these agents may, in part, arise from outdoor sources (e.g., pollen and mold). As noted, indoor sources of biogenic particles include dust mites, fungi, and cat and dog saliva and dander. Both allergy and asthma have been linked with indoor exposure to biogenic particles. Although the risk levels for most indoor allergens have not been defined, it is generally agreed that the risk of sensitization increases as the level of exposure increases (1).

As with other agents discussed above, source control is of the greatest importance. Since one of the major limiting factors in both mite and mold survival and growth is the availability of moisture, the relative humidity should be less than 50% or as low as possible. Local sources of excess moisture in kitchens and bathrooms should be controlled by fans vented to the outdoors. Water-damaged carpets should either be removed or cleaned and dried. Home humidification devices, particularly spray humidifiers, are a source of contamination with biogenic parti-cles. General measures for mite control and mold abatement are shown in Tables 28-7 and 28-8 (1).

Although ventilation is still generally applicable as a means of control for biogenic particles of indoor origin, the same may not be true of air cleaning. In particular, there is some possibility that bacteria collected from the air may thrive in and later escape from certain types of air-handling or -cleaning systems. Moreover, dust mite antigen appears to be airborne for a relatively short time, primarily with bed-making and cleaning activities. It is not effectively removed by air-cleaning devices. Room air-cleaning devices, therefore, may be an adjunct to other more primary methods of reducing antigen production (1). It is noteworthy that in the face of high concentrations of airborne particles, such as would arise from a cat, residential air-cleaning devices can quickly become ineffective.

Finally, and perhaps most important, the amount of biological material of indoor origin can be reduced substantially by rather ordinary household functions, including routine vacuuming and airing of a home. In some cases, the levels can even be reduced by modifying the form of heating or by incorporating an improved filter system. And, as is obvious, mere cleaning or improved hygienic practices can affect the availability of bacteria and other viable particles.

TABLE 28-7.   Mite Control Measures[a]

Proved actions	Rationale or effect
House	
Weekly vacuum cleaning of carpets and upholstered furniture	Removes surface dust and fecal pellets but not live mites
Decrease absolute humidity below 7 g/kg or relative humidity <50% at 22° C	Controls mite growth (also effective for molds)
If possible, remove and do not install any fixed (wall-to-wall) carpet over cement slab	Mites grow in carpets with high humidity
Bedroom	
Cover mattress and pillows with plastic zippered covers	Isolates mites and prevents rapid reinfestation of bedding
Regular (every 1 to 2 weeks) washing of bedding, including pillows and mattress pads at ≥55° C	Kills mites—removes allergen. Bedding must be suitable for hot washing
Regular hot washing (every 1 to 2 weeks) of soft toys	Kills mites—removes allergen
Remove carpets	Reduces mite habitat and allows rapid drying of flooring
Removing curtains, toys, and books	May reduce accumulation of dust in a room, and thus reduce airborne levels
Unproved methods	
Daily vacuum cleaning	Vacuum cleaning increases airborne allergen; little or no effect on living mites
Washing in cool cycles, dry cleaning, and most insecticides	Live mites are not killed by these procedures
Methods under experimental study	
Acaricides: solidified benzoic acid esters, pirimiphos methyl, liquid nitrogen	Kills mites in carpets, furniture, or bedding; does not denature allergens
Tannic acid	Denatures mite antigen; no effect on mite numbers

[a]From American Thoracic Society (1).

TABLE 28-8. Mold Abatement in Domestic Interiors[a]

Problem	Solution
Basements are usually contaminated	Prevent intrusion of basement air into living space.
	Clean basement; use 10% chlorine bleach on smooth surface; do not use carpeting on damp basement floors
	Ventilate basement and dehumidify
Every uncorrected moisture incursion causes mold contamination	Correct situation causing water incursion
	Remove all water-damaged soft material
	Disinfect hard surfaces with 10% chlorine bleach
Water-containing appliances are usually contaminated with microorganisms	Do not use water-spray humidifying devices in areas with asthmatics or immunocompromised persons
	Clean humidifiers/vaporizers with chlorine bleach before each use
Elevated relative humidity is associated with surface mold growth	Keep relative humidity below 50%
	Insulate well to prevent cold surfaces
	Clean moldy surfaces with 10% chlorine bleach
Outdoor fungus spores and pollen can cause symptoms	Prevent intrusion of the outdoor aerosol with air conditioning and closed windows

[a]From American Thoracic Society (1).

SUMMARY

Control of pollutants at their source is the most effective means of promoting indoor air quality. Increasing ventilation, often simply by opening windows, is the next consideration. Finally, air cleaning is appropriate to circumstances where other means fail and where effective and affordable cleaning devices are available. It is noteworthy that changing behavior is often one of the most effective means of reducing pollution at its source, e.g., environmental tobacco smoke. The potential for reducing indoor air pollutant levels depends substantially on the pollutant class, the particular circumstances, and the control methods available. Moreover, depending on the situation, the amount of exposure reduction required may be large, modest, or undetermined.

This chapter has focused on the improvement of indoor air quality, especially in relation to excessive pollutant concentrations. An alternative view might consider the de novo creation of an indoor environment with low pollutant levels. At present, this is ordinarily only a secondary consideration. However, as more and more information becomes available, it becomes increasingly straightforward to lower the indoor concentrations of pollutants whose sources are well understood. Thus, by selection of building materials, furnishings, and appliances and by specific attention to building features that affect either pollutants in general or such specific pollutants as radon, it becomes increasingly possible, and indeed realistic, to construct and furnish buildings that carry a low pollutant load.

REFERENCES

1. American Thoracic Society: Environmental controls and lung disease. Am Rev Respir Dis 142:915, 1990.
2. Centers for Disease Control: Preventing Lead Poisoning in Young Children, A Statement by the Centers for Disease Control, CDC, Atlanta, 1991.
3. Committee on Passive Smoking, National Research Council: Environmental Tobacco Smoke: Measuring Exposures and Assessing Health Effects. National Academy Press, Washington, 1986.
4. Consumer Reports: Air cleaners: Some really did clear the air of smoke and dust, but ones that worked aren't cheap. Consumer Rep 50:7, 1985.
5. Electric Power Research Institute: Manual on Indoor Air Quality. Prepared by Lawrence Berkeley Laboratory, Berkeley, CA, for the Energy Management and Utilization Division, Electric Power Research Institute, Palo Alto, CA, 1984.
6. Fisk WJ, Turiel I: Residential air-to-air exchangers: Performance, energy savings, and economics. Energy Buildings 5:197, 1983.
7. Girman JR, Hodgson AT, Newton A, et al: Emissions of volatile organic compounds from adhesives with indoor applications. In: Proceedings of the Third International Conference on Indoor Air Quality and Climate. Vol. 4, p 271, Swedish Council for Building Research, Stockholm, 1984.
8. Girman J, Alevantis L, Kullasingam G, et al: Bake-out of an office building. In: Indoor Air '87: Proceedings of the 4th International Conference on Indoor Air Quality and Climate, p. 22, Seifert B, Esdorn H, Fischer M, et al., eds., Institute for Water, Soil and Water Hygiene, Berlin, 1987.
9. Godish T: Indoor Air Pollution Control, Lewis Publishers, Chelsea, Michigan, 1989.
10. Godish T, Rouch J: Mitigation of residential formaldehyde contamination by indoor climate control. Am Ind Hyg Assoc J 47:729, 1986.
11. Jewell RA: Reducing Formaldehyde Levels in Mobile Homes Using 29% Aqueous Ammonia Treatment or Heat Exchanges, Weyerhauser Corp., Tacoma WA, 1984.
12. Krause C, Mailahn W, Nagel R, et al: Occurrence of volatile organic compounds in the air of 500 homes in the Federal Republic of Germany. In: Indoor Air '87:

Proceedings of the 4th International Conference on Indoor Air Quality and Climate, p 102, Seifert B, Esdorn H, Fischer M, et al. (eds.), Institute for Water, Soil and Water Hygiene, Berlin, 1987.

13. Leaderer BP: Air pollutant emissions from kerosene space heaters. Science 218:1113, 1982.

14. Mahajan BM: A method for measuring the effectiveness of gaseous contaminant removal filters, National Institute of Standards and Technology, US Department of Commerce, Gaithersburg, MD, 1989.

15. National Council on Radiation Protection and Measurement: Control of Radon in Houses, NCRP Report #103, National Council on Radiation Protection and Measurements, Bethesda, 1989.

16. Nero AV Jr: The indoor radon story. Technol Rev 89:28, 1986.

17. Nero AV Jr: Elements of a strategy for control of indoor radon. In: Radon and Its Decay Products in Indoor Air, p 459, Nazaroff WW, Nero AV Jr. (eds.), John Wiley & Sons, New York, 1988.

18. Nero AV, Nazaroff WW: Characterising the source of radon indoors. Radiat Prot Dos 7:23, 1984.

19. Nero AV, Berk JV, Boegel ML, et al: Radon concentrations and infiltration rates measured in conventional and energy-efficient houses. Health Phys 45:401, 1983.

20. Nero AV, Gadgil AJ, Nazaroff WW, et al: Indoor Radon and Decay Products: Concentrations, Causes, and Control Strategies, DOE/ER-048OP, US Department of Energy, Washington, 1990.

21. Offerman FJ, Sextro RG, Fisk WJ, et al: Control of respirable particles in indoor air with portable air cleaners. Atmos Environ 19:1761, 1985.

22. Rittfeldt L, Sandberg M: Indoor air pollutants due to vinyl floor tiles. In: Proceedings of the Third International Conference on Indoor Air Quality and Climate, Vol. 3, p 297, Swedish Council for Building Research, Stockholm, 1984.

23. Samet JM, Marbury MC, Spengler JD: Health effects and sources of indoor air pollution. Part I. Am Rev Respir Dis 136:1486, 1987.

24. Samet JM, Marbury MC, Spengler JD: Health effects and sources of indoor air pollution. Part II. Am Rev Respir Dis 137:221, 1988.

25. Samet JM, Nero AV Jr: Indoor Radon and Lung Cancer, N Engl J Med 320:591, 1989.

26. Traynor GW, Allen JR, Apte MG, et al: Pollutant emissions from portable kerosene-space heaters. Environ Sci Technol 17:369, 1983.

27. US Consumer Product Safety Commission, US Environmental Protection Agency: Asbestos in the Home, US Government Printing Office, Washington, 1982.

28. US Department of Health and Human Services, Public Health Service, Office on Smoking and Health: The Health Consequences of Involuntary Smoking. A Report of the Surgeon General, DHHS (CDC) 87-8398, US Government Printing Office, Washington, 1986.

29. US Environmental Protection Agency: A Citizen's Guide to Radon—What It Is and What to Do about It, OPA 86-004, USEPA, Washington, 1986.

30. US Environmental Protection Agency: Radon Reduction in New Construction, An Interim Guide, OPA-87-009, USEPA, Washington, 1987.

31. US Environmental Protection Agency: The Inside Story—A Guide to Indoor Air Quality, EPA/400/1-88/004, USEPA, Washington, 1988.

32. US Environmental Protection Agency: Radon Reduction Methods—A Homeowner's Guide, 3rd ed., USEPA, Washington, 1989.

33. US Environmental Protection Agency: Indoor Air Facts No. 3: Ventilation and Air Quality in Offices, 20A-4402, USEPA, Washington, 1990.

34. US Environmental Protection Agency: Residential Air-Cleaning Devices—A Summary of Available Information, EPA 400/1-90-002, USEPA, Washington, 1990.

35. Wadden RA, Scheff PA: Indoor Air Pollution, John Wiley & Sons, New York, 1983.

36. Wallace LA: Total exposure assessment methodology (TEAM) study: Summary and analysis, Vol 1, US Environmental Protection Agency, Washington, 1987.

RECOMMENDED READINGS

American Thoracic Society: Environmental controls and lung disease. Am Rev Respir Dis 142:915, 1990.

Godish T: Indoor Air Pollution Control, Lewis Publishers, Boca Raton, 1989.

Nero AV Jr, Gadgil AJ, Nazaroff WW, et al: Indoor Radon and Decay Products: Concentrations, Causes, and Control Strategies, DOE/ER-048OP, US Department of Energy, Washington, 1990.

US Consumer Product Safety Commission, US Environmental Protection Agency: Asbestos in the Home, US Government Printing Office, Washington, 1982.

US Environmental Protection Agency: The Inside Story—A Guide to Indoor Air Quality, EPA/400/1-88/004, USEPA, Washington, 1988.

US Environmental Protection Agency: Radon Reduction Methods—A Homeowner's Guide, 3rd ed., USEPA, Washington, 1989

29. PERSONAL METHODS OF CONTROLLING EXPOSURE TO CHEMICAL CONTAMINANTS IN FOOD

Sushma Palmer and Kulbir S. Bakshi

INTRODUCTION

Any attempt to advise individuals on steps to reduce exposure to environmental pollutants in food is hampered by a dearth of applicable data and by the variety of treatments that may be required for removing different chemical substances from the same food. The reduction of overall exposure is also complicated by the finding that in some cases, the means employed to minimize exposure to one compound may inadvertently increase exposure to another.

This chapter focuses primarily on those categories of compounds that are discussed in Chapter 3, which deals with contaminants in food, i.e., polycyclic aromatic hydrocarbons (PAHs), pesticide residues, toxic metals, and polychlorinated biphenyls (PCBs). Food-packaging materials are not discussed. One reason is lack of reliable data about their presence in specific categories of foods. Another is that common sense would dictate that the most effective means of reducing exposure is to minimize the use of plastic containers and plastic films and to select fewer foods packaged in material containing acrylonitrile or polyvinyl chloride (see Chapter 3).

Principles and Practice of Environmental Medicine, edited by Alyce Bezman Tarcher. Plenum Medical Book Company, New York, 1992.

The methods of reducing exposure suggested below are general and exploratory. Their success cannot be guaranteed because their effectiveness depends too much on factors requiring more study or better documentation.

There are four stages at which exposure to environmental pollutants may be reduced: during the selection of foods, during processing and storage, during preparation prior to cooking, and during cooking.

SELECTION OF FOODS

Although information may be difficult to obtain, knowledge of the source and conditions under which food (particularly fresh produce and seafood) is grown and brought to market will help in the selection of food less likely to contain pollutants (28). The following are some of the conditions affecting the content of PAHs, pesticides, toxic metals, and PCBs.

Polycyclic Aromatic Hydrocarbons

Vegetables and fruit cultivated in heavily industrialized areas are likely to have a high PAH content. Air pollution particulates, which contain significant amounts of pyrolytically generated PAHs, can contaminate the surface of growing fruits, vegetables, and grain. Only a small proportion of this PAH may be removed by washing, probably because of its incorporation into the waxes on the leaf surface or penetration into the plant tissues (6). Howard and

549

Fazio (10) have reviewed studies in Germany indicating a strong correlation between air pollution and the benzo[a]pyrene (BaP) content of grain and vegetables (BaP constitutes 1–20% of the total carcinogenic PAHs in the environment). These investigators also noted that the PAH content of produce grown in heavily industrialized areas may be ten times greater than that of produce grown in less industrialized areas. Similarly, seafood from petroleum-contaminated waters, especially oysters, clams, and mussels, may have a high PAH content. In one study, maintenance of contaminated shellfish in clean water for 24 to 52 days was sufficient to cleanse the tissues of clams and oysters of detectable PAHs, and 2 weeks was sufficient for mussels. However, short depuration periods of 1 to 3 days, commonly used to eliminate bacterial contamination from edible shellfish before marketing, are likely to have little effect on lowering the BaP content of shellfish (10).

Pesticides

In recent decades there has been considerable focus on the possible merits of organic farming, primarily with the intent of reducing exposure to pesticides and other environmental pollutants. The assessment of the potential advantages of organically grown foods is limited by the difficulty in clearly distinguishing between organically and conventionally grown foods, by the problem of unintentional pesticide contamination from aerial spraying of pesticides, and by the absence of regular monitoring of the pesticide content of organic foods (12). Clearly, more research is needed before any conclusion can be reached about pesticide residues in organic foods. Thorough washing or peeling, however, is likely to remove considerable pesticide residue from the surface of plants.

Toxic Metals

The application of municipal sludge and waste water plant sewage sludge to agricultural land is known to increase the content of certain heavy metals, especially cadmium and possibly lead, in the soil (4). The limited translocation of most metals prevents their reaching excessive foliar levels in crops and thus prevents phytotoxicity. Cadmium, however, appears to be an exception (1). Aquatic food species including fish, crabs, oysters, and shrimp and organ meats such as liver, kidneys, and pancreas tend to bioconcentrate cadmium. Similarly, vegetables grown in land after the application of municipal sewage sludge may contain excessive cadmium. However, contrary to expectations, data from a study conducted by the Loma Linda University of California concerning dietary patterns of Seventh-Day Adventists indicated that the lacto-ovo-vegetarian diet is no higher in cadmium than the average diet. In this study, substitution of potatoes for legumes and fruits increased the average cadmium intake by about 13 μg/day, whereas replacing potatoes with fruit could decrease cadmium intake by 8 μg/day (17).

Although the use of municipal sludge may not significantly affect the lead content of produce, fruits and vegetables grown in gardens near a street with heavy traffic may have a higher lead content (8). Hemphill et al. (8), Motto et al. (19), and Preer et al. (22) have reported that the lead content of garden vegetables (e.g., lettuce) grown near heavy traffic or industrialized areas is higher than that of those grown in areas removed from traffic. No consistent correlation was found between the cadmium content of vegetables and proximity to traffic.

Seafood from both fresh and marine waters contains mercury, and seafood derived from polluted waters is the only regular source of methyl mercury in the diet. In the United States, health warnings by numerous states are indicative of the extent of concern about exposure to methyl mercury in fish, especially halibut, red snapper, rockfish, shrimp, and larger marine fish, e.g., swordfish and tuna (21).

Efforts to reduce personal exposure to methyl mercury may primarily consist of determining the source of the seafood. A 1977 listing of the status of individual state and commercial fisheries is provided by the National Academy of Sciences (21). Distribution of methyl mercury evenly throughout the tissues precludes the effectiveness of selective trimming or other home preparation techniques to reduce the intake of methyl mercury.

Polychlorinated Biphenyls

As pointed out in Chapter 3, freshwater fish from contaminated lakes and streams are the predominant source of dietary exposure to PCBs. In the Wisconsin area, for example, larger and more mature lake trout and salmon (22 to 30 inches long) may contain up to five times the amount of PCBs as fish that are less than 22 inches long. Carp and catfish from certain lakes in Wisconsin may also be contaminated with PCBs (14). Table 29-1 provides a partial list of lakes and rivers in the United States where at least one sample of seafood has been found to have PCB residues greater than 5 ppm (2).

As noted, toxic chemicals discharged into fresh and marine waters can accumulate in fish that, when eaten, can pose a health hazard. In the United States, when states find levels of toxic substances in fish that exceed established safety standards, fishing advisories or bans are issued. Although there is a great deal of variability in the criteria and monitoring programs used by the various states, in 1988 a

TABLE 29-1.   Areas Where at Least One Sample with High PCB Residue Levels (>5 ppm) Has Been Reported in the Listed Species[a]

Species	Location
Striped bass	Hudson River, NJ
Chub	Lake Michigan
Carp	Mississippi River, MN; Lake Onandaga, NY
Chain pickerel, alewife	Hudson River
Coho salmon	Lake Michigan, Lake Ontario, Hudson River
Chinook salmon	Lake Michigan, Lake Ontario, Hudson River
Steelhead trout	Lake Michigan, Lake Ontario
Lake trout	Lake Michigan, Lake Ontario, Lake George, NY
Smallmouth bass	Lake Onandaga, Genessee River, NY, Hudson River, Mohawk River, St. Lawrence River
White perch	Lake Onandaga, Hudson River
Alewife	Hudson River
White sucker	Hudson River, Mohawk River
Walleye	Hudson River, Mohawk River, Black River, NY
Largemouth bass	Hudson River, Mohawk River
Yellow perch	Hudson River
American eel, crabs, sturgeon	Hudson River
Rock bass, catfish	Hudson River
Bluefish	Long Island Sound (muscle from one large oil fish contained 8 ppm)

[a]The Hudson River above Fort Edward, NY, is not contaminated with PCBs, and the residue levels in fish are quite low. From Cordle et al. (2).

total of 135 advisories or bans were reported by 21 states (26). The pollutants most commonly cited in the advisories or bans included PCBs, chlordane, mercury, dioxin, and DDT (26) (Fig. 29-1). Industrial discharges, hazardous waste sites, agricultural activities, spills, and atmospheric deposition account for these pollutants.

METHODS OF PROCESSING AND STORAGE

The method of processing and storage can have a substantial impact on the dietary levels of environmental contaminants (27).

Polycyclic Aromatic Hydrocarbons

Fresh vertebrate fish are not generally found to have detectable levels of PAHs. Canned fish, however, especially if processed with vegetable oil, may be contaminated, probably because of the vegetable oil itself (6). The PAH content of vegetable oils varies with the technological treatment, the heating process, usage of solvents, and the process of refining and oxidation. There is no consensus regarding the major sources of contamination. In one study, heating destroyed about 70% of PAHs in edible vegetable oils (10).

Smoking of foods is associated with increasing the PAH content of foods. However, the amount of BaP appears to vary with the method of smoking. In general, commercially smoked foods are likely to

have a lower BaP content than home-smoked foods. For example, in one study 107 µg/kg of BaP was measured in meat hung over a stove compared to 1 µg/kg of BaP in meat or fish smoked commercially. A large percentage (60–70%) of BaP resides in the superficial tissues. The use of protective coverings such as a cotton fabric or cellophane or cellulose casing (for smoked bologna or bacon) is therefore likely to significantly reduce the BaP content. Furthermore, products smoked with liquid smoke solutions (a condensate produced from wood smoke that, being cleansed, is thought to contain smaller amounts of PAHs) are likely to contain substantially less BaP—but not necessarily other PAHs—than those smoked with traditional wood smoke (10). Unfortunately, food labels in the United States do not generally provide information on the method of smoking.

Pesticide Residues

In Germany, Stobwasser et al. (24) conducted a series of long-term storage studies with pesticide-treated fresh and processed fruits and vegetables. They demonstrated a substantial reduction in pesticide residues in many foods stored at temperatures above 0°C and suggested that higher temperatures may accelerate the loss of pesticide residues. Conversely, during storage at low temperatures, pesticide residues may remain constant for long periods. The exception may be malathion residues, which, in one series of experiments by the National Canners

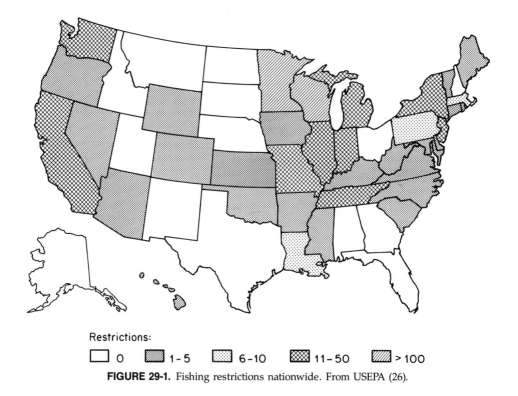

Restrictions:

☐ 0   ▨ 1–5   ▩ 6–10   ▨ 11–50   ▨ >100

FIGURE 29-1. Fishing restrictions nationwide. From USEPA (26).

Association Research Foundation (20) decreased during storage of raw products at low temperatures.

Canned produce, with some exceptions, has been reported to contain considerably lower levels of pesticide residues. Pressure cooking and cooking or blanching may also lower pesticide residues, especially when the cooking temperature is increased. In the studies of Stobwasser et al. (24), processing of fruits into juices considerably reduced pesticide residues, probably because most of the residue remained in the peels.

Stobwasser et al. (24) reported that production of oils (from olives or peppermint) tended to concentrate the lipid-soluble chlorinated pesticide residues. Special refining of oils, however, tended to eliminate the residue, possibly because of dehalogenation. Liska and Stadelman (15) have reviewed a series of experiments suggesting that some reduction in residues of organochlorine pesticides takes place during the processing of milk. For example, drastic heat treatment of milk, such as in the manufacture of dried whole milk, may reduce the levels of chlorinated pesticides. In one study, the preparation of evaporated milk led to a greater than 50% reduction in residues of dieldrin, about 82% in lindane and DDT, and a 40% to 50% reduction in dieldrin. In comparison, there was only a 10% to 20% reduction

in the same residues during the preparation of dried whole milk (25). In the separation of milk from cream, these residues tend to concentrate mainly in the cream. Therefore, an effective way to reduce exposure would be to use low-fat or skim-milk products more frequently. Similarly, egg yolks rather than the whites tend to contain most of the organochlorine compounds. Organophosphates, however, are more evenly distributed in milk and eggs (15).

Toxic Metals

The method of handling, processing, and storing of foods may substantially affect their content of lead. For example, such meats as hamburger and frankfurters, produced by grinding in contact with metal grinders, tend to have a higher lead level than other meats (11).

Canned foods are thought to contribute significantly to exposure to lead in the diet because of the lead used in some cans. Levels of lead in canned produce are frequently higher than in raw fruits and vegetables. They also tend to increase with storage because of leaching of lead from the solder of cans into the food, especially under acidic conditions. Moran (18) compared the lead content of canned pickled foods containing vinegar (such as cucumbers, sauerkraut, mixed pickles, leeks, and mustard greens) with fresh produce or produce pickled or stored in glass jars. They reported that fresh and bottled vinegar produce has lead levels that are well below the FDA's legal limit of 2 ppm compared to 5 to 10 ppm in all foods canned in vinegar. Once opened, foods should not be stored in cans.

The use of glass jars for packaging infant foods has resulted in about 90% reduction in the lead levels in infant foods between 1971 and 1980. Also, a recent trend toward packing foods in seamless two-piece cans or in cans with an electrically welded side seam is expected to lead to further reduction in lead exposure (Fig. 29-2) (3).

In general, storage of foods in glazed pottery, ceramic, or pewter dishes should be avoided. Some glazes contain lead, which can leach out when they come in contact with such acidic foods as citrus juices and tomatoes (7).

PREPARATION PRIOR TO COOKING

Thorough washing with water, selective trimming, peeling, and scraping appear to be effective means to reduce exposure to several environmental pollutants. However, many factors determine their effectiveness, including the chemical nature of the compound and the type of food.

Polycyclic Aromatic Hydrocarbons

On the basis of limited data it appears that only a small proportion of PAHs from contaminated fruits and vegetables may be removed by washing. This is probably because the PAHs penetrate into the tissues of the food or are incorporated into the waxes on leaf surfaces. Peeling fruits and vegetables or removing the outer leaves of such head crops as lettuce and cabbage would tend to reduce their PAH content further (6).

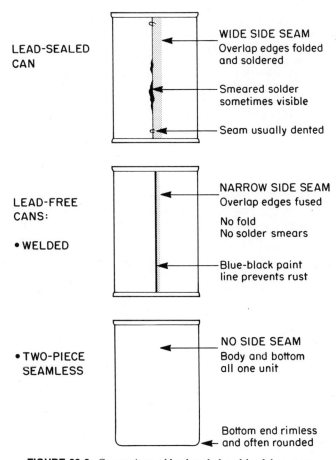

LEAD-SEALED CAN

WIDE SIDE SEAM
Overlap edges folded and soldered

Smeared solder sometimes visible

Seam usually dented

LEAD-FREE CANS:

• WELDED

NARROW SIDE SEAM
Overlap edges fused

No fold
No solder smears

Blue-black paint line prevents rust

• TWO-PIECE SEAMLESS

NO SIDE SEAM
Body and bottom all one unit

Bottom end rimless and often rounded

FIGURE 29-2. Comparison of lead-sealed and lead-free cans.

Pesticides

Washing with water has generally been found to be effective in reducing the residues of many pesticides in fruits and vegetables. The degree of removal, however, ranges from 0 to 79%. It appears to depend on whether the pesticide is on the surface or has penetrated into the interior of the plant, on the solution properties of the pesticide, and on the age of the residue. In a series of experiments conducted in Germany, washing pesticide-treated fresh produce with water for a short period of time resulted in maximal removal of residues. The use of detergents afforded no major additional advantage (24). Nonsystemic pesticides, which tend to remain principally in the peels or in the leaves of produce, may be removed by washing, scraping, and peeling. The scraping process can completely eliminate aldrin and dieldrin residues, both of which are now banned in the United States. In some foods (e.g., carrots), oil-soluble pesticides such as diazinon or parathion are only partially removed by scraping.

The National Canners Association Research Foundation (20) tested the effectiveness of home preparation methods in the removal of residues of DDT, malathion, parathion, and carbaryl applied to field-grown crops of spinach, green beans, tomatoes, potatoes, and broccoli. In the case of DDT, surface residues appeared to be easily removed by washing and, in most cases, were practically eliminated by peeling. Blanching with hot water and cooking led to no major additional removal. For malathion, however, a small but significant amount appeared to penetrate into the plant and was difficult to remove. The peeling of tomatoes removed almost all of the malathion residue. Parathion was the least readily removed by home preparation, only 20% being removed by washing and blanching with water. A large proportion of carbaryl in these experiments was easily removed by washing with water, and an additional amount was removed by peeling, especially in the case of tomatoes (20).

In another series of experiments to study the removal of pesticide residues in fruits and vegetables, washing with water removed 78% to 90% of DDT from tomatoes but only 10% to 15% from apples. However, peeling of apples removed an additional 30% to 40% DDT, suggesting that the wax in apples tends to absorb DDT (15).

Toxic Metals

The washing of fruits and vegetables tends to remove a large percentage of their initial metal burden, and washing with detergent may slightly increase the amount of metal removed. Preer et al. (22) reported that the washing of lettuce grown in industrialized areas resulted in a reduction of 70% in the level of lead and 50% in the level of cadmium.

Polychlorinated Biphenyls

Selective trimming of fish obtained from contaminated lakes and streams appears to be an effective means to lower its PCB content. Since PCBs are fat soluble, they are generally deposited in fatty tissue. According to the Wisconsin Department of Natural Resources (14), a substantial reduction (about 30%) in PCB intake can be achieved by removing the fatty belly flap and the dorsal fat line along the back. Further reduction will occur if the skin and the dark lateral line along the side are also removed. Trimming should be done prior to cooking to prevent the PCBs in the rendered fat from being absorbed by the previously lean tissue. The juices and rendered fat from cooked fish should be discarded (14).

METHODS OF COOKING

Polycyclic Aromatic Hydrocarbons

The method of cooking foods, especially meats, has a significant impact on their PAH content. For example, Lijinsky and Ross (13) observed a significant correlation between the fat content and the BaP content of charcoal-grilled meats and between the proximity of meat to the heat source and its BaP content. The authors theorized that the meat fat dripping onto hot coals is pyrolyzed, giving rise to the BaP, which is then deposited on the surface of the meat. Levels of BaP as high as 50 µg/kg were found in thick T-bone steaks cooked close to the coals for long periods. A significant reduction was noted in similar steaks that were as well cooked but at a greater distance from the coals.

DeSogra and Groll (5) have suggested several means to reduce the BaP content of meats. Short of avoiding barbecuing to decrease dietary exposure to BaP, the authors suggest selecting lean meats or trimming all fat from meats, longer cooking at lower temperatures, and avoiding contact with flames. For a charcoal grill, the temperature can be lowered by sprinkling water on the coals or, in the case of a gas barbecue, by setting it low. Electric or gas heat or a microwave oven may be preferable to a charcoal grill. Broiling should be done under the heat source.

Food may be further protected by wrapping it in aluminum foil or by using a pan and keeping it far away from the coals. Skin from chicken should be discarded prior to cooking to reduce PAH content. In addition, basting with oil or fat should be avoided. The skin can also be removed after cooking, since BaP is mostly on the skin. In the case of fish, however, the skin should be removed before cooking if there is reason to suspect that the fish is contaminated with PCBs. In addition, instead of grilling or broiling, foods may be cooked longer at lower temperature by baking, poaching, or steaming (5).

To minimize PAH formation during the baking or heating of bread, it is advisable to avoid baking at a high temperature or browning or burning the crust. Similarly, coffee roasted at high temperatures may have a substantially higher BaP content than coffee roasted at normal temperatures (10).

Pesticides

Chlorinated pesticides tend to concentrate in the lipid portion of foods. They may be substantially removed during cooking when the fatty tissues are rendered out (e.g., in the fat from meat, chicken, or fish) or concentrated in one fraction of the food (e.g., in cream from milk or in yolks rather than the whites of eggs). Other possible means of destroying pesticide residues are heat processing, irradiation, or bacterial fermentation. These methods are not applicable, however, to home preparation (15). Ritchey et al. (23) achieved only a minor reduction in the level of chlorinated pesticide residues by cooking chicken (baking, frying, or steaming) for 30, 60, and 90 min. The reduction was attributed primarily to leaching of pesticides with fat and water, although some destruction of lindane and heptachlor epoxide occurred as a result of heating.

Toxic Metals

The uptake of lead by foods from lead-contaminated water may be an additional source of dietary exposure to lead. Little et al. (16) observed that lead initially became adsorbed onto the surface of saucepans, especially in an acidic medium. This may be significant if vegetables are cooked in a small amount of water. In Little et al.'s experiments, the amount of lead adsorbed depended on many factors. These include the hardness of the water, the amount of salt used in cooking, the duration of cooking, and the surface area of the vegetables. For heavily lead-contaminated foods, boiling may decrease the lead content. Overall, the authors concluded that there is likely to be a net gain in lead content during cooking in contaminated water (16).

In recent years, questions have arisen about the safety of certain metal cookware, especially cookware made with aluminum, copper, pottery, and lead glaze. According to the Food and Drug Administration, aluminum cookware appears to be safe for cooking but may not be suitable for prolonged storage (5 h or more) of acidic foods. In the case of copper, the FDA advised the use of only tin-lined copper pans to avoid migration of copper into

foods. Although some imported enameled cookware may contain cadmium, in the United States enameled ceramic and glass cookware is generally considered to be safe because it does not contain lead or cadmium (9). Similarly, Teflon®-coated utensils are considered safe because the Teflon® coating is made of inert fluorocarbons. If the coating remains intact, it is thought that no migration of toxic chemicals will result (Kodasky and Shibko, 1984, personal communication).

Polychlorinated Biphenyls

Compared to selective trimming, the cooking or other processing of fish is not very effective in reducing its PCB content. For example, according to studies by the Wisconsin Department of Natural Resources, deep frying, pan frying, baking, or boiling of fish led to only a 5% to 15% reduction in PCBs. Processing and canning reduced the PCB content by only 8% to 25% (14).

ORGANIC PRODUCE
CERTIFICATION PROGRAMS

In the United States a number of states including California, Montana, North Dakota, South Dakota, Nebraska, Iowa, Wisconsin, Connecticut, and Maine have organic labeling laws and rules in place. Twelve other states have organic labeling laws pending (25). In general, state organic certification programs define organic produce in terms of allowable fertilizers and pest control methods. Farmers are generally required to wait at least a year after their last application of synthetic fertilizers and pesticides before they can successfully apply for organic certification. Some programs, however, require a waiting period of 2 to 3 years. Organic food standards and regulations are defined within each state and are of relatively recent origin (25).

SUMMARY

Several steps may be suggested to individuals in an attempt to reduce dietary exposure to environmental pollutants in foods. Because of the scarcity of precise data, no guarantee can be offered about the success of these methods.

For vegetables and fruits, knowledge of the source of foods appears to be particularly important. Fruits and vegetables grown in industrialized areas are potentially high in PAH content, and those grown near highways or other areas with heavy traffic also have the potential for a high lead content. Produce from agricultural lands using municipal sludge is likely to be high in cadmium, but the degree of risk from such exposure has not been determined. Although it is reasonable to assume that organically grown produce is lower in pesticide residues, there are thus far no reliable data to support this assumption.

Thorough washing of produce is likely to remove a substantial amount of pesticide residue, some of the toxic metal burden, and some of the PAH content. Peeling fruits and vegetables or removing the outer leaves of head crops (such as lettuce and cabbage) will further reduce residues of pesticides, metals, and PAHs. Blanching and such further processing as canning and pureeing may lower the levels of pesticides. However, canned produce, especially if canned in vinegar or other acidic medium, is likely to be higher in lead than are fresh produce, foods pickled in glass jars, or foods canned in either lead-free two-seamed cans or cans with electrically welded seams. Foods should not be stored in opened cans.

For dairy products, the selection of low-fat or skim-milk products is likely to lower the exposure to chlorinated pesticides and PCBs.

Seafood from petroleum-contaminated waters is likely to be contaminated with PAH, which is not easily removed during the usual cleansing practices followed prior to marketing. In general, salt-water fish is lower in PCBs than is freshwater fish taken from PCB-contaminated lakes and streams. In some parts of Wisconsin, PCBs may be particularly high in carp, lake trout, salmon, and catfish. Younger fish less than 22 inches in length are likely to contain considerably less PCBs than older, larger fish. The PCB content of fish may be reduced by removing the skin and trimming the fatty tissues prior to cooking and by discarding the fat and the juices rendered during cooking. Fish and shellfish tend to bioconcentrate cadmium as well as PCBs. Fish packed in lead-containing cans, although lower in PCBs, may be higher in lead than is fresh fish. If the can contains PAH-contaminated vegetable oil, the fish may also have a higher PAH content than does the fresh fish.

Exposure to environmental contaminants in meat and poultry may be substantially decreased by several methods. These are the selection of leaner meats, the removal of skin from poultry, and cooking at lower temperatures for longer periods, i.e., baking, poaching, and steaming. Because charcoal grilling of meats contributes substantially to their PAH content, it has been suggested that exposure may be reduced by trimming all fat prior to cooking, by covering meats with aluminum foil or using a pan, by cooking longer at a lower temperature, i.e., reducing the temperature of coals if using a charcoal grill or using a gas or electrical grill, by maintaining greater distance from the source of heat, by not basting with fat, and by discarding the rendered fat.

Selecting smoked foods less frequently, using commercially smoked rather than home-smoked foods, and using meats prepared with a liquid smoke solution rather than conventional wood smoke are also likely to reduce exposure to PAHs. Finally, certain fresh or processed meats (e.g., ground hamburger, frankfurters, sausages, and canned meats) are likely to be higher in lead than minimally processed fresh meat.

Personal measures of reducing exposure to contaminants in grain products are primarily limited to storing in a cool, dry place and avoiding cooking at high temperatures or browning to prevent the formation of PAHs.

REFERENCES

1. Chaney RL: Health risks associated with toxic metals in municipal sludge. In: Sludge—Health Risks of Land Application, p 59, Bitton G, Damron BL, Edds GT, et al. (eds.), Ann Arbor Science Publishers/Butterworth Group, Ann Arbor, 1980.
2. Cordle F, Corneliussen P, Jelinek C, et al: Human exposure to polychlorinated biphenyls and polybrominated biphenyls. Environ Health Perspect 24: 157, 1978.
3. Corwin E: On getting the lead out of food. FDA Consumer 16:18, 1982.
4. Council for Agricultural Science and Technology: Application of Sewage Sludge to Cropland: Appraisal of Potential Hazards of the Heavy Metals to Plants and Animals, General Services Administration, Denver, 1976.
5. DeSogra C, Groll L: Nutrition and Cancer Prevention: A Guide to Food Choices, Northern California Cancer Program, Palo Alto, CA, 1981.
6. Dunn BP: Polycyclic aromatic hydrocarbons. In: Carcinogens and Mutagens in the Environment: Vol. 1, Food Products, p. 175, Stitch HF (ed.), CRC Press, Boca Raton, 1982.
7. Groth E III: The Child in the Leaded Environment, Consumers Union, Mt. Vernon, NY, undated.
8. Hemphill DD, Marienfeld CJ, Reddy RF, et al: Toxic heavy metals in vegetables and forage grasses in Missouri's lead belt. J Assoc Off Anal Chem 56:994, 1973.
9. Henderson D: Cookware as a source of additives. FDA Consumer 16:10, 1982.
10. Howard JW, Fazio T: Review of polycyclic aromatic hydrocarbons in foods. Analytical methodology and reported findings of polycyclic aromatic hydrocarbons in foods, J Assoc Off Anal Chem 63:1077, 1980.
11. Jelinek CF: Levels of lead in the United States food supply. J Assoc Off Anal Chem 65:942, 1982.
12. Knorr P: Natural and organic foods: Definitions, quality, and problems. Cereal Foods World 27:163, 1982.
13. Lijinsky W, Ross AE: Production of carcinogenic polynuclear hydrocarbons in the cooking of food. Food Cosmet Toxicol 5:343, 1967.
14. Lindsay RC, Myrdal GR, Daubert JP: Can We Remove PCBs from Fish? Publication 12-3600(76), Department of Natural Resources, Madison, WI, 1976.

15. Liska BJ, Stadelman WJ: Effects of processing on pesticides in foods. Residue Rev 29:61, 1969.
16. Little P, Fleming RG, Heard MJ: Uptake of lead by vegetable foodstuffs during cooking. Sci Total Environ 17:111, 1981.
17. Loma Linda University: Average Daily Intake of Vegetarians by Food Class, Department of Biostatistics and Epidemiology, Loma Linda University School of Health, Loma Linda, CA, 1978.
18. Moran JJ: Lead content in canned foods containing vinegar. J Food Sci 47:322, 1981.
19. Motto HL, Daines RH, Chilko DM, et al: Lead in soils and plants: Its relationship to traffic, volume, and proximity to highways. Environ Sci Technol 4:231, 1970.
20. National Canners Association Research Foundation: Investigations on the Effect of Preparation and Cooking on the Pesticide Residue Content of Selected Vegetables. Final Report, May 13, 1965 to November 13, 1967, Agricultural Research Service, US Department of Agriculture, Washington, 1967.
21. National Research Council: An Assessment of Mercury in the Environment, Panel on Mercury, Environmental Studies Board, National Academy of Sciences, Washington, 1977.
22. Preer JR, Sekhon H, Stephens B, et al: Factors affecting heavy metal content of garden vegetables. Environ Pollut [B] 1:95, 1980.
23. Ritchey SJ, Young RW, Essary EO: Effects of heating and cooking method on chlorinated hydrocarbon residues in chicken tissues. J Agr Food Chem 20:291, 1972.
24. Stobwasser H, Rademacher B, Lange E: Einfluss von Nacherntefaktoren auf die Ruckstande von Pflanzenschutzmitteln in Obst, Gemuse und einigen Sonderkulturen. Residue Rev 22:106, 1968.
25. US Environmental Protection Agency: Pesticides and food safety. EPA J 16(3):2–54, 1990.
26. US Environmental Protection Agency: The Quality of Our Nation's Water. A Summary of the 1988 National Water Quality Inventory, EPA 440/4-90-005, USEPA, Washington, 1990.
27. Williams S: Effects of Washing, Cooking, and Other Processing on Residues of Organochlorine Pesticides, International Union of Pure and Applied Chemistry, Pesticide Section, Oxford, 1969.
28. Winter CK, Seiber JN, Nuckton CF (eds.): Chemicals in the Human Food Chain, Van Nostrand Reinhold, New York, 1990.

RECOMMENDED READING

US Environmental Protection Agency: Pesticides and food safety. EPA J 16(3):2–54, 1990.
Winter CK, Seiber JN, Nuckton CF (eds.): Chemicals in the Human Food Chain, Van Nostrand Reinhold, New York, 1990.

30. PERSONAL METHODS OF CONTROLLING EXPOSURE TO CHEMICAL CONTAMINANTS IN DRINKING WATER

Frank Bell, Ervin Bellack, and Joseph A. Cotruvo

INTRODUCTION

Public water suppliers have a legal responsibility to provide safe drinking water for the public. Consumers have an obligation as well. If their drinking water comes from from an individual well, they have almost all of the responsibility for maintaining the quality of the water. But even if their drinking water comes from a public supply, consumers should be actively interested in the quality of water being delivered and in the problems the water utility may face in providing that water.

Since drinking water contributes to the patients' exposure to a number of chemicals, physicians must also maintain an awareness of the local water supply, its source(s), composition, and potential routes of contamination. Physicians, for example, should know if the local drinking water comes from ground water that is high in sodium or is located near a hazardous waste site. They must be aware of local industrial and agricultural practices that may affect the quality of the drinking water.

About 214 million persons receive their drinking water from the approximately 60,000 water systems designated as "public water systems." Under the provisions of the Safe Drinking Water Act, such systems serve 25 or more persons on a regular basis

Disclaimer: The contents do not necessarily reflect the views and policies of the Environmental Protection Agency, nor does the mention of trade names of products constitute endorsement or recommendation for use.

Principles and Practice of Environmental Medicine, edited by Alyce Bezman Tarcher. Plenum Medical Book Company, New York, 1992.

or have 15 or more service connections. The balance of the United States population, or about 20 million persons, receive their drinking water from smaller water systems or from individual home water supplies. Water supplied by public water systems must meet minimum primary (health-related) standards of bacteriological, chemical, and radiological quality (see Chapter 4). The secondary (esthetic) standards—taste, odor, color—are advisory. Some states, however, include esthetic factors in their enforceable standards for public supplies. The water supplied by nonpublic systems or by individual sources (usually home wells) is not subject to federal health regulation. Frequently individual water supplies are not subject to any regulation at all.

Most, but certainly not all, public water systems are in compliance with health-related standards. In the complying systems, excessive exposure of consumers to contaminants is generally limited to substances that affect the esthetic quality of water or to substances (health-related or otherwise) that are not yet included in drinking water regulations. In contrast, consumers using individual water supplies can be, and often are, exposed to bacteriological, chemical, or radiological contaminants, and sometimes to all of these.

Consumers are able to recognize esthetic problems (i.e., undesirable taste, odor, or color) in drinking water but are generally unaware of contaminants having possible adverse health effects unless they are linked to an undesirable appearance, odor, or taste. The most common complaints of consumers about public water supplies include turbidity (cloudiness) and taste and odor related to algae or chlorination. Although components that impart an undesirable appearance, taste, or smell to water may not have health implications at the levels commonly found, they may provide a clue to the presence of contaminants having adverse health effects. At worst, esthetically inferior drinking water may cause consumers to use alternative drinking water sources that are less safe. This is true whether the water comes from a public system or from an individual well.

The following discussion focuses on methods of controlling both the esthetic contaminants, i.e., taste, odor, and appearance, and health-related chemical and radioactive contaminants in drinking water.

DRINKING WATER CONTAMINATION AND METHODS OF CONTROL

Esthetic Contaminants

Discolored Water

The presence of iron and manganese in drinking water is the most common esthetic problem (7). "Rusty" water, or the formation of a gelatinous yellow to orange-red to brown precipitate in water, particularly when the water has been allowed to stand in the open air, commonly indicates the presence of iron. Similar deposits may also indicate the presence of iron-reducing bacteria. Black deposits signify the presence of manganese. Frequently both iron and manganese occur in the same water. Besides the unesthetic appearance and "metallic" taste these agents give to water, they may also impart colored stains to plumbing fixtures and "ruin" laundry by leaving colored deposits.

Iron and manganese as natural constituents of ground water of mineral origin may go unnoticed until the water is exposed to air. Air oxidation converts the soluble iron and manganese salts to insoluble colored oxides. Iron in water may also arise from the corrosive action of water on galvanized iron piping, on iron pump components, or on iron fixtures.

Iron and manganese in public water supplies are among the most frequent causes of consumer complaints. The volume of complaints frequently determines the water utility's institution of corrective measures. Some individual water supplies rely primarily on untreated ground water sources, and iron and manganese problems are even more frequent in such supplies.

The question of the health significance of consuming water containing iron and manganese often arises. Although adverse reactions to bad taste might occur, the amount of iron generally ingested from potable water is only a fraction of that consumed in food. The concentration of manganese found in water is generally much lower than that observed to have adverse health effects (13).

Control measures, particularly for iron, are dictated by the source of contamination. If iron is the result of corrosion of plumbing, the problem can be solved by stabilizing the water. Stabilizers include "calcite filters" (also called marble chip filters), caustic feeders, and "water conditioners" (6). If iron or manganese comes from the water source, chlorination or other oxidizing treatment will convert these agents into insoluble oxides, which can be removed by filtration (6,8). If the iron stems from the action of "iron bacteria," shock treatment of the entire home plumbing system with a strong chlorine solution followed by flushing usually eliminates the problem.

Taste and Odor

Disagreeable taste and odor are commonly perceived problems of drinking water quality. "Off" tastes or objectionable odors stem from inorganic or organic chemicals and from natural or man-made substances. Inorganic sources of taste and odor problems include chlorination (the chlorine odor), sulfides (rotten egg odor), sodium, chlorides, sulfates (salty taste), and a number of metals, e.g., iron, manganese, and copper (metallic taste). Organic substances producing objectionable tastes include gasoline or oils, phenols, which impart a medicinal taste, and a number different algae, which impart a fishy, earthy, musty, or perfumy taste. Synthetic organic chemicals may be detected in drinking water if present in sufficient concentrations to exceed the taste and odor threshold. This, however, is seldom the case. Except in instances of extreme contamination with chlorinated phenols, mercaptans, or gasoline, the presence of synthetic organic contaminants in drinking water is seldom detected by taste and odor.

Undesirable taste and odor are problems in both public and individual water supplies. In public supplies, consumer complaints usually result in corrective action. In some cases, however, as with the salty taste from natural minerals, regular water consumers become so accustomed to the taste that they fail to notice it. Similarly, some consumers of individual well supplies become accustomed to a particular taste or odor, even that of sulfide, and either accept it or ignore it. A taste or odor suggesting the presence of organic chemicals in the drinking water should immediately be identified and corrected.

Treatment to eliminate objectionable tastes or odors is geared to the type of substance creating the problem. Mineral salts are difficult to remove; only reverse osmosis and distillation are effective. Sulfides and some organic tastes and odors (and colors) are amenable to such oxidation processes as aeration, chlorination, or permanganate treatment. Many synthetic organic chemicals, as well as organic chemicals of natural origin, can be removed with activated carbon or other adsorbents. Most commonly advertised units, however, are designed to remove the chlorine taste rather than to remove significant amounts of synthetic organic chemicals.

Turbidity

Turbidity, or cloudiness of water, is a physical characteristic that can have both esthetic and biological implications. The appearance of cloudy water is usually objectionable. In addition, the suspended particles responsible for the cloudiness are capable of masking the detection of bacteria and of shielding them from disinfecting agents. Turbidity in public water supplies is regulated for these reasons.

Turbidity in individual water supplies is most common when surface supplies are being used. It may be quite variable as, for example, when heavy rains or winds introduce particulate matter into surface waters. For individual surface water supplies, filtration and disinfection are recommended in order to remove protozoan cysts, viruses, or other pathogenic organisms that may be present.

Turbidity in public supplies is removed by sedimentation, coagulation, and filtration. It is nonetheless a common complaint of consumers receiving public supplies. Turbidity and red-colored water generally result from distribution system upsets that cause sediment to be flushed into home taps. This condition usually clears spontaneously or is remedied by water utility maintenance actions.

Corrosion

Corrosive water, per se, may not be perceived to be objectionable, but its effects are readily apparent. Rusty-appearing stains on fixtures or laundry indicate the presence of iron corrosion (or the presence of iron in the water source); blue-green stains on fixtures or discolored water indicates copper corrosion. Corrosion of lead (from pipe or lead-containing solder) is not usually visible but is potentially significant. In some locations the useful life of plumbing and hot water tanks is materially shortened by highly corrosive drinking water.

Water can exhibit corrosive properties because of the presence of oxygen or acidity or the relative absence of minerals. Iron is attacked by oxygenated water. Iron, copper, and lead are corroded by water having a low pH or a very high pH. Because of water's solvent properties, soft water (low calcium and magnesium) or relatively mineral-free water is corrosive toward many substances. Galvanic action from contact between dissimilar metals also causes corrosion.

Public water systems are responsible for providing noncorrosive water to consumers (1). Corrosion control practices for public water systems include pH adjustment (e.g., raising pH by adding lime or sodium carbonate) and the addition of corrosion inhibitors (e.g., polyphosphates or silicates). For individual water supplies, the usual practice is to install a stabilizer (i.e., calcite filters, caustic feeder, water conditioners).

Corrosion is largely an esthetic and economic problem unless the plumbing system contains lead (from pipe or solder), cadmium (from galvanizing), or other toxic metals. Under certain conditions, such as when water remains in contact with metal for extended periods of time (overnight or longer) without flowing, sufficient metal can be dissolved by corrosive water to constitute a potential health risk. Thus, the water first drawn from the tap, especially that standing overnight, should not be consumed, and hot water from the tap should not be used for cooking or beverages.

Hardness

In many parts of the country, the available water is classified as "hard." Hardness is defined in terms of calcium and magnesium content and is recognized by the difficulty in producing lather with soap. Accumulation of deposits in water heater tanks and subsequent failure of the water heater can also be attributed to hard water. Although the advent of nonsoap detergents has made hard water less of a problem than in the past, hard-water problems lead many consumers to seek corrective measures.

Most hard-water problems are associated with the use of ground water as a water source. Since many public water systems and most individual water supplies use ground water, hard water is a frequently encountered problem.

Softeners remove the calcium and magnesium responsible for hardness. The softening of hard water is therefore a common water treatment practice. It is achieved in municipal water systems by precipitating calcium and magnesium through the addition of excess calcium (lime) and then filtering the water. Lime and sodium hydroxide (lime–soda) are also used. For individual systems, and occasionally for public systems, ion-exchange treatment is used. In this process, water passes through a bed of zeolite (a natural or synthetic mineral) or resin. These materials have the capability of exchanging hardness (calcium and magnesium) ions for sodium ions. When the capacity of the bed is exhausted, it is regenerated with brine (sodium chloride solution).

The softening process, particularly ion-exhange, has health significance in that as hardness is removed, sodium is added. The National Heart Association and EPA recommend 20 mg/L of sodium ion in drinking water as a guide to avoid excess exposure for individuals on a low-sodium diet. Some softening processes use resin that exchanges hydrogen ions for calcium and magnesium ions. When installing a home water softener, the homeowner can avoid adding sodium to the drinking water by making certain that only the water supplied to the water heater is softened.

Salinity or Residue

Excess salinity is manifested by a salty or mineral taste and by heavy encrustations in vessels used to heat water. Where the salinity is extremely high, mineral deposits composed primarily of calcium and magnesium carbonates and sodium chlorides and sulfates can be found in pipelines or fixtures, particularly where water has had the opportunity to evaporate.

In some parts of the United States, particularly those that are arid, the only available drinking water is highly mineralized. The minerals are usually derived from the ground through which the water has passed. But sometimes, particularly in coastal areas, sea water intrusion occurs, with a resultant increase in the salinity of well water. Salinity is usually considered to be an esthetic and economic problem rather than a health problem. The consumption of heavily mineralized water (especially with sulfates), however, can cause transient gastrointestinal effects in individuals unaccustomed to such water.

Distillation, reverse osmosis, and electrodialysis are the principal methods available for reducing salinity. All of these methods have been used to some degree for the treatment of municipal systems, but only reverse osmosis and distillation are available to individual homeowners (8). Inorganic salts of all kinds, including those that contribute to taste problems and those that constitute objectionable residues, can be removed, in varying degrees, by small reverse-osmosis units that operate on home water pressure (8).

Health-Related Contaminants

Inorganic Substances

A number of inorganic substances appear in drinking water as a result of its percolation through mineral deposits. Many inorganic substances are either adopted or proposed for the primary (health-related) drinking water regulations. Metals, including lead, copper, cadmium, chromium, and mercury, can occur in drinking water as the result of corrosion or contamination of the water source. Zinc usually enters drinking water as a result of the corrosion of galvanized iron. Silver may occur in drinking water through the use of silver as a bacteriostat in small carbon filters. Nitrate usually enters

surface and ground water from surface runoff, animal wastes, and/or the application of fertilizer. Sodium, usually derived from natural sources, may also enter the water supply from highway salting. The adverse effects of most inorganic chemicals included in the national primary (health-related) drinking water regulations are not immediately or readily apparent. In most cases their adverse effects may not be manifested for many years (15). For example, excess fluoride exposure in early childhood may not be evident until staining and pitting of the permanent teeth is noted (15). The exception is nitrate, which can cause methemoglobinemia in infants after only a single episode of excessive exposure. In some cases fatalities have occurred (see Chapter 21).

The presence of undesirable inorganic ions in drinking water usually is determined by specific testing. Public water systems are required to periodically test their water and reduce the levels of health-related substances to values below the maximum contaminant levels (MCLs) established by regulation. The treatment process varies with the type of water source (surface or ground), the source of the contaminant (natural or as the result of industrial pollution or corrosion), and the chemical nature of the specific ion to be removed. Some metals are removed by conventional coagulation and filtering. Others are removed by softening processes (lime softening on surface sources and zeolite softening on ground-water sources). Nonmetals (arsenic as arsenite or arsenate, fluoride, selenium as selenite or selenate) are removed by reverse osmosis or activated alumina. Metals introduced into drinking water by corrosion are sequestered by polyphosphates for stabilization. Some inorganic ions, such as sodium, sulfate, and chloride, can be removed only by distillation, reverse osmosis, or electodialysis. Nitrate can be removed by anion exchange. However, protecting the water supply from excessive nitrate contamination is the preferred approach.

Homeowners' concerns about the presence of inorganic ions in their well water may be stimulated by news reports of contamination in their vicinity, by an episode of illness, by the birth of a baby, or by conditions attached to the sale or purchase of property. Such concerns often result in having the water tested. Testing should always be conducted by state-certified laboratories.

Treatment processes available to the individual homeowner for removing undesirable inorganic agents in drinking water are limited. Conventional coagulation and filtration, as practiced on municipal surface water systems, are not practical for individual systems. Ion exchange is available, but the maintenance of an ion exchanger may require professional assistance. Softening, activated alumina, and stabilization are processes that have been adapted for home use. Reverse osmosis, which is effective for the removal of nearly all the inorganic ions, is available for home application.

Radionuclides

Radium and other natural radionuclides frequently occur naturally in drinking water supplies (especially from ground water); man-made radionuclides are seldom present. Both public and individual ground-water systems can be affected. Specialized monitoring techniques are required to detect radionuclides in drinking water. The principal concern is radon, a gas that can be transported by ground water. It can volatilize into the indoor air from showering and other high-volume water uses.

Treatment to remove radionuclides is based on the chemical nature of the specific substance. Radium, a divalent cation, responds to softening treatment, as do calcium and barium. Radon gas can be removed with an activated carbon filter or, if feasible, by aeration. Uranium can be removed by anion exchange (11).

Organic Compounds: Trihalomethanes and Synthetic Organic Chemicals

Natural organic matter, which includes humic substances and their degradation products, comprises by far the largest portion of organic chemicals in drinking water. The regulated organic chemicals in drinking water are primarily synthetic chemicals, e.g., pesticides and trihalomethanes (THM). The THMs are contaminants produced along with other chemicals during the process of disinfecting water. These water treatment byproducts, which include chloroform, bromodichloromethane, dibromochloromethane, and bromoform, are formed by the reaction of chlorine with natural organic matter. Sensitive analytical techniques such as gas chromatography are required to measure the concentrations of organic chemicals present in drinking water.

The monitoring and control of THMs are required for large public water systems in the United States (9). All public water systems now monitor the presence of other synthetic organic chemicals. Some states have established requirements for the monitoring and control of selected organic chemicals of regional importance. In public water systems, treatment to control THMs usually involves measures to reduce the formation of these compounds. Other organic chemicals can be controlled by aeration (if the specific substance is readily volatile) or by adsorption with activated carbon or resins (18). Activated carbon treatment is widely used for public water supply treatment in Europe. It is less commonly used in the United States.

As with other classes of contaminants, no monitoring is required for organic chemicals in individual water supplies. Therefore, the homeowner whose drinking water comes from an individual well will be unaware that his water supply is contaminated with synthetic organic chemicals unless the nature and quantity of the contaminants give the water an offensive taste or smell. As previously mentioned, the presence of organic chemicals in drinking water is rarely detected by abnormal taste.

Toxic organic compounds, those producing taste and odor problems, and chlorine-related tastes and odors can be removed in most cases with activated carbon filters. Users of contaminated individual water supplies frequently employ activated carbon treatment. Small, single-faucet activated carbon devices are commonly used for this purpose. Since most of these devices are designed for taste and odor control, they are not particularly effective in removing synthetic organic chemicals. As shown by an EPA-sponsored study, some of the larger, under-the-sink models containing activated carbon are effective in removing certain synthetic organic chemicals (4).

Experimental work by EPA has shown that the homeowner can remove essentially 100% of selected volatile organic chemicals in drinking water by boiling or electric mixing (20). Open standing, aeration, and pouring were all less effective, and faucet aeration had a negligible effect. The homeowner should be aware that volatilization methods may drive the contaminant into his breathing zone.

The National Academy of Sciences (NAS), under contract to EPA's Office of Drinking Water, produced a series of comprehensive reports on drinking water contaminants and health (13–19,22,23). These reports examine the health effects associated with microbial, chemical, and radioactive contaminants in drinking water. Other topics considered include the distribution and treatment technology available to public water systems, the assessment of human health effects of current practices of water disinfection, and the risk assessment of drinking water contaminants on human health.

HOME WATER TREATMENT UNITS

Design and Efficiency

Home water treatment units are available to remove contaminants in drinking water. Point-of-use water treatment systems are installed on single or multiple taps, whereas point-of-entry systems are installed on the main water line entering the building (5,12). Regunathan et al. (12) has described the basic designs and application of these units (Figs. 30-1 and 30-2). All of the designs shown in Figures

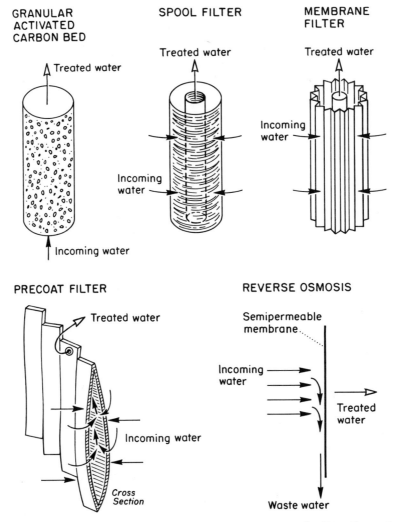

FIGURE 30-1. Basic designs of common home drinking water treatment units. From Regunathan et al. (12).

30-1 and 30-2 treat only drinking water. When a chemical presents a tactile or respiratory hazard, it is possible to treat all of the water entering the house by a whole-house filter unit.

The basic water treatment methods used in the home units and the reasons for their use are outlined in Table 30-1. Most of the home water treatment devices depend on carbon filtration. Activated carbon removes the organic impurities in water by a process of contact adsorption. The filter's effectiveness depends on the amount of carbon present. The longer the water is in contact with the carbon, the more contaminants are trapped. In order to maintain the efficiency of the unit, the carbon must be replaced on a regular basis.

Some home units contain spool or membrane devices that remove organic impurities in water by barrier filtration. The spool filter is designed to remove relatively large particles, i.e., greater than 20 μm, whereas the membrane filter removes particles between 0.5 and 0.05 μm. Some home water treatment units contain precoat filters, which remove organic impurities by a combination of barrier filtration and contact adsorption (Fig. 30-1).

Reverse osmosis is also used in some home units to remove contaminants from drinking water. Reverse osmosis is based on the following principle: When two water solutions having differing concentrations of dissolved solids are separated by a semipermeable membrane, water will pass through the

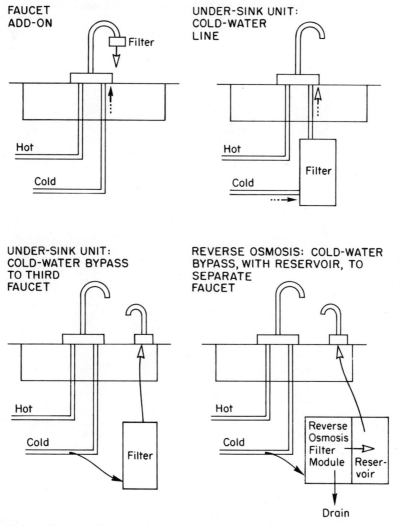

FAUCET
ADD-ON

Filter

Hot

Cold

UNDER-SINK UNIT:
COLD-WATER
LINE

Hot

Filter

Cold

UNDER-SINK UNIT:
COLD-WATER BYPASS
TO THIRD
FAUCET

Hot

Cold

Filter

REVERSE OSMOSIS: COLD-WATER
BYPASS, WITH RESERVOIR, TO
SEPARATE
FAUCET

Hot

Cold

Reverse
Osmosis
Filter
Module   Reser-
voir

Drain

FIGURE 30-2. Basic applications of common home drinking water treatment units. From Regunathan et al. (12).

membrane from the side with lower concentration to the side with the higher concentration. This process of osmosis causes the liquid level on the side of greater concentration to be higher than that on the other side. When the system comes to equilibrium, such that there is no net passage of water across the membrane, the pressure corresponding to the difference in the liquid levels is the osmotic pressure. If pressure greater than the osmotic pressure is applied to the side with higher concentration of dissolved solids, the passage of water will be reversed. Thus, the term "reverse" osmosis is used. Because ions do not pass as easily through the membrane, reverse osmosis selectively admits only purified

water while sending a waste stream to the drain. Since reverse osmosis works continuously but very slowly, a service reservoir is required to provide water for the tap on demand. Reverse osmosis will concurrently remove beneficial ions such as calcium and magnesium and may make the water more corrosive.

Table 30-2 shows the relative abilities of different types of home units containing activated carbon to remove trihalomethane and volatile organic chemicals from water. The units were tested against a limited array of toxic organics. Relative carbon adsorption indices indicate that many organic compounds are less readily removed from water [e.g.,

TABLE 30-1. Home Water Treatment Units

Separation process	Treatment method	Removal capabilities
Adsorption	Activated carbon	Tastes, odors, some organic colors, some organic chemicals, i.e., endrin, lindane, methoxychlor, toxaphene, phenoxyherbicides, i.e., 2,4-D[a], 2,4,5-T[b], THMs (Trihalomethanes), solvents
Filtration	Spool, membrane, and precoat filters (some precoat filters also contain activated carbon and will reduce tastes, odors, and some organic compounds)	Sand, sediment, turbidity, fine particles, fibers
Reverse osmosis	Reverse osmosis	Metals, TDS (total dissolved solids), radionuclides, inorganic compounds, i.e., fluoride, sulfates, chlorides

[a]2,4-Dichlorophenoxyacetic acid.
[b]2,4,5-Trichlorophenoxyacetic acid.

benzene, n-dimethylnitrosamine, bis(2-chloroethyl)ether] while others (e.g., chlordane, DDT, PCB) are more readily removed (2).

The carbon cartridges in the home units remove residual chlorine and foreign material as well as organic chemicals from the water. High concentrations of bacteria are therefore commonly present in the initial water drawn from such home units. The health effects of ingesting these organisms is unknown. National voluntary standards for the reduction of health and esthetic constituents by water filters have been established by the National Sanitation Foundation (3).

The National Sanitation Foundation, a nonprofit third-party testing and certification organization, has a certification program for drinking water treatment systems. Certified point-of-use and point-of-entry devices include carbon, softening, mechanical filtration, distillation, and reverse osmosis systems. Once a system is certified, the company and the system are included in the published and electronically accessed National Sanitation Foundation Listings for Drinking Water Treatment Systems (10).

Water treatment units that contain silver are registered by EPA as bacteriostatic units. However, the bacteriostatic effectiveness of silver against heterotrophic bacteria in these units is questionable. The main requirement of the registration is that units do not release excessive amounts of silver. Registration does not imply that EPA has examined the effectiveness of bacteriostatic units. A few units, containing a chemical disinfectant, are designed to

TABLE 30-2. Removal Capabilities of Home Water Treatment Units Containing Carbon Filtration, by Type of Unit[a]

Type of unit	Trihalomethanes		Volatile organic chemicals[b]	
	Number of units tested	Removal efficiency (%)	Number of units tested	Removal efficiency (%)
Faucet bypass units, attached to faucet with bypass valve for drinking water	6	6–69	2	76–97
Faucet no-bypass units, attached to faucet with no bypass valve	1	6	Not tested	
Line bypass units: a bypass takes cold water through the filter unit to a separate tap	14	23–99	6	97–99
Stationary units filter all water coming to the cold water tap	5	15–46	1	90
Portable pour-through units: water is poured through the unit into a container below	3	19–74	1	94
Portable—other: other potable unit operates with a hand pump	1	4	Not tested	

[a]From Gulf South Research Institute (4).
[b]Composite efficiencies (selected units) for reduction of simultaneous challenges of carbon tetrachloride (20 ppb), trichloroethylene (50 ppb), tetrachloroethylene (50 ppb), and 1,1,1-trichloroethane (50 ppb).

be microbiological purifiers. Such units would be subject to registration by EPA and would be required to prove the microbiological and other claims made. Manufacturers of water treatment units are required to obtain an establishment (Est.) registration number to identify their plant. Some manufacturers seem to use their establishment number to make it appear that EPA has endorsed or approved their product.

Monitoring and Maintenance

For the control of esthetic properties, the principal monitoring tool will be the consumer's senses. Her nose, mouth, and eyes will inform her when a water treatment unit has ceased to function properly. Home treatment is not the recommended method for the control of health-related contaminants in drinking water. However, where home treatment is used, sophisticated measurements are usually required to monitor performance. The individual home user with highly contaminated water should proceed with home treatment only after obtaining advice from public health officials. Reliance on a home treatment unit to protect against a health risk rather than an esthetic problem dictates the need for a water-quality-monitoring program and for a plan to replace or regenerate filter media on a routine basis. Field observations have also shown the need for ongoing maintenance to correct problems of leakage and intermittent flow in some home units.

Bottled Water

Bottled water that is shipped interstate is under the control of the Food and Drug Administration (FDA). The FDA applies EPA national primary maximum contaminant limits in determining acceptable bottled water quality. Intrastate bottled water is subject to state laws and controls. No current independent national survey is available on bottled water quality.

THE INDIVIDUAL'S ROLE IN MAINTAINING WATER QUALITY

For consumers using a public water supply, drinking water problems should first be checked by the responsible water utility or public health department. The utility will usually answer questions and provide water quality data. If the problem is not readily resolved, a maintenance worker may make a local investigation and take remedial action. If this investigation does not resolve an esthetic complaint (i.e., chlorine taste or odor) and the consumer decides to buy a treatment unit, he should review

verified test data (10). Such data should be provided by the unit's producer or seller, and performance should be guaranteed. Information on several different units should be obtained before a purchase is made. Further information may also be available from the local health department or state water supply agency.

For persons having a contaminated individual water supply, the first step should be to contact the local health department. Frequently the local agency will provide bacterial sampling and analysis of the water as well as a site visit by a sanitary inspector. To remedy a contaminated well or spring, consideration should be given first to arresting the contamination at the source, only later to treatment.

When the problem involves chemical contamination of the drinking water, the consumer should try to determine the nature of the problem. This involves an assessment of the type and source(s) (e.g., septic tanks, agriculture, industry, hazardous waste sites) of the chemical contamination. It is critical that the assessment be done properly, since it provides a guide to which specific chemicals should be analyzed in the water. Testing for specific chemicals clearly requires some perception of which chemicals to look for, since it is impossible to survey all known chemicals. The local health agency should be helpful in assessing the problem, in deciding on what tests should be done, and in selecting a certified laboratory. The levels of contaminants found can be compared to the national primary drinking water regulations (see Chapter 4). In the absence of drinking water standards for a particular contaminant, a review of the federal drinking water health advisories may be helpful. Information on the nature, degree, and source(s) of the chemical contaminants provides the basis for the proper correction of the problem.

In general, the public should rely on the local water supplier and public health authorities to assure the quality of their drinking water in public water systems. Consumers may sometimes choose to deal independently with esthetic matters such as an undesirable taste or odor in their home well or public water supply. If a question arises about the healthfulness of drinking water from a private home well or other source, the assistance of local public health officials should be sought immediately (21). Any proposed solution should be considered in concert with these officials and other public health professionals.

REFERENCES

1. Amendments to the Interim Primary Drinking Water Regulations, 40 CFR, Part 141, Federal Register 45(168), 1980.

2. Dobbs RA, Cohen JM: Carbon Adsorption Isotherms for Toxic Organics. EPA-600/8-80-023, Municipal Environmental Research Laboratory, USEPA, Washington, 1980.

3. Drinking Water Treatment Units: Health Effects (Standard 53) and Aesthetic Effects (Standard 42), National Sanitation Foundation, Ann Arbor, 1990.

4. Gulf South Research Institute: Development of Basic Data and Knowledge Regarding Organic Removal Capabilities of Commercially Available Home Water Treatment Units Utilizing Activated Carbon: Seven Reports to the Office of Drinking Water, Order No. PB82-159-583, National Technical Information Service, Springfield, VA, 1981.

5. Lykins BW Jr, Clark RM, Goodrich JA: Point-of-Use/Point-of-Entry Water Manual, Lewis Publishers, Boca Raton, 1991.

6. Manual of Individual Drinking Water Supply Systems, Office of Drinking Water, EPA-570/9-82-004, US Government Printing Office, Washington, 1982.

7. McCabe LJ, Symons, JM, Lee RD, et al: Survey of community water supply systems. J Am Water Works Assoc 62:680, 1970.

8. McGowan W: Sensitivity: A key water conditioning skill. Water Technol 5:20, 1982.

9. National Interim Primary Drinking Water Regulations, Control of Trihalomethanes in Drinking Water; Final Rule, Federal Register, November 29, Vol. 44(231), 1979.

10. National Sanitation Foundation: Listings for Drinking Water Treatment Systems, National Sanitation Foundation, Ann Arbor, September 1, 1991.

11. Radioactivity in Drinking Water, Criteria and Standards Division, EPA 570/9-81-002, USEPA, Washington, 1981.

12. Regunathan P, Beauman WH, Kreusch EG: Efficiency of point-of-use treatment devices. J Am Water Works Assoc 75:1, 1983.

13. Safe Drinking Water Committee, National Research Council: Drinking Water and Health, Vol 1, National Academy Press, Washington, 1977.

14. Safe Drinking Water Committee, National Research Council: Drinking Water and Health, Vol 2, National Academy Press, Washington, 1980

15. Safe Drinking Water Committee, National Research Council: Drinking Water and Health, Vol 3, National Academy Press, Washington, 1980.

16. Safe Drinking Water Committee, National Research Council: Drinking Water and Health, Vol 4, National Academy Press, Washington, 1982.

17. Safe Drinking Water Committee, National Research Council: Drinking Water and Health, Vol 5, National Academy Press, Washington, 1983

18. Safe Drinking Water Committee, National Research Council: Drinking Water and Health, Vol 6, National Academy Press, Washington, 1986.

19. Safe Drinking Water Committee, National Research Council: Drinking Water and Health, Vol 9, National Academy Press, Washington, 1989.

20. Sorrell RK, Daly EM, Weisner MJ, et al: Effectiveness of in-home treatment methods for the removal of volatile organic chemicals. J Am Water Works Assoc 77:5, 1985.

21. Standard Methods for the Examination of Water and Wastewater, 16th ed., American Public Health Association, Washington, DC, 1985.

22. Subcommittee on Disinfectants and Disinfectant By-Products, National Research Council: Drinking Water and Health, Disinfectants and Disinfectant By-Products, Vol 7, National Academy Press, Washington, 1987.

23. Subcommittee on Pharmacokinetics and Risk Assessment. Drinking Water and Health, National Research Council: Pharmacokinetics and Risk Assessment, Vol 8, National Academy Press, Washington, 1987.

RECOMMENDED READINGS

Lykins BW Jr, Clark RM, Goodrich JA: Point-of-Use/Point-of-Entry Water Manual, Lewis Publishers, Chelsea, Michigan, 1991.

National Sanitation Foundation: Listings for Drinking Water Treatment Systems, National Sanitation Foundation, Ann Arbor, September 1, 1991.

31. GOVERNMENTAL REGULATION OF EXPOSURE TO ENVIRONMENTAL CHEMICALS AND PHYSICAL AGENTS

James M. Kawecki and Si Duk Lee

INTRODUCTION

All over the world, environmental regulations have been promulgated in response to public health problems—often long-brewing problems that suddenly erupted into crises. This has certainly been our historical experience in the United States. The evolution of the government's regulatory role began in the 19th century. Steamboat boilers were exploding with alarming frequency, taking lives and releasing hazardous substances. The public response to this crisis led to the earliest environmental regulations by the United States government.

In the 1960s, following a decade of frequent oil spills, incidences of mercury poisoning, episodes of highly visible air pollution, and the publication of Rachel Carson's *Silent Spring*, legislation related to air and water quality was passed. In 1970, the Environmental Protection Agency (EPA) was established as a direct result of rising political pressure for a coordinated federal policy on regulating the quality of the environment.

Congressional expansion of agency responsibilities and detailed requirements for health, safety, and environmental regulation vastly expanded agency rulemaking and increased the number of challenges to regulatory action in federal courts. Rules and regulations published in the *Federal Register*, for instance, increased from 8902 in 1947 to 65,603 in 1977.

The yearly and total increases in the number of published regulatory notices and rules were largely the result of the surge in rulemaking on health, safety, and environmental matters. The 1970s are notable for numerous new federal regulations applicable to the environment, both in the workplace and in the community. These laws reflect a dramatic and relatively rapid shift in public priorities toward the protection of health. This shift was stimulated by scientific advances that revealed the potential extent of environmental health problems.

As an introduction to this very complex and active area of environmental regulation, the interested reader is directed to the references and recommended readings at the end of this chapter. The citations were selected because of their broad and comprehensive coverage of the bases for environmental legislation.

REGULATED SUBSTANCES

Pollutants and other chemical substances that pose risk to human health and safety and to the environment are properly designated "hazardous"* and are subject to government regulation. Risks stem from the manufacture or processing, transport, consumer use, and planned or inadvertent release of hazardous agents. Adverse health effects may occur as a result of exposure to hazardous chemicals, wastes, and consumer products (1,22, 30,32).

When deemed necessary to protect public health, legislative action by the U.S. Congress has given federal agencies authority to restrict such pri-

Principles and Practice of Environmental Medicine, edited by Alyce Bezman Tarcher. Plenum Medical Book Company, New York, 1992.

*In the United States, hazard means the nature and likelihood of an adverse effect, and risk reflects the likelihood of the effect. In Europe, the terms are usually reversed.

vate actions as the production, use, and disposal of chemicals. The federal agencies given this authority include the Environmental Protection Agency (EPA), Food and Drug Administration (FDA), Occupational Safety and Health Administration (OSHA), Consumer Product Safety Commission (CPSC), Department of Transportation (DOT), Department of Agriculture (USDA), and the Nuclear Regulatory Commission (NRC).

Early regulatory efforts were limited to controlling the risk of poisoning and other acute effects of toxic chemicals. Policy making directed to acute effects was usually based on the results of short-term animal studies designed to establish no-observed-effect doses. From such studies, the allowable human exposure was calculated based on the application of uncertainty (safety) factors to relatively uncomplicated and unsophisticated scientific findings. Problems such as cancer and birth defects, which may be associated with low long-term exposures, were seldom seen as preventable by government regulations. In the past 20 years, however, scientific advances have revealed the interrelationship between toxic exposure and chronic health effects (1,22,30,32). These findings resulted in a flurry of legislative activity oriented to protect human health and safety and the environment. Unfortunately, such regulation often rests on a foundation of judgment more than on fact.

Federal regulatory legislation recognized that hazardous chemicals may be encountered in air, food, and water and in drugs and consumer products. Chemical hazards are found in the workplace and in the general environment. Toxic chemicals may be inhaled, ingested, or absorbed. Exposure may be direct or mediated. Toxic substances may move through the food chain and migrate from storage lagoons and hazardous waste sites into surface and ground water. Fugitive emissions, emergency releases, and unintentional spills all contribute to possible exposures and to the need for regulation.

REGULATORY DECISION-MAKING PROCESS

Despite the broad range of pollutants subject to regulation by a variety of agencies, the regulatory decision-making process usually follows the same model. Regulatory actions are based on two distinct elements: risk assessment and risk management (24,27). Risk assessment is the use of a factual or scientific base to define the health effects of exposure of individuals or populations to hazardous materials. Risk management is the process of weighing policy alternatives and selecting the appropriate regulatory action. By integrating the results of risk assessment with engineering data and with social, economic, and polital concerns, regulatory decisions are made. The often-voiced concern that regulatory decisions are made on the basis of political pressures rather than scientific analysis refers to the risk management component of regulation. For scientists, the focus has been on improving the process of risk assessment (9–15,25,27).

Risk Assessment

Risk assessment can be divided into four major steps: hazard identification, dose–response assessment, exposure assessment, and risk characterization (27).

Hazard Identification

Hazard identification is defined as the process of determining whether exposure to an agent can be linked to an increased incidence of an adverse health effect (cancer, birth defects, etc.) (27). It is a qualitative assessment characterizing the nature and strength of the evidence of causation. Hazard identification is necessary to sort through the vast numbers of substances to which people are exposed. Over 70,000 chemicals are commercially in use in the United States and thousands more are introduced every year (5,7,8). The United States and other industrial countries produce literally millions of raw materials, materials in process, and final goods and services. Many of these substances offer potential risks to health (1,22,30,32).

The scientific basis for much of hazard identification is well established. It draws on epidemiologic data, animal bioassays, in vitro studies, comparisons of molecular structures (structure–activity relationship), and other biomedical research areas. A risk assessment might stop with the step of hazard identification. This can occur if no adverse effect is found or if an agency, for policy or statutory reasons, takes regulatory action without further analysis.

Epidemiologic Data Epidemiologic studies that reveal a relationship between an agent and a disease provide the most convincing evidence of risk to humans. This evidence is usually difficult to obtain for the following reasons: the latent period between an exposure and the onset of the disease is often long, exposures are mixed and multiple, and the number of exposed persons in a particular group is often small. An important limitation of epidemiologic studies is that they provide evidence of an adverse effect(s) only after an agent(s) has been released into the environment. This limitation requires that other methods be used to predict the presence of a health hazard before it is released into the environment. Except for agents found in the workplace, few environmental chemicals have been studied using epidemiological approaches.

Animal Bioassays Although epidemiologic data may be the most convincing means of identifying health hazards, data obtained from animal bioassays are the most commonly available. The extrapolation of animal data to humans remains a topic of considerable debate. Despite their shortcomings, however, animal tests have generally been reliable indicators of such adverse health effects as the development of cancer. Animal studies will undoubtedly continue to play a role in our efforts to identify carcinogens.

The species of animals tested, the type of chemical, the amount, the route of administration, the length of exposure, the sex, age, and numbers of species, the adverse biological endpoint, and the complementary information from other health investigations are all important parameters in assessing the potential hazards a chemical may pose to human populations. Consistently positive results in both sexes and in several species and evidence of a dose–response effect constitute the best evidence that an adverse effect such as carcinogenicity will also occur in humans. More often than not, however, such data are not available.

In general, there is no consistent and uniform approach to evaluating the nature of adverse effects for noncancer endpoints. This situation is understandable for the following reasons: first, it requires the measurement of multiple medically significant endpoints and graded responses; second, the variety of testing procedures used to determine systemic health effects of a particular agent result in chemical-specific criteria that vary in completeness, content, and comparability; third, a threshold in the dose-response curve may exist for noncarcinogenic effects. Unlike EPA's policy on cancer, which assumes a linear, nonthreshold dose–response at low doses, the EPA generally assumes that there is a threshold for noncarcinogenic effects. The hazard identification of noncarcinogenic agents must thus consider the adverse effect at the dose threshold.

Traditionally, the appearance of overt effects, also referred to as "frank" effect levels, was used to determine the adverse effects of chemicals on an organism. The types of severity that constitute an adverse effect included permanent organ injury, LD_{50} levels, or injury leading to incapacitating illness. These reactions were used by toxicologists to determine the degree of toxicity. However, as toxicologists became increasingly concerned about the less obvious effects of chemical exposure, their observations turned to the working parts of the organ or organ system. Under these conditions it becomes important to examine the biochemical, cellular, and

structural components as well as the overall integrity of the biological system.

In Vitro Studies Evidence of the close association between mutagens and carcinogens leads to a presumption that most mutagenic substances will also be carcinogenic. As a result, a positive response in an in vitro mutagenicity assay provides supportive evidence that the agent tested is likely to be carcinogenic. Although quick, low-cost tests are valuable for screening potential carcinogens, they afford insufficient evidence to conclude that the agent in question is carcinogenic (27).

Comparison of Molecular Structure It is thought that by comparing an agent's chemical structure with those of known carcinogens, some evidence of potential carcinogenicity may be obtained. This area of investigation is called structure–activity relationships (SAR). Experimental data support this association for a few structural classes, but this method has so far provided little help in identifying carcinogens (26).

Dose–Response Assessment

The second step in assessing risk is the dose–response assessment. This process characterizes the relationship between the dose of a pollutant administered or received and the incidence of an adverse health effect in exposed animals or populations. The incidence of the adverse effect is then estimated as a function of exposure to the agent. Dose–response assessment considers the intensity of exposure, age, pattern of exposure, and other mitigating factors such as gender, socioeconomic status, etc. (27).

Useful human data are commonly lacking for most chemicals being assessed for their adverse health effects. The dose–response assessment therefore usually depends on tests performed on rats or mice. Current testing practices include one group of animals that is given the highest dose tolerable, a second that is exposed at half that dose, and an unexposed control group. The evidence that increased exposure leads to an increased incidence of an adverse effect has been used primarily to corroborate hazard identification.

The use of high doses of chemicals in animal testing has been challenged. It has been argued that the high doses used under experimental conditions may overpower the normal detoxication mechanisms and lead to adverse effects in animals that would not appear in humans who are exposed to lower doses (26). The validity of animal data has also been questioned because of the metabolic differences among animal species. Another consideration in evaluating dose–response information is that the actual dose of a chemical reaching the affected tissue or organ is usually not known. Such information is therefore based on administered dose, not on the dose reaching the tissues (27).

In the process of risk assessment, decisions are related to the levels of human exposure. Such doses are usually much lower than those administered to animals. The dose–response assessment, therefore, often requires that the dose–response curve be extrapolated from the high doses to which animals were exposed to the lower doses to which humans may be exposed. Such extrapolation is often done from one or two actual data points. Differences in the size and metabolic rates between man and laboratory animals also require that the doses used experimentally be adjusted to reflect these differences. A dose–response assessment should describe and justify the methods of extrapolation used to predict the incidence of the adverse effect. Statistical and biological uncertainties should be characterized as well.

Exposure Assessment

The third major step in risk assessment is exposure assessment. This step involves measuring or estimating the intensity, frequency, and duration of human exposures to an agent present in the environment or estimating the exposures that might arise from the release of new chemicals into the environment. In its most complete form, exposure assessment describes the magnitude, duration, schedule, and route of exposure; the size, nature, and population groups exposed; and the uncertainties inherent in these estimates. Exposure assessment is often used to identify technical options for controlling exposure and for predicting their effects on exposure.

The prime objective of an exposure assessment is to use direct measurement for determining actual human exposure or, more typically, to make estimates of exposure. Models are used to estimate exposure. Such models are often complex, even in so structured a setting as the workplace. Measuring exposure often can be difficult and costly because an agent may be present in varying concentrations in diverse occupational and environmental settings (26).

In community environments, exposure assessment is particularly complex. Estimating exposure is complicated not only by the number of hazards but also by their varied sources. Pollutants occur as mixtures from natural, industrial, transportation, and residential sources. The concentration of pollutants within a community may vary widely. When no direct measurements are available, indirect estimates of exposure must be made. The ambient concentrations of chemicals to which people may be exposed can be estimated from emission rates only if transport and conversion processes are known. Current research is attempting to improve the indirect estimates of exposure and to resolve the discrepancies of such estimates with the results obtained by direct measurements.

One of the most important factors in exposure assessment is determining which groups in the population may be exposed to a chemical agent. Certain groups are recognized to have enhanced susceptibility to hazardous exposure. These include the fetus, the very young, the elderly, and those with impaired health. The effects of exposure to a mixture of chemicals must also be considered. Data on the synergistic effects of exposure to multiple pollutants are rarely available. This important parameter is therefore commonly ignored.

For new chemicals with no measurement data, rough estimations of exposure are necessary. The assessment of such exposure must often take into account variations in personal habits and diet. For example, some chemical agents cause concern because they are contaminants in foods (34). The assessment of exposure to such agents is affected by the particular dietary patterns and personal habits of particular groups of the population.

Discussion of specific components in exposure assessment is complicated by the fact that current methods and approaches to exposure assessment appear to be medium specific or route specific. In contrast with hazard identification and dose–response assessment, exposure assessment has very few components that could be applicable to all media. Yet the scientist gathering data in support of regulatory efforts is concerned with a multimedia health assessment, that is, the adverse health effect of the total dose received through air, water, and food. The total dose received should equal the fractional contributions via inhalation, ingestion, dermal absorption, etc. A thorough exposure assessment may consider several different assumptions about the frequency and duration of human exposure to an agent or medium, the rates of intake or contact, and the rates of absorption.

Risk Characterization

The final step in risk assessment is risk characterization, which involves integration of information from the various components of risk assessment, discussed above. It is defined as the estimate of the magnitude of the public health problem. Risk characterization is derived from combining the outcome of exposure and dose–response assessments. The subjectivity introduced in aggregating population groups with varied susceptibility and different exposure may affect the estimate (27). In addition, there is no clinical agreement on whether adverse health effects can be aggregated and, if so, how they should be aggregated.

The process of risk characterization, by dealing with the effects of various types of exposure on various groups, provides much information. However, the need to handle so many numbers can make their interpretation impossible. In addition, the physiological and perceived effects of exposure among many groups is fraught with estimation difficulties. Not only are the data often spotty, but the results are rarely comparable, and the figures are subject to errors of observation and to problems of extrapolation.

The formidable obstacles and inherent uncertainties cause some individuals to throw up their hands and decide that the task of regulation is impossible. As a result, regulators often choose to ignore uncertainty, treating estimates as facts and basing regulatory decisions on the estimates. Ideally, however, regulation explicitly recognizes uncertainty and, in full light of these uncertainties, makes decisions based on the current state of scientific knowledge.

Risk Management

As stated, risk management is the process of weighing policy alternatives and selecting the appropriate regulatory action. Risk management decisions take into account the results of risk assessment, of engineering data, and of social, economic, and political factors. Though risk management may in large part be implemented by environmental legislation, it is also subject to the constraints of particular statutes. Risk management comes under the egis of a number of regulatory agencies.

REGULATORY AGENCIES

In the United States most authority for regulating activities and substances that pose health risks rests with four federal agencies: Environmental Protection Agency (EPA), Food and Drug Administration (FDA), Occupational Safety and Health Admintration (OSHA), and Consumer Product Safety Commission (CPSC) (6,9,27) (Table 31-1).

The Environmental Protection Agency is responsible for administering the greatest number of statutes protecting human health and the environment. The Agency is headed by a single administrator appointed by the President and confirmed by the Senate. Established in 1970, the EPA resembles a loosely knit federation of relatively discrete regulatory programs that are coordinated and overseen by a central management. These programs deal with air and water pollution, solid waste management, pesticides, radiation, toxic substances, and hazardous wastes. The principal laws administered by the EPA are noted in Table 31-1.

The Food and Drug Administration, a component of the Department of Health and Human Services, is headed by the Commissioner of Food and Drugs. It has regulatory powers over the toxicity of drugs, foods, and cosmetics (see Chapter 3). The basic food and drug law, the Federal Food, Drug and Cosmetic Act (FDCA), was enacted in 1938. It has been amended many times since that time. The FDA is organized in product-related bureaus, each of which employs its own scientists, technicians, compliance officers, and administrators. Among its responsibilities, the FDA, in conjunction with the EPA, is charged with establishing tolerances for pesticides (see Chapter 3).

TABLE 31-1. Agencies and Laws Regulating Chemicals in the United States

Agency	Law (year passed)
Food and Drug Administration (FDA)	Federal Food, Drug and Cosmetic Act (1938)
Occupational Safety and Health Administration (OSHA)	Occupational Safety and Health Act (1970)
Environmental Protection Agency (EPA)	Clean Air Act (1970)
	Clean Water Act (1977)
	Federal Insecticide, Fungicide and Rodenticide Act (FIFRA) (1972)
	Safe Drinking Water Act (1974)
	Resource Conservation and Recovery Act (RCRA) (1976)
	Comprehensive Environmental Response, Compensation and Liability Act (CERCLA) (1980)
	Toxic Substances Control Act (TSCA) (1976)
Consumer Product Safety Commission (CPSC)	Consumer Product Safety Act (1972)
	Federal Hazardous Substance Act (1960)
	Poison Prevention Packaging Act (1970)
	Flammable Fabrics Act (1953)

The Occupational Safety and Health Act of 1970 was passed "to assure so far as possible every working man and woman in the nation safe and healthful working conditions." Its passage resulted in the creation of two important agencies: the Occupational Safety and Health Administration (OSHA) and the National Institute for Occupational Safety and Health (NIOSH). OSHA is the regulatory agency concerned with occupational exposures to hazardous substances; NIOSH is the government research organization in the occupational safety and health field. The Occupational Safety and Health Administration is part of the Department of Labor and is headed by an Assistant Secretary of Labor. Until recently, OSHA derived its scientific support for the regulation of workplace hazards largely from the National Institute of Occupational Safety and Health and other agencies. Congress mandated this division in the hope that regulatory decisions would be more likely to be based on scientific inquiry and less vulnerable to political influence.

The Consumer Product Safety Commission enforces statutes that empower it to regulate unreasonable risk of injury from exposure to products used by consumers in the home, in schools, or in recreation. Of the four agencies responsible for regulating chemicals in the United States, the CPSC is the newest and smallest. It is governed by five commissioners appointed for fixed terms by the President. The commissioners can make major regulatory decisions only by majority vote.

REGULATORY DECISIONS

The Process

Regulatory decisions, the subject of much discussion, depend on the integration of many complex parts, each having its distinctive strengths and weaknesses (3,4,17,18,20,23–25,27–29,31,40). According to Clifford Grobstein, the scientific contribution to policy and decision making, whether in regulation or other areas, has three components (17). The first is substantive, having to do with the assembly and interpretation of relevant and scientifically valid information. The second is transitional in the sense that it proceeds beyond the strictly substantive but is not truly decisional. The third component is the policy-making process itself. This process occurs within the complex context of the social arena, with conflicting values and interests playing their roles in a structured political framework.

A general consensus has emerged in recent years that the first component, involving risk assessment, is essential to much current policy making

and requires the participation of highly competent scientists. There is also a consensus that policy-making decisions that affect risk management, though influenced by scientifically valid information, are not a matter of science. They are not, therefore, the business of scientists qua scientists. There is uncertainty and controversy among scientists and nonscientists alike with respect to the second component: whether it exists and, if so, what role scientists can and should play in policy-making decisions. Clearly, the relative importance of the components involved in policy-making decisions may vary from issue to issue.

The National Research Council has recommended that risk assessment and risk management be clearly distinguished (27) (Fig. 31-1). This separation was deemed desirable because it delineates risk assessment, which is primarily a scientific exercise, from risk management, which involves technical, social, economic, and political considerations. It is generally agreed, however, that risk assessment cannot be completely free of policy consideration and that some interaction between assessment and management activities is inescapable (27).

In an attempt to promote quality, consistency, and orderliness and to deal openly with uncertainty in the risk assessment process, the EPA has published a number of guidelines. The guidelines published thus far deal with carcinogens and mutagenicity risk assessment, with health assessment of suspected developmental toxicants, with the effects of chemical mixtures, and with exposure assessment (35–39).

The guidelines provide general directions for analyzing and organizing the available data when making a risk assessment. They represent the consensus of scientists within EPA and the EPA's Science Advisory Board about salient principles to be used in evaluating the quality of the data and in formulating judgments to be used in the process of risk assessment. As scientific advances are constantly being made, the guidelines are considered working documents subject to change as necessary.

Considerable effort is now directed to quantitative risk assessment (3,18,20,24). Although quantitative risk assessment may not always be feasible, it can be useful in setting regulatory priorities. To date, however, in EPA's regulatory activities, there are no guidelines for factoring the severity of effects into the decision-making process. The approaches developed by the EPA's Environmental Criteria and Assessment Office are beginning to address this issue. Currently, determinations of an acceptable daily intake (AID), or reference dose (RfD), do include guidelines on whether the effects are adverse or not adverse. In this case, adverse effects are defined as effects that result in functional impair-

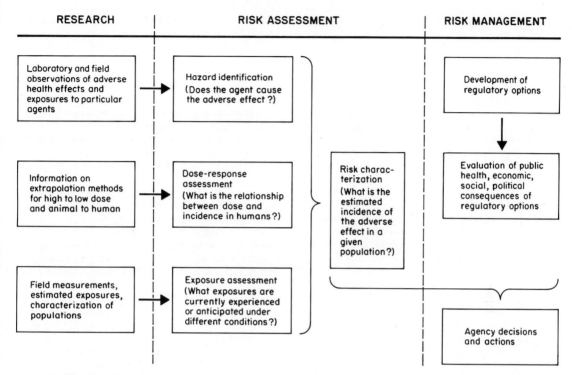

FIGURE 31-1. Elements of risk assessment and risk management. From National Research Council (27).

ment and/or pathological lesions that may affect the performance of an organism or reduce its ability to respond to an additional challenge.

The only risk assessment guidelines developed by the EPA that make use of a ranking system to evaluate health risks are the cancer guidelines (18,21,23,30,35). These guidelines provide for the ranking of potentially cancer-causing agents according to the type of data available. The proposed or drafted risk assessment guidelines for developmental toxicants, systemic/target organ toxicants, male reproductive toxicants, and neurotoxicants stress the need to use all pertinent data in the evaluation of a chemical's potential for causing developmental toxicity in humans. Existing, proposed, or published guidelines do not include schemes that allow chemicals to be ranked according to the level of concern for toxicity or to the level of confidence in the data base.

Changing Goals

As some problems are mediated by pollution control programs, and as others take their place, it is natural that the directions of many regulatory pro-

grams will change. Environmental problems that are currently the focus of attention, particularly in industrialized nations, include nontraditional and nonpoint sources of pollution, cross-media transfer of pollutants, ground-water contamination, and indoor air pollution.

In the industrialized countries, pollution control programs have, in many cases, checked the release of major industrial pollutants coming from point sources. As a number of large-volume conventional pollutants such as sulfur dioxide and nitrogen dioxide come under greater control, more attention is directed to controlling the release of such toxic and carcinogenic substances as organic chemicals and metals. In addition, nonpoint sources of pollution, derived from urban areas and the field application of pesticides, herbicides, and fertilizers, are receiving regulatory scrutiny.

The importance of maintaining a cross-media perspective is currently receiving greater emphasis. Although it has long been recognized that many pollutants are released into air, water, and food, these releases traditionally have been dealt with under separate laws, implemented independently, often by different government agencies. A cross-media perspective means that an environmental-control agency must consider the risks caused by the presence of pollutants in all media. A cross-media perspective considers the interrelationships among various pollution abatement programs. Current air and water pollution abatement programs, which often provide an important source of hazardous waste, reflect the need of cross-media analysis.

Protecting ground water from contamination is the preeminent environmental issue arising in the 1980s. Over the past decade, it has become apparent that contamination of ground water threatens both drinking water supplies and the availability of clean water for agricultural and industrial uses (7,8). The future promises increased regulatory action in this area even though most of the early environmental statutes designed to prevent contamination of air or surface water also provided the EPA with authority to protect ground water.

The issue of exposure to indoor air pollutants has recently become a public health concern. It is now well recognized that typical Americans spend about 80% of their time indoors. Reports of dangerously high asbestos levels in schools, high radon levels in some homes, and general complaints of irritating air quality in many office buildings provide a major stimulus for legislative initiatives (see Chapter 2).

The Radon Gas and Indoor Air Research Act of 1986 (Title IV of the Superfund Amendents and Reauthorization Act) gives the EPA, for the first time, a clear mandate to consider indoor air research priorities and to direct attention to exposures that are peculiar to indoor environments. This legislation directs EPA to establish a research program with respect to indoor air quality generally and radon gas in particular. Although no regulatory program is explicitly authorized, EPA is directed to undertake a comprehensive effort of research and development. Previously, EPA's indoor air research efforts were tied closely to ambient pollutants regulated under the Clean Air Act. Other industrial nations have energetically studied the problem of indoor air pollution and have developed programs to deal with this issue (16).

An important concept that has recently influenced environmental legislation deals with the "right to know" (19). The concept that citizens of a community have a "right to know" about hazardous chemicals stored, treated, manufactured, used, or disposed of in their vicinity has been brewing at the state and local level since about 1980 (2,33). The community "right-to-know" effort is closely tied to union and labor efforts to obtain more information about potential workplace hazards. Both movements sprang from a common concern that many supposedly harmless chemicals to which workers and the public had been exposed might actually cause acute or chronic diseases.

In 1988, under the Toxic Substances Control Act (TSCA), U.S. industries were required to disclose their storage and use of more that 300 hazardous substances and their releases of hazardous chemicals into the environment. The importance of communities having the Toxic Release Inventory (TRI) and other right-to-know information is that they will be able to access it, understand it in context, and use it. Some of the information, for example, should be of help to those who must respond in an emergency. The Toxic Release Inventory will allow priority setting and long-range planning. The usefulness of the information will depend largely on how it is processed through data-base systems.

The concept of community "right to know" when applied to the workplace is termed "hazard communication." This is the name the Occupational Safety and Health Administration (OSHA) has given to its efforts to ensure that workers are informed of the physical and health hazards of the chemical substances to which they are exposed. OSHA's authority and duty to concern itself with informing employees of chemical hazards is derived from amendments to the Occupational Safety and Health Act of 1970. Since 1986, chemical manufacturers and importers have been required to conduct comprehensive analyses of the hazards of their products and to provide downstream users with chemical hazard labels and highly detailed material safety data sheets (MSDSs). In the manufacturing sector, employees are required to have MSDSs for the hazardous chemicals at their workplaces. In addition, employee training and information programs regarding chemical hazards are to be implemented. OSHA has announced plans to extend the requirements of the hazard communication program to employers in all sectors of the economy. Hazard communication is therefore of considerable actual and potential significance to all those who produce, import, distribute, or use hazardous chemicals.

Regulatory Problems and Shortcomings

Despite the undeniable progress made in regulation of hazardous chemicals, the regulatory process remains subject to serious problems and shortcomings. Decision makers commonly face three major difficulties: (1) the vastness and complexity of the problem and the associated difficulty in designing and integrating the various regulatory programs, (2) the inherent limitations of knowledge and resources, and (3) the external constraints imposed by the fact that regulation is a public function.

Vastness and Complexity of the Pollution Problem and the Associated Difficulty in Regulation

In scale and complexity, the pollution problem is clearly overwhelming. Regulatory agencies are called on to control food contamination, air and water pollution, and hazardous waste production and dispersion. The varied sources of environmental pollution include manufacturing processes, mining activities, the field application of herbicides and pesticides, and the disposal of hazardous wastes. In sheer numbers, regulators encounter staggering figures. There are over 70,000 chemicals in commercial use with about 5000 showing some evidence of toxicity. It has been estimated that, in the United States alone, about 162 million metric tons of air pollutants were emitted in 1981, and about 638,000 metric tons of pesticides were manufactured in 1981 (7,8). The EPA has estimated that about 247 million metric tons of hazardous waste and 200 million metric tons of municipal solid waste are produced annually. It has also been estimated that there are about 22,000 inactive or abandoned waste sites, with approximately 2000 of these requiring cleanup action (8).

To carry out the complex task of regulating hazardous pollutants, the U.S. Congress has passed numerous laws and created an army of regulatory agencies, sometimes with conflicting and overlapping mandates. For example, there are nearly two dozen federal statutes governing toxic substances as well as a comparable number of federal agencies responsible for the research, regulatory, and advisory provisions of these various acts.

The approach to regulation varies considerably among the agencies, primarily as a result of variations in agency structure and differences in statutory mandates and their interpretation. The statutes accord different weights to such criteria as risk, costs of control, and technical feasibility. In addition, different modes of regulation vary in their capacity to generate the scientific data necessary to perform comprehensive risk assessments.

Several laws require agencies to balance regulatory costs and benefits. These include the Safe Drinking Water Act and the section on fuel additives in the Clean Air Act. Other statutes, including portions of the clean water program, involve the establishment of technology-based exposure controls. Still others mandate control techniques to reduce risks to zero whenever a hazard is affirmed. The Delaney clause in the Federal Food, Drug, and Cosmetic Act, for example, bans the addition to food of any substance shown to cause cancer in man or animals.

In an effort to expedite the resolution of many complex environmental problems, extensive collaborations occur among the various agencies. Approximately three-fourths of the environmental research in the United States is performed by agencies other than the EPA. Although some overlap occurs, most is avoided through formal or ad hoc ties between EPA and other agencies or interagency commissions.

Inherent Limitations in the Regulatory Decision-Making Process

The regulatory process draws on scientific findings that link chemical exposure to chronic health effects. Nevertheless, the overwhelming problem in the assessment of a health hazard is pervasive uncertainty. Data may be incomplete, and conclusive direct evidence of a threat to human health is rare. Although some 1500 substances are reportedly carcinogenic in animal tests, fewer than 50 chemicals, groups of chemicals, and industrial processes are clearly linked with cancer in humans (22,30,32). We know very little about most other chemicals, and even less about chronic health effects other than cancer.

Although our knowledge is steadily increasing, our often incomplete understanding of the nature and extent of the health risks for many pollutants leads to high levels of uncertainty in risk assessment. An important element in reducing this uncertainty is having information on the relative severity of the adverse health effect induced by the chemical in question. The severity of a particular effect constitutes an important factor in defining the term "adverse" and, as such, provides more "weight of evidence" in reducing the uncertainty of the risk analysis. Ultimately, standardized methods to rank severity would provide regulatory agencies with a common, explicit, and consistent approach for determining what would be medically significant as health criteria.

Limited analytic resources further hamper the quality of regulation. The existence of more than four million chemicals, with new ones produced each day, strains our analytical powers. About 3500 chemicals are under some sort of active consideration by various programs in EPA. The FDA must cope with more than 2000 food-related chemicals and 12,000 indirect additives. Although there is little doubt that a significant number of chemical substances pose a threat human health, an agency cannot consider acting on too many agents without stretching its scientific resources too thin.

External Influences on the Regulatory Decision-Making Process

Because regulation is a public function, it is subject to political and economic forces that can outweigh the purely scientific aspect of a decision. When risks from exposure to pollutants involve a serious disease, affected groups may insist that regulatory action need not await conclusive evidence of cause and effect. Conversely, although it is rarely known who will be saved from adverse health effects by a new regulation that reduces exposure, those who bear the economic costs of such restrictions can identify themselves easily. They can often offer concrete evidence of economic damage from regulation and can even point out the victims, such as unemployed workers. Because of their immediacy, such political and economic forces easily influence regulatory action (25).

CONCLUSION

The regulatory decision-making process is stalked by dominant and pervasive uncertainty. What is certain, however, is that regulation will remain central to the mediation between hazardous chemicals and human health. Above all, the reader should be aware that all regulatory decisions are complicated; they involve questions that are at or beyond the current frontiers of science. Each involves areas where measurement is difficult, theory is incomplete, and judgment is required.

REFERENCES

1. Andelman JB, Underhill DW (eds.): Health Effects from Hazardous Waste Sites, Lewis Publishers, Boca Raton, 1987.
2. Ashford NA, Caldart CC: The "right to know" toxics information transfer in the workplace. Annu Rev Public Health 6:383, 1985.
3. Brown SL: Quantitative risk assessment of environmental hazards. Annu Rev Public Health 6:247, 1985.
4. Burger EJ: Health Risks: The Challenge of Informing the Public, The Media Institute, Washington, 1984.
5. Cannon JD: Regulation of toxic air pollutants. J Air Pollut Control Assoc 36:562, 1986.
6. Colle J: Federal Activities in Toxic Substances, EPA-560/13-80-15, United States Environmental Protection Agency, Washington, 1980.
7. Council on Environmental Quality: Environmental Quality, 13th Annual Report, Council on Environmental Quality, Washington, 1982.
8. Council on Environmental Quality: Environmental Quality, 16th Annual Report, Council on Environmental Quality, Washington, 1985.
9. Crandal RW, Lave LB (eds.): The Scientific Basis of Health and Safety Regulations, Brookings Institution, Washington, 1981.
10. Crump KS: Fundamental carcinogenic processes and their implications for low dose risk assessment. Cancer Res 36:2973, 1976.

11. Crump KS: Dose–response problems in carcinogenesis. Biometrics 35:157, 1979.
12. Crump KS: The scientific basis for health risk assessment. Conference on Science, Technology, and Public Policy, sponsored by George Washington University, United States Environmental Protection Agency, Washington, 1982.
13. Crump KS: An improved procedure for low dose carcinogenic risk assessment from animal data. J Environ Pathol Toxicol Oncol 5:339, 1984.
14. Fusfeld HI, Haklisch CS (eds.): Science and Technology Policy: Perspectives for the 1980s. Annals of the New York Academy of Sciences, Vol 334, New York Academy of Sciences, 1979.
15. Gage SJ: Research for protection of our environment. In: Nitrogen Oxides and Their Effects on Health, p. 1, Lee SD (ed.), Ann Arbor Science, Ann Arbor, 1980.
16. Gammage RB, Kaye SV (eds.): Indoor Air and Human Health, Lewis Publishers, Chelsea, Michigan, 1985.
17. Grobstein C: The role of the National Academy of Sciences in public policy and regulatory decision making. In: Law and Science in Collaboration, p. 115, Nyart JD, Carrow MM (eds.), Lexington Books, Lexington, MA, 1983.
18. Hallenbeck WH, Cunningham KM: Quantitative Risk Assessment for Environmental and Occupational Health, Lewis Publishers, Boca Raton, 1986.
19. Himmelstein JS, Frumkin H: The right to know about toxic exposures. N Engl J Med 312:687, 1985.
20. Hoel DG, Merrill RA, Perera FP (eds.): Risk Quantitation and Regulatory Policy, Banbury Report 19, Cold Spring Harbor Laboratory, New York, 1985.
21. International Agency for Research on Cancer: Classification of Weight-of-Evidence for Carcinogencity of a Suspected Carcinogen, World Health Organization, Lyon, 1982.
22. International Agency for Research on Cancer: IARC Monographs on the Evaluation of Carcinogenic Risk of Chemicals to Humans, IARC Monographs, Vols. 1–42, Supplement 7, IARC, Lyon, 1987.
23. Krewski D, Brown C: Carcinogenic risk assessment: A guide to the literature. Biometrics 37:353, 1981.
24. Lave LB: Quantitative Risk Assessment in Regulation, Brookings Institution, Washington, 1982.
25. Lowrance WW: Of Acceptable Risk. Science and the Determination of Safety, William Kauffman, Los Altos, CA, 1976.
26. National Academy of Sciences: Principles for Evaluating Chemicals in the Environment, National Academy of Sciences. Washington, 1975.
27. National Research Council: Risk Assessment in the Federal Government: Managing the Process, National Academy Press, Washington, 1983.
28. Nyart JD, Carrow MM (eds.): Law and Science in Collaboration, Lexington Books, Lexington, MA, 1983.
29. O'Brien M: Marbury, the APA, science-policy disputes: The alluring and elusive judicial administrative partnership. Harvard Law Public Policy 7:443, 1984.
30. US Congress Office of Technology Assessment: Identifying and Regulating Carcinogens, Lewis Publishers, Chelsea, Michigan, 1988.
31. Oftedal P, Brogger A (eds.): Risk and Reason—Risk

Assessment in Relation to Environmental Mutagens and Carcinogens, Alan R Liss, New York, 1986.

32. Sharp DS, Eskenszi B, Harrison R, et al: Delayed health hazards of pesticide exposure. Annu Rev Public Health 7:441, 1986.

33. Tapscott G: Community right-to-know: A new environmentalist agenda. Environ Forum 3:8, 1984.

34. US Environmental Protection Agency: Updated Mutagenicity and Carcinogenicity Assessment of Cadmium. Addendums to Health Assessment Document for Cadmium, USEPA, Washington, 1981.

35. US Environmental Protection Agency: Guidelines for carcinogen risk assessment. Fed Register 51:33992, 1986.

36. US Environmental Protection Agency: Guidelines for mutagenicity risk assessment. Fed Register 51:34006, 1986.

37. US Environmental Protection Agency: Guidelines for the health assessment of suspect developmental toxicants, Fed Register 51:34028, 1986.

38. US Environmental Protection Agency: Guidelines for the health risk assessment of chemical mixtures. Fed Register 51:34014, 1986.

39. US Environmental Protection Agency: Guidelines for estimating exposures. Fed Register 51:34042, 1986.

40. Woodhead AD, Shellabarger CJ, Pond V, et al. (eds.): Assessment of Risk from Low-Level Exposure to Radiation and Chemicals, Plenum Press, New York, 1985.

RECOMMENDED READINGS

Grant L, Lee SD (eds.): US-Dutch expert workshop on health and environmental hazards from toxic chemicals in air, an international symposium, Toxicology and Industrial Health, Vol. 6, No. 5, Princeton Scientific Publishing Co, Princeton, 1990.

Hart RW, Hoerger FD (eds.): Carcinogen Risk Assessment: New Directions in the Qualitative and Quantitative Aspects, Banbury Report 31, Cold Spring Harbor Laboratory, New York, 1988.

National Research Council: Risk Assessment in the Federal Government: Managing the Process, National Academy Press, Washington, DC, 1983.

Sheilds J: Environmental Health: New Directions, Princeton Scientific Publishing Co, Princeton, 1990.

Tardiff RG, Rodricks JV (eds.): Toxic Substances and Human Risk, Plenum Press, New York, 1987.

US Congress Office of Technology Assessment Task Force: Identifying and Regulating Carcinogens, Lewis Publishers, Chelsea, Michigan, 1988.

US Environmental Protection Agency, Science Advisory Board: Reducing Risks: Setting Priorties and Strategies for Environmental Protection, SAB-EC-90-021, USEPA, Washington, DC, 1990.

US Environmental Protection Agency: Preserving Our Future Today, 21K-1012, Washington, DC, 1991.

Part VIII

APPENDIXES

APPENDIX A SELECTED TOXIC CHEMICALS AND THEIR ADVERSE HEALTH EFFECTS

Principles and Practice of Environmental Medicine, edited by Alyce Bezman Tarcher. Plenum Medical Book Company, New York, 1992.

Agent	Exposure	Route of entry	System(s) affected	Primary manifestation	Aids in diagnosis[a]	Remarks
Metals and metallic compounds						
Arsenic	Alloyed with lead and copper for hardness; manufacturing of pigments, glass, pharmaceuticals; byproduct in copper smelting; insecticides; fungicides; rodenticides; tanning	Inhalation and ingestion of dust and fumes	Neuromuscular Gastrointestinal Skin	Peripheral neuropathy, sensory > motor Nausea and vomiting, diarrhea, constipation Dermatitis, finger and toenail striations, skin cancer, nasal septum perforation Lung cancer	Arsenic in urine	
Arsine	Accidental byproduct of reaction of arsenic with acid; used in semiconductor industry	Inhalation of gas	Pulmonary Hematopoietic	Intravascular hemolysis: hemoglobinuria, jaundice, oliguria or anuria	Arsenic in urine	
Beryllium	Hardening agent in metal alloys; special use in nuclear energy production; metal refining or recovery	Inhalation of fumes or dust	Pulmonary (and other systems)	Granulomatosis and fibrosis	Beryllium in urine (acute) Beryllium in tissue (chronic) Chest x ray Immunologic tests (such as lymphocyte transformation) may also be useful	Pulmonary changes virtually indistinguishable from sarcoid on chest x ray
Cadmium	Electroplating; solder for aluminum; metal alloys, process engraving; nickel–cadmium batteries	Inhalation or ingestion of fumes or dust	Pulmonary Renal	Pulmonary edema (acute) Emphysema (chronic) Nephrosis	Urinary protein	Also a respiratory tract carcinogen
Chromium	In stainless and heat-resistant steel and alloy steel; metal plating; chemical and pigment manufacturing; photography	Percutaneous absorption, inhalation, ingestion	Pulmonary Skin	Lung cancer Dermatitis, skin ulcers, nasal septum perforation	Urinary chromate (questionable value)	

(Continued)

Agent	Exposure	Route of entry	System(s) affected	Primary manifestation	Aids in diagnosis[a]	Remarks
Lead	Storage batteries; manufacturing of paint, enamel, ink, glass, rubber, ceramics, chemical industry	Ingestion of dust, inhalation of dust or fumes	Hematologic Renal Gastrointestinal Neuromuscular CNS Reproductive	Anemia Nephropathy Abdominal pain("colic") Palsy ("wrist drop") Encephalopathy, behavioral abnormalities Spontaneous abortions (?)	Blood lead Urinary ALA Zinc protoporphyrin (ZPP); free erythrocyte protophyrin (FEP)	Lead toxicity, unlike that of mercury, is believed to be reversible, with the exception of late renal and some CNS effects.
Mercury Elemental	Electronic equipment; paint; metal and textile production; catalyst in chemical manufacturing; pharmaceutical production	Inhalation of vapor; slight percutaneous absorption	Pulmonary CNS	Acute pneumonitis Neuropsychiatric changes (erethism); tremor	Urinary mercury	Mercury illustrates several principles. The chemical form has a profound effect on its toxicology, as is the case for many metals. Effects of mercury are highly variable. Though inorganic mercury poisoning is primarily renal, elemental and organic mercury poisoning are primarily neurological. The responses are difficult to quantify, so dose-response data are generally unavailable. Classic tetrad of gingivitis, sialorrhea, irritability, and tremor is associated with both elemental and inorganic mercury poisoning; the four signs are not generally seen together. Many effects of mercury toxicity, especially those in CNS, are irreversible.
Inorganic		Some inhalation and GI and percutaneous absorption	Pulmonary Renal CNS	Acute pneumonitis Proteinuria Variable	Urinary mercury	
Organic	Agricultural and industrial poisons	Efficient GI absorption, percutaneous absorption, and inhalation	Skin CNS	Dermatitis Sensorimotor changes, visual field constriction, tremor	Blood and urine mercury, but ? sensitivity	

Agent	Uses/Sources	Route of Exposure	Target Organ	Effects	Biological Monitoring	Comments
Nickel	Corrosion-resistant alloys; electroplating; catalyst production; nickel–cadmium batteries	Inhalation of dust or fumes	Skin Pulmonary	Sensitization dermatitis ("nickel itch") Lung and paranasal sinus cancer		
Zinc oxide[b]	Welding byproduct; rubber manufacturing	Inhalation of dust or fumes that are freshly generated		"Metal fume fever" (fever, chills, and other symptoms)	Urinary zinc (useful as an indicator of exposure, not for acute diagnosis)	A self-limiting syndrome of 24–48 h with apparently no sequelae
Hydrocarbons						
Benzene	Manufacturing of organic chemicals, detergents, pesticides, solvents, paint removers; used as a solvent	Inhalation of vapor; slight percutaneous absorption	CNS Hematopoietic Skin	Acute CNS depression Leukemia, aplastic anemia Dermatitis	Urinary phenol	Note that benzene, as with toluene and other solvents, can be monitored via its principal metabolite.
Toluene	Organic chemical manufacturing; solvent; fuel component	Inhalation of vapor, percutaneous absorption of liquid	CNS Skin	Acute CNS depression Chronic CNS problems such as memory loss Irritation dermatitis	Urinary hippuric acid	
Xylene	A wide variety of uses as a solvent; an ingredient of paints, lacquers, varnishes, inks, dyes, adhesives, cements; an intermediate in chemical manufacturing	Inhalation of vapor; slight percutaneous absorption of liquid	Pulmonary Eyes, nose, throat CNS	Irritation, pneumonitis, acute pulmonary edema (at high doses) Irritation Acute CNS depression	Methylhippuric acid in urine, xylene in expired air, xylene in blood	
Ketones Acetone Methyl ethyl ketone (MEK) Methyl n-propyl ketone (MPK) Methyl n-butyl ketone (MBK) Methyl isobutyl ketone (MIBK)	A wide variety of uses as solvents and intemediates in chemical manufacturing	Inhalation of vapor, percutaneous absorption of liquid	CNS PNS Skin	Acute CNS depression MBK has been linked with peripheral neuropathy Dermatitis	Acetone in blood, urine, expired air (used as an index for exposure, not for diagnosis)	The ketone family demonstrates how a pattern of toxic responses (that is, CNS narcosis) may feature exceptions (that is, MBK peripheral neuropathy).

(Continued)

Agent	Exposure	Route of entry	System(s) affected	Primary manifestation	Aids in diagnosis[a]	Remarks
Formaldehyde	Widely used as a germicide and a disinfectant in embalming and histopathology, for example, and in the manufacture of textiles, resins, and other products	Inhalation	Skin Eye Pulmonary	Irritant and contact dermatitis Eye irritation Respiratory tract irritation, asthma	Patch testing may be helpful for dermatitis	Recent animal tests have shown it to be a respiratory carcinogen. Confirmatory epidemiologic studies are in progress
Trichloroethylene (TCE)	Solvent in metal degreasing, dry cleaning, food extraction; ingredient of paints, adhesives, varnishes, inks	Inhalation, percutaneous absorption	Nervous Skin Cardiovascular	Acute CNS depression Peripheral and cranial neuropathy Irritation, dermatitis Arrhythmias	Breath analysis for TCE	TCE is involved in an important pharmacological interaction. Within hours of ingesting alcoholic beverages, TCE workers experience flushing of the face, neck, shoulders, and back. Alcohol may also potentiate the CNS effects of TCE. The probable mechanism is competition for metabolic enzymes.
Carbon tetrachloride	Solvent for oils, fats, lacquers, resins, varnishes, other materials; used as a degreasing and cleaning agent	Inhalation of vapor	Hepatic Renal CNS Skin	Toxic hepatitis Oliguria or anuria Acute CNS depression Dermatitis	Expired air and blood levels	Carbon tetrachloride is the prototype for a wide variety of solvents that cause hepatic and renal damage. This solvent, like trichloroethylene, acts synergistically with ethanol.
Carbon disulfide	Solvent for lipids, sulfur, halogens, rubber, phosphorus, oils, waxes, and resins; manufacturing of organic chemicals, paints, fuels, explosives, viscose rayon	Inhalation of vapor, percutaneous absorption of liquid or vapor	Nervous Renal Cardiovascular Skin Reproductive	Parkinsonism, psychosis, suicide Peripheral neuropathies Chronic nephritic and nephrotic syndromes Acceleration or worsening of atherosclerosis; hypertension Irritation; dermatitis Menorrhagia and metorrhagia	Iodine–azide reaction with urine (nonspecific since other bivalent sulfur compounds give a positive test); CS_2 in expired air, blood, and urine	A solvent with unusual multisystem effects, especially noted for its cardiovascular, renal, and nervous system actions.

Substance	Uses	Route of exposure	Target organs	Signs and symptoms	Comments
Stoddard solvent	Degreasing, paint thinning	Inhalation of vapor, percutaneous absorption of liquid	Skin CNS	Dryness and scaling from defatting; dermatitis Dizziness, coma, collapse (at high levels)	A mixture of primarily aliphatic hydrocarbons, with some benzene derivatives and naphthenes.
Ethylene glycol ethers	The ethers are used as solvents for resins, paints, lacquers, varnishes, gum, perfume, dyes, and inks; the acetate derivatives are widely used as solvents and ingredients of lacquers, enamels, and adhesives. Exposure occurs in dry cleaning, plastic, ink, and lacquer manufacturing, and textile dying, among other processes.				Ethylene glycol ethers, as a class of chemicals, have been shown in animals to have adverse reproductive effects, including reduced sperm count and spontaneous abortion, as well as CNS, renal, and liver effects.
Ethylene glycol monoethyl ether (Cellosolve®)		Inhalation of vapor, percutaneous absorption of liquid	Reproductive, CNS, renal, liver		
Ethylene glycol monoethyl ether acetate (cellosolve acetate)					
Methyl- and butyl-substituted compounds such as ethylene glycol monomethyl ether (Methyl Cellosolve®)			Hematopoietic CNS	Pancytopenia Fatigue, lethargy, nausea, headaches, anorexia, tremor, stupor (from encephalopathy)	Effects primarily associated with ethylene glycol monomethyl ether (Methyl Cellosolve®)
Ethylene oxide	Used in the sterilization of medical equipment, in the fumigation of spices and other foodstuffs, and as a chemical intermediate	Inhalation	Skin Eye Respiratory tract Nervous system	Dermatitis and frostbite Severe irritation; possibly cataracts with prolonged exposure Irritation Peripheral neuropathy	Recent animal tests have shown it to be carcinogenic and to cause reproductive abnormalities. Epidemiologic studies indicate that it may cause leukemia in exposed workers.
Dioxane	Used as a solvent for a variety of materials, including cellulose acetate, dyes, fats, greases, resins, polyvinyl polymers, varnishes, and waxes	Inhalation of vapor, percutaneous absorption of liquid	CNS Renal Liver	Drowsiness, dizziness, anorexia, headaches, nausea, vomiting, coma Nephritis Chemical hepatitis	Dioxane has caused a variety of neoplasms in animals.

(Continued)

Agent	Exposure	Route of entry	System(s) affected	Primary manifestation	Aids in diagnosis[a]	Remarks
Polychlorinated biphenyls (PCBs)	Formerly used as a dielectric fluid in electrical equipment and as a fire retardant coating on tiles and other products. New uses were banned in 1976, but much of the electrical equipment currently used still contains PCBs	Inhalation, ingestion, skin absorption	Skin Eye Liver	Chloracne Irritation Toxic hepatitis	Serum PCB levels for chronic exposure	Animal studies have demonstrated that PCBs are carcinogenic. Epidemiologic studies of exposed workers are inconclusive.
Irritant gases[c] Ammonia	Refrigeration; petroleum refining; manufacturing of nitrogen-containing chemicals, synthetic fibers, dyes, and optics	Inhalation of gas	Upper respiratory tract	Upper respiratory irritation		Also irritant of eyes and moist skin
Hydrochloric acid	Chemical manufacturing; electroplating; tanning; metal pickling; petroleum extraction; rubber, photographic, and textile industries	Inhalation of gas or mist	Upper rspiratory tract	Upper respiratory irritation		Strong irritant of eyes, mucous membranes, and skin
Hydrofluoric acid	Chemical and plastic manufacturing; catalyst in petroleum refining; aqueous solution for frosting, etching, and polishing glass	Inhalation of gas or mist	Upper respiratory tract	Upper respiratory irritation		In solution, causes severe and painful burns of skin and can be fatal
Sulfur dioxide	Manufacturing of sulfur-containing chemicals; food and textile bleach; tanning; metal casting	Inhalation of gas, direct contact of gas or liquid phase on skin or mucosa	Middle respiratory tract	Bronchospasm (pulmonary edema or chemical pneumonitis in high dose)	Chest x ray, pulmonary function tests[d]	Strong irritant of eyes, mucous membranes, and skin
Chlorine	Paper and textile bleaching; water disinfection; chemical manufacturing; metal fluxing; detinning and dezincing iron	Inhalation of gas	Middle respiratory tract	Tracheobronchitis, pulmonary edema, pneumonitis	Chest x ray, pulmonary function tests	Chlorine combines with body moisture to form acids, which irritate tissues from nose to alveoli.

Agent	Source/Use	Route	Site affected	Effect	Diagnostic tests	Comments
Fluorine	Uranium processing; manufacturing of fluorine-containing chemicals; oxidizer in rocket fuel systems	Inhalation of gas	Middle respiratory tract	Laryngeal spasm, bronchospasm, pulmonary edema	Chest x ray, pulmonary function tests	Potent irritant of eyes, mucous membranes, and skin
Ozone	Inert gas-shielded arc welding; food, water, and air purification; food and textile bleaching; emitted around high-voltage electrical equipment	Inhalation of gas	Lower respiratory tract	Delayed pulmonary edema (generally 6–8 h following exposure)	Chest x ray, pulmonary function tests	Ozone has a free radical structure and can produce experimental chromosome aberrations; it may thus have carcinogenic potential.
Nitrogen oxides	Manufacturing of acids, nitrogen containing chemicals, explosives, and more; byproduct of many industrial processes	Inhalation of gas	Lower respiratory tract	Pulmonary irritation, bronchiolitis fibrosa obliterans ("silo filler's disease"), mixed obstructive-restrictive changes	Chest x ray, pulmonary function tests	
Phosgene	Manufacturing and burning of isocyanates, and manufacturing of dyes and other organic chemicals; in metallurgy for ore separation; burning or heat source near trichloroethylene	Inhalation of gas	Lower respiratory tract	Delayed pulmonary edema (delay seldom longer than 12 h)	Chest x ray, pulmonary function tests	
Isocyanates TDI (toluene diisocyanate) MDI (methylene diphenyldiisocyanate) Hexamethylene diisocyanate and others	Polyurethane manufacture; resin-binding systems in foundries; coating materials for wires; used in certain types of paint	Inhalation of vapor	Predominantly lower respiratory tract	Asthmatic reaction and accelerated loss of pulmonary function	Chest x ray, pulmonary function tests	Isocyanates are both respiratory tract "sensitizers" and irritants in the conventional sense.
Asphyxiant gases Simple asphyxiants: nitrogen hydrogen, methane, and others	Enclosed spaces in a variety of industrial settings	Inhalation of gas	CNS	Anoxia	O$_2$ in environment	No specific toxic effect; act by displacing O$_2$

(Continued)

Agent	Exposure	Route of entry	System(s) affected	Primary manifestation	Aids in diagnosis[a]	Remarks
Chemical asphyxiants						
Carbon monoxide	Incomplete combustion in foundries, coke ovens, refineries, furnaces, and more	Inhalation of gas	Blood (hemoglobin)	Headache, dizziness, double vision	Carboxyhemoglobin	
Hydrogen sulfide	Used in manufacturing of sulfur-containing chemicals; produced in petroleum production; byproduct of petroleum product use; decay of organic matter	Inhalation of gas	CNS Pulmonary	Respiratory center paralysis, hypoventilation Respiratory tract irritation	PaO_2	
Cyanides	Metallurgy, electroplating	Inhalation of vapor, percutaneous absorption, ingestion	Cellular metabolic enzymes (especially cytochrome oxidase)	Enzyme inhibition with metabolic asphyxia and death	SCN^- in urine	
Pesticides						
Organophosphates: malathion, parathion, and others		Inhalation, ingestion, percutaneous absorption	Neuromuscular	Cholinesterase inhibition, cholinergic symptoms: nausea and vomiting, salivation, diarrhea, headache, sweating, meiosis, muscle fasciculations, seizures, unconsciousness, death	Refractoriness to atropine; plasma or red cell cholinesterase	As with many acute toxins, rapid treatment of organophosphate toxicity is imperative. Thus, diagnosis is often made based on history and a high index of suspicion rather than on biochemical tests. Treatment is atropine to block cholinergic effects and 2-PAM (2-pyridine-alsoxine methiodide) to reactivate cholinesterase.
Carbamates: carbaryl (Sevin) and others		Inhalation, ingestion, percutaneous absorption	Neuromuscular	Same as organophosphates	Plasma cholinesterase; urinary 1-naphthol (index of exposure)	Treatment of carbamate poisoning is the same as that of organophosphate poisoning except that 2-PAM is contraindicated.

Agent	Route	System	Effect	Test	Comments
Chlorinated hydrocarbons: chlordane, DDT, heptachlor, chlordecone (Kepone), aldrin, dieldrin, uridine	Ingestion, inhalation, percutaneous absorption	CNS	Stimulation or depression	Urinary organic chlorine, or p-chlorophenyl acetic acid	The chlorinated hydrocarbons may accumulte in body lipid stores in large amounts.
Bipyridyls: paraquat, diquat	Inhalation, ingestion, percutaneous absorption	Pulmonary	Rapid massive fibrosis, only following paraquat ingestion		An interesting toxin in that the major toxicity, pulmonary fibrosis, apparently occurs only after ingestion

[a]Occupational and medical histories are, in most instances, the most important aids in diagnosis.
[b]Zinc oxide is a prototype of agents that cause metal fume fever.
[c]The less water-soluble the gas, the deeper and more delayed its irritant effect.
[d]Pulmonary function tests are useful aids in diagnosis of irritant effects if the patient is subacutely or chronically ill.
*Data compiled by H. Frumkin and J. Melius; reprinted with permission from Levy BS, Wegman DH (eds.): Occupational Health: Recognizing and Preventing Work-Related Disease, 2nd ed., Little, Brown, Boston, 1988.

APPENDIX B   SELECTED WORK-RELATED DISEASES

Condition	Industry or occupation	Agent
Infections		
Anthrax	Shepherds, farmers, butchers, handlers of imported hides or fibers, veterinarians, veterinarian pathologists, weavers	*Bacillus anthracis*
Brucellosis	Farmers, shepherds, vets, lab and slaughterhouse workers	*Brucella abortus, suis*
Plague	Shepherds, farmers, ranchers, hunters, field geologists	*Yersinia pestis*
Hepatitis		
A	Day-care center, orphanage, and mental retardation institution staff, medical personnel	Hepatitis A virus
B	Nurses and aides, anesthesiologists, orphanage and mental institution staffs, medical lab workers, general dentists, oral surgeons, physicians	Hepatitis B virus
C (formerly included in non-A, non-B)	Same as hepatitis A and B	Hepatitis C virus
Ornithosis	Psittacine bird breeders, pet shop and zoo workers, poultry producers, veterinarians	*Chlamydia psittaci*
Rabies	Veterinarians, game wardens, lab workers, farmers, ranchers, trappers	Rabies virus
Rubella	Medical personnel	Rubella virus
Tetanus	Farmers, ranchers	*Clostridium tetani*
Tuberculosis		
Pulmonary	Physicians, medical personnel, medical lab workers	*Mycobacterium tuberculosis*
Silicotuberculosis	Quarrymen, sandblasters, silica processors, miners, foundry workers, ceramic industry	Silicon dioxide (silica), *M. tuberculosis*
Tularemia	Hunters, fur handlers, sheep industry, cooks, veterinarians, ranchers, veterinarian pathologists	*Francisella tularensis*
Malignant neoplasms		
Bladder	Rubber and dye workers	Benzidine, 1- and 2-naphthylamine, auramine, magenta, 4-aminobiphenyl, 4-nitrophenyl
Bone	Dial painters, radium chemists and processors	Radium
Kidney and other urinary organs	Coke oven workers	Coke oven emissions
Liver hemangiosarcoma	Vinyl chloride polymerization industry	Vinyl chloride monomer
	Vintners	Arsenical pesticides
Lung, bronchial, tracheal	Asbestos industry, users	Asbestos
	Topside coke oven workers	Coke oven emissions
	Uranium and fluorspar miners	Radon daughters
	Chromium producers, processors, users	Chromates
	Smelters	Arsenic
	Mustard gas formulators	Mustard gas
	Ion-exchange resin makers, chemists	Bis(chloromethyl)ether, chloromethyl methyl ether

(Continued)

Principles and Practice of Environmental Medicine, edited by Alyce Bezman Tarcher. Plenum Medical Book Company, New York, 1992.

Condition	Industry or occupation	Agent
Nasal cavity	Woodworkers, furniture makers	Hardwood dusts
	Boot and shoe industry	Unknown
	Radium chemists and processors, dial painters	Radium
	Chromium producers, processors, users	Chromates
	Nickel smelting and refining	Nickel
Peritoneal, pleural mesothelioma	Asbestos industry, users	Asbestos
Scrotal	Automatic lathe operators, metalworkers	Mineral, cutting oils
	Coke oven workers, petroleum refiners, tar distillers	Soots and tars, tar distillates
Hematological disorders		
Agranulocytosis or neutropenia	Workers exposed to benzene	Benzene
	Explosives, pesticide industries	Phosphorus
	Pesticide, pigment, pharmaceutical industries	Inorganic arsenic
Anemia		
Aplastic	Explosives manufacturing	TNT
	Workers exposed to benzene	Benzene
	Radiologists, radium chemists, dial painters	Ionizing radiation
Hemolytic, nonautoimmune	Whitewashing and leather industry	Copper sulfate
	Electrolytic processes, arsenical ore smelting	Arsine
	Plastics industry	Trimellitic anhydride
	Dye, celluloid, resin industries	Naphthalene
Leukemia		
Acute lymphoid	Rubber industry	Unknown
	Radiologists	Ionizing radiation
Acute myeloid	Workers exposed to benzene	Benzene
	Radiologists	Ionizing radiation
Erythroleukemia	Workers exposed to benzene	Benzene
Methemoglobinemia	Explosives, dye industries	Aromatic amino and nitro compounds (e.g., aniline, TNT, nitroglycerin)
Cardiovascular disorders		
Angina	Auto mechanics, foundry workers, wood finishers, traffic control, driving in heavy traffic	Carbon monoxide
Arrhythmias	Metal cleaning, solvent use, refrigerator maintenance	Solvents, fluorocarbons
Raynaud's phenomenon (secondary)	Lumberjacks, chain sawyers, grinders, chippers	Whole-body or segmental vibration
	Vinyl chloride polymerization	Vinyl chloride monomer
Pulmonary disorders		
Alveolitis (extrinsic, allergic)	Farmer's lung bagassosis, bird-breeder's lung, suberosis, maltworker's lung, mushroom worker's lung, maple bark disease, cheese-washer's lung, coffee-worker's lung, fish-meal-worker's lung, furrier's lung, sequoiosis, woodworker's lung, miller's lung	Various agents
Asbestosis	Asbestos workers, users	Asbestos
Asthma (extrinsic)	Jewelry, alloy, catalyst makers	Platinum
	Polyurethane, adhesive, paint workers	Isocyanates
	Alloy, catalyst, refinery workers	Chromium, cobalt
	Solderers	Aluminum soldering flux
	Plastic, dye, insecticide makers	Phthalic anhydride
	Foam workers, latex makers, biologists	Formaldehyde
	Printing industry	Gum arabic
	Nickel platers	Nickel sulfate
	Bakers	Flour
	Plastics industry	Trimellitic anhydride
	Woodworkers, furniture makers	Red cedar, other wood dusts
	Detergent formulators	Bacillus-derived exoenzymes
	Animal handlers	Animal dander

Condition	Industry or occupation	Agent
Beryllium disease (chronic)	Beryllium alloy, ceramic, cathode-ray tube, nuclear reactor workers	Beryllium
Bronchitis, pneumonitis, pulmonary edema (acute)	Refrigeration, fertilizer, oil-refining industries	Ammonia
	Alkali, bleach industries	Chlorine
	Silo fillers, arc welders, nitric acid workers	Nitrogen oxides
	Paper, refrigeration, oil-refining industries	Sulfur dioxide
	Cadmium smelters, processors	Cadmium
	Plastics industry	Trimellitic anhydride
Byssinosis	Cotton industry	Cotton, flax, hemp, cotton–synthetic dusts
Pneumoconiosis	Coal miners, bauxite workers	Coal dust, bauxite fumes
Silicosis	Mining, metal, and ceramic industries, quarrymen, sandblasters, silica processors	Silica
Talcosis	Talc processors	Talc
Neurological disorders		
Cerebellar ataxia	Chemical industry	Toluene
	Electrolytic chlorine production, battery manufacturing, fungicide formulators	Organic mercury
Encephalitis (toxic)	Battery, smelter, foundry workers	Lead
	Electrolytic chlorine production, battery manufacturing, fungicide formulators	Organic, inorganic mercury
Neuropathy (toxic and inflammatory)	Pesticide, pigment, pharmaceutical industries	Arsenic, arsenic compounds
	Furniture refinishers, degreasers	Hexane
	Plastic-coated-fabric workers	Methyl butyl ketone
	Explosives industry	TNT
	Rayon manufacturing	Carbon disulfide
	Plastics, hydraulics, coke industries	Tri-o-cresyl phosphate
	Battery, smelter, foundry workers	Inorganic lead
	Dentists, chloralkali workers	Inorganic mercury
	Chloralkali, fungicide, battery workers	Organic mercury
	Plastics, paper manufacture	Acrylamide
Parkinson's disease (secondary)	Manganese processors, battery manufacturing, welders	Manganese
	Internal combustion engine industries	Carbon monoxide
Miscellaneous		
Abdominal pain	Battery manufacturing, enamelers, smelter, painters, ceramics workers, plumbers, welders	Lead
Cataract	Microwave, radar technicians	Microwaves
	Explosives industry	TNT
	Radiologists	Ionizing radiation
	Blacksmiths, glass blowers, bakers	Infrared radiation
	Moth repellent formulators, fumigators	Naphthalene
	Explosives, dye, herbicide, pesticide industries	Dinitrophenol, dinitro-o-cresol
Dermatitis (contact, allergic)	Adhesives, sealants, and plastics industries, leather tanning, poultry dressing, fish packing, boat building and repair, electroplating, metal cleaning, machining, housekeeping	Irritants (cutting oils, solvents, phenol, acids, alkalies, detergents, fibrous glass), allergens (nickel, epoxy resins, chromates, formaldehyde, dyes, rubber products)
Headache	Firefighters, foundry workers, wood finishers, dry cleaners, traffic control, driving in heavy traffic	Carbon monoxide, solvents
Hepatitis (toxic)	Solvent users, dry cleaners, plastics industry	Carbon tetrachloride, chloroform, tetrachloroethane trichloroethylene
	Explosives and dye industries	Phosphorus, TNT
	Fire- and waterproofing additive formulators	Chloronaphthalene
	Plastics formulators	4,4-Methylene-dianiline
	Fumigators, gasoline and fire-extinguishers formulators	Ethylene dibromide

(Continued)

Condition	Industry or occupation	Agent
Hepatitis (toxic) (*Continued*)	Disinfectant, fumigant, synthetic resin formulators	Cresol
Inner ear damage	Various	Excessive noise
Infertility (male)	Formulators	Kepone
	Producers, formulators, applicators	1,2-Dibromo-3-chloropropane
Psychosis (acute)	Gasoline, seed, and fungicide workers, wood preservation, rayon manufacturing	Lead (especially organic), mercury, carbon disulfide
Renal failure (acute, chronic)	Battery manufacturing, plumbers, solderers	Inorganic lead
	Electrolytic processes, arsenical ore smelting	Arsine
	Battery manufacturing, jewelers, dentists	Inorganic mercury
	Fluorocarbon, fire-extinguisher formulators	Carbon tetrachloride
	Antifreeze manufacturing	Ethylene glycol

*Reprinted from Uncovering Occupational Illness, Emergency Medicine 22(3):22, 1990. Adapted from Rutstein DD, Mullan RJ, Frazier TM, et al: Sentinel health events (occupational): A basis for physician recognition and public health surveillance. Am J Public Health 73:1054, 1983.

APPENDIX C SELECTED JOB CATEGORIES, EXPOSURES, AND WORK-RELATED DISEASES

Job categories	Exposures	Work-related diseases
Agricultural workers	Pesticides, infectious agents, gases, sunlight	Pesticide poisoning, "farmers' lung," skin cancer
Anesthetists	Anesthetic gases	Reproductive effects, cancer
Animal handlers	Infectious agents, allergens	Asthma
Automobile workers	Asbestos, plastics, lead, solvents	Asbestosis, dermatitis
Bakers	Flour	Asthma
Battery makers	Lead, arsenic	Lead poisoning, cancer
Butchers	Vinyl plastic fumes	"Meat wrappers' asthma"
Caisson workers	Pressurized work environments	"Caisson disease," "the bends"
Carpenters	Wood dust, wood preservatives, adhesives	Nasopharyngeal cancer, dermatitis
Cement workers	Cement dust, metals	Dermatitis, bronchitis
Ceramic workers	Talc, clays	Pneumoconiosis
Demolition workers	Asbestos, wood dust	Asbestosis
Drug manufacturers	Hormones, nitroglycerin, etc.	Reproductive effects
Dry cleaners	Solvents	Liver disease dermatitis
Dye workers	Dyestuffs, metals, solvents	Bladder cancer, dermatitis
Embalmers	Formaldehyde, infectious agents	Dermatitis
Felt makers	Mercury, polycyclic hydrocarbons	Mercuralism
Foundry workers	Silica, molten metals	Silicosis
Glass workers	Heat, solvents, metal powders	Cataracts
Hospital workers	Infectious agents, cleansers, radiation	Infections, accidents
Insulators	Asbestos, fibrous glass	Asbestosis, lung cancer, mesothelioma
Jack hammer operators	Vibration	Raynaud phenomenon
Lathe operators	Metal dusts, cutting oils	Lung disease, cancer
Laundry workers	Bleaches, soaps, alkalis	Dermatitis
Lead burners	Lead	Lead poisoning
Miners (coal, hard rock, metals, etc.)	Talc, radiation, metals, coal dust, silica	Pneumoconiosis, lung cancer
Natural gas workers	Polycyclic hydrocarbons	Lung cancer
Nuclear workers	Radiation, plutonium	Metal poisoning, cancer
Office workers	Poor lighting, poorly designed equipment	Joint problems, eye problems
Painters	Paints, solvents, spackling compounds	Neurologic problems
Paper makers	Acids, alkalis, solvents, metals	Lung disorders, dermatitis
Petroleum workers	Polycyclic hydrocarbons, catalysts, zeolites	Cancer, pneumoconiosis
Plumbers	Lead, solvents, asbestos	Lead poisoning
Railroad workers	Creosote, sunlight, oils, solvents	Cancer, dermatitis
Seamen	Sunlight, asbestos	Cancer, accidents
Smelter workers	Metals, heat, sulfur dioxide, arsenic	Cancer
Steel workers	Heat, metals, silica	Cataracts, heat stroke
Stone cutters	Silica	Silicosis
Textile workers	Cotton dust, fabrics, finishers, dyes, carbon disulfide	Byssinosis, dermatitis, psychosis
Varnish makers	Solvents, waxes	Dermatitis
Vineyard workers	Arsenic, pesticides	Cancer, dermatitis
Welders	Fumes, nonionizing radiation	Lead poisoning, cataracts

From Environmental and Occupational Medicine, Rom WN (ed.), Table 3-1, p. 24, Little, Brown, 1983. Reprinted by permission.

Principles and Practice of Environmental Medicine, edited by Alyce Bezman Tarcher. Plenum Medical Book Company, New York, 1992.

APPENDIX D INFORMATION RESOURCES IN THE FIELD OF ENVIRONMENTAL AND OCCUPATIONAL MEDICINE

Compiled by
Alyce Bezman Tarcher

GENERAL REFERENCES

Amdur MO, Doull J, Klaassen CD (eds.): Casarett and Doull's Toxicology: The Basic Science of Poisons, 4th ed., Pergamon Press, London, 1991.

Committee on Animals as Sentinels of Environmental Health Hazards, National Research Council: Animals as Sentinels of Environmental Health Hazards, National Academy, Press, 1991.

Emmett EA, Brooks SM, Harris RL, et al: Year Book of Occupational and Environmental Medicine, Mosby-Year Book Inc., St. Louis, Missouri, 1992.

Goldsmith JR (ed.): Environmental Epidemiology: Epidemiological Investigation of Community Environmental Health Problems, CRC Press, Boca Raton, 1986.

Gordis L (ed.): Epidemiology and Health Risk Assessment, Oxford University Press, Oxford, 1988.

Guthrie FE, Perry JJ (eds.): Introduction to Environmental Toxicology, Elsevier, Amsterdam, 1980.

Hernberg S: Introduction to Occupational Epidemiology, Lewis Publishers, Chelsea, Michigan, 1992.

Jeyaratnam J (ed.): Occupational Health in Developing Countries, Oxford Medical Publications, Oxford University Press, Oxford, 1992.

LaDou J (ed.): Occupational Medicine, Appleton & Lange, Norwalk, Connecticut, 1990.

Last JM: Public Health and Human Ecology, Appleton & Lange, Norwalk, Connecticut, 1990.

Last JM, Wallace R.B. (eds.): Maxcy-Rosenau-Last Public Health & Preventive Medicine, 13th ed., Appleton & Lange, Norwalk, Connecticut, 1992.

Lave LB (ed.): Quantitative Risk Assessment in Regulation, The Brookings Institution, Washington, 1982.

Lave LB, Upton AC (eds.): Toxic Chemicals, Health, and the Environment, The Johns Hopkins Press, Baltimore, 1987.

Levy BS, Wegman DH (eds.): Occupational Health: Recognizing and Preventing Work-Related Disease, 2nd ed., Little, Brown, Boston, 1988.

Kimbrough R, Mahaffey K, Grandjean P, et al: Clinical Effects of Environmental Chemicals: A Guide to Etiologic Diagnosis, Hemisphere, Washington, 1989.

Murdock BS (ed.): Environmental Issues in Primary Care, Minnesota Department of Health, Minneapolis, 1991.

Raffle PAB, Lee WR, McCallum RI, et al: Hunter's Diseases of Occupations, Hodder and Stoughton, London, 1987.

Rom WN (ed.): Environmental and Occupational Medicine, Little, Brown, Boston, 1983.

Rosenstock L, Cullen MR (eds.): Clinical Occupational Medicine, Blue Books Series, WB Saunders, Philadelphia, 1986.

Shields J: Environmental Health: New Directions, Princeton Scientific Publishing Co., Princeton, 1990.

Upton AC (guest ed.): Environmental medicine. Med Clin North A 74(2):235–546, 1990.

Principles and Practice of Environmental Medicine, edited by Alyce Bezman Tarcher. Plenum Medical Book Company, New York, 1992.

Weeks JL, Levy BS, Wagner GR (eds.): Preventing Occupational Disease and Injury, American Public Health Association, Washington, 1991.

World Health Organization: Our Planet, Our Health. Report of the WHO Commission on Health and Environment. World Health Organization, Geneva, 1992.

Zenz C (ed.): Occupational Medicine: Principles and Practical Applications, Year Book Medical Publishers, Chicago, 1988.

Schardein J: Chemically Induced Birth Defects, Marcel Dekker, New York, 1985.

Shepard TH: Catalog of Teratogenic Agents, 7th ed., The Johns Hopkins University Press, Baltimore, 1992.

Sittig M: Handbook of Toxic and Hazardous Chemicals and Carcinogens, 3rd ed., Noyes Data Corporation, Park Ridge, New Jersey, 1990.

Tver DF, Anderson KA: Industrial Medicine Desk Reference, Chapman and Hall, London, 1986.

HANDBOOKS AND MANUALS

Baselt RC, Cravey RH: Disposition of Toxic Drugs and Chemicals in Man, 3rd ed., Year Book Medical Publishers, Chicago, 1989.

California Department of Health Services: The Toxics Directory, References and Resources on the Health Effects of Toxic Substances, California Department of Health Services, Berkeley, California, 1990.

Centers for Disease Control: Preventing Lead Poisoning in Young Children, A Statement by the Centers for Disease Control, CDC, Atlanta, 1991.

Dreisbach RH: Handbook of Poisoning: Prevention, Diagnosis and Treatment, 12th ed., Appleton and Lange, Norwalk, Connecticut, 1987.

Forum for Scientific Excellence: Index of Hazardous Contents of Commercial Products in Schools and Colleges, American Chemical Society, Washington, 1990.

Forum for Scientific Excellence: Compendium of Hazardous Chemicals in Schools and Colleges, American Chemical Society, Washington, 1990.

Gosselin RE, Smith RP, Hodge HC: Clinical Toxicology of Commercial Products, 5th ed., Williams & Wilkins, Baltimore, 1984.

Hathaway GJ, Proctor NH, Hughes JP, et al. (eds.): Proctor and Hughes' Chemical Hazards of the Workplace, 3rd ed., Van Nostrand Reinhold, New York, 1991.

Hayes WJ, Laws ER Jr (eds.): Handbook of Pesticide Toxicology, Academic Press, Orlando, 1990.

Mackison FW, Stricoff RS, Partridge LJ Jr. (eds.): NIOSH/OSHA Pocket Guide to Chemical Hazards, US Department of Health and Human Services and US Department of Labor, Washington, 1978; reprinted US Government Printing Office, Washington, 1980.

Morgan DP: Recognition and Management of Pesticide Poisonings, 4th ed., EPA-540/9-88-001, USEPA, Washington, 1989.

Rossol M: The Artist's Complete Health and Safety Guide, Allworth Press, New York, 1990.

Sax I, Lewis RJ: Hazardous Chemicals Desk Reference, Van Nostrand Reinhold, New York, 1987.

PERIODICALS

American Journal of Epidemiology: Society of Epidemiologic Research, 624 N Broadway, Baltimore, MD 21205.

American Journal of Industrial Medicine: Alan R Liss. 41 E 11 Street, New York, NY 10003.

American Journal of Public Health: American Public Health Association, 1015 Fifteenth Street, NW, Washington, DC, 20005.

Annals of Occupational Hygiene, Pergamon Press, Headington Hill Hall, Oxford, United Kingdom, or Maxwell House, Fairview Park, Elmsford, New York, New York 10523.

Archives of Environmental Contamination and Toxicology: Springer-Verlag, 175 Fifth Avenue, New York, New York 10010.

Archives of Environmental Health: Society for Occupational and Environmental Health, Heldref Publications, 4000 Albermarle Street NW, Washington, DC 20016.

British Journal of Industrial Medicine: British Medical Association, Tavistock Square, London WC1 H9JR, England.

Environmental and Occupational Health Sciences Institute INFOletter: Public Education and Risk Communication Division, University of Medicine and Dentistry of New Jersey, Robert Wood Johnson Medical School, 675 Hoes Lane, Piscataway, NJ 08854.

Environmental Health Perspectives: National Institute of Environmental Health Sciences, US Government Printing Office, Washington, DC 20202.

Environmental Research: Academic Press, 1250 Sixth Avenue, San Diego, CA 92101.

Hazardous Substances & Public Health: Agency for Toxic Substances and Disease Registry, 1600 Clifton Road, NE, Mail Stop E33, Atlanta, GA 30333.

Health & Environmental Digest: 2500 Shadywood Road, Box 90, Navarre, MN 55392.

International Archives of Occupational and Environmental Health, Springer-Verlag, 175 Fifth Avenue, New York, New York 10010.

Journal of Occupational Medicine: American College of Occupational Medicine, 428 East Preston Street, Baltimore, MD 21202.

Journal of Toxicology, Clinical Toxicology: Marcel Dekker, 270 Madison Avenue, New York, New York 10016.

Journal of Toxicology and Environmental Health: Taylor & Francis/Hemisphere Publishing Corp., 1900 Frost Road, Bristol, PA.

Occupational Health, Bailliere Tindall, 24-28 Oval Road, London, England.

Scandinavian Journal of Work, Environment & Health: Topeliuksenkatu 41aA, SF-00250 Helsinki, Finland.

U.S. GOVERNMENT AGENCIES, INTERNATIONAL AND PRIVATE AGENCIES AND ORGANIZATIONS

For U.S. agencies, the material has been extracted from the U.S. Government Manual. The reader is urged to consult this publication, which is updated regularly, for more extensive and detailed information.

Agency for Toxic Substances and Disease Registry (ATSDR)
1600 Clifton Road, NE, Mail Stop E33, Atlanta, GA 30333
The Agency for Toxic Substances and Disease Registry operates within the U.S. Public Health Service. The Agency was developed to protect the public and workers from exposure and the adverse health effects of hazardous substances present in storage sites or released in fires, explosions, or transportation accidents. Its activities include health professional training and the development of educational materials for physicians in the form of case studies. These case studies provide a guide to the diagnosis, treatment, and surveillance of patients exposed to hazardous agents.

Centers for Disease Control (CDC)
1600 Clifton Road, Atlanta, GA 30333
The Centers for Disease Control, as part of its function, administers, develops, and implements national programs to deal with environmental health problems, including response to environmental, chemical, and radiation emergencies in the United States. The Center for Environmental Health and Injury Control is one of the nine major operating components of the Centers for Disease Control.

Chemical Manufacturers Association
2501 M Street, NW, Washington, DC 20037
The Chemical Manufacturers Association operates the National Chemical Response and Information Center. The Center includes CHEMTREC, the Chemical Transportation Emergency Center, CHEMNET, the Chemical Mutual Aid Network, Emergency Response Training, and the Chemical Referral Center. CHEMTREC offers 24-h communications with emergency response personnel, chemists, product specialists, and medical departments. CHEMNET offers access to chemical industry emergency response teams trained to mitigate chemical spills, leaks, and fires. The Chemical Referral Center is designed to help the public, transportation workers, and users of chemicals obtain health and safety information about chemicals and chemical products for nonemergency aspects of chemical hazards.

Consumer Product Safety Commission (CPSC)
5401 Westbard Ave, Washington, DC 20257
The Consumer Product Safety Commission is responsible for the protection of the U.S. public from the hazards of consumer products. It also develops uniform safety standards for consumer products.

Environmental Protection Agency (EPA)
401 M Street, SW, Washington, DC 20460
The U.S. Environmental Protection Agency is responsible for administering legislative acts protecting humans or the environment from the unwanted effects of chemical and physical agents. The Agency is involved in research, monitoring, standard setting, and enforcement activities. Hotlines provide the public with access to EPA programs, technical capabilities, and services. Recent publications provide the public with information about avoiding environmental risks. See the section on referral and consultation sources for additional information.

European Chemical Industry Ecology and Toxicology Centre (ECETOC)
250, avenue Louise, boite 63, B-1050 Brussels, Belgium
The Centre collects information related to the health of individuals working with chemicals. It also disseminates scientific, ecological, and toxicological information.

Food and Agricultural Organization of the United Nations (FAO)
Via delle Terme di Caracalla, 00100 Rome, Italy
The Food and Agricultural Organization aims to raise nutritional levels and living standards and increase the efficiency of production and distribution of foods and agricultural products.

Food and Drug Administration (FDA)
5600 Fishers Lane, Rockville, MD 20857
The U.S. Food and Drug Administration's activities are directed toward assessing safety and providing protection against impure and unsafe foods, drugs, and cosmetics and other potential hazards.

International Agency for Research on Cancer (IARC)
    150, cours Albert Thomas, F-69372 Lyon Cedex 08
France

The International Agency for Research on Cancer has a program that evaluates the carcinogenic risk of chemicals to humans. The program's objective is to elaborate and publish monographs that critically evaluate data on carcinogenicity for agents to which humans are known to be exposed and on specific exposure situations.

International Programme on Chemical Safety (IPCS)
    Division of Environmental Health
    World Health Organization, Ch-1211 Geneva 27,
Switzerland

The aims of the International Programme on Chemical Safety, which represents the cooperative efforts of the International Labour Organization, the United Nations Environmental Program, and the World Health Organization, include evaluating health risks posed to humans and the environment by exposure to chemicals and providing guidelines on safe levels of chemical exposure.

National Cancer Institute (NCI)
    Bethesda, MD 20892

The National Cancer Institute supports various types of investigative approaches to cancer, including molecular biology, immunology, epidemiology, and radiotherapy. The Institute developed the National Cancer Program, which is aimed at expanding knowledge on the causes and prevention of cancer.

National Institute for Occupational Safety and Health (NIOSH)
    Building 1, Room 3007, Centers for Disease Control
    1600 Clifton Road, Atlanta, GA 30333

The National Institute for Occupational Safety and Health has a broad range of responsibilities related to worker health in the United States. This includes research on occupational disease and the development and recommendations for limits of exposure to potentially hazardous substances or conditions in the workplace. NIOSH publishes numerous documents including specific workplace hazards.

National Institutes of Environmental Health Sciences (NIEHS)
    P.O. Box 12233, Research Triangle Park, NC 27709

The National Institutes of Environmental Health Sciences is the principal federal agency for biomedical research on the health effects of environmental chemicals and physical agents.

National Toxicology Program (NTP)
    M.D. B2-04, P.O. Box 12233, Research Triangle Park, NC 27709

The major function of the National Toxicology Program is the selection and testing of chemicals for toxicity.

Nuclear Regulatory Commission (NRC)
    Washington, DC 20555

The U.S. Nuclear Regulatory Commission regulates the commercial use of nuclear materials and issues licenses for such use.

Occupational Safety and Health Administration (OSHA),
US Department of Labor
    200 Constitution Avenue NW, Washington, DC 20010

The Occupational Safety and Health Administration is the primary regulatory agency for occupational safety and health in the United States.

Organisation for Economic Co-operation and Development (OECD)
    2, rue Andre-Pascal, 75775 Paris Cedex 16, France

The Organisation for Economic Co-operation and Development, with 24 members, includes representatives of western European governments, Australia, Canada, Japan, New Zealand, Turkey, Norway, Sweden, Denmark, Finland, Portugal, Spain, and the United States. Environmental information and reporting are important activities of the OECD member countries. The OECD Chemicals Programme, concerned with the problem of existing chemicals, is producing a priority list and action program.

The Center for Safety in the Arts (CSA)
    5 Beekman Place, Suite 1030
    New York, New York 10038

The Center for Safety in the Arts is a national clearinghouse for research and education on hazards in the visual arts, performing arts, museums, and school art programs. It is funded with public support from the National Endowment for the Arts and from New York State and New York City agencies.

United Nations Environment Programme (UNEP)
    P.O. Box 300552, Nairobi, Kenya

The United Nations Environment Programme encourages and coordinates sound environmental practices worldwide. This includes publishing documents and sponsoring a variety of programs. It monitors changes in the environment through a worldwide surveillance system that collects data and offers information. The Programme is also concerned with transboundary environmental problems such as ozone depletion and global warming.

World Health Organization
    1211 Geneva 27, Switzerland

The World Health Organization offers a wide range services in environmental and occupational health and safety. This includes publishing documents and sponsoring a variety of programs.

REFERRAL AND CONSULTATION SOURCES

American College of Occupational Medicine
55 W Seegers Street
Arlington Heights, IL 60005

American Board of Medical Toxicology
National Office, New York Poison Center
Bellevue Hospital, 27th Street and First Ave
New York, NY 10016

Teratogen Exposure Registry and Surveillance (TERAS)
The Teratogen Exposure Registry and Surveillance is a network of 20 centers where pathologists and geneticists study human embryos and fetuses exposed to potentially teratogenic agents. Physicians who have concerns about possible teratogenic effects of environmental exposures may consult with TERAS. For referral, contact Frederick Bieber, PhD, Harvard Medical School, Boston, MA 02115.

Organization of Teratology Information Services (OTIS)
Massachusetts Teratogen Information Service
National Birth Defects Center, Franciscan Children's
Hospital
30 Warren Street, Boston, MA 02135
Organization of Teratology Information Services is a network of teratology information services in the United States, Canada, France, Germany, Israel, Italy, The Netherlands, Switzerland, and the United Kingdom that provides current information to the public and health care professionals regarding possible reproductive risks from environmental exposures.

INFOTERRA Network
INFORTERRA/US
Environmental Protection Agency (EPA)
401 M Street, SW, Washington, DC 20460
INFOTERRA is an international environmental research and referral system sponsored by the United Nations Environment Programme. INFOTERRA supports a network of 137 participating countries. In the United States, the INFOTERRA office is administered by the Office of Information Resources Management. The INFOTERRA reference and referral services utilize the EPA library and information services network. An international directory of sources of expertise is available. Data-base and communication services include a pathfinder to international environmental data bases.

Association of Occupational and Environmental Clinics
1030 15th Street NW, Suite 410, Washington, DC 20005
The Association of Occupational and Environmental Clinics was established to enhance the practice of occupational and environmental medicine through information sharing and research. The Clinics have a multidisciplinary staff that provides clinical and consultative services and professional training. There is a strong commitment to the prevention of environmental and occupational disease. The following clinics are members of the Association of Occupational and Environmental Clinics (AOEC):

California
  Occupational Health Clinic
    San Francisco General Hospital
    1001 Potrero Avenue
    San Francisco, CA 94110

  Occupational and Environmental Medicine Clinic
    University of California at San Francisco
    400 Parnassus Avenue
    San Francisco, CA 94143

Colorado
  National Jewish Center for Immunology and
    Respiratory Medicine
    1400 Jackson Street
    Denver, CO 80206

Connecticut
  Yale Occupational Medicine Program
    School of Medicine
    333 Cedar Street
    New Haven, CT 06510

  University of Connecticut
    Occupational Medicine Program
    Farmington Avenue
    Farmington, CT 06032

District of Columbia
  Division of Occupational and Environmental
    Medicine
    George Washington University of Medicine
    2300 K Street NW, Suite 201
    Washington, DC 20037

Illinois
  MacNeal Occupational Medicine Clinic at Bridgeview Medical Center
    7217 West 84th Street
    Bridgeview, IL 60455

  Occupational Medicine Clinic
    Cook County Hospital
    720 South Wolcott
    Chicago, IL 60612

Iowa
  Pulmonary Disease Division
    Department of Internal Medicine
    University of Iowa College of Medicine
    Iowa City, IA 52242

Maryland
  Johns Hopkins Occupational Medicine Program
    615 North Wolfe Street
    Baltimore, MD 21205

Occupational Health Project
Division of General Internal Medicine
University of Maryland, School of Medicine
405 Redwood Street
Baltimore, MD 21202

Massachusetts
Occupational and Environmental Health Center
Cambridge Hospital
1493 Cambridge Avenue
Cambridge, MA 02139

Occupational Health Service
Massachusetts Respiratory Hospital
2001 Washington Street
South Braintree, MA 02184

Occupational Health Services
Department of Family and Community Medicine
University of Massachusetts Medical Center
55 Lake Avenue North
Worcester, MA 01655

Massachusetts General Hospital
Occupational Medicine Clinic
32 Fruit Street
Boston, MA 02114

Michigan
Occupational Health Program
Department of Occupational Health
School of Public Health
University of Michigan
1420 Washington Heights
Ann Arbor, MI 48109

Division of Occupational Health
Wayne State University
Department of Family Medicine
4201 St Antoine
Detroit, MI 48420

Michigan State University
Department of Medicine
B338 Clinical Center
East Lansing, MI 48824

Minnesota
Occupational Health Services and Occupational Residency Training Program
Ramsey Clinic
640 Jackson Street
St Paul, MN 55101

New Jersey
Occupational and Environmental Medicine Clinic
Department of Environmental and Community Medicine
University of Medicine and Dentistry of New Jersey–Robert Wood Johnson Medical School
675 Hoes Lane
Piscataway, NJ 08845

New York
Mount Sinai Irving J. Selikoff Occupational Health Clinical Center
P.O. Box 1058, 1 Gustave Levy Place
New York, NY 10029

Occupational Medicine Clinic
Department of Community and Preventive Medicine
Division of Occupational Medicine
State University of New York
Stony Brook, NY 11794

Central New York Occupational Health Clinical Center
550 Harrison Center
Syracuse, NY 13202

Eastern NY Occupational Health Program
1201 Troy Schnenectady Road
Latham, NY 12110

North Carolina
Duke University Medical Center
Division of Occupational and Environmental Medicine
Box 2914
Durham, NC 27710

Ohio
Center for Occupational Health
Holmes Hospital
Eden and Bethesda Avenue
Cincinnati, OH 45267

Greater Cincinnati Occupational Health Center
10475 Reading Road
Cincinnati, OH 45241

Occupational/Environmental Health Clinic
Department of Family Practice–MetroHealth Medical Center
3395 Scranton Road
Cleveland, OH 44109

Oklahoma
University Occupational Health Services
Oklahoma Memorial Hospital
800 NE 13th Street
Oklahoma City, OK 73104

Pennsylvania
Occupational Health Service
Department of Community and Preventive Medicine
Medical College of Pennsylvania
3300 Henry Avenue
Philadelphia, PA 19129

Occupational and Environmental Medicine Program
University of Pittsburgh School of Medicine
130 DeSoto Street
Pittsburgh, PA 15261

Rhode Island
  Memorial Hospital of Rhode Island
    Occupational Health Service
    Brown University Program in Occupational
      Medicine
    Division of General Internal Medicine
    111 Brewster Street
    Pawtuckett, RI 02860

Washington
  Occupational Medicine Program
  University of Washington
  Harborview Medical Center
  325 Ninth Avenue
  Seattle, WA 98104

West Virginia
  Division of Occupational and Environmental
      Health
  Department of Family and Community Health
  Marshall University School of Medicine
  Huntington, WV 25755

Environmental Protection Agency
  The U.S. Environmental Protection Agency operates a number of telephone hotlines. In addition
to the hotlines, the EPA has a variety of clearinghouses, libraries, and dockets. An updated *Guide
to EPA Hotlines, Clearinghouses, Libraries, and
Dockets* is published regularly.
  General information about the Agency's programs can be obtained from any of the regional
offices and from the EPA's Public Information Center:

  Public Information Center
  U.S. EPA (PM-211B)
  401 M Street, SW
  Washington, DC 20460

  Selected National EPA Hotlines and Clearinghouses are listed below:

Center for Environmental Research Information
  (513) 569-7391
Asbestos Programs (800) 368-5888
Emergency Planning and Community Right-to-
  Know (800) 535-0202
National Pesticides Telecommunications Network
  Hotline (800) 858-7378
Pollution Prevention Information Clearinghouse
  (800) 424-9346
Radon Information (202) 475-9605
RCRA/CERCLA (Superfund) Hotline (800) 424-9346
Safe Drinking Water Hotline (800) 426-4791

State Health Departments
  State Health Departments in the United States
may be consulted with issues related to environmental and occupational health.

CONTINUING EDUCATION IN ENVIRONMENTAL AND OCCUPATIONAL MEDICINE

*National Institute for Occupational Safety and Health
(NIOSH)*
  Educational Resource Centers
  NIOSH has established centers of learning for
occupational safety and health throughout the United
States. Courses on a variety of topics in occupational
and environmental medicine are presented. A sched-
ule of courses may be obtained from NIOSH Divi-
sion of Training and Manpower Development, 4676
Columbia Parkway, Cinncinnati, OH 45226.

COMPUTER DATA-BASE INFORMATION

  Computer data-base information, both bibliographic and full text, is produced for public access
by various national and international government
agencies and by private publishing companies. Ac-
cessing these systems is possible through direct
agency contact or by commercial vendor. Major ven-
dors have extensive collections that include both
government and privately produced data bases.
  The National Library of Medicine (NLM) com-
puter-based Medical Literature Analysis and Retrieval System (MEDLARS) provides rapid bibliographic access to NLM's vast store of biomedical
information. MEDLARS now represents a family of
data bases, some of which provide information in
the field of environmental and occupational medicine. Only a few of these data bases are listed below.
For assistance and information on data bases and on
various software packages available for access to
MEDLARS, the reader may consult:

  National Library of Medicine
  Specialized Information Services
  8600 Rockville Pike
  Bethesda, MD 20894

The following data bases are included in the MED-
LARS system:
  MEDLINE contains all citations indexed in *Index Medicus* and selected titles from other indexes. It
indexes articles from over 3200 biomedical journals
published in the United States and abroad. MED-
LINE currently contains some 6 million references
going back to 1966.
  TOXLINE (Toxicology Information Online) and
TOXLIT (Toxicology Literature from Special Sources)
are bibliographic data bases covering the pharmacological, biochemical, physiological and toxicological effects of drugs and other chemicals.
  CCRIS (Chemical Carcinogenesis Research Information System) is a factual data bank sponsored
by the National Cancer Institute. It contains data

derived from both short- and long-term bioassays on approximately 1200 chemicals.

ETICBACK (Environmental Teratology Information Center Backfile) is a bibliographic data base covering teratology and development toxicology.

TRI (Toxic Chemical Release Inventory) contains information on the annual estimated releases of toxic chemicals to the environment in the United States. These data include the names and addresses of the facilities and the amounts of certain toxic chemicals they release to the air, water, or land or transfer to waste sites.

HSDB (Hazardous Substances Data Bank) is a comprehensive data base containing records for over 4100 toxic or potentially toxic chemicals. It contains information in such areas as toxicity, environmental fate, human exposure, chemical safety, waste disposal, emergency handling, and regulatory requirements.

IRIS (Integrated Risk Information System) is an online data base built by the Environmental Protection Agency (EPA). It contains EPA carcinogenic and noncarcinogenic health risk and regulatory information on about 400 chemicals.

RTECS (Registry of Toxic Effects of Chemical Substances) contains toxic effects data for approximately 100,000 chemicals. It is built and maintained by the National Institute of Occupational Safety and Health (NIOSH). Acute and chronic effects are covered in such areas as skin/eye irritation, carcinogenicity, mutagenicity, and reproductive consequences.

INDEX